Handbook of VETERINARY NEUROLOGY

Handbook of VETERINARY NEUROLOGY

FIFTH EDITION

MICHAEL D. LORENZ, BS, DVM, DACVIM

Professor of Small Animal Internal Medicine
Dean, College of Veterinary Clinical Sciences
Center for Veterinary Health Sciences
Oklahoma State University
Stillwater, Oklahoma

JOAN R. COATES, BS, DVM, MS, DACVIM

Associate Professor of Neurology and Neurosurgery
Department of Small Animal Medicine and Surgery
College of Veterinary Medicine
University of Missouri
Columbia, Missouri

MARC KENT, DVM, BA, DACVIM

Associate Professor and Neurologist
Department of Small Animal Medicine
College of Veterinary Medicine
University of Georgia
Athens, Georgia

With 261 illustrations

ELSEVIER
SAUNDERS

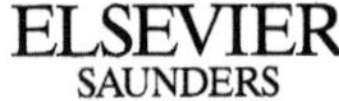

SAUNDERS

3251 Riverport Lane
St. Louis, Missouri 63043

HANDBOOK OF VETERINARY NEUROLOGY

ISBN: 978-1-4377-0651-2

Notice

Knowledge and best practice in this field are constantly changing. As new research and experience broaden our understanding, changes in research methods, professional practices, or medical treatment may become necessary.

Practitioners and researchers must always rely on their own experience and knowledge in evaluating and using any information, methods, compounds, or experiments described herein. In using such information or methods they should be mindful of their own safety and the safety of others, including parties for whom they have a professional responsibility.

With respect to any drug or pharmaceutical products identified, readers are advised to check the most current information provided (i) on procedures featured or (ii) by the manufacturer of each product to be administered, to verify the recommended dose or formula, the method and duration of administration, and contraindications. It is the responsibility of practitioners, relying on their own experience and knowledge of their patients, to make diagnoses, to determine dosages and the best treatment for each individual patient, and to take all appropriate safety precautions.

To the fullest extent of the law, neither the Publisher nor the authors, contributors, or editors, assume any liability for any injury and/or damage to persons or property as a matter of products liability, negligence or otherwise, or from any use or operation of any methods, products, instructions, or ideas contained in the material herein.

Library of Congress Cataloging-in-Publication Data

Lorenz, Michael D.
Handbook of veterinary neurology / Michael D. Lorenz, Joan R. Coates, Marc Kent. — 5th ed.
p. ; cm.
Includes bibliographical references and index.
ISBN 978-1-4377-0651-2 (hardcover : alk. paper) 1. Veterinary neurology—Handbooks, manuals, etc. 2. Nervous system—Diseases—Diagnosis—Handbooks, manuals, etc. I. Coates, Joan R. II. Kent, Marc. III. Title.
[DNLM: 1. Nervous System Diseases—veterinary—Handbooks. 2. Animal Diseases—diagnosis—Handbooks. 3. Neurologic Examination—veterinary—Handbooks. SF 895]
SF895.O44 2012
636.089'680475—dc22 2010034818

Vice President and Publisher: Linda Duncan
Publisher: Penny Rudolph
Senior Developmental Editor: Shelly Stringer
Associate Developmental Editor: Brandi Graham
Publishing Services Manager: Catherine Jackson
Senior Project Manager: Rachel E. McMullen
Design Direction: Jessica Williams

Printed in the United States of America

Last digit is the print number: 9 8 7 6 5

We dedicate this edition to our mentors who helped train and inspire each of us in the discipline of clinical neurology. We are especially indebted to Alexander deLahunta, John Oliver, Joe Kornegay, and Joe Mayhew who have paved our way for the fifth edition of the Handbook of Veterinary Neurology. *We are sincerely grateful to our current and past colleagues who have continued to foster our knowledge of veterinary neurology and neurosurgery and who have mentored us during our career endeavors. We dedicate this book to our students, past, present, and future, whose curiosity and questions have inspired us to develop better methods of teaching. And, we dedicate this book to our families for their support and understanding that enabled us to spend the extra time required to complete this edition.*

PREFACE

The fifth edition of *Handbook of Veterinary Neurology* has been substantially updated, providing students and practitioners with up-to-date information on small and large animal neurology. The new edition is in full color, enhancing the learning experience and providing a stronger knowledge of neuroanatomy. We have continued to use the problem-oriented format from previous editions. The emphasis remains on lesion localization because one cannot diagnose what is wrong if one does not know where the lesion(s) is (are) located.

Handbook of Veterinary Neurology is simple and easy to use by veterinary students and practitioners. Numerous algorithms are included that diagram the logic necessary to localize lesions and to formulate diagnostic plans. Each chapter has been extensively reviewed, updated, and heavily referenced.

A unique feature of our book is the Appendix. The Appendix lists breed-associated, breed-specific, or inherited neuromuscular diseases in domestic animals. The Appendix has been substantially updated to include new diseases reported since the fourth edition was published. It contains more than 1000 references.

Veterinary Neurology Cases

veterinaryneurologycases.com

The fifth edition has an accompanying website that can be found at www.veterinaryneurologycases.com. The website includes 20 video case studies that correlate to all of the cases presented in Chapters 2 and 15 of the book. Each case study on the website is presented as a narrated PowerPoint presentation with videos highlighting important aspects of each case, such as symptoms, lesion localization, and diagnosis.

Michael D. Lorenz
Joan R. Coates
Marc Kent

ACKNOWLEDGMENTS

We are grateful for the assistance of the Elsevier team, Shelly Stringer, Brandi Graham, Penny Rudolph, and Rachel McMullen. We acknowledge the College of Veterinary Medicine at Cornell University for permitting use of neurologic images posted to their website.

We would like to especially acknowledge Philip J. Johnson, G. Diane Shelton, and William F. Fales, who have assisted us with their areas of expertise in preparation of this book.

Finally, we thank all of you, our colleagues, for making the fifth edition necessary.

CONTENTS

PART I

Fundamentals

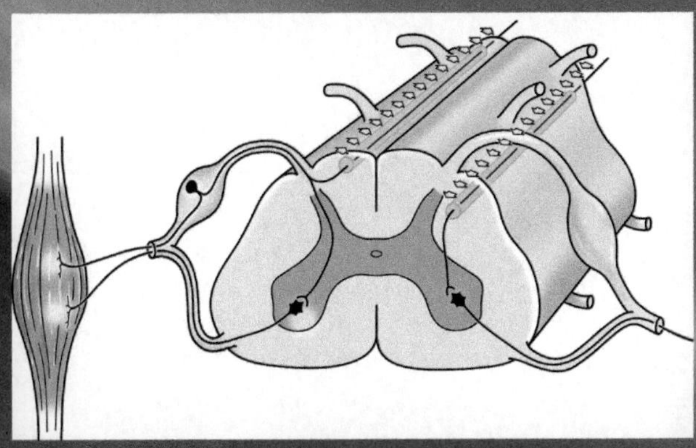

CHAPTER 1

Neurologic History, Neuroanatomy, and Neurologic Examination

The objectives in the management of an animal with a problem that may be related to the nervous system are to (1) confirm that the problem is caused by a lesion in the nervous system, (2) localize the lesion in the nervous system, (3) estimate the severity and extent of the lesion in the nervous system, (4) determine the cause or the pathologic process or both, and (5) estimate the prognosis with no treatment or with various alternative methods of treatment.

Many diseases may be accompanied by a complex combination of clinical signs and laboratory data. Diagnosis of these diseases may seem impossible. Weed demonstrated the value of starting the diagnostic process by independently listing and analyzing all the patient's problems.[1] A minimum set of data (minimum database) is necessary to solve any medical problem. The minimum database may be modified because of risk, cost, or accessibility as balanced against the severity of the disease. Priorities should be established for collecting data that evaluate the most probable causes of a problem. Tests for rare diseases and those that are dangerous are reserved until last.

Weed's problem-oriented system is eminently suited for neurologic diagnosis. The steps necessary for the management of a neurologic problem are listed in Box 1-1.

MINIMUM DATABASE

The initial evaluation of a patient, including a history and a physical examination, usually provides evidence that a neurologic problem is present (Table 1-1).

Some problems are difficult to classify, for example, syncope versus epileptic seizures, or weakness (loss of muscle strength) versus paresis (loss of motor control). The initial physical examination of every patient should include a screening neurologic examination designed to detect the presence of any neurologic abnormality. The screening examination is described later in the section on neurologic examination.

The minimum database recommended for an animal with a neurologic problem is listed in Box 1-2.

Because chemistry panels are usually available at less cost than individual tests, selection of tests is usually not necessary. Otherwise, the selection of chemistry profiles should be based on the problems presented. Additions to the database are recommended for specific problems.

PROBLEM LIST

A problem list is formulated from information obtained from the minimum database. For each problem, a diagnostic plan is formulated. A diagnostic plan for a neurologic problem includes the following steps:

1. The level of the lesion is localized with a neurologic examination. Confirmation of the lesion may require diagnostic imaging.
2. The extent of the lesion is estimated both longitudinally and transversely (e.g., L4-6 spinal cord segments, left

BOX **1-1**

Plan for Neurologic Diagnosis

Collect minimum database
Identify problems
Identify one or more problems related to nervous system
Localize level of lesion
Estimate extent of lesion within that level
List most probable causes (rule-outs or differential diagnosis)
Construct diagnostic plan to determine cause or pathologic injury
Determine prognosis with and without therapy

Modified from Oliver JE Jr: Localization of lesions in the nervous system. In Hoerlein BF, editor: Canine neurology, ed 3, Philadelphia, 1978, WB Saunders.

TABLE 1-1

Clinical Problems in the Nervous System

Problem	Localization
Usually of CNS Origin	
1. Epileptic seizures	Cerebrum, diencephalon
2. Altered mental status	Cerebrum, limbic system, diencephalon
a. Stupor or coma	Brainstem reticular activating formation
b. Abnormal behavior	Limbic system
3. Paresis, paralysis, proprioceptive deficit	See Tables 2-2 to 2-4
4. Ataxia	
a. Head tilt, nystagmus	Vestibular system
b. Intention tremor, dysmetria	Cerebellum
c. General proprioceptive deficits, no brain signs	Spinal cord
5. Hypesthesia, anesthesia	See Figures 1-36,1-38, and 1-39; CN V
Possibly of CNS Origin	
1. Syncope	Usually cardiovascular, metabolic
2. Weakness	See Figure 2-1 and Table 2-2; metabolic or muscular
3. Lameness	Orthopedic: see Table 1-5
4. Pain, hyperesthesia	
a. Generalized	Thalamus, meningitis, lesions affecting multiple joints muscles, bones
b. Localized	See Figures 1-37 to 1-40; CN V
5. Blindness	
a. Pupils normal	Diencephalon or occipital lobe of cerebrum (contralateral)
b. Pupils abnormal	Retina, optic nerve, optic chiasma
6. Hearing deficit	
a. No vestibular signs	Cochlear labyrinth
b. Vestibular signs	CN VIII, vestibular labyrinth, rostral medulla
7. Anosmia	Nasal passages, CN I
8. Urinary incontinence	Pudendal/pelvic nerves, spinal cord, brainstem (see Chapter 3)

Modified from Oliver JE Jr: Localization of lesions in the nervous system. In Hoerlein BF, editor: Canine neurology, ed 3, Philadelphia, 1978, WB Saunders.

side). The neurologic examination provides most of this information, but ancillary diagnostic procedures may be of assistance.

3. The cause of the pathologic process is determined. The history is most useful for establishing the class of disease (neoplasia, infectious disease, trauma, and so forth). Laboratory, diagnostic imaging, or electrophysiologic tests are usually required to substantiate the diagnosis. From this information, the clinician can establish a prognosis with and without appropriate therapy, based on information available about the disease.

BOX 1-2

Minimum Database: Neurologic Problem

History
Physical examination
Neurologic examination
Clinical pathology:
- Complete blood count
- Urinalysis
- Chemistry profile
- Creatine kinase activity

Modified from Oliver JE Jr: Localization of lesions in the nervous system. In Hoerlein BF, editor: Canine neurology, ed 3, Philadelphia, 1978, WB Saunders.

This chapter describes the fundamentals for making a correct neurologic diagnosis. It includes the neurologic history, construction of a sign-time graph, neuroanatomy and organization of the nervous system, and the neurologic examination. Lesion localization is discussed in Chapter 2.

THE HISTORY

Traditionally, the history is taken by the veterinarian. Paraprofessional personnel (e.g., registered veterinary technician, veterinary assistant, nurse) assist the process by obtaining a defined database that is used in conjunction with a problem-oriented medical record system.[1] If one establishes a minimum base of necessary information about every patient or about every patient with a certain problem, then one can obtain that information in a number of ways.

Owner-Supplied History

A basic history can be obtained by use of a well-designed questionnaire. The receptionist gives the questionnaire to the client, who completes it in the reception area. A paraprofessional can assist the client in answering difficult questions. The general medical history is available for review by the veterinarian, who notes important items that may need further clarification. Problem-specific owner histories can be used to supplement the general history.

Role of the Veterinarian

The veterinarian should review most of the important parts of the history with the client. Misinterpretation of terminology, a course of events, or clinical signs occurs frequently. The veterinarian may need to rephrase questions several times before receiving a meaningful answer. The manner in which a question is phrased is important. Questions that imply negligence or ignorance on the part of the client may lead to defensive answers. Questions that suggest a correct answer may lead the client to interpret events incorrectly. All questions should be framed so that the answer "I don't know" is an acceptable alternative; otherwise the client may hypothesize rather than relate facts.[2]

Neurologic History

Signalment

The species, breed, age, and sex of the patient may provide important clues to the diagnosis. Although few diagnoses can be positively ruled in or out on the basis of the signalment, many diseases are more or less likely to occur among certain groups of animals.

The prevalence of some diseases varies greatly among species and breeds. Many infectious diseases are species specific, such as canine distemper, feline infectious peritonitis, and equine protozoal encephalomyelitis. Known inherited diseases must be considered, especially in cases involving multiple offspring of the same litter or lineage. The Appendix lists many of the diseases with a species or breed predilection. Infectious diseases are discussed in Chapter 15.

Young animals are more likely to have congenital and inherited disorders and infectious diseases. Older animals are more likely to have degenerative and neoplastic diseases. Although these criteria are not absolute, the probability is much greater that a 8-year-old brachycephalic dog experiencing seizures will have a neoplasm of the central nervous system (CNS) rather than a congenital anomaly. In the preliminary assessment, and sometimes in the final assessment, a diagnosis is an ordering of probabilities.

Sign-Time Graph

Construction of a sign-time graph is useful for evaluating the course of a disease (Figure 1-1).

The sign-time graph plots the severity of clinical signs (on the vertical axis) against time (on the horizontal axis). A complete history allows the clinician to construct a graph that has no major gaps.[3] The sign-time graph is not usually drawn and entered on the case record. Rather, it is a useful tool for the clinician to construct mentally.

The time of onset of some problems may be exact (e.g., an automobile accident), or it may be difficult to determine, as in the case of neoplastic disease. The first time the client recognizes a problem must be taken as the starting point. Sometimes seemingly unrelated episodes may be the earliest signs and are recognized as such only as the complete history unfolds. For example, an animal with degenerative spinal cord disease may have been observed to stumble or to have difficulty with stairs for some time before clear manifestations of paresis were evident.

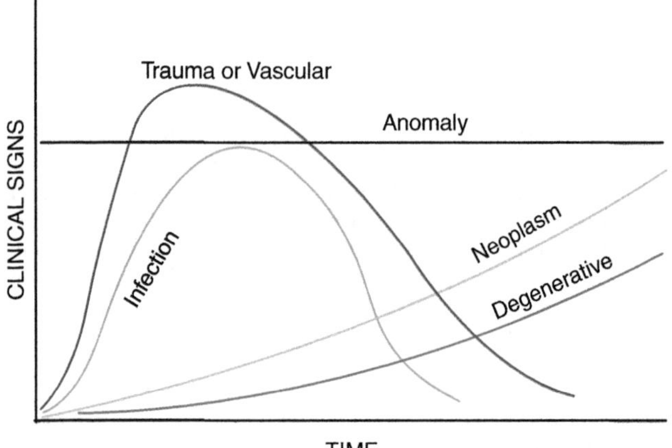

Figure 1-1 Sign-time graph of neurologic diseases. Progression of metabolic, nutritional, and toxic diseases is variable, depending on the cause.

The course of the disease as revealed by the sign-time graph provides important information about the cause of the disease (see Figure 1-1). Slowly progressive diseases with an unrelenting course are immediately distinguished from acute diseases. The first step in making an etiologic diagnosis is classifying the problem as acute or chronic and progressive or nonprogressive. With this information, the problem logically falls into a group of diseases (Figures 1-1 and 1-2 and Table 1-2).

The neurologic examination can further narrow the choice of diseases by indicating whether the problem is focal or diffuse (see Figure 1-2). After a general etiologic or pathologic diagnosis is considered, the diagnostic plan can be established so that one can investigate each probable cause (see discussion of diagnostic methods in Chapter 4).

Prognosis

Providing the owner with a reasonably accurate prognosis is an essential part of clinical neurology. The prognosis is influenced by many variables. The major variables are the location, extent, and cause of the lesion.

The clinical course provides significant insight into the prognosis. Slowly progressive diseases such as neoplastic or degenerative conditions have a much poorer prognosis than those that have passed peak severity and are improving (see Figure 1-1).

Clinical signs are also valuable clues to prognosis. Spinal cord compression produces signs that vary with increasing compression (Figure 1-3).

The signs are not related to the location of the tracts in the spinal cord but do correlate with the diameter of the fibers. With spinal cord compression, large fibers lose function before small fibers are affected. Functional recovery is possible until pain perception is lost. An animal with no response to a painful stimulus for more than 48 hours has a low probability of recovery. Animals that do recover still may have severe motor deficits.

The duration of the lesion is also a significant factor in prognosis because nervous tissue tolerates injury for only a short time. Spinal cord compression has been studied more thoroughly than most CNS injuries. Spinal cord compression severe enough to abolish voluntary motor function but not severe enough to abolish the response to a noxious stimulus is associated with a reasonably good prognosis for recovery if decompression is achieved within 5 to 7 days. The longer the duration of compression, the slower the recovery.

The location and character of the lesion are also important. An infarction of the spinal cord can range from mild to severe. Equally severe lesions have different prognoses, depending on the location. For example, an animal with an infarct primarily affecting gray matter at the L1 segment, with intact sensation

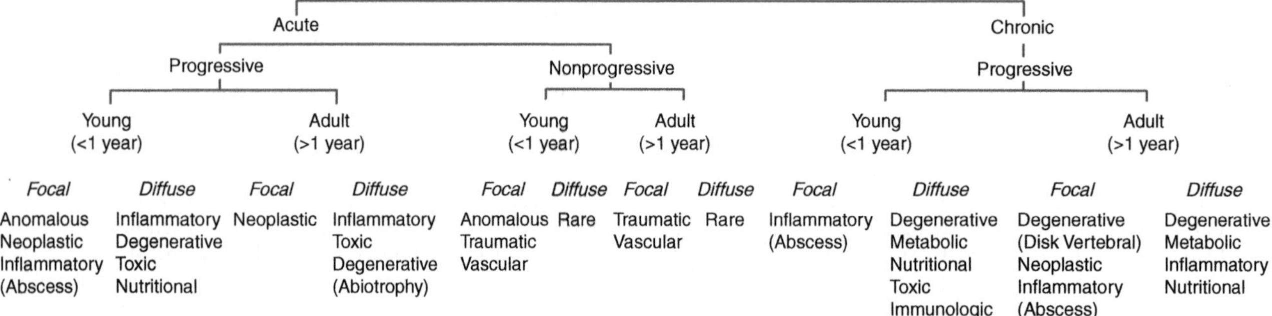

Figure 1-2 Classification of neurologic diseases in approximate order of frequency.

to the pelvic limbs, has a reasonably good prognosis. The same degree of injury at the L5 segment is likely to produce permanent dysfunction because of destruction of the lower motor neurons supplying the femoral nerve.

ANATOMIC AND FUNCTIONAL ORGANIZATION OF THE NERVOUS SYSTEM—AN OVERVIEW

Neurologic examination and lesion localization are dependent on understanding basic concepts of neuroanatomy and neurophysiology and the terminology commonly used in clinical neurology. Although considerable debate exists over the amount of neuroanatomy that must be learned, for practitioners and students, it is much less than the total body of information currently available. The following sections present an overview of the organization and function of the nervous system.

TABLE 1-2

Checklist for Differential Diagnosis

Category of Disease	Examples
D = Degenerative	Primary axonal degeneration
	Storage disorders
	Myelin disorders
	Neuronopathy
	Intervertebral disk disease
	Spondylosis
	Spondylopathy
A = Anomalous	Congenital defects
M = Metabolic	Nervous system disorders secondary to an abnormality of other organ systems (e.g., hypoglycemia, uremia, hypoxia, hepatic)
N = Neoplastic	All tumors
Nutritional	All nutritional disorders
I = Idiopathic	Epilepsy
	Facial nerve paralysis
	Vestibular dysfunction
	Trigeminal nerve
Immune	Myasthenia gravis (acquired)
	Polyradiculoneuritis
	Myositis
Inflammatory	Infectious and noninfectious diseases
	Immune mediated
T = Traumatic	Physical injury
Toxic	Exposure to all toxic agents (may include tetanus and botulism)
V = Vascular	Infarct
	Ischemia
	Hemorrhage

Central Nervous System

The CNS consists of the brain and spinal cord. Embryologically, the CNS develops from ectoderm that forms the neural tube. The brain is divided into the cerebral hemispheres, brainstem, and cerebellum. The five major areas of the brain are the telencephalon (cerebrum), diencephalon, mesencephalon, metencephalon, and myelencephalon (Figure 1-4).

Telencephalon (Cerebrum)

This large area includes the lobes of the cerebral hemispheres, subcortical basal nuclei, olfactory bulbs (cranial nerve I [CN I]), cerebral peduncles, and hippocampus. In general, distinct gross landmarks separating the various lobes are absent. From a clinical standpoint, lesions cannot be reliably localized to a specific lobe of the cerebrum. The following are the lobes of the cerebral cortex:

Frontal: This lobe includes the neurons responsible for voluntary motor functions, especially learned or skilled responses. The major motor pathways are the corticospinal tracts.

Piriform: This lobe is the termination site for tracts that relay information for smell.

Parietal: This lobe largely functions for conscious perception of touch, pressure, temperature, and noxious stimuli.

Temporal: This lobe functions for conscious perception of sound (hearing) and shares some functions with the parietal lobe.

Occipital: This lobe contains vision centers.

The following are the three types of axons (fibers) from cortical neurons:

Association fibers: axons that communicate with other neurons in the same cerebral hemisphere.

Projection fibers: axons that leave the cerebrum via the internal capsule to enter the brainstem (e.g., the corticospinal tracts). These fibers have important clinical application to lesion localization and will be described further in the section on Motor Functions.

Commissural fibers: axons that cross from one cerebral hemisphere to the other.

Diencephalon

The diencephalon includes the thalamus and hypothalamus. The rostral-ventral border is demarcated by the optic chiasm. The optic tracts lie on the lateral surfaces. The thalamus contains nuclei that receive sensory information from many areas.

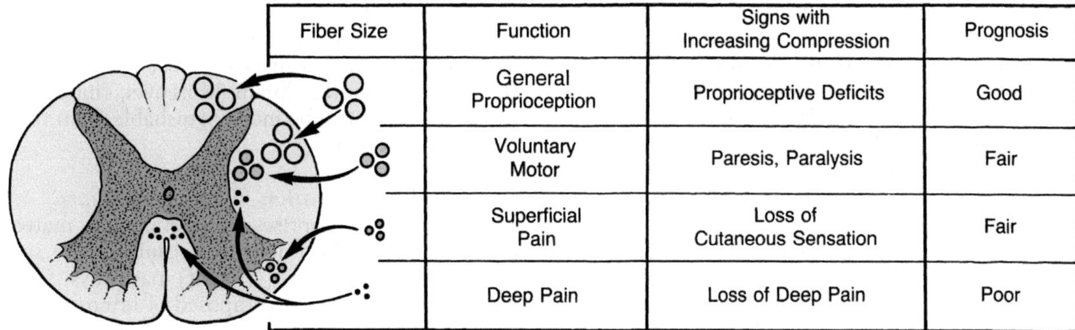

Figure 1-3 Progression of signs in spinal cord compression.

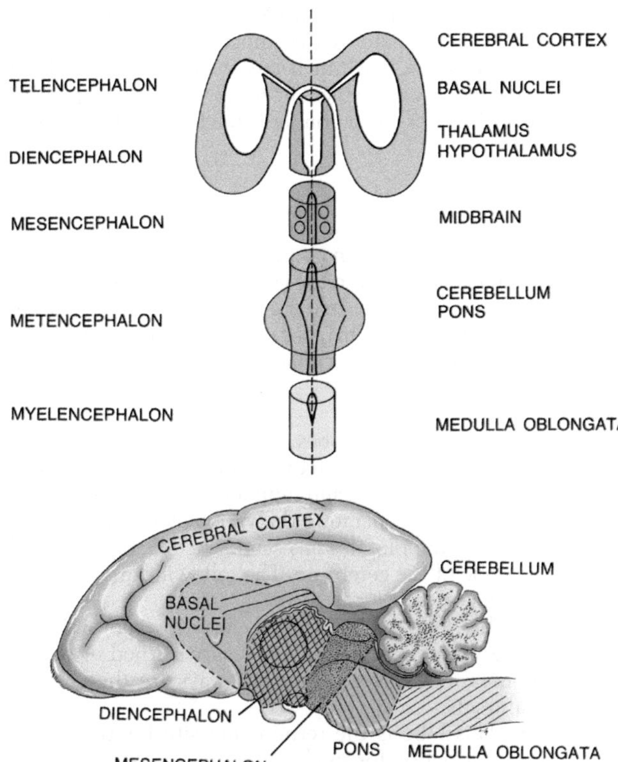

Figure 1-4 Segmental organization of the brain. Five major regions are significant clinically: the cerebrum, including the cerebral cortex, cerebral white matter, and the basal nuclei; the diencephalon, including the thalamus and the hypothalamus; the brainstem, including the midbrain, the pons, and the medulla oblongata; the vestibular system, including the labyrinth (peripheral) and the vestibular nuclei (central) in the rostral medulla; and the cerebellum. (From Hoerlein BF: Canine neurology, ed 3, Philadelphia, 1978, WB Saunders.)

It serves as the major relay center for afferent (sensory) fibers projecting to the cerebral cortex. The hypothalamus lies ventral to the thalamus and has neuroendocrine and autonomic functions. It connects to the pituitary gland via the infundibular stalk.

Mesencephalon (Midbrain)

The mesencephalon contains the neurons for CN III (oculomotor) and CN IV (trochlear), which innervate extraocular muscles. The rostral and caudal colliculi, located in the tectum (roof) or dorsal aspect of the midbrain, are associated with visual and auditory reflexes, respectively, and relay information to the cerebellum. The centers for pupillary light reflexes (parasympathetic-pupillary constriction) (parasympathetic motor nucleus of CN III) and motor to extraocular muscles (oculomotor nuclei of CN III) also are located in the dorsal aspect of the midbrain. Beneath the tectum lies the tegmentum, the origin of the tectotegmentospinal tract, which provides the upper motor neurons (UMNs) pathway for the sympathetic innervations. Finally, centers (red nucleus) for motor control of gait are located here.

Metencephalon

The metencephalon contains the pons and cerebellum. The pons contains neurons for CN V (trigeminal), whose axons innervate the muscles of mastication. It also provides sensory innervation to the face (maxillary and ophthalmic regions) and mandible and is the location of the center for micturition. The ascending reticular activating system (ARAS) arises in the pons and is responsible for consciousness. The pons contains motor pathways from the cerebrum that synapse in the cerebellum. The cerebellum composes the dorsal metencephalon. It coordinates motor activity and helps regulate muscle tone.

Myelencephalon (Medulla Oblongata)

The myelencephalon contains the neurons of CN VI through XII (Figure 1-5) and central components of the vestibular system. Motor tracts (medullary reticulospinal) also arise from within this area. The major centers for respiratory and vasomotor (cardiac) function lie mostly in the medulla.

Forebrain

The forebrain contains the telencephalon and diencephalon. Lesions affecting these areas generally create contralateral clinical signs and generally are similar. Forebrain signs include blindness, depression, seizures, contralateral loss of postural reactions, and contralateral sensory deficits.

Midbrain

The midbrain has been described already (see section on Mesencephalon). Lesions in the midbrain produce abnormal mentation, disorders of ocular movement (nystagmus [oculocephalic reflex]) and position (strabismus), dilated (parasympathetic dysfunction) or constricted (sympathetic dysfunction) pupil(s), poor or absent pupillary light reflexes, gait deficits, and contralateral or ipsilateral postural reaction deficits.

Hindbrain

These three structures lie in the caudal cranial fossa (caudal to the osseous tentorium) of the skull. The hindbrain includes the pons, medulla, and cerebellum. The pons and medulla also contain upper motor neurons responsible for the generation of gait. Lesions in the pons and medulla cause ipsilateral motor and sensory deficits, vestibular dysfunction, deficits in cranial nerve function (CN V-XII), and abnormal mentation. Clinical signs of cerebellar dysfunction include incoordination, cerebellar ataxia predominated by hypermetria in which there is overflexion of the joints of the limbs during the swing phase of the gait. The overall impression is that the animal is overreaching as it advances the limb. Additionally, intention tremors may be present. Because the cerebellum has direct connections with the vestibular system, cerebellar disorders also can cause signs of vestibular dysfunction. Lesions in the cerebellum also can cause menace deficits with normal vision; the pathway for this is still unknown.

Brainstem

Anatomically, the brainstem contains the diencephalon, mesencephalon, metencephalon, and myelencephalon. Functionally, it includes all structures except the diencephalon. Functionally, most clinicians restrict the brainstem to the pons and medulla. Clinical signs are those previously described for the midbrain and hindbrain. Moreover, clinical signs of diencephalic lesions can be indistinguishable from those involving the telencephalon.

Anatomic Organization of the Spinal Cord

The spinal cord comprises peripheral white matter composed of nerve tracts. The tracts are organized into specific motor (efferent) and sensory (afferent) pathways. Gray matter is located centrally and is composed of interneurons and motor neurons that innervate muscle. Specific structures are discussed in sections on functional organization of the CNS.

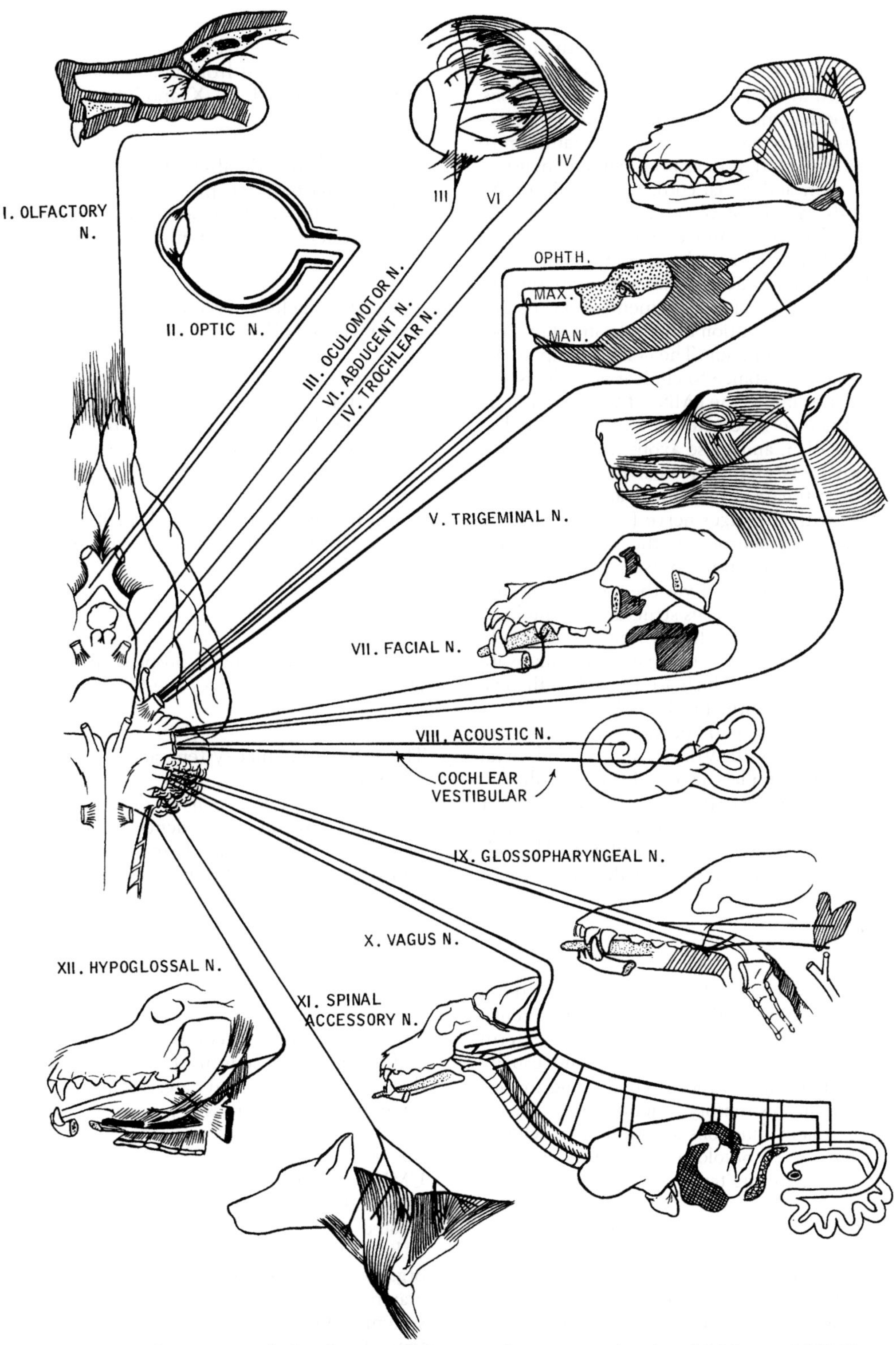

Figure 1-5 The origin and distribution of the cranial nerves in the dog. *N,* Nerve; *OPHTH,* ophthalmic nerve; *MAX,* maxillary nerve; *MAN,* mandibular nerve. (From Hoerlein BF: Canine neurology, ed 3, Philadelphia, 1978, WB Saunders.)

Peripheral Nervous System

The peripheral nervous system contains the axons of the spinal and cranial nerves and their receptors and effector organs. It includes both general and autonomic components. Peripheral nerves may contain fibers that are motor, sensory, or both. The motor neuron cell body is typically located in the CNS. The neuronal cell body, its axon, junction between the axon and muscle (neuromuscular junction), and muscle are known as the lower motor neuron unit (LMN unit). The anatomic distribution and function of spinal nerves are discussed later (see section on lower motor neurons, or LMNs) and in Chapters 3 and 5. Cranial nerves are further discussed in Chapters 8, 9, and 11.

Autonomic Nervous System

The autonomic nervous system contains sympathetic and parasympathetic divisions. It is a multineuron system. Central neurons are located in the hypothalamus, midbrain, pons, and medulla. The hypothalamus is the primary center for integrating autonomic functions. Axons traverse the brainstem to affect autonomic LMNs, referred to as preganglionic neurons, located in the brainstem and spinal cord. Autonomic LMNs innervate the smooth muscle of blood vessels and visceral structures, glands, and cardiac muscle. Sensory fibers from body viscera are included in the peripheral component.

The LMNs of the sympathetic nervous system are distributed in the thoracolumbar spinal cord segments and generally use the spinal nerves for distribution to muscle and skin. Specific nerves control visceral function. The cranial sympathetic nerve has considerable importance to clinical neurologists in lesion localization. For example, the LMNs of the sympathetic nervous system destined to innervate the eye are located in spinal cord segments T1-3, and these axons leave the spinal cord associated with roots of the brachial plexus. The cranial sympathetic nerve traverses the thorax and the cervical region in association with the vagus nerve (vagosympathetic trunk). Axons synapse on neurons in the cranial cervical ganglion. Axons from these neurons course near the middle ear and are distributed to the head via the vasculature and other cranial nerves. Of the numerous structures of the head innervated by sympathetic fibers, clinical signs are typically appreciated because of the effect of the axons that innervate the dilator muscle of the pupil, which are carried to the eye along with fibers of CN V (ophthalmic branch).

The LMNs of the parasympathetic nervous system are located in the brainstem (CN III, VII, IX, and X) and sacral spinal cord segments. The pupillary light reflex is described in following sections. The vagus nerve (CN X) is the major motor nerve for innervation of the muscles of the larynx, esophagus, and thoracic and abdominal viscera (see Chapter 9). The pelvic nerve innervates the detrusor muscle of the bladder (see Chapter 3).

Functional Organization of the Central Nervous System

Functionally, the CNS can be classified in several ways, but a simple scheme includes motor (efferent), sensory (afferent), and autonomic systems (efferent and afferent). The term *efferent* means conducting away from a center and usually indicates motor function. *Afferent* means conducting toward a center and usually indicates sensory function. Neuroanatomists may divide the major functions according to a scheme that relates function to embryologic development. That scheme is presented because the terms are still used in clinical literature.[4]

General Somatic Efferent System

The general somatic efferent (GSE) system includes motor neurons that innervate voluntary striated muscle of the head and skeleton. These neurons are found in CN III, IV, VI, and XII and all spinal nerves.

General Visceral Efferent System

The general visceral efferent (GVE) system includes motor neurons of the autonomic nervous system. It includes neurons in CN III, VII, IX, X, and (for parasympathetic division) XI and all spinal nerves. It includes sympathetic and parasympathetic divisions. The thoracic and lumbar spinal cord regions contain preganglionic neurons for the sympathetic division. The cranial (CN III, VII, IX, and X) and the sacral regions contain preganglionic neurons for the parasympathetic division.

Special Visceral Efferent System

Neurons in the special visceral efferent (SVE) innervate striated muscle derived from brachial arch mesoderm. They are found in CN V, VII, IX, X, and XI.

General Somatic Afferent System

The general somatic afferent (GSA) system includes sensory neurons that have receptors in the surface of the head, body, and limbs. The neurons are located in CN V and all spinal nerves. It detects touch, temperature, and noxious stimuli.

Special Somatic Afferent System (SSA)

This system includes vision and hearing, and neurons are associated with CN II and VIII.

General Visceral Afferent System (GVA)

This system includes sensory neurons from visceral structures of the head, body cavities, and blood vessels. Neurons are located in CN VII, IX, and X, and in spinal nerves.

Special Visceral Afferent (SVA)

This is the system for taste and smell. Taste receptors are associated with CN VII, IX, and X, and smell is associated with CN I.

General Proprioception (GP)

Proprioception is detection of changes in position of the trunk, limbs, and head. General proprioception neurons are associated with all spinal nerves and CN V.

Special Proprioception (SP)

This is the vestibular system, and neurons are associated with CN VIII.

Over the years we have determined that this "classic" scheme is difficult for students and practitioners to remember. Therefore we use a scheme that describes function based on motor, GP, vestibular, general sensory (touch, temperature, pressure, and response to noxious stimuli), special sensory (smell, taste, vision, and hearing), cerebellar, and cognitive systems. These major systems are described in subsequent sections.

Motor Systems

The motor system is composed of two divisions, the upper and lower motor neurons. Lesions of the motor system produce clinical signs called paresis or paralysis, depending on the severity or completeness of lesions.

Upper Motor Neurons

UMNs are responsible for initiating voluntary motor functions and modulating the activity of the LMN units. They are located in the cerebral cortex and brainstem and are found in both the somatic and autonomic systems. Their axons are organized into specific tracts, and they synapse in spinal cord gray matter on interneurons or directly on LMNs. The UMN system is divided into the pyramidal and extrapyramidal systems (Figure 1-6).

The pyramidal system allows animals to perform finely skilled movements but is not necessary for initiation of gait in animals. Neurons are located in the frontal/parietal lobe of the cerebral cortex (caudal cruciate gyrus) and the axons are contained in the corticospinal tracts. Axons cross in the pyramids located in the caudal medulla and descend on the contralateral side. Axons synapse on LMNs in the spinal cord and cranial nerve LMNs in the brainstem. Lesions of the motor cortex or section of the pyramids produce little gait deficit but will cause postural reaction deficits in contralateral limbs.

The extrapyramidal system allows animals to gait and to initiate voluntary movement. Neurons are located in nuclei in all divisions of the brain. Some of the more clinically important motor pathways include the tectospinal, reticulospinal, rubrospinal, and vestibulospinal tracts. Caudal to the midbrain, lesions generally produce signs in ipsilateral limbs and severe gait deficits. Lesions rostral to the midbrain produce signs in contralateral limbs and less gait involvement.

Upper motor neurons may stimulate or inhibit motor actions. For instance, the UMN is necessary for voluntary motor action and at the same time exerts inhibitory action on other functions, such as spinal cord reflexes. Animals with UMN lesions caudal to the midbrain may have exaggerated reflexes (hyperreflexia) and increased muscle tone (hypertonia).

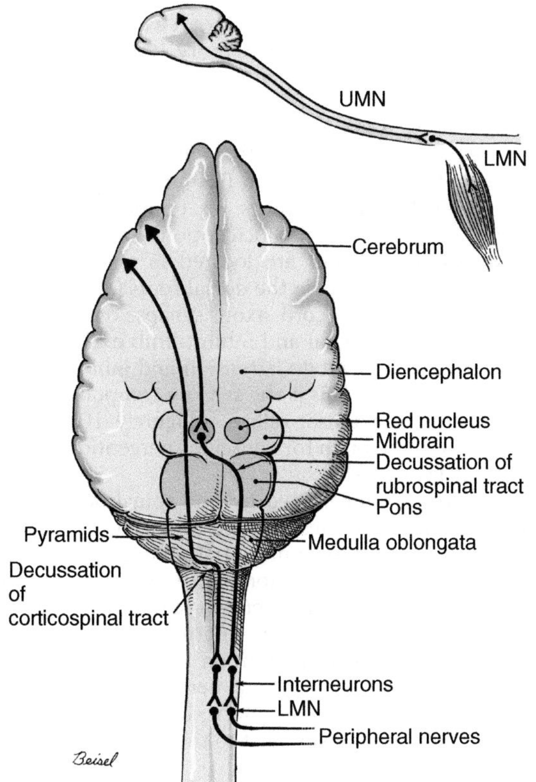

Figure 1-6 Neurons in the cerebral cortex and the brainstem send axons to the lower motor neurons (LMNs) in the brainstem and the spinal cord. The upper motor neurons (UMNs) provide voluntary control of movement. Two of the major voluntary motor pathways, the corticospinal (pyramidal) pathway and the corticorubrospinal pathway, are illustrated.

Signs of Upper Motor Neuron Lesions

UMN lesions produce a characteristic set of clinical signs caudal to the level of the injury. These signs are summarized in Table 1-3 and are compared with signs of LMN lesions.

The primary sign of motor dysfunction is paresis. With disease of the UMN system, the paresis or paralysis is associated with normal or increased extensor tone and normal or exaggerated reflexes. Abnormal reflexes (e.g., a crossed extensor reflex) may be seen in some cases. Loss of descending inhibition on the LMN produces these findings. Disuse muscle atrophy may occur and is slow to appear, is not complete, and includes the entirety of the affected limb(s) in most cases.

Because lesions at many different levels of the CNS may produce UMN signs, localization of a lesion to a specific segment usually is not possible when only UMN signs are considered. Proper interpretation of UMN signs and other associated signs, however, allows one to localize a lesion to a region. For example, UMN paresis of the pelvic limbs indicates a lesion cranial to L4 spinal cord segment. If the lesion were at L4-S2 spinal cord segments, LMN paresis of the pelvic limbs would be present. If the thoracic limbs are normal, the lesion must be caudal to T2 spinal cord segment. Therefore pelvic limb paresis (UMN) with normal thoracic limbs indicates a lesion between the T3 and L3 spinal cord segments.

Lower Motor Neurons

The lower motor neurons (LMN) connect the CNS with muscles and glands. All motor activity of the nervous system ultimately is expressed through LMNs. The LMNs are located in all spinal cord segments in the intermediate and ventral horns of the gray matter and in cranial nerve nuclei (CN III-VII, IX-XII) in the brainstem. The axons extending from these cells form the spinal (see Figure 1-6) and cranial nerves.

The nervous system is arranged in a segmental fashion. A spinal cord segment is demarcated by a pair of spinal nerves. Each spinal nerve has a dorsal (sensory) and a ventral (motor) root (Figure 1-7).

The muscle or group of muscles innervated by one spinal nerve is called a myotome. Myotomes are arranged segmentally in the paraspinal muscles but are more irregular in the limbs. Dysfunction of a specific muscle is localizing to a spinal nerve or a ventral root (Figures 1-8 and 1-9). The approximate

TABLE 1-3

Summary of Lower Motor Neuron (LMN) and Upper Motor Neuron (UMN) Signs

	LMN: Segmental Signs	UMN: Long-Tract Signs
Motor function	Paresis to paralysis: flaccid muscles	Paresis to paralysis: spastic muscles
Reflexes	Hyporeflexia to areflexia	Normal to hyperreflexia (especially myotatic reflexes)
Muscle atrophy	Early and severe: neurogenic; limb contracture	Late and mild: disuse
Muscle tone	Decreased	Normal to increased
Electromyographic changes	Abnormal potentials (fibrillation potentials, no positive sharp waves) after 5 to 7 days	No changes
Associated sensory signs	Anesthesia of innervated area (dermatomes); paresthesia or hyperesthesia of adjacent areas; decreased to absent proprioception	Decreased to absent proprioception, decreased perception of noxious stimuli caudal to the lesion

relationship of spinal cord segments to vertebrae is illustrated in Figure 1-8.

Signs of LMN Lesions

Lesions of the LMN, whether of the cell body, the axon, motor end plate, or muscle produce a characteristic group of clinical signs summarized in Table 1-3. Signs of LMN lesions are easily recognized on neurologic examination. Paresis or paralysis, loss of muscle tone, and reduced or absence of reflexes occur immediately after the LMN unit is damaged. Rapid muscle atrophy is detectable within 1 week and becomes severe. Atrophy is limited to denervated muscles. Proper interpretation of LMN signs allows the clinician to localize accurately lesions to a specific segment of the CNS from which the affected LMN unit arises. For example, LMN signs affecting the thoracic limb are localized to the C6-T2 spinal cord segments, peripheral nerves, or muscles.

Most muscles are innervated by nerves that originate in more than one spinal cord segment. For example, the quadriceps muscle is innervated by neurons originating in spinal cord segments L4-6. Loss of one segment or one root causes partial loss of the innervation of the muscle. The clinical sign is paresis, but not paralysis, of the affected muscles. The reflexes may be depressed. Lesions of peripheral nerves are more likely to cause severe loss of function, and all muscles innervated by the nerve are affected. The reflexes are usually absent in these lesions (see Figure 1-9).

Differentiating UMN and LMN signs is extremely important for localizing lesions in the spinal cord and brainstem. UMN signs localize lesions to spinal cord *regions*, whereas LMN signs help localize lesions to specific nerves, nerve roots, or spinal cord *segments*.

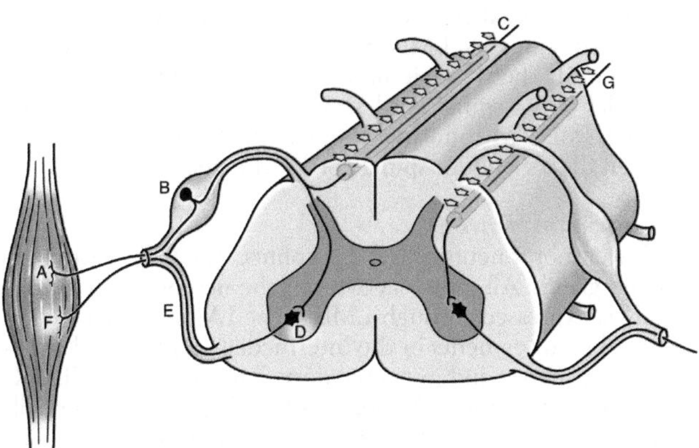

Figure 1-7 Components of the spinal reflex. **A,** Muscle spindle. **B,** Dorsal root ganglion. **C,** Ascending sensory pathway in the dorsal column. **D,** Ventral horn motor neuron (lower motor neuron). **E,** Ventral (motor) root. **F,** Neuromuscular junction. **G,** Descending motor pathway in the lateral column (upper motor neuron). The dorsal and ventral roots join to form the peripheral nerve. (From Oliver JE: Neurologic examination, Vet Med Small Anim Clin 68:151–154, 1973.)

Sensory Systems

In our organizational scheme, sensory systems are divided into general proprioception, general sensory (segmental and long tract), and special sensory systems.

Segmental Sensory Neurons

Sensory neurons are located in the spinal ganglia within the dorsal roots along the spinal cord (see Figure 1-7) and in the ganglia of CN V. The receptors for temperature, pressure, touch, and noxious stimuli (nociception) are located on or near body surfaces. Axons are located in peripheral nerves and enter the spinal cord via the dorsal roots (see Figure 1-7). After entering the spinal cord, axons synapse on interneurons that stimulate limb flexion and inhibit limb extension in the ipsilateral limb and facilitate extension and inhibit flexion in the contralateral limb. This is the sensory component of withdrawal and crossed extensor reflexes (Figure 1-10). Fibers are also projected to the brain for conscious perception of sensory information (Figure 1-11).

The area of skin innervated by one spinal nerve is called a dermatome. Dermatomes also are arranged in regular segmental fashion, except for some variation in the limbs (Figure 1-12). Alterations in the sensation of a dermatome can be used to localize a lesion to a spinal nerve or a dorsal root. The area of skin innervated by the sensory neurons of a named peripheral nerve has a different distribution (Figure 1-13), allowing localization of lesions of peripheral nerves.

Cranial nerve V is the major nerve for facial sensation (see Figure 1-5). Sensory fibers project to the contralateral cerebral cortex.

Signs of Segmental Sensory Neuron Lesions

Lesions of the sensory neurons also produce characteristic clinical signs. Segmental sensory signs include (1) anesthesia (complete lesion), (2) hypesthesia (decreased perception of noxious stimuli, partial lesion), (3) hyperesthesia (increased

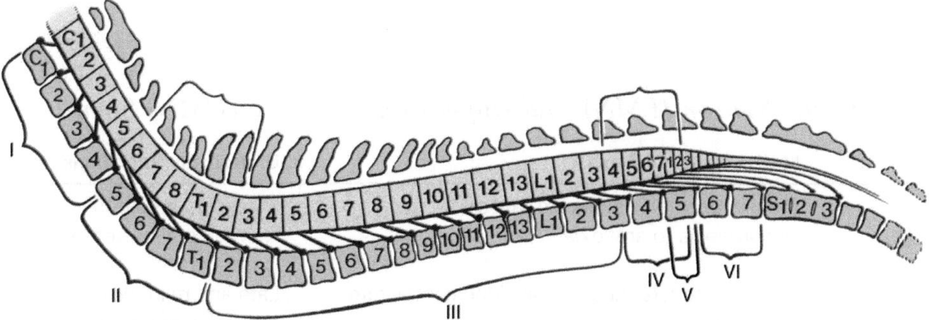

Figure 1-8 The spinal cord has a segmental arrangement; each segment has a pair of spinal nerves. The approximate relationship of spinal cord segments and vertebrae in the dog is illustrated here. Regions of the spinal cord that give rise to characteristic clinical signs when damaged are labeled. I, C1-5, Upper motor neuron (UMN) to all limbs; II, C6-T2, lower motor neuron (LMN) to thoracic, UMN to pelvic limbs; III, T3-L3, normal thoracic, UMN to pelvic limbs; IV, L4-S2, normal thoracic, LMN to pelvic limbs; V, S1-3, partial LMN to pelvic limbs, absent perineal reflex, atonic bladder; VI, caudal nerves, atonic tail.

sensitivity of nociception, irritative lesion), and (4) loss of reflexes. Increased or decreased sensation of a dermatome can be mapped by pinching the skin. Mapping the distribution of sensory loss is accurate to within three spinal cord segments. Similarly, the alteration of sensitivity in the distribution of a named peripheral nerve localizes the lesion accurately.

Long-Tract Sensory Pathways

Sensory pathways of clinical significance include those responsible for general proprioception (position sense) and general somatic afferent information (specifically, response to noxious stimuli). In animals, two types of fibers relaying information regarding noxious stimuli traverse the spinal cord. Based on the location of receptors, these are called superficial and deep pathways. Superficial nociceptive pathways (for perception of discrete noxious stimuli in the skin [e.g., a pinprick]) are located primarily in the ventrolateral (primate) or dorsolateral (cat) portion of the spinal cord, with a relay in the thalamus. The pathway primarily projects to the contralateral cerebral cortex for conscious recognition of pain. The deep nociceptive pathway (for perception of severe pain in the bones, the joints, or the viscera [e.g., a crushing pain]) is a bilateral, multisynaptic system that projects to the reticular formation, the thalamus, and the cerebral cortex. In general, damage must be bilateral and severe to block conscious perception of noxious stimuli distal to lesions.

General Proprioception

Proprioception means "sense of position." The clinical sign of proprioception dysfunction is ataxia (incoordination). General proprioception describes the position of muscles, joints, and tendons because proprioceptors are located in neuromuscular spindles and Golgi tendon organs. Axons project within peripheral nerves and enter the spinal cord via dorsal roots. Neurons are located in the spinal ganglia. On entering the spinal cord, axons may (1) synapse directly on alpha motor neurons for initiation of extensor reflexes such as the patellar or knee jerk reflex (monosynaptic reflex arc) (Figure 1-14), (2) synapse on interneurons to indirectly influence alpha motor neurons, or (3) synapse on interneurons and then send afferent fibers via the spinal cord to the brainstem, cerebellum, and cerebrum (Figure 1-15).

Proprioception is transmitted to the cerebellum via spinocerebellar tracts. This information is used by the cerebellum to regulate muscle tone, posture, locomotion, and equilibrium. Lesions involving these tracts have a profound effect on gait and may create clinical signs similar to cerebellar dysfunction (i.e., truncal swaying, hypermetria). Spinocerebellar tracts activate Purkinje neurons in the cerebellum that inhibit protraction (flexion) of limbs. This facilitates limb extension for weight bearing. Lesions in spinocerebellar tracts result in overflexion of limbs, known as hypermetria. Clinical signs are ipsilateral to lesions.

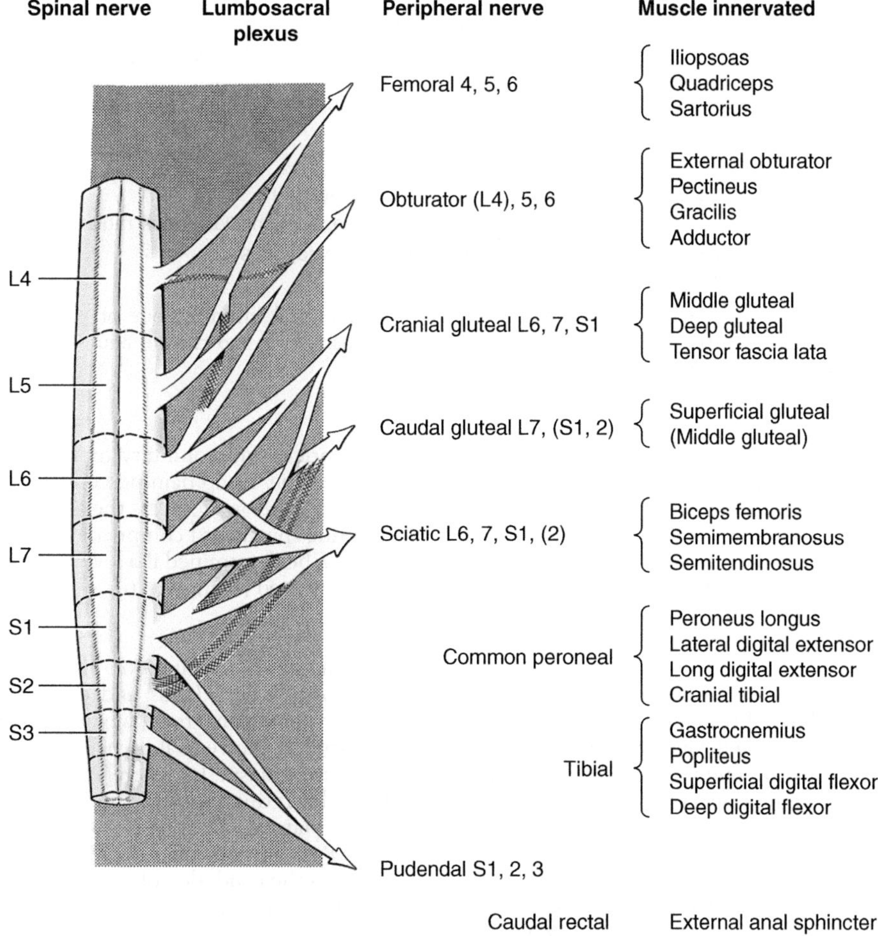

Figure 1-9 **A,** Segmental innervation from cervical intumescence of thoracic limb muscles in the dog.

Continued

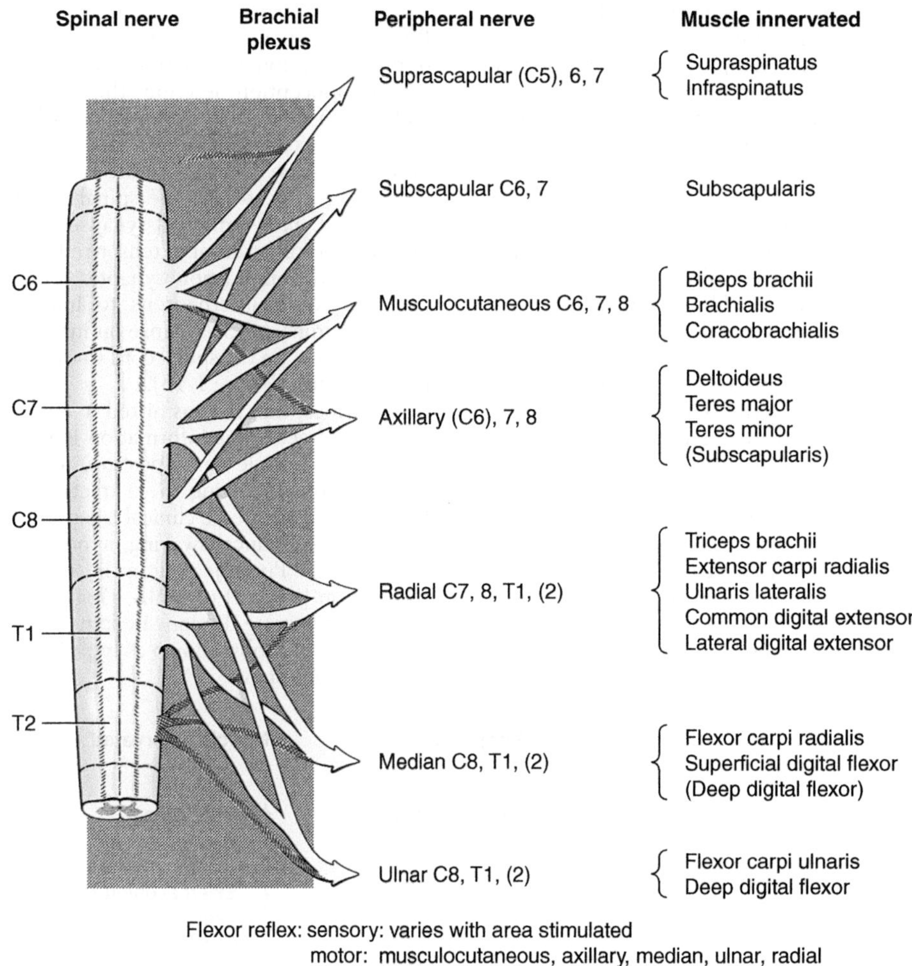

Figure 1-9—cont'd **B,** Segmental innervation from lumbosacral intumescence of pelvic limb muscles in the dog. (From de Lahunta A: Veterinary neuroanatomy and clinical neurology, ed 3, St Louis, 2009, Elsevier.)

Conscious proprioception is carried to the medulla via the dorsal columns (fasciculus gracilis [from pelvic limbs] and cuneatus [from thoracic limbs]), whose fibers first synapse in medullary nuclei (nuclei gracilis and cuneatus, respectively). Axons from these nuclei cross to the opposite side via the deep arcuate fibers and then traverse the brainstem in the medial lemniscus to the thalamus. Ultimately, fibers are projected to the contralateral parietal lobe of the cerebral cortex.

Lesions of these pathways are associated with general proprioceptive ataxia and delayed responses in the initiation of postural reactions (hopping, knuckling-paw placement). Lesions rostral and caudal to the midbrain create deficits in contralateral and ipsilateral limbs, respectively.

Signs of Long-Tract Sensory Lesions

The signs of sensory long-tract lesions are valuable for the formulation of a prognosis of CNS disorders and for localization. Spinal cord lesions frequently cause decreased sensation caudal to the level of the lesion. Proprioceptive deficits usually are the first signs observed with compressive lesions of the spinal cord. Abnormal positioning of the feet and ataxia may be present before any significant loss of voluntary motor activity occurs. Superficial pain perception (the conscious perception of a pinprick) and voluntary motor activity are often lost at the same time. Deep pain perception (perception of a strong pinch of a bone or a joint) is the last neurologic function to be lost during spinal cord compression. The level of a spinal cord lesion can be determined if a level of hypesthesia or anesthesia can be detected (Figure 1-16).

Special Sensory: Vision

The retina serves the function of a digital scanner. It contains photosensitive cells (rods and cones), bipolar neurons, and ganglion cells. Axons from ganglion cells form the optic nerve. Just rostral to the ventral diencephalon, the optic nerves join at the optic chiasm. In general, fibers from the medial (nasal) half of the retina cross at the optic chiasm, whereas fibers from the lateral (temporal) half of the retina remain ipsilateral. Post chiasm, fibers continue in bilateral optic tracts located on the caudodorsolateral surface of the diencephalon. Most optic-tract fibers involved in vision synapse in the lateral geniculate nucleus of the thalamus; however, about 20% to 25% of fibers pass over the geniculate nucleus and terminate in the pretectal area of the midbrain and participate in pupillary light reflexes. Visual fibers project from the lateral geniculate nucleus to the contralateral occipital cortex, where the image is perceived.

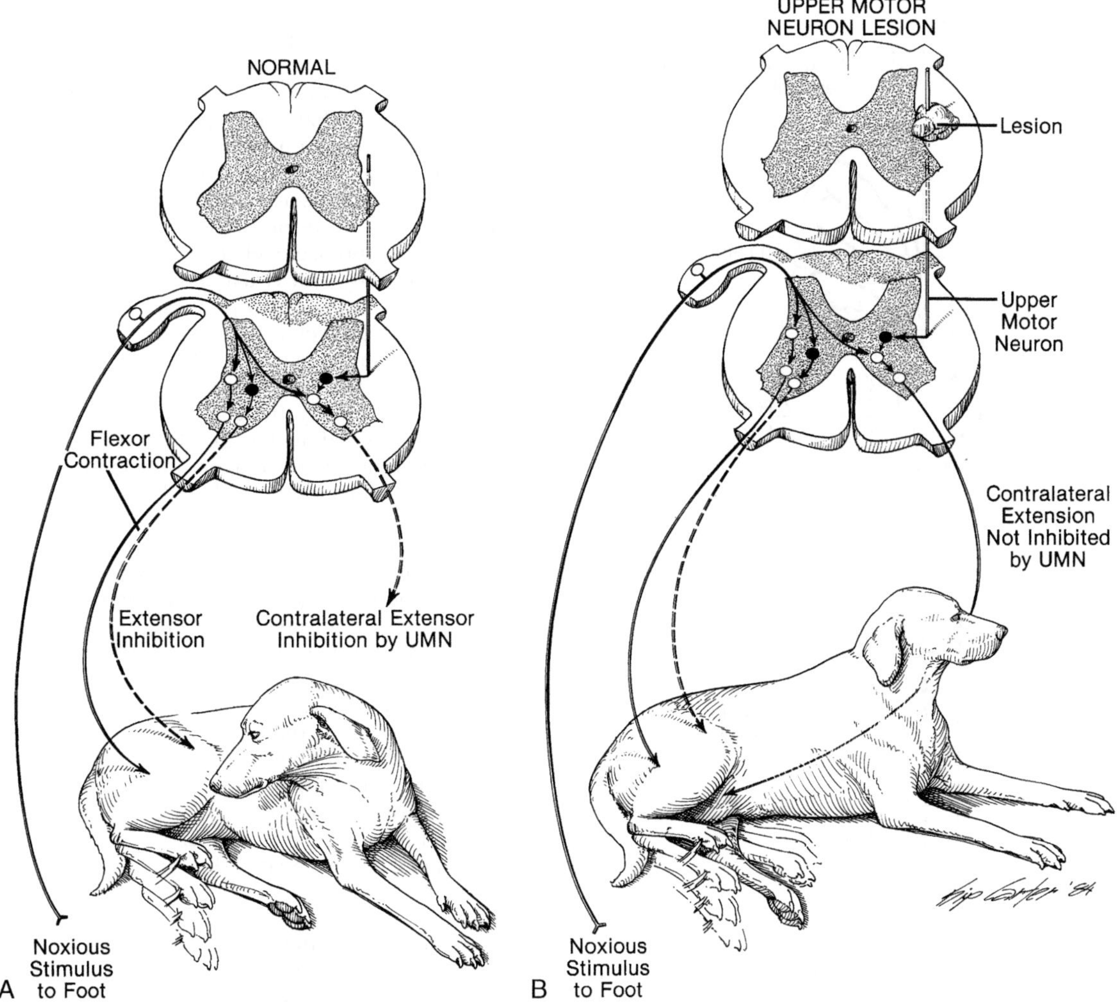

Figure 1-10 Flexor and crossed extension reflexes. **A,** The animal is positioned in lateral recumbency and a noxious stimulus is applied to a digit. The limb is immediately withdrawn. Sensory fibers enter the spinal cord through the dorsal root to synapse on interneurons. Flexor motor neurons are activated, causing flexion of the limb. Simultaneously, inhibitory interneurons cause relaxation of the antagonistic extensor muscles. Other interneurons cross the spinal cord to activate contralateral extensor muscles—the crossed extensor reflex. **B,** The crossed extensor reflex is inhibited unless damage to UMN systems has occurred. Sensory fibers also project to the brain, causing a conscious awareness of pain and subsequently a behavioral reaction **(A)**. The reflex is not dependent on a behavioral reaction. The behavioral reaction may be absent if sensory pathways are damaged. (From Oliver JE, Hoerlein BF, Mayhew IG: Veterinary neurology, Philadelphia, 1987, WB Saunders.)

Pupillary Light Reflexes

Axons that pass over the lateral geniculate nucleus enter the midbrain and synapse on parasympathetic nuclei in the pretectal area. A second neuron then synapses on the parasympathetic motor nucleus of CN III. This is a bilateral pathway that influences both nuclei. Parasympathetic axons follow CN III and synapse in the ciliary ganglion. The short ciliary nerve synapses on the iris sphincter muscle, resulting in both direct and consensual pupillary light reflexes. Disorders of vision (blindness), pupil size (anisocoria), and ocular movement (nystagmus) and position (strabismus) are discussed in Chapter 11.

Special Sensory: Hearing

The cochlea is the receptor organ for hearing and is located in the inner ear. Movement of special hair cells in the cochlea activates fibers in the cochlear nerve. The cochlear nerve joins the vestibular nerve to form CN VIII, the vestibulocochlear nerve, which enters the rostral medulla. The cochlear nerve neurons are located in nuclei just inside the medulla. Numerous pathways and synapses are available for reflex activity and conscious perception of sound. Conscious perception of sound is bilateral and resides in the temporal lobes of the cerebral cortex. These pathways provide little help in localizing lesions within the brain. Deafness is discussed in Chapter 9.

Vestibular System

This is a special proprioception system that maintains an animal's orientation relative to gravity and position in face of linear or rotatory acceleration or tilting of the head. It maintains proper position of the eyes, trunk, and limbs relative to head position or movement. Neurons are located in the vestibular nuclei of the brainstem and connect to receptors

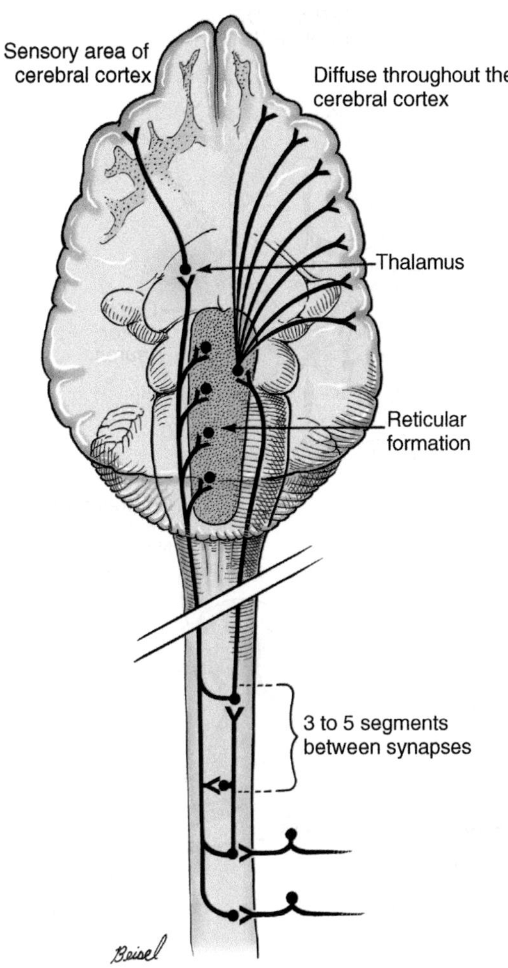

Figure 1-11 The pain pathway in animals is bilateral and multisynaptic (see also Figure 1-15). The deep pain pathway apparently has synapses every three to five segments, with projections continuing cranially on both sides of the spinal cord.

in the inner ear via CN VIII. The receptors for balance are located in the semicircular canals. To maintain proper posture and coordinated (conjugate) eye movements, vestibular stimuli are projected from vestibular nuclei to the cerebellum and rostrally via the medial longitudinal fasciculus (MLF) to nuclei of CN III, IV, and VI. Motor fibers from vestibular nuclei project to all levels of the spinal cord via vestibulospinal tracts and synapse on interneurons in ventral gray matter. The net effect is facilitation of ipsilateral (same side) extensor muscles and inhibition of ipsilateral flexor muscles and contralateral extensor muscles. This is important for maintenance of extensor tone and facilitation of the stretch reflex mechanism. Both are important components of the animal's antigravity system.

Vestibular syndromes are characterized by ataxia, head tilt, circling, nystagmus, and falling toward the side of the lesion (Figure 1-17). Vestibular syndromes are classified as peripheral (inner ear, vestibular nerve) or central (medulla and cerebellum) and are discussed in Chapter 8.

Cerebellum

The cerebellum functions as a coordinator of movements that originate in the UMN system. It also functions to help maintain equilibrium, posture, body support against gravity, and eye movements. The cerebellum receives sensory information and compares or measures where body parts are in relationship to the action required to perform coordinated movements. It contains both efferent and afferent pathways, which enter or leave the cerebellum via three pairs of peduncles that connect the brainstem to the cerebellum. For the cerebellum to function, it must receive sensory information related to position of the head, trunk, and limbs. The most important sensory pathways are the spinocerebellar tracts (unconscious proprioception from the limbs, trunk, and neck), vestibulocerebellar tracts (special proprioception for head position), and visual and auditory sensation via the colliculi and tectocerebellar processes. Extrapyramidal motor information is projected to the cerebellum via the olivary nuclei located in the caudal medulla. Axons from all areas of the cerebral cortex project fibers to the cerebellum via the pontine nuclei. Finally, the cerebellum receives motor information from the red nucleus (midbrain) and reticular formation. No efferent cerebellar axons project into the spinal cord and directly influence the LMNs. The cerebellum exerts its regulatory functions via efferent fibers that influence UMNs in the brainstem.

In general, cerebellar disease causes severe ataxia, dysmetria (both hypermetria and hypometria, and affects the rate and force with which movement is made), tremors (both generalized and intention), and sometimes vestibular signs. Because the cerebellum does not initiate motor action, paresis and paralysis are not signs of cerebellar disease. Movements may be uncoordinated to the point where severely affected animals are unable to ambulate but these animals are not paretic because they can initiate movement and can support their weight against gravity. Postural reactions and gait can be initiated, and muscle tone is normal. Cerebellar syndromes are discussed in Chapters 8 and 10.

Cerebrum: Cognitive Function

Sensory and motor functions that involve specific areas of the cerebral cortex have been previously described. The cerebrum contains areas for cognitive (thought, thinking) function, learned responses, and behavior. Generalized disease of the cerebrum may cause alterations of mental status (dullness, stupor, coma), loss of learned responses such as house training, and aimless pacing or walking. Seizures can be a sign of cerebral disease.

NEUROLOGIC SIGNS

Signs that are likely to be associated with an abnormality of the nervous system are listed in Table 1-1.

Seizures always indicate a neuroanatomic localization to the forebrain, although the problem (etiology) may be secondary to a metabolic or toxic condition. Differentiation between seizures and syncope may be difficult and may require wording the questions carefully and interpreting the answers even more carefully.

Stupor and coma are manifestations of abnormal cerebral or brainstem function. Behavioral changes may be caused by primary brain abnormalities or may be secondary to environmental factors.

Paresis and paralysis, signs of primary motor dysfunction, are caused by a neurologic abnormality. Lameness of musculoskeletal origin is differentiated from these signs by the physical and neurologic examinations.

Sensory deficits such as loss of proprioception or hypesthesia (decreased sensation) are always a result of an abnormality in the nervous system.

Pain (one's subjective response to a noxious stimulus) may be related to neural lesions. For example, nerve-root irritation

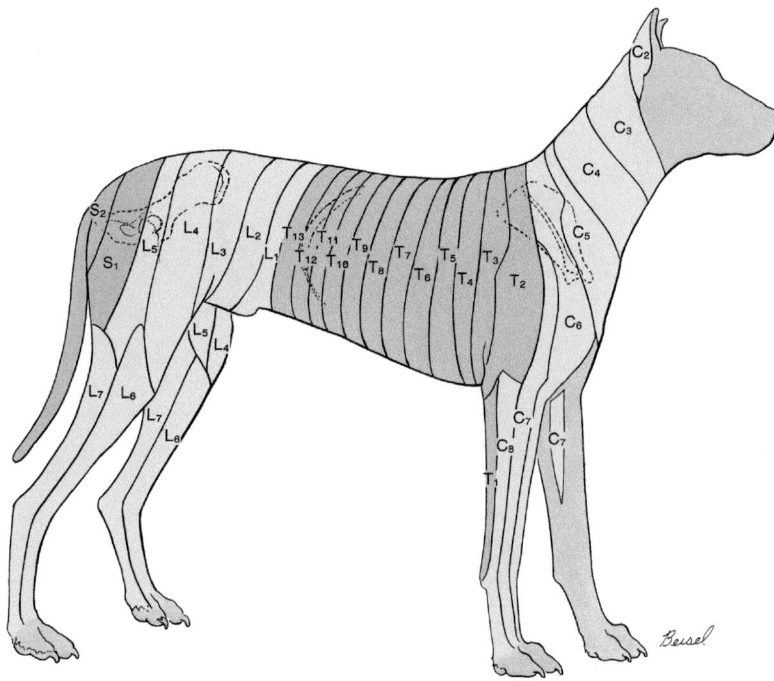

Figure 1-12 Dermatomes of the dog. This illustration represents the results of several studies. Dermatomes differ among individuals, and overlapping innervation of approximately three segments is present in most areas. The distribution to thoracic limbs is tentative. (From Oliver JE, Hoerlein BF, Mayhew IG: Veterinary neurology, Philadelphia, 1987, WB Saunders.)

may cause localized pain and lameness, sometimes called root signature. The client's observations may be helpful in localizing the animal's pain. A careful physical and neurologic examination is essential to verify the signs.

Visual deficits may be caused by an abnormality of the eye or of the nervous system. Thorough ophthalmologic and neurologic examinations are necessary to make a diagnosis. Historical information may be deceptive in the case of visual abnormalities. Animals in their usual surroundings may function normally even though they may be completely blind.

Deficits in hearing usually are not recognized unless they are bilateral. Bilateral hearing loss is usually caused by abnormalities of the inner ear. Brain lesions causing deafness are rare.

Loss of sense of smell (anosmia) is rarely recognized except in working dogs. Anorexia occasionally may be associated with anosmia.

NEUROLOGIC EXAMINATION

In the neurologic examination, the clinician systematically evaluates the functional integrity of the various components of the nervous system. The examination can be conveniently divided into the following parts: observation; palpation; examination of postural reactions, spinal reflexes, and cranial nerve responses; and sensory evaluation (Box 1-3).

In every complete neurologic examination, each of these categories is investigated to assess any problem possibly related to the nervous system. An abbreviated neurologic examination might include the items marked with an asterisk in Box 1-3. Positive findings on any of these tests indicate the need for a more complete neurologic examination. Neurologic responses of neonatal dogs are outlined in Table 1-4.

The neurologic examination is usually described as a complicated process that is wholly separate from the physical examination. In reality, much of the neurologic examination is done as a routine part of the physical examination. The examiner needs only to be aware of what is being observed. The addition of a few extra steps completes the examination. A brief description of integration of the neurologic examination with the physical examination of a small animal patient is presented as an example. This is followed by detailed discussion of each of the components. The process of completing the neurologic examination differs depending on the examiner's routine in a physical examination.

Efficient Neurologic Examination

A simple numeric grading scheme may be used to record results of the examination. Grades are assigned as follows: 0 = no response (reflex, reaction); +1 = a decreased response; +2 = a normal response; +3 = an exaggerated response; and +4 = a myotatic reflex with clonus.

1. Observation: Completed while taking the history.
2. Palpation: Usually done early in a physical examination.
3. Postural reactions: Require special tests. Hopping and proprioceptive positioning (paw replacement) of each limb are usually all that are necessary. Proprioceptive positioning can be done during palpation; when the examiner's hand reaches the foot, the foot is knuckled under and the response observed.
4. Spinal reflexes: Require special tests. Patellar (quadriceps, knee jerk), extensor carpi radialis, and flexion reflexes are adequate. If gait and postural reactions are normal, spinal reflexes are usually normal.
5. Cranial nerves (CN): Can be examined during the general physical examination when the head is examined. While observing the head, the examiner notes symmetry of the face (CN VII) and symmetry of eye

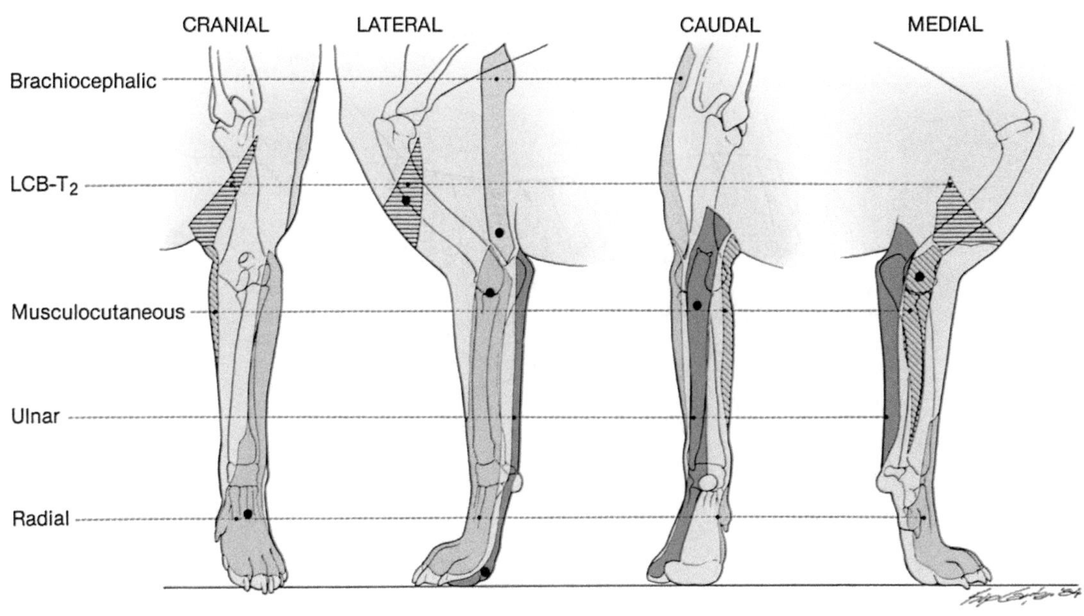

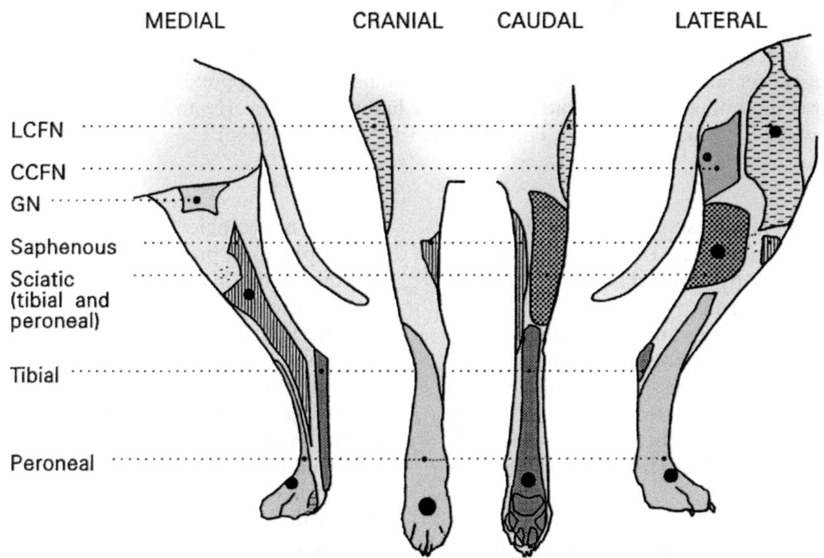

Figure 1-13 **A,** Cutaneous innervation of the left thoracic limb of the dog. Autonomous zones, innervated by only one nerve, are shown along with recommended sites for testing of sensation *(dots)*. The median nerve does not have an autonomous zone. LCB-T_2, Lateral cutaneous branch of the second thoracic nerve. **B,** Cutaneous innervation of the right pelvic limb of the dog. Autonomous zones and testing sites are shown as in **A.** *LCFN,* Lateral cutaneous femoral nerve L3, L4 (L5); *CCFN,* caudal cutaneous femoral nerve (L7), S1-2; *GN,* genitofemoral nerve L(2), L3-4. (**A** is based on Kitchell RL, et al: Electrophysiological studies of cutaneous nerves of the thoracic limb of the dog, Am J Vet Res 41:61, 1980 and Bailey CS, Kitchell RL: Clinical evaluation of the cutaneous innervation of the canine thoracic limb, J Am Anim Hosp Assoc 20:939, 1984. **B** is based on Haghighi SS, et al: Electrophysiologic studies of cutaneous innervation of the pelvic limb of male dogs, Am J Vet Res 52:352, 1991 and Bailey CS, Kitchell RL: Cutaneous sensory testing in the dog, J Vet Intern Med 1:128, 1987.)

position and pupils (CN III, IV, VI, and sympathetic nerves). A menacing gesture is made at each eye, provoking a blink (CN II and VII). The medial and lateral canthus is touched on each eye, provoking a blink (CN V-ophthalmic [medial] and maxillary [lateral] branches; CN VII). The examiner turns the head from side to side, observing conjugate eye movements (CN III, IV, VI, and VIII) and then shines a light in each eye, observing the pupillary light reflex (CN II and III). The nose and lower jaw are touched or pinched, eliciting facial or behavioral movements (CN V-maxillary and mandibular; CN VII). The temporal and masseter muscles are palpated and the mouth opened, with the examiner noting jaw tone (CN V–mandibular). With the patient's mouth open, while assessing mucous membranes and tonsils, the examiner notes symmetry

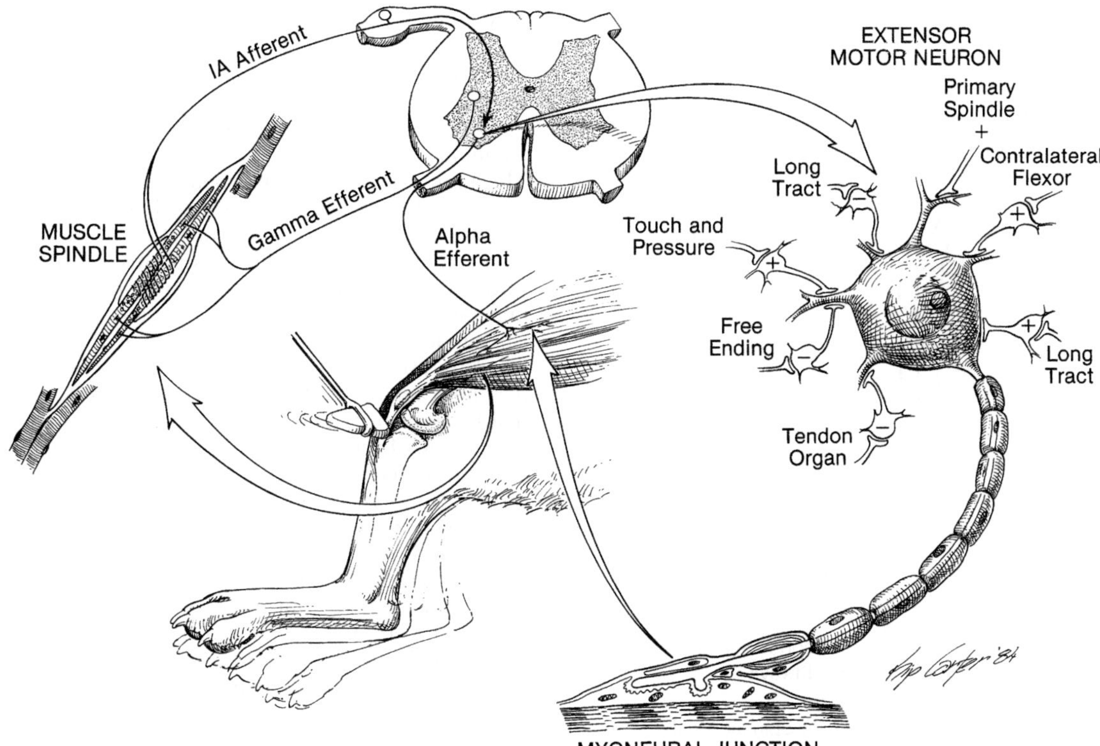

Figure 1-14 Myotatic (stretch) reflex. Percussion of the tendon or muscle stretches the muscle spindle. IA afferent fibers are activated and synapse directly on motor neurons of the muscle. The motor neuron discharges when a threshold level of excitation is reached. The level of excitation of the motor neuron is related to synapses from a variety of sources, as illustrated. The impulse travels down the axon (alpha efferent) to the neuromuscular junction, causing a release of acetylcholine. Acetylcholine binds to receptors on the muscle, causing depolarization and contraction of the muscle. Gamma motor neurons maintain tension on the muscle spindle regardless of the state of contraction of the muscle. (From Oliver JE, Hoerlein BF, Mayhew IG: Veterinary neurology, Philadelphia, 1987, WB Saunders.)

of the larynx and pharynx and touches the pharynx, causing a gag reflex (CN IX X, and XI). The examiner observes symmetry of the tongue and, as the mouth is closed, rubs the nose; most animals will lick, illustrating symmetry of tongue movements (CN XII). During palpation of the animal, the trapezius and brachiocephalicus muscles are observed for atrophy (CN XI). The only cranial nerve not tested is CN I–olfactory, which can be assessed by an aversive response to alcohol. It is not tested unless a forebrain deficit is suspected. This assessment of cranial nerves adds less than 2 minutes to the usual examination of the head.

6. Sensory examination: Hyperesthesia may have been detected during palpation. Response to noxious stimuli can be assessed during flexion reflex testing and cranial nerve evaluation. Areas of suspicion are pursued last to avoid upsetting the animal early in the examination. Testing for deep pain perception (response to noxious stimuli) is done only if the animal is not responsive to superficial stimulation and when there is no motor movement.

The complete neurologic examination adds only a minimal amount of time to the total physical examination.

Components of the Neurologic Examination

Observation

During every physical examination, the veterinarian should observe the animal's mental status, posture, and movement. The animal should be allowed to move around the examination room or in an open area while the history is being taken.[5-7]

Mental Status

Technique. The examiner can obtain a general impression of the animal's level of consciousness and behavior by observing its response to environmental stimuli or to people. Natural variations such as the aggressive curiosity of puppies, the indifference of older hounds, and the withdrawal of cats must be recognized as normal behavior. Overt aggression and fear-biting usually can be recognized.

Anatomy and Physiology. Consciousness is a function of the cerebral cortex and the brainstem. Sensory stimuli from the body, such as touch, temperature, and response to noxious stimuli, and from outside the body, such as sight, sound, and odors, provide input to the reticular formation. Consciousness is maintained by diffuse projections of the reticular formation to the cerebral cortex (Figure 1-18).

This arousal system is termed the ascending reticular activating system (ARAS).[4] A common cause of decreased levels of consciousness is a disruption of the pathways between the reticular formation and the cerebral cortex. The limbic system, consisting of portions of the cerebrum and diencephalon, constitutes the substrate for behavior.

Assessment. An animal's mental status may be recorded as alert, dull, stuporous, or comatose depending on its level of consciousness (see Chapter 12). Behavioral changes

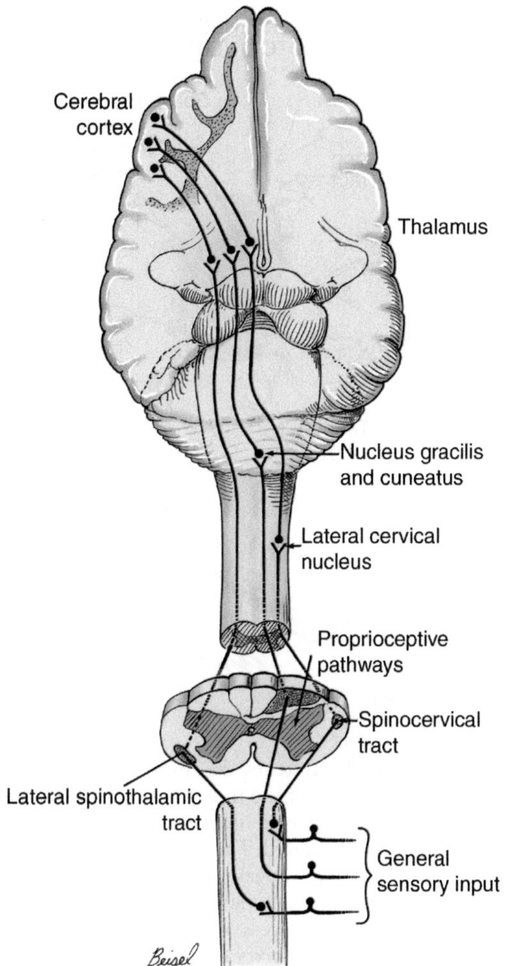

Figure 1-15 Somatic sensory innervation is transmitted to the brain through several pathways. General proprioception is a function of the spinomedullothalamic pathway (near the spinocervical tract) for the pelvic limbs and of the fasciculus cuneatus of the dorsal columns for the thoracic limbs. Pain is transmitted by several tracts (see also Figure 1-11), including the spinothalamic, spinocervical, and spinoreticular tracts and the dorsal columns.

may include aggression, fear, withdrawal, and disorientation. Other signs related to abnormal behavior include yawning, head pressing, compulsive walking, circling, and "stargazing."

Dullness, also denoted as obtundation or depression in an animal, is characterized by a conscious but inactive state. The animal is relatively unresponsive to the environment and tends to sleep when undisturbed. Dullness may be caused by systemic problems (extracranial), such as fever, anemia, or metabolic disorders. When associated with primary brain (intracranial) problems, dullness usually indicates diffuse cerebral cortical disease or a brainstem lesion.

Stupor is exemplified by an animal that tends to sleep when undisturbed. Innocuous stimuli such as touch or noise may not cause arousal, but a noxious stimulus causes the animal to awaken. Stupor usually is associated with partial disconnection of the reticular formation and the cerebral cortex, as in diffuse cerebral edema with herniation of the cerebrum causing compression of the brainstem.

Coma is a state of deep unconsciousness. The animal cannot be aroused even with noxious stimuli, although simple reflexes may be intact. For example, pinching the foot produces a flexor reflex but does not cause arousal. Coma indicates complete disconnection of the reticular formation and the cerebral cortex. The most common cause in small animals is acute head injury with hemorrhage in the pons and the midbrain.[8] Animals that are unable to stand because of spinal cord dysfunction are alert.

Behavioral disorders are often functional, that is, related to environment and training. Primary brain disease, however, also can cause alterations in behavior. These are indicative of a cerebral or diencephalic lesion.

Posture

Technique. Abnormalities in posture may be noticed while the history is being recorded and the animal is free to move about. Further observations may necessitate moving the animal to different positions so that its ability to regain normal posture can be evaluated.

Anatomy and Physiology. Normal posture is maintained by coordinated motor responses to sensory inputs from receptors in the limbs and body, the visual system, and the vestibular system. Vestibular receptors sense alterations in the position of the animal's head in relation to

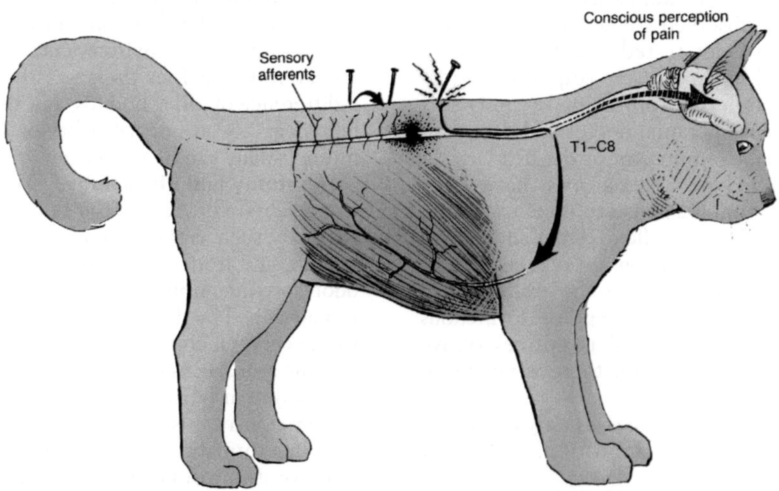

Figure 1-16 The cutaneous trunci (panniculus) reflex is the contraction of cutaneous trunci muscle, producing a skin twitch from stimulation of cutaneous sensory fibers. (From Greene CE, Oliver JE: Neurologic examination. In Ettinger SJ, editor: Textbook of veterinary internal medicine, ed 2, Philadelphia, 1982, WB Saunders.)

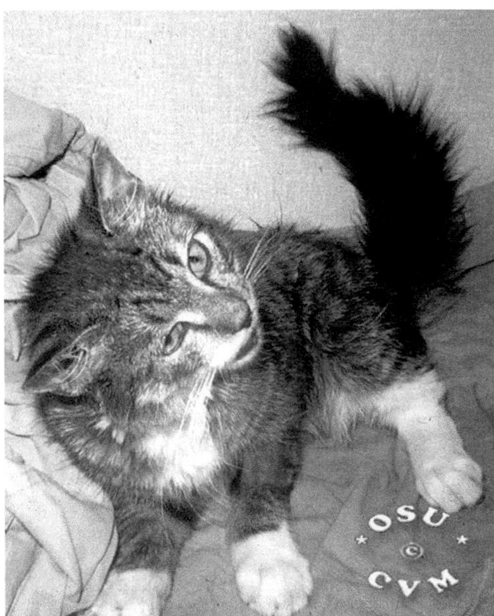

Figure 1-17 A cat with a head tilt and falling, signs typical of vestibular disease.

BOX 1-3

Neurologic Examination

- I. Observation*
  - Mental status
  - Posture
  - Movement
- II. Palpation*
  - Integument
  - Muscles
  - Skeleton
- III. Postural Reactions
  - Proprioceptive positioning*
  - Wheelbarrowing
  - Hopping*
  - Extensor postural thrust
  - Hemistanding and hemiwalking
  - Placing (tactile)
  - Placing (visual)
  - Sway test
  - Tonic neck
- IV. Spinal Reflexes
  - Myotatic
    - Pelvic limb
      - Quadriceps femoris muscle*
      - Cranial tibial muscle
      - Gastrocnemius muscle
    - Thoracic limb
      - Extensor carpi radialis muscle
      - Triceps
      - Biceps brachii muscle
  - Flexor*
  - Extensor thrust
  - Perineal*
  - Crossed extensor
  - Extensor toe
- V. Cranial Nerves
  - Olfactory
  - Optic*
  - Oculomotor*
  - Trochlear
  - Trigeminal*
  - Abducent*
  - Facial*
  - Vestibulocochlear*
  - Glossopharyngeal*
  - Vagus*
  - Accessory
  - Hypoglossal*
- VI. Sensation
  - Touch
  - Hyperesthesia*
  - Superficial pain*
  - Deep pain†

*Included in a screening examination.
†If superficial pain perception is absent.

gravity and detect motion. Sensory information is processed through the brainstem, cerebellum, and cerebrum. The cerebellum and vestibular system are especially important. The integrated output through motor pathways to the muscles of the neck, trunk, and limbs maintains normal posture. All domestic animals can maintain an erect posture shortly after birth; however, they vary in their ability to stand and walk.

Assessment

Head. The most common abnormality is a tilt or a twist to one side (see Figure 1-17). Intermittent head tilt, especially if associated with rubbing of the ear, may be due to otitis externa or ear mites. A continuous head tilt with resistance to straightening of the head by the examiner is almost always due to vestibular system dysfunction. Signs range from tilting of the head (roll) or turning of the head and neck (yaw) to twisting and rolling of the head, neck, and body. A yaw may indicate brainstem or cerebral disease; a roll or tilt is usually vestibular in origin. Both must be differentiated from spasms of cervical muscles caused by spinal cord or nerve root disease.

The head and neck may be held in a fixed position when cervical pain is present. Dogs with caudal cervical pain and weakness of the thoracic limb often arch their back and put their nose to the ground, apparently in an effort to keep weight off the thoracic limbs.

Trunk. Abnormal posture of the trunk may be associated with congenital or acquired lesions of the vertebrae or abnormal muscle tone from brain or spinal cord lesions. Deviations in vertebral contour consist of (1) scoliosis, lateral deviation; (2) lordosis, ventral deviation (swayback); and (3) kyphosis, dorsal deviation.

Limbs. Abnormal posture of the limbs includes improper positioning and increased or decreased extensor tone. A wide-based stance is common to all forms of ataxia and is also seen in cases of generalized weakness. Proprioceptive or motor deficits may cause the animal to stand with a foot knuckled over. With LMN or UMN lesions, the animal often makes repeated attempts to reposition the limb. Uneven distribution of weight on the limbs may provide a clue to weakness or pain. Animals try to carry most of their weight on the thoracic limbs when the pelvic limbs are weak or painful and on the pelvic limbs when the thoracic limbs are affected.

Decreased tone in limb muscles is often associated with LMN lesions and causes abnormal posture. The limbs are positioned passively, often with the toes knuckled.

Decerebrate rigidity is characterized by extension of all four limbs and the trunk. It is caused by a lesion in the rostral brainstem (midbrain or pons). Opisthotonos may be associated with decerebrate rigidity if the rostral lobes of the cerebellum are damaged. Opisthotonos is extension of the head and the neck. Mentation is often altered.

Decerebellate rigidity is similar, but the pelvic limbs are usually flexed. It is seen only in association with an acute lesion of the cerebellum.

Increased tone in the extensor muscles is a sign of UMN disease (see Table 1-3). Partial lesions may produce an exaggerated straightness in the stifle and hock joints. Decerebrate rigidity is an extreme form of increased extensor tone. Increased tone in the forelimbs with flaccid paralysis of the hind limbs is called the Schiff-Sherrington phenomenon and is associated with spinal cord lesions between T2 and L4 spinal

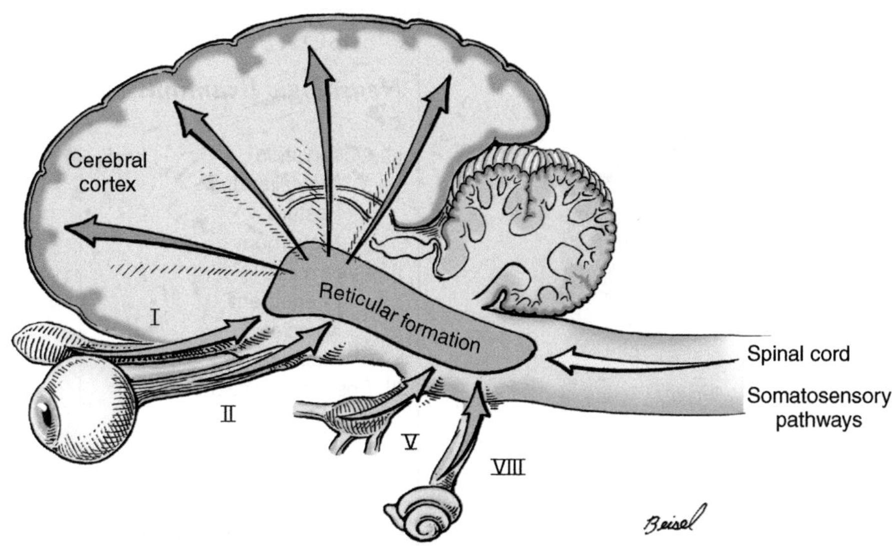

Figure 1-18 The ascending reticular activating system in the brainstem receives sensory information from the spinal cord and cranial nerves. It projects, through thalamic relays, diffusely to the cerebral cortex, thus maintaining consciousness.

TABLE 1-4

Neurologic Evaluation of the Neonatal Dog

	EXPECTED RESPONSE (Age in Days)		
	Strong	**Weak, Variable**	**Absent or Adultlike**
Motor			
Crossed extensor reflex	1-16	16-18	18+ (absent)
Magnus	1-17	17-21	21+ (absent)
Neck extension posture	Flexion 1-4	Hyperextension 4-21	Normotonia 21+
Forelimb placing	4+	2-4	0-2 (absent)
Hind limb placing	8+	6-8	0-6 (absent)
Forelimb supporting	10+	6-19	0-6 (absent)
Hind limb supporting	15+	11-15	0-11 (absent)
Standing on all limbs	21+	18-21	1-18 (absent)
Body righting (cutaneous)	1+	0-1	—
Sensory			
Rooting reflex	0-14	14-25	25+ (absent)
Nociceptive withdrawal reflex	0-19	19-23	23+ (adult)
Cutaneous trunci reflex	0-19	19-25	25+ (adult)
Reflex urination	0-22	22-25	25+ (absent)
Visual and Auditory			
Blinking response to light	16+	4-16	0-4 (absent)
Visual orientation	25+	20-25	0-20 (absent)
Auditory startle reflex	24+	15-24	0-15 (absent)
Sound orientation	25+	18-25	0-18

Modified from Fox MW: The clinical behavior of the neonatal dog, J Am Vet Med Assoc 143:1331-1335, 1963.

cord segments. Increased tone in both extensors and flexors is seen in tetanus and strychnine poisoning.

Movement

The animal should be observed for abnormal movements while resting and at gait. Careful observation is important because movement may be the most significant part of the neurologic examination, especially in large animals, in which postural reaction testing is more difficult.

Gait

Technique. The gait should be observed with the animal on a surface that offers adequate traction (carpet, synthetic turf, grass).[7] Gaits vary among species and breeds, and the examiner must be knowledgeable of these differences. Some breeds of dogs have been selectively developed for characteristic gaits. Because of this breeding, neurologic diseases may have inadvertently been genetically selected. The gait should be observed from the side and while the animal is moving toward and away from the examiner. Each limb should be evaluated while the animal is walking and trotting. The animal should be turned in wide, tight circles and should be backed up. Large animals are walked up and down a slope and with the head and neck extended.[9] The examiner may exaggerate minimal abnormalities in gait by blindfolding the animal.

Anatomy and Physiology. The neural organization of gait and posture is complex, involving all levels of the nervous system. Limbs are maintained in extension for supporting weight by spinal cord reflexes. Stepping movements also are programmed at the spinal level (Figure 1-19).

Organization of the various gaits used in normal locomotion occurs at the brainstem level in the reticular formation, probably in the subthalamic or pretectal areas. Removal of the input from the forebrain does not abolish the capacity for locomotion, including all normal gaits (trot, gallop, walk, and so forth). Cerebellar regulation of this system makes locomotion smooth and coordinated. Vestibular input maintains balance. Cerebral cortical input to the system is necessary for purposeful movement, voluntary control, and fine coordination, especially of learned movements.[10-12]

An animal with a lesion in the cerebrum or diencephalon is able to walk but does not have the precision of movement of a healthy animal. However, postural reactions are abnormal. Severe rostral brainstem lesions (of the midbrain and the pons) cause decerebrate rigidity because the voluntary motor pathways that inhibit extensor muscle activity are lost. Lesions in the pons or the medulla abolish integrated locomotion. Acute lesions of the cerebellum produce severe incapacitating dysmetria in which the animal may not be able to gait, whereas chronic lesions produce dysmetria evident in gait.

Assessment. Abnormalities of gait may include paresis and general proprioceptive, vestibular, or cerebellar ataxia or lameness as is observed with orthopedic disease.

General proprioception, or position sense, is the ability to recognize the location of the limbs in relation to the rest of

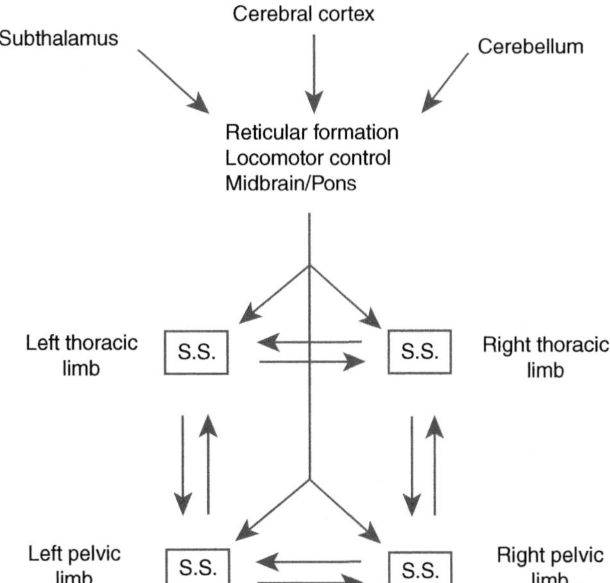

Figure 1-19 Schematic diagram of automatic control of locomotion. Spinal stepping reflexes are controlled by the brainstem centers for locomotion. Voluntary control is imposed from the cerebral cortex. The cerebellum and other areas coordinate the movements. S.S., Spinal stepping circuit in spinal cord.

the body. A deficit appears as a misplacement or a knuckling of the foot that may not occur with every step. The general proprioceptive pathways in the spinal cord are in the dorsal and dorsolateral columns and project to both the cerebellum (unconscious) and the cerebral cortex (conscious).

Paresis is a deficit of motor function. Affected limbs are unable to support weight appropriately. In addition, the affected limbs have inadequate or absent voluntary motion, which may be described as monoparesis-paresis of one limb; paraparesis-paresis of both pelvic limbs; tetraparesis or quadriparesis-paresis of all four limbs; or hemiparesis-paresis of the thoracic and the pelvic limb on the same side.

The suffix -plegia may be used to denote complete loss of voluntary movements and is used by some to indicate both motor and sensory loss. In this text, paresis indicates partial deficit of motor function, whereas paralysis (-plegia) indicates a complete loss of voluntary movements. In general, the only difference in the two is the severity of the lesion; the localization is the same.

Paresis only is evident clinically with disruption of the descending UMN tract originating from caudal to the midbrain and spinal cord or with lesions affecting the LMN unit. Therefore, paresis may be of the UMN or the LMN type (see Table 1-3), the determination of which is made through evaluation of the reflexes, and muscle mass and tone.

A neurologic disease may cause an animal to circle. Circling may range from a tendency to drift in wide circles to forced spinning in a tight circle. Circling usually is not a localizing sign except that tight circles usually are caused by vestibular or caudal brainstem lesions and wide circles usually are caused by forebrain lesions. A head turn is usually seen with forebrain lesions. The direction of the circling is usually toward the side of the lesion, but exceptions occur, especially in lesions rostral to the midbrain. Twisting or head tilt associated with circling usually indicates involvement of the vestibular system.

Ataxia is a lack of coordination without spasticity, paresis, or involuntary movements, although each of these conditions may be seen in association with ataxia. Given the close anatomic relationship of the UMN tracts with the general proprioceptive tracts, most naturally occurring lesions affect both systems. As a result, it is often difficult to separate ataxia from paresis in many clinically affected animals. Truncal ataxia is characterized by poorly controlled swaying of the body. Movement of the limbs is uncoordinated. The feet may be crossed or placed too far apart. Ataxia can be exaggerated by elevating the head or walking the animal on a slope. Ataxia may be caused by lesions of the cerebellum, the vestibular system, or the general proprioceptive pathways (see Chapters 2 and 8).

A characteristic of cerebellar dysfunction, dysmetria is characterized by movements that are too long (overreaching or hypermetria) in which there is overflexion of the joints during the swing phase of the gait or too short (hypometria). Goose-stepping is the most common sign of dysmetria. The stride may be abruptly stopped, forcing the animal to lurch from side to side. Dysmetria of the head and the neck may be most apparent when the animal tries to drink or eat and overshoots or undershoots the target. Dysmetria usually is caused by cerebellar or cerebellar pathway lesions and may be associated with ataxia and intention tremors (see Chapters 2 and 8).

Involuntary Abnormal Movement

Technique. Abnormal movements may occur when the animal is at rest or when it is moving and may be intermittent or continuous. The most frequently recognized movement disorder is myoclonus, which if occurs repetitively, appears clinically as a tremor (see Chapter 10).

Assessment. A tremor is produced by alternating contractions of opposing groups of muscles. The oscillatory movements may result in small or large excursions (fine or coarse tremors). Tremor from neurologic causes must be differentiated from those induced by fatigue, fear, chilling, drug reactions, or primary muscle disease (see Chapter 10).

An intention tremor is one that is more pronounced when movements are initiated. It is an important sign of cerebellar disease. A continuous tremor usually is associated with an abnormality of the motor system.

Myoclonus is a coarse, jerking of muscle groups. Myoclonus associated with canine distemper encephalomyelitis is usually a rhythmic jerking of one muscle group, such as the flexors of the elbow or the temporal muscle. The myoclonus of distemper has been called chorea; however, chorea more accurately describes irregular, purposeless movements that are brief and that often change in location from one part of the body to the other. Two forms of myoclonus may be seen in the dog. In acute encephalitis, the lesion is probably related to destruction of areas in the basal nuclei. The more common chronic form is related to the interneurons or the LMN at the segmental level.[13] Cataplexy is a sudden, complete loss of muscle tone that causes the animal to fall limp. It is usually seen in association with narcolepsy (see Chapter 13). Athetosis is a "pill rolling" movement of the hands in people with Parkinson disease. A similar movement disorder has been produced in cats with lesions of the basal nuclei but has not been described in clinical patients.

Palpation

Technique. After the mental status, posture, and gait of the animal have been assessed, the physical examination is initiated. Careful inspection and palpation of the musculoskeletal and integumentary systems should be performed at one time or on a regional basis in conjunction with other parts of the examination. Comparison of one side with the other for symmetry is best done as one step in the examination.[14]

Assessment

Integument. Although the skin is not often involved in neurologic disease, careful inspection may reveal clues to the diagnosis. Scars may indicate previous trauma. Worn nails may be associated with paresis or with proprioceptive deficits. Coat and eye color may be related to a hereditary abnormality. For example, a white coat and blue eyes are associated with deafness in cats. A myelomeningocele may be palpated as it attaches to the skin in the lumbosacral region. The temperature of the extremities may be significantly lowered with arterial occlusion. Dermatomyositis is an inflammatory disease of the skin and muscle of collies and Shetland sheepdogs. Cutaneous lesions are present on the face, lips, and ears, and over bony prominences.

Skeleton. Careful palpation of the skeletal system may reveal masses, deviation of normal contour, abnormal motion, or crepitation. Tumors involving the skull or the vertebral column may be palpable as a mass. The spinous processes of the vertebrae should be palpated for irregularities of contour. Deviations may indicate a luxation, fracture, or congenital anomaly. Depressed or elevated skull fractures often can be palpated, especially in animals with minimal temporal muscle mass. Persistent fontanelles and suture lines in the skull may indicate congenital hydrocephalus. Abnormal motion or crepitation may be detected in fractures and luxations. When vertebral luxations or fractures are suspected, manipulation should not be attempted because additional displacement may cause serious spinal cord damage. Peripheral nerve injuries may be associated with fractures of the long bones.

Muscles. Muscles are evaluated for size, tone, and strength. All muscle groups should be systematically palpated, starting with the head, extending down the neck and the trunk, and continuing down each limb.

Changes in muscle size may be apparent from observation and from palpation. Loss of muscle mass (atrophy) is the most frequent finding. Atrophy may indicate LMN disease or disuse. Criteria for differentiating the two are presented in Chapter 2. Localized muscle atrophy, which usually accompanies LMN disease, is an important localizing sign.

Muscle tonus is maintained through the spinal stretch (myotatic) reflex. Alterations in tone, either increased or decreased, can be detected by palpation and passive manipulation of the limb. Increased tone of the extensor muscles, a common finding in UMN disease, manifests as increased resistance to passive flexion of the limb.

Muscle strength is difficult to evaluate even in the most cooperative patients. The extensor muscles can be evaluated during postural reactions such as hopping, in which the animal must support all of its weight on one limb (see the section on hopping in this chapter). The flexor muscles can be evaluated by comparing the relative strength of pull during a flexor reflex (see the section on the flexor reflex in this chapter). Loss of muscle strength is usually a sign of LMN disease but is occasionally observed with UMN disease.

Postural Reactions

The complex responses that maintain an animal's normal, upright position are known as postural reactions. If an animal's weight is shifted from one side to the other, from front to rear, or from rear to front, the increased load on the supporting limb or limbs requires increased tone in the extensor muscles to keep the limb from collapsing. Part of the adjustment in tone is accomplished through spinal reflexes, but for the changes to be smooth and coordinated, the sensory and motor systems of the brain must be involved.

Abnormalities of complex reactions such as the hopping reaction do not provide precise localizing information because lesions in any one of several areas of the nervous system may affect the reaction. The assessment of postural reactions, however, is an important part of the neurologic examination. Minimal deficits in the function of a key component such as the cerebrum may cause significant alterations in postural reactions that are not detected when one observes the gait.

Two major types of postural reactions are used. The first consists of hopping, wheelbarrowing, and extensor postural thrust; these require movement of the limb to correct for displacement of the body and differ only in which limbs are tested. Weight bearing occurs, and so weakness has a significant impact on the performance of the reaction. The second type includes proprioceptive positioning and placing; these usually are performed with some support of the animal's weight. Therefore weakness has less influence on performance. Both types of reactions are useful. Because the pathways for the postural reactions are similar, interpretation is essentially the same for all reactions.

The following postural reactions are listed in a sequence convenient for performing an examination. In an initial screening examination, hopping and proprioceptive positioning reactions (see Box 1-3) should be tested. If they are normal, abnormalities are unlikely to be found in the other reactions.

Proprioceptive Positioning Reaction (Foot/Limb Placement Test)

Technique. This reaction tests more than general proprioception: light touch and pressure are also evaluated.[15] Although sensory functions are evaluated, the reactions described in this section also require motor responses. It is incorrect to assume that abnormalities observed are strictly due to proprioceptive dysfunction.

The simplest method of evaluation entails flexing the foot so that the dorsal surface is on the floor (Figure 1-20).

The animal should return the foot to a normal position immediately. Most animals do not allow weight bearing to occur in the abnormal position. In large animals, the foot or hoof is placed on a sheet of cardboard that is slowly pulled laterally. As the limb reaches an abnormal position, the animal should reposition it for normal weight bearing. The first test is the most sensitive for proprioception in the distal extremity, whereas the second test is more sensitive for detecting abnormalities in the proximal portion of the limb. With either method, the examiner should test each foot separately.

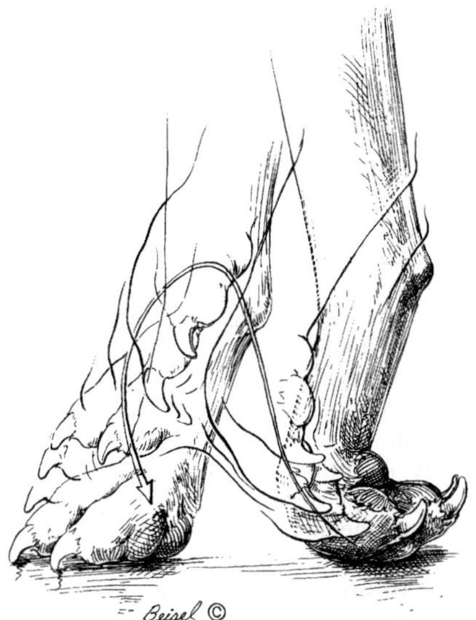

Figure 1-20 Proprioceptive positioning response. Proprioceptive function is tested by placing the dorsal surface of the animal's foot on the floor. The animal should immediately replace it to the normal position. (From Greene CE, Oliver JE: Neurologic examination. In Ettinger SJ (ed): Textbook of veterinary internal medicine, ed 2, Philadelphia, 1982, WB Saunders.)

Anatomy and Physiology. General proprioceptive information is carried in the dorsal columns and the spinomedullothalamic tract in the dorsolateral funiculus of the spinal cord, through the brainstem, to the sensorimotor cortex and fibers that project to the cerebellum (see Figure 1-15). The motor response is initiated by the cerebral cortex and is transmitted to the LMN in the spinal cord (see the section on sensation).

Assessment. Because the proprioceptive pathways are sensitive to compression, abnormalities in proprioceptive positioning may occur before motor dysfunction (paresis) can be detected. The response is abnormal if significant paresis exists, but other postural reactions such as hopping are also affected. Proprioceptive positioning is less useful in large animals because many do not respond. Observation of abnormal positioning of the limbs at rest may be interpreted similarly.[9] Some normal dogs will not reposition the paw after it is knuckled over. In this situation, the hopping reaction should always be evaluated.

Hopping Reaction

Technique. The hopping reaction is a reliable postural reaction test. It evaluates all components involved in voluntary limb movements. Normal hopping responses require intact sensory receptors, peripheral nerves, ascending long tracts in the spinal cord and brainstem, sensory cortex, UMN systems, and integration with LMNs in the spinal cord.

The hopping reaction of the thoracic limbs is tested with one thoracic limb lifted from the ground (Figure 1-21).

Although it is easy to pick up three limbs in small dogs and cats, this is not necessary in larger animals. The animal's pelvis should be supported sufficiently to increase weight bearing on the extended limb. As weight is increased on the extended limb, the ability of the animal to maintain full limb

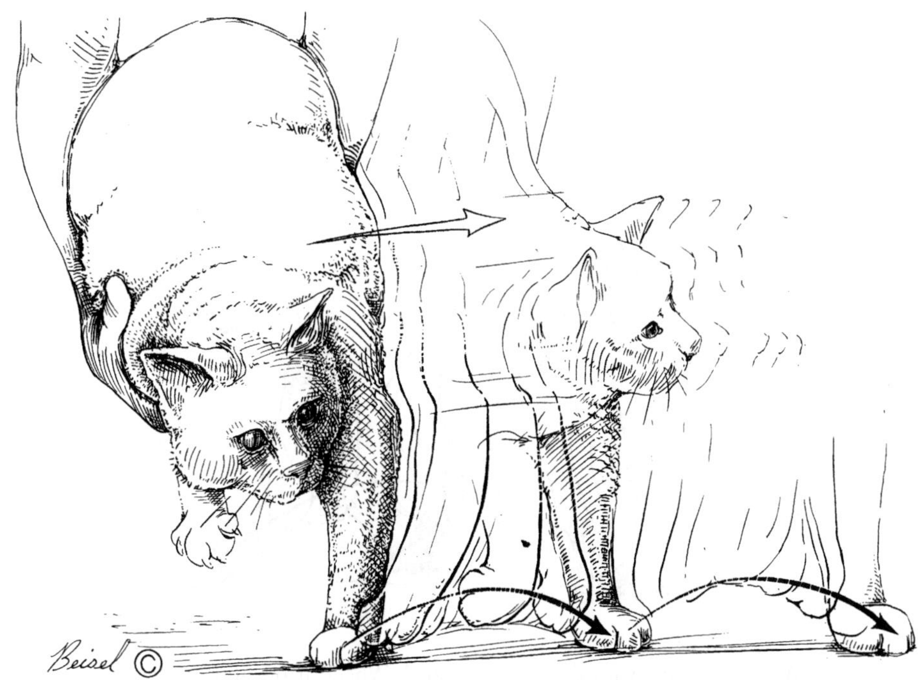

Figure 1-21 The hopping reaction. The normal animal responds to hopping by quickly replacing the limb under the body as it moves laterally. Large animals can be tested by picking up one limb and pushing the body laterally. (From Greene CE, Oliver JE: Neurologic examination. In Ettinger SJ (ed): Textbook of veterinary internal medicine, ed 2, Philadelphia, 1982, WB Saunders.)

extension is assessed. With the animal facing away from the examiner, the patient's weight is then shifted laterally over the limb being tested, and initiation, movement, and support during hopping are assessed. Medial hopping is much more difficult, and more subtle abnormalities may be detected with this maneuver. Hopping of the pelvic limbs is accomplished by supporting the thorax and lifting one pelvic limb. With the patient facing toward the examiner, weight is shifted laterally over the limb being evaluated and initiation, movement, and support are assessed. A large animal, such as a giant-breed dog, a horse, and a cow, can be tested by lifting one limb and shifting the weight of the animal so that it hops on the opposite limb. Alternatively, large animals can be pulled by the tail or pushed laterally (sway reaction) to elicit movements similar to the hopping reaction.

Assessment. The hopping reaction is more sensitive than other postural reactions for detecting minor deficits. Poor initiation of the hopping reaction suggests sensory (proprioceptive) deficits, whereas poor follow-through suggests a motor system abnormality (paresis). Asymmetry is easily seen and helps to lateralize lesions.

Wheelbarrowing Reaction

Technique. The animal is supported under the abdomen with all of the weight on the thoracic limbs (Figure 1-22).

The normal animal can walk forward and sideways with coordinated movements of both thoracic limbs. The examiner should not lift the pelvic limbs so high that the animal's posture is grossly abnormal. If movements appear normal, the maneuver is repeated with the head lifted and the neck extended. This position prevents visual compensation, making the animal mostly dependent on proprioceptive information. A tonic neck reaction, which causes slightly increased extensor tone in the thoracic limbs, is also elicited. When the neck is extended, subtle abnormalities of the thoracic limbs may be seen in animals that otherwise appear normal. This reaction is especially useful for detecting compressive lesions in the caudal cervical region that predominantly cause paraparesis.

Assessment. Weakness in the thoracic limbs may be detected when the wheelbarrowing reaction is tested because the animal is forced to carry most of its weight on two limbs while standing on only one limb while moving.

Slow initiation of movement may be a sign of a proprioceptive deficit or of paresis that is caused by a lesion of the cervical spinal cord, the brainstem, or the cerebral cortex. Exaggerated movements (dysmetria) may indicate an abnormality of the cervical spinal cord, the caudal brainstem, or the cerebellum.

Extensor Postural Thrust Reaction

Technique. Extensor postural thrust is elicited by supporting the animal by the thorax caudal to the thoracic limb and lowering the pelvic limbs to the floor (Figure 1-23).

When the limbs touch the floor, they should move caudally in a symmetric walking movement to achieve a position of support. As the animal is lowered to the floor, it extends its limbs, anticipating contact. This is a vestibular reaction and may be lacking or uncoordinated in animals with lesions of the vestibular system.

Assessment. Asymmetric weakness, lack of coordination, and dysmetria can be seen in the extensor postural thrust reaction as in the wheelbarrowing reaction. Extensor postural thrust reaction is difficult or impossible to perform on larger animals. In cats, this reaction may be more easily elicited than hopping or proprioceptive placing.

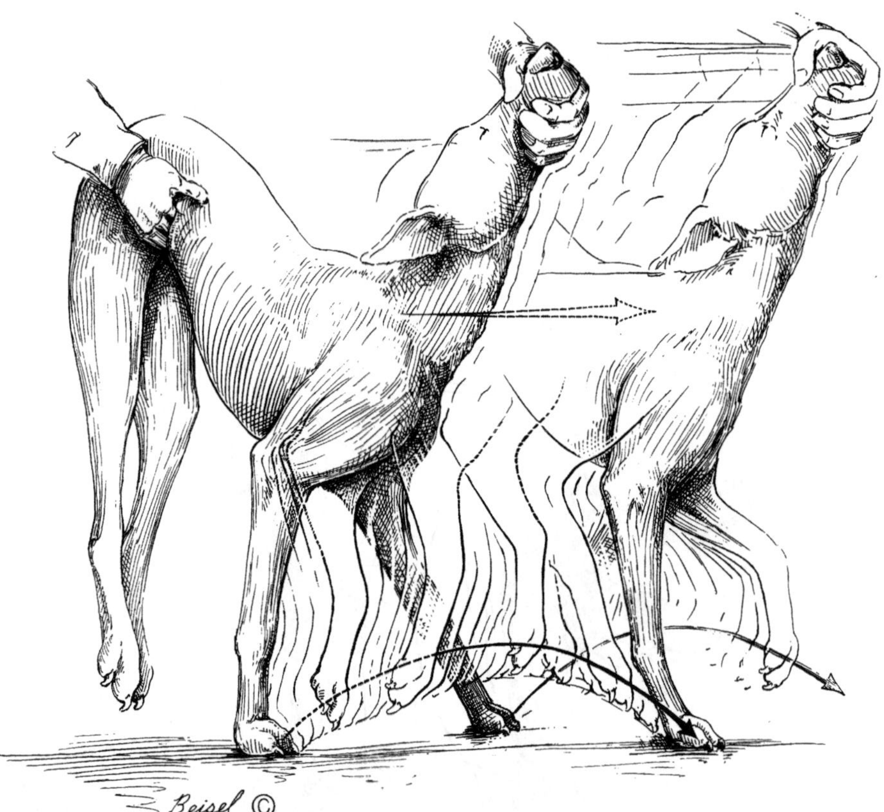

Figure 1-22 Wheelbarrowing with the neck extended. Wheelbarrowing is performed with the pelvic limbs elevated. The body should be in a position as close to normal as possible. The head may be elevated to accentuate abnormalities, as illustrated here. (From Greene CE, Oliver JE: Neurologic examination. In Ettinger SJ (ed): Textbook of veterinary internal medicine, ed 2, Philadelphia, 1982, WB Saunders.)

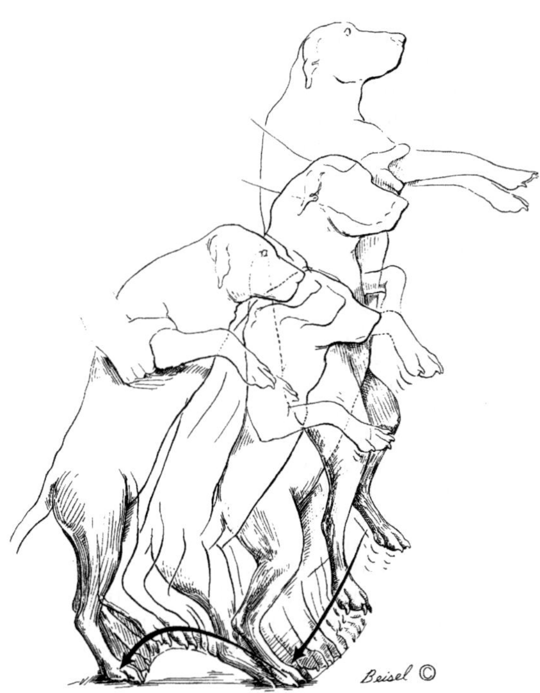

Figure 1-23 The extensor postural thrust reaction. The animal responds by stepping backward when its feet make contact with the floor. (From Greene CE, Oliver JE: Neurologic examination. In Ettinger SJ [ed]: Textbook of veterinary internal medicine, ed 2, Philadelphia, 1982, WB Saunders.)

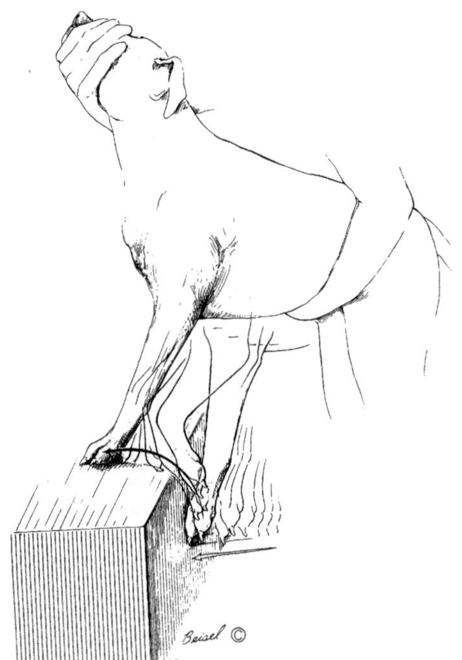

Figure 1-24 The tactile placing reaction is elicited with the animal's eyes covered. When the carpus makes contact with the edge of the surface, the animal should immediately place its foot on the surface. Similar responses can be elicited from large animals by leading them over a curb or up steps. (From Greene CE, Oliver JE: Neurologic examination. In Ettinger SJ [ed]: Textbook of veterinary internal medicine, ed 2, Philadelphia, 1982, WB Saunders.)

Hemistanding and Hemiwalking Reactions

Technique. The thoracic and pelvic limbs on one side are lifted from the ground so that all of the animal's weight is supported by the opposite limbs. Forward and lateral walking movements are then evaluated.

Assessment. Abnormal signs may be seen in hemistanding and hemiwalking as in the other postural reactions. They are most useful in animals with forebrain lesions. These animals have relatively normal gaits but have deficits of postural reactions in both the thoracic and the pelvic limbs contralateral to the side of the lesion. This reaction should be performed with caution in large dogs with obvious weakness as they can easily fall and potentially exacerbate their clinical signs.

Placing Reaction

Technique. Placing is evaluated first without vision (tactile placing) and then with vision (visual placing). The examiner supports the animal under the thorax and covers its eyes with one hand or with a blindfold. The thoracic limbs are brought in contact with the edge of a table at or ventral to the carpus (Figure 1-24).

The normal response is immediate placement of the feet on the table surface in a position that supports weight. Care must be taken not to restrict the movement of either limb. When one limb is consistently slower to respond, the animal should be held in the examiner's other hand to ensure that its movements are not being restricted.

Visual placing is tested by allowing the animal to see the table surface. Normal animals reach for the surface before the carpus touches the table. Peripheral visual fields can be tested by making a lateral approach to the table. The veterinarian can evaluate giant-breed dogs and large animals such as horses and cows by leading them over a curb or a step, with and without vision. Some dogs and cats that are accustomed to being held may ignore the table. These animals usually respond if they are held in a less secure or less comfortable position away from the body of the examiner.

Anatomy and Physiology. Tactile placing requires touch receptors in the skin, sensory pathways through the spinal cord and the brainstem to the cerebral cortex, and motor pathways from the cerebral cortex to the LMN of the thoracic limbs. Visual placing requires normal visual pathways to the cerebral cortex, communication from the visual cortex to the motor cortex, and motor pathways to the LMN of the forelimbs.[16]

Assessment. A lesion of any portion of the pathway may cause a deficit in the placing reaction. Normal tactile placing with absent visual placing indicates a lesion of the visual pathways. Normal visual placing with abnormal tactile placing suggests a sensory pathway lesion. Forebrain lesions produce a deficit in the contralateral limb. Lesions caudal to the midbrain usually produce ipsilateral deficits.

Tonic Neck Reaction

Technique. With the animal in a normal standing position, the head is elevated and the neck is extended. The normal reaction is a slight extension of the thoracic limbs and a slight flexion of the pelvic limbs. Lowering the head causes the thoracic limbs to flex and the pelvic limbs to extend. Turning the head to the side causes a slight extension of the ipsilateral thoracic limb and a slight flexion of the contralateral thoracic limb. The normal reactions are easy to remember if one considers the usual movements of an animal. For example, a cat about to jump onto a table extends the head and the neck, extends the thoracic limbs, and flexes the pelvic limbs. A dog crawling under a bed lowers the head and the neck and flexes the thoracic limbs as it extends the pelvic limbs for propulsion. A horse making a sharp turn leads with the head and the neck, plants the ipsilateral limb in extension, and flexes the contralateral limb to take a step.[17] Tonic eye reactions also may be observed. They are discussed in the section on cranial nerves.

Assessment. The tonic neck reactions are initiated by receptors in the cranial cervical area and are mediated by brainstem reticular formation. The responses are subtle in normal animals and often are inhibited volitionally through cortical control. Abnormalities in sensory (proprioception) or motor systems may produce abnormal reactions. Lesions in the cerebellum cause exaggerated tonic neck reactions. The tonic neck reactions are not usually helpful in detecting abnormality.

Spinal Reflexes

Examination of the spinal reflexes tests the integrity of the sensory and motor components of the reflex arc and the influence of descending motor pathways on the reflex. Three kinds of reactions may be seen. Absence or depression of a reflex indicates complete or partial loss of either sensory or motor (LMN) components of the reflex; a normal reaction indicates that both sensory and motor components are intact; and an exaggerated response indicates an abnormality in the motor pathways (UMN) that normally have an inhibitory influence on the reflex or a deficit that results in paresis of the antagonistic muscles is present.

The examination should be performed with the animal in lateral recumbency. Muscle tone, previously evaluated with the animal in a standing position, should be evaluated again at this time. The pelvic limbs are tested first. Passive manipulation of the limb assesses the degree of muscle tone, especially in the extensor muscles. Spreading the toes with slight pressure on the footpads elicits the extensor thrust reflex. The myotatic (stretch) reflexes then are evaluated. Routinely, only the patellar (knee jerk or quadriceps) reflex is tested. The cranial tibial and gastrocnemius muscles can also be evaluated, but the reflexes are more difficult to elicit and quantify. Next, the flexor reflex is tested by gently pinching the toes. To maintain cooperation of the patient, the examiner should apply the mildest stimulus that elicits a response. If flexion is induced by touching the foot, one need not crush the toe with a hemostat.

The most predictable myotatic reflex in the thoracic limb is elicited when the extensor carpi radialis muscle (tendons over the carpus in large animals) is struck, producing a slight extension of the carpus. The triceps and biceps reflexes are difficult to elicit and evaluate in many normal animals. After examining the limbs on one side, the veterinarian turns the animal and examines the opposite limbs. With the exception of the flexor reflex, thoracic limb reflexes are inconsistently elicited even in normal animals.

The perineal reflex is a contraction of the anal sphincter in response to a touch, a pinprick, or a pinch in the perineal area. Flexion of the tail may occur simultaneously.

Myotatic (Stretch) Reflexes

Patellar (Knee Jerk, Quadriceps) Reflex

Technique. With the animal in lateral recumbency, the limb is supported under the femur with the left hand (by a right-handed examiner) and the stifle is flexed slightly (see Figure 1-14). The patellar ligament is struck crisply with the plexor. The response is a single, quick extension of the stifle. The plexor is recommended for performing myotatic reflex testing, but other instruments such as bandage scissors may be used. Nose tongs or similar heavy instruments are useful for testing large animals. The examiner should use the same type of instruments in each examination to obtain consistent results.

Anatomy and Physiology. The myotatic or stretch reflexes are basic to the regulation of posture and movement. The reflex arc is a simple two-neuron (monosynaptic) pathway. The sensory neuron has a receptor in the muscle spindle and its cell body in the spinal ganglion. The motor neurons have their cell bodies in the ventral horn of the gray matter of the spinal cord. The axons form the motor components of peripheral nerves that end on the muscle (the neuromuscular junction) (see Figure 1-14).

The muscle spindle is the stretch receptor of the muscle. The spindle has three to five striated muscle fibers (intrafusal muscle fibers) at each end, with a nonstriated portion in the middle (see Figure 1-14). The spindles are located in the belly of the skeletal muscle (extrafusal muscle fibers). These sensory fibers are large and have a spiral ending, called the primary ending, around the nonstriated portion of each fiber. Small sensory fibers have secondary endings. Primary endings are of greatest importance in phasic responses (e.g., patellar reflex). Secondary endings respond primarily to tonic activation (e.g., extensor thrust). The small intrafusal muscle fibers of the spindle are innervated by small (gamma) motor neurons.

Stretching a muscle depolarizes the nerve endings of the spindle, producing a burst of impulses in the sensory fibers. The sensory fibers directly activate the large (alpha) motor neuron in the spinal cord. The alpha motor neuron discharges impulses through its axon, causing a contraction of the extrafusal muscle fibers of the same muscle. Thus a sudden stretch of the muscle causes a reflex muscle contraction, as seen in the patellar reflex. A more tonic stretch of the muscle causes a slower discharge of sensory activity and a slower, steadier muscle contraction.

Contraction of the extrafusal muscle fibers causes relaxation of the intrafusal fibers because they are parallel. Loss of tension on the intrafusal fibers stops the sensory input from the spindle. To prevent this situation from occurring, gamma motor fibers adjust the length of the intrafusal fibers. Thus tension is maintained on the spindle through the range of motion of the limb.

Gamma motor neuron activation of the intrafusal fibers also can stretch the primary spindle endings directly and thus can elicit a response indirectly in the alpha motor neuron. Alpha and gamma motor neurons are facilitated or inhibited by a variety of segmental and long spinal pathways. The output of the motor neurons is a summation of their facilitatory and inhibitory inputs. For example, the motor neuron that innervates the quadriceps responds to a sudden stretch by a quick contraction (patellar reflex), but the reaction can be modulated by voluntary inhibition (see Figure 1-14). This occurs in animals that are nervous and maintain a pronounced tone in the limb as the examiner is performing the test. In such cases, the patellar reflex may appear blunted.

The spindle sensory fibers also facilitate interneurons in the spinal cord, which in turn inhibit motor neurons of antagonistic muscles. This activity is called reciprocal innervation. For example, spindle sensory fibers from the quadriceps muscle inhibit antagonistic flexor motor neurons, allowing the limb to extend. Spindle sensory fibers also contribute collaterals to ascending pathways, which provide information to the brain regarding activity in the muscles.

Assessment. The patellar reflex is the most reliably interpreted myotatic reflex. The reflex should be recorded as absent (0), depressed (+1), normal (+2), exaggerated (+3), or exaggerated with clonus (+4). Normal responses vary widely among species and among breeds within a species. In large dogs the response is less brisk than in small dogs. The examiner should become familiar with these natural variations.

Absence (0) of a myotatic reflex indicates a lesion of the sensory or motor component of the reflex arc—an LMN or segmental sign (see Table 1-3). In general, loss of the reflex in one muscle group suggests a peripheral nerve lesion; for example, a lesion of the femoral nerve. Bilateral loss of the reflex suggests a segmental spinal cord lesion affecting the motor neurons to both limbs located in spinal cord segments L4-6 in the dog. Ultimately, differentiation between peripheral nerve

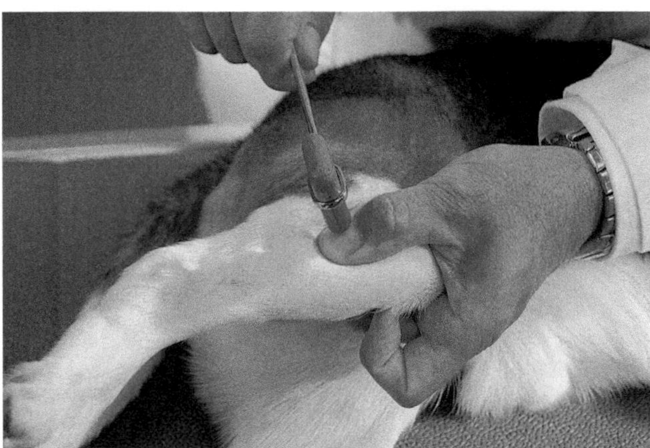

Figure 1-25 The cranial tibial reflex is elicited with the animal in lateral recumbency, with both stifle and hock slightly flexed. The cranial tibial muscle is percussed just distal to the stifle.

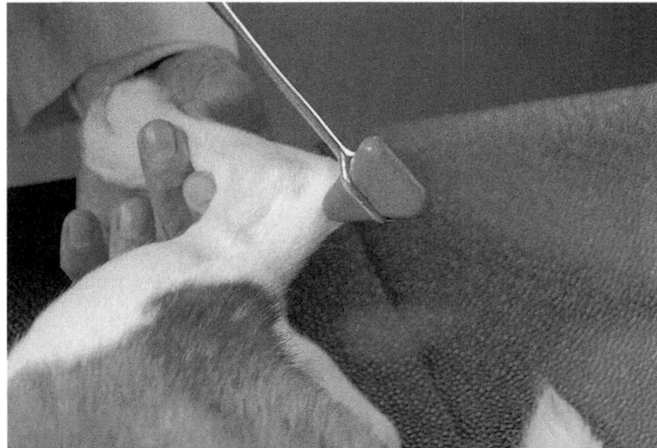

Figure 1-26 The gastrocnemius reflex is elicited with the animal in the same position as for testing of the cranial tibial reflex. The tendon of the gastrocnemius muscle is percussed proximal to the tarsus.

and spinal cord lesions may require assessment of the sensory examination and the presence or absence of other neurologic signs.

Depression (+1) of the reflex has the same significance as absence of the reflex, except the lesion is incomplete. Depression of the reflex is more common with spinal cord lesions in cases in which some, but not all, of the segments (L4-6) are affected. Other reflexes also must be tested because generalized depression of reflexes may be seen in polyneuropathies or in abnormalities of the neuromuscular junction (botulism, tick paralysis).

Animals that are tense and keep the limb in extension commonly have depressed or absent reflexes. Sometimes the reflex is hard to elicit in normal dogs in the recumbent or nonrecumbent limb. You only have to elicit the normal reflex one time to be sure the reflex arc is intact.

Normal (+2) or exaggerated reflexes (+3, +4) and increased tone result from loss of descending inhibitory pathways. The voluntary motor pathways are facilitatory to flexor muscles and inhibitory to extensor muscles. Damage to these pathways releases the myotatic reflex, causing an exaggerated reflex and increased extensor tone. Clonus (+4) is a repetitive contraction and relaxation of the muscle in response to a single stimulus. Clonus often is seen with chronic (weeks to months) loss of descending inhibitory pathways. Clonus has the same localizing significance as exaggerated reflexes. Bilateral exaggerated reflexes most often are associated with damage to descending inhibitory pathways cranial to the level of the reflex. UMN injury causing exaggerated myotatic reflexes also causes paresis. If gait and postural reactions are normal, the "exaggerated reflex" is then likely to be an examiner error or normal for the animal being tested. Exaggerated reflexes should not be overinterpreted. If gait and postural reactions are normal, the only concern is that the reflex be at least normal.

Cranial Tibial Reflex

Technique. With the animal in lateral recumbency, the examiner tests the cranial tibial reflex. The belly of the cranial tibial muscle is struck with the plexor just distal to the proximal end of the tibia (Figure 1-25). The response is flexion of the hock.

Anatomy and Physiology. The cranial tibial muscle is a flexor of the hock and is innervated by the peroneal branch of the sciatic nerve (with origin in the L6-7 segments of the spinal cord in the dog).

Assessment. The cranial tibial reflex is more difficult to elicit in a normal animal than is the patellar reflex. Absent or decreased reflexes should be interpreted with caution. Exaggerated reflexes indicate a lesion cranial to the spinal cord segments L6-7.

Gastrocnemius Reflex

Technique. The gastrocnemius reflex is tested after the cranial tibial reflex. The tendon of the gastrocnemius muscle is struck with the plexor just dorsal to the tibial tarsal bone (Figure 1-26).

Slight flexion of the hock is necessary for some tension of the muscle to be maintained. The response is extension of the hock. Contraction of the caudal thigh muscles may also occur.

Anatomy and Physiology. The gastrocnemius is primarily an extensor of the hock and is innervated by the tibial branch of the sciatic nerve (with origin in the L7-S1 segments of the spinal cord in the dog).

Assessment. The gastrocnemius reflex is interpreted in the same manner as the cranial tibial reflex but is even less reliable.

Extensor Carpi Radialis Reflex

Technique. The animal is in lateral recumbency while the reflexes of the thoracic limb are evaluated. The limb is supported under the elbow, with flexion of the elbow and the carpus maintained. The extensor carpi radialis muscle is struck with the plexor just distal to the elbow (Figure 1-27).

The response is a slight extension of the carpus. The carpus must be flexed, and the digits must not touch the floor or the other limb or the reflex will be mechanically inhibited.[19] The extensor tendons crossing the carpal joint are struck in large animals.

Anatomy and Physiology. The extensor carpi radialis muscle is an extensor of the carpus and is innervated by the radial nerve (with origin in the C7-T1 segments of the spinal cord in the dog).

Assessment. The extensor carpi radialis reflex is more difficult to elicit than the patellar reflex but usually can be recognized in dogs. Absent or decreased reflexes should be evaluated with caution. Strong reflexes are usually exaggerated (+3) and indicate a lesion cranial to C7.

Triceps Reflex

Technique. The animal is held in the same position as that for the extensor carpi radialis reflex. The triceps brachii muscle is struck with the plexor just proximal to the olecranon (Figure 1-28).

The response is a slight extension of the elbow or a visible contraction of the triceps muscle. The elbow must be maintained in flexion for a response to be elicited.

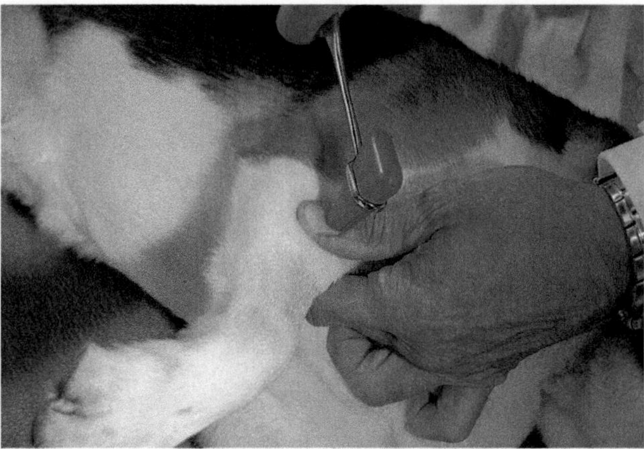

Figure 1-27 The extensor carpi radialis reflex is the most reliable myotatic reflex in the thoracic limb. With the animal in lateral recumbency and the elbow and carpus flexed, the extensor muscle group is percussed distal to the elbow. The digital extensor tendons can be percussed at the carpus in large animals.

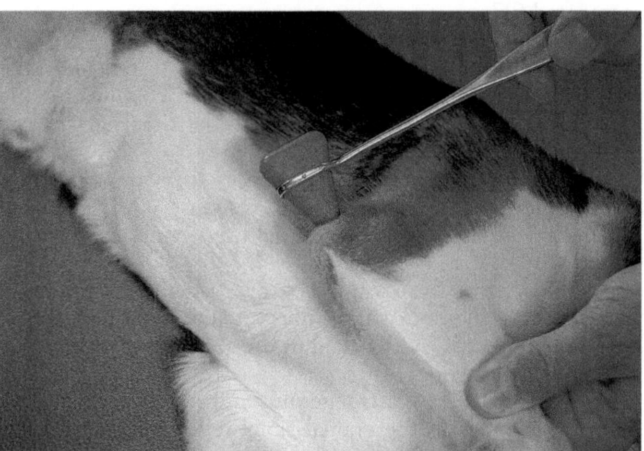

Figure 1-28 The triceps reflex is elicited with the animal in the same position as for the extensor carpi radialis reflex. The triceps tendon is percussed proximal to the elbow.

Anatomy and Physiology. The triceps brachii muscle extends the elbow and is essential for weight bearing in the forelimb. Innervation is through the radial nerve (with the origin from spinal cord segments C7-T1 in the dog).

Assessment. The triceps reflex is difficult to elicit in the normal animal. Absent or decreased reflexes should not be interpreted as abnormal. Lesions of the radial nerve can be recognized by a loss of muscle tone and an inability to support weight. Exaggerated reflexes are interpreted in the same way as for the extensor carpi radialis reflex.

Biceps Reflex

Technique. The index or middle finger of the examiner's hand that is holding the animal's elbow is placed on the biceps and the brachialis tendons cranial and proximal to the elbow. The elbow is slightly extended, and the finger is struck with the plexor (Figure 1-29).

The response is a slight flexion of the elbow. Movement of the animal's elbow must not be blocked by the examiner's restraining hand. In this case, movement of the skin overlying the biceps brachii muscle may be observed.

Anatomy and Physiology. The biceps brachii and brachialis muscles are flexors of the elbow. They are innervated by the musculocutaneous nerve, which originates from spinal cord segments C6-8 in the dog.

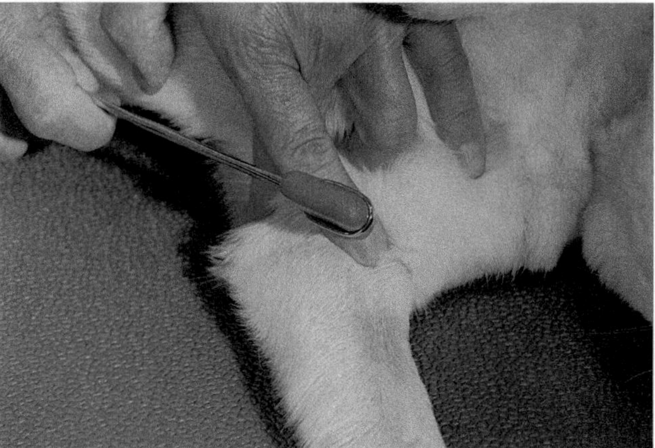

Figure 1-29 The biceps reflex is elicited with the elbow slightly extended. The examiner's finger is placed on the biceps tendon proximal to the elbow, and the finger is percussed.

Assessment. The biceps reflex is difficult to elicit in the normal animal. Absent or decreased reflexes should not be interpreted as abnormal. Flexion of the elbow on the flexor reflex provides a better assessment of the musculocutaneous nerve. An exaggerated (+3) reflex is indicative of a lesion cranial to C6.

Flexor (Pedal, Withdrawal) Reflexes

Pelvic Limb

Technique. The animal is maintained in lateral recumbency, the same position as that for examination of the myotatic reflexes. A noxious stimulus is applied to the foot. The normal response is a flexion of the entire limb, including the hip, stifle, and hock (see Figure 1-10). The least noxious stimulus possible should be used. If an animal flexes the limb when the digit is touched, the digit need not be crushed. If a response is not easily elicited, a hemostat should be used to squeeze across a digit. Pressure should not be so great as to injure the skin. Both medial and lateral digits should be tested on each limb. The limb should be in a slightly extended position when the stimulus is applied to allow the limb to flex. The opposite limb also should be free to extend.[18]

Anatomy and Physiology. The flexor reflex is more complex than the myotatic reflex. The response involves all of the flexor muscles of the limb and thus requires activation of motor neurons in several spinal cord segments (see Figures 1-9, *B* and 1-10).

The receptors for the flexor reflex are primarily free nerve endings in the skin and other tissues that respond to noxious stimuli, such as pressure, heat, and cold. A stimulus that produces a sensory discharge in these nerves ascends to the spinal cord through the dorsal root. The sensory nerves from the digits of the pelvic limbs are primarily branches of the sciatic nerve, the superficial peroneal nerve on the dorsal surface, and the tibial nerve on the plantar surface. The sciatic nerve originates from spinal cord segments L6-S1. The medial digit is partially innervated by the saphenous nerve, a branch of the femoral nerve that originates from spinal cord segments L4-6. Interneurons are activated at these segments and at adjacent segments both cranially and caudally. The interneurons activate sciatic motor neurons, which stimulate flexor muscle contraction (see Figure 1-10). The net result is withdrawal of the limb from the noxious stimulus. Inhibitory interneurons to the extensor motor neurons also are activated, resulting in decreased activity in the extensor muscles. Relaxation of the extensor muscles and contraction of the flexor muscles allow complete flexion of the limb.

The flexor reflex is a spinal reflex and does not require any activation of the brain. If an animal steps on a sharp piece of glass, it immediately withdraws the foot before consciously perceiving pain. If the spinal cord is completely transected cranial to the segments that are responsible for the reflex, the reflex is present even though the animal has no conscious perception of pain.

Assessment. Absence (0) or depression (+1) of the reflex indicates a lesion of L6-S1 segments or the branches of the sciatic nerve. Unilateral absence of the reflex is more likely the result of a peripheral nerve lesion, whereas bilateral absence or depression of the reflex is more likely the result of a spinal cord lesion. A normal (+2) flexor reflex indicates that the spinal cord segments and the nerves are functional. An exaggerated (+3) flexor reflex rarely is seen with acute lesions of descending pathways. Chronic and severe descending pathway lesions may cause exaggeration of the reflex. This exaggeration is manifested as a sustained withdrawal after release of the stimulus. A mass reflex (+4) occasionally is seen as a sustained flexion of both pelvic limbs, with contraction of the tail and perineal muscles in response to a stimulus applied to only one limb. Exaggerated flexor reflexes usually reflect chronicity rather than severity of the lesion.

The crossed extensor reflex and the conscious perception of pain also are evaluated while the flexor reflex is performed, but these assessments are discussed later.

Thoracic Limb

Technique. The thoracic limb flexor reflex is tested in the same manner as the pelvic limb flexor reflex. Cranial and palmar surfaces and medial and lateral digits should be tested.

Anatomy and Physiology. Branches of the radial nerve innervate the cranial surface of the foot and arise from spinal cord segments C7-T1. The medial palmar surface is innervated by the ulnar and median nerves, which originate from spinal cord segments C8-T1. The lateral palmar surface and most of the lateral digit are innervated by branches of the ulnar nerve. The organization of the flexor reflex of the thoracic limb is similar to that previously described for the pelvic limb. Flexor muscles of the thoracic limb are innervated by the axillary, musculocutaneous, median, and ulnar nerves and by parts of the radial nerve. These nerves originate from spinal cord segments C6-T1, with small contributions from C5 and T2 in some animals (see Figure 1-8, *A*).

Assessment. Depressed reflexes indicate a lesion of the C6-T1 segments of the spinal cord or the peripheral nerves. Exaggerated reflexes indicate a lesion cranial to C6.

Extensor Thrust Reflex. The extensor thrust reflex is important for maintaining posture and is a component of more complex reactions such as hopping.[17]

Technique. The reflex may be elicited with the animal in lateral recumbency (the same position as that for the myotatic reflex) or with the animal suspended by the shoulders with the pelvic limbs hanging free (Figure 1-30).

The toes are spread, and slight pressure is applied between the pads. The response is a rigid extension of the limb.[19]

Anatomy and Physiology. The extensor thrust reflex is initiated by a stretching of the spindles in the interosseous muscles of the foot.[16] Simultaneously, the cutaneous sensory receptors are stimulated. The extensors predominate, forcing the limb into rigid extension. The sensory fibers are in the sciatic nerve (spinal cord segments L6-S1), and the response involves both femoral and sciatic nerves (spinal cord segments L4-S1). Excessive stimulation of the flexor reflex sensory fibers (e.g., with a noxious stimulus) causes the flexor reflex to predominate and withdrawal occurs.

Assessment. The extensor thrust reflex is difficult to elicit in normal animals, especially when they are in lateral recumbency. Elicitation of the reflex generally indicates a lesion cranial to L4.

Perineal (Bulbocavernosus, Anal) Reflex

Technique. The perineal reflex is elicited by light stimulation of the perineum with forceps. Noxious stimuli that are painful usually are not necessary. The reaction is a contraction of the anal sphincter muscle and a flexion of the tail (Figure 1-31).

One can obtain a similar reaction by squeezing the penis or the vulva (bulbocavernosus reflex). If the anal sphincter appears weak or if the response is questionable, the examiner can insert a gloved digit into the anus because minimal responses often can be felt in this manner.

Anatomy and Physiology. Sensory innervation occurs through the pudendal nerves and spinal cord segments S1-2 (sometimes S3) in the dog and the cat. Motor innervation of the anal sphincter also occurs through the pudendal nerves. Tail flexion is mediated through the caudal nerves. The organization of the reflex is similar to that of the flexor reflex.

Assessment. The perineal reflex is the best indication of the functional integrity of the sacral spinal cord segments and nerve roots. Evaluation of this reflex is especially important in animals with urinary bladder dysfunction (see Chapter 3). Absence (0) or depression (+1) of the reflex indicates a sacral spinal cord or pudendal nerve lesion.

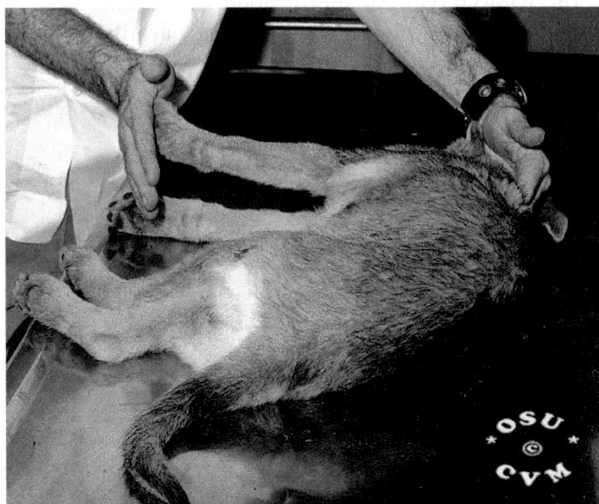

Figure 1-30 The extensor thrust reflex is elicited by spreading the phalanges.

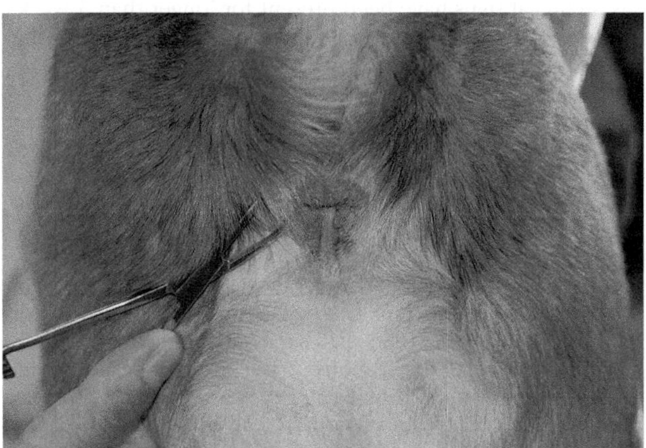

Figure 1-31 The perineal reflex is a contraction of the anal sphincter and a ventral flexion of the tail in response to tactile stimulation of the perineum.

Crossed Extensor Reflex

Technique. The crossed extensor reflex may be observed when the flexor reflex is elicited. The response is an extension of the limb opposite the stimulated limb.[18]

Anatomy and Physiology. The crossed extensor reflex is a part of the normal supporting mechanism of the animal. The weight of an animal in a standing position is evenly distributed among the limbs. If one limb is flexed, increased support is required of the opposite limb. The flexor reflex sensory fibers send collaterals to interneurons on the opposite side of the spinal cord, which excite extensor motor neurons (see Figure 1-10).

Assessment. The crossed extensor reflex generally is considered an abnormal reflex except in the standing position. In the normal recumbent animal, the extension response is inhibited through descending pathways. Crossed extensor reflexes result from lesions in ipsilateral descending pathways, a sign of UMN disease. The crossed extensor reflex has been considered evidence of a severe spinal cord lesion. However, it is not a reliable indicator of the severity of the lesion. Animals that are still ambulatory may have crossed extensor reflexes, especially when the lesion is in the cervical spinal cord or the brainstem.

Extensor Toe (Babinski) Reflex

Technique. The animal is positioned in lateral recumbency (the same position as that for the myotatic reflex). The pelvic limb is held proximal to the hock, with the hock and the digits slightly flexed. The handle of the plexor or a forceps is used to stroke the limb on the caudolateral surface from the hock to the digits.

The normal animal exhibits no response or a slight flexion of the digits. The abnormal response is an extension and a fanning of the digits.[20]

Anatomy and Physiology. The extensor toe reflex has been compared with the Babinski reflex in human beings.[21] The two reflexes are not strictly analogous because the Babinski reflex includes elevation and fanning of the large toe, which is not present in domestic animals; it is reported to be a sign of pyramidal tract damage in human beings. The extensor toe reflex has been produced by lesions in the brainstem.[21] It has been seen clinically in dogs with chronic UMN pelvic limb paresis.[20] Acute experimental lesions of the sensorimotor cortex, the dorsal columns, the lateral columns, or the ventral columns of the spinal cord have not produced an extensor toe reflex. Some investigators have considered this reflex to be an abnormal form of the flexor reflex.

Assessment. The extensor toe reflex has been observed in dogs with paralysis of the pelvic limbs associated with extensor hypertonus and exaggerated myotatic reflexes. In most cases clinical signs have been present for longer than 3 weeks. The reflex should be interpreted in the same manner as other exaggerated reflexes.

Cranial Nerves

Examination of the CNs is an important part of the neurologic examination, especially when disease of the brain is suspected. An abnormality of a CN constitutes evidence of a specific, localized area of disease not provided by postural reactions. The cranial nerve examination is not difficult, and the most commonly affected CNs can be evaluated quickly (see Figure 1-5). The majority of the evaluation of cranial nerves is done through testing reflexes. Two assessments differ and are denoted by the term "response": the menace response and response to noxious stimulation of the nasal mucosa. The term *response* is used to specifically imply that the response observed to the stimulus requires normal forebrain function. This is in contradistinction to other cranial nerve reflexes, which analogous to spinal reflexes, only need normal functional integrity of a specific segment of the brainstem to be normal. The general outline of the cranial nerve examination was discussed in the section on The Efficient Neurologic Examination at the beginning of this chapter. Detection of any abnormalities on the screening examination may be followed by a more complete examination to define the abnormality further.

Olfactory Nerve (CN I). The olfactory nerve is the sensory path for the conscious perception of smell.

Technique. A behavioral response to a pleasurable or a noxious odor, either inferred from the history or assessed by direct testing, may be used (Figure 1-32).

Alcohol, cloves, xylol, benzol, or cat food containing fish appears to stimulate the olfactory nerves. Irritating substances such as ammonia or tobacco smoke cannot be used because they stimulate the endings of the trigeminal nerve in the nasal mucosa.

Anatomy and Physiology. Chemoreceptors in the nasal mucosa give rise to axons, which pass through the cribriform plate to synapse in the olfactory bulb. Axons from the olfactory bulb course through the olfactory tract to the ipsilateral olfactory cortex. Behavioral reactions to odors are controlled by connections to the limbic system.

Assessment. Deficiencies in the sense of smell are difficult to evaluate. Rhinitis is the most common cause of anosmia (loss of olfaction). Tumors of the nasal passages and diseases of the cribriform plate also must be considered. Only rarely are structural lesions such as tumors of importance. Olfaction is also impaired by inflammatory diseases such as canine distemper and parainfluenza virus infection.[22]

Optic Nerve (CN II). The optic nerve is the sensory path for vision and pupillary light reflexes.

Technique. The optic nerve is tested in conjunction with the oculomotor nerve (CN III), which provides the motor pathway for the pupillary light reflex, and the facial nerve, which provides the motor pathway for the menace reflex. Vision can be assessed by observation of the animal's movements in unfamiliar surroundings, avoidance of obstacles, and following of moving objects. More objective evaluation requires three tests. The examiner elicits the menace response by making a threatening gesture with the hand at one eye. The normal response is a blink and, sometimes, an aversive movement of the head (Figure 1-33).

The visual placing reaction (see the section on postural reactions) is an excellent method of assessing vision. The examiner induces the pupillary light reflex by shining a light in each eye and observing for pupillary constriction in both eyes.

Anatomy and Physiology. See Chapters 2 and 11.

Assessment. See Chapters 2 and 11.

Oculomotor Nerve (CN III). The oculomotor nerve contains the parasympathetic motor fibers for pupillary constriction and innervates the following extraocular muscles: dorsal,

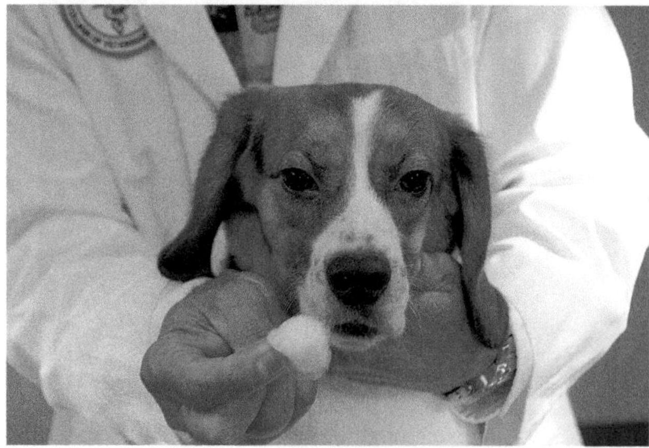

Figure 1-32 Noxious odors that are nonirritating cause an aversion or licking reaction.

medial, and ventral recti and ventral oblique. This nerve also innervates the levator palpebrae muscle of the upper eyelid.

Technique. The examiner tests the pupillary light reflex by shining a light in the animal's eye and observing for pupillary constriction in both eyes (Figure 1-34, *A*). One can assess eye movement by observing the eyes as the animal looks in various directions voluntarily or in response to movements in the peripheral fields of vision. A more direct method is to elicit vestibular eye movements (normal nystagmus) by moving the head laterally (see Figure 1-34, *B*).

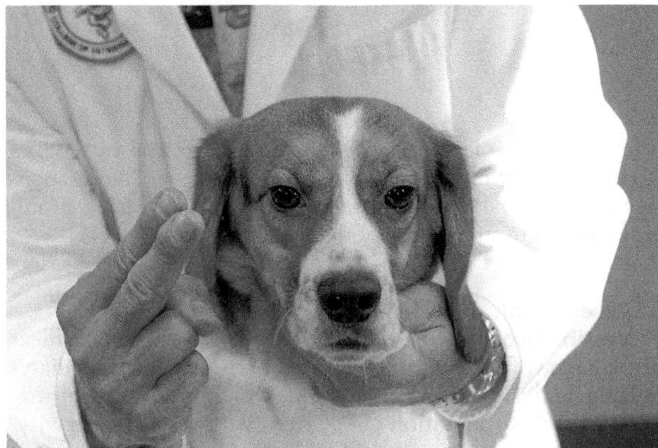

Figure 1-33 The menace response is elicited by making a threatening gesture at the eye, which should result in a blink. The examiner must avoid creating wind currents or touching the hairs around the eye, which will cause a palpebral reflex. The sensory pathway is in the optic nerve and the visual pathway. The motor pathway is in the facial nerve.

The fast beat of the nystagmus is in the direction of the head movement. The eyes should move in coordination with each other (conjugate movements). One can easily test the rectus muscles by this method.

A drooping upper lid (ptosis) is indicative of paresis of the levator palpebrae muscle. Lesions of the oculomotor nerve cause a fixed ventrolateral deviation (strabismus) of the eye and a dilated pupil. In cattle, the eye usually remains horizontal regardless of the head position. The function of each of the extraocular muscles can be assessed in the same manner if the examiner bears this difference in mind. The functions of the extraocular muscles of large animals have not been directly established, but presumably they are similar to the functions of the corresponding muscles in other species.

Anatomy and Physiology. See Chapters 2 and 11.

Assessment. See Chapters 2 and 11.

Trochlear Nerve (CN IV). The trochlear nerve is the motor pathway to the dorsal oblique muscle of the eye.

Technique. The trochlear nerve is difficult to assess. Lesions may cause a lateral rotation of the eye, which can be seen most clearly in animals with a horizontal pupil (cow) or a vertical pupil (cat) or by ophthalmoscopic examination of the dorsal retinal vein. A slight deficit is present in dorsomedial gaze.

Anatomy and Physiology. See Chapters 2 and 11.

Assessment. See Chapters 2 and 11.

Trigeminal Nerve (CN V). The trigeminal nerve is the motor pathway to the muscles of mastication and the sensory pathway to the face.

Technique. The motor branch of the trigeminal nerve is in the mandibular nerve and innervates the masseter, temporal, rostral digastric, pterygoid, and mylohyoid muscles. Bilateral paralysis produces a dropped jaw that cannot be closed voluntarily. Unilateral lesions may cause decreased jaw tone.

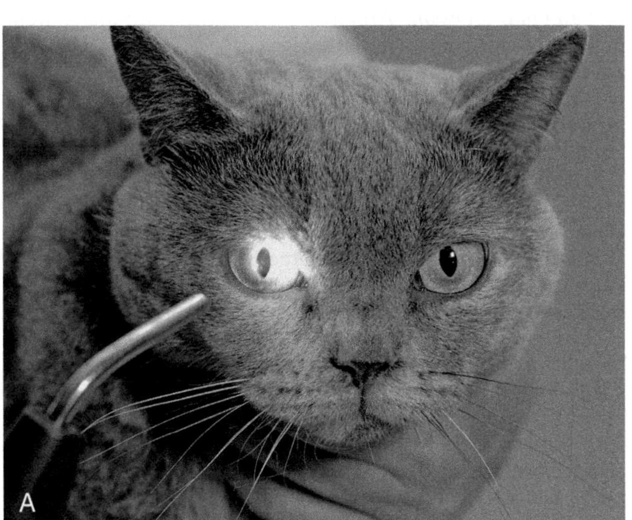

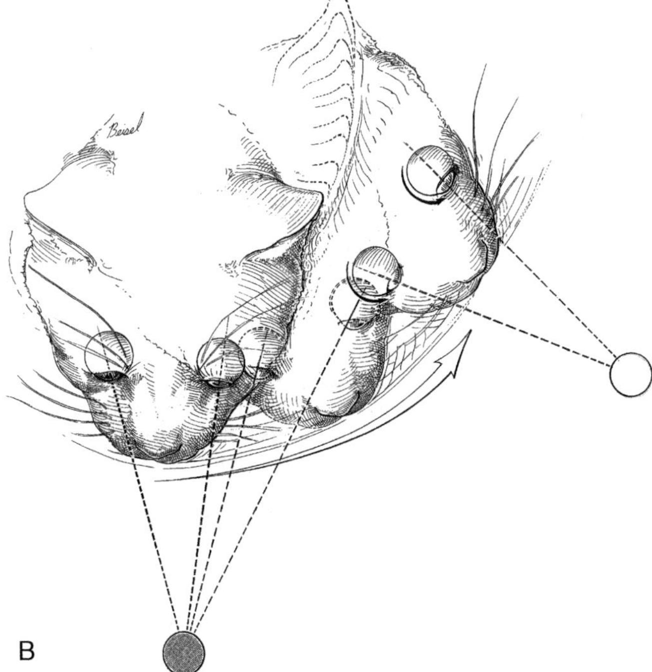

Figure 1-34 **A,** The pupillary light reflex (PLR) is evaluated by using a bright light source directed from a temporal to nasal position and observing for direct and consensual pupillary constriction. **B,** Vestibular eye movements are elicited by turning the animal's head from side to side. The eyes lag behind the head movement and then rotate to return to the center of the palpebral fissure. Both visual (oculokinetic or physiologic nystagmus) and vestibular pathways are active in this response, but vestibular pathways predominate and produce these movements in the absence of vision. (**A,** from August: Consultations in feline internal medicine, Vol 6, 2010, Saunders.)

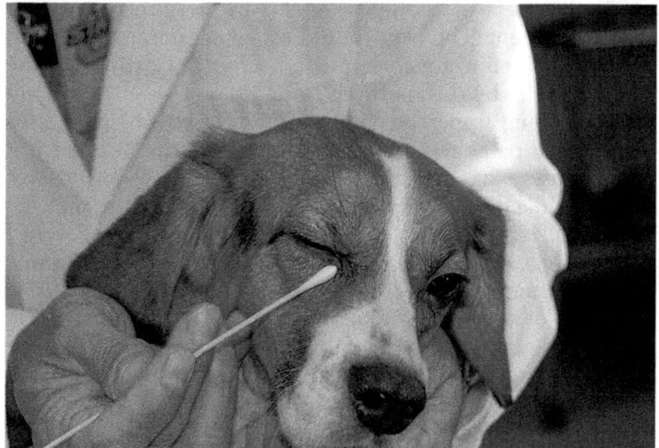

Figure 1-35 The palpebral reflex is checked by touching the eyelid and observing for a blink. The sensory pathway is in the trigeminal nerve; the motor pathway is in the facial nerve.

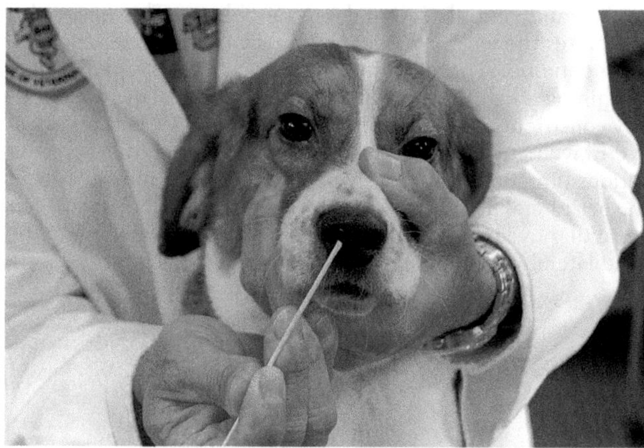

Figure 1-36 Tactile stimulation on the head rostral to the ears tests the sensory branches of the trigeminal nerve. The reactions may be behavioral or reflex. Even dull or obtunded and stoic animals respond to stimulation of the nasal mucosa.

Atrophy of the temporal and masseter muscles is recognized by careful palpation approximately 1 week after the onset of paralysis. Sensation should be tested over the distribution of all three branches: ophthalmic, maxillary, and mandibular. A touch of the skin may be an adequate stimulus in some animals, whereas a gentle pinch with a forceps may be needed in others. The palpebral reflex is a blink response to a touch at the medial canthus of the eye that tests the ophthalmic branch (Figure 1-35).

Touching the lateral canthus tests the maxillary branch. The blink response is dependent on innervation of the muscles by the facial nerve.

Response to stimulation of the nasal mucosa tests the maxillary and ophthalmic branches and should elicit a response even in dull or obtunded and stoic animals (Figure 1-36).

Pinching the jaw tests the mandibular branch.

Anatomy and Physiology. See Chapters 2 and 9.

Assessment. See Chapters 2 and 9.

Abducent Nerve (CN VI). The abducent nerve innervates the lateral rectus and the retractor bulbi muscles.

Technique. Eye movements are tested by the method described for the oculomotor nerve. The retractor bulbi muscles can be tested with a palpebral or a corneal reflex. Normally, the globe is retracted, allowing extrusion of the third eyelid. Lesions of the abducent nerve cause a loss of lateral (abducted) gaze and medial strabismus combined with inability to retract the globe.

Anatomy and Physiology. See Chapters 2 and 11.

Assessment. See Chapters 2 and 11.

Facial Nerve (CN VII). The facial nerve is the motor pathway to the muscles of facial expression and the sensory pathway for taste to the palate and the rostral two thirds of the tongue. It also provides sensory innervation to the inner surface of the pinna.

Technique. Asymmetry is usually seen in cases of facial paralysis. The lips, eyelids, and ears may droop. The nose may be slightly deviated to the normal side, and the nostril may not flare on inhalation. The palpebral fissure may be slightly widened and fails to close when a palpebral or a corneal reflex is attempted (see Figure 1-35). Pinching the lip produces a behavioral response, but the lip may not retract. The examiner can test the animal's sense of taste by moistening a cotton-tipped applicator with atropine and touching it to the rostral part of the tongue. The affected side is tested first. Normal dogs react immediately to the bitter taste. Delayed reactions may occur as the atropine spreads to normal areas of the tongue.

Anatomy and Physiology. See Chapters 2 and 9.

Assessment. See Chapters 2 and 9.

Vestibulocochlear Nerve (CN VIII). The vestibulocochlear nerve has two branches: the cochlear division, which mediates hearing, and the vestibular division, which provides information about the orientation of the head with respect to gravity.

Technique

Cochlear Division. Most tests for hearing are dependent on behavioral reactions to sound and therefore are subject to misinterpretation. No good test exists for unilateral deficits other than those involving electrophysiologic systems. Crude tests involve startling the animal with a loud noise (clap, whistle). Similar responses may be monitored by an electroencephalogram (EEG) or by observation or direct measurement of the respiratory cycle. Human audiometry equipment can also be adapted for animals. The most precise equipment involves a signal-averaging computer, which measures electrical activity of the brainstem in response to auditory stimuli (brainstem auditory-evoked response [BAER]). BAER not only detects auditory deficits but also may indicate the location of the lesion (see Chapter 4).

Vestibular Division. Abnormalities of the vestibular system produce several characteristic signs. Most vestibular lesions are unilateral except in congenital anomalies and occasionally in inflammatory diseases. Unilateral vestibular disease usually produces ataxia, nystagmus, and a head tilt to the side of the lesion.[7]

The head tilt should be apparent on observation (see Figure 1-17). The examiner can accentuate the head tilt by removing visual compensation or by removing tactile proprioception. Vestibular ataxia (an uncoordinated, staggering gait) usually is accompanied by a broad-based stance and a tendency to fall or to circle to the side of the lesion.

Nystagmus is involuntary rhythmic movement of the eyes. Two forms of nystagmus are recognized. Jerk nystagmus has a slow phase in one direction and a rapid recovery phase to return. Pendular nystagmus is small oscillations of the eyes with no slow or fast components. Pendular nystagmus is associated with visual defects and cerebellar diseases. Jerk nystagmus is associated with vestibular and brainstem diseases. See Chapter 11 for a more complete discussion of nystagmus. Nystagmus should be observed with the head held in varying positions. The direction of the fast component is noted (e.g., left horizontal nystagmus). Jerk nystagmus may be horizontal, vertical, or rotatory. Forced deviation of the globe (strabismus) also may be seen when the head is elevated or lowered. Typically, in small animals, the ipsilateral eye deviates ventrally when the head is elevated. Producing eye movements by moving the animal's head from side to side, physiologic nystagmus (see the section on CN III) also tests the vestibular system (see Figure 1-34). Vestibular lesions may alter the direction or may abolish the response. In some cases, the eyes do not move together (dysconjugate movement).

Lesions of the receptors or the vestibular nerve cause a horizontal or rotatory nystagmus that does not change with varying head positions. Lesions of the vestibular nuclei and associated structures may cause nystagmus in any direction that may change that direction with varying head positions. We have observed a few relatively rare instances of nystagmus that changes direction with confirmed peripheral disease and no evidence of central disease.

Postrotatory nystagmus may help to evaluate vestibular disease. As an animal is rotated rapidly, physiologic nystagmus is induced. When rotation is stopped, nystagmus (postrotatory) occurs in the opposite direction and is observed for a short time. The receptors opposite the direction of rotation are stimulated more than the ipsilateral receptors because they are farther from the axis of rotation. Unilateral lesions produce a difference in the rate and duration of postrotatory nystagmus when the animal is tested in both directions. The test is performed in the following manner: The animal is held by an assistant, who rapidly turns 360 degrees 10 times and then stops. The examiner counts the beats of nystagmus. After several minutes, the test is repeated in the opposite direction. Normal animals have three or four beats of nystagmus, with the fast phase opposite the direction of rotation. Peripheral lesions usually depress the response when the animal is rotated away from the side of the lesion. Central lesions may depress or prolong the response.

The caloric test is a specific test for vestibular function. This test has the advantage of assessing each side independently. It is difficult to perform in many animals, however, and may be unreliable if the patient is uncooperative. Negative responses occur in many normal animals. The examiner performs the test by holding the animal's head securely in one position, irrigating the ear canal with ice water, and observing for nystagmus. A rubber ear syringe should be used for the irrigation. Usually, 50 to 100 mL of cold water is adequate, and the infusion takes approximately 3 minutes. The test should not be performed if the tympanic membrane is ruptured or if the ear canal is plugged. Nystagmus is induced with the fast phase away from the side being tested. Warm water also produces the same effect, except that the nystagmus is in the opposite direction. Warm water is even less reliable. If the animal resists and shakes its head, the response usually is abolished. The test is helpful for the evaluation of brainstem function in comatose animals but has been replaced by the BAER test at most institutions.

Anatomy and Physiology. See Chapters 2 and 8.

Assessment. See Chapters 2 and 8.

Glossopharyngeal Nerve (CN IX), Vagus Nerve (CN X), and Accessory Nerve (CN XI). Cranial nerves IX, X, and XI are considered together because of their common origin and intracranial pathway. The glossopharyngeal nerve innervates the muscles of the pharynx along with some fibers from the vagus nerve. The glossopharyngeal nerve also supplies parasympathetic motor fibers to the zygomatic and parotid salivary glands. It is sensory to the caudal one third of the tongue and the pharyngeal mucosa, including the sensation of taste. The vagus nerve innervates the pharynx, the larynx, and the palate and supplies parasympathetic motor fibers to the viscera of the body, except for the pelvic viscera, which are innervated by sacral parasympathetic nerves. Gastric abnormalities are common in vagus nerve problems in ruminants. The vagus nerve is the sensory pathway to the caudal pharynx, the larynx, and the viscera. The accessory nerve has two roots, cranial and spinal. The cranial roots originate in the same nucleus as the vagus and glossopharyngeal nerves, the nucleus ambiguus. As the accessory nerve exits the cranial cavity, fibers join with the vagus to innervate the pharyngeal and laryngeal musculature. The spinal roots of the accessory nerve are discussed separately (see later discussion).

Technique. Taste can be evaluated by the method described for CN VII, although making an accurate assessment of the caudal part of the tongue is more difficult. The simplest test for function is to observe the palate and the larynx for asymmetry and to elicit a gag or a swallowing reflex by inserting a tongue depressor to the pharynx. The laryngeal region also can be externally palpated, and a swallowing reflex and tongue movements are observed. Stertorous breathing may be observed with laryngeal paralysis. Endoscopic observation of the larynx is useful in the horse. The laryngeal adductor response (slap test) is performed during endoscopic observation. The skin caudal to the dorsal part of the scapula is slapped gently with the hand during expiration. The normal response is brief adduction of the contralateral arytenoid cartilage.[9]

Historical evidence of an inability to swallow may be suggestive of an abnormality in CNs IX, X, and XI. The clinician should be cautious when examining animals with swallowing problems because dysphagia is one of the signs of rabies.

Anatomy and Physiology. See Chapters 2 and 9.

Assessment. See Chapters 2 and 9.

Accessory Nerve. The spinal roots of the accessory nerve are the motor pathway to the trapezius muscle and parts of the sternocephalicus and brachiocephalicus muscles.

Technique. The detection of an abnormality in an accessory nerve injury may be difficult, except by careful palpation for atrophy of the affected muscles. Passive movement of the head and the neck may demonstrate a loss of resistance to lateral movements in a contralateral direction.

Anatomy and Physiology. The spinal roots of the accessory nerve arise from fibers in the ventral roots of the C1-7 spinal cord segments. The fibers course cranially as the spinal root of the accessory nerve, which lies between the dorsal and the ventral spinal nerve roots and enters the cranial cavity via the foramen magnum. The accessory nerve emerges from the skull by way of the tympanooccipital fissure and then courses caudally in the neck to innervate the trapezius and portions of the sternocephalicus and brachiocephalicus muscles. These muscles elevate and advance the limb and fix the neck laterally.[4]

Assessment. Lesions of the accessory nerve are either rare or rarely recognized. An injury to the nerve in the vertebral canal or the cranial cavity probably would be masked by other, more severe signs of paresis. The course of the nerve in the neck is well protected by muscle but could be damaged by deep penetrating wounds, injections, or contusions. Atrophy of the affected muscles would be the most obvious sign of injury. Electromyography (EMG) may be necessary for diagnosis. Lesions in the vertebral canal should produce other signs of spinal cord dysfunction.

Hypoglossal Nerve. The hypoglossal nerve is the motor pathway to the intrinsic and extrinsic muscles of the tongue and the geniohyoideus muscle.

Technique. The muscles of the tongue protrude and retract it. Each side is innervated independently. Protrusion is tested by wetting the animal's nose and observing the ability to extend its tongue forward (Figure 1-37).

The strength of retraction can be tested by grasping the tongue with a gauze sponge. Atrophy can be observed if a lesion has been present for 5 to 7 days.

Anatomy and Physiology. See Chapters 2 and 9.

Assessment. See Chapters 2 and 9.

Sensory Testing

The sensory examination provides information relative to the anatomic location and severity of the lesion. At this point in the neurologic examination, sensation has been tested by assessment of the cranial nerves, spinal reflexes, and proprioceptive positioning. Sensory modalities still to be tested include hyperesthesia, superficial pain, and deep pain from the limbs and the trunk.

Technique. Testing for sensation is usually done last in the examination to avoid losing cooperation of the patient. The objective of the sensory examination is threefold: (1) map areas of increased sensation (hyperesthesia), (2) map any areas of decreased sensation (hypesthesia), and (3) ensure that the animal has a conscious response to a noxious stimulus. The first two are accomplished by testing for hyperesthesia and the ability to perceive superficial pain, respectively. Evaluation of the animal's conscious response to a noxious stimulus should only be tested in animals that display paralysis. Given the orderly and predictable manner in which function is lost with a compressive lesion affecting the spinal cord, an animal displaying voluntary movement (even if not able to support weight or walk) should be able to perceive a noxious stimulus. Always apply the minimum stimulus that elicits a reaction.

Hyperesthesia is an increased sensitivity to stimulation. For a comprehensive discussion of hyperesthesia and pain, see Chapter 14. Behavioral reactions to what should be a non-noxious stimulus are interpreted as "pain." Testing should be done first from distal to proximal or caudal to cranial. Lesions of the nervous system decrease sensation caudal or distal to the lesion, sometimes increase sensation at the lesion site, and leave sensation normal proximal to the lesion. Therefore testing from distal to proximal or caudal to cranial goes from decreased sensation through increased sensation to normal sensation. The direction can be reversed to define more clearly the boundaries of abnormality. The pelvic limbs are palpated first, followed by the vertebral column. Beginning with L7 and progressing cranially, the examiner squeezes the transverse processes. Alternatively, one can press each spinous process firmly. The severity of the stimulus is increased from light touch to deep palpation. Proper palpation causes no reaction in normal areas and a behavioral reaction in areas that are painful. Animals that are in extreme pain may react regardless of where they are palpated. Localization of the source of pain in these patients may be more accurate if the animal is sedated before examination. Increased muscle tension may be noticed when the painful area is palpated, even under light anesthesia. By placing one hand on the abdomen during palpation of the vertebral column, one can detect splinting of the abdominal muscles when pain is experienced (Figure 1-38).

At the opposite extreme, some hounds may almost let you amputate a leg without flinching.

Sometimes the animal's reaction can be increased by mashing a toe until it reacts. One or two repetitions often overcome the animal's reluctance to protest, and they then react when you palpate the painful areas. During palpation of the animal, areas of increased sensitivity (hyperesthesia) are noted.

Testing for superficial pain or eliciting the cutaneous trunci (panniculus) reflex is best done with a small hemostat. Gently grasp a fold of skin, then pinch (Figure 1-39).

Needles may be applied, but they are less reliable and may cause injury. As in palpating, testing should be done from distal

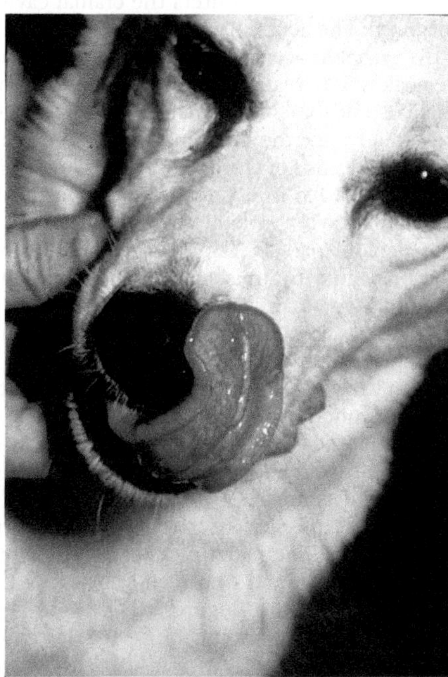

Figure 1-37 Most animals can be induced to lick if their noses are moistened. The tongue should be extended without forced deviation to the side.

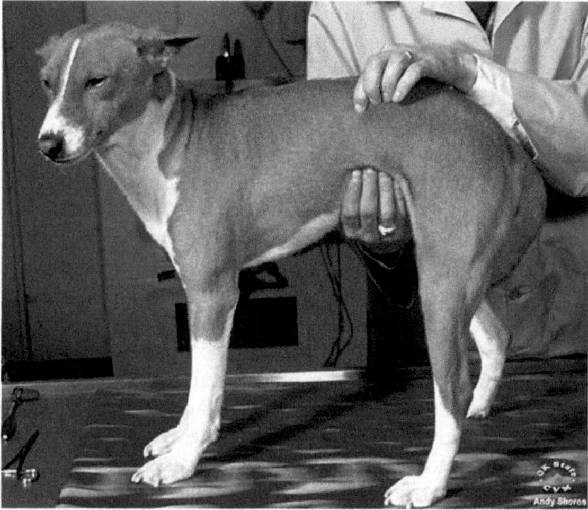

Figure 1-38 Deep palpation may elicit areas of hyperesthesia. Minimal response may be detected by simultaneously palpating adjacent areas for changes in muscle tone (guarding reaction).

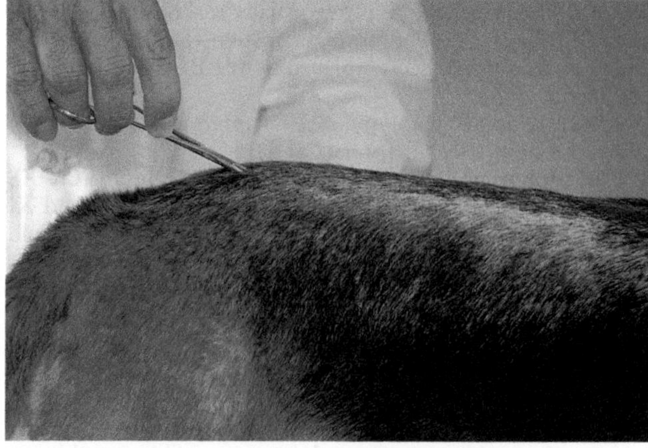

Figure 1-39 Gentle pricking or pinching of the skin can be used to outline the area of hyperesthesia more precisely. Both behavioral reactions and the cutaneous reflex may be elicited. The skin should be stimulated dorsally and laterally for the examiner to develop a map of abnormal reactions.

to proximal or caudal to cranial. The examiner tests the skin just lateral to the midline and then repeats on a line lateral to the site of the first evaluation. The opposite side is tested similarly. Three responses may be observed: a behavioral response, a reflex withdrawal of a limb, or a twitch of the skin (the cutaneous trunci or panniculus reflex). A behavioral response such as a display of anxiety, an attempt to escape, a turning of the head, or a vocalization indicates perception of superficial pain. Withdrawal of a limb is a reflex and only indicates an intact reflex arc (see section on flexor reflexes). The cutaneous reflex is a contraction of the cutaneous trunci muscle, causing a twitch of the skin along the dorsal and lateral areas of the trunk. A significant behavioral response at any step indicates the presence of sensation, and more severe stimuli are not needed once sensation has been established. If a dog turns and snaps when its toe is touched, one need not squeeze the toe with a hemostat.[23]

The caudal margins of normal superficial pain can be determined bilaterally. Spinal cord or nerve root lesions produce an area of hyperesthesia or a transition from decreased to normal sensation in a pattern conforming to the dermatomal distribution of the nerves (see Figure 1-12). Testing of cutaneous sensation of the neck is unreliable for localizing cervical lesions. Manipulation of the head and the neck and deep palpation of the cervical vertebrae are more useful for localizing pain in this area.

A noxious stimulus that elicits any behavioral response is adequate for determining the presence of deep pain. When a response is difficult to elicit, a hemostat is used to squeeze a digit. Withdrawal of the limb is not a behavioral response (see the section on the flexor reflexes).

Anatomy and Physiology. Newer concepts emphasize the integration and interaction of all sensory systems and the effect of descending pathways that modify sensation. The concepts presented in this section are in general agreement with current research and are adequate for the clinical interpretation of sensory signs.[24-26]

Sensory fibers from the skin, the muscles, the joints, and the viscera enter the spinal cord at each segment by way of the dorsal nerve root. Fibers that innervate the skin are arranged in regular patterns called dermatomes. A dermatome is the area of skin innervated by one spinal nerve root. Because of overlap, each strip of skin has some innervation from three segments.[27-31]

Proprioceptive fibers entering the spinal cord may ascend in the dorsal columns and the spinomedullothalamic tract to relay information to nuclei in the medulla (see Figure 1-15). Other fibers synapse on neurons in the dorsal horn of the gray matter. The neurons then send axons cranially along one of several named pathways, both ipsilaterally and contralaterally. The primary functions of these pathways include unconscious proprioception and sensitivity to touch, temperature, and superficial pain.

The deep pain pathway (spinoreticular and propriospinal tracts) is interrupted at three- to five-segment intervals to synapse on neurons in the spinal cord gray matter. These neurons give rise to axons, which rejoin the pathway on the same side or on the opposite side. The deep pain system is bilateral and multisynaptic and is composed of small-diameter unmyelinated fibers (see Figure 1-11).[25]

The cutaneous trunci or panniculus reflex is a twitch of the cutaneous muscle in response to a cutaneous stimulus. The sensory nerves from the skin enter by way of the dorsal root. The ascending pathway is probably the same as that for superficial pain. The synapse occurs bilaterally at the C8, T1 segments with motor neurons of the lateral thoracic nerve that innervates the cutaneous trunci muscle (see Figure 1-16).[4]

Assessment. Alterations in a sensory modality are described as absent (0), decreased (+1), normal (+2), or increased (hyperesthesia, +3). Absent or decreased sensation indicates damage to a sensory nerve or a pathway. Increased sensitivity may indicate irritation of a nerve or, more commonly, irritation of adjacent structures (e.g., disk herniation with irritation of meninges).

The cutaneous trunci reflex is most prominent in the "saddle" area of the trunk. It cannot be elicited from stimulation over the sacrum or the neck. The reflex is absent caudal to the level of a lesion that disrupts the superficial pain pathway. For example, a severe compression of spinal cord segment L1 results in a normal reflex when stimulation is applied to the T13 dermatome but no response caudal to that point.

When alterations in touch, superficial pain, or hyperesthetic areas are found, the pattern of abnormality is carefully mapped. The pattern generally conforms to one of three possibilities:

1. Transverse spinal cord lesions cause an abnormality in all areas caudal to the lesion. The line of demarcation between normal and abnormal areas follows the pattern of a dermatome (see Figure 1-12).
2. Hyperesthesia, reflecting an irritation at a spinal cord segment or a nerve root, follows the distribution of one or more dermatomes but usually no more than three.
3. Lesions of a peripheral nerve produce a pattern of abnormality conforming to the distribution of that peripheral nerve (see Figure 1-13).

One of these three patterns localizes the lesion to a peripheral nerve (e.g., sciatic nerve, radial nerve) or to a spinal cord segment accurate to within three segments (e.g., L1-3).

The presence or absence of pain perception provides an important assessment of the extent of neural damage, especially in compressive lesions. When nerves are compressed, large nerve fibers are the first to lose function. With greater compression, small nerve fibers may be affected. In the spinal cord, loss of function develops in the following sequence: (1) loss of proprioception, (2) loss of voluntary motor function, (3) loss of superficial pain perception, and (4) loss of deep pain perception (see Figure 1-3). An animal with a spinal cord compression that has lost proprioception and voluntary motor function (paralyzed) but still has superficial and deep pain perception therefore has less spinal cord damage than one that has lost all four functions. A loss of deep pain perception indicates a severely damaged spinal cord and a guarded prognosis.

REFERENCES

1. Weed LL: Medical records, medical education and patient care, Chicago, 1971, Year Book Medical Publishers.
2. Osborne CA, Low DG: The medical history redefined: idealism vs. realism, Denver, 1976, AAHA. In Proceedings of the American Animal Hospital Association.
3. Oliver JE: Neurologic examinations: taking the history, Vet Med Small Anim Clin 67:433–434, 1972.
4. de Lahunta A: Veterinary neuroanatomy and clinical neurology, ed 3, St Louis, 2009, Elsevier.
5. Oliver JE: Neurologic examinations: observations on mental status, Vet Med Small Anim Clin 67:654–659, 1972.
6. Oliver JE: Neurologic examinations: observations on posture, Vet Med Small Anim Clin 67:882–884, 1972.
7. Oliver JE: Neurologic examinations: observations on movement, Vet Med Small Anim Clin 67:1105–1106, 1972.
8. Oliver JE, Hoerlein BF, Mayhew IG: Veterinary neurology, Philadelphia, 1987, WB Saunders.
9. Mayhew IG: Large animal neurology: a handbook for veterinary clinicians, ed 2, Ames, IA, 2009, Wiley-Blackwell.
10. Grillner S: Neurobiological bases of rhythmic motor acts in vertebrates, Science 228:143–149, 1985.

11. Grillner S: Locomotion in vertebrates: central mechanisms and reflex interaction, Physiol Rev 55:247–304, 1975.
12. Willis JB: On the interaction between spinal locomotor generators in quadrupeds, Brain Res Rev 2:171–204, 1980.
13. Breazile JE, Blaugh BS, Nail N: Experimental study of canine distemper myoclonus, Am J Vet Res 27:1375–1379, 1966.
14. Oliver JE: Neurologic examinations: palpation and inspection, Vet Med Small Anim Clin 67:1327–1328, 1972.
15. Oliver JE: Neurologic examinations-sensation: proprioception and touch, Vet Med Small Anim Clin 67:295–298, 1972.
16. Holliday TA: The origins of the neurological examination: the postural and attitudinal, placing and righting reactions. In Proceedings of the Seventh Annual Veterinary Medical Forum, San Diego, 1989, American College of Veterinary Internal Medicine.
17. Roberts TDM: Neurophysiology of postural mechanisms, New York, 1967, Plenum Press.
18. Oliver JE: Neurologic examinations: flexion and crossed extension reflexes, Vet Med Small Anim Clin 68:383–385, 1973.
19. Oliver JE: Neurologic examinations-spinal reflexes: extensor thrust reflex, Vet Med Small Anim Clin 68:763, 1973.
20. Kneller S, Oliver J, Lewis R: Differential diagnosis of progressive caudal paresis in an aged German shepherd dog, J Am Anim Hosp Assoc 11:414–417, 1975.
21. Hoff H, Breckenridge C: Observations on the mammalian reflex prototype of the sign of Babinski, Brain 79:155–167, 1966.
22. Myers LJ, Nusbaum KE, Swango LJ, et al: Dysfunction of sense of smell caused by canine parainfluenza virus infection in dogs, Am J Vet Res 49:188–190, 1988.
23. Oliver JE: Neurologic examinations-sensation: pain, Vet Med Small Anim Clin 69:607–610, 1974.
24. Willis WD, Coggeshall RE: Sensory mechanisms of the spinal cord, ed 2, New York, 1991, Plenum Press.
25. Willis WD Jr: The pain system: the neural basis of nociceptive transmission in the mammalian nervous system, Basel, Switzerland, 1985, S Karger.
26. Willis W, Chung J: Central mechanisms of pain, J Am Vet Med Assoc 191:1200–1202, 1987.
27. Kirk E: The dermatomes of the sheep, J Comp Neurol 134:353–370, 1968.
28. Bailey C, Kitchell R, Haghighi S, et al: Cutaneous innervation of the thorax and abdomen of the dog, Am J Vet Res 45:1689–1698, 1984.
29. Fletcher T, Kitchell R: The lumbar, sacral and coccygeal tactile dermatomes of the dog, J Comp Neurol 128:171–180, 1966.
30. Kirk E, Kitchell R, Johnson R: Neurophysiologic maps of cutaneous innervation of the hind limb of sheep, Am J Vet Res 48:1485–1492, 1987.
31. Hekmatpanah J: Organization of tactile dermatomes, C1 through L4, in cat, J Neurophysiol 24:129–140, 1961.

CHAPTER 2

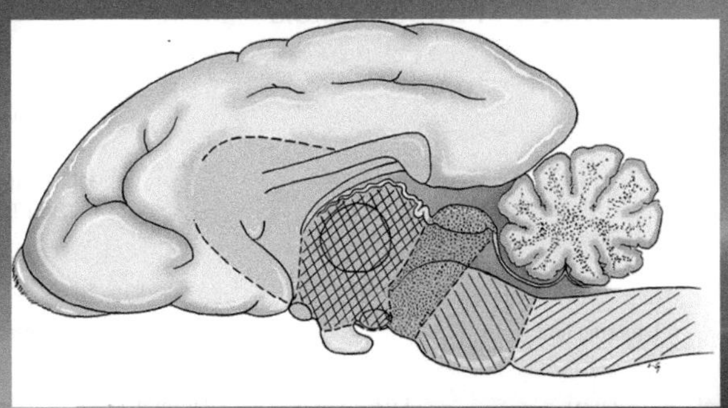

Localization of Lesions in the Nervous System

In Chapter 1, the fundamentals of organizing a diagnosis, neuroanatomy, and neurologic examination were described. In this chapter, the principles of lesion localization will be described using the anatomic information described in Chapter 1.

LOCALIZATION TO A REGION OF THE SPINAL CORD OR THE BRAIN

Upper Motor Neuron (UMN) and Lower Motor Neuron (LMN) Signs

Examination of the motor system should allow the clinician to localize the lesion to one of five levels of the spinal cord or to the brain (Figure 2-1 and Table 2-1).

Gait and postural reactions detect paresis or paralysis; spinal reflexes detect LMN abnormality. The thoracic and pelvic limbs should be classified as normal or as exhibiting LMN or UMN signs (see Table 1-3). Briefly, LMN signs are paresis or paralysis, a loss of reflexes, and a loss of muscle tone. UMN signs are a loss of voluntary motor activity (paresis or paralysis), an increase in muscle tone, and normal or exaggerated reflexes. Note that with both UMN and LMN signs, paresis or paralysis is the primary finding. The status of the reflexes distinguishes between the two.

The examiner can localize a lesion to a region of the spinal cord or the brain by using these findings and the material presented in Figure 2-1, which is an algorithm that explains the logic of the diagnosis. For example, paresis in the pelvic limbs with normal thoracic limbs indicates that the brain and spinal cord as far caudal as T2 are functioning. Therefore, a lesion is caudal to T2. To determine whether the lesion is in the T3-L3 or L4-S2 region, the reflexes of the pelvic limb must be evaluated. If they are normal or exaggerated, the L4-S2 segments must be functioning and the lesion is between T3 and L3. If the reflexes are decreased or absent, the lesion is in the L4-S2 segments. Paresis or paralysis of all four limbs indicates a lesion cranial to T3. Reflexes are tested in all four limbs. Normal or exaggerated reflexes of all limbs indicate a lesion cranial to C6. Other findings are used to localize the lesion further. With a lesion cranial to C6, one should examine the cranial nerves and mentation to rule out brain disease. The sensory examination is further reviewed for possible signs related to the neck (e.g., C1-5).

Using only the information related to LMN and UMN signs of the limbs, the examiner can localize the lesion to one of the following regions: (1) the brain, (2) C1-5, (3) C6-T2-brachial plexus (thoracic limb), (4) T3-L3, (5) L4-S2-lumbosacral plexus (pelvic limb), or (6) S3-Cd5.

LOCALIZATION TO A SEGMENTAL LEVEL OF THE SPINAL CORD

Lower Motor Neuron Signs

If LMN signs are present in the limbs, the examiner can localize the lesion further by identifying the affected muscles. Table 2-2 lists spinal cord segments (roots) and peripheral nerves for the most commonly tested reflexes.

The examiner can localize within two to four segments or to a peripheral nerve if LMN signs are present. Spinal cord segments do not correlate directly with vertebral levels. When the examiner has determined the spinal cord level, Figure 1-8 can be referred to for an estimation of the vertebral level. As a general rule, the sacral segments overlie L5. This can be remembered because S (for sacral) resembles the number 5.

Peripheral nerve lesions usually cause monoparesis (paresis of one limb) because the most common lesions are the result of injury to a limb or a specific nerve. Localization of lesions in monoparesis is reviewed in Chapter 5. The primary exception is generalized peripheral neuropathies, which affect all of the limbs. These conditions are discussed in Chapter 7.

Sensory Perception

Hyperesthesia (increased sensitivity to noxious stimuli) is a useful localizing sign and may be present with little or no motor deficit. The animal's limbs and trunk, especially the

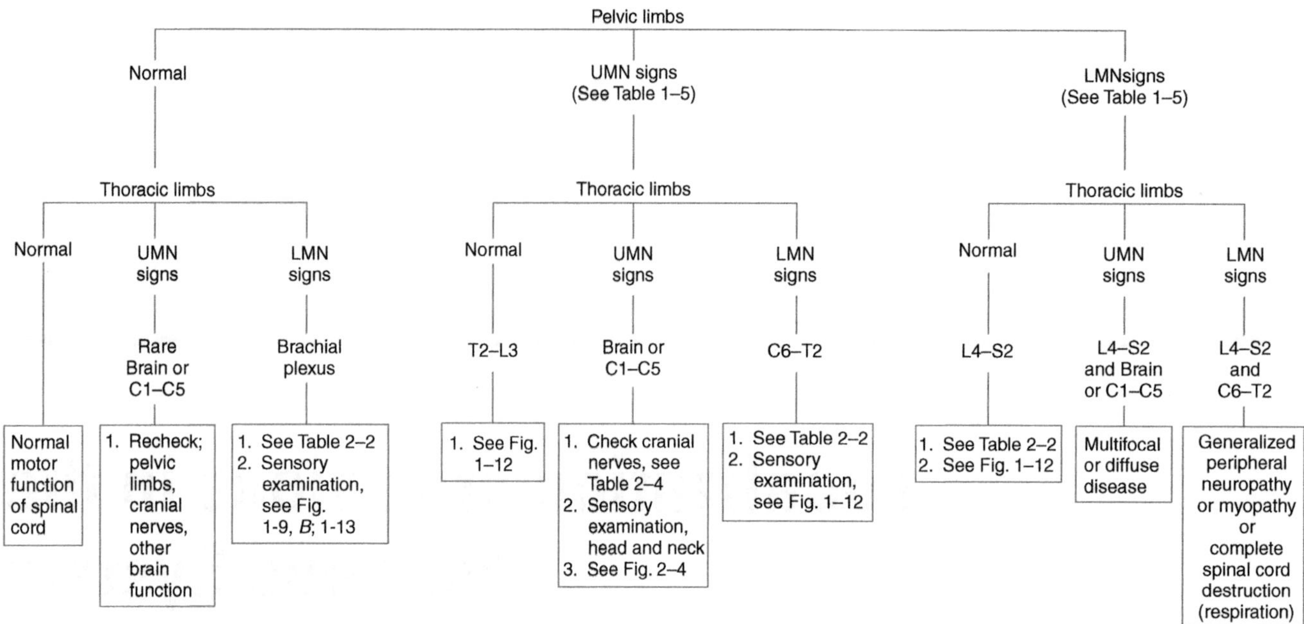

Figure 2-1 Localization of lesions based on motor function. *UMN,* Upper motor neuron; *LMN,* lower motor neuron; C, cervical; *T,* thoracic; *L,* lumbar; *S,* sacral spinal cord segments. (From Hoerlein BF: Canine neurology, ed 3, Philadelphia, 1978, WB Saunders.)

TABLE 2-1

Signs of Lesions in the Spinal Cord

Site of Lesion	Sign
Cd1-5	LMN—tail
S1-3	UMN—tail
Pelvic plexus	LMN—bladder
Pudendal nerve	LMN—anal sphincter, urethral external sphincter
L4-S2	UMN—tail
Lumbosacral plexus	LMN—hind limbs
	UMN or LMN—bladder, anal sphincter
T3-L3	UMN—hind limbs, bladder, anal sphincter
	LMN—segmental spinal muscles
C6-T2	UMN—hind limbs, bladder
Brachial plexus	LMN—forelimbs
C1-5 or brainstem	UMN—all four limbs, bladder

LMN, Lower motor neuron; *UMN,* upper motor neuron.

vertebral column, are palpated and manipulated while the examiner observes for signs of pain. Obvious reactions may include resistance to movement and tensing of the muscles. If the clinician places one hand on the animal's abdomen while squeezing each vertebral segment with the other hand, increased tension of the abdominal muscles may be felt as painful areas are palpated. The skin is pinched with a hemostat after palpation is completed. A fold of skin is grasped gently with the hemostat, and the skin is pinched lightly so that no significant behavioral reaction is elicited from normal areas. Pinching areas of hyperesthesia may elicit an exaggerated skin twitch or a behavioral response.

The superficial pain examination should be performed in a caudal to cranial direction because areas caudal to a lesion usually have decreased sensory perception (see Figures 1-16 and 1-39). A level of normal or increased sensory perception can be ascertained by this method. If a spinal lesion is present, the sensory level should have the conformation of a dermatome (see Figure 1-12). Peripheral nerves have a different pattern of sensory distribution (see Figure 1-13).

The cutaneous trunci (panniculus) reflex is elicited with a hemostat in the same manner as that just described for detecting hyperesthesia. Cutaneous sensation enters the spinal cord at each segment (dermatomes) and ascends to the brachial plexus (C8-T1) to the lateral thoracic nerve, which innervates the cutaneous trunci (panniculus carnosus) muscle. Contraction of the cutaneous trunci muscle causes a skin twitch. A segmental lesion blocks the ascending afferent stimulus, abolishing the reflex. Pinching the skin in a caudal to cranial direction identifies the first level at which the reflex can be elicited. This segment is normal, and the lesion is one segment caudal to this level. The superficial pain pathways must be damaged to abolish the reflex. Normally the cutaneous trunci reflex is most apparent in the thoracolumbar (saddle) area. A minimal response is obtained from a stimulus applied to the sacral or caudal regions, and no response is obtained from a stimulus applied to the cervical region. Cervical spinal hyperesthesia is assessed by manipulation of the neck and deep palpation of the vertebrae. Although defining the location of the pain precisely may be difficult, determining whether it is in the cranial, middle, or caudal cervical segments is usually possible by performing palpation carefully and gently.

Hypesthesia (decreased sensory perception) and anesthesia (lack of sensory perception) also are good localizing signs. Single nerve root lesions usually do not produce a clinically detectable area of decreased sensation because of the overlapping pattern of cutaneous innervation (see Figure 1-12). Multiple nerve roots may be involved in some lesions, especially in the area of the cauda equina. Lesions of the spinal cord may result in decreased perception of pain caudal to the lesion. Determining the level of sensory loss was discussed earlier, and the prognostic implications of the loss of sensation are discussed later. A carefully performed sensory examination localizes the lesion to within three segments of the spinal cord

TABLE 2-2

Spinal Reflexes

Reflex	Muscle(s)	Peripheral Nerve	Segments*
Myotatic (stretch)	Biceps brachii	Musculocutaneous	(C6), C7-8, (T1)
	Triceps brachii	Radial	C7-8, T1, (T2)
	Extensor carpi radialis	Radial	C7-8, T1, (T2)
	Quadriceps	Femoral	(L3), L4-5, (L6)
	Cranial tibial	Peroneal (sciatic)	L6-7, S1
	Gastrocnemius	Tibial (sciatic)	L6-7, S1
Flexor (withdrawal)	Thoracic limb	Radial, ulnar, median, musculocutaneous	C6-T2
	Pelvic limb	Sciatic	L6-S1, (S2)
Cutaneous trunci	Cutaneous trunci	Lateral thoracic	C8, T1
Perineal	Anal sphincter	Pudendal	S1-2, (S3)

Modified with permission from Oliver JE Jr: Localization of lesions in the nervous system. In Hoerlein BF, editor: Canine neurology, ed 3, Philadelphia, 1978, WB Saunders.
*Parentheses indicate segments that sometimes contribute to a nerve.

TABLE 2-3

Signs of Lesions in the Brain and Peripheral Vestibular System

Lesion Site	Mental Status	Posture	Movement	Postural Reactions	Cranial Nerves
Cerebral cortex	Abnormal behavior, and mentation, seizures	Normal; head turned toward side of lesion	Gait normal to slight hemiparesis (contralateral)	Deficits (contralateral)	Normal (vision may be impaired contralateral side)
Diencephalon (thalamus and hypothalamus)	Abnormal behavior and mentation, endocrine and autonomic dysfunction	Normal	Gait normal to hemiparesis or tetraparesis	Deficits (contralateral)	CN II, abnormal pupillary light reflex
Brainstem (midbrain, pons, medulla)	Dullness, stupor, coma	Normal, turning, falling	Hemiparesis or tetraparesis, ataxia	Deficits (ipsilateral or contralateral)	CN III-XII
Vestibular, central (cranial medulla)	Normal to depressed	Head tilt, falling (usually toward side of lesion)	Ipsilateral hemiparesis, vestibular ataxia	Deficits usually ipsilateral	CN VIII, may involve CN V and VII; nystagmus
Vestibular, peripheral	Normal	Head tilt, circling, falling, rolling	No paresis, severe vestibular ataxia	Normal	CN VIII, sometimes CN VII; Horner's syndrome, nystagmus
Cerebellum	Normal	Wide-based stance or normal unless paradoxical vestibular disease is present, decerebellate posture	No paresis; severe cerebellar ataxia, dysmetria, and resting and intention tremors	No paresis; dysmetria present	Usually normal. May see depressed menace response nystagmus, or vestibular signs

or to a peripheral nerve. For additional details on pain, see Chapter 14.

LOCALIZATION IN THE BRAIN

If the lesion has been localized to the brain, the next step is to determine what part of the brain is involved. Localization to one of five regions of the brain or to the peripheral vestibular apparatus (labyrinth) is made on the basis of clinical signs (Table 2-3).

BRAINSTEM

For our purposes, the functional brainstem includes the midbrain, pons, and medulla oblongata. Lesions of the brainstem produce UMN signs in all four limbs (tetraparesis) or in the

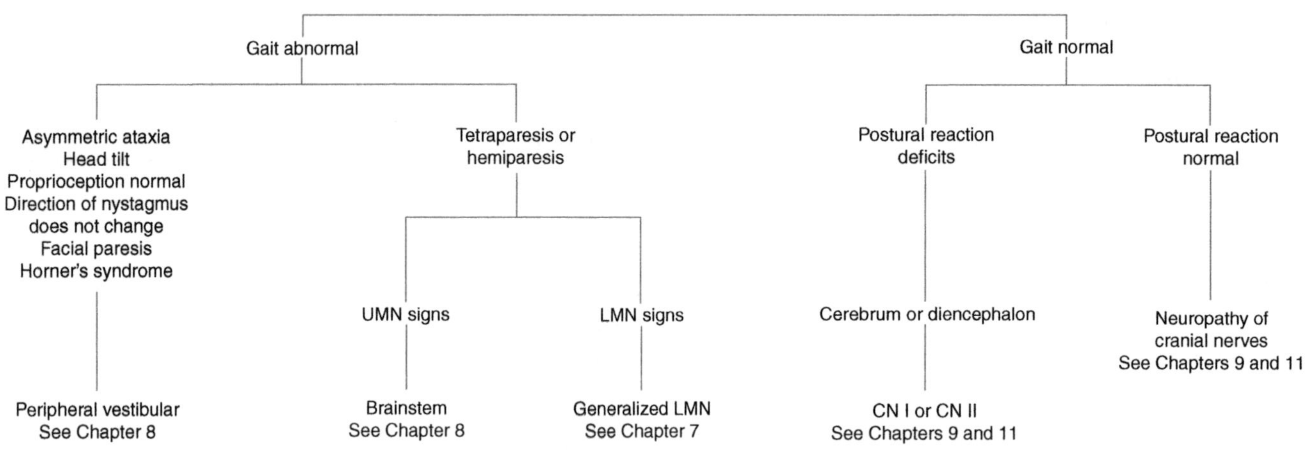

Figure 2-2 Localization of lesions causing cranial nerve signs.

thoracic and pelvic limbs on one side (hemiparesis). The paresis or paralysis produced by brainstem lesions is obvious both in the gait and in postural reactions. Cerebral or forebrain lesions affect postural reactions with minimal change in gait, although compulsive walking and circling may be seen. Brainstem or hindbrain lesions can cause abnormal posture resulting from vestibular involvement. Cranial nerve signs (CN III-XII) are present with larger or extensive brainstem lesions and provide important localizing signs (LMN or sensory) (Figure 2-2). The evaluation of cranial nerves is outlined in Table 2-4 (see Chapters 1, 9, 10, and 11).

Cranial nerve dysfunction with brainstem disease is ipsilateral to the lesion, whereas motor dysfunction may be ipsilateral or contralateral, depending on the level and the pathways involved. The animal's mental status may be altered, especially in lesions of the midbrain and the pons, which disrupt the ascending reticular activating system. Signs vary from dullness to coma (see Chapter 12).

Diencephalon

Diencephalic lesions (lesions of the thalamus or hypothalamus) may produce UMN signs in all four limbs (tetraparesis) or in the thoracic and pelvic limbs on one side (hemiparesis), depending on the symmetry of the lesion. The gait is not severely affected (similar to cerebral lesions), but postural reaction deficits may be present. The animal may circle in either direction depending upon lesion symmetry. CN II (optic) may be affected in diencephalic lesions with evidence of visual and pupillary light reflex abnormalities. Space-occupying lesions (e.g., tumors, abscesses) of the diencephalon also may affect CN III, IV, and VI depending on lesion extent (see Table 2-3). Cranial nerve signs are ipsilateral to the lesion, whereas postural reaction deficits can be ipsilateral or contralateral to the lesion. It is not uncommon for signs of diencephalic lesions to be vague and may include only mentation changes.

The most characteristic signs of diencephalic lesions are related to abnormal function of the hypothalamus and its connections with the pituitary gland. The hypothalamus is the control center for the autonomic nervous system and most of the endocrine system. If the hypothalamus is not affected, distinguishing diencephalic from cerebral lesions is difficult.

All sensory pathways of the body, with the exception of those serving olfaction, relay in the thalamus (diencephalon) en route to the cerebral cortex. Clinical signs of lesions in these systems in the diencephalon usually are not localizing. A rare generalized hyperesthesia has been described as a result of an abnormality in the relay nuclei of the pain pathways. Large lesions in the diencephalon may produce alterations in the level of consciousness (stupor, coma) because of interference with the ascending reticular activating system (see Chapter 12).

Vestibular System

Vestibular signs may be the result of central (brainstem) or peripheral (labyrinth) disease. Distinguishing central disease from peripheral disease is important because of the differences in treatment and prognosis. General signs of vestibular disease include falling, rolling, head tilting, circling, nystagmus, positional strabismus (deviation of one eye in certain positions of the head), and asymmetric ataxia (Figures 2-3 and 2-4). Vestibular ataxia is observed with other signs of vestibular dysfunction. Pathologic nystagmus (jerk nystagmus) seen with vestibular dysfunction can be spontaneous (at rest) or induced with change in head position. Jerk nystagmus consists of a slow phase that is followed by a fast phase. The direction of the fast phase of nystagmus is noted and recorded as rotary, horizontal, and vertical. A reliable technique to elicit a pathologic nystagmus is to decompensate the animal (if small) by rapidly flipping it on its back or in larger animals by rapidly elevating the head. Congenital nystagmus (pendular nystagmus) and strabismus occur in some breeds of exotic cats as a result of an anomaly in routing of the visual pathway from the retina to the contralateral visual cortex but cause no visual impairment.

Peripheral lesions involve the labyrinth within the petrosal bone. Middle-ear lesions (bulla ossea) may produce a head tilt with no other signs, presumably through pressure changes on the windows of the inner ear. Horizontal or rotatory nystagmus may be seen occasionally. Inner-ear disease, which actually involves the receptors and the vestibular nerve, usually produces one or more of the signs listed earlier in addition to the head tilt. In either case, the head tilt is ipsilateral to the lesion. Horner's syndrome (miosis, ptosis, enophthalmos) of the ipsilateral eye may be present with either middle- or inner-ear disease in the dog and cat because the sympathetic nerves pass through the middle ear in proximity to the petrosal bone. The facial nerve (CN VII) may be affected in inner-ear disease as it courses through the petrosal bone in contact with the vestibulocochlear nerve (CN VIII). The primary characteristics of peripheral vestibular disease are an asymmetric ataxia without deficits in postural reactions and a horizontal, or rotatory, nystagmus that usually maintains a constant direction with different head positions. The quick (jerk) phase of the nystagmus is away from the side of the lesion.

Any signs of brainstem disease in association with vestibular signs indicate that central involvement is present. The

TABLE 2-4

Cranial Nerves

Number and Name	Origin or Termination in Brain	Course	Function	Test	Normal Response	Abnormal Response	Occurrence
CN I olfactory	Pyriform cortex	Nasal mucosa, cribriform plate, olfactory bulbs, olfactory tract, olfactory stria, pyriform cortex	Sense of smell	Smelling of nonirritating volatile substances (food)	Behavioral reaction; aversion or interest	No reaction	Rare: nasal tumors and infections (evaluation difficult)
CN II optic	Lateral geniculate nucleus (vision), pretectal nucleus (pupillary reflex)	Retina, optic nerve, optic chiasma optic tract, lateral geniculate nucleus, optic radiation, visual cortex, optic tract, pretectal nucleus, parasympathetic nucleus of CN III, oculomotor nerve	Vision, pupillary light reflexes	Menace response, obstacle test and behavior, placing reaction, following movement, pupillary light reflex, ophthalmoscopy	Blinks, avoids obstacles and responds to visual cues, placing good, follows objects, pupillary light reflexes present, retina normal	No blink, poor avoidance of obstacles, no visual placing, direct pupillary light reflex absent, retina or optic disk may be abnormal	Optic neuritis, neoplasia, orbital trauma, orbital mass
CN III oculomotor	Midbrain, tegmentum (level of rostral colliculus)	Nucleus ventral to mesencephalic aqueduct, exits ventral to midbrain between cerebral peduncles, runs in cavernous and CN VI, exits orbital fissure	Constriction of pupil; ciliary muscle for accommodation reaction of lens; extraocular muscles: dorsal, ventral, and medical rectus and ventral oblique	Pupillary size, pupillary light reflex, eye position, eye movements, physiologic nystagmus	Pupils symmetric, pupils constrict to light, eyes centered in palpebral fissure, eyes move in all directions	Mydriasis, ipsilateral, no direct pupillary reflex, ventrolateral strabismus, no movement except laterally (CN VI)	Orbital lesions, tentorial herniation, midbrain lesion
CN IV trochlear	Midbrain, tegmentum (level of caudal colliculus)	Nucleus ventral to mesencephalic aqueduct, exits dorsal to tectum, caudal to caudal colliculus, contralateral to origin, courses along ridge of petrosal bone, follows course of CN III	Dorsal oblique muscle, rotates dorsal portion of eye medioventrally	Eye position, eye movements, physiologic nystagmus	Eye centered in palpebral fissure, eyes move in all directions	Normal; rotation may be detected in animal with elliptical pupil or by position of vessels	Rare, difficult to evaluate; reported in polioencephalomalacia of cattle, but eyes move
CN V trigeminal ophthalmic, maxillary, and mandibular nerves	Motor nucleus: Pons Sensory nucleus: Pons, medulla, C1 spinal cord segment	Motor: Pons, exits at cerebellopontine angle, trigeminal canal of petrosal bone, oval foramen, mandibular nerve Sensory: Same except trigeminal ganglion in trigeminal canal; ophthalmic, maxillary, and mandibular nerves	Motor: Muscles of mastication Sensory: Face rostral to ears	Motor: Ability To close mouth, jaw tone Sensory: Palpebral reflex, pinch face, touch nasal mucosa	Closed mouth, good jaw tone; no atrophy of temporal or masseter muscles; palpebral reflex present; behavioral response to noxious stimulus	Jaw hangs open (bilateral), poor jaw tone, atrophy, loss of palpebral reflex or behavioral response to noxious stimulus (check all three branches)	Idiopathic mandibular paralysis, trigeminal neuritis, cerebellopontine angle tumors,nerve sheath tumors, rabies, trauma

Continued

TABLE 2-4
Cranial Nerves—cont'd

Number and Name	Origin or Termination in Brain	Course	Function	Test	Normal Response	Abnormal Response	Occurrence
CN VI abducent	Medulla (rostral and dorsal)	Medulla, lateral to pyramid, exits orbital fissure	Lateral rectus and retractor bulbi muscles, lateral movement of eye, retraction of globe	Eye position, eye movements	Eye moves laterally and retracts corneal reflex	Medial strabismus, lack of lateral eye movements or retraction of globe	Orbital trauma, orbital mass, brainstem disease
CN VII facial	Medulla (rostral and ventrolateral)	Motor: Axons leave nucleus, loop around abducent nucleus, and exit ventrolateral medulla ventral to CN VIII to internal acoustic meatus, facial canal in petrosal bone, and stylomastoid foramen to muscles of facial expression Taste: Solitary tract and nucleus, medulla follows course of trigeminal nerve Sensory: Geniculate ganglion and branches from vagus nerve	Muscles of facial expression and taste, rostral two thirds of tongue, and cutaneous sensation of inner surface of pinna	Facial symmetry, palpebral reflex, ear movements Taste: Atropine applied to rostral two thirds of tongue with cotton swabs Sensory: Touch inner surface of pinna	Face symmetric; normal movements of lips, ears, eyelids; palpebral reflex present; ears move in response to stimulation Taste: Aversive reaction immediately Sensory: Behavioral and ear twitch response	Asymmetry of face, ptosis, lip drops, deviation of nasal philtrum, palpebral reflex absent (check CN V), ears do not move Taste: No reaction until mouth is closed and material reaches caudal portion of tongue Sensory: No behavioral or ear twitch response	Idiopathic facial paralysis, polyneuropathies, inner ear infections, brainstem lesions
CN VIII vestibulocochlear	Vestibular nuclei medulla; cochlear nuclei medulla; cerebellomedullary angle, medulla	Inner ear, petrosal bone, internal acoustic meatus to medulla (nestibular nuclei)	Equilibrium, hearing	Vestibular: Posture and gait, eye movements, rotatory and caloric tests Hearing: Startle reaction, electrophysiology (EEG alerting, brainstem-evoked response)	Vestibular: Normal posture and gait, oculocephalic reflex, normal, brief postrotatory nystagmus and caloric-induced nystagmus Hearing: Startled reaction to handclap, evoked response present	Vestibular: Head tilt, head twist, circling, nystagmus, prolonged or absent postrotatory nystagmus, abnormal or absent caloric response Hearing: Poor startle reaction, no evoked response	Otitis media and otitis interna, idiopathic vestibular disease, polyneuropathy, brainstem disease

CN IX glossopharyngeal	Medulla (caudal)	Sensory: Solitary tract and nucleus Motor: Parasympathetic, ambiguus nucleus, exit together along lateral surface of medulla, exit through jugular foramen	Sensory and motor to pharynx and palate, parasympathetic to zygomatic and parotid salivary glands (in CN V); sensory to carotid body and sinus	Gag reflex	Swallowing	Poor gag reflex, dysphagia	Rare; common in rabies; brainstem disease
CN X vagus	Medulla (caudal)	Same as CN IX	Sensory and motor to pharynx and larynx, thoracic and abdominal viscera	Gag reflex, laryngeal reflex, slap test, oculocardiac reflex	Swallowing, coughing, bradycardia	Poor gag reflex, dysphagia, inspiratory dyspnea, no abduction of laryngeal folds, regurgitation	Rare, except in laryngeal paralysis; polyneuropathy
CN XI accessory	Medulla (caudal) and cervical spinal cord	Ambiguus nucleus of medulla and cervical gray matter, axons run rostrally from cervical cord to join cranial roots, exit jugular foramen	Trapezius and parts of sternocephalicus and brachiocephalicus muscles	Palpate for atrophy of muscles; EMG	Normal muscles	Atrophied muscles, denervation	Rare
CN XII hypoglossal	Medulla (caudal)	Axons exit medulla lateral to pyramid, hypoglossal canal to tongue	Movements of tongue	Protrusion of tongue (wet nose), retraction of tongue	Tongue protrudes symmetrically and can lick in both directions, strong withdrawal of tongue	Tongue deviates to side of lesion, atrophy, weak withdrawal	Brainstem disease, polyneuropathy

CN, Cranial nerve; *EEG,* electroencephalography; *EMG,* electromyography.

most important differentiating feature is a deficit in postural reactions. Peripheral vestibular disease does not cause paresis or loss of proprioception, whereas central disease frequently does (due to involvement of sensory and motor long tracts in the brainstem). Postural reactions must be evaluated critically because an animal with peripheral vestibular disease has deficits in equilibrium, which make the performance of tests such as hopping awkward. An evaluation of proprioceptive positioning is an excellent method for discrimination. Alterations in mental status or deficits in CN V and CN VII also are indicative of central vestibular disease (see Figure 2-3); however, some polyneuropathies may affect the cranial nerves, including CN V, VII, and VIII.

Lesions near the caudal cerebellar peduncle may produce what has been called a paradoxical vestibular syndrome. The signs are usually similar to those of central vestibular disease except that the direction of the head tilt is contralateral to the side of the lesion.[6] Additional signs of cerebellar disease, such as dysmetria and ataxia, may be seen.

Bilateral vestibular disease, which can be peripheral or central, produces a more symmetric ataxia. The animal walks with the limbs flexed and spread apart to maintain balance. The head often sways with wide excursions from side to side. No nystagmus is present, and vestibular eye movements are usually absent.[7]

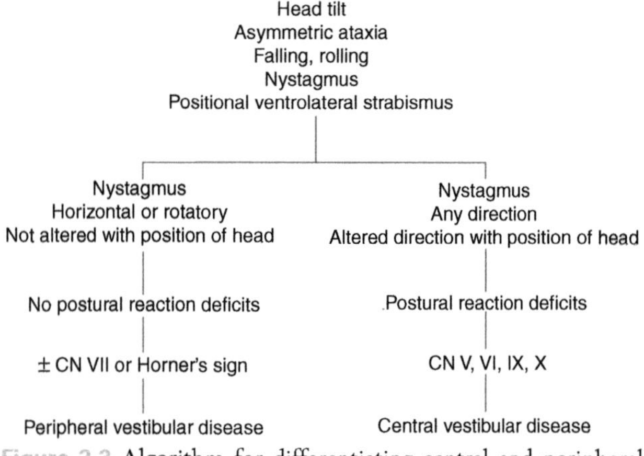

Figure 2-3 Algorithm for differentiating central and peripheral vestibular diseases.

Cerebellum

The cerebellum coordinates movements. It controls the rate and range of movements without actually initiating motor activity. Cerebellar lesions may be unilateral or bilateral, depending on cause. Characteristic signs include spastic ataxia, wide-based stance, dysmetria, intention tremor, and no obvious signs of weakness. Cerebellar ataxia is often characterized by dysmetria, which denotes stride lengths that are too short (hypometria) or too long (hypermetria). Head movement abnormalities differentiates cerebellar lesions from spinocerebellar tract lesions, which may produce similar signs in the limbs. For example, head dysmetria usually is recognized as a severe head drop when the head is elevated and suddenly released. Intention tremors are uncoordinated movements that become much worse as the animal initiates an activity, such as eating or drinking (see Figure 2-4).[8] The animal may stick its nose too far into its water dish when drinking or may even hit the edge of the dish.

Nystagmus may occur in cerebellar disease but is usually more of a tremor of the globe than the slow-quick (jerk) movements associated with vestibular disease. Cerebellar nystagmus is most pronounced as the animal shifts its gaze and fixates on a new field (an intention tremor). A down-beat vertical nystagmus may be seen upon dorsal extension of the head.

Acute injury to the cerebellum can cause a decerebellate posture, typically extensor hypertonus in the thoracic limbs, flexion in the pelvic limbs, and opisthotonos.[6] Isolated cerebellar trauma is unusual because of the protected location of the cerebellum. These signs are most pronounced when combined with brainstem lesions at the level of the midbrain or the pons.

Lesions of the flocculonodular lobes of the cerebellum produce signs similar to those of vestibular disease, including loss of equilibrium, nystagmus, and tendency to fall (see Chapter 8).

Diffuse cerebellar lesions may cause the menace response to be absent with vision remaining normal.

Cerebrum

Cerebral lesions (including the cerebral hemispheres and basal nuclei) usually cause alterations in behavior or mental status, seizures, loss of vision with intact pupillary light reflex, contralateral decrease in facial sensation, and mild contralateral hemiparesis and deficits in postural reactions.[9] Only one or two of these signs may be present because the cerebrum is a relatively large structure with well-localized functional areas. Signs are generally contralateral to the lesion.

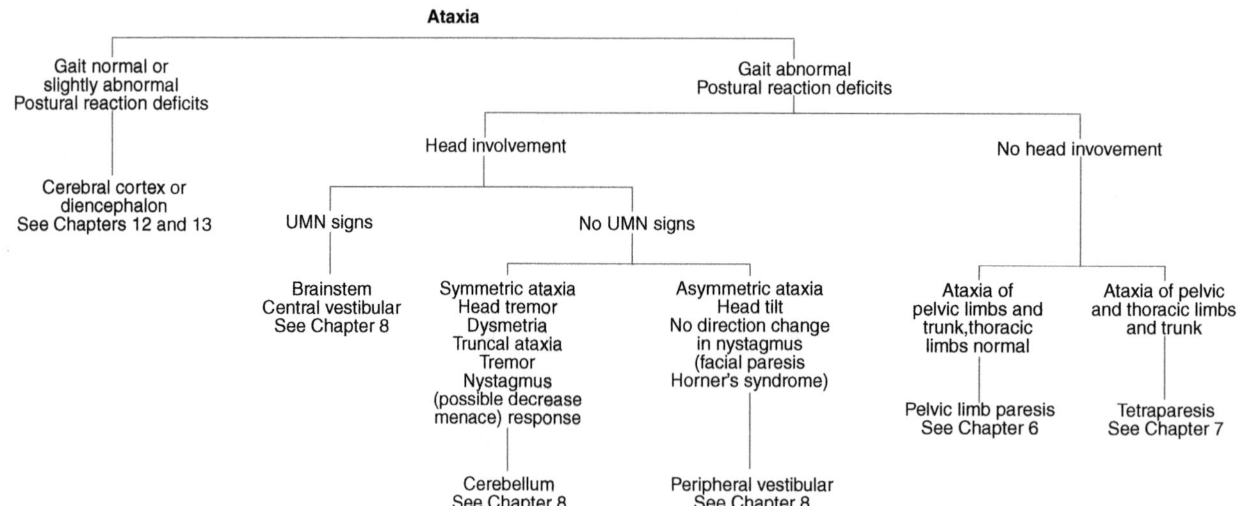

Figure 2-4 Algorithm for the diagnosis of ataxia based on gait, head involvement, and motor function of the limbs.

Behavioral changes usually reflect a lesion of the limbic system or the frontal or temporal lobes of the cortex. Frontal-lobe lesions often cause a disinhibition that results in excessive pacing. Compulsive pacing may continue until the animal walks into a corner and stands with its head pressed against the obstruction. If the lesion is unilateral or asymmetric, the animal may circle. Circling in an animal with a cerebral lesion is usually to the same side as the lesion. The animal's movement tends to be in large circles. The gait is reasonably normal, although obstacles may not be perceived. Circling is not a localizing sign because it can be caused by lesions in the forebrain, brainstem, and vestibular system.

Dullness, stupor, and coma represent decreasing levels of consciousness caused by a separation of the cerebral cortex from the ascending reticular activating system of the brainstem. Mentation abnormalities are usually more severe with brainstem lesions and diffuse cerebrocortical disease (see Chapter 12). Conscious visual perception requires intact visual pathways to the occipital lobes of the cerebral cortex. Occipital cortical lesions cause blindness with intact pupillary reflexes (see Chapter 11).

The sensorimotor cortex is important for voluntary motor activity but is not necessary for relatively normal gait and posture. Animals with lesions in this area can stand, walk, and run with minimal deficits. The animal's ability for fine discrimination is lost, however, and it is unable to avoid obstacles smoothly or to perform fine maneuvers, such as walking on the steps of a ladder. Markedly abnormal postural reactions are found.

Localization to one of the five regions of the brain is usually adequate for a clinical diagnosis. Cranial nerve signs provide positive evidence for precise localization within the brainstem. Clinical signs referable to several parts of the nervous system indicate diffuse or multifocal disease, such as infection, metabolic disorder, or malignant neoplasia (see Chapter 15).

CASE STUDIES

The following case studies use the information presented in chapters 1 and 2. The reader is encouraged to review the case, localize the lesion(s), and develop a diagnostic plan. Case summaries are listed at the end of the case studies section.

Key: *0*, Absent; *+1*, decreased; *+2*, normal; *+3*, exaggerated; *+4*, very exaggerated or clonus: *PL*, pelvic limb; *TL*, thoracic limb; *NE*, not evaluated.

CASE STUDY 2-1 *TURBO*

veterinaryneurologycases.com

▪ Signalment

German shepherd dog, male, 8 years old

▪ History

CC: seizures and paraparesis

Cluster seizures for 1 year. Treated with phenobarbital and potassium bromide. One month ago had a seizure and developed paraparesis immediately on recovery. Paraparesis was progressive and somewhat responsive to corticosteroid therapy.

▪ Physical Examination

Normal except for neurologic signs

▪ Neurologic Examination

Mental status: alert and responsive
Posture: normal
Gait: marked paraparesis with ataxia; occasionally crosses front feet
Palpation: negative; no perispinal pain noted

Postural reactions

Left	Reactions	Right
	Proprio (positioning) ceptive	
+1	PL	+1
+2	TL	+2
+2	Wheelbarrowing	+2
	Hopping	
+1	PL	+2
+2	TL	+2−+2
	Extensor postural	
NE	thrust	NE
NE	Hemistand-hemiwalk	NE
+1−+2	Tonic neck	+1−+2
	Placing, tactile	
NE	PL	NE
NE	TL	NE
	Placing, visual	
NE	PL	NE
NE	TL	NE

Spinal reflexes

Left	Reflex, Spinal Segment	Right
	Quadriceps	
+3	L4-6	+2−+3
	Extensor carpi radialis	
+2	C7-T1	+2
	Triceps	
+2	C7-T1	+2
	Flexion–PL	
+2	L5-S1	+2
	Flexion–TL	
+2	C6-T1	+2
Absent	Crossed extensor	Absent
	Perineal	
+2	S1-2	+2

Cranial nerves: normal

Sensory evaluation

1. Hyperesthesia: none
2. Superficial pain perception: normal
3. Deep pain perception: NE

Complete the sections below before reviewing the case summary.

Assessment (lesion localization and estimation of prognosis)

Diagnostic plan

▪ Rule-outs

1.
2.
3.
4.

CASE STUDY 2-2 BIRK

veterinaryneurologycases.com

▪ Signalment
Weimaraner, male castrated, 6 years old

▪ History
CC: Lameness—left pelvic limb; circles to right, leans to right, and has right head tilt
Referring veterinarian had diagnosed severe degenerative joint disease of the left coxofemoral joint. The dog seemed to respond to corticosteroids and nonsteroidal antiinflammatory drugs. The head tilt and circling have been present for several weeks and are slowly getting worse. Dog has been referred for total hip replacement surgery.

▪ Physical Examination
Pain and crepitus in right coxofemoral joint

▪ Neurologic Examination
Mental status: Alert and responsive
Posture: Right head tilt
Gait: Circles and falls to the right; no obvious paresis at gait
Palpation: Pain and crepitus in right coxofemoral joint

Postural reactions

Left	Reactions	Right
	Proprioceptive positioning	
+2	PL	+2
+2	TL	+2
+2	Wheelbarrowing	+2
	Hopping	
+2	PL	+1
+2	TL	+1−+2
	Extensor postural	
NE	thrust	NE
+2	Hemistand-hemiwalk	+1−+2
+2	Tonic neck	+2
	Placing, tactile	
NE	PL	NE
NE	TL	NE
	Placing, visual	
NE	PL	NE
NE	TL	NE

Spinal reflexes

Left	Reflex, Spinal Segment	Right
	Quadriceps	
+2	L4-6	+2−+3
	Extensor carpi radialis	
+2	C7-T1	+2
	Triceps	
+2	C7-T1	+2
	Flexion-PL	
+2	L5-S1	+2
	Flexion-TL	
+2	C6-T1	+2
Absent	Crossed extensor Perineal	Absent
+2	S1-2	+2

Cranial nerves: normal

Sensory evaluation

1. Hyperesthesia: none
2. Superficial pain perception: normal
3. Deep pain perception: NE

Complete the sections below before reviewing the case summary.

Assessment (lesion localization and estimation of prognosis)

Diagnostic plan

▪ Rule-outs
1.
2.
3.
4.

CASE STUDY 2-3 DOSSIE BOY

veterinaryneurologycases.com

▪ Signalment
Mixed breed canine, male, 5-6 years old,

▪ History
CC: comatose condition
Obtained as stray 1 year ago Rabies vaccination unknown. One month ago, coughing and microfilaria were found on blood smear. Referring veterinarian gave 0.5 mL levamisole SC. That evening, dog was acutely recumbent and may have had a seizure. Since then, dog has been in comatose state. Dog has been given atropine, antibiotics, and fluids prior to admission.

▪ Physical Examination
See neurologic examination (performed about 3 days post onset of signs)

▪ Neurologic Examination*
Mental status: Comatose and cannot be aroused
Posture: At times demonstrates opisthotonos and extension of the thoracic limbs
Gait: Severe tetraplegia, limbs are hypotonic
Palpation: Negative

Continued

CASE STUDY 2-3 DOSSIE BOY—cont'd

Postural reactions

Left	Reactions	Right
	Proprioceptive positioning	
0	PL	0
0	TL	0
0	Wheelbarrowing	0
	Hopping	
0	PL	0
0	TL	0
0	Extensor postural thrust	0
0	Hemistand-hemiwalk	0
NE	Tonic neck	NE
	Placing, tactile	
NE	PL	NE
NE	TL	NE
	Placing, visual	
NE	PL	NE
NE	TL	NE

Spinal reflexes

Left	Reflex, Spinal Segment	Right
+2–+3	Quadriceps L4-6	+2–+3
NE	Extensor carpi radialis C7-T1	NE
NE	Triceps C7-T1	NE
+2	Flexion-PL L5-S1	+2
+2	Flexion-TL C6-T1	+2
Present	Perineal crossed extensor	Present
+2	S1-2	+2

*Dog is comatose and cannot be roused. Severe tetraplegia. Limbs are hypotonic. Sometimes demonstrates decerebrate posture. Patellar reflexes are +2-+3. Bilateral miosis with response to light, 0 menace, horizontal nystagmus that changes direction. Response to noxious stimuli is reduced.

Cranial nerves

1. No menace response in either eye
2. Horizontal jerk nystagmus that changes direction depending on which side dog is lying (lying on right side, jerk phase is to the right; lying on left side, jerk phase is to the left)
3. Normal (+2) palpebral reflexes (CN V and VII)
4. Decreased facial sensation (CN V)
5. Bilateral miosis with pupillary constriction to strong light

Sensory evaluation

1. Hyperesthesia: none
2. Superficial pain perception: Difficult to assess; marked decrease response to noxious stimuli
3. Deep pain perception: present but hard to elicit cerebral response

Complete the sections below before reviewing the case summary.

Assessment (anatomic diagnosis and estimation of prognosis)

Diagnostic plan

■ **Rule-outs**

1.
2.
3.
4.

CASE STUDY 2-4 BRANDY

 veterinaryneurologycases.com

■ **Signalment**

Malamute-shepherd cross, female spayed approximately 7-8 years old

■ **History**

Since a puppy, dog has been clumsy. The signs are not progressive. Dog has been treated by several veterinarians for coxofemoral degenerative joint disease. Owner wants to know what is causing the gait problem in her dog. Local veterinarian sends owner-provided video tape for consultation.

■ **Physical Examination**

See neurologic examination

■ **Neurologic Examination**

1. Mental status: normal
2. Posture: base wide; no head tilt or circling
3. Gait: generalized ataxia, truncal ataxia, intention tremors, hypermetria, no paresis
4. Palpation: NE

Postural reactions: not provided

Spinal reflexes: not provided

Cranial nerves: NE

Sensory evaluation: NE

Complete the sections below before reviewing the case summary.

Assessment (anatomic diagnosis and estimation of prognosis)

Diagnostic plan

■ **Rule-outs**

1.
2.
3.
4.

CASE STUDY 2-5 *RUDY*

veterinaryneurologycases.com

▪ Signalment

Canine, Labrador retriever, male castrated, 2 years old

▪ History

Acute onset of clinical signs. Became base wide in pelvic limbs and falling when walking. Taken to RDVM that morning and four injections of dexamethasone SP were administered. Spinal, radiographs were taken but no lesions found. There has been no change in neurologic status over the past 3 days. Dog is not painful and the bladder is easily expressed. Dog has difficulty moving his tail.

▪ Physical Examination

No systemic signs noted

▪ Neurologic Examination

Mental status: alert and responsive
Posture: normal; see gait
Gait: paraparesis with signs more severe in the right pelvic limb. Dog dribbles urine and does not move his tail.
4. *Palpation:* normal

Postural reactions

Left	Reactions	Right
	Proprioceptive positioning	
+2	PL	0
+2	TL	+2
	Wheelbarrowing	
	Hopping	
+1	PL	0
+2	TL	+2
	Extensor postural	
NE	thrust	NE
	Hemistand-hemiwalk	
NE	Tonic neck	NE
	Placing, tactile	
NE	PL	NE
NE	TL	NE
	Placing, visual	
NE	PL	NE
NE	TL	NE

Spinal reflexes

Left	Reflex, Spinal Segment	Right
	Quadriceps	
+2	L4-6	0
	Extensor carpi radialis	
+2	C7-T1	+2
	Triceps	
+2	C7-T1	+2
	Flexion-PL	
+2	L5-S1	0
	Flexion-TL	
+2	C6-T1	+2
	Crossed extensor	
0	Perineal	0
+1	S1-2	0

Cranial nerves: normal
Sensory evaluation

1. Hyperesthesia: none
2. Superficial pain perception: normal from all areas except for localized area of hypalgesia in caudal lumbar area on the right side
3. Deep pain perception: normal

Complete the sections below before reviewing the case summary.

Assessment (anatomic diagnosis and estimation of prognosis)
Diagnostic plan

▪ Rule-outs

1.
2.
3.
4.

CASE STUDY 2-6 *DUSTY*

veterinaryneurologycases.com

▪ Signalment

Whippet, female, 8 years old.

▪ History

3 months ago, acute onset of paraplegia. Dog was running and went around a farm building. Dog cried out and when owner found Dusty, she was paralyzed in her pelvic limbs and in considerable pain. She was seen by local veterinarian who provided symptomatic therapy. Signs are not progressive and dog is not in pain. Dusty can urinate and defecate but has no cerebral control over either. Owner is seeking second opinion and prognosis.

▪ Physical Examination

No systemic signs noted

▪ Neurologic Examination

Mental status: normal
Posture: normal
Gait: paraplegia
Palpation: generalized atrophy of lumbar and pelvic limb muscles

CASE STUDY 2-6 DUSTY—cont'd

Postural reactions

Left	Reactions	Right
	Proprioceptive positioning	
0	PL	0
+2	TL	+2
	Wheelbarrowing	
	Hopping	NE
0	PL	0
+2	TL	+2
0	Extensor postural thrust	0
NE	Hemistand-hemiwalk	NE
NE	Tonic neck	NE
	Placing, tactile	
NE	PL	NE
NE	TL	NE
	Placing, visual	
NE	PL	NE
NE	TL	NE

Spinal reflexes

Left	Reflex, Spinal Segment	Right
	Quadriceps	
+4	L4-6	+4
	Extensor carpi radialis	
+2	C7-T1	+2
	Triceps	
+2	C7-T1	+2
	Flexion-PL	
	Quadriceps	
+2	L5-S1	+2
	Flexion-TL	
+2	C6-T1	+2
Brisk	Crossed extensor (PL)	Brisk
	Perineal	
+2	S1-2	+2

Cranial nerves: normal

Sensory evaluation

1. Hyperesthesia: none
2. Superficial pain perception: poor caudal to T_{13}; the cutaneous trunci reflex is absent behind caudal to T_{13} vertebrae
3. Deep pain perception: good

Complete the sections below before reviewing the case summary.

Assessment (anatomic diagnosis and estimation of prognosis)

Diagnostic plan

▪ Rule-outs

1.
2.
3.
4.

CASE STUDY 2-7 ANGEL

veterinaryneurologycases.com

▪ Signalment

Feline, DSH, FS, 1 year old

▪ History

Cat was left in garage for 3 days while owners were out of town. When owners returned home, they noted ataxia, left head tilt, and salivation. Another cat at home is fine.

▪ Physical Examination

T 103° F, dehydrated 8% and tense abdomen on palpation

▪ Neurologic Examination

Observation

Mental status: alert; constantly vocalizes

Posture: Left head tilt and circles to the left; crouched posture and very reluctant to walk. Tends to swing head in wide excursions from side to side. Occasionally circles to the right.

Gait: asymmetric ataxia; no paresis detected

Palpation: normal

Postural reactions

Left	Reactions	Right
	Proprioceptive positioning	
+2	PL	+2
+2	TL	+2
+2	Wheelbarrowing	+2
	Hopping	
+2	PL	+2
+2	TL	+2
+2	Extensor postural thrust	+2
NE	Hemistand-hemiwalk	NE
NE	Tonic neck	NE
	Placing, tactile	
NE	PL	NE
NE	TL	NE
	Placing, visual	
NE	PL	NE
NE	TL	NE

Spinal reflexes: not examined

Cranial nerves

1. Menace: decreased in right eye; normal in left eye
2. Left pupil is constricted; slight protrusion of left membrana nictitans
3. Normal pupillary light reflexes
4. Normal palpebral reflexes
5. No spontaneous nystagmus
6. Normal facial sensation

Continued

CASE STUDY 2-7 ANGEL—cont'd

Sensory evaluation
1. Hyperesthesia: none
2. Superficial pain perception: normal
3. Deep pain perception: normal

Complete the sections below before reviewing the case summary.

Assessment (anatomic diagnosis and estimation of prognosis)
Diagnostic plan

▪ Rule-outs
1.
2.
3.
4.

CASE STUDY 2-8 CHLOE

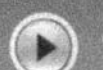 veterinaryneurologycases.com

▪ Signalment
Golden retriever, female, 20 months old

▪ History
Dog presented with severe tetraparesis. Clinical signs developed at 10:00 AM on July 10. Dog became weak in all four legs and over a period of a few hours, she lost the ability to stand and walk. She has been in excellent health and Chloe is primarily an indoor dog that lives in a rural area and spends time outdoors unsupervised. She was eating fine until 2 days ago. Dog gags, coughs, and retches when eating and drinking. Several small "seed" ticks have been noted on the dog. She was in estrus 6 months ago. No treatment has been given. Dog was observed eating a dead rabbit about 2 days before onset of clinical signs. Another dog with her has developed similar but less severe clinical signs.

▪ Physical Examination Findings

Vital signs:	T: 101.5° F Pulse: 116 RR: 32 Wt: 28.4 kg.
General appearance	Dog is recumbent and unable to stand. She is very depressed.
Integument	Several small ticks are present. No engorged ticks are found.
Musculoskeletal	Mild muscle atrophy present in limbs. No hyperesthesia is noted.
Circulatory	No abnormalities noted.
Respiratory	Rapid shallow respiration noted.
Digestive	Abdomen is distended, nonpainful, and firm feces are present on rectal palpation.
Genitourinary	Bladder is distended with urine and easily expressed
Eyes	Left pupil is normal to dilated. Right pupil is small and third eyelid is prolapsed.
Ears	Normal
Nervous	See neurologic examination
Lymph nodes	Normal
Mucous membranes	Normal

▪ Neurologic Examination
Mental status: The dog is alert and responsive to her name. She has very shallow respirations.
Posture: No head tilt is noted. Dog is recumbent.
Gait: Dog is tetraplegic. She can wag her tail voluntarily and she can lift her head. Voluntary motor movements in the limbs are weak.
Palpation: Muscle tone is reduced in all limbs.

Postural reactions

Left	Reactions	Right
	Proprioceptive positioning	
0	PL	0
0	TL	0
	Wheelbarrowing	
	Hopping	
0	PL	0
0	TL	0
0	Extensor postural thrust	0
NE	Hemistand-hemiwalk	NE
NE	Tonic neck	NE
	Placing, tactile	
NE	PL	NE
NE	TL	NE
	Placing, visual	
NE	PL	NE
NE	TL	NE

Spinal reflexes

Left	Reflex, Spinal Segment	Right
	Quadriceps	
0–+1/2	L4-6	0
	Extensor carpi radialis	
0	C7-T1	0
	Triceps	
0	C7-T1	0
	Flexion-PL	
+1/2	L5-S1	+1/2
	Flexion-TL	
+1/2	C6-T1	+1/2
None	Crossed extensor	None
	Perineal	
+2	S1-2	+2

Cranial nerves
1. Menace: slightly delayed in left eye and normal in right eye.
2. Pupils: Left pupil is dilated compared to right.

Continued

CASE STUDY 2-8 CHLOE—cont'd

3. Pupillary light reflexes: decreased in left eye but normal in right eye.
4. Palpebral: normal
5. Facial sensation: normal
6. Gag reflex: decreased
7. Voice: decreased

Sensation: location
1. Hyperesthesia: none
2. Superficial pain perception: +2
3. Deep pain perception: +2

Complete the sections below before reviewing the case summary.

Assessment (anatomic diagnosis and estimation of prognosis)
Diagnostic plan

▪ Rule-outs
1.
2.
3.
4.

CASE STUDY 2-9 DUFFY

veterinaryneurologycases.com

▪ Signalment

DSH cat, spayed female, 7 years old

▪ History

Owner found cat dragging its right pelvic limbs. Cat is inside and owner denies any possibility of trauma. Signs are not progressive and cat is normal in all respects.

▪ Physical Examination

Nothing abnormal except monoparesis

▪ Neurologic Examination

Mental status: alert and responsive
Posture: normal
Gait: paralysis of right pelvic limb
Palpation: painful in right caudal thigh

Postural reactions

Left	Reactions	Right
	Proprioceptive positioning	
+2	PL	0
+2	TL	+2
	Wheelbarrowing	
	Hopping	
+2	PL	0
+2	TL	+2
+2	Extensor postural thrust	0
NE	Hemistand-hemiwalk	NE
NE	Tonic neck	NE
	Placing, tactile	
NE	PL	NE
NE	TL	NE
	Placing, visual	
NE	PL	NE
NE	TL	NE

Spinal reflexes

Left	Reflex, Spinal Segment	Right
	Quadriceps	
+2	L4-6	+2
	Extensor carpi radialis	
NE	C7-T1	NE
	Triceps	
NE	C7-T1	NE
	Flexion-PL	
+2	L5-S1	0
	Flexion-TL	
+2	C6-T1	+2
Absent	Crossed extensor	Absent
	Perineal	
+2	S1-2	+2

Cranial nerves: normal
Sensory evaluation
1. Hyperesthesia: very painful in caudal thigh region
2. Superficial and deep pain perception: cat does not perceive noxious stimuli from the right pelvic paw (tibial and peroneal nerves). Deep pain is perceived in the distribution of the superficial saphenous nerve. Normal perception of noxious stimuli from the tail and others of the body.

Complete the sections below before reviewing the case summary.

Assessment (anatomic diagnosis and estimation of prognosis)
Diagnostic plan

▪ Rule-outs
1.
2.
3.
4.

CASE STUDY 2-10 *BRITTANY*

veterinaryneurologycases.com

▪ Signalment
Brittany spaniel dog, female spayed, 2 years old

▪ History
Presented a few hours after being injured by an automobile. At the time of admission, the dog was non ambulatory in the pelvic limbs. Depression, bilateral epistaxis, and conjunctival hemorrhage in the right eye were noted. One hour after admission, the dog was noted to fall on the right thoracic and pelvic limbs and tended to circle to the left. Thoracic and abdominal radiographs were negative.

▪ Physical Examination: see neurologic examination

▪ Neurologic Examination
Examination performed the following morning and after dog was stable and improving.
Mental status: Dog is alert and responsive. She explores her environment.
Posture: No head tilt is present.
Gait: Dog tends to aimlessly walk in wide circles to the left and sometimes to the right. No paresis or knuckling of the paws are noted.
Palpation: normal

Postural reactions

Left	Reactions	Right
	Proprioceptive positioning	
+2	PL	+1
+2	TL	+1
+2	Wheelbarrowing	+1
	Hopping	
+2	PL	+1
+2	TL	+1
+2	Extensor postural thrust	+1
+2	Hemistand-hemiwalk	+1
NE	Tonic neck	NE
	Placing, tactile	
NE	PL	NE
NE	TL	NE
	Placing, visual	
NE	PL	NE
NE	TL	NE

Spinal reflexes

Left	Reflex, Spinal Segment	Right
	Quadriceps	
+2	L4-6	+2–+3
	Extensor carpi radialis	
+2	C7-T1	+2
	Triceps	
+2	C7-T1	+2
	Flexion-PL	
+2	L5-S1	+2
	Flexion-TL	
+2	C6-T1	+2
Absent	Crossed extensor	Absent
	Perineal	
+2	S1-2	+2

Cranial nerves
1. Decreased menace response in right eye but normal palpebral reflex is present
2. Decreased perception of noxious stimuli to right side of face
3. PLRs are normal and pupils are normal size and equal

Sensory evaluation
1. Hyperesthesia: none
2. Superficial pain perception: decreased right side of face
3. Deep pain perception: normal

Complete the sections below before reviewing the case summary.

Assessment (anatomic diagnosis and estimation of prognosis)
Diagnostic plan

▪ Rule-outs
1.
2.
3.
4.

CASE STUDY 2-11 *LINUS*

veterinaryneurologycases.com

▪ Signalment
Golden retriever, male, 9 years old

▪ History
Owner reports progressive difficulty eating and drinking for several weeks. Dog has trouble closing its mouth and is becoming more depressed and lethargic. There is recent weight loss and partial anorexia. Owner reports no gait abnormalities.

▪ Physical Examination: see neurologic examination

▪ Neurologic Examination
Mental status: subdued
Posture: normal
Gait: normal
Palpation: atrophy of left temporalis muscle

CASE STUDY 2-11 *LINUS—cont'd*

Postural reactions: normal

Spinal reflexes: normal

Cranial nerves

1. Olfaction is decreased on right side compared to the left side
2. Difficulty closing mouth; atrophy of left temporalis muscle
3. Palpebral reflex: absent right eye; normal left eye
4. Menace response: normal left eye; right eye: no blink but dog moves head to avoid hand
5. Facial sensation: decreased on the right side and mandible but present on left side

Sensation: location

1. Hyperesthesia: none
2. Superficial pain perception: decreased right facial area
3. Deep pain perception: NE

Complete the sections below before reviewing the case summary.

Assessment (anatomic diagnosis and estimation of prognosis)
Diagnostic plan

▪ Rule-outs

1.
2.
3.
4.

CASE SUMMARIES

CASE STUDY 2-1 *ASSESSMENT*

▪ Lesion Localization (anatomic diagnosis and estimation of prognosis)

1. The neurologic examination is consistent with a bilateral lesion T3-L3. One cannot exclude a caudal cervical lesion.
2. The seizures are most likely due to a forebrain lesion.

▪ Diagnostic plan

The history supports a progressive myelopathy. Given the history, categories of disease to consider are degenerative, neoplastic, inflammatory/infectious.

Rule-outs

Spinal cord disease (see Chapters 6 and 7)

1. Henson type 2 intervertebral disk disease—Cervical and TL radiographs, myelography, and CT
2. Neoplasia—See type 2 disk disease
3. Degenerative myelopathy—rule out compressive myelopathy
4. Inflammation—CSF

▪ Rule-outs

Seizures (see Chapter 13): Given the dog's age, acquired (secondary) epilepsy is most likely. While there are several causes in this category, neoplasia would be a prime rule-out.

1. Extracranial (metabolic) causes—Complete small animal profile (see Chapter 4)
2. Intracranial causes—Advanced imaging (MR, CT) should be performed (see Chapter 4)

▪ Case Summary

Myelogram and CT—large disk protrusion at C6-7. Compression persists with cervical distraction. Mild compression at C5-6 but disappears with distraction. CT of brain reveals large mass in left frontal lobe displacing frontal bone of sinus. Owner elected cervical decompressive surgery (ventral slot) for the Henson type 2 invertebral disk disease and continued to manage the seizures medically. The paraparesis improved but the seizures became increasingly difficult to control.

CASE STUDY 2-2 ASSESSMENT

▪ Assessment (lesion localization and estimation of prognosis)

Dog is presented with clinical signs of a vestibular syndrome (circling, falling, head tilt). The decreased hopping reactions on the right side are consistent with "central vestibular disease." The lesion most likely is located in the right rostral medulla. The sign-time graph is slowly progressive. Neoplastic, degenerative, and inflammation are the primary categories to consider. The musculoskeletal problem is most likely unrelated to the neurologic signs.

▪ Diagnostic plan

Rule-outs

1. Neoplasia: MR or CT of the brain is recommended.
2. Inflammation: CSF; MRI of brain
3. Neurodegenerative disease: brain biopsy, MRI of brain

▪ Case Summary

- CSF—Normal
- CT—Enhancing mass in right cranial dorsal brainstem and right ventral cerebellum. A meningioma was suspected.
- Pelvic radiographs—severe degenerative joint disease (DJD) of left coxofemoral joint
- Treatment—The owner declined surgery for the mass. No follow up was recorded.
- Final diagnosis—DJS left coxofemerol joint (CFJ); mass right cranial dorsal brainstem

CASE STUDY 2-3 ASSESSMENT

▪ Assessment (anatomic diagnosis and estimation of prognosis)

Bilateral, severe brainstem and forebrain disease (medulla, pons, and maybe midbrain). The sign-time graph in this case is acute and progressive over a few hours. Inflammation, toxicity, and vascular infarction are the major categories to consider (see Chapters 12, 13, and 15).

▪ Diagnostic plan

Rule-outs

1. Rabies (dumb form)—observation and strict rabies precautions
2. Levamisole toxicity—symptomatic therapy
3. GME—CSF, MRI brain
4. Brainstem infarction—MRI of brain

▪ Case Summary

CSF and brain scan would be beneficial. Given dog's condition, possibility of rabies and poor anesthetic risk, dog was managed symptomatically with fluids. Dog made a wonderful recovery. A vascular lesion affecting the rostral brainstem was suspected. Dog did not receive a toxic dose of levamisole. Suspect levamisole killed microfilaria that caused a brainstem vascular occlusion. Rabies was discounted when dog began to improve. The dog was treated as a rabies suspect for several days. He began to walk in 10 days, remained cortically blind and continued to demonstrate forebrain signs. He was nearly normal in 60 days.

CASE STUDY 2-4 ASSESSMENT

▪ Assessment (anatomic diagnosis and estimation of prognosis)

The clinical signs are very suggestive of generalized cerebellar disease. The sign-time graph is nonprogressive. One can assume the signs were present at birth.

▪ Diagnostic plan

Rule-outs

1. Cerebellar hypoplasia, MRI of brain
2. Cerebellar trauma at birth
3. Cerebellar abiotrophy (unlikely since signs are not progressive)

▪ Case Summary

No diagnostic procedures were performed. Given the history and clinical signs, cerebellar hypoplasia is a reasonable clinical diagnosis. There is no treatment and the prognosis is good for this dog. Cerebellar diseases are discussed in Chapter 8.

CASE STUDY 2-5 ASSESSMENT

▪ Assessment (anatomic diagnosis and estimation of prognosis)

The lesion is located L4-S2 and is more severe on the right side (tends to lateralize). There are LMN signs in right pelvic limb with normal perception of noxious stimuli the limb. This suggests that the lesion is within the ventral gray matter of the spinal cord. The sign-time graph is acute and nonprogressive. Traumatic, and vascular categories of disease should be considered.

▪ Diagnostic plan

Rule-outs

1. Spinal cord infarction: MRI of lumbar spinal cord; rule out other etiologies
2. Intervertebral disk disease: spinal radiographs, myelogram, CT, MRI
3. Trauma: vertebral fracture or subluxation; lumbosacral fracture, subluxation: spinal radiographs, CT, MRI

▪ Case Summary

CaseSpinal radiographs, myelography, and CT of lumbosacral spine are normal. CSF examination is normal. By exclusion, spinal cord infarction was the clinical diagnosis. The dog was given physical therapy and bladder care (assisted urination with gentle manual expression). Within 10 days, dog was more than 50% improved. In 90 days, dog was 90% improved and urinary incontinence resolved. Spinal cord infarction (fibrocartilagenous emboli) is discussed in Chapters 6 and 7.

CASE STUDY 2-6 ASSESSMENT

▪ Assessment (anatomic diagnosis and estimation of prognosis)

The dog has paraplegia with increased reflexes in pelvic limbs and normal thoracic limbs. The lesion is bilateral and located in spinal cord segments T3-L3. Sensory examination further localizes the lesion to the caudal thoracic spinal cord segments. The sign-time graph is acute and nonprogressive. Disease categories to consider are trauma and vascular. Thoracolumbar spinal cord diseases are presented in Chapter 6.

▪ Diagnostic plan

Rule-outs

1. Trauma (vertebral fracture/subluxation): spinal radiographs
2. Intervertebral disk disease (type 1): spinal radiographs, myelography, CT
3. Spinal cord infarction: MRI of spinal cord

▪ Case Summary

After 3 months, the dog is stable and may be slightly improved. Spinal radiographs are normal. Given the history and clinical signs, it is very unlikely that the dog will benefit from more in-depth diagnostic tests. The prognosis for recovery of motor function is poor. The owner was instructed to continue her physical therapy and bladder care.

CASE STUDY 2-7 ASSESSMENT

▪ Assessment (anatomic diagnosis and estimation of prognosis)

The clinical signs are those of a vestibular syndrome (see Chapter 8). The postural reactions are normal, which would support a peripheral vestibular disorder. The signs are bilateral but much worse on the left side. The left sympathetic nerve is affected (often found in otitis media-interna).

▪ Diagnostic plan

The clinical signs are acute and progressive. Categories of disease to consider include inflammation, idiopathic, and toxic.

Rule-outs

1. Bacterial otitis media-interna: otoscopic examination, skull radiographs, and CT of skull / brain
2. Idiopathic feline vestibular disease: exclude other rule-outs

▪ Case Summary

Otoscopic examination revealed inflammation of both tympanic membranes. No exudate was apparent in the middle ear. A clinical diagnosis of bacterial otitis media-interna was made. The cat was placed on amoxicillin and rechecked in 5 days. Cat was clinically improved in 10 days. She had slight head tilt to the left but her gait was remarkably improved.

CASE STUDY 2-8 ASSESSMENT

■ Assessment (anatomic diagnosis and estimation of prognosis)

The neurologic examination defines a generalized LMN disorder. Given the findings, one suspects a disease affecting motor neurons or motor end plates. The sign-time graph is acute and progressive over several hours. Disease categories to consider are inflammation and toxicity. Generalized LMN disorders are discussed in Chapter 7.

■ Diagnostic plan

Rule-outs

1. Botulism is the number 1 rule-out given the combination of autonomic and LMN involvement
2. Tick paralysis—usually no autonomic involvement. No engorged female ticks found on the dog.
3. Polyradiculoneuritis—usually no autonomic involvement

Diagnostic procedures

1. Assess dog for megaesophagus and aspiration pneumonia—thoracic radiographs, CBC
2. Assess dog for intestinal ileus and detrusor atony—abdominal radiographs
3. Assess dog for systemic inflammation—CBC
4. Rule out any metabolic consequences of vomiting—biochemical profile, UA
5. Botulism—consider mouse inoculation or immunologic testing of feces for botulinum toxin.
6. EMG

The CBC, biochemical profile, and urinalysis were normal. Thoracic radiographs: dilation of entire intrathoracic esophagus with a mixture of air and fluid. Early alveolar pulmonary opacity involving the ventral aspects of the right cranial, right middle, and left cranial lung lobes. Radiographic diagnosis: generalized megaesophagus and aspiration pneumonia involving the right cranial, right middle, and left cranial lung lobes.

■ Case Summary

The differential diagnosis included botulism, tick paralysis, and polyradiculoneuritis. Organophosphate intoxication was also considered but excluded early in the case evaluation.

Diagnosis: Given the history of multiple dog involvement, exposure to carrion 4 days before development of clinical signs and the presence of autonomic nervous system involvement, botulism was the most likely diagnosis. While several seed ticks were present on the dog, no engorged female ticks were identified and the dog did not improve when ticks were removed. Polyradiculoneuritis does not cause autonomic signs and was deemed less likely.

Treatment: Aspiration pneumonia: IV antibiotics (ampicillin, enrofloxacin), terbutaline SC, thoracic coupage and nasal O_2

Regurgitation: metoclopramide SC q8h

Physical therapy: Passive manipulation of limbs several times a day. Sterile indwelling urinary catheter. Manual evacuation of feces and enemas.

The dog began to improve in 6 days. Over several months, she gradually recovered normal motor function.

CASE STUDY 2-9 ASSESSMENT

■ Assessment (anatomic diagnosis and estimation of prognosis)

The lesion is localized to the right lower sciatic nerve involving the tibial and peroneal nerves. The sign-time graph is acute and nonprogressive. Categories of disease to consider are trauma and vascular. Peripheral nerve disorders are discussed in Chapter 5.

■ Diagnostic plan

Rule-outs

1. Sciatic nerve trauma: pelvis and right pelvic limb radiographs
2. Ischemic myoneural necrosis (vascular occlusion): check for other evidence of thrombosis (cardiac radiographs, echocardiography, thoracic radiographs)

■ Case Summary

Radiographs of the pelvis and right pelvic limb were normal. Evaluation of the heart and lungs were normal. Owner agreed to surgical exploration of the sciatic nerve in the caudal thigh region. A small, dark mass was found around the sciatic nerve just above the bifurcation into the peroneal and tibial nerves. The mass was an organized hematoma. Following surgery, the cat improved about 50% over the next 6 months.

CASE STUDY 2-10 ASSESSMENT

▪ Assessment (anatomic diagnosis and estimation of prognosis)

The dog has a right forebrain lesion (compare the gait and with the postural reactions). We know that trauma is the etiology in this case. The dog most likely has a contusion affecting the right cerebral cortex. The prognosis is good. The dog should be observed for seizures in the future. Head trauma is discussed in Chapter 12.

▪ Diagnostic plan

At this point, the dog is recovering following treatment for head trauma. No further diagnostics are indicated.

CASE STUDY 2-11 ASSESSMENT

▪ Assessment (anatomic diagnosis and estimation of prognosis)

Cranial nerves I (right), V (right and left), and VII (right) are affected. The sign-time graph is chronic and progressive. Categories of disease to consider include neoplasia, degeneration, and inflammation/infection. Prognosis is guarded.

▪ Diagnostic plan

Rule-outs

1. Meningioma (and other tumors) affecting base of brain—MRI of brain
2. Fungal infection—MRI of brain, CSF, serology
3. Abscess—MRI of brain, CSF
4. Neurodegenerative disease—MRI of brain

▪ Case Summary

Owner elected euthanasia. Necropsy revealed a large expanding meningioma extending from the olfactory tracts on the right side to the medulla on both sides. Cranial nerves were involved after their exit from the brainstem. This explains the normal gait and posture but multiple cranial nerve involvement. Cranial nerve disorders are discussed in Chapters 9 and 11.

REFERENCES

1. De Lahunta A: Veterinary neuroanatomy and clinical neurology, ed 3, St Louis, 2009, Elsevier.
2. Willis W, Chung J: Central mechanisms of pain, J Am Vet Med Assoc 191:1200–1202, 1987.
3. Breazile JE, Kitchell RL: A study of fiber systems within the spinal cord of the domestic pig that subserve pain, J Comp Neurol 133:373–382, 1968.
4. Kennard MA: The course of ascending fibers in the spinal cord of the cat essential to the recognition of painful stimuli, J Comp Neurol 100:511–524, 1954.
5. Tarlov IM: Spinal cord compression: mechanism of paralysis and treatment, Springfield, Ill, 1957, Charles C Thomas.
6. Holliday T: Clinical signs of acute and chronic experimental lesions of the cerebellum, Vet Res Commun 3:259–278, 1980.
7. Holliday TA: Clinical signs caused by experimental lesions in the vestibular system. In Proceedings of the Eighth Annual Veterinary Medical Forum, Washington, DC, 1990, American College of Veterinary Internal Medicine.
8. Kornegay JN: Ataxia of the head and limbs: cerebellar diseases in dogs and cats, Prog Vet Neurol 1:255–274, 1990.
9. Oliver JE: Localization of lesions in the nervous system. In Hoerlein BF, editor: Canine neurology, ed 3, Philadelphia, 1978, WB Saunders.

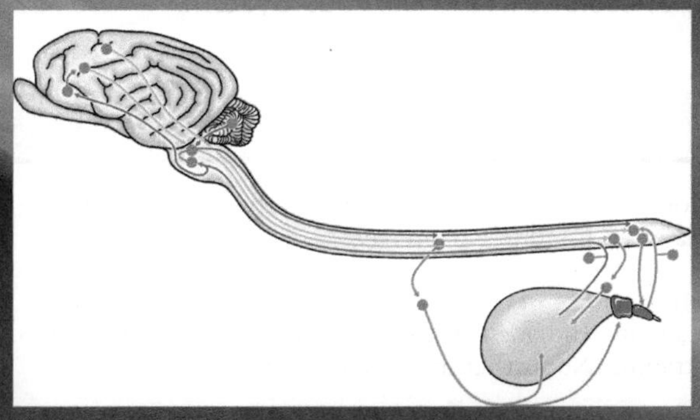

CHAPTER 3

Disorders of Micturition

Abnormal visceral function may reflect a pathologic change in the nervous system; however, the importance of nervous control of the viscera is often overlooked.

The classic view of the autonomic nervous system as one with discrete boundaries is giving way to a concept of a more integrated system with no limits. For example, conventional theory held that the autonomic system controlled functions that the individual could not modify voluntarily; however, the fact that one can regulate blood pressure, heart rate, micturition, and many other autonomic activities has been proven. In conventional theory, the sympathetic *(adrenergic)* system functions as an antagonist to the parasympathetic *(cholinergic)* system. This simplistic view, which separates the autonomic system from the somatic system, does not explain well-defined somatovisceral and viscerosomatic reflexes.

Problems associated with micturition are common in neurologic disorders. Other forms of visceral dysfunction traditionally have been the concern of cardiologists and internists, and these are discussed in books on cardiology and internal medicine. This chapter reviews the anatomy, physiology, and clinical syndromes of micturition.

ANATOMY AND PHYSIOLOGY OF MICTURITION

The normal function of the lower urinary tract includes both storage and expulsion of urine. Micturition is the reaction that ultimately occurs if a bladder is gradually distended, leading to the coordinated expulsion of its contents.[1] Two major reflexes are involved in the normal function of the lower urinary tract, the detrusor and micturition reflexes. The detrusor reflex is specifically involved with the evacuation of urine in response to stretch of the bladder whereas the micturition reflex involves both the storage and evacuation of urine of which the detrusor reflex plays a role. The micturition reflex is a complex integration of parasympathetic, sympathetic, and somatic pathways extending from the sacral segments of the spinal cord to the brainstem and cerebral cortex.[2,3] The components of the micturition reflex are discussed in functional groups before a complete description of the micturition reflex is discussed.

Urinary Bladder

The urinary bladder is divided into a neck (trigone) and body, and serves as a low pressure reservoir. The urinary bladder, also called the detrusor muscle, consists of three interwoven layers of smooth muscle. Adrenergic and muscarinic cholinergic receptors lie within the detrusor smooth muscle (Figure 3-1). The emptying phase of micturition is mediated by cholinergic fibers of the pelvic nerve. The pelvic nerve innervates all regions of the bladder and conveys both sensory and motor information.

Sympathetic fibers found in the pelvic plexus, the pelvic ganglia, and the urinary bladder serve to enhance the storage phase of micturition. The preganglionic sympathetic neurons to the bladder are located in the lumbar spinal cord (L2-5 in the cat, L1-4 in the dog).[2,4-6] The preganglionic fibers course as the lumbar splanchnic nerves to synapse with nicotinic cholinergic receptors in the caudal mesenteric ganglion and the postganglionic fibers continue as the hypogastric nerve to the bladder, urethra, and the pelvic plexus (see Figure 3-1). Both α- and β-adrenergic (sympathetic postganglionic) synapses have been found on neurons in the pelvic ganglia, in the bladder wall, and on the detrusor muscle, especially in the area of the trigone.[7,8] Stimulation of the β-adrenergic receptors causes detrusor muscle relaxation and allows bladder filling at constant pressure. Sensory receptors lie within muscle fascicles and connective tissue of the smooth muscle layers. They mediate sensory information conveyed by distention (stretch) and pain of the detrusor muscle. The filling threshold triggers the micturition reflex.

Pharmacologic studies have demonstrated that α-adrenergic receptors are located primarily in the trigone area, bladder neck, and proximal urethra, causing contraction of the smooth muscle.[9,10] β-adrenergic receptors are found in all parts of the detrusor muscle and cause relaxation of smooth muscle. The presence of adrenergic synapses on cholinergic ganglion cells suggests that the sympathetic pathways can also modulate the activity of the parasympathetic pathway, but this effect has not been demonstrated in naturally occurring sympathetic firing.[11-13] Adrenergic innervation of the bladder neck and the trigone has been demonstrated to have major significance in the prevention of retrograde ejaculation.

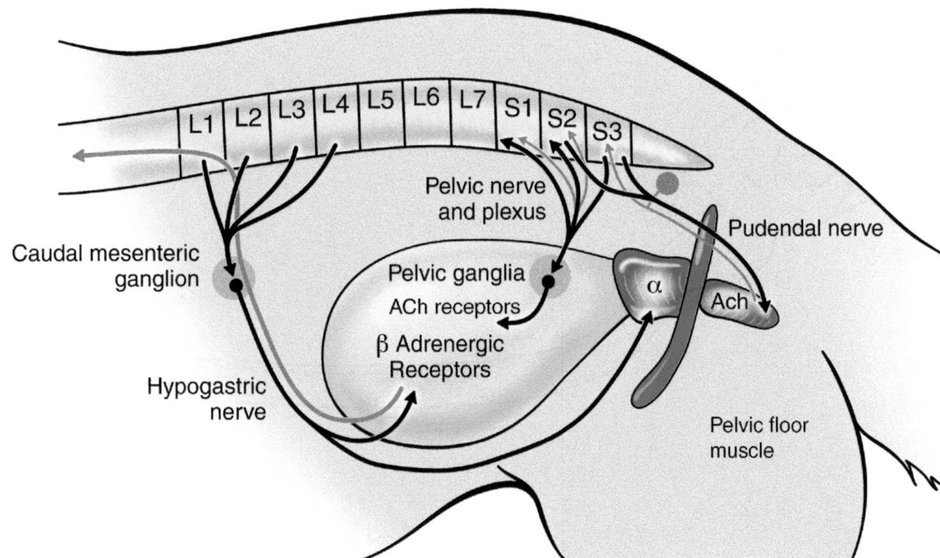

Figure 3-1 Anatomic organization of the local innervations of the bladder and urethra. Motor innervations are represented by the darker lines; sensory innervations are represented by the lighter lines. *Motor innervation*—The preganglionic neurons for the sympathetic innervation originate from L1-4 (dog) and L2-5 (cat) and leave the spinal cord as the splanchnic nerves to synapse in the caudal mesenteric ganglion. Postganglionic sympathetic fibers (hypogastric nerve) innervate the bladder wall (β-adrenergic receptors) and the proximal smooth muscle of the urethral sphincter (α-adrenergic receptors). These fibers are active during the storage phase of micturition. The preganglionic neurons for the parasympathetic innervation orginate from S1-3 spinal cord segments. The preganglionic fibers from S1-3 leave the spinal cord as the pelvic (splanchnic) nerve to synapse in the pelvic ganglia located within the bladder wall and innervate the detrusor muscle via cholinergic synapses for bladder contraction during the voiding phase of micturition. The pudendal nerve arises from the ventral branches of the S1-3 sacral nerves to supply the striated external urethral sphincter muscle. *Sensory innervation*—Sensory fibers from the urinary bladder reach the cord via both pelvic (stretch receptors) and hypogastric (nociceptive receptors) nerves. Sensory input from the urethra reaches the cord via the pudendal nerve. These pathways ascend to the center for micturition located in the pons. (Courtesy Dennis P. O'Brien, DVM, PhD, University of Missouri.)

Lesions of the sympathetic pathways apparently do not have a major effect on micturition; however, there is increasing acceptance of the theory that the sympathetic pathways play an important role in animals and humans with lesions of the parasympathetic pathways.[8,14-16] Evidence for this is supported by patients with neurogenic bladder dysfunction complicated by a narrowing of the bladder neck or spasms of the urethra, which may be helped by α-adrenergic blockade.[8]

Sensory Pathways from the Urinary Bladder

Sensory fibers originating in the bladder run in both the pelvic and the hypogastric nerves. Stretch receptors in the bladder wall give rise to fibers that run through the pelvic nerve into the sacral spinal cord (S1-3 in the cat and the dog) and ascend to the pontine reticular formation to initiate the detrusor reflex.[17] Sensory fibers in the hypogastric nerve reach the spinal cord at the lumbar segments (L2-5 in the cat, L1-4 in the dog).[6,18] Afferent fibers from both pelvic and hypogastric nerves reach the cerebral cortex in the cat, whereas only hypogastric neural activity is relayed to the cortex in the dog.[19] The hypogastric fibers respond to overdistention of the bladder. Activation of these fibers is perceived as pain.[20] A lesion of the caudal lumbar or sacral spinal cord could abolish micturition, although the animal would still perceive overdistention of the bladder as a painful sensation mediated through the hypogastric nerve.

Motor Innervation of the Urinary Bladder

Each motor branch of the pelvic nerve in the bladder wall innervates many muscle cells, although not all muscle cells have direct innervation. Muscarinic cholinergic receptors are located within the body and base of the bladder musculature. They mediate information conveyed by postganglionic parasympathetic fibers of pelvic nerve. Stimulation causes detrusor muscle contraction and bladder emptying.

The neuromuscular junction is characterized by a varicosity of the axon-containing synaptic vesicles, a thinning of the Schwann cell layer, and a close apposition to specialized areas of the detrusor muscle fibers. Excitation of the innervated muscle cell (pacemaker cell) initiates a spread of excitation and contraction through adjacent cells by means of "tight junctions."[11] The spread of excitation has also been hypothesized to occur by diffusion of a neurotransmitter in the extracellular space to adjacent detrusor muscle fibers.

Disruption of tight junctions between muscle fibers may occur when the bladder is overdistended (e.g., obstruction of the urethra). If tight junctions are disrupted, the wave of excitation cannot spread and a flaccid bladder results. Reconnection of the junction occurs in 1 to 2 weeks if the distention is relieved early. If the bladder remains distended too long or if infection is present, fibrosis develops between the cells, preventing restoration of function.

Urethral Sphincter

The urethral musculature consists of two sphincters that are considered outlets for urine from the urinary bladder.[21-24] Internal smooth muscle (internal urethral sphincter) is composed of outer and inner longitudinal and middle circular layers and begins at the bladder neck and extends distally. External striated muscle (external urethral sphincter) is interwoven with the proximal urethral smooth muscle, but is more

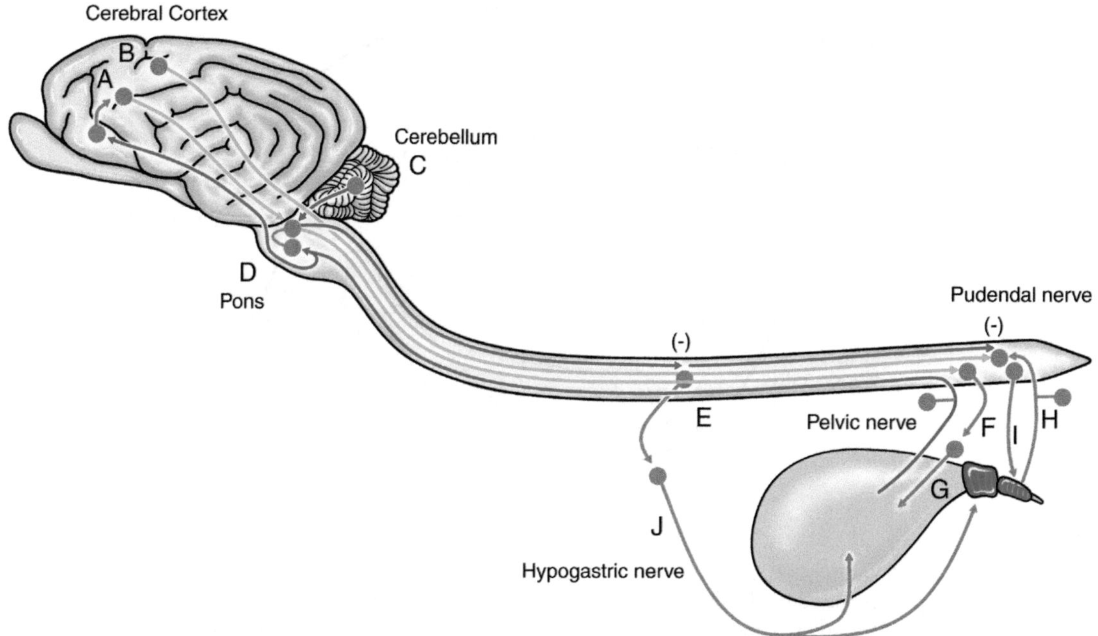

Figure 3-2 Anatomic organization of micturition. **A,** Cortical neurons for voluntary control of micturition *(green line)*. **B,** Cortical neurons for voluntary control of sphincters *(green line)*. **C,** Cerebellar neurons that have an inhibitory influence on micturition. **D,** Pontine reticular neurons (center for micturition) that are necessary for the detrusor reflex. **E,** Afferent (sensory) pathway *(blue line)* for the detrusor reflex. **F,** Preganglionic pelvic (parasympathetic) neuron to the detrusor. **G,** Postganglionic pelvic (parasympathetic) neuron to the detrusor. **H,** Afferent (sensory) neuron from the urethral sphincter, pudendal nerve. **I,** Efferent (motor) neuron to the urethral sphincter, pudendal nerve. During voiding the pontine reticular neurons also send descending inhibitory pathways *(red line)* to the hypogastric nerve *(J)* and the pudendal nerve *(I)* to inhibit urethral sphincter contraction. (From Oliver JE Jr, Osborne CA: Neurogenic urinary incontinence. In Kirk RW, editor: Current veterinary therapy, VII, Philadelphia, 1980, WB Saunders.)

prominent in the distal half of the urethra. Adrenergic and nicotinic cholinergic receptors are located on the internal smooth and external striated muscles, respectively. α-Adrenergic receptors predominate at the base of the detrusor muscle and internal sphincter of proximal urethra. They mediate information relayed by postganglionic sympathetic fibers, the *hypogastric nerve*. Stimulation causes contraction of smooth muscles of the bladder neck and proximal urethra to counter urine flow and facilitate bladder filling.

The skeletal muscle surrounding the urethra contains spindles that discharge in response to stretch, as do other skeletal muscles. The skeletal muscle in the urethral sphincter is innervated by the pudendal nerve of the general somatic nervous system (see Figure 3-1). The motor neurons that give rise to the urethral branches of the pudendal are located in spinal cord segments L7-S3 in the dog and the cat, although they are found primarily in S1 and S2 in both species.[18,25] Sensory discharges ascend in the pudendal nerves to the sacral segments. Monosynaptic activation of the motor neurons is transmitted back down the pudendal nerve to innervate the nicotinic cholinergic receptors located within these skeletal muscle fibers (see Figure 3-1). Stimulation causes external sphincter muscle contraction, which counters urine flow and facilitates bladder filling. Afferent discharge through the pelvic nerves also activates the pudendal nerve. These pathways produce urethral contraction in response to a sudden stretch, maintaining continence during a cough, a sneeze, and so forth. Voluntary control of the urethral sphincter is provided by cortical pathways to the sacral segments.

Lesions of the sacral segments or the pudendal nerve cause a hypotonic paralysis of the sphincter. Cortical or spinal lesions may abolish voluntary control of the sphincter and may produce increased sphincter tone, which increases outflow resistance.[11] Typically, T3-L3 lesions of the spinal cord abolish the long-routed detrusor reflex and cause increased tone in the sphincter.

Detrusor Reflex

The primary component of micturition is the *detrusor* (the muscle of the urinary bladder) *reflex* (Figure 3-2). Detrusor reflex is a pathway for urination via a brainstem/spinal cord reflex arc. As the bladder fills with urine, a slight increase in bladder pressure occurs with each increase in volume until the limit of elasticity of the smooth muscle is reached. The sensory nerve endings in the bladder wall are tension receptors and are arranged in a series with the muscle fibers. As the bladder nears its capacity, these nerves begin to discharge. The sensory fibers from the bladder are located in the pelvic nerve and project to the sacral segments of the spinal cord (see Figure 3-1).[6,18] The sensory discharge ascends in the spinal cord to the pontine reticular formation in the brainstem, centers for micturition (see Figure 3-2, *E*).[26] Integration occurs at this level, eventually giving rise to activation of descending upper motor neuron (UMN) pathways that stimulate the preganglionic parasympathetic neurons in the intermediate horn of the sacral segments (see Figure 3-2, *F* and *G*).

The detrusor reflex is mediated through the parasympathetic nervous system (sacral spinal cord segments). The preganglionic parasympathetic neurons are located in segments S1-3 in the cat and the dog.[4,17,18] They have not been located precisely in other species, but gross dissections indicate that they are in the sacral segments. The preganglionic

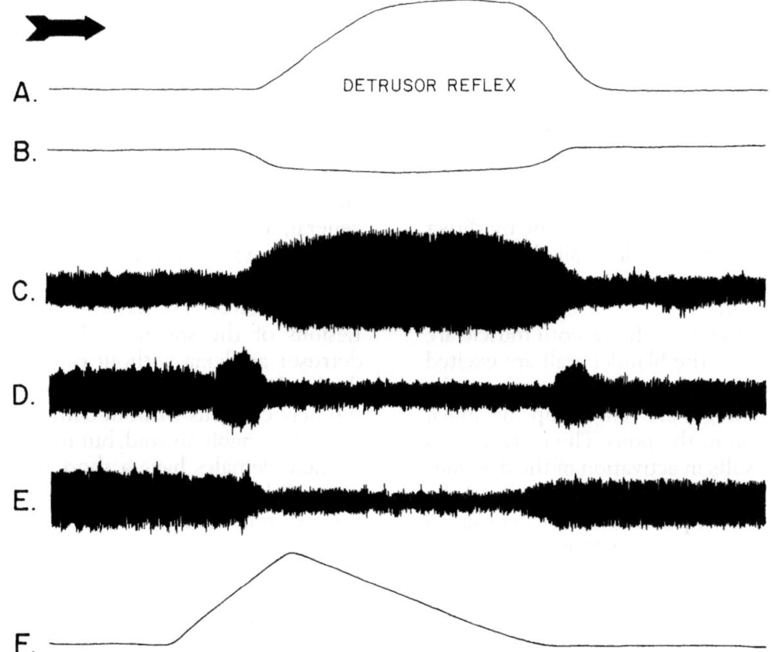

Figure 3-3 Schematic representation of sequential pressure *(A–B)* and neural discharges *(C-E)* over time during micturition (not drawn to scale). **A,** Intravesical pressure. **B,** Urethral pressure. **C,** Pelvic nerve. **D,** Hypogastric nerve. **E,** Pudendal nerve. **F,** Bladder volume. (Modified from Jonas U, Tanagho EA: Studies on vesicourethral reflexes, Invest Urol 12:357–373, 1975; Bradley WE, Teague CT: Hypogastric and pelvic nerve activity during the micturition reflex, J Urol 101:438–440, 1969.)

neurons discharge and activate postganglionic neurons, which are located in the pelvic ganglia, along the course of the pelvic nerves, and in the wall of the bladder. Some integration of activity apparently takes place in the ganglia. Ultimately, the postganglionic neurons synapse on detrusor muscle fibers and cause a contraction—the detrusor reflex (see Figure 3-2).

Integration of the brainstem is necessary for the detrusor reflex to be coordinated and sustained long enough for bladder evacuation (see Figure 3-2). Complete lesions of any portion of this pathway abolish the detrusor reflex and therefore result in a micturition disorder.

Voluntary Control of the Detrusor Reflex

The sensory pathway to the brainstem that signals distention of the bladder also sends collaterals to the cerebral cortex (see Figure 3-2). Integration at the cortical level allows voluntary initiation (e.g., in territorial marking) or inhibition (e.g., in house training) of micturition. The precise location of the control center of the cerebral cortex is not clear. Stimulation and evoked-response studies indicate that several areas of the cortex influence the detrusor reflex.[27] Lesions of the cerebral cortex may cause a loss of voluntary control of micturition and may reduce the capacity of the bladder.[28] For example, animals with cerebral tumors may start voiding in the house for no apparent reason. From the owner's perspective, the animal can initiate voiding normally and void completely but does so in inappropriate places (e.g., cat that voids outside the litter box).

Cerebellar Inhibition of the Detrusor Reflex

The cerebellum can inhibit the detrusor reflex (see Figure 3-2). Stimulation of the fastigial nucleus abolishes detrusor reflex contraction.[29] Lesions of the cerebellum, such as cerebellar hypoplasia, may produce increased frequency of voiding with a reduced bladder capacity.[1]

Reflex Integration

The micturition reflex involves a coordinated and sustained contraction of the detrusor muscle (the detrusor reflex) along with simultaneous relaxation of the urethra.[20] Moreover, depending on the size of the bladder, the micturition reflex may also result in urine storage. Pelvic sensory neurons that produce the detrusor reflex also send collaterals to inhibitory interneurons in the sacral spinal cord.[30] The inhibitory interneurons synapse on the pudendal motor neurons, which are also in the sacral segments, to reduce motor activity in the pudendal nerves and the periurethral striated muscle (Figure 3-3, *B* and *E*). As the detrusor muscle contracts, the urethra relaxes, allowing urine to pass. If the long pathways are intact, voluntary activation of the pudendal neurons by the corticospinal pathways can override this effect and block micturition. Lesions of the long tracts or at the segmental level may interfere with reflex integration. Detrusor contraction without urethral relaxation is called *reflex dyssynergia*.[31]

Reflex connections between the pelvic *(parasympathetic)* nerve afferents and the lumbar *(sympathetic)* motor neurons also have been demonstrated.[6,20,32] The effect seems similar to that observed in the pudendal (somatic) nerve—that is, as the pelvic motor neuron begins to fire to initiate a detrusor contraction, the hypogastric nerve becomes silent (see Figure 3-3, C and *D*). When the pelvic nerve stops firing as the bladder is emptied, the hypogastric nerve discharges once more. Presumably, the effect of the hypogastric nerve is on bladder relaxation and urethral contraction.

Micturition Reflex

Integration of filling, storage, and emptying of the bladder with contraction and then relaxation of the sphincters is the *micturition reflex* (see Figure 3-3).[6] The following discussion presents each of the components for a more complete picture.

Urine is transported from the kidneys to the bladder through the ureters. Peristaltic waves move the urine into the bladder in spurts. Vesicoureteral reflux is prevented by the oblique course of the ureter through the bladder wall, resulting in the formation of a flap valve. The detrusor muscle spirals around the ureter, assisting in the maintenance of the valve effect.

Initially, the bladder fills without a significant increase in pressure as the smooth muscle stretches (see Figure 3-3, *A* and *F*). The sympathetic *(adrenergic)* pathways may assist by inhibiting parasympathetic *(cholinergic)* neurons or by direct relaxation of smooth muscle. If the bladder fills beyond the normal elasticity of the smooth muscle, pressure increases linearly with the increase in volume.

Normally, as the limits of stretch of the smooth muscle are approached, stretch receptors in the bladder wall are excited and send sensory discharges through the pelvic nerves to the sacral spinal cord. These discharges are relayed up the spinal cord to the reticular formation in the pons. The activation of neuronal pools in the pons results in activation of the descending UMN pathways that project to the sacral segments of the spinal cord. Preganglionic parasympathetic motor neurons in the intermediate horn of the sacral gray matter are activated. The motor discharge passes down the pelvic nerves to activate postganglionic neurons in the pelvic ganglia and in the wall of the bladder, which in turn activates the bladder smooth muscle *(detrusor)*. The sustained discharge of neurons through these pathways produces a coordinated, sustained contraction of the detrusor muscle (see Figure 3-3, *A* and *C*).[6]

The fibers of the detrusor muscle spiral into the neck of the bladder and help to maintain continence in the relaxed state. As the fibers contract, the bladder neck is pulled open into a funnel shape. Simultaneously, sensory discharges from the pelvic nerves are relayed to the lumbar segments (inhibiting the output of the sympathetic pathway) and to the pudendal motor neurons in the ventral horn of the sacral segments (inhibiting the tonic output in the nerves to the skeletal sphincter) (see Figure 3-3, *C* to *E*).

The result is a coordinated contraction of the bladder and a relaxation of the sphincter, which is maintained until voiding is complete (see Figure 3-3, *A* and *B*). Sustaining the contraction also is enhanced by sensory fibers in the urethra that respond to the flow of urine.

When the bladder is empty, sensory discharges in the pelvic nerve stop. Motor discharges in the pelvic nerve cease and activity in the sympathetic and pudendal nerves returns. The bladder relaxes, and the sphincters close.

DISORDERS OF MICTURITION

The neurogenic disorders of micturition are caused by abnormal detrusor muscle or sphincter function or both (Table 3-1). Detrusor or sphincter activity may be decreased, increased, or normal. Typical syndromes include inappropriate voiding; inadequate voiding with an overflow of urine; increased frequency, reduced urinary bladder capacity, or both; and incomplete voiding when normal voiding reactions are interrupted by abrupt contractions of the urethral sphincter.[11]

Clinical Signs

The clinical signs of abnormal micturition are summarized in Table 3-2.

Detrusor Areflexia with Sphincter Hypertonus

The most frequently recognized disorder of micturition is a loss of the detrusor reflex with increased tone in the urethral sphincter. Lesions from the pontine reticular formation to the L7 spinal cord segments may cause these complications. The animal is unable to void and the bladder becomes greatly distended, and expressing the bladder manually is difficult or impossible. The perineal reflex is intact. The most common cause is compression of the spinal cord, such as occurs with intervertebral disk herniation, which disrupts the long pathways that are responsible for the detrusor reflex and the UMN pathways to the skeletal muscle of the urethral sphincter. Loss of voluntary control of micturition occurs with lesions severe enough to disrupt voluntary motor function of the limbs. In general, as voluntary motor function of the limbs returns, so does voluntary control of micturition.

Detrusor Areflexia with Normal Sphincter Tone

Lesions of the spinal cord or the brainstem may produce detrusor areflexia without causing increased tone in the urethral sphincter. Traumatic injuries of the pelvis may damage the pelvic plexus without damage to the pudendal nerve. The animal is unable to void, but manual expression can be accomplished. Females have a short skeletal sphincter so that even with UMN lesions, sphincter tone may not be excessive.[33] Perineal reflexes are intact.

Detrusor Areflexia with Sphincter Hypotonia

Lesions of the sacral spinal cord or the nerve roots, such as fractures of the L6 or L7 vertebra or fibrocartilaginous embolism (FCE) affection the sacral spinal cord segments, cause a loss of the detrusor reflexes and urethral sphincter reflexes and tone. The bladder is easily expressed and may leak urine continuously. Perineal reflexes are diminished or absent. Dysautonomia *(Key Gaskell syndrome)* produces clinical signs of urinary incontinence attributable to loss of parasympathetic and sympathetic innervations.[34] Somatic innervation of the anus (absent perineal reflex) is affected, but generalized paresis is not a clinical feature of the disease (see Chapter 15).

Detrusor Areflexia from Overdistention

Loss of excitation-contraction coupling in the detrusor muscle (detrusor atony) may occur as a result of severe overdistention of the bladder. Manual expression of the bladder may be difficult because the sphincter is normal. The animal may empty the bladder partially by abdominal contraction. Attempts to void indicate that sensory pathways are intact and suggest a primary detrusor muscle abnormality. The most frequent cause is obstruction of the urethral outflow tract (e.g., calculi). Detrusor areflexia from overdistention also may occur because it is too painful to stand or posture to urinate. This scenario is not uncommon following pelvic fractures and prolonged recumbency.

Detrusor Hyperreflexia

Frequent voiding of small quantities of urine, often without warning, may be caused by partial lesions of the long pathways or of the cerebellum.[1] Inflammation of the bladder (cystitis) may produce similar signs. Little or no residual urine is present, the capacity of the bladder is reduced, and perineal reflexes are intact.

The so-called UMN bladder as seen in chronic paraplegic human beings is rare in animals.[35] In animals, chronic spinal cord lesions severe enough to affect voluntary micturition cause detrusor areflexia, not hyperreflexia. The bladder may have small uncoordinated contractions, but these are inadequate to empty the bladder. Animals with partial lesions, especially in the recovery phase, may have spastic detrusor contractions as they approach normal.

Reflex Dyssynergia

Functional urethral obstruction results from neurogenic or nonneurogenic causes (obstructive calculi). A lesion affecting the UMN pathways is the most common neurogenic cause

TABLE 3-1

Effect of Lesions on the Neural Pathways of Micturition

		BLADDER					SPHINCTER			
Location of Lesion	**Normal Function**	**Voluntary Control**	**Sustained Detrusor Reflex**	**Tone**	**Volume**	**Residual Urine**	**Voluntary Control**	**Perineal Reflex**	**Tone**	**Synergy with Detrusor**
Forebrain	Voluntary control	Absent	N	N	↑, N, ↓	None	Absent	N to ↑	N to ↑	N
Cerebellum	Inhibition of detrusor reflex	Normal, ↑ frequency	May be hyperreflexic	N	↓	None	N	N	N	N
Brainstem to sacral spinal cord	Sustained detrusor reflex	Absent	None early; small unsynchronized contractions late	Atonic early, may be ↑≠ late	↑	↑	Absent	N to ↑	N to ↑	Absent
Partial lesions; brainstem to sacral spinal cord (reflex dyssynergia)	Coordination of detrusor and sphincter	May be present	May be present	↑ to ↓	↑	↑ to ↓	May be present	N	N to ↑	Absent
Sacral spinal cord or roots	LMN to detrusor and sphincter	Absent	Absent	↓	↑	↑	Absent	Absent	↓	Absent
Detrusor muscle (tight junctions)	Spread of excitation in detrusor	Absent	Absent	↓	↑	↑	N	N	N	N (impossible to evaluate)

Modified from Oliver JE Jr, Osborne CA: Neurogenic urinary incontinence. In Kirk RW, editor: Current veterinary therapy, VI, Philadelphia, 1977, WB Saunders.
↑, Increased; ↓, decreased; *N*, normal; *LMN*, lower motor neuron.

TABLE 3-2

Signs of Abnormal Micturition

Problem	Voiding	Attempts to Void	Expression of Bladder	Residual Urine	Perineal Reflex	Probable Lesion
Detrusor areflexia, sphincter hypertonus	Absent	No	Difficult	Large amount	Present	Brainstem to L7 spinal cord
Detrusor areflexia, normal sphincter tone	Absent	No	Possible, some resistance	Large amount	Present	Brainstem to L7 spinal cord
Detrusor areflexia, sphincter areflexia	Absent	No	Easy, often leaks urine	Large to moderate amounts	Absent	Sacral spinal cord or nerve roots
Detrusor areflexia (overdistention)	Absent	Yes	Possible, some resistance	Large amount	Present	Detrusor muscle
Detrusor hyperreflexia	Frequent, small quantity	Yes	Possible, some resistance	None	Present	Brainstem to L7, partial, or cerebellum; also inflammation of bladder
Reflex dyssynergia	Frequent, spurting, unsustained	Yes	Difficult	Small to large amount	Present	Brainstem to L7, partial lesions
Normal detrusor reflex, incompetent sphincter	Normal, but with leakage of urine with stress or full bladder	Yes	Easy	None	May or may not be present	Pudendal nerves, sympathetic nerves, hormone deficiency

of reflex dyssynergia, where there is a loss of coordination between the detrusor and the urethral sphincter muscles.[31,36] The term *dyssynergia* refers to simultaneous contraction of muscles whose activity is opposite in direction. Often with reflex dyssynergia, normal initiation of voiding is followed by interruption of the stream through an involuntary contraction of the urethral sphincter. The stream of urine is normal at first, followed by short spurts, and then by a complete cessation of the flow. Frequently the animal continues to strain with no success. Reflex dyssynergia is seen primarily in male dogs and rarely in cats.[31,36,37] The pathogenesis is not certain but is presumed to be the result of a partial lesions in the UMN pathways causing a loss of the normal inhibition of the pudendal nerves during the detrusor reflex. The detrusor reflex is present, and the perineal reflex is often hyperactive.

Increased sensory input from abnormal structures innervated by the sacral nerves may also play a role. Examples include prostatic disease, perineal trauma, and surgical wounds in this area. Excessive sympathetic stimulation can cause dyssynergia. We have observed an abnormality clinically similar to reflex dyssynergia in a male dog recovering from tetanus. Diagnosis of idiopathic detrusor-urethral sphincter dyssynergia is based on exclusion of pathologic causes of urine outflow obstruction.[38,39] A dyssynergic-like condition has been seen in dogs with a cauda equina lesion.[40]

Normal Detrusor Reflex with Decreased Sphincter Tone

Loss of normal urethral resistance with a normal detrusor reflex causes leaking of urine when voiding is delayed. The animal can empty the bladder, but as soon as a small amount of urine accumulates, leakage occurs. The leakage may occur during an abdominal press (barking, coughing) or during complete rest. The most frequent cause is the lack of sex hormones in a neutered animal. Hormone-responsive incontinence has been well documented in ovariectomized bitches and less frequently in neutered male dogs.[41-45] Both are responsive to hormone replacement therapy with or without supplementation with adrenergic agents. A similar clinical picture may be seen in some animals that are not responsive to hormone therapy. The lesion may be a structural abnormality of the urethra, a loss of pudendal innervation, or a loss of sympathetic innervation to the urethra.[46-48]

Diagnosis

The minimum database recommended for the evaluation of an animal with a problem associated with micturition is presented in Box 3-1. The minimum database is designed to reveal any additional problems and to provide the information necessary to make a diagnosis and to formulate a prognosis. Figure 3-4 outlines the process of establishing a diagnosis. Specific steps in the process are discussed in the following sections.

History

In addition to the usual items in the history, the examiner should obtain some specific information pertinent to micturition.

Previous History. The clinician should determine the animal's pattern of micturition habits from as early an age as possible. Age when house trained, frequency of micturition at various ages, and changes in habits may provide insight into the onset of a problem before the owner's recognition of its significance.

BOX 3-1

Minimum Database for Diagnosis of Disorders of Micturition

History

Physical examination

Includes: Observation of voiding (stream size, dysuria, duration, urine color), measurement of residual urine, palpation of external genitalia, observation of urine scald, abdominal palpation, vaginal examination, rectal palpation (masses, anal sphincter tone, urethra)

Neurologic examination

Includes: Evaluation of sphincter reflexes (perineal, bulbocavernosus), tail tone, low lumbar spinal pain

Clinical pathology

Includes: Complete blood cell count, urinalysis, urine culture, (blood urea nitrogen or creatinine concentration)

Radiologic examination

Includes: Survey of abdomen and pelvis, contrast cystography and urethrography, intravenous pyelogram, advanced imaging (CT, MRI).

Modified from Oliver JE Jr, Osborne CA: Neurogenic urinary incontinence. In Kirk RW, editor: Current veterinary therapy, VI, Philadelphia, 1977, WB Saunders.

Signs of abnormality in the nervous system or the urinary tract and previous trauma are important. Previous surgical procedures, especially neurologic, abdominal, or pelvic (e.g., ovariohysterectomy), should be analyzed in relation to the time of onset of the problem.

History of the Problem. Information regarding the onset and the chronologic course of the problem allows the examiner to construct a sign-time graph, which is useful for determining the cause of the disease (see Chapter 1).

Voluntary control of micturition is often best established by the owner's perceptions, which are supplemented and confirmed by direct observations of the animal in natural surroundings (e.g., outside on the grass). If the animal can volitionally initiate voiding, the detrusor reflex is probably present. Voluntary control also implies that micturition can be withheld for a reasonable length of time (house training) and can be interrupted if necessary. Interruption of micturition is difficult to evaluate. A dog that is lead-trained can be interrupted by a pull on the lead and a command to "come." Individual interpretation of this interruption is quite subjective.

Dyssynergia begins with a normal initiation of voiding followed by a narrowing of the stream and a sudden interruption of the flow. The animal often strains and may continue voiding in brief spurts. Dyssynergia must be differentiated from *partial anatomic obstruction* (e.g., that is caused by urethral calculi), which can be demonstrated by catheterization and urethral contrast-enhanced radiography or urethroscopy.

Various types of incontinence may be described by the owner. *Detrusor hyperreflexia*, in which the animal voids suddenly in inappropriate places without apparent warning, called precipitate voiding, is characteristic of cerebellar lesions and some partial spinal cord or brainstem lesions (see Table 3-2). Differentiation between precipitate voiding and loss of normal voluntary micturition, as in forebrain lesions or behavioral disorders, may be difficult on the basis of the history alone. In these instances, other neurologic signs may help localize a lesion to the cerebellum or forebrain. History also may help define the disorder as behavioral in nature (e.g., behavioral marking of territory). Dribbling of urine may result from anatomic anomalies (e.g., ectopic ureters), loss of urethral resistance, or overflow from an areflexic bladder (see Table 3-2).

Physical Examination

Observation of the animal may confirm the characteristics of micturition as described in the history. The differences in the various abnormalities of micturition may be subtle; therefore the problem described by the owner must be verified by the examiner.

The presence of a detrusor reflex can be assumed if voiding is sustained (see Figure 3-4); however, bladder contractions with incomplete voiding are common in neurologic disorders. Such contractions are not the result of a true detrusor reflex. The residual urine must therefore be measured in every animal with a problem associated with micturition. After the animal has voided, preferably outside in natural surroundings and to avoid any influence of the animal's reluctance because of house training, the bladder is catheterized and the residual urine is measured. Residual urine should be less than 10% of the normal volume. Dogs will have less than 10 mL remaining (0.2 to 0.4 mL/kg) and less than 2 mL remaining in cats.[8]

Except for some dogs with prostatic enlargement due to benign prostatic hypertrophy or prostatic tumors, or as occurs with urethral flaps (rare), obstructions in the urethra can be detected when a catheter is passed. A flap can be demonstrated only by excretory urethrography.[41]

Palpation of the bladder before and after the animal voids provides some information regarding bladder tone. The tone of the detrusor muscle is intrinsic and is not directly related to innervation; however, a normal bladder contracts to accommodate the volume of urine present. An overdistended bladder with disruption of the tight junctions does not contract. A chronically infected bladder is often small and has a thickened and fibrotic wall. A small, contracted bladder with infection may not be the primary problem because bladder infection is a common sequela of urine retention from neurogenic disorders.[8,49,50] Some of the nonneurogenic causes of incontinence, such as tumors or calculi, may be identified by palpation, radiography, or ultrasonography.[47]

Manual expression of the bladder provides some information regarding urethral sphincter tone. Normally, expression of the bladder is more difficult in the male than in the female. Urethral sphincter tone is decreased in lesions of the sacral spinal cord, the sacral roots, or the pudendal nerve (lower motor neuron [LMN]) and is increased in lesions between the L7 spinal cord segment and the brainstem (see Table 3-2). The sacral spinal cord segments lie within the body of the fifth lumbar vertebra in the dog so that lesions of the vertebrae from L5-6 caudad can affect the sacral roots. In large animals, lesions at the level of the midsacrum affect the sacral segments and nerve roots.

Neurologic Examination

The complete neurologic examination is described in Chapter 1. Reflexes related to the sacral spinal cord segments are especially important in evaluating micturition disorders.

The anal and urethral sphincters are innervated by the pudendal nerve, primarily from sacral segments 1 and 2 but occasionally with fibers from S3. Anal sphincter function is easy to observe or to palpate, whereas the urethral sphincter is evaluated best by electrodiagnostic procedures.

Tone of the anal sphincter can be observed, or the sphincter can be palpated with a gloved digit. Two other sacral reflexes also can be evaluated to help assess function of the pudendal and sacral spinal cord segments. The *bulbocavernosus reflex* is a sharp contraction of the sphincter in response to a squeeze of the bulb of the penis or the clitoris. The *perineal reflex* is a

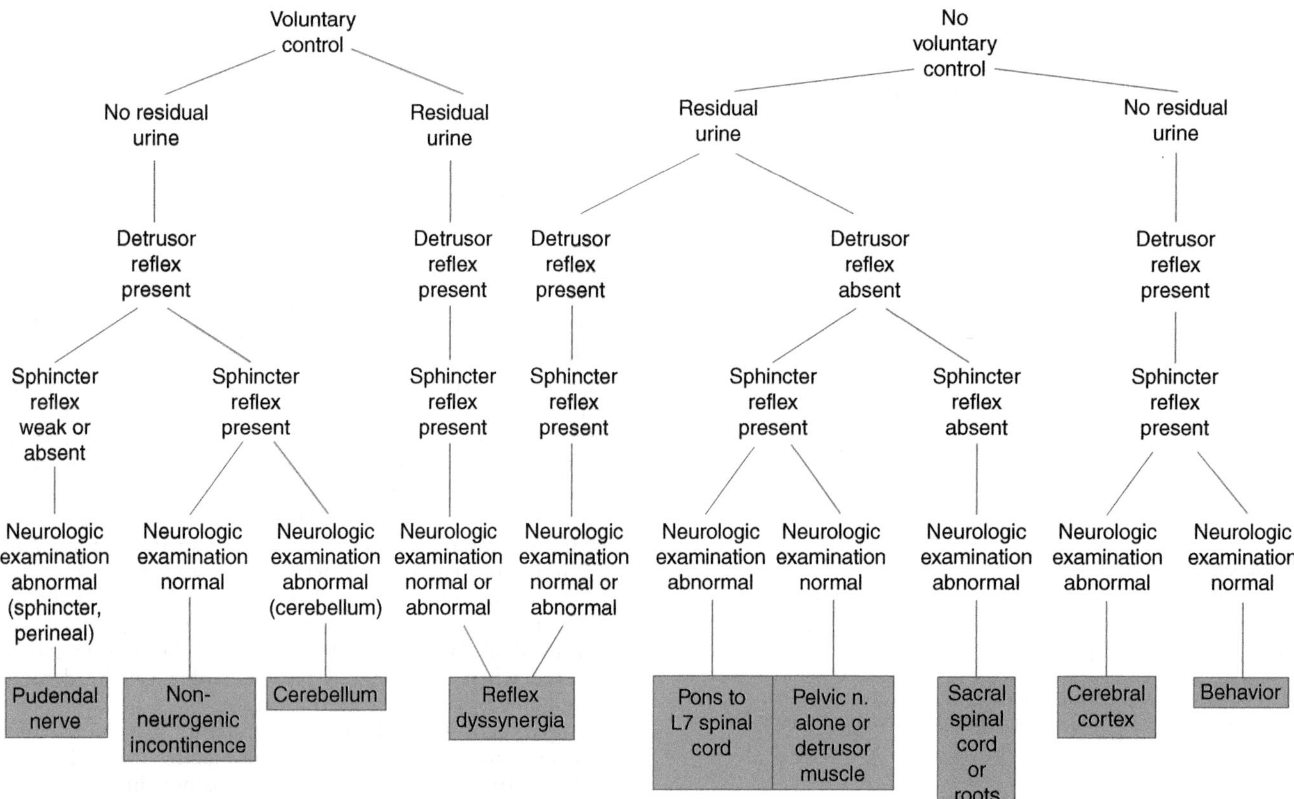

Figure 3-4 Algorithm for diagnosis of disorders of micturition. (From Oliver JE Jr, Osborne CA: Neurogenic urinary incontinence. In Kirk RW, editor: Current veterinary therapy, VII, Philadelphia, 1980, WB Saunders.)

contraction of the sphincter in response to a pinch or pinprick of the perineal region. The perineal reflex also is used to test sensory distribution in the perineal region. Because each side of the perineum can be tested individually, unilateral lesions can be identified.

Lesions of the sacral spinal cord, sacral roots, or pudendal nerves abolish these reflexes, and the anal sphincter is atonic. Frequently, there is a concurrent history of fecal incontinence.

The history, physical examination, and neurologic examination provide sufficient data to differentiate neurogenic from nonneurogenic bladder disorders and to localize the lesion in the nervous system if a neurogenic disorder is present (see Tables 3-1 and 3-2). Additional data are necessary for the formulation of diagnosis and prognosis.

Clinical Pathology

The minimum database includes a complete blood cell count, chemistry analysis, and urinalysis. Each is essential to the formulation of a prognosis of urinary tract dysfunction, and each may assist in the diagnosis of nonneurogenic problems of micturition.

Animals with neurogenic bladder disorders are likely to have urinary tract infections. Constant surveillance and appropriate treatment, when indicated, are imperative if a favorable outcome is to be expected.[49] Ureteral reflux is also a frequent complication of neurogenic bladder dysfunction. Reflux of infected urine may lead to chronic pyelonephritis and renal failure.

Imaging Studies of the Urinary Tract

Radiography and ultrasonography are important for the identification of nonneurogenic problems, for the evaluation of the extent of urinary tract disease (which may be a complication of neurogenic disorders), and for the assessment of the primary

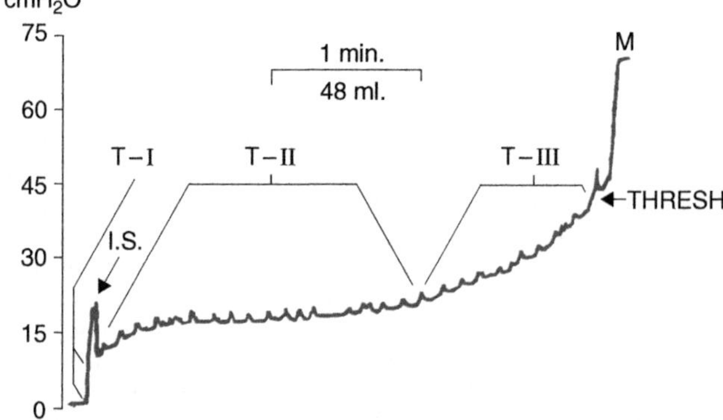

Figure 3-5 Cystometrogram of a dog showing segments of the tonus limb. *T-I*, Resting pressure; *T-II*, bladder filling pressure change (smooth muscle elasticity); *T-III*, bladder filling pressure change after capacity is reached. Scale indicates time and volume. *THRESH*, Threshold of detrusor reflex; *M*, maximal contraction; *I.S.*, initial spike, an artifact.

$$T-II = \frac{(\text{Pressure at inflection} - \text{Resting pressure}) \times 100}{\text{Volume}}$$

(From Oliver JE Jr, Young WO: Air cystometry in dogs under xylazine-induced restraint, Am J Vet Res 34:1433, 1973.)

neurologic problem. Survey abdominal and pelvic radiography including the entire urethra to assess for bony or soft tissue abnormalities of the lumbosacral spine and pelvis, and detect radiopaque urinary calculi. Contrast-enhanced cystourethrography, especially when performed in conjunction with cystometry, augments assessment of the functional morphology of the lower urinary tract.[41] Intravenous pyelogram evaluates

TABLE 3-3

*Normal Values for Cystometrograms (CMGs) Using Xylazine for Restraint**

	VALUES OF CMG	
Measurement	**Dog**	**Horse**
Tonus limb I	9.7 ± 4.3	1.9 ± 1.6
Tonus limb II	12.6 ± 12.2	1.0 ± 0.7
Threshold pressure	24.4 ± 10.0	22.0 ± 7.5
Threshold pressure minus tonus limb I	14.4 ± 8.7	14.4 ± 10.6
Threshold volume	206.6 ± 184.4	2554 ± 1087
Maximal contraction pressure	77.6 ± 33.8	100.1 ± 5.9

Data from Oliver JE Jr, Young WO: Air cystometry in dogs under xylazine-induced restraint, Am J Vet Res 34:1433–1435, 1973; and Clark ES et al: Cystometrography and urethral pressure profiles in healthy horse and pony mares, Am J Vet Res 48:552–555, 1987.
*All values are means ± SD and are given in centimeters of H_2O except for threshold volume, which is given in milliliters of air (see Figure 3-5).

the renal architecture. Ultrasonography assesses integrity of the bladder wall and lower urinary tract anatomy. Computed tomography gives anatomic detail on bony structures of the lumbosacral spine and pelvis. Magnetic resonance imaging provides detail on soft tissue structures associated with the spinal cord and pelvic region.

Urodynamic and Electrophysiologic Examinations

Urodynamic and electrophysiologic testing were not included in the minimum database described in Chapter 1 because they currently are not widely available. In some cases, however, these tests are needed to make a definitive diagnosis and assist with anatomic localization.[51]

The *cystometrogram* (CMG) measures intravesical pressure during a detrusor reflex (Figure 3-5).[41,52-54] A sustained detrusor reflex is difficult to document clinically in most cases. Additionally, the CMG provides data on threshold volume and pressure, capacity, ability of the bladder to fill at a normal pressure (a measure of elasticity of the bladder wall), and presence of uninhibited bladder contractions (a sign of denervation). Normal data from the CMG of the dog and horse are presented in Table 3-3.

The *urethral pressure profile* measures the pressure along the length of the urethra.[52,55-60] An EMG of the striated urethral sphincter can be recorded simultaneously. The maximum urethral closure pressure and the functional profile length are the most important parameters (Figure 3-6). Normal values are listed in Table 3-4. *Stress leak point pressure* is a functional technique used to simulate urethral compliance associated with an external abdominal press.[61]

Ideally, the CMG, urethral pressure profile, and stress leak point pressure recordings should be performed in awake animals without chemical restraint. However, it is often necessary to sedate animals due to their fractious nature, difficulty in catheterizing female animals, or the painful nature of their disease. Consequently, measurements are often recorded using chemical restraint or general anesthesia.[52,54,58,62-67] All anesthetic agents affect these urodynamic tests; however, propofol (0.8 mg/kg/min) may have a minimal impact on UPP recordings, whereas xylazine may be used for CMG recordings.[68] Alternatively, the animal may be anesthetized

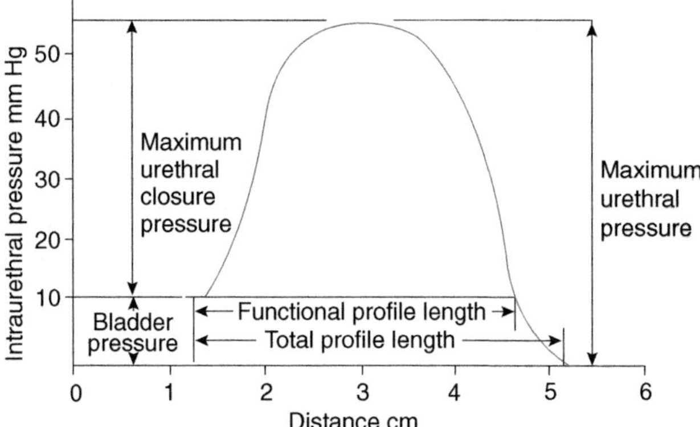

Figure 3-6 Schematic representation of the urethral closure pressure profile. (From Rosin A, Rosin E, Oliver JE Jr: Canine urethral pressure profile, Am J Vet Res 41:1113–1116, 1980.)

(using short-acting anesthetics such as propofol) for urethral catheter placement, allowed to recover, and then a recording can be made.[68]

Simultaneous measurement of the CMG and urinary flow allows more complete assessment of the function of the bladder and urethra, especially in disorders of coordination of bladder contraction and urethral relaxation.[69,70] An electromagnetic flow transducer records the flow of urine collected in a funnel. Intravesical pressure is measured simultaneously. The major disadvantage of this technique is the necessity of placing two catheters through the abdominal wall into the bladder. Normal dogs have minimal problems, but we have had leakage from cystocentesis with 22-gauge needles in animals with neurogenic bladders. This procedure must therefore be used with caution.[51]

Electromyography (EMG) of the skeletal muscles of the anal and urethral sphincters and other muscles in the pelvic diaphragm provides direct evidence of the status of innervation. The perineal or bulbocavernosus reflex also can be tested while a recording is being taken directly from these muscles in cases in which clinical evaluation is equivocal. To perform this, the animal must be maintained under a light plane of anesthesia to evoke the reflex contraction of the anal sphincter.

An EMG recorded from the anal sphincter while the urethra or the bladder is stimulated with a catheter electrode is termed an *electromyelograph* (EMyG).[51] Urethral stimulation evokes a response similar to the bulbocavernosus reflex. Stimulation of the bladder wall evokes a comparable response, except that the sensory pathway is in the pelvic nerves. The evoked bladder response is difficult to record in most animals. An EMyG from bladder stimulation provides evidence of the integrity of the pelvic nerves. The main advantages of these evoked tests are the following: (1) the response is objective, (2) the response can be measured accurately, and (3) the latencies are recorded that provide information about partial denervation.

Averaged *somatosensory-evoked responses* can be recorded from the scalp (cortex) or the spinal cord during stimulation of the bladder or the urethra (see the section on the somatosensory-evoked response in Chapter 4). The cortical-evoked response is a method of evaluating the sensory pathways. Results of these tests are useful for lesion localization. Table 3-5 summarizes data provided by physical examination findings and electrophysiologic tests.

The final diagnosis should include (1) location of the lesion in the nervous system, (2) cause of the lesion, (3) functional central nervous system (CNS) deficit, and (4) functional deficit related to micturition.

TABLE 3-4

*Normal Values for Urethral Pressure Profiles**

Study Animal (Condition)	Maximal Urethral Pressure (cm H_2O)	Maximal Urethral Closure Pressure (cm H_2O)	Functional Profile Length (cm)
Female dogs (xylazine)	35.2 ± 16.2	31.0 ± 15.3	7.2 ± 1.9
Male dogs (xylazine)	42.5 ± 5.3	36.79 ± 5.2	28.3 ± 3.9
Female dogs (medetomidine)	NA	25.4 ± 11.6	6.1 ± 1.1
Male dogs (medetomidine)	23.9 ± 3.2	29.5 ± 6.0	23.4 ± 1.8
Female dogs (no sedation)	90.18 ± 4.48	79.72 ± 4.61	8.68 ± 0.57
Male dogs (no sedation)	109.77 ± 11.52	99.77 ± 11.71	24.00 ± 0.9
Female cats, intact (xylazine)	76.6 ± 26.7	71.4 ± 25	4.4 ± 1.5
Female cats, ovariohysterectomized (xylazine)	81.3 ± 31.7	77.5 ± 31.3	5.78 ± 0.9
Male cats (xylazine)	163.2 ± 47.5	161.6 ± 47.1	10.53 ± 0.5
Female horse (xylazine)		43.4 ± 21.6	3.7 ± 1.4
Female horse (no sedation)		49.1 ± 19.4	5.0 ± 1.8

Data sources: Female and male dogs (xylazine)—Rosin A, Rosin E, Oliver JE Jr: Canine urethral pressure profile, Am J Vet Res 41:1113–1116, 1980 (values converted from mm Hg). Female and male dogs, no sedation—Richter KP, Ling GV: Effects of xylazine on the urethral pressure profile of healthy dogs, Am J Vet Res 46:1881–1886, 1985. Female cats, intact versus ovariohysterectomized (xylazine)—Gregory CR, Willits NH: Electromyographic and urethral pressure evaluations: assessment of urethral function in female and ovariohysterectomized female cats, Am J Vet Res 47:1472–1475, 1986. Male cats (xylazine)—Gregory CR et al: Electromyographic and urethral pressure profilometry: assessment of urethral function before and after perineal urethrostomy in cats, Am J Vet Res 45:2062–2065, 1984. Female and male dogs (medetomidine) — Rawlings CA, Barsanti JA, Chernosky AM: Results of cystometry and uretral pressure profilometry in dogs sedated with medetomidine or xylazine, Am J Vet Res 62:167–170, 2001. Female horse, xylazine or no sedation—Clark ES et al: Cystometrography and urethral pressure profiles in healthy horse and pony mares, Am J Vet Res 48:552–555, 1987.

*Values are means ± SD.

TABLE 3-5

Diagnostic Tests of Micturition

Test	Detrusor Reflex	Detrusor Tone and Capacity	Complete Voiding	Sensation to Bladder	Urethral Resistance/ Obstruction	Synchrony of Bladder and Urethra
Cystometrogram	+	+		+		
Urethral pressure profile					+	
Stress leak point pressure		+			+	
Flow	+	+			+	+
Evoked potentials				+		
Observation of voiding	+	+	+	+	+	+
Palpate bladder			+			
Measure residual urine			+			
Resistance to expression and catheterization					+	

+, Test evaluates this function or this anatomic component.

Treatment

Management of a case depends on the final diagnosis. The treatment of primary neurologic disease is described throughout this text. Functional deficits of micturition secondary to neurologic disease may be temporary or permanent, depending on the reversibility of the neurologic lesion and the maintenance of the integrity of the urinary system. If the bladder is severely infected and secondary fibrosis of the bladder wall occurs, normal function cannot be restored even if the neurologic lesion is corrected. This section presents management of the urinary tract based on the functional disorder of micturition. Table 3-6 lists the most common drugs used in the pharmacologic management of disorders of micturition.

Medical therapy includes control of the urinary tract infection and management of the functional abnormality of the bladder and urethra.[71-73] Treatment of urinary tract infections is described in detail in most general veterinary medical books.

Detrusor Areflexia with Sphincter Hypertonus

Lesions from the pons to the L7 spinal cord segments may abolish the detrusor reflex and may produce a UMN-type sphincter characterized by hyperreflexia and increased tone (see Table 3-2). The animal is unable to void, and the bladder is difficult if not impossible to express manually.

The primary consideration in all neurogenic bladder disorders is to evacuate the bladder completely at least three times daily. When tone in the urethra is exaggerated, manual expression is not only ineffective but also dangerous. Aseptic catheterization is required. Indwelling urethral catheters are associated with a higher risk of infection, and their long-term

TABLE 3-6

Drugs Used in Treating Disorders of Micturition

Drug Action	Drug	Dosage	Side Effects
Increase detrusor contractility	Bethanechol (Urecholine)	2.5-15 mg PO or SQ q8h (dog) 1.25-5 mg PO q12h (cat)	Cholinergic: GI hypermotility, bronchoconstriction
Decrease detrusor contractility	Propantheline (Pro-Banthine)	0.25-0.5 mg/kg PO q8-12h	Anticholinergic: decreased GI motility, decreased salivation, tachycardia
	Oxybutynin (Ditropan)	0.5 mg PO q8-12h	
Increase urethral resistance	Phenylpropanolamine	1.5 mg/kg PO q8-12h (dog and cat)	Sympathomimetic: urine retention, hypertension
	Diethylstilbestrol (in female)	0.1-1 mg/day PO for 3-5 days, then 1 mg/wk (dog)	Estrus, bone marrow toxicity
	Testosterone cypionate (male)	2 mg/kg IM at intervals of weeks to months	Caution in animals with prostatic hyperplasia, perineal hernia, perianal adenoma
Decrease urethral resistance	Phenoxybenzamine (Dibenzyline)	0.25-0.5 mg/kg PO q12h	Nonspecific α-adrenergic blocker: hypotension
	Prazosin	1 mg/15 kg PO q8-12h (dog) 0.25-0.5 mg q12-24h (cat)	α_1-adrenergic blocker: hypotension, salivation, sedation
	Acepromazine	up to 3 mg IV (dogs) 1-2 mg/kg PO q12-24h (cat)	hypotension, sedation
	Diazepam (Valium)	0.25-1 mg/kg PO q8-12h (dog) 1-2 mg/kg PO q12h (cat)	Centrally acting tranquilizer and skeletal muscle relaxant: sedation, hepatocellular necrosis in cats
	Dantrolene	1-5 mg/kg PO q8h (dog) 0.5-2 mg/kg PO q8h (cat)	Direct acting skeletal muscle relaxant: weakness, hepatoxicity, vomiting, hypotension

Modified from Oliver JE, Hoerlein BF, Mayhew IG: Veterinary neurology, Philadelphia, 1987, WB Saunders.
GI, Gastrointestinal; *PO*, orally; *q8h*, every 8 hours; *SQ*, subcutaneous.

use should be avoided if possible.[74] Female dogs often are at higher risks for developing urinary tract infection. Detrusor areflexia from overdistention (described later) requires an indwelling urethral catheter or intermittent catheterization.[75] An aseptic closed urine collection system is required for all animals with indwelling urethral catheters. Indiscriminant use of antibiotics in animals with indwelling urinary catheters should be avoided.

Urethral tone may be reduced pharmacologically with α-adrenergic blocking agents and skeletal muscle relaxants, making management easier (see Table 3-6).[66,76-78] Phenoxybenzamine, a nonspecific α-adrenergic blocking agent, is sometimes effective at a dosage of 0.5 mg/kg of body weight daily divided into two doses (small animals). Prazosin is an α_1-adrenergic blocking agent administered in dogs at 1 mg per every 15 kg of body weight once to three times daily and administered 30 minutes before bladder expression.[78] Hypotension is the most common side effect of α-adrenergic blocking agents. Diazepam is used for relaxation of the striated external urethral sphincter.

Bethanechol, a cholinergic agent, can be given to stimulate bladder contraction. We have not found it effective if the bladder is areflexic, however. If bladder contractions are present but are inadequate for good voiding, bethanechol in doses of 2.5 to 10 mg given subcutaneously three times daily may be beneficial. Side effects include increased motility of the gastrointestinal tract, salivation, and rarely bronchoconstriction. Oral doses of up to 50 mg also may be effective. Because bethanechol is a nonspecific cholinergic-acting agent (also will act on the nicotinic receptors of the preganglionic neurons), pretreatment with an α-adrenergic blocking agent may be necessary to prevent further contraction of the urethral sphincter.[14,71]

Urinalysis is performed weekly or anytime the urine appears abnormal. At the first sign of infection, urine is obtained for quantitative culture and sensitivity tests.[41] Appropriate antibiotic therapy should be continued until the urinalysis verifies resolution of the problem. Animals with urinary tract infections secondary to neurologic disease should be considered to have a "complicated" urinary tract infection and should receive a longer course of therapy than a dog with an "uncomplicated" or simple urinary tract infection. Caution should be exercised when using antibiotics in dogs with permanent neurologic disease. In these animals the probability of reinfection is great. Therefore the chronic use of antibiotic therapy may lead to the development of reinfection with multidrug-resistant organisms. Animals receiving antiinflammatory drugs such as corticosteroids are at increased risk of urinary tract infection. In addition, corticosteroids can suppress the inflammatory response to infection. Risk factors for urinary tract infection in dogs surgically treated for intervertebral disk disease include females, dogs that cannot ambulate or voluntarily urinate, dogs not administered perioperative cefazolin, and dogs whose body temperature falls to less than 35° C during anesthesia.[49] Asymptomatic infection may go undetected unless urine is cultured repeatedly for microorganisms.

If the detrusor reflex returns with good voiding of urine, the bladder is catheterized or ultrasounded periodically to ensure that minimal residual urine is present. Voiding is often incomplete in the early stages, and residual urine in quantities of 10 to 20 mL or more can result in a urinary tract infection.

Detrusor Areflexia With Normal Sphincter Tone

Some lesions of the spinal cord and brainstem may abolish the detrusor reflex without producing hypertonus of the urethral sphincter. The bladder can be expressed manually in many of these cases. The urethra of the female dog is short and has less resistance than observed with male dogs.[33,59,79,80] Manual expression may be effective even in the context of sphincter hypertonus. Manual expression, if adequate, and intermittent catheterization is less likely to produce infection than is indwelling urethral catheterization.[75] Other aspects of management are the same as when sphincter tone is increased.

Detrusor Areflexia With Sphincter Hypotonia

Lesions of the sacral spinal cord or nerve roots produce a deficit of the LMNs of both the bladder and sphincter. Management of the bladder is the same as that described previously.

Constant leakage of urine through an incompetent sphincter leads to soiling of the skin, irritation, and ulceration. Frequent evacuation of the bladder reduces the problem but does not eliminate it. Hydrotherapy, dry and padded bedding, and protective emollients are useful adjuncts.

Long-term management of the patient with sphincter atonia is problematic. Surgical reconstruction of the bladder neck and the urethra is sometimes successful. Prosthetic urethral sphincters have been successfully used in people, but the cost of these devices currently limits their applicability in animals.

Detrusor Areflexia from Overdistention

Severe overdistention of the bladder can disrupt the tight junctions between the detrusor muscle fibers, which prevents excitation-contraction coupling. Neural elements may be normal.

Complete evacuation of the bladder must be accomplished early and maintained for 1 to 2 weeks.[71,72] Manual expression is not recommended because of the increased stress on the detrusor muscle. Intermittent aseptic urethral catheterization can be performed at least three times a day. Long-term closed-system indwelling urethral catheterization should be avoided if possible. When necessary, the system should be used for several days, followed by intermittent catheterization. Function should return in 1 to 2 weeks. Bethanechol may be of benefit, especially if partial contractions are present. In some cases of chronic overdistention, return to function may not occur.

Frequent urinalysis with cultures when indicated, is mandatory. Infection in the overdistended bladder leads to fibrosis of the detrusor muscle, and adequate function cannot be restored in this case.

Detrusor Hyperreflexia

Frequent voiding of small volumes of urine, often without much warning and with little or no residual urine, is characteristic of detrusor hyperreflexia.[81] Partial long-tract lesions or abnormalities of the cerebellum may produce these signs. The condition is not usually detrimental to the patient, but it may be an early sign of a progressive disease of the nervous system. Additionally, it is socially unacceptable in the house pet. The condition must be differentiated from the small, contracted, irritable bladder associated with chronic cystitis.

Anticholinergic medication may be of benefit. Propantheline (Pro-Banthine) is used in dosages of 0.25 to 0.5 mg/kg of body weight every 8 to 12 hours. The lowest dose should be tried first, and the dose should be increased in small increments until a response is obtained. Oxybutynin may be more effective than propantheline in some cases. Overdosage may result in urine retention in addition to the other side effects characteristic of this group of drugs.[81]

Reflex Dyssynergia

Initiation of a detrusor reflex with voiding followed by an uncontrolled reflex contraction of the urethral sphincter is termed *reflex dyssynergia*. Partial lesions of the long tracts are presumed to be responsible.[31,37] The problem may be related to uninhibited reflexes of the external urethral sphincter (skeletal muscle) or to increased tone in the smooth muscle related to adrenergic innervation.

Limited reports in humans and dogs have not yet provided a definitive therapeutic regimen.[37,71,72] Skeletal muscle reflexes may be reduced with diazepam (centrally acting muscle relaxant) or dantrolene.[77,82] Sympathetic (adrenergic) activity can be reduced with an α-adrenergic blocking agent.[38,78]

Normal Detrusor Reflex With Decreased Sphincter Tone

Medical treatment is aimed at increasing urethral closure pressure.[43,73,83,84] Many incontinent female dogs respond well to hormonal supplementation.[73,83] If hormone therapy is ineffective in an animal with normal voiding but leakage, an α-adrenergic stimulating drug, such as phenylpropanolamine in combination or alone may be effective.[85] The dosage is 1.5 mg/kg of body weight administered orally every 8 to 12 hours.[84] Side effects include restlessness and irritability. Surgical management using colposuspension, cystourethropexy, and intraurethral injection procedures may be of benefit in cases refractory to medical management.[16,86-88] Colposuspension is a technique that moves the bladder neck from an intrapelvic to an intraabdominal position to restore continence by transferring the pressure to the proximal urethra and bladder neck.

CASE STUDIES

For the following cases, the reader should concentrate on the problem related to micturition, even though it may be only a part of the total deficit. Using Table 3-2, decide the location of the lesion causing the problem.

CASE STUDY 3-1 *HANS*

 veterinaryneurologycases.com

▪ Signalment

Canine, dachshund, male, 5 years old.

▪ History

The dog became paralyzed in the pelvic limbs last night. The dog was alone in a fenced-in backyard when the owners found him.

▪ Physical Examination

The bladder is large and easily palpated. It cannot be manually expressed, even with considerable pressure. The dog makes no attempt to initiate urination.

▪ Neurologic Examination

Mental status

Alert

Continued

CASE STUDY 3-1 *HANS—cont'd*

Gait and posture
Paraplegic

Postural reactions
Normal in the thoracic limbs and absent in the pelvic limbs

Spinal reflexes
The spinal reflexes are normal in the thoracic limbs. In the pelvic limbs the patellar reflexes are exaggerated (+3) bilaterally, and the flexion reflexes are normal (+2). The perineal and bulbocavernosus reflexes are present. The anal sphincter has good tone. The cutaneous trunci reflex is absent caudal to L1.

Cranial nerves
Normal

Spinal palpation
Palpation of the spine reveals paraspinal hyperesthesia from T13 to L2.

Sensory evaluation
Deep pain perception is present in the pelvic limbs

▪ Lesion Localization
The neurologic examination indicates an UMN paralysis of the pelvic limbs and a T3 to L3 myelopathy. The sensory examination localizes the lesion to T13-L2. The bladder problem can be characterized as detrusor areflexia with sphincter hypertonia, which is typical of a lesion cranial to L7. Cystometry confirms detrusor areflexia.

▪ Diagnosis
The dog has a herniated intervertebral disk, which is decompressed by hemilaminectomy. Seven days after surgery, voluntary movements of the pelvic limbs are seen, and voiding begins with minimal pressure of the abdomen.

▪ Diagnostic Plan and Treatment
Management of the bladder should include intermittent urinary catheterization and attempts with manual bladder expression. Administration of an α-adrenergic blocking agent relaxes the urethral sphincter for easier manual bladder expression. Voiding returned to normal in 10 days. Urinalysis is normal upon discharge.

CASE STUDY 3-2 *TWINKIE*

 veterinaryneurologycases.com

▪ Signalment
Canine, Pekingese, female, 6 years old.

▪ History
The dog suddenly became paralyzed in the pelvic limbs while playing with the owners' children. When first seen by the referring veterinarian 4 hours later, the dog was unable to ambulate with increased muscle tone in the pelvic limbs, had exaggerated patellar reflexes but decreased flexion reflexes bilaterally, and no sensation caudal to L4 vertebra.

▪ Physical Examination
The dog is seen 12 hours after the onset of paralysis. Urine is leaking during the trip to the clinic, and the dog is obviously in pain. The bladder is large and is easily expressed on palpation.

▪ Neurologic examination
Mental status
The dog is alert and anxious.

Gait and posture
The dog is recumbent and unable to ambulate in the pelvic limbs.

Postural reactions
The thoracic limbs are normal. Postural reactions are absent in both pelvic limbs.

Spinal reflexes
Spinal reflexes are absent in the pelvic limbs. The perineal reflex is absent, and the anal sphincter is dilated.

Cranial nerves
Normal

Sensory evaluation
No deep pain perception exists caudal to T13.

▪ Lesion Localization
The dog has LMN paralysis of the pelvic limbs and the sphincters. This finding indicates a lesion from L4 through S3. Initially the lesion spared the L4-6 segments because the patellar reflex was intact and extension of the limb occurred. The loss of pain perception has progressed from L4 to T13 in 8 hours, and the patellar reflex has been lost, indicating a progressive lesion. Detrusor areflexia and sphincter areflexia are present, consistent with a lesion of the sacral segments of the spinal cord.

▪ Diagnosis
The dog has a herniated disk with ischemic myelomalacia.

▪ Diagnostic Plan and Treatment
The prognosis is so poor based on examination findings that no other tests are performed. Cystometry would confirm the detrusor areflexia. The urethral pressure profile would be expected to show pressures below normal. EMG would demonstrate no voluntary or reflex activity, but fibrillation potentials would not be present this early. If management were attempted, manual evacuation of the bladder probably would be effective.

CASE STUDY 3-3 CHI-CHI

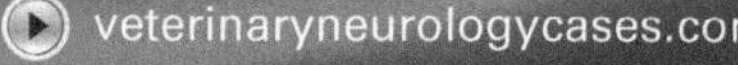

Signalment
Canine, Chihuahua, male, 3 years old.

History
The dog has had generalized seizures at least three times in the past 2 weeks. The previous medical history is noncontributory. The dog started urinating in the house within the past 3 months, although he was well house-trained since a puppy. The dog has not been administered any medications.

Physical Examination
The skull is dome shaped, and the fontanelle is 1.5 cm in diameter. The bladder is empty on palpation.

Neurologic Examination
Mental status
The dog is alert.

Gait and posture
Normal

Postural reactions
The postural reactions are judged to be a bit slow.

Spinal reflexes
Normal

Cranial nerves
Normal

Sensory evaluation
Normal

Lesion Localization
The seizures indicate abnormality of the forebrain. This may represent a primary problem involving the forebrain or a metabolic problem resulting in seizures. The change in urination habits also could be either forebrain or metabolic (polyuria).

Ruleouts
1. Hydrocephalus
2. Encephalitis
3. Tumor (unlikely)
4. Idiopathic epilepsy

Diagnostic Plan
A laboratory evaluation is indicated to rule out metabolic diseases. Brain imaging would assess presence of a structural lesion in the brain. Cystometry would assess detrusor muscle function.

Results and Diagnosis
A CBC, chemistry profile, and urinalysis were within normal limits. Computed tomography confirmed hydrocephalus. The cystometrogram was normal and showed adequate capacity and a good detrusor reflex. The voiding behavior was related to cerebral dysfunction.

Treatment
The dog was treated with corticosteroids and complete remission of signs resulted (see Chapter 12 for a discussion of hydrocephalus).

REFERENCES

1. Oliver JE, Selcer RR: Neurogenic causes of abnormal micturition in the dog and cat, Vet Clin North Am 4(3):517–524, 1974.
2. Fletcher TF, Bradley WE: Neuroanatomy of bladder-urethra, J Urol 119:153–160, 1978.
3. Petras JM, Cummings JF: Sympathetic and parasympathetic innervation of the urinary bladder and urethra, Brain Res 153:363–369, 1978.
4. Oliver JE Jr, Bradley WE, Fletcher TF: Identification of preganglionic parasympathetic neurons in the sacral spinal cord of the cat, J Comp Neurol 137(3):321–328, 1969.
5. Morgan C, deGroat WC, Nadelhaft I: The spinal distribution of sympathetic preganglionic and visceral primary afferent neurons that send axons into the hypogastric nerves of the cat, J Comp Neurol 243:23–40, 1986.
6. Oliver JE Jr, Bradley WE, Fletcher TF: Spinal cord representation of the micturition reflex, J Comp Neurol 137(3):329–346, 1969.
7. Elbadawi A, Schenk EA: A new theory of the innervation of bladder musculature. Part 4. Innervation of the vesicourethral junction and external urethral sphincter, J Urol 111(5):613–615, 1974.
8. Moreau PM: Neurogenic disorders of micturition in the dog and cat, Compend Contin Educ Vet 4(1):12–22, 1982.
9. Rohner TJ, Raezer DM, Wein AJ: Contractile responses of dog bladder neck muscle to adrenergic drugs, J Urol 105:657–661, 1971.
10. Sundin T, Dahlström A, Norlén L: The sympathetic innervation and adrenoreceptor function of the human lower urinary tract in the normal state and after parasympathetic denervation, Invest Urol 14(4):322–328, 1977.
11. Oliver JE: Disorders of micturition. In Hoerlein BF, editor: Canine neurology, ed 3, Philadelphia, 1978, WB Saunders.
12. deGroat WC: Booth AM: Physiology of the urinary bladder and urethra, Ann Intern Med 92(2):312–315, 1980.
13. Sundin T, Dahlström A: The sympathetic innervation of the urinary bladder and urethra in the normal state and after parasympathetic denervation at the spinal root level. An experimental study in cats, Scand J Urol Nephrol 7(2):131–149, 1973.
14. O'Brien D: Neurogenic disorders of micturition, Vet Clin North Am Small Anim Pract 18(3):529–544, 1988.
15. O'Brien DP: Disorders of the urogenital system, Semin Vet Med Surg (Small Anim) 5(1):57–66, 1990.
16. Rawlings CA, Coates JR, Purinton PT: Evaluation of a selective neurectomy model for low urethral pressure incontinence in female dogs, Am J Vet Res 66:695–699, 2005.
17. Samson MD, Reddy VK: Localization of the sacral parasympathetic nucleus in the dog, Am J Vet Res 43(10):1833–1836, 1982.
18. Purinton PT, Oliver JE: Spinal cord origin of innervation to the bladder and urethra of the dog, Exp Neurol 65(2):422–434, 1979.
19. Purinton PT, Oliver JE Jr, Bradley WE: Differences in routing of pelvic visceral afferent fibers in the dog and cat, Exp Neurol 73(3):725–731, 1981.

20. Fowler CJ, Griffiths D, deGroat WC: The neural control of micturition, Nat Rev Neurosci 9:453–466, 1970.
21. Cullen WC, Fletcher TF, Bradley WE: Histology of the canine urethra II. Morphometry of the male pelvic urethra, Anat Rec 199(2):187–195, 1981.
22. Cullen WC, Fletcher TF, Bradley WE: Histology of the canine urethra. I. Morphometry of the female urethra, Anat Rec 199(2):177–186, 1981.
23. Cullen WC, Fletcher TF, Bradley WE: Morphometry of the male feline pelvic urethra, J Urol 129:186–189, 1983.
24. Cullen WC, Fletcher TF, Bradley WE: Morphometry of the female feline urethra, J Urol 29:190–192, 1983.
25. Oliver J, Bradley W, Fletcher T: Spinal cord distribution of the somatic innervation of the external urethral sphincter of the cat, J Neurol Sci 10(1):11–23, 1970.
26. Kuru M, Iwanaga T: Ponto-sacral connections in the medial reticulospinal tract subserving storage of urine, J Comp Neurol 127:2–41, 1966.
27. Gjone R, Setekleiv J: Excitatory and inhibitory bladder responses to stimulation of the cerebral cortex in the cat, Acta Physiol Scand 59:337–348, 1963.
28. Langworthy OR, Hesser FH: An experimental study of micturition released from cerebral control, Am J Physiol 115:694–700, 1936.
29. Bradley WE, Teague CT: Cerebellar influence on the micturition reflex, Exp Neurol 23:399–411, 1969.
30. deGroat WC: Nervous control of the urinary bladder of the cat, Brain Res 87:201–211, 1975.
31. Oliver JE: Dysuria caused by reflex dyssynergia. In Kirk RW, editor: Current veterinary therapy, ed 8, Philadelphia, 1983, WB Saunders.
32. Bradley WE, Timm GW: Physiology of micturition, Vet Clin North Am 4(3):487–500, 1974.
33. Augsburger HR, Cruz-Orive LM, Arnold S: Morphology and stereology of the female canine urethra correlated with the urethral pressure profile, Acta Anat (Basel) 148(4):197–205, 1993.
34. O'Brien DP, Johnson GC: Dysautonomia and autonomic neuropathies, Vet Clin North Am Small Anim Pract 32:251–265, 2002.
35. Kaplan SA, Chancellor MB, Blaivas JG: Bladder and sphincter behavior in patients with spinal cord lesions, J Urol 146(1):113–117, 1991.
36. Galeano C, Jubelin B, Germain L: Micturitional reflexes in chronic spinalized cats: the underactive detrusor and detrusor-sphincter dyssynergia, Neurourol Urodyn 5:45–63, 1986.
37. Barsanti JA, Coates JR, Bartges JW: Detrusor-sphincter dyssynergia, Vet Clin North Am Small Anim Pract 26(2):327–338, 1996.
38. Diaz Espineira MM, Viehoff FW: Nickel RF: Idiopathic detrusor-urethral dyssynergia in dogs: a retrospective analysis of 22 cases, J Small Anim Pract 39(6):264–270, 1998.
39. Gookin JL, Bunch SE: Detrusor-striated sphincter dyssynergia in a dog, J Vet Intern Med 10(5):339–344, 1996.
40. Coates JR: Urethral dyssynergia in lumbosacral syndrome, Proc ACVIM, Chicago, pp 299–302, 1999.
41. Barsanti JA: Diagnostic procedures in urology, Vet Clin North Am Small Anim Pract 14(1):3–14, 1984.
42. Arnold S: Relationship of incontinence to neutering. In Kirk RW, Bonagura JD, editors: Kirk's current veterinary therapy XI: small animal practice, Philadelphia, 1992, WB Saunders.
43. Gregory SP: Developments in the understanding of the pathophysiology of urethral sphincter mechanism incompetence in the bitch, Br Vet J 150(2):135–150, 1994.
44. Holt PE: Urinary incontinence in the bitch due to sphincter mechanism incompetence: prevalence in referred dogs and retrospective analysis of sixty cases, J Small Anim Pract 26(4):181–190, 1985.
45. Aaron A, Eggleton K, Power C: Urethral sphincter mechanism incompetence in male dogs: a retrospective analysis of 54 cases, Vet Rec 139(22):542–546, 1996.
46. Keane DP, O'Sullivan S: Urinary incontinence: anatomy, physiology, and pathophysiology, Baillieres Clin Obstet Gynaecol 14:207–226, 2000.
47. Lane IF, Lappin MR: Urinary incontinence and congenital urogenital anomalies in small animals. In Bonagura JD, Kirk RW, eds: Kirk's current veterinary therapy XII, Philadelphia, 1995, Saunders, pp 1022–1026.
48. Guilford WG, Shaw DP, O'Brien DP: Fecal incontinence, urinary incontinence, and priapism associated with multifocal distemper encephalomyelitis in a dog, J Am Vet Med Assoc 197(1):90–92, 1990.
49. Stiffler KS, Stevenson MAM, Sanchez S: Prevalence and characterization of urinary tract infections in dogs with surgically treated type 1 intervertebral disc extrusion, Vet Surg 35:330–336, 2006.
50. Lane IF: A diagnostic approach to micturition disorders, Vet Med Small Anim Clin 98:49–57, 2003.
51. Oliver JE: Urodynamic assessment. In Oliver JE, Hoerlein BF, editors: Veterinary neurology, Philadelphia, 1987, WB Saunders.
52. Barsanti JA, Finco DR, Brown J: Effect of atropine on cystometry and urethral pressure profilometry in the dog, Am J Vet Res 49(1):112–114, 1988.
53. Johnson CA, Beemsterboer JM, Gray PR: Effects of various sedatives on air cystometry in dogs, Am J Vet Res 49(9):1525–1528, 1988.
54. Oliver JE, Young WO: Air cystometry in dogs under xylazine-induced restraint, Am J Vet Res 34(11):1433–1435, 1973.
55. Clark ES, Semrad SD, Bichsel P: Cystometrography and urethral pressure profiles in healthy horse and pony mares, Am J Vet Res 48(4):552–555, 1987.
56. Kay AD, Lovoie JP: Urethral pressure profilometry in mares, J Am Vet Med Assoc 191:212–216, 1987.
57. Gregory CR, Willits NH: Electromyographic and urethral pressure evaluations: assessment of urethral function in female and ovariohysterectomized female cats, Am J Vet Res 47(7):1472–1475, 1986.
58. Richter KP, Ling GV: Effects of xylazine on the urethral pressure profile of healthy dogs, Am J Vet Res 46(9):1881–1886, 1985.
59. Rosin A, Rosin E, Oliver J: Canine urethral pressure profile, Am J Vet Res 41(7):1113–1116, 1980.
60. Rosin AE, Barsanti JA: Diagnosis of urinary incontinence in dogs: role of the urethral pressure profile, J Am Vet Med Assoc 178(8):814–822, 1981.
61. Rawlings CA, Coates JR, Chernosky A: Stress leak point pressures and urethral pressure profile tests in clinically normal female dogs, Am J Vet Res 60(6):676–678, 1999.
62. Oliver JE Jr, Young WO: Evaluation of pharmacologic agents for restraint in cystometry in the dog and cat, Am J Vet Res 34(5):665–668, 1973.
63. Rawlings CA, Barsanti JA, Chernosky A: Results of cystometry and urethral pressure profilometry in dogs sedated with medetomidine or xylazine, Am J Vet Res 62:167–170, 2001.
64. Combrisson H, Robain G, Cotard JP: Comparative effects of xylazine and propofol on the urethral pressure profile of healthy dogs, Am J Vet Res 54(12):1986–1989, 1993.
65. Gregory SP, Holt PE: Comparison of stressed simultaneous urethral pressure profiles between anesthetized continent and incontinent bitches with urethral sphincter mechanism incompetence, Am J Vet Res 54(2):216–222, 1993.

66. Straeter-Knowlen IM, Marks SL, Speth RC: Effect of succinylcholine, diazepam, and dantrolene on the urethral pressure profile of anesthetized, healthy, sexually intact male cats, Am J Vet Res 55(12):1739–1744, 1994.
67. Barsanti JA, Mahaffey MB, Crowell WA: Cystometry in dogs under oxymorphone and acepromazine restraint, Am J Vet Res 45(10):2152–2153, 1984.
68. Goldstein RE, Westropp JL: Urodynamic testing in the diagnosis of small animal micturition, Clin Tech Small Anim Pract 20:65–72, 2005.
69. Moreau PM, Lees GE, Gross DR: Simultaneous cystometry and uroflowmetry (micturition study) for evaluation of the caudal part of the urinary tract in dogs: studies of the technique, Am J Vet Res 44(9):1769–1773, 1983.
70. Moreau PM, Lees GE, Gross DR: Simultaneous cystometry and uroflowmetry (micturition study) for evaluation of the caudal part of the urinary tract in dogs: reference values for healthy animals sedated with xylazine, Am J Vet Res 44(9):1774–1781, 1983.
71. Fischer JR, Lane IF: Medical treatment of voiding dysfunction in dogs and cats, Vet Med 98:67–73, 2003.
72. Lane IF: Diagnosis and management of urinary retention, Vet Clin North Am Small Anim Pract 30:25–57, 2000.
73. Lane IF: Treating urinary incontinence, Vet Med 98:58–63, 2003.
74. Bubenik LJ, Hosgood GL, Waldron DR: Frequency of urinary tract infection in catheterized dogs and comparison of bacterial culture and susceptibility testing results for catheterized and noncatheterized dogs with urinary tract infections, J Am Vet Med Assoc 231:893–899, 2007.
75. Bubenik LJ, Hosgood G: Urinary tract infection in dogs with thoracolumbar intervertebral disc herniation and urinary bladder dysfunction managed by manual expression, indwelling catheterization or intermittent catheterization, Vet Surg 37:791–800, 2008.
76. Khanna OP, Gonick P: Effects of phenoxybenzamine hydrochloride on canine lower urinary tract: clinical implications, Urology 6(3):323–330, 1975.
77. Straeter-Knowlen IM, Marks SL, Rishniw M: Urethral pressure response to smooth and skeletal muscle relaxants in anesthetized, adult male cats with naturally acquired urethral obstruction, Am J Vet Res 56(7):919–923, 1995.
78. Fischer JR, Lane IF, Cribb AE: Urethral pressure profile and hemodynamic effects of phenoxybenzamine and prazosin in non-sedated male beagle dogs, Can J Vet Res 67:30–38, 2003.
79. Arnold S, Chew DJ, Hubler M: Reproducibility of urethral pressure profiles in clinically normal sexually intact female dogs by use of microtransducer catheters, Am J Vet Res 54(8):1347–1351, 1993.
80. Awad SA, Downie JE: The effect of adrenergic drugs and hypogastric nerve stimulation on the canine urethra. A radiologic and urethral pressure study, Invest Urol 13(4):298–301, 1976.
81. Lappin MR, Barsanti JA: Urinary incontinence secondary to idiopathic detrusor instability: cystometrographic diagnosis and pharmacologic management in two dogs and a cat, J Am Vet Med Assoc 191(11):1439–1442, 1987.
82. Teague CT, Merrill DC: Effect of baclofen and dantrolene on bladder stimulator-induced detrusor-sphincter dyssynergia in dogs, Urology 11(5):531–535, 1978.
83. Holt PE: Pathophysiology and treatment of urethral sphincter mechanism incompetence in the incontinent bitch, Vet Med Int 3:15–26, 1992.
84. Richter KP, Ling GV: Clinical response and urethral pressure profile changes after phenylpropanolamine in dogs with primary sphincter incompetence, J Am Vet Med Assoc 187(6):605–611, 1985.
85. Creed KE: Effect of hormones on urethral sensitivity to phenylephrine in normal and incontinent dogs, Res Vet Sci 34(2):177–181, 1983.
86. Arnold S, Hubler M, Lott-Stolz G: Treatment of urinary incontinence in bitches by endoscopic injection of glutaraldehyde cross-linked collagen, J Small Anim Pract 37(4):163–168, 1996.
87. Arnold S, Jager P, DiBartola SP: Treatment of urinary incontinence in dogs by endoscopic injection of Teflon, J Am Vet Med Assoc 195(10):1369–1374, 1989.
88. White RN: Urethropexy for the management of urethral sphincter mechanism incompetence in the bitch, J Small Anim Pract 42:481–486, 2001.

CHAPTER 4

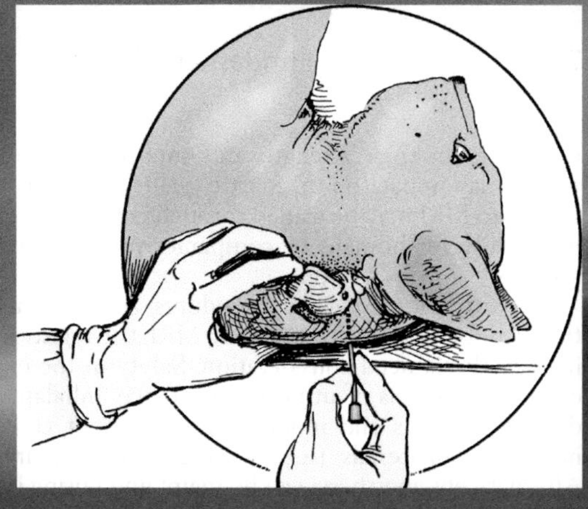

Confirming a Diagnosis

After the history has been taken and the physical and neurologic examinations have been completed, a list of neurologic problems is made. From this list of problems, a specific and accurate anatomic diagnosis must be established. Chapters 1 and 2 provide the information necessary for identifying neurologic problems and for making an anatomic diagnosis. Once an anatomic diagnosis is made, a systematic and ordered list of potential disease processes that can manifest with problems similar to that of the animal being examined, a differential diagnosis, is constructed. Chapters 5 through 15 elaborate on each problem in terms of arriving at a definitive diagnosis through appropriate diagnostic tests. The differential diagnosis is ordered from most likely to least likely diseases. This chapter discusses the tests available; indicates the feasibility of performing them; suggests references for further reading on techniques and interpretation; and outlines the indications, contraindications, and limitations of the tests.

CLINICAL LABORATORY STUDIES: HEMATOLOGY, BLOOD CHEMISTRY ANALYSIS, AND URINALYSIS

Availability

All clinical practices have access to routine hematology studies, chemistry analysis, and urinalysis.

Indications

A laboratory database is required for all ill animals so that common diseases are not overlooked and the general status of the animal can be assessed. Clinical laboratory studies are especially important in evaluating animals with brain disorders, seizures, signs of multisystem disease, and where general anesthesia is required for diagnostic procedures or surgery. Occasionally, blood gas analysis is required to assess aspects such as ventilation, oxygenation, and acid-base status of the patient not appreciated with routine blood chemistry analysis. Similarly, concentrations of electrolytes in their ionized states (i.e., ionized calcium) may be useful in assessing the metabolic status of the patient.

In recent years, disorders of inborn errors of metabolism have been identified antemortem through measurement of the concentration of organic acids in specimens such as blood and urine.[1,2] These disorders are discussed in Chapter 15. Few specialized laboratory perform these tests. It is important to use a laboratory experienced in the evaluation of animal samples.

DIAGNOSTIC IMAGING

Unlike all other body systems, normal neurologic function is largely predicated on normal structure. As such, for many neurologic problems much of the diagnostic workup entails the use of diagnostic imaging to establish the presence of an abnormal structure of the nervous system. For this reason, it is essential that an accurate anatomic diagnosis is established so that the appropriate region of the nervous system is evaluated. An incorrect anatomic diagnosis may lead to misdiagnosis or errors in judgment regarding the clinical relevancy of imaging findings.

Magnetic Resonance Imaging

Availability

With ever greater frequency, magnetic resonance imaging (MRI) is becoming more available to veterinarians in general and specialty practice. Imaging centers dedicated to MRI for small animals are becoming established throughout the United States and other parts of the world. Many of these facilities have an onsite board-certified veterinary anesthesiologist to anesthetize animals and access via telemedicine to board-certified radiologists to provide interpretation of studies. In most instances, prior screening of suitable cases should be done in concert with a neurologist to ensure the appropriate region (i.e., correct anatomic diagnosis) of the nervous system is imaged. For many general practitioners these facilities provide ready access for those owners willing to pursue diagnostic evaluation. MRI units also are becoming more commonplace for large and small animal specialty veterinary hospitals depending on the individual hospital's ability to support the expense. Likewise, most veterinary schools have MRI capabilities. MRI units vary in their strength and sophistication of software, which may impact on diagnostic quality. Alternatively, accessibility to MRI may be gained through contracts with an imaging facility for humans or companies providing mobile MRI services.

As with many imaging procedures, animals must be anesthetized for MRI. When pursuing MRI, the logistics of providing anesthesia need consideration. Safety in the environment of an MRI unit is of utmost importance. Inhalant anesthesia delivery systems and monitoring equipment constructed of nonferrous materials (e.g., MRI compatible) are available. Alternatively, anesthesia can be maintained using intermittent boluses or constant rate infusion of anesthetics.

Indications

Without question, the advent of MRI in veterinary medicine has revolutionized the diagnostic acumen in examining neurologic animals. The primary reason for this is related to the superior soft tissue contrast that MRI provides, allowing differentiation of anatomic structures. No other imaging procedure provides similar soft tissue discrimination along with exceptional resolution. Moreover, imaging can be performed in different planes (axial, sagittal, dorsal) without a loss of resolution enabling examination of complex anatomic regions. Consequently, MRI is the preferred imaging modality for the assessment of nearly all neurologic problems regardless of the site of the lesion (i.e., brain, spinal cord, and to a lesser degree, the peripheral nervous system [PNS]).

MRI is based on the magnetic properties of hydrogen atoms, which are extremely abundant in tissues containing water, protein, and lipids. With its unpaired electron, the positively charged hydrogen atoms spin around their axis, similar to a planet, and create small magnetic fields. Placed within the external magnetic field of the MRI unit, the orientation of the hydrogen atoms align together, akin to the needle of a compass placed beside a magnet. Energy in the form of a radiofrequency pulse changes the alignment of the atoms. Once the radiofrequency pulse is removed, the perturbed atoms return to their previous orientation and in doing so release energy, a radiofrequency pulse, back to the environment. It is this radiofrequency pulse that helps form the resultant image. The rate at which this occurs differs for different tissues based on inherent tissue characteristics. Two time constants, termed T1 and T2, describe this process. The T1 and T2 constants vary between different tissues more greatly than tissue density, which explains the better soft tissue contrast provided by MRI over computed tomography (CT).[3] A series of images, called a pulse sequence, can be acquired based or "weighted" on the T1 or T2 properties, referred to as T1-weighted (T1W) or T2-weighted (T2W) images. These two image types form the backbone of MRI. The resultant images are gray scale images in which the degree of relative darkness or lightness is referred to as intensity. Dark or relative black areas are called hypointense and light or relatively white areas are called hyperintense. Typically, the T1W images have excellent resolution, which allows identification of anatomic structures. In general, nervous tissues are homogeneously gray while structures containing fluids with low protein content such as cerebrospinal fluid (CSF) are hypointense or black. T2W images are capable of delineating gray and white matter structures whereas fluids such as CSF are hyperintense or white. Often T2W images are used to identify pathology. Moreover, T1W sequences are performed after intravenous administration of gadolinium-based contrast media. Postcontrast T1W images are compared with T1W images before administration of contrast media. The use of intravenous administration of contrast media can increase the conspicuity of a lesion and better define its borders by creating greater contrast between the lesion and surrounding tissue.[4] Contrast media accomplishes this by altering the local magnetic environment, causing the T1 constant to shorten, which increases the signal intensity.[4] In tissues where contrast media may accumulate related to an abnormal vascular supply such as a tumor, the lesion becomes hyperintense on T1W images (Figure 4-1). In addition, a variety of sequences have been designed that aim to suppress the signal from certain tissues, such as CSF and fat. Many of these sequences are referred to as "inversion recovery" sequences. Fluid attenuated inversion recovery (FLAIR) can be obtained as a T2W sequence, which maintains the contrast between gray and white matter, yet it suppresses the signal from fluid with low or no protein content such as CSF so that it is hypointense rather than hyperintense (Figure 4-2). This sequence allows improved identification of pathologies, such as tissue edema, and aids in identifying those lesions anatomically adjacent to areas such as a ventricle.[5,6] Short tau inversion recovery (STIR) is another sequence with characteristics of a T2W image, yet the normal hyperintense signal of fat is suppressed.[7] Alternatively, the normal signal intensity of fat can be suppressed on any sequence using a different technique (chemical fat suppression pulse). Many times fat suppression is used in sequences performed after intravenous administration of contrast media to make lesions more conspicuous. Some sequences are designed to highlight blood products as are found in hemorrhage. One such sequence is called T2*-weighted (T2 "star" weighted) (Figure 4-3). This sequence takes advantage of the magnetic properties of hemosiderin, oxy-, deoxy-, and methemoglobin and their location intracellularly or extracellularly to identify areas of accumulation of these blood products in hemorrhage.[8] Whereas most sequences take several minutes to acquire, sequences taking several seconds are available to allow rapid identification of lesions or pathology such as increased CSF protein content in meningitis, which is often not observed with conventional sequences.[9] Lastly, sequences can be performed to investigate functional disturbances, such as blood flow (MR angiography), ischemia (diffusion weighted imaging), dynamic contrast enhancement, and MR spectroscopy, which defines the molecular makeup of a lesion.

Proper patient positioning is crucial. Animals should be positioned with the long axis (i.e., vertebral column) in straight alignment. Likewise, precise transverse alignment allows for comparison between affected and normal structures at the same anatomic site. Some disease processes necessitate that the animal be positioned in a particular manner to observe lesions and help define potential surgical interventions. Such lesions are referred to as dynamic lesions. Repeated imaging of an animal in differing position is often performed in large-breed dogs with caudal cervical spondylomyelopathy or with degenerative lumbosacral stenosis.

To effectively communicate the results of imaging studies with other veterinarians for consultation or referral, a standard approach to describe lesions should be performed. One such approach is described here. Lesions should be characterized based on number (single or multiple), intensity (hypointense, hyperintense, isointense [terms differ based on imaging modality in relationship to an adjacent normal area]), distribution of the intensity (homogeneous or heterogeneous), lesion borders (well or poorly defined), anatomic location of the lesion and lesion location in reference to the central nervous system (CNS) and meninges (intracranial lesions are considered intraaxial or extraaxial based on location within the brain parenchyma or not, respectively). Lesions affecting the spinal cord are considered extradural (outside the dura), intradural/extramedullary (contained within the subarachnoid space), or intramedullary (within the spinal cord parenchyma). Similarly, lesions are characterized based on pattern of contrast enhancement. Descriptions should detail degree and distribution of contrast enhancement. Finally, secondary consequences to the surrounding anatomy, such as

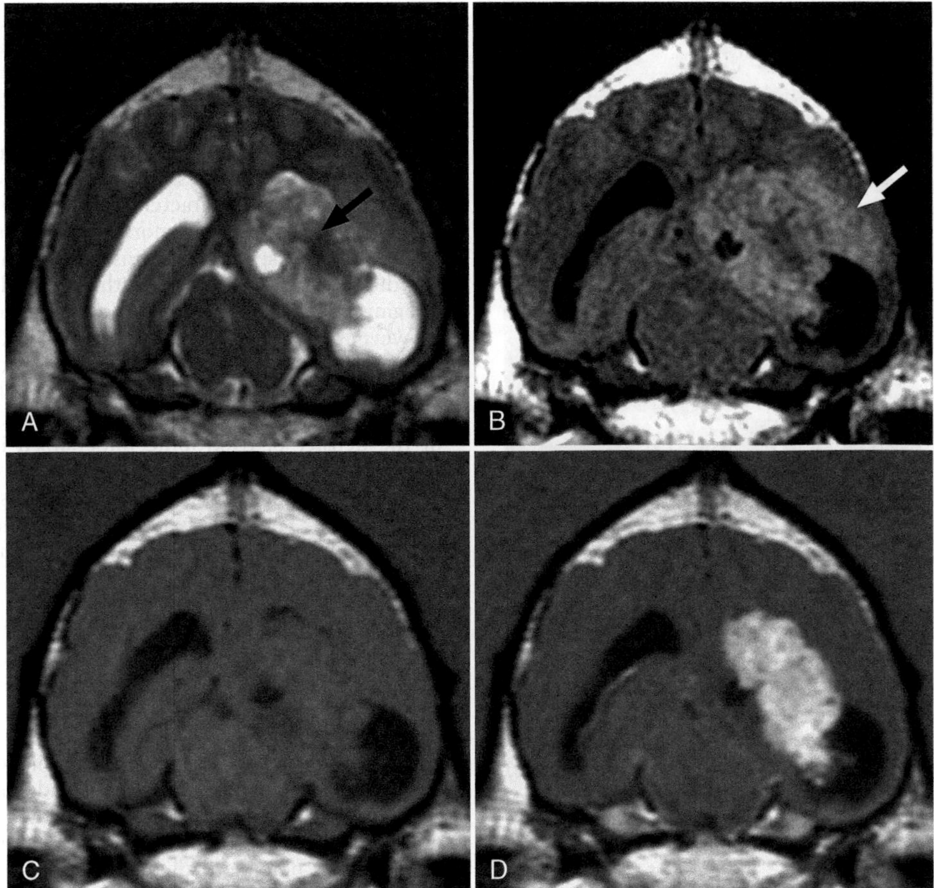

Figure 4-1 Magnetic resonance images of the brain of a 10-year old male neutered, mixed-breed dog that was evaluated for a 1-month history of recurrent seizures and a change in mental state. **A,** Axial T2W images were obtained at the level of the midbrain. There is a single, well-circumscribed, lobulated intraaxial mass within the left lateral ventricle of the cerebrum. The mass has a heterogenous intensity with areas of hyperintensity and isointensity compared with the normal cerebrum *(black arrow)*. The mass has expanded the left cerebrum, causing compression of the midbrain. The ventral portion of the left lateral ventricle is dilated. **B,** Axial T2W FLAIR image at the same level as in A. Edema in the overlying cerebrum is more conspicuous as a result of suppression of the signal intensity in the lateral ventricle *(white arrow)*. **C,** T1W image at the same level as in **A.** The mass is isointense compared with the normal cerebrum, which makes it difficult to appreciate its borders. **D,** T1W images obtained after intravenous administration of a gadolinium-based contrast media. The mass displays strong, homogeneous contrast enhancement. (Copyright 2010 University of Georgia Research Foundation, Inc.)

compression or distortion of local anatomy, should be characterized. Using a combination of sequences depicting lesion characteristics combined with contrast enhancement patterns, MRI may provide a relatively accurate presumptive antemortem diagnosis in many cases.

Contraindications

There are very few contraindications for MRI. As with all diagnostic procedures that necessitate general anesthesia, the clinician must weigh the anesthetic risk to the animal against the value of the information gained with the imaging procedure. Consequently, before imaging, careful consideration should be given to animals that are a poor anesthetic risk. One such risk is increased intracranial pressure. During anesthesia, animals with increased intracranial pressure may lose the ability to compensate with additional increases in intracranial pressure (ICP) from the anesthesia itself, leading to deleterious effects or even death. Intracranial pressure is uncommonly measured in neurologic animals. However, the presence of an increase in intracranial pressure should be considered in animals with severe alterations in sensorium. Before general anesthesia for imaging, therapeutic measures should be taken to lower intracranial pressure in animals with suspected or confirmed increases in ICP. For details, see Chapter 12. From a technical standpoint, whereas generally inconsequential to the animal, image quality may be adversely affected in animals with a metallic implant, gun shot or pellets, and microchips. Animals with cardiac pacemakers or other implantable electronic devices cannot undergo MRI imaging.

Computed Tomography

Availability

The expanded utility of CT in animals beyond its use in evaluating the nervous system combined with the relative inexpensiveness of new or refurbished CT units has put the feasibility of acquiring and maintaining CT technology within the realm of many veterinary specialty practices. As with MRI, access to CT also can be obtained through veterinary imaging centers, local hospitals or imaging facilities for humans, or through contracts with companies providing mobile CT services.

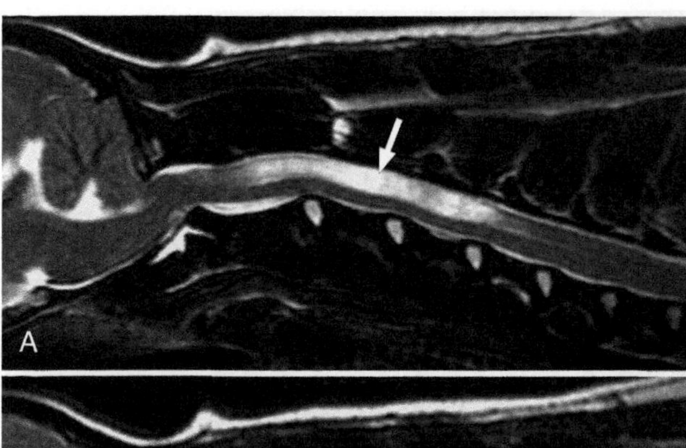

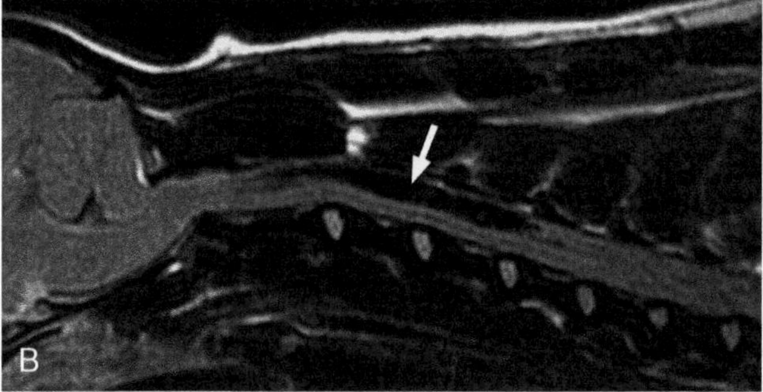

Figure 4-2 Sagittal images of the cervical spinal cord of a Brussel Griffon dog presented for evaluation of GP ataxia and tetraparesis. **A,** T2W sagittal image: There is an intramedullary hyperintensity in the spinal cord contained in the C2-4 vertebrae *(arrow)*. **B,** The hyperintense signal demonstrates suppressions (signal void) *(arrows)* on FLAIR images consistent with water containing a low protein content. (Copyright 2010 the University of Georgia Research Foundation, Inc.)

Indications

Similar to that which occurs with conventional radiography, CT is a cross-sectional imaging modality in which images are constructed based on the attenuation of x-rays through tissue. The main benefit of CT over conventional radiography is that with CT there is greater soft tissue differentiation and lack of superimposition of overlying structures, which greatly improves the evaluation of complex anatomy such as the calvaria or the vertebral column.[10] An additional benefit to CT is that images can be acquired within minutes.

Images are constructed as an x-ray tube rotates 360 degrees around the animal and emits x-ray photons. As these pass through the patient, attenuation of x-ray photons occurs through absorption and scatter, in large part, related to tissue density. Opposite the x-ray tube, detectors absorb the remaining x-rays and convert them into a digital signal. As the animal is passed through the gantry, which houses the x-ray tube and detectors, information regarding a cross section or "slice" is obtained. Through a process called back projection, computer-generated images of each slice of the anatomy scanned are constructed. The resultant image is a highly accurate cross-sectional image displayed in black, white, and shades of gray based on the attenuation of the x-ray beam. Dark or relative black areas are hypodense or hypoattenuating whereas light or relative white areas are hyperdense or hyperattenuating. Administration of iodinated intravenous or contrast media can improve visualization of pathology. Iodinated contrast media accumulation due to a breakdown in the blood-brain barrier or abnormal vasculature of a tumor causes an increase in tissue density that attenuates the x-ray beam and results in a hyperdense or hyperattenuating lesion.

The computer is able to define hundreds to thousands of shades of gray, which enables differentiation of tissues. Unfortunately the human eye is only able to perceive approximately 20 shades of gray.[11] Postacquisition manipulation of images allows the operator to center (level) and select the range (window width) over which the 20 shades of gray are displayed to highlight different tissues in the image.[11] In doing so, images can be displayed to enhance bone (bone window) or soft tissues (soft tissue window) (Figure 4-4).

Image interpretation should be done similar to that with MRI (see previous discussion). Although likely not as specific as with MRI, lesion characterization may provide a relatively accurate presumptive antemortem diagnosis.

Despite the speed of acquisition and improved soft tissue differentiation obtained with CT, MRI remains the best imaging modality for investigating most neurologic diseases. However, CT has some advantages over MRI in the evaluation of bony lesions. For example, CT may provide more useful information over MRI in cases of vertebral fractures or subluxation where bony details are important. Taking advantage of the density of dystrophic mineralized intervertebral disk material, CT can be used in the evaluation of chondrodystrophic dogs with suspected intervertebral disk disease (Figures 4-5 and 4-6). The sensitivity of CT in evaluating spinal cord disease is improved with the addition of subarachnoid iodinated contrast media (CT/myelography).[12,13]

Contraindications

See contraindications for MRI.

Radiography

Availability

Radiography is the most frequently employed imaging modality. Most veterinary practices have radiographic capabilities adequate for the investigation of neurologic animals. Radiography can be performed with conventional film screen or digital systems. The benefit to digital radiography over film screen systems is the ability to acquire diagnostic quality images over a wide range of exposures without negatively impacting the diagnostic quality of the images.[14] Likewise, image quality is not impaired by processing errors that can occur during film development.[14] Unfortunately the main drawback to radiography is the inability to discriminate soft tissues. Nervous tissue essentially has the same opacity as other soft tissues. Lesions of nervous tissue such as hemorrhage, tumors, or degenerative lesions are detected only rarely when calcification of the lesion or lytic change in adjacent bone is present. In general, radiographic evaluation of neurologic animals is restricted to identification of lesions involving the vertebral column. Due to the size of large animals, penetration of x-ray photons limits its evaluation to primarily the cervical vertebral column. Even with definitive identification of pathologic changes to the axial skeleton, nervous system involvement can only be inferred using plain radiography. In addition, radiographs represent the summation of anatomy into a two-dimensional image, which limits accurate identification of a lesion affecting the complex anatomy of the calvaria or vertebral column. With the increased access to cross-sectional imaging, radiography of the cranial cavity has been replaced by MRI and CT. As a result, radiographic evaluation is primarily performed on the vertebral column. The most common radiographic changes and their causes are listed in Table 4-1. Examples of radiographic changes associated with specific disease processes are included in the discussion of each disease (see Chapters 5 through 15).

Meticulous technique, collimation, and proper patient positioning are essential for detection of subtle changes that are often the key for a diagnosis.[15] Sedation or anesthesia may be necessary for proper positioning. Beyond these aspects, the only limitation is the interpretive skill of the veterinarian. Interpretive skill is developed through practice. Although many lesions are obvious with cursory inspection, subtle changes may be difficult to appreciate. If possible, radiographs should be made with the lesion in the center of the field of

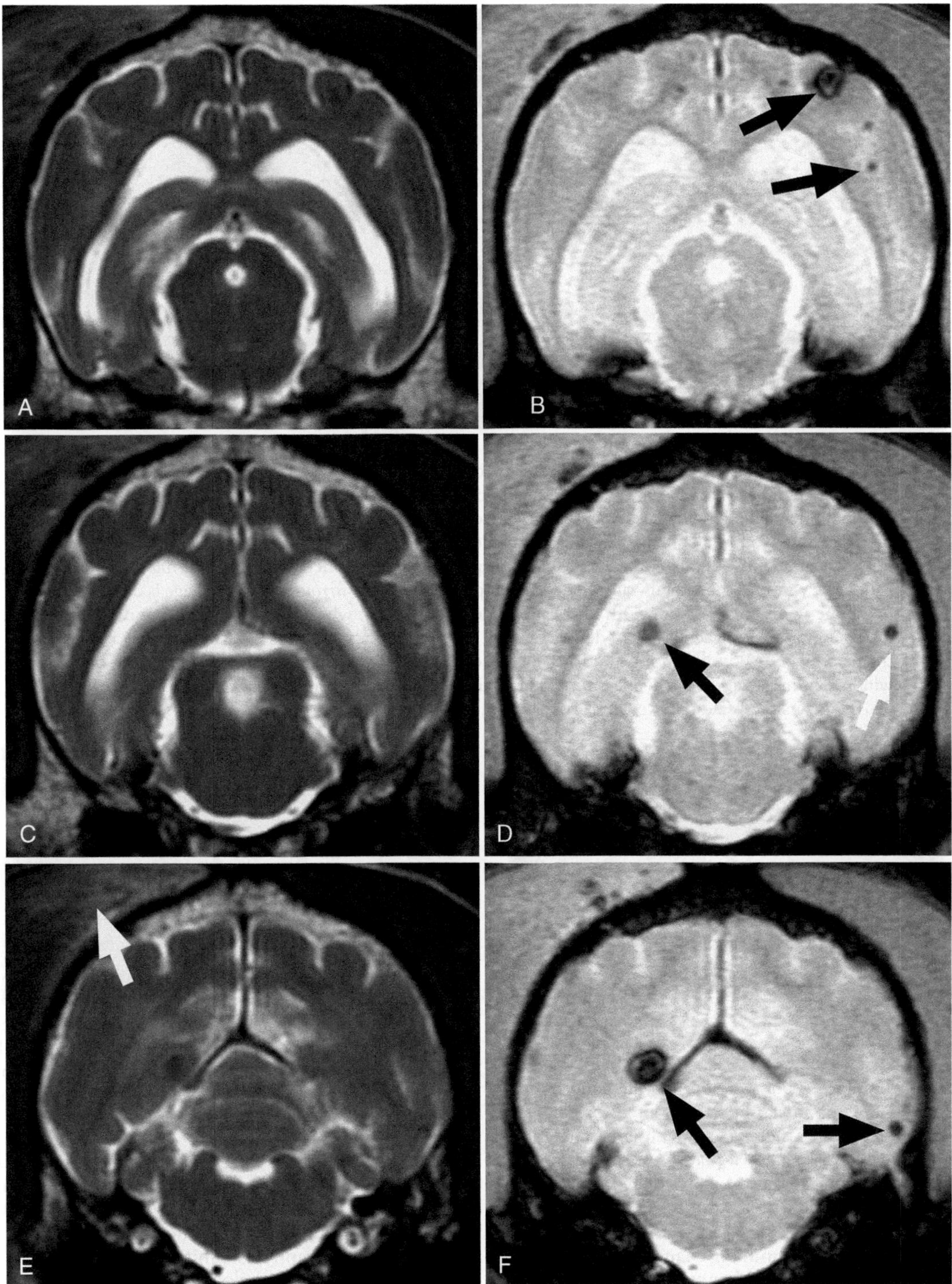

Figure 4-3 Axial MRI images of a 16-year-old Jack Russell terrier presented for evaluation of a change in behavior. Pictures **A, C,** and **E** are axial T2W images obtained at the level of the midbrain, pons, and rostral medulla oblongata, respectively. Pictures **B, D,** and **F** are T2*W images acquired at the corresponding levels of pictures **A, C,** and **E.** While it is difficult to appreciate any abnormalities in **A, C,** and **E,** pictures **B, D,** and **F** show multiple variable sized round hypointense lesions consistent with blood products (i.e., hemorrhage) *(black arrows)*. Additionally, in picture **E**, the temporal muscle is hyperintense consistent with edema of the muscle *(white arrow)*. (Copyright 2010 University of Georgia Research Foundation, Inc.)

view to reduce distortion of anatomy present at the edges of the image. An approach to the interpretation of radiographic evaluation of the vertebral column is as follows:

1. Scan the entire radiograph for quality of exposure, positioning, and the presence of artifacts or motion. Recognize the limitations imposed by these factors.
2. Scan the structures on the radiograph that are not of primary interest, such as the soft tissue, abdomen, and chest.
3. Systematically evaluate the area of primary interest.
4. Scan the entire vertebral column for contour: the ventral surface of the vertebral bodies, the floor of the vertebral canal, and the lamina, articulations, and spinous processes (see Table 4-1).

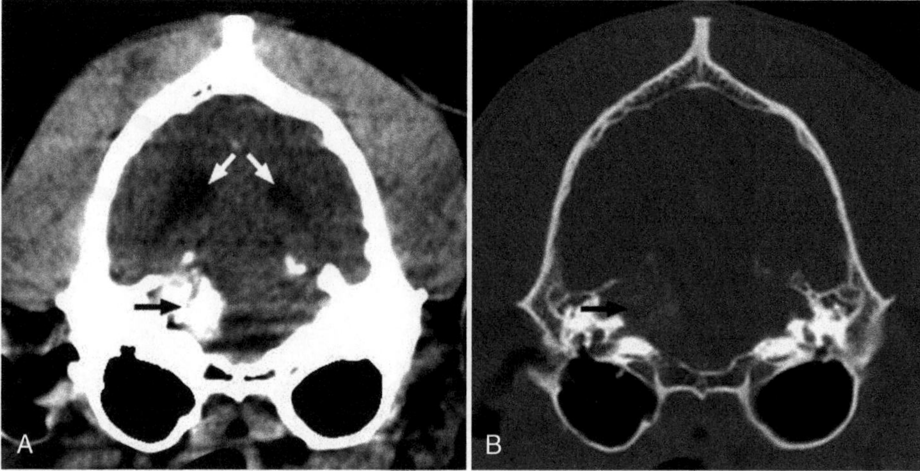

Figure 4-4 Computed tomography images of the brain of a 7-year-old male neutered collie dog that was evaluated for right-sided vestibular dysfunction. Axial images were obtained at the level of the rostral medulla. There is a single, irregularly contoured extraaxial mass at the level of the left cerebellopontine angle. The mass is hyperattenuating compared with normal brain parenchyma. **A,** The image is displayed in a soft tissue window (window width 140 and window level 60). On images obtained after intravenous contrast, the mass displays strong enhancement *(black arrow)*. Using a soft tissue window, the lateral ventricles can be appreciated *(white arrows)*. **B,** The image is displayed in a bone window (window width 2800 and widow level 350), which highlights the fine detail of the spongy bone between layers of dense compact bone of the calvaria. This is particularly evident in the parietal bone dorsally and the petrous portion of the temporal bone ventrolaterally. On the bone window, mineralization of the mass results in a faintly visible appearance *(black arrow)*. (Copyright 2010 University of Georgia Research Foundation, Inc.)

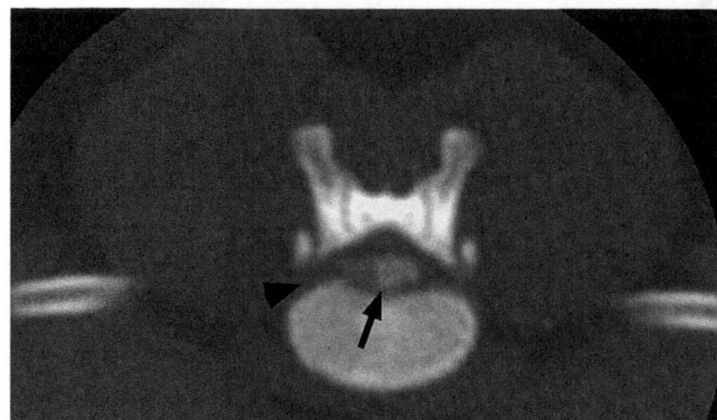

Figure 4-5 Axial CT image (bone window) of the caudal endplate of the T12 vertebra of a dachshund presented for paraplegia. Within the vertebral canal, there is a hyperattenuating lesion consistent with herniated disk material *(black arrow)*. The lesion extends to the intervertebral foramen on the right *(arrowhead)*. (Copyright 2010 University of Georgia Research Foundation, Inc.)

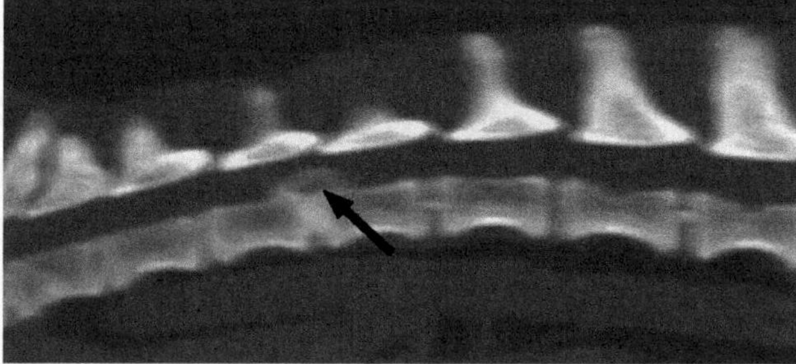

Figure 4-6 Reconstruction of the CT images of the dog in Figure 4-5. The lesion occupies the ventral aspect of the vertebral canal centered over the T12-13 intervertebral disk space *(arrow)*. (Copyright 2010 University of Georgia Research Foundation, Inc.)

5. Scan the entire vertebral column for changes in bone opacity, such as lytic or proliferative changes (see Table 4-1).
6. Scan the vertebral canal for changes in opacity, especially at the intervertebral foramina and the intervertebral disk spaces.
7. Compare the size of adjacent intervertebral disk spaces and foramina and the joint spaces between articular processes. A narrowing of one or more of these spaces is suggestive of intervertebral disk disease.
8. Stand back and scan the vertebral column again. Changes in contour or spacing are sometimes more apparent from a distance.

Indications

Given the availability, ease in performing, and cost, plain radiographic evaluation of the vertebral column should be considered in most animals demonstrating signs of spinal cord dysfunction. In particular, animals with suspected or known trauma should undergo radiographic evaluation to definitively establish the existence of fractures or luxations. However, in the majority of instances, the diagnostic capabilities of plain radiography is limited. The diagnostic capabilities are improved with myelography (from injection of iodinated contrast media into the subarachnoid space). Injections of iodinated contrast media are made in either the lumbar area at L5-6 or L6-7 or at the cerebellomedullary cistern. In our experience, compressive lesions are better defined when the contrast media are injected into the lumbar area. The injection pressure attained there forces the media past lesions. Media injected from the cerebellomedullary cistern may be blocked by compressive lesions and may flow cranially into the cranial cavity. Seizures are the most common complication of myelography. Factors that predispose animals to seizures include body weight of 20 kg, multiple injections, and injections made at the cerebellomedullary cistern.[16,17] Iatrogenic trauma or hemorrhage/hematoma formation also can occur, which can exacerbate clinical signs.[18] Inadvertent trauma to

TABLE 4-1

Radiographic Findings and Interpretation Involving the Vertebrae*

Radiographic Change	Possible Causes
Proliferation	*Degenerative:* Spondylosis, dural ossification (linear opacity in vertebral canal), diffuse/disseminated idiopathic skeletal hyperostosis (DISH), caudal cervical spondylomyelopathy, degenerative lumbosacral stenosis *Neoplastic:* Primary or metastatic vertebral tumor *Nutritional:* Ankylosing spondylosis, hypervitaminosis A *Inflammatory:* Osteomyelitis, discospondylitis (osteomyelitis usually is proliferative and lytic) *Traumatic:* Healing fracture
Lysis	*Neoplastic:* Primary or metastatic vertebral tumor, widening of vertebral canal (spinal cord tumor), widening of intervertebral foramen (nerve sheath tumor) *Nutritional:* Generalized loss of bone opacity, hypocalcemia, hyperparathyroidism *Inflammatory:* Osteomyelitis, discospondylitis (osteomyelitis usually is proliferative and lytic)
Abnormal shape of vertebrae	*Degenerative:* Caudal cervical spondylomyelopathy *Anomalous:* Hemivertebrae, spina bifida, fused vertebrae *Traumatic:* Fracture
Displacement	*Degenerative:* Caudal cervical spondylomyelopathy, degenerative lumbosacral stenosis, intervertebral disk herniation (narrowing of intervertebral disk space, foramen, and facet space) joint space between articular processes *Anomalous:* Hemivertebrae, agenesis/hypoplasia of dens (atlantoaxial luxation) *Neoplastic:* Pathologic fractures *Nutritional:* Pathologic fractures *Inflammatory:* Pathologic fractures *Traumatic:* Fractures, luxations

*Radiographic changes are rarely diagnostic. In most cases, advanced imaging is necessary to establish a definitive diagnosis. Definitive diagnosis based on radiographic changes alone is limited to vertebral fracture or luxation, discospondylitis, or vertebral lysis secondary to neoplasia.

the nervous tissue at the cerebellomedullary cistern can cause severe (or worsen) clinical signs and even death.

Masses that occupy space in the vertebral canal (e.g., tumors, abscesses, disc herniations) cause alterations in the myelographic contrast column. The extradural, intradural-extramedullary, or intramedullary location can be determined by the type of distortion occurring in the contrast column (Figures 4-7 and 4-8).[19] Evaluating both the lateral and ventrodorsal views are critical to avoid misdiagnosis. As an example, asymmetric extradural lesions may cause a pattern similar to of intradural-extramedullary lesions on lateral radiographic views. Similarly, midline extradural lesions may appear as intramedullary lesions on ventrodorsal radiographic views. Focal spinal cord atrophy causes narrowing of the spinal cord with widening of the contrast column. Severe myelomalacia may allow the contrast media to pool in the spinal cord parenchyma. The central canal may be filled by the contrast medium in some cases, without apparent clinical consequences, particularly when injections are made cranial to L5 in small dogs.[20]

Myelography for the diagnosis of lumbosacral lesions is limited by the fact that the spinal cord terminates at L5 in most dogs. This varies among breed size. In one study, the spinal cord extended further caudally in dachshunds than in German shepherd dogs.[21]

Contraindications

The same contraindications should be considered for plain radiography or myelography as with any imaging procedure requiring general anesthesia. However, in those animals in which radiography can be performed, there are few contraindications associated with obtaining plain radiographs. In animals with suspected or confirmed increased ICP, myelography is a contraindication to spinal tap; hence, myelography should not be performed in such cases. Because contrast medium is irritating, myelography is usually not done in the presence of meningitis except when a focal mass is suspected. When the puncture is made for myelography, a CSF analysis should be performed before injection of the contrast agent. If the cell count indicates active inflammation, myelography is not performed unless it is considered essential to diagnosis and treatment.

Ultrasonography

Because the CNS is contained within bone, there is a limited role of ultrasonography in the evaluation of the neurologic patients. Ultrasonography can be used when a fontanelle of the calvaria is persistent or during brain or spinal surgery once the overlying bone has been removed[22-26] (Figure 4-9). Precise localization of masses is best accomplished using MRI or CT. However, ultrasonography can be helpful in delineating lesions at surgery. Masses tend to be hyperechoic and cause shifts in the ventricular system or other local anatomic structures.[23] Hydrocephalus can be diagnosed in dogs with persistent fontanelles.[25]

Cerebrospinal Fluid Analysis

Availability

The equipment and technique necessary for collection of CSF for analysis are not beyond the means of general practitioners. Clinicians wanting to perform the procedure should acquire training and expertise and perform CSF collection often enough to maintain confidence and accuracy. However, CSF collection is not routinely performed by most veterinarians in general practice for several reasons. Although a sensitive test for detecting abnormalities of the CNS, CSF analysis rarely

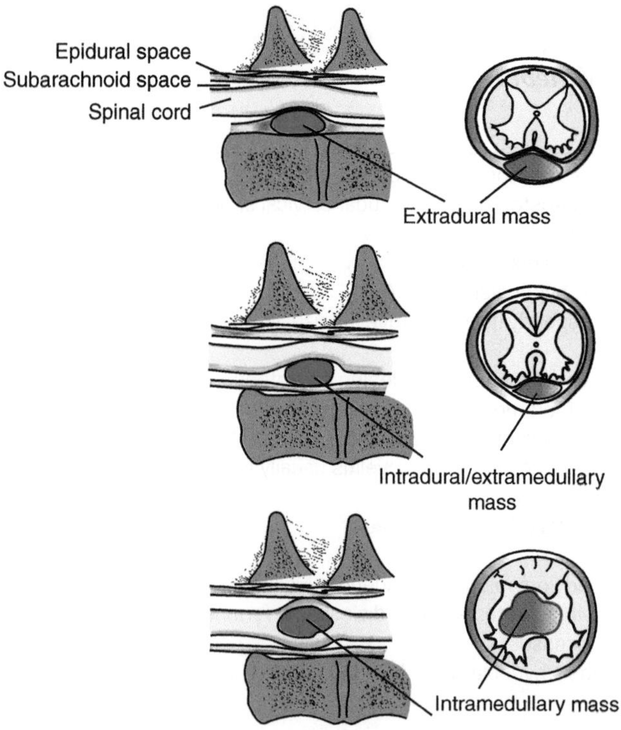

Figure 4-7 **A,** Myelogram of a cat with malacia in the spinal cord caused by an infarct. Note the contrast media pooled in the area of the malacia *(arrowheads)*. **B,** Spinal cord showing the area of malacia. (Copyright 2010 University of Georgia Research Foundation, Inc.)

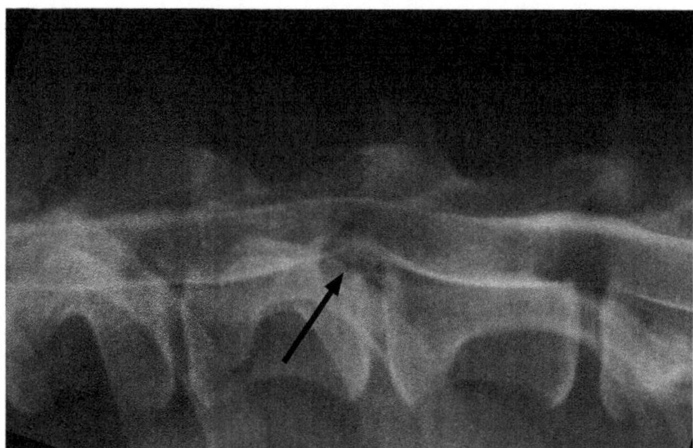

Figure 4-8 Lateral radiographic view of the vertebral column at the thoracolumbar junction after administration of iodinated contrast media into the subarachnoid space (myelogram). There is dorsal deviation of the ventral contrast column and attenuation of the dorsal contrast column consistent with an extradural myelographic pattern. The lesion is consistent with intervertebral disk herniation.(Copyright 2010 University of Georgia Research Foundation, Inc.)

provides a definitive diagnosis. Instead, CSF analysis may help limit the differential diagnosis by excluding conditions from consideration (Table 4-2). Results of CSF analysis most often are interpreted in light of imaging findings. Secondly, CSF collection should be performed immediately after imaging studies if possible, as contraindication to spinal tap may be apparent on imaging studies. Lastly, CSF analysis needs to be done immediately after collection. The cells in the fluid begin to degenerate within 30 minutes from time of collection. Consequently, the diagnostic information gained from CSF analysis, logistics

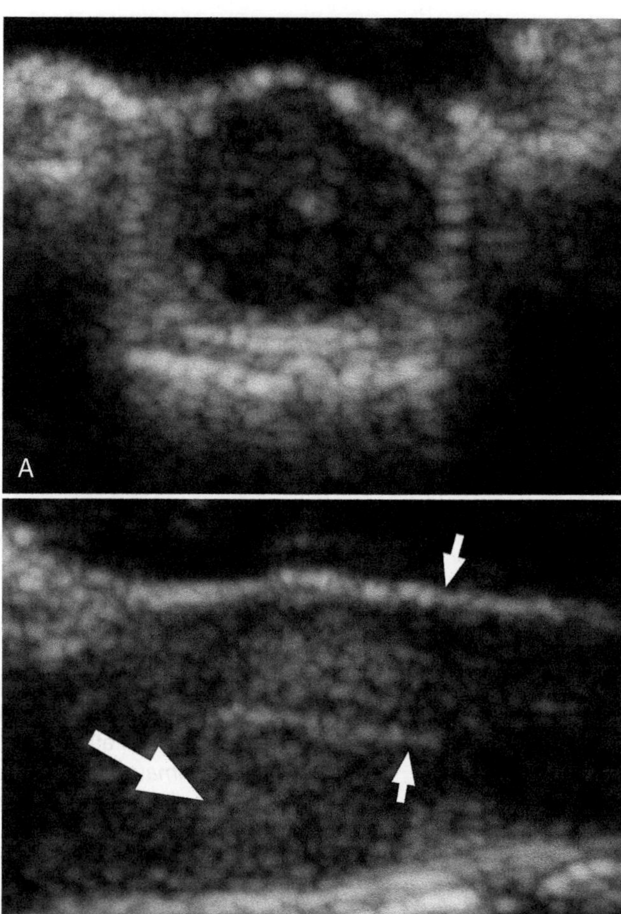

Figure 4-9 **A,** Intraoperative ultrasound (US) image in the axial plane. A dorsal laminectomy has been performed; the surgical site was filled with saline. The ultrasound probe has been placed in a sterile sleeve. The normal spinal cord can be seen as a round structure. Surrounding the spinal cord is the dura, which is hyperechoic. The central canal is seen as a hyperechoic central area. **B,** Sagittal US image of the same dog, the dorsal and ventral aspects of the dura are hyperechoic and demarcate the spinal cord *(small arrows)*. Cranially the spinal cord is deviated dorsally by a mass *(large arrow)*. (Copyright 2010 University of Georgia Research Foundation, Inc.)

in performing and analyzing it, and the low frequency in performing the procedure in general practice has resulted in the procedure being largely performed by veterinarians in specialty practice.

A CSF sample is collected routinely by cerebellomedullary cisternal puncture. CSF can also be obtained, with somewhat greater difficulty, from the subarachnoid space at L5-6 or L6-7 in dogs and at the lumbosacral interspace in cats and large animals.[27,28] As a general rule, CSF is obtained from the site closest to the lesion. Consequently, lumbar CSF is more likely to disclose abnormalities in animals with thoracolumbar spinal cord disease.[29]

In dogs and cats, CSF is collected under general anesthesia with the animal intubated to avoid movement of the animal during needle placement. In food animals and horses, lumbar puncture can be accomplished with sedation and the animal standing. The hair is clipped and the skin is prepared for an aseptic procedure. The needle (a 22-gauge, 1.5-inch disposable spinal needle with a stylet for most small animals; a 20-gauge, 3.5-inch needle for most large animals) should be handled

TABLE 4-2
Cerebrospinal Fluid

Disease	Appearance	White Blood Cells* Per mm³	Cell Type	Protein (mg/dL)	Other
Normal dog	Clear	<5	Mononuclear	<25[†]	
Normal cat	Clear	<5	Mononuclear	<25	
Normal horse	Clear	<6	Mononuclear	<100	
Normal cow	Clear	<10	Mononuclear	<40	
Normal pig	Clear	<30	Mononuclear	<40	
Normal sheep	Clear	<10	Mononuclear	<40	
Inflammatory, Noninfectious					
Steroid responsive meningitis arteritis	Clear to turbid	Increased, usually >100	Mostly neutrophils (nondegenerative appearance)	Increased	Measure IgA levels, serum C-reactive protein and α_2- macroglobulin levels
Granulomatous meningoencephalomyelitis	Clear to turbid	Increase (wide range)	Mostly mononuclear, sometimes neutrophils	Increased	PCR, serology for infectious disease (e.g., *Toxoplasma gondii, Neospora caninum, Cryptococcus neoformans, and conine distemper virus*)
Inflammatory, Infectious					
Bacterial	Clear to turbid	Increased, usually >100	Mostly neutrophils (± degenerative appearance)	Increased, usually >100	PCR, culture; organisms may be seen
Viral	Clear	Increased, usually	Mostly mononuclear[‡]	Increased, usually <100	PCR, antibody titer, EM (viral particles)
Fungal	Clear to turbid	Increased variable	Mixed, Sometimes eosinophils	Increased, usually < 100	PCR, antibody or antisen titers, culture
Protozoal	Clear	Increased, may be >100	Mononuclear, sometimes neutrophils	Increased, usually >100	Antibody titer
Parasitic	Clear to xanthochromic	Increased, variable	Mixed, sometimes eosinophils	Increased, usually >100	Parasitic
Degenerative, including compression	Clear	Normal to slight increase	Mononuclear or neutrophilic sometimes mixed	Increased, usually <100	Degenerative, including compression
Neoplastic	Clear	Normal to increased	Mononuclear sometimes neutrophils	Increased, usually <100	Tumor cells may be seen if tumor adjacent to subarachnoid space (hematopoietic, ependymoma, choroid plexus tumors); PCR for antigen receptor rearrangement (lymphoma)
Traumatic	Xanthochromic	Normal to increased	RBCs, WBCs	Increased, variable	Usually contraindicated
Vascular	Xanthochromic	Normal to Increased	RBCs, WBCs	Increased, variable	Vascular

Data from Hoerlein BF: Canine neurology: diagnosis and treatment, ed 3, Philadelphia, 1978, WB Saunders; Kornegay JN: Cerebrospinal fluid collection, examination, and interpretation in dogs and cats, Compend Contin Educ Pract Vet 3:85–92, 1981; deLahunta A, Glass EN: Veterinary neuroanatomy and clinical neurology, ed 3, Philadelphia, 2009, Saunders Elsevier; Mayhew IG, Whitlock RH, Tasker JB: Equine cerebrospinal fluid: reference values of normal horses, Am J Vet Res 38:1271–1274, 1977; Bailey CS, Higgins RJ: Comparison of total white blood cell count and total protein content of lumbar and cisternal cerebrospinal fluid of healthy dogs, Am J Vet Res 46:1162–1165, 1985; Bailey CS, Higgins RJ: Characteristics of cisternal cerebrospinal fluid associated with primary brain tumors in the dog: a retrospective study, J Am Vet Med Assoc 188:414–417, 1986; Dickinson PJ, Sturges BK, Kass PH, et al: Characteristics of cisternal cerebrospinal fluid associated with intracranial meningiomas in dogs: 56 cases (1985-2004), J Am Vet Med Assoc 228:564–567, 2006; Bohn AA, Wills TB, West CL, et al: Cerebrospinal fluid analysis and magnetic resonance imaging in the diagnosis of neurologic disease in dogs: a retrospective study, Vet Clin Pathol 35:315–320, 2006; Windsor RC, Vernau KM, Sturges BK, et al: Lumbar cerebrospinal fluid in dogs with type I intervertebral disc herniation, J Vet Intern Med 22:954–960, 2008; Bailey CS, Higgins RJ: Characteristics of cerebrospinal fluid associated with canine granulomatous meningoencephalomyelitis: a retrospective study, J Am Vet Med Assoc 188:418–421, 1986; Windsor RC, Sturges BK, Vernau KM, et al: Cerebrospinal fluid eosinophilia in dogs, J Vet Intern Med 23:275–281, 2009.

*White blood cell counts may be normal in animals with encephalitis; this is particularly true of some viral and protozoal infections.

†Protein is normally higher in lumbar versus cerebellomedullary CSF and may exceed 25 mg/dL.

‡Neutrophils may predominate in some viral diseases (e.g., feline infectious peritonitis and eastern equine encephalomyelitis).

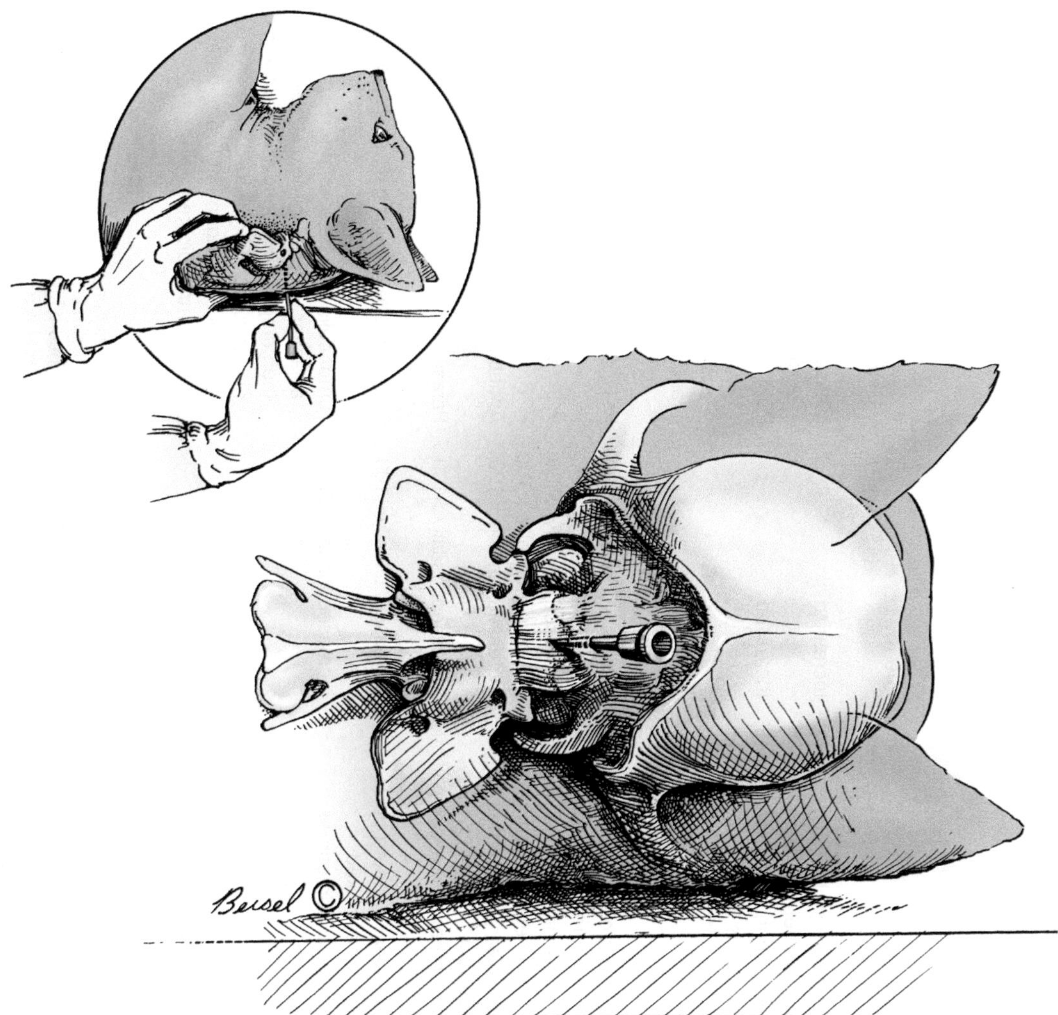

Figure 4-10 Landmarks for cerebrospinal fluid collection. (From Greene CE, Oliver JE Jr: Neurologic examination. In Ettinger SJ, editor: Textbook of veterinary internal medicine, ed 2, Philadelphia, 1982, WB Saunders.)

with sterile gloves. For cerebellomedullary puncture, the landmarks for the midline are the external occipital protuberance and the spinous process of the axis (C2) (Figure 4-10). The needle is inserted on the midline near the cranial border of the wings of the atlas (C1). A slight loss of resistance is felt as the needle penetrates the dorsal atlantooccipital membrane and enters the subarachnoid space. The stylet is withdrawn, and fluid is allowed to flow from the hub of the needle into sterile tubes. Alternatively, once the skin is punctured, the stylet can be removed before advancing the needle. Using this technique, there is less risk of iatrogenic injury to the nervous tissue as CSF should flow once the needle enters the subarachnoid space. With this technique, CSF samples contain little to no red blood cell (RBC) contamination. The CSF sample should be divided into two or three aliquots collected in separate tubes. The initial collection may contain RBCs from trauma, but subsequent aliquots may be devoid of this contamination. In horses, three or four 2-mL samples should be collected in separate tubes and analyzed. Total protein concentration and red cell contamination are significantly lower in samples 2, 3, and 4, whereas sample 1 may not be suitable for serologic or cytologic examinations.[30] Aspiration of the needle with a syringe should not performed as this may "draw" the nervous tissue toward the needle, resulting in iatrogenic injury or blood contamination.

Total and differential white blood cell (WBC) counts are the most important parts of a CSF analysis. Unless specific steps are taken to preserve cells, cell counts must be determined within 30 minutes of collection because WBCs deteriorate rapidly. Total cell counts should be done with a hemocytometer. A differential WBC count and cytologic evaluation is performed on a sample prepared using a cytocentrifuge to concentrate cells. Several methods exist for determining the differential count, including sedimentation and centrifugation techniques that can be done in practice. Techniques for RBC and WBC counts and differentials are described in the references. The addition of cell-free autologous serum protects cellular morphology for up to 48 hours when samples are stored at 4° C.[31] To make an 11% serum concentration, 30 μL of serum is added to 250 μL of CSF. Alternatively, a 1:1 mixture of CSF and 6% hydroxyethyl starch in 0.9% NaCl (hetastarch) can be used to preserve cells in CSF.[32] The disadvantage of these techniques is that a separate, undiluted CSF sample also must be submitted for protein determination.

The examiner should observe the appearance of the CSF. Hemorrhage caused by the puncture produces a red tinge to the fluid that decreases as the fluid continues to flow. WBC counts may be corrected for hemorrhage by subtracting approximately 1 WBC for each 500 RBCs; however, the validity of correction formulas has been questioned.[33] High CSF nucleated cell counts and protein concentrations correlate with the presence of neurologic disease, even when samples contain moderate amounts of blood contamination.[34] Centrifugation should leave a clear, colorless fluid. A yellowish tinge to the CSF is called xanthochromia and is caused by free bilirubin. Previous subarachnoid hemorrhage is the usual cause, although prolonged icterus can produce xanthochromia. Turbidity is caused by an increase in the cell content of the fluid to more than 500 cells/mm.[29]

Often changes identified in CSF are nonspecific. The ability to identify a definitive diagnosis using CSF can be improved using a variety of specialized tests, including microbiologic testing, measurement of antibody or antigen titers, polymerase chain reaction (PCR) testing, and immunocytochemistry. Due to the high diagnostic sensitivity and specificity, molecular techniques, such as PCR and reverse transcription PCR, have greatly improved the ability to identify infection in the CNS. A variety of infectious agents, including bacterial, viral, protozoal, and fungal agents, have been identified using molecular techniques.[35] PCR technology can also be used in the diagnosis of lymphoma.[36] Immunophenotyping of nucleated cells has been performed on normal canine CSF.[37] Characterization of specific immunophenotypes of nucleated cells in CSF can lead to a definitive diagnosis.[38]

Along with advanced techniques, traditional methods of identifying infectious agents should be pursued in animals in which an infectious etiology is considered. If bacterial infection is strongly suspected based on clinical findings or if neutrophils are increased in the CSF, culture and sensitivity testing should be done. Fluid should be obtained in two sterile containers, one for laboratory analysis and one for culture.

Titers to agents such as viruses,[39,40] fungi,[41] and protozoa[42,43] also may be indicated when meningoencephalitis or meningomyelitis is suspected. The CSF titer is compared with the serum titer because serum antibodies may cross the blood-brain barrier in inflammatory diseases. Indirect fluorescent antibody testing for canine distemper virus may be positive in 60% to 82% of dogs with noninflammatory and inflammatory distemper, respectively.[44]

Measurement of CSF protein levels is necessary for a complete examination. Simple qualitative studies such as the Pandy test are adequate, although quantitative methods are preferred. The Pandy test can be performed in the practice; it qualitatively estimates globulin concentrations. Quantitative analysis also can be done in the practice, or the sample can be sent to a reference laboratory. Electrophoresis is used to determine quantitatively the levels of protein fractions or immunoglobulins in CSF. Increased protein levels in CSF is a nonspecific indicator of CNS pathology. Increased albumin indicates a disturbance of the blood-brain barrier, whereas significant increased immunoglobulin indicates synthesis intrathecally.[45-48]

Indications

Increased WBC counts and protein levels are expected with active CNS inflammatory diseases and in any disease process that disrupts the blood-brain barrier. In general, the WBCs are predominantly polymorphonuclear leukocytes in bacterial diseases and predominantly lymphocytes in viral diseases. Fungal and protozoal diseases may produce mixed populations of leukocytes. An eosinophilic pleocytosis is found in some protozoal, parasitic, or idiopathic diseases such as granulomatous or eosinophilic meningoencephalomyelitis.[49-51] Mixed populations of neutrophils, lymphocytes, and monocytes (pyogranulomatous pleocytosis) are characteristic of granulomatous meningoencephalomyelitis of dogs and the neurologic form of feline infectious peritonitis. The CSF may be completely normal in animals with inflammatory diseases.[39,42,44]

Primary degenerative or demyelinating diseases, neoplasia, infarction, or CNS compression may produce an increase in CSF protein with little or no increase in cells (albuminocytologic dissociation) (see Table 4-2).

Free blood or xanthochromia may be seen after subarachnoid hemorrhage. Hemorrhage may be caused by trauma, primary vascular disease, or vascular lesions secondary to inflammation or neoplasia. Blood contamination may also occur at the time of CSF collection.

Contraindications

General anesthesia is required for CSF collection; therefore, if anesthesia is contraindicated, CSF should not be obtained. When the animal is positioned for cerebellomedullary cisternal puncture, the anesthetist should be certain that the airway is patent and ventilation is adequate. All animals should be intubated for collection of CSF.

Cerebrospinal fluid should not be collected if increased ICP is suspected. Removal of CSF from the cerebellomedullary cistern or lumbar subarachnoid space causes a pressure gradient, and the cerebrum or cerebellum may be displaced caudally. Herniation of the cerebellum through the foramen magnum may lead to apnea and death because of compression of the medullary respiratory centers or pathways (see Chapter 12). The occipital lobes of the cerebrum may herniate through the tentorial notch and compress the midbrain, with resultant pupillary dilation. Either foramen magnum of the cerebellum or transtentorial herniation of the cerebrum may also lead to tetraplegia and stupor or coma because of involvement of the descending pathways and the reticular activating system, respectively. Increased pressure from generalized brain inflammation, tumors, large abscesses, or intracranial trauma also predisposes the animal to brain herniation. The information obtained from the CSF analysis may not be worth the risk to the animal in these cases. Pressure shifts may occur with either cerebellomedullary or lumbar puncture. Herniation of the cerebellum, however, compromises the cerebellomedullary cistern. For this reason, if CSF collection is deemed necessary in animals with the potential for herniation, collection from a lumbar site is preferred. Steps should be taken to reduce CSF pressure before collecting fluid (see Chapter 12).

Electrophysiology

Availability

Electrophysiologic techniques require expensive equipment and extensive training and experience for valid interpretation of results. These factors generally limit electrophysiologic studies to specialty practices and institutional settings. Electromyography (EMG), direct nerve stimulation tests, nerve conduction studies, and evoked potentials are the most widely used techniques. Many of the available tests are listed in Table 4-3. Unlike other diagnostic tests used in neurology, electrophysiologic techniques test the functional integrity of the peripheral and central nervous systems. The majority of the tests evaluate the peripheral nervous system allowing clinicians the ability to document functional abnormalities. Many electrophysiologic tests are sensitive for identification of functional defects; however, many tests lack specificity, making it difficult to delineate a definitive diagnosis because many disease processes result in abnormal function. Consequently, electrophysiologic data often complement structural assessment of the nervous system through imaging.

Indications

Electromyography, the measurement of the electrical activity of muscle, and direct nerve stimulation and conduction studies, the measurement of nerve function, are the best diagnostic tools for the evaluation of myopathies and neuropathies.

TABLE 4-3

Electrophysiology*

Test	Indications	Probable Usefulness	Contraindications
Electromyography (EMG)	Lower motor neuron (LMN) diseases	High (typically not specific but supportive of LMN disorders)	None; signs may occasionally worsen with anesthesia
Direct nerve stimulation, conduction velocity, F-wave test, cord dorsum potential	LMN diseases	High (not specific for disorder)	None; signs may occasionally worsen with anesthesia
Repetitive nerve stimulation, single fiber EMG	Neuromuscular junction diseases	High	None; signs may occasionally worsen with anesthesia
Electroretinography	Retinal disease	High	None
Evoked response (cortical, brain-stem, and spinal)	Localization of lesions in pathways	Low in most cases	None
Auditory-evoked response	Test of hearing, location of brainstem lesions	High (mainly used to guide breeding recommendations or to diagnosis congenital deafness)	
Visual-evoked response	Cortical function	Low	
Somatosensory-evoked response	Spinal cord, plexus lesions	Low	
Urodynamics (cystometrogram, urethral pressure, sphincter reflexes)	Neurogenic bladder disorders (see Ch. 3)	Low	Detrus or muscle atony and overfilling
Electroencephalography (EEG)	Seizures (see Ch. 13)	Moderate (may be useful when not certain if abnormal behavior is related to a seizure)	None
	Sleep disorders (see Ch. 13)	Moderate	
	Structural brain disease	Low (not specified or sensitive)	

CV, Conduction velocity.
*Many electrophysiologic tests require general anesthesia to perform. Technical expertise and specialized equipment are required, which limits testing to specialty practices.

These tests are performed with the same equipment, usually during the same examination. The information provided by these procedures regarding the location and the extent of the abnormality may support a presumptive diagnosis. EMG examination entails recording the electrical potential of the extracellular fluid surrounding myofibers using a small gauge, Teflon-coated needle (recording electrode) inserted into the muscle. Examination is typically performed under anesthesia. In large animals and in certain conditions in small animals, EMG examination may be performed with heavy sedation. Under anesthesia, voluntary muscle contractions should not occur because the muscles are relaxed. Consequently, muscle fibers are considered electrically silent. During EMG examination, the recording needle measures the resting membrane potential of myofibers reflected in the extracellular fluid and compares these to the extracellular potential measured by a reference electrode. As such, the potential difference between the recording and the reference electrode is minimal to none. This is depicted as a horizontal ("flat") line on the tracing. With depolarization of the muscle, a potential difference exists between the recording and reference electrode and is manifested as a deflection of the tracing. The EMG examination includes evaluation of the electrical activity of the muscle at the following times: (1) during insertion or movement of the recording electrode (insertion activity), (2) when the muscle is resting (resting activity), (3) during muscle contraction (voluntary or reflex), and (4) in response to electrical stimulation of a motor nerve (primarily used in testing nerve conduction). The basis of EMG involves analysis of insertion activity and the recognition of three abnormalities occurring at rest, fibrillation potentials, positive sharp waves, and complex repetitive discharges. The observation of any of these signifies a disorder of the muscle or nerve. However, EMG alone cannot distinguish between these pathologies. Importantly, the number of abnormal potentials observed at rest does not directly translate to degree of dysfunction because with severe fibrosis as an endstage of disease, abnormal potentials may not be observed.

Mechanical distortion of the muscle membrane by the insertion of the recording electrode causes the membrane to depolarize, producing a brief burst of electrical activity (i.e., insertion activity). A reduction in insertional activity may signify a loss of functional myofibers due to fibrosis or severe atrophy. Increased insertional activity (essentially activity lasting longer than placement of the needles) signifies myofiber hyperexcitability. Most often this occurs with damage or disease affecting the muscle membrane as occurs with myopathies or loss of nerve supply to a muscle (denervation), causing an increase in the excitability of the muscle membrane within 7 to 10 days. In addition, at rest, fibrillation potentials, small triphasic waves, and positive sharp waves are produced spontaneously. These are produced by *individual* myofibers depolarizing at random. Complex repetitive discharges are a series of abnormal potentials generated by *multiple* myofibers in which the complex morphology of each potential is constant. Complex repetitive discharges sound like dive bombers or motorcycles on the speaker of the EMG unit. At one time thought specific for myopathies, complex repetitive discharges also can occur with neuropathies. Contraction of the muscle voluntarily, by activation of a reflex or by direct stimulation of a nerve, usually is reduced because of denervation.

Direct nerve stimulation tests and nerve conduction studies include motor-nerve-conduction (MNCV) or sensory-nerve-conduction (SNCV) evaluations. For SNCV, the nerve to be tested is stimulated and a potential is recorded directly from the nerve proximal to the site of stimulation.[52] The distance between the recording and stimulation sites is divided by the latency of the potential (the time from stimulation to onset of the recorded potential) to give a conduction velocity in meters per second (m/s).[53] For MNCV, the nerve to be evaluated is stimulated and the subsequent depolarization of the innervated muscles is recorded. The waveform recorded is called the compound muscle action potential (CMAP) or M-wave. Measurement of the latency from stimulation to onset of the CMAP reflects the conduction velocity of the nerve, the time required to release ACh from the nerve terminal, and the time required for depolarization of the muscle. To define only the MNCV, latencies are recorded from two stimulation sites. By measuring the distance between stimulation sites and dividing that by the difference in latencies between the two sites, MNCV of that segment of nerve can be obtained. Decreased conduction velocity (MNCV or SNCV) is associated with demyelination.

The stimulus used is supramaximal to ensure depolarization of all functional axons. Consequently, all functional myofibers will depolarize producing the CMAP. Analysis of the CMAP amplitude, duration, and area under the curve of the waveform is a reflection of functional axon numbers. With axonal loss, there is a reduction in the amplitude of the CMAP. Alternatively, a reduction in CMAP can occur with severe muscle disease or atrophy. In dogs, adult MNCV is reached between 6 months to 1 year of age.[54] MNCV remains stable until age 7 after which there is a gradual decline; by age 10 MNCV is reduced by approximately 10% to 15%.[54] In cats, adult MNCV is reached at approximately 3 months.[55] Conduction velocity also declines with body temperature. For each decrease in degree (Celsius), MNCV decreases 1.7 m/s.[56] Typically, recordings are measured in the palmar and plantar interosseous muscles, which are innervated by the ulnar nerve in the thoracic limb and the tibial branch of the sciatic nerve in the pelvic limb. Recordings from the extensor carpi radialis muscle are used for evaluation of radial nerve function. Stimulation of the ulnar nerve can be performed at the axilla, the groove formed by the medial epicondyle of the humerus and olecranon, and medial to the accessory carpal bone. Stimulation of the sciatic-tibial nerve can be performed dorsomedial to the greater trochanter, caudal to the lateral femoral condyle, and caudal to the tibia at the hock. Stimulation of the radial nerve is performed just proximal and distal to the elbow.

Nerve stimulation also elicits smaller, more delayed secondary action potentials in muscle.[57] Orthodromic stimulation of sensory fibers produces the H-wave or reflex, whereas antidromic stimulation of motor fibers produces the F-wave. Evaluation of these secondary waves provides information about the integrity of reflex arcs and the nerve roots, respectively. Evaluation of the F-wave may allow identification of subtle abnormalities that may not be detected using nerve conduction tests. With direct stimulation of the nerve and measurement of conduction velocity over small segments, mild reductions may not be recorded outside of the wide reference range of normal conduction velocity. As the F-wave tests a greater length of the nerve, mild reduction in conduction velocity is exaggerated by having to conduct over a longer length of the nerve and therefore will more likely be detected given the more narrow reference range.[58] Moreover, F-ratio, the ratio of conduction velocity proximal to and distal to the stimulation site can be used to determine whether the lesion primarily affects the proximal or distal aspect of the nerve.[58]

Repetitive motor nerve stimulation evaluates neuromuscular transmission. The test involves the generation of a train of 10 motor nerve stimulations at rates less than 5 Hz; for each stimulus a CMAP is recorded. Comparison of the amplitude of the first CMAP with the amplitudes of subsequent stimuli is described as a percent difference. A decrement greater than 10% is suggestive of myasthenia gravis.[57,59] Single-fiber electromyography (SFEMG) also is used to evaluate neuromuscular transmission. Delayed neuromuscular conduction, as with myasthenia gravis, causes latency variability termed jitter.[60] Table 4-4 details the electrophysiologic tests used to evaluate the peripheral nervous system.

Several electrophysiologic tests require the use of a technique termed signal averaging. Signal averaging is a method for eliminating unwanted data and variability in measurements. Essentially, multiple measurements of the same evoked response (the measurement of the depolarization of myofibers, axons, or neurons) are averaged over numerous time points, which provides a mean value at a given time point. In doing so, artifacts in recordings are reduced. Typically, various evoked responses necessitate signal averaging to obtain accurate evaluation. The following are electrophysiologic tests that use signal averaging.

The brainstem auditory-evoked response (BAER) entails the recording of brainstem potentials in response to a noise (click) stimulus in the ear canal. A signal-averaging computer is necessary to record this response.[61-64] The peripheral auditory system can be evaluated rapidly and accurately with this technique. Partial hearing loss requires pure tone stimuli, which present more difficult technical problems. Brainstem function also can be evaluated. The recording consists of a series of waves that represent electrical activity at successive levels of the brainstem. A lesion at one level of the brainstem blocks the responses at that level and at all succeeding levels. The BAER has been used most commonly to diagnose inherited unilateral or bilateral deafness in susceptible breeds such as the dalmatian.[65,66] Brainstem lesions also cause BAER abnormalities.[67] BAER can confirm a diagnosis of complete loss of brainstem function in brain death.

Analogous to the F-wave, cord dorsum potentials can be evaluated to assess the functional integrity of the proximal sensory nerves, dorsal roots, and dorsal gray matter of the spinal cord.[58] Sensory or mixed nerves are stimulated and the resultant incoming action potential of the sensory axons and depolarization of the dorsal gray matter of the spinal cord is recorded with electrodes placed over the dorsal lamina of the vertebral column at the C7-T1 or L4-5 vertebrae for thoracic or pelvic limb nerves, respectively.[58] Normative data has been described in dogs.[68] Limited data have been described in clinically affected animals. Cord dorsum potentials have been used in the assessment of cats with neuropathies related to diabetes mellitus.[69]

Somatosensory-evoked potentials (SEPs) are the potentials recorded from the spinal cord, brainstem, or brain in response to a stimulus administered to a peripheral nerve.[70,71] The SEP is used to determine the functional integrity of sensory pathways, as with a paraplegic animal with questionable

TABLE 4-4

Electrophysiologic Testing Procedures Used to Evaluate the Peripheral Nervous System

Testing Procedure	Anatomy	Expected Abnormalities
Electromyography (EMG)*	Abnormalities with myopathy or neuropathy	Increase insertional activity, Fibrillation potentials, PSW, CRD
Direct motor nerve stimulation*	Motor neuropathies/mixed neuropathies Differentiate disorders of myelin Decreased CMAP amplitude (axonal disorders)	Decreased CV (myelin disorders) Increased duration of CMAP (myelin disorders) from axonal disorders involving motor nerves Decreased AUC (axonal disorders)
F-wave testing* (minimal latency and F-ratio)	Identification of mild motor neuropathies Allows assessment of proximal aspect of nerves (from spinal cord to most proximal aspect of the nerve which can be directly stimulated)	Increased minimal latency (neuropathies)
Calculation of F-ratio	Allows determination of which aspect of the nerve is most affected (proximal, distal or diffuse)	Increased F-ratio (proximal nerve disease) Decreased F-ratio (distal nerve disease) Normal F-ratio (diffuse nerve disease)†
Repetitive nerve stimulation*	Neuromuscular junction Used primarily in the diagnosis of myasthenia gravis	Decremental reduction in successive CMAP
Single fiber EMG	Neuromuscular junction Used primarily in the diagnosis of myasthenia gravis	Increased latency variability; jitter
Direct sensory nerve stimulation*	Sensory neuropathies/mixed neuropathies Differentiate disorder of myelin from axonal disorders involving sensory nerves	Decreased CV (myelin disorders) Decreased amplitude (axonal disorders)
Cord dorsum potential (CDP)	Assessment of the sensory nerve and dorsal gray matter of the spinal cord	Increased latency of the onset and onset to peak of the CDP

PSW, Positive sharp waves; *CRD,* complex repetitive discharges; *CV,* conduction velocity; *CMAP,* compound muscle action potential; *AUC,* area under the curve.

*Most commonly used tests.

†Provided minimal F-wave latency or motor nerve conduction velocity is prolonged, the finding of a normal F-ratio suggests diffuse involvement of the motor nerve.

sensory function on neurologic examination.[72] Recordings are made by measuring the potentials with the shortest latencies (those of the faster pathways [e.g., the dorsal and dorsolateral funiculi of the spinal cord]). Unfortunately, these axons also are the first to be affected even in animals with minimal clinical signs. Therefore, the utility of SEP in assessment of animals with structural CNS lesions is questionable. Similar motor-evoked potentials (MEPs) can be recorded from either muscle or the spinal cord in response to either magnetic or electrical stimulation of the motor cortex.[73-77] Limited reports have been performed to evaluate the utility of MEPs. In dogs and horses, MEP may correlate with severity of clinical signs.[78-80]

Electroretinography (ERG) is the recording of the electrical potential of the retina in response to light. The light stimulus may be single or multiple flashes of light. The intensity and frequency of stimulation along with dark or light adapted enables assessment of rods and cones.[81] The ERG is helpful for differentiating diseases of the retina from lesions occurring in the visual pathway caudal to the retina (optic nerve, chiasm, optic tract, optic radiation, and occipital cortex).[82]

The visual-evoked response (VER) is the cortical electrical activity that occurs in response to a light stimulus administered to the eye. The response provides an objective evaluation of central visual pathways.[83,84] Although rarely performed, pattern stimuli, light-emitting diode goggles, or a red filter has made this technique more useful.[85,86]

Electroencephalography (EEG), the graphic recording of the electrical activity of the cerebral cortical neurons, may be used in assessment of cerebral disease.[87,88] Although its utility has been largely supplanted by MRI, EEG may still have a role in the diagnosis of seizure activity and monitoring of anticonvulsant effects. The EEG varies with the level of consciousness. Low voltage and fast activity are seen in the alert animal. Higher voltage and slower activity occur during drowsiness and sleep. Drugs such as sedatives, tranquilizers, and anesthetics produce higher voltage and slower activity similar to sleep patterns. Results of the EEG may indicate that cerebral disease is present and whether it is focal or diffuse, acute or chronic, and inflammatory or degenerative.

The following general principles of EEG changes have been listed by Klemm and Hall[89]:

1. Low voltage, fast activity (LVFA), and spikes (very fast activity) indicate irritation from any cause (usually inflammatory disease).
2. High voltage and slow activity (HVSA) suggest neuronal death or compression.
3. Neither change is diagnostic of a disease but rather reflects the kind of process occurring (e.g., inflammation or degeneration).
4. A focal EEG abnormality indicates a focal cerebral cortical lesion.
5. A generalized EEG abnormality indicates a diffuse cerebral cortical disease or a subcortical abnormality that alters the activity of the majority of the cerebral cortex.
6. The EEG can change with time, suggesting progression or resolution of the disease process.

Quantitative electroencephalography provides more objective data on the spectral frequency content and amplitudes of the EEG recording.[90]

Urodynamics studies includes cystometrography, urethral pressure profiles, and electrophysiologic testing of bladder and sphincter reflexes (see Chapter 3 for details).

Contraindications

No significant contraindications exist to any of the electrophysiologic tests unless anesthesia or tranquilization is necessary and is contraindicated.

Biopsy

Availability

Biopsies of the CNS primarily are confined to the cerebrum (brain biopsy). Generally, biopsies are performed with CT guidance.[91-95] Alternatively, ultrasonographic guidance can be used during surgical procedures.[23]

Biopsies of nerve and muscle can be performed by any veterinary surgeon; however, the difficulties in obtaining good diagnostic samples generally limit this procedure to specialty practices and institutions. Paramount to obtaining a histologic diagnosis is adequate sample submission, proper sample preservation (i.e., unfixed muscle tissue submitted on ice or nerve fascicles preserved in glutaraldehyde) and evaluation by a pathologist specialized in neuropathology.

Indications

A biopsy or a fine-needle aspirate of lesions in the CNS is used to confirm a diagnosis of an intracranial neoplasia or a diffuse encephalopathy, such as viral inflammation or storage disease.[92,96] Many of the diseases cannot be definitively diagnosed antemortem with other procedures. Because of the invasive nature of the procedure and potential for morbidity and mortality, it is not generally pursued except with focal lesions identified with CT or MRI.

Cytologic diagnosis can be obtained with the use of fine-needle aspirate procedures. Fine-needle aspiration of epidural or spinal cord masses can be accomplished with fluoroscopy.[97] Lymphoma may be readily identified using this technique. Fine-needle aspirate also may allow cytologic diagnosis of intracranial lesions.[98,99]

Biopsy of a nerve is indicated in neuropathies. Excision of a few fascicles of a mixed nerve is preferred if a motor neuropathy is suspected, but small sensory nerves may be sampled in many disorders.[100,101] A muscle biopsy usually is performed simultaneously with a nerve biopsy to differentiate neuropathies from myopathies. Proximal and distal muscles should ideally be sampled because pathologic changes may differ widely among muscles. Tissues must be handled properly for satisfactory histopathologic evaluation. The nerve or muscle specimen must be maintained straight, without excess tension, during fixation. This positioning usually is attained by tying or pinning the ends of the nerve to a tongue depressor or using double clamps on the muscle.[100] The histochemical staining necessary to diagnose or better characterize most muscle diseases must be done on unfixed muscle. The pathologist should be consulted regarding the proper handling of the tissues before obtaining samples.

Contraindications

The invasive nature of these procedures must be weighed against the benefits of the information to be gained. The brain biopsy does require specialized equipment and expertise. Misdiagnosis can result from nondiagnostic samples. A spinal cord biopsy is contraindicated because the procedure causes seriously compromised spinal cord function; however, fine-needle aspiration of mass lesions in the vertebral canal is useful and produces little damage. Nerve and muscle biopsies are performed more commonly and do not produce serious deficits if care is exercised in the selection of the nerve undergoing the biopsy.

REFERENCES

1. Jezyk PF, Haskins ME, Patterson DF: Screening for inborn errors of metabolism in dogs and cats, Prog Clin Biol Res 94:93–116, 1982.
2. Sewell AC, Haskins ME, Giger U: Inherited metabolic disease in companion animals: searching for nature's mistakes, Vet J 174:252–259, 2007.
3. Edelman RR, Warach S: Magnetic resonance imaging: first of two parts, N Engl J Med 328:708–716, 1993.
4. Kuriashkin IV, Losonsky JM: Contrast enhancement in magnetic resonance imaging using intravenous paramagnetic contrast media: a review, Vet Radiol Ultrasound 41:4–7, 2000.
5. Cherubini GB, Platt SR, Howson S, et al: Comparison of magnetic resonance imaging sequences in dogs with multi-focal intracranial disease, J Small Anim Pract 49:634–640, 2008.
6. Benigni L, Lamb CR: Comparison of fluid-attenuated inversion recovery and T2-weighted magnetic resonance images in dogs and cats with suspected brain disease, Vet Radiol Ultrasound 46:287–292, 2005.
7. Armbrust LJ, Hoskinson JJ, Biller DS, et al: Low-field magnetic resonance imaging of bone marrow in the lumbar spine, pelvis, and femur in the adult dog, Vet Radiol Ultrasound 45:393–401, 2004.
8. Tidwell AS, Specht A, Blaeser L, et al: Magnetic resonance imaging features of extradural hematomas associated with intervertebral disc herniation in a dog, Vet Radiol Ultrasound 43:319–324, 2002.
9. Pease A, Sullivan S, Olby N, et al: Value of a single-shot turbo spin-echo pulse sequence for assessing the architecture of the subarachnoid space and the constitutive nature of cerebrospinal fluid, Vet Radiol Ultrasound 47:254–259, 2006.
10. Perry RL: Principles of conventional radiography and fluoroscopy, Vet Clin North Am 23:235–252, 1993.
11. Tidwell AS, Jones JC: Advanced imaging concepts: a pictorial glossary of CT and MRI technology, Clin Tech Small Anim Pract 14:65–111, 1999.
12. Sharp NJH, Cofone M, Robertson ID, et al: Computed tomography in the evaluation of caudal cervical spondylomyelopathy of the Doberman pinscher, Vet Radiol Ultrasound 36:100–108, 1995.
13. Drost WT, Love NE, Berry CR: Comparison of radiography, myelography and computed tomography for the evaluation of canine vertebral and spinal cord tumors in sixteen dogs, Vet Radiol Ultrasound 37:28–33, 1996.
14. Armbrust LJ: Digital images and digital radiographic image capture. In Thrall DE, editor: Textbook of veterinary diagnostic radiology, St Louis, 2007, Saunders Elsevier.
15. Middleton DL: Radiographic positioning for the spine and skull, Vet Clin North Am 23:253–258, 1993.
16. Barone G, Ziemer LS, Shofer FS, et al: Risk factors associated with development of seizures after use of iohexol for myelography in dogs: 182 cases (1998), J Am Vet Med Assoc 220:1499–1502, 2002.
17. Lewis DD, Hosgood G: Complications associated with the use of iohexol for myelography of the cervical vertebral column in dogs: 66 cases (1988-1990), J Am Vet Med Assoc 200:1381–1384, 1992.
18. Platt SR, Dennis R, Murphy K, et al: Hematomyelia secondary to lumbar cerebrospinal fluid acquisition in a dog, Vet Radiol Ultrasound 46:467–471, 2005.
19. Suter PF, Morgan JP, Holliday TA, et al: Myelography in the dog: diagnosis of tumors of the spinal cord and vertebrae, Vet Radiol Ultrasound 12:29–44, 1971.

20. Kirberger RM, Wrigley RH: Myelography in the dog: review of patients with contrast medium in the central canal, Vet Radiol Ultrasound 34:253–258, 1993.
21. Morgan JP, Atilola M, Bailey CS: Vertebral canal and spinal cord mensuration: a comparative study of its effect on lumbosacral myelography in the dachshund and German shepherd dog, J Am Vet Med Assoc 191:951–957, 1987.
22. Finn-Bodner ST, Hudson JA, Coates JR, et al: Ultrasonographic anatomy of the normal canine spinal cord and correlation with histopathology after induced spinal cord trauma, Vet Radiol Ultrasound 36:39–48, 1995.
23. Gallagher JG, Penninck D, Boudrieau RJ, et al: Ultrasonography of the brain and vertebral canal in dogs and cats: 15 cases (1988-1993), J Am Vet Med Assoc 207:1320–1324, 1995.
24. Hudson JA, Cartee RE, Simpson ST, et al: Ultrasonographic anatomy of the canine brain, Vet Radiol Ultrasound 30:13–21, 1989.
25. Rivers WJ, Walter PA: Hydrocephalus in the dog: utility of ultrasonography as an alternate diagnostic imaging technique, J Am Anim Hosp Assoc 28:333–343, 1992.
26. Spaulding KA, Sharp NJH: Ultrasonographic imaging of the lateral cerebral ventricles in the dog, Vet Radiol Ultrasound 31:59–64, 1990.
27. Kornegay JN: Cerebrospinal fluid collection, examination, and interpretation in dogs and cats, Compend Contin Educ Pract Vet 3:85–94, 1981.
28. Mayhew IG: Collection of cerebrospinal fluid from the horse, Cornell Vet 65:500–511, 1975.
29. Thomson CE, Kornegay JN, Stevens JB: Analysis of cerebrospinal fluid from the cerebellomedullary and lumbar cisterns of dogs with focal neurologic disease: 145 cases (1985-1987), J Am Vet Med Assoc 196:1841–1844, 1990.
30. Sweeney CR, Russell GE: Differences in total protein concentration, nucleated cell count, and red blood cell count among sequential samples of cerebrospinal fluid from horses, J Am Vet Med Assoc 217:54–57, 2000.
31. Bienzle D, McDonnell JJ, Stanton JB: Analysis of cerebrospinal fluid from dogs and cats after 24 and 48 hours of storage, J Am Vet Med Assoc 216:1761–1764, 2000.
32. Fry MM, Vernau W, Kass PH, et al: Effects of time, initial composition, and stabilizing agents on the results of canine cerebrospinal fluid analysis, Vet Clin Pathol 35:72–77, 2006.
33. Wilson JW, Stevens JB: Effects of blood contamination on cerebrospinal fluid analysis, J Am Vet Med Assoc 171:256–258, 1977.
34. Hurtt AE, Smith MO: Effects of iatrogenic blood contamination on results of cerebrospinal fluid analysis in clinically normal dogs and dogs with neurologic disease, J Am Vet Med Assoc 211:866–867, 1997.
35. Sellon RK: Update on molecular techniques for diagnostic testing of infectious disease, Vet Clin North Am 33:677–693, 2003.
36. Burnett RC, Vernau W, Modiano JF, et al: Diagnosis of canine lymphoid neoplasia using clonal rearrangements of antigen receptor genes, Vet Pathol 40:32–41, 2003.
37. Duque C, Parent J, Bienzle D: The immunophenotype of blood and cerebrospinal fluid mononuclear cells in dogs, J Vet Intern Med 16:714–719, 2002.
38. Schwartz M, Moore PF, Tipold A: Disproportionally strong increase of B cells in inflammatory cerebrospinal fluid of dogs with steroid-responsive meningitis-arteritis, Vet Immunol Immunopathol 125:274–283, 2008.
39. Thomas WB, Sorjonen DC, Steiss JE: A retrospective evaluation of 38 cases of canine distemper encephalomyelitis, J Am Anim Hosp Assoc 29:129–133, 1993.
40. Vandevelde M, Zurbriggen A, Steck A, et al: Studies on the intrathecal humoral immune response in canine distemper encephalitis, J Neuroimmunol 11:41–51, 1986.
41. Berthelin CF, Legendre AM, Bailey CS, et al: Cryptococcosis of the nervous system in dogs, part 2: diagnosis, treatment, monitoring, and prognosis, Prog Vet Neurol 5:136–146, 1994.
42. Dunigan CE, Oglesbee MJ, Podell M, et al: Seizure activity associated with equine protozoal myeloencephalitis, Prog Vet Neurol 6:50–54, 1995.
43. Muñana KR, Lappin MR, Powell CC, et al: Sequential measurement of Toxoplasma gondii-specific antibodies in the cerebrospinal fluid of cats with experimentally induced toxoplasmosis, Prog Vet Neurol 6:27–31, 1995.
44. Tipold A: Diagnosis of inflammatory and infectious diseases of the central nervous system in dogs: a retrospective study, J Vet Intern Med 9:304–314, 1995.
45. Bichsel P, Vandevelde M, Vandevelde E, et al: Immunoelectrophoretic determination of albumin and IgG in serum and cerebrospinal fluid in dogs with neurological diseases, Res Vet Sci 37:101–107, 1984.
46. Kristensen F, Firth EC: Analysis of serum proteins and cerebrospinal fluid in clinically normal horses, using agarose electrophoresis, Am J Vet Res 38:1089–1092, 1977.
47. Rand JS, Parent J, Jacobs R, et al: Reference intervals for feline cerebrospinal fluid: biochemical and serologic variables, IgG concentration, and electrophoretic fractionation, Am J Vet Res 51:1049–1054, 1990.
48. Sorjonen DC: Total protein, albumin quota, and electrophoretic patterns in cerebrospinal fluid of dogs with central nervous system disorders, Am J Vet Res 48:301–305, 1987.
49. Smith-Maxie LL, Parent JP, Rand J, et al: Cerebrospinal fluid analysis and clinical outcome of eight dogs with eosinophilic meningoencephalomyelitis, J Vet Intern Med 3:167–174, 1989.
50. Sorjonen DC: Clinical and histopathological features of granulomatous meningoencephalomyelitis in dogs, J Am Anim Hosp Assoc 26:141–147, 1990.
51. Windsor RC, Sturges BK, Vernau KM, et al: Cerebrospinal fluid eosinophilia in dogs, J Vet Intern Med 23:275–281, 2009.
52. Redding RW, Ingram JT: Sensory nerve conduction velocity of cutaneous afferents of the radial, ulnar, peroneal, and tibial nerves of the cat: reference values, Am J Vet Res 45:1042–1045, 1984.
53. Tuler SM, Bowen JM: Measurement of conduction velocity of the peroneal nerve based on recordings from extensor digitorum brevis muscle, J Am Anim Hosp Assoc 26:164–168, 1990.
54. Swallow JS, Griffiths IR: Age related changes in the motor nerve conduction velocity in dogs, Res Vet Sci 23:29–32, 1977.
55. Pillai SR, Steiss JE, Wright JC: Age-related changes in peripheral nerve conduction velocities of cats, Prog Vet Neurol 2:95–104, 1991.
56. Lee AF, Bowen JM: Effect of tissue temperature on ulnar nerve conduction velocity in the dog, Am J Vet Res 36:1305–1307, 1975.
57. Sims MH, McLean RH: Use of repetitive nerve stimulation to assess neuromuscular function in dogs. A test protocol for suspected myasthenia gravis, Prog Vet Neurol 1:311–319, 1990.

58. Cuddon PA: Acquired canine peripheral neuropathies, Vet Clin North Am 32:31–62, 2002.
59. Gödde T, Jaggy A, Vandevelde M, et al: Evaluation of repetitive nerve stimulation in young dogs, J Small Anim Pract 34:393–398, 1993.
60. Hopkins AL, Howard JF, Wheeler SJ, et al: Stimulated single fibre electromyography in normal dogs, J Small Anim Pract 34:271–276, 1993.
61. Holliday TA, Te Selle ME: Brain stem auditory-evoked potentials of dogs: wave forms and effects of recording electrode positions, Am J Vet Res 46:845–851, 1985.
62. Rolf SL, Reed SM, Melnick W, et al: Auditory brain stem response testing in anesthetized horses, Am J Vet Res 48:910–914, 1987.
63. Strain GM, Olcott BM, Thompson DR, et al: Brainstem auditory-evoked potentials in Holstein cows, J Vet Intern Med 3:144–148, 1989.
64. Sims MH, Moore RE: Auditory-evoked response in the clinically normal dog: early latency components, Am J Vet Res 45:2019–2027, 1984.
65. Holliday TA, Nelson HJ, Williams DC, et al: Unilateral and bilateral brainstem auditory-evoked response abnormalities in 900 Dalmatian dogs, J Vet Intern Med 6:166–174, 1992.
66. Strain GM, Kearney MT, Gignac IJ, et al: Brainstem auditory-evoked potential assessment of congenital deafness in Dalmatians: associations with phenotypic markers, J Vet Intern Med 6:175–182, 1992.
67. Steiss JE, Cox NR, Hathcock JT: Brain stem auditory-evoked response abnormalities in 14 dogs with confirmed central nervous system lesions, J Vet Intern Med 8:293–298, 1994.
68. Cuddon PA, Delauche AJ, Hutchison JM: Assessment of dorsal nerve root and spinal cord dorsal horn function in clinically normal dogs by determination of cord dorsum potentials, Am J Vet Res 60:222–226, 1999.
69. Mizisin AP, Shelton GD, Burgers ML, et al: Neurological complications associated with spontaneously occurring feline diabetes mellitus, J Neuropath Exp Neurol 61:872–884, 2002.
70. Strain GM, Taylor DS, Graham MC, et al: Cortical somatosensory-evoked potentials in the horse, Am J Vet Res 49:1869–1872, 1988.
71. Oliver JE, Purinton PT, Brown J: Somatosensory evoked potentials from stimulation of thoracic limb nerves of the dog, Prog Vet Neurol 1:433–443, 1990.
72. Shores A, Redding RW, Knecht CD: Spinal-evoked potentials in dogs with acute compressive thoracolumbar spinal cord disease, Am J Vet Res 48:1525–1530, 1987.
73. Nollet H, Deprez P, van Ham L, et al: Transcranial magnetic stimulation: normal values of magnetic motor evoked potentials in 84 normal horses and influence of height, weight, age and sex, Equine Vet J 36:51–57, 2004.
74. Nollet H, Van Ham L, Deprez P, et al: Transcranial magnetic stimulation: review of the technique, basic principles and applications, Vet J 166:28–42, 2003.
75. Strain GM, Prescott-Mathews JS, Tedford BL: Motor potentials evoked by transcranial stimulation of the canine motor cortex, Prog Vet Neurol 1:321–331, 1990.
76. Sylvestre AM, Cockshutt JR, Parent JM, et al: Magnetic motor evoked potentials for assessing spinal cord integrity in dogs with intervertebral disc disease, Vet Surg 22:5–10, 1993.
77. van Ham LML, Mattheeuws DRG, Vanderstraeten GGW: Transcranial magnetic motor evoked potentials in anesthetized dogs, Prog Vet Neurol 6:5–12, 1995.
78. da Costa RC, Poma R, Parent JM, et al: Correlation of motor evoked potentials with magnetic resonance imaging and neurologic findings in Doberman pinschers with and without signs of cervical spondylomyelopathy, Am J Vet Res 67:1613–1620, 2006.
79. Nollet H, Deprez P, Van Ham L, et al: The use of magnetic motor evoked potentials in horses with cervical spinal cord disease, Equine Vet J 34:156–163, 2002.
80. Poma R, Parent JM, Holmberg DL, et al: Correlation between severity of clinical signs and motor evoked potentials after transcranial magnetic stimulation in large-breed dogs with cervical spinal cord disease, J Am Vet Med Assoc 221:60–64, 2002.
81. Komaromy AM, Smith PJ, Brooks DE: Electroretinography in dogs and cats. Part I. Retinal morphology and physiology, Compend Contin Educ Pract Vet 20:343–345, 348–350, 1998.
82. Komaromy AM, Smith PJ, Brooks DE: Electroretinography in dogs and cats. Part II. Technique, interpretation, and indications, Compend Contin Educ Pract Vet 20:355–359, 362–366, 1998.
83. Strain GM, Claxton MS, Olcott BM, et al: Visual-evoked potentials and electroretinograms in ruminants with thiamine-responsive polioencephalomalacia or suspected listeriosis, Am J Vet Res 51:1513–1517, 1990.
84. Sims MH, Laratta LJ, Bubb WJ, et al: Waveform analysis and reproducibility of visual-evoked potentials in dogs, Am J Vet Res 50:1823–1828, 1989.
85. Bichsel P, Oliver JE Jr, Coulter DB, et al: Recording of visual-evoked potentials in dogs with scalp electrodes, J Vet Intern Med 2:145–149, 1988.
86. Sims MH, Laratta LJ: Visual-evoked potentials in cats, using a light-emitting diode stimulator, Am J Vet Res 49:1876–1881, 1988.
87. Redding RW: Electroencephalography, Prog Vet Neurol 1:181–188, 1990.
88. Redding RW, Knecht CD: Atlas of electroencephalography in the dog and cat, ed, New York, 1984, Praeger.
89. Klemm WR, Hall CL: Current status and trends in veterinary electroencephalography, J Am Vet Med Assoc 164:529–532, 1974.
90. Moore MP, Greene SA, Keegan RD, et al: Quantitative electroencephalography in dogs anesthetized with 2.0% end-tidal concentration of isoflurane anesthesia, Am J Vet Res 52:551–560, 1991.
91. Giroux A, Jones JC, Bohn JH, et al: A new device for stereotactic CT-guided biopsy of the canine brain: design, construction, and needle placement accuracy, Vet Radiol Ultrasound 43:229–236, 2002.
92. Koblik PD, LeCouteur RA, Higgins RJ, et al: CT-guided brain biopsy using a modified Pelorus Mark III stereotactic system: experience with 50 dogs, Vet Radiol Ultrasound 40:434–440, 1999.
93. Moissonnier P, Blot S, Devauchelle P, et al: Stereotactic CT-guided brain biopsy in the dog, J Small Anim Pract 43:115–123, 2002.
94. Moissonnier P, Bordeau W, Delisle F, et al: Accuracy testing of a new stereotactic CT-guided brain biopsy device in the dog, Res Vet Sci 68:243–247, 2000.
95. Troxel MT, Vite CH: CT-guided stereotactic brain biopsy using the Kopf stereotactic system, Vet Radiol Ultrasound 49:438–443, 2008.

96. Swaim SF, Vandevelde M, Faircloth JC: Evaluation of brain biopsy techniques in the dog, J Am Anim Hosp Assoc 15:627–633, 1979.
97. Irving G, McMillan MC: Fluoroscopically guided percutaneous fine-needle aspiration biopsy of thoracolumbar spinal lesions in cats, Prog Vet Neurol 1:473–475, 1990.
98. Platt SR, Alleman AR, Lanz OI, et al: Comparison of fine-needle aspiration and surgical-tissue biopsy in the diagnosis of canine brain tumors, Vet Surg 31:65–69, 2002.
99. Vernau KM, Higgins RJ, Bollen AW, et al: Primary canine and feline nervous system tumors: intraoperative diagnosis using the smear technique, Vet Pathol 38:47–57, 2001.
100. Braund KG: Nerve and muscle biopsy techniques, Prog Vet Neurol 2:35–56, 1991.
101. Braund KG, Walker TL, Vandevelde M: Fascicular nerve biopsy in the dog, Am J Vet Res 40:1025–1030, 1979.

PART II

Clinical Problems: Signs and Symptoms

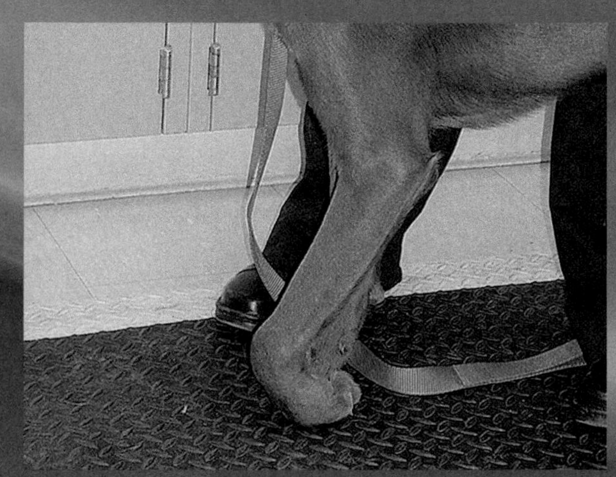

CHAPTER 5

Paresis of One Limb

The term *monoparesis*, or *monoplegia*, denotes partial or complete loss of voluntary motor function in one limb, resulting from a neurologic lesion. Monoparesis must be distinguished from lameness that is due to musculoskeletal involvement. Severe neural lesions cause characteristic sensory and motor deficits (see Lesion Localization section). Peripheral nerve and nerve root compression and neoplastic involvement, however, often initially cause lameness and pain (*nerve root signature*) suggestive of musculoskeletal disease (Figure 5-1). Results of the neurologic examination must be reviewed critically in these animals to identify typical deficits. Electrodiagnostic testing may be particularly helpful in localizing lesions to the peripheral nerve or nerve root in such cases (see Chapter 4).

Peripheral or spinal nerves may be injured owing to skeletal fractures or luxations. Thus both systems must be critically evaluated in animals with monoparesis after trauma. In general, the prognosis for recovery is better with skeletal than with neurologic injuries.

LESION LOCALIZATION

The basic anatomic and physiologic principles that enable a clinician to localize lesions based on motor or sensory deficits are presented in Chapter 2. Concepts related to the localization of lesions producing monoparesis or monoplegia are reviewed here (Figure 5-2).

Monoparesis usually is caused by disease or injury to the lower motor neurons (LMNs) innervating the affected limb. Thus dysfunction of the motor neuron (motor nerve cell body), axon (ventral root, spinal nerve, peripheral nerves), or neuromuscular endplate results in motor dysfunction and denervation atrophy. Monoparesis can also be the result of a lesion affecting specific muscle groups of the thoracic limb. Monoparesis most commonly occurs because of involvement of axons of either peripheral or spinal nerves but less frequently results from lesions affecting neuronal cell bodies in the ventral gray matter of the spinal cord. Rarely, monoparesis is a consequence of a disease process affecting the neuromuscular junction. Most disorders of the neuromuscular junction are diffuse (see Chapter 7). In most cases, unilateral spinal cord lesions cranial to T3 cause hemiparesis, and bilateral lesions cause tetraparesis. Unilateral spinal cord lesions caudal to T2 produce paresis or paralysis of the ipsilateral pelvic limb, whereas bilateral lesions produce paraparesis or paraplegia. Thus in animals with thoracic limb monoparesis and no involvement of the other limbs, primary consideration is given to the spinal roots and nerves, brachial plexus, or the peripheral nerves (Table 5-1). Spinal cord lesions at C6-T2 confined entirely to the ventral gray matter could cause thoracic limb monoparesis but more commonly these lesions also involve general proprioceptive (GP) and upper motor neuron (UMN) pathways to the ipsilateral pelvic limb. Pelvic limb monoparesis may occur because of unilateral spinal cord lesions between the T3 and S1 segments or more commonly because of involvement of spinal roots and nerves, or nerves

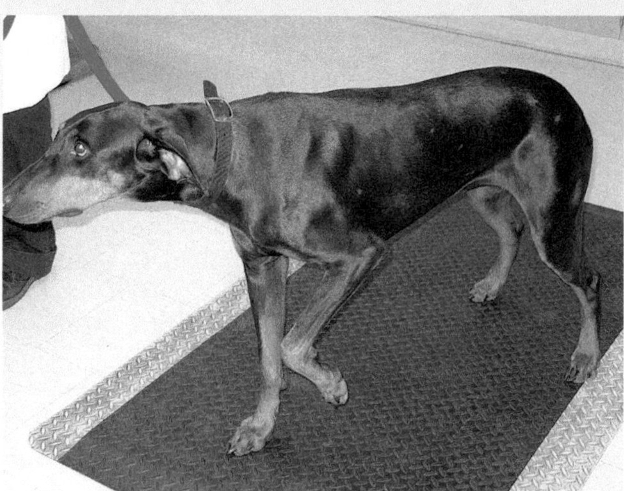

Figure 5-1 Doberman pinscher with "nerve root signature" involving the left thoracic limb, resulting from compression of the left C6 nerve root by foraminal entrapment of a laterally extruded disk. The dog held the limb off the floor and had pain when the limb was manipulated.

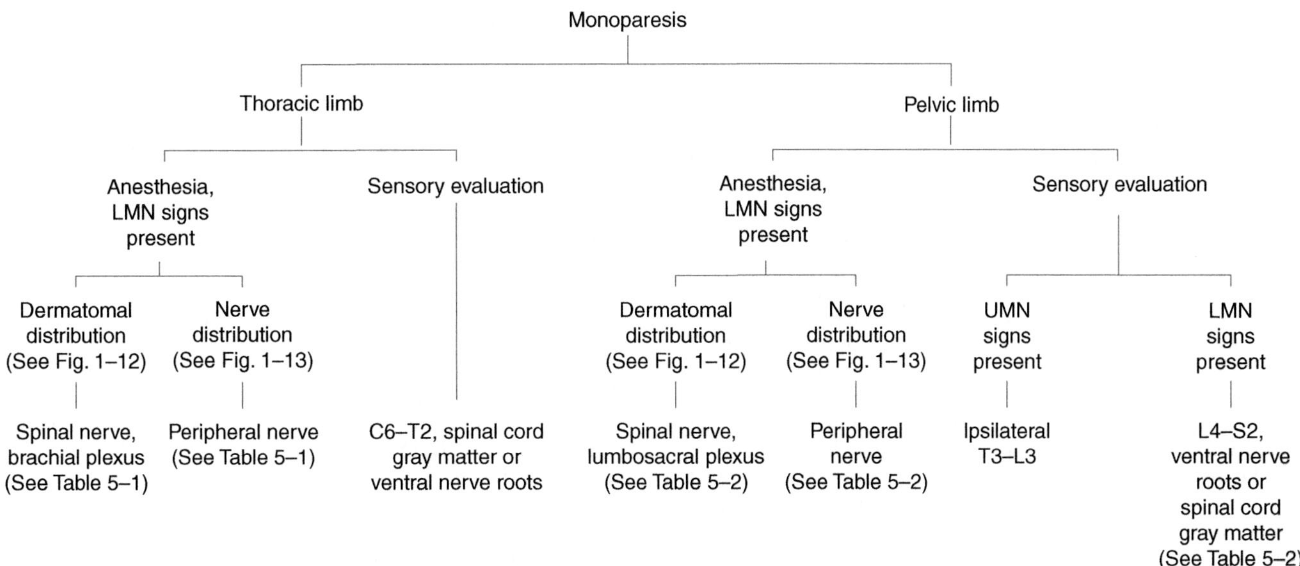

Figure 5-2 An algorithm for localization of lesions that produce monoparesis.

TABLE 5-1

Nerves of the Brachial Plexus

Nerve	Spinal Cord Segments*	Motor Function	Cutaneous Sensory Distribution	Signs of Dysfunction
Suprascapular	***C6***, C7	Extension and lateral support of the shoulder	None	Little gait abnormality, pronounced atrophy of supraspinatus and infraspinatus muscles (sweeney)
Brachiocephalicus	***C6***, C7	Advance limb	Cranial surface of brachium	Little gait abnormality, anesthesia of cranial brachium
Musculocutaneous	C6, ***C7***, C8	Flexion of the elbow	Medial antebrachium	Little gait abnormality, weakened flexion of the elbow; anesthesia of medial antebrachium
Axillary	C6, ***C7***, C8	Flexion of the shoulder	Dorsolateral brachium	Little gait abnormality, decreased shoulder flexor reflex; anesthesia of lateral side of brachium
Radial	***C7, C8, T1***, T2	Extension of the elbow, the carpus, and the digits	Dorsal surface of the foot and dorsal, and lateral parts of the antebrachium	Loss of weight bearing, knuckling of pes, decreased extensor carpi radialis and triceps reflexes, anesthesia of dorsal surface distal to elbow
Median and ulnar	***C8, T1***, T2	Flexion of the carpus and the digits	Palmar surface of the foot; caudal antebrachium	Little gait abnormality, slight sinking of the carpus; loss of carpal flexion on flexor reflex; partial loss of pain perception of the palmar surface of the foot and caudal antebrachium
Lateral thoracic	***C8***, T1	Cutaneous muscle of the trunk	None	Absent ipsilateral cutaneous trunci reflex, normal sensory evaluation
Sympathetic†	T1, T2, T3	Dilation of the pupil	None	Miosis, ptosis, enophthalmos, and protrusion of third eyelid

*The major spinal cord segments that form the peripheral nerves are italicized and bolded.
†The sympathetic nerve is not considered part of the brachial plexus; however, its nerve fibers travel along the roots of the brachial plexus as they exit the vertebral column.

of the lumbosacral plexus. Unilateral T3-L3 spinal cord lesions cause GP/UMN signs in the ipsilateral limb, whereas lesions between the L4 and S2 spinal cord segments, or spinal nerves and roots cause LMN signs.

Disease of the spinal or peripheral nerves results in both sensory and motor dysfunction distal to the lesion because most nerves contain both sensory and motor fibers. In contrast, lesions confined to the ventral gray matter of the spinal cord produce only motor dysfunction. Unilateral T3 to L3 spinal cord lesions do not cause anesthesia of the affected limb because deep pain perception is transmitted over bilateral, multisynaptic pathways (see Chapter 1). Anesthesia occurring in a single affected limb therefore suggests peripheral nerve or nerve root involvement. If sensory loss cannot be detected in the affected limb, lesions in the spinal cord gray matter or the ventral spinal nerve roots should be considered. Figure 5-2 outlines the localization of lesions that produce monoparesis of the thoracic and pelvic limbs.

The distribution of sensory loss in an affected limb has great localizing value because lesions can be pinpointed to a particular nerve or within two to three spinal cord segments (see Figure 1-12).[1,2] The total area innervated by a particular cutaneous nerve is termed its *cutaneous area*.[3] The cutaneous area includes a peripheral *overlap zone* innervated by other cutaneous nerves and a central *autonomous zone* innervated solely by that nerve (Figure 5-3). These zones can be detected clinically using a method termed the "two-step pinch technique." Using a mosquito hemostat, a small fold of skin is lifted and gently grasped, activating mechanoreceptors in adjacent cutaneous areas. After the animal is quiet, a small fold of skin is pinched, stimulating only the autonomous zone of the particular nerve. Either a conscious response or reflex withdrawal indicates functional integrity of the particular nerve. The degree of sensory loss also influences the prognosis for functional recovery.

The pattern of denervation atrophy (see Figure 5-4) facilitates localization of lesions to a particular nerve or nerve group. Tables 5-1 and 5-2 outline the motor and sensory distribution of the brachial and lumbosacral plexus and the neurologic signs associated with lesions in each major nerve. Animals with peripheral nerve disease or injury also may mutilate the area normally innervated by the affected nerves.[4] This behavior apparently occurs because of *dysesthesia (paresthesia)* caused by ectopic excitation of axonal sprouts in the neuroma or sensory neurons in the dorsal spinal ganglion of the injured nerve. Self-mutilation can become particularly problematic and necessitate amputation of the involved digits, limb, or tail.

Lesions in the gray matter of the spinal cord at T1-3 segments or in the roots of the brachial plexus may injure the LMNs of the sympathetic nerve fibers that form the cranial sympathetic trunk. Loss of sympathetic stimulation to the ipsilateral eye produces signs of miosis, enophthalmos with elevation of the third eyelid (membrana nictitans), and ptosis (Horner's syndrome). In the horse, miosis is not as obvious and sweating is seen on the face and neck to the level of C2 on the side of the lesion.[5] Horner's syndrome commonly is associated with traumatic injuries of the brachial plexus. Similarly, lesions of the C8-T1 gray matter, nerve roots, or spinal nerves affect the lateral thoracic nerve, which is the motor component of the cutaneous trunci (panniculus) reflex. Therefore, lesions of the brachial plexus may cause LMN paresis of the limb, Horner's syndrome, and loss of the cutaneous trunci reflex on the same side.

Mononeuropathy refers to a disease or an injury of a specific peripheral nerve or its nerve roots. If a large nerve such as the sciatic or radial nerve is injured, severe monoparesis may occur. In most cases, mononeuropathies result from physical injury secondary to compression, laceration, or contusion or from intramuscular injection of drugs. In addition to motor dysfunction and atrophy, variable degrees of sensory loss are encountered because peripheral nerves innervating the limbs contain both motor and sensory fibers.

Polyneuropathy refers to a disease or an injury of several peripheral nerves or their nerve roots. The term is generally used to indicate involvement of many nerves. Those diseases are described in Chapter 7.

In regard to monoparesis, polyneuropathy suggests an injury or a disease of the brachial plexus, the lumbosacral plexus, or the cauda equina. Alternatively, a polyneuropathy resulting in monoparesis also may be due to injury or disease affecting multiple spinal nerve roots or spinal nerves giving rise to the brachial plexus, lumbosacral plexus, or cauda equina. As for mononeuropathies, physical injury is the most common cause of polyneuropathy and subsequent monoparesis. Occasionally, monoparesis occurs because of neoplastic involvement of a specific peripheral nerve, nerve root, or nerve plexus. Resulting clinical signs progress insidiously, in

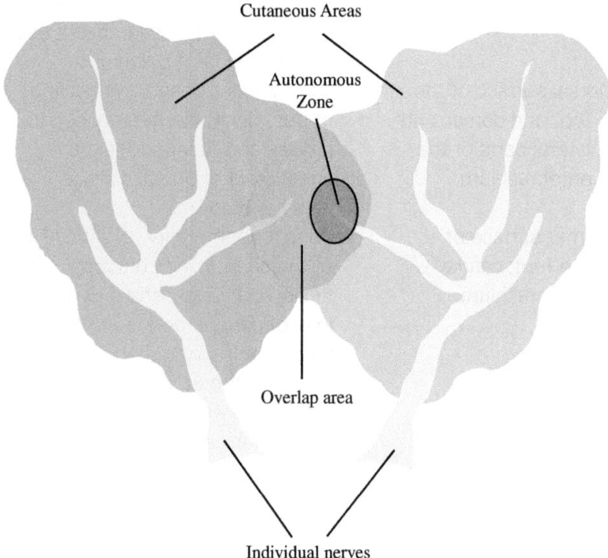

Figure 5-3 A schematic illustrating the cutaneous area innervated by a nerve to include its overlap zone and autonomous zone.

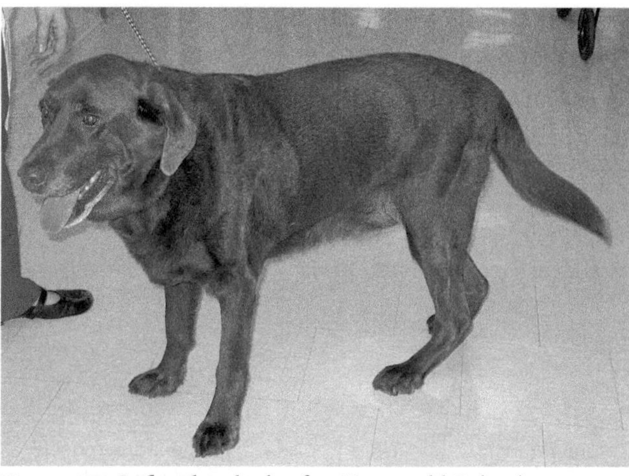
Figure 5-4 Left pelvic limb of a 10-year-old Labrador retriever ("nerve root signature") that progressed to monoparesis with associated hyporeflexia and neurogenic muscle atrophy. Atrophy of the biceps femoris and gastrocnemius muscles is shown here. Note the dropped hock. Magnetic resonance imaging revealed a mass involving the proximal sciatic nerve. A presumptive diagnosis of a nerve sheath tumor was made.

TABLE 5-2

Nerves of the Lumbosacral Plexus

Nerve	Spinal Cord Segments*	Motor Function	Cutaneous Sensory Distribution	Signs of Dysfunction
Obturator	L4, ***L5***, L6	Adduction of pelvic limb	None	Little gait abnormality, abduction on slick surface
Femoral	L3, ***L4, L5***, L6	Extension of stifle, flexion of hip	Saphenous branch supplies medial surface of limb and medial digit	Severe gait dysfunction, no weight bearing, decreased or absent patellar reflex, loss of sensation in medial limb and medial digit
Sciatic	***L6, L7, S1***, S2	Extension of hip, extension and flexion of stifle (see tibial and peroneal branches)	Caudal and lateral surfaces of limb distal to stifle (see tibial and peroneal branches)	Severe gait dysfunction; paw is knuckled, but weight bearing occurs; hip cannot be extended, hock cannot be flexed or extended (in more proximal lesions, hip is flexed and drawn toward the midline); loss of cutaneous sensation distal to stifle (except for areas supplied by saphenous nerve); absent flexor reflex
Peroneal	***L6, L7***, S1,S2	Flexion of hock, extension of digits	Cranial surface of limb distal to stifle	Hock is straightened and foot tends to knuckle; loss of sensation on cranial surface to limb distal to stifle, poor hock flexion on flexor reflex†
Tibial	L6, ***L7, S1***, S2	Extension of hock, flexion of digits	Caudal surface of limb distal to stifle	Hock is dropped, loss of sensation on caudal surface of limb distal to stifle†

*The major spinal cord segments that form the peripheral nerves are italicized and bolded.

†Peroneal and tibial nerve paralysis commonly occurs in association with each other. Signs of peroneal nerve damage tend to predominate.

contrast to the acute, nonprogressive course typical of physical injuries. Specific diseases that cause monoparesis are discussed in greater detail next.

DISEASES

The disorders or diseases that cause monoparesis and focally affect the LMN system are classified in Table 5-3. This table uses the logic for the formulation of a neurologic diagnosis, discussed in Chapter 1. The etiologic categories are organized according to the DAMNITV scheme described in Table 1-2. The diseases are further divided into acute nonprogressive, acute progressive, and chronic progressive disease categories based on the clinical course. The most important disorders that primarily present as monoparesis or plegia are described in sections of this chapter based on anatomic location.

Acute Nonprogressive Diseases, Monoparesis of the Pelvic Limbs

Peripheral Nerve Injuries

Traumatic peripheral nerve injuries are classified into three categories based on the degree of injury. *Neurapraxia* refers to transient interruption of nerve function and conduction, sometimes associated with a lesion of the myelin but without physical disruption to the axon and therefore no evidence that Wallerian degeneration exists. Neurapraxia is usually caused by a loss of blood supply, such as that produced by application of a tourniquet or by pressure from the weight of the animal during anesthesia. The condition can last for days to months. Demyelination will probably occur if signs persist for more than a few days. A period of 3 to 4 weeks is required for remyelination. *Axonotmesis* denotes separation of the axon from the neuronal cell body with subsequent degeneration of the distal axon (Wallerian degeneration) and loss of conduction in 3 to 5 days. The endoneurium and the Schwann cell sheath supporting structures remain intact. Regeneration of the axon usually begins in about 1 week and progresses at a rate of approximately 1 mm per day (1 inch per month). *Neurotmesis* refers to complete severance of the nerve (physical disruption of the axons and the myelin sheaths). Regeneration may occur, but neuroma formation is likely. The degree of nerve injury dictates the relative likelihood of regeneration, with restoration of function being most likely with neurapraxia and least likely with neurotmesis.

Electromyography (EMG) and nerve conduction studies are useful for confirming a diagnosis and determining the distribution of the nerve injury. Changes on EMG appear about 1 week after injury in dogs and 2 weeks after injury in horses (see Chapter 4 for details). The presence of voluntary motor-unit action potentials indicates an incomplete injury. The EMG and nerve conduction studies also can be used to monitor the progress of recovery.

Sciatic Nerve. The sciatic nerve is a mixed nerve that arises from spinal cord segments L6-S2 (see Table 5-2). The sciatic nerve is the extrapelvic continuation of the lumbosacral trunk. Because caudal lumbar and sacral spinal cord segments lie cranial to the corresponding vertebrae, nerve fibers that become the sciatic nerve must course caudally before exiting from the vertebral canal. As a result, these nerve fibers are particularly subject to injury from lumbosacral fractures and subluxations, lumbosacral stenosis, and pelvic or femoral fractures. Traumatic injuries of the lumbosacral area rarely result in a true mononeuropathy because fibers forming the pudendal, pelvic, and caudal nerves are also injured. In degenerative lumbosacral stenosis, however, the L7 nerve root may be entrapped in the L7-S1 foramen, causing lameness or monoparesis. Sciatic nerve paralysis is common in cows during dystocia. Damage to the fibers within the pelvic canal near the ventral surface of the cranial sacrum usually

TABLE 5-3

Diseases Causing Paresis of One Limb: Differential Diagnosis Based on Clinical Course and Etiologic Categories*

Etiologic Category	Acute Nonprogressive	Acute Progressive	Chronic Progressive
Degenerative disease (6)	None	Horner's type I disk disease (6)	Foraminal stenosis from lumbosacral disease (6) Infraspinatus muscle contracture (5)
Anomalous	None	None	None
Metabolic	None	None	None
Neoplastic (6)	None	Lymphoreticular	Primary—nerve sheath tumor (5) Hematopoietic Skeletal Metastatic
Nutritional	None	None	None
Inflammatory	None	Myelitis/meningomyelitis (15) Focal tetanus (10) Protozoal neuritis (15) Brachial plexus neuritis (5)	Myelitis/meningomyelitis (15)
Immune	None	Brachial plexus neuritis (5)	
Toxic	None	None	None
Traumatic	Fractures (6) Brachial plexus injury (5) Radial nerve injury (5) Sciatic nerve injury (5) Horner's type I intervertebral disk herniation (6) Iatrogenic injury	Horner's type I intervertebral disk herniation (6)	None
Vascular	Fibrocartilaginous embolism (6) Arterial thromboembolism (6)	None	None

*Numbers in parentheses refer to chapters in which the entities are discussed.

results in bilateral injury and paraparesis. Occasionally the injury is asymmetric, involving only the fibers of one sciatic nerve.

After giving off branches within the pelvis, the major portion of the sciatic nerve exits at the greater ischiatic foramen and courses caudally to the coxofemoral joint, between and deep to the tuber ischii and the greater trochanter of the femur. The nerve then continues distally between the semimembranosus and biceps femoris muscles. Branches of the sciatic nerve supply muscles that extend the hip and flex the stifle. Between the hip and the stifle, the sciatic nerve bifurcates to form the common peroneal (fibular) and tibial nerves, which supply all muscles distal to the stifle and provide sensory innervations to all areas of the foot except the medial digit, which is innervated by the saphenous branch of the femoral nerve.

Injuries below the distal third of the femur cause signs of peroneal and/or tibial nerve dysfunction. These injuries are described later. Damage to the proximal sciatic nerve results in severe monoparesis because the extensor muscles of the stifle (innervated by the femoral nerve) are the only group that remains functional. Although the animal can bear weight due to the ability of the stifle to extend related to intact femoral nerve function, the stifle does not flex. The hock and the digits do not extend or flex because of tibial and peroneal nerve involvement. The animal stands on the dorsum of the foot, "knuckled over," and assumes a plantigrade stance; the hock usually is "dropped." Sensation distal to the stifle is severely compromised laterally (peroneal), caudally (tibial), and cranially (peroneal), but it is preserved medially if the saphenous branch of the femoral nerve is intact (see Figure 1-13). The dorsal surface of the foot frequently is ulcerated if the animal drags or walks on the affected paw (Figure 5-5).

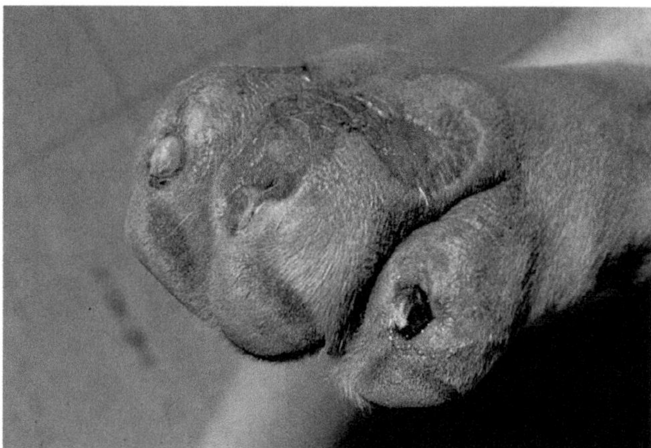

Figure 5-5 Ulcerated digits of the pelvic limb in a dog with peroneal nerve paralysis.

The sciatic nerve is the major nerve contributing to the pelvic limb flexor reflex. In proximal sciatic nerve injuries, the digits, hock, and stifle do not flex when the toes are stimulated. Stimulation of the medial digit or the medial aspect of the distal limb elicits a conscious response and flexion of the hip due to saphenous innervation, but the remainder of the joints of the affected limb do not flex. Atrophy of the caudal thigh muscles and the muscles distal to the stifle may be severe. Dogs with nerve entrapment may have severe pain. Self-mutilation also may occur. Clinical deficits usually are acute but may be delayed if fibrosis leads to nerve entrapment.

The proximal portion of the sciatic nerve is most frequently damaged by fractures of the shaft of the ilium, acetabulum, and proximal femur and during calving injuries in cows.[6-9] Proximity of the sciatic nerve to the pelvic bone predisposes it to iatrogenic injury during surgical procedures involving the ilium, acetabulum, sacroiliac joint, and the coxofemoral joint.[10] Iatrogenic injury of the sciatic nerve is more common with retrograde placement of intramedullary pins in the femur and during treatment of pelvic orthopedic diseases.[11-13] Less common causes include severe hip dysplasia and total hip replacement surgery.[14-16] Peripheral nerve regeneration after iatrogenic injury is determined by the degree of nerve injury with crushing lesions having a worse prognosis.[10] The prognosis for return of function is poor if sciatic injuries are complete.

Surgical relief of compression injury may be rewarding. Clinical outcome was studied in one series of 34 dogs with nerve injury subsequent to pelvic fractures and dislocations. Nerve entrapment was noted at surgery in 13 dogs.[9] Return of limb function was considered good or excellent 2 to 16 weeks after surgery in 11 dogs in which the nerve was decompressed and internal fixation was applied. Return of function was also good to excellent 2 to 12 weeks after injury in 10 of 12 dogs that did not undergo surgery. Many dogs in both groups had decreased cutaneous sensory loss. The authors suggested that surgery is indicated in dogs with severe pain or "signs of moderate to severe peripheral nerve injury." Markedly blunted or absence of pain perception suggests severe involvement.

The sciatic nerve, or the peroneal or tibial nerves along the caudal aspect of the femur, can be injured by injections or femoral fractures. Injected materials intended for the biceps femoris or semimembranosus muscles may go instead into the fascial plane between these muscles.[17] Injury can occur from direct laceration of the nerve by the needle, from the irritating nature of the agent being injected directly into the nerve, or from secondary scarring around the nerve. Injection injuries may be prevented by using another site for intramuscular injections, such as the quadriceps or lumbar muscles. The diagnosis is based on the history (paresis or paralysis typically occurs immediately after injection) and the lack of another explanation for the deficits. Establishing a direct cause-and-effect relationship is usually difficult but may be important from a medicolegal standpoint.

Prognosis and management depend on the severity of injury. Careful assessment of motor and sensory function determines whether both peroneal and tibial components are affected. Functionally, dogs with tibial nerve paralysis can accommodate better. If both nerves are affected, sensory evaluation is important to determine whether the lesion is complete (see Fig. 1-13). If function remains, especially in the peroneal nerve distribution, conservative treatment is recommended and a fairly good prognosis is given. Many of these injuries are due to neurapraxia or axonotmesis and limb function often returns. If the lesion is complete, more aggressive treatment may be indicated. Conservative treatment includes protecting the foot from injury by using an orthotic or splint and physical therapy to maintain muscle mass and range of motion.[18] Boots for dogs are available from several sources such as physical rehabilitation facilities and as advertised in hunting magazines or over the Internet. Surgical exploration of the nerve with débridement of surrounding tissues, neurolysis, resection of neuromas, and anastomosis of the nerve segments is indicated with severe injuries but requires specialized training to perform.[19]

Peroneal Nerve. The peroneal nerve supplies the muscles that flex the hock and extend the digits. It provides cutaneous sensory innervation to the dorsal aspect of the foot and the cranial surface of the hock and the tibia. This nerve is subject to injury where it crosses the lateral aspect of the stifle joint. In large animals, prolonged recumbency may injure the nerve at this site. In small animals and calves, injuries usually result from intramuscular injection of drugs into or near the nerve.

The foot tends to "knuckle over," and the hock may be overextended. The cranial tibialis and the digital extensor muscles are atrophied in small animals. Loss of sensation occurs on the dorsal areas of the foot and the cranial surface overlying the hock and the tibia. The flexor reflex is severely depressed when the dorsal aspects of the foot or the digits are stimulated. Pinching the plantar surface of the digits or the foot elicits a definite conscious response, and the flexor reflex is present, but the animal may not actively flex the hock joint. The examiner must exercise care in evaluating the flexor reflex because some passive flexion of the hock may occur as the stifle actively flexes. Although the foot tends to knuckle over, the dorsal surface usually does not become so severely abraded or ulcerated as it does in more proximal sciatic nerve lesions (see Figure 5-5). Dogs soon learn to place the foot by greater flexion of the hip and extension of the stifle. This gives the impression of a "high-stepping gait," which should not be confused with hypermetria associated with GP/UMN or cerebellar lesions. Transfer of tendons of muscles that are not denervated to affected muscles may be beneficial.[20] Horses reportedly have minimal gait deficits 3 months after injury.[5]

Tibial Nerve. The tibial nerve supplies the muscles that extend the hock and flex the digits. It provides cutaneous sensory innervation to the plantar surface of the foot and the caudal surface of the limb. In most animals, tibial nerve lesions occur in association with peroneal nerve injuries, and a mixture of neurologic signs occurs. In a pure tibial nerve injury, the hock joint is dropped when the animal walks or supports weight (Figure 5-6). The gastrocnemius muscle is atrophied. Loss of sensation occurs from the plantar aspect of the foot. The flexor reflex is severely depressed when the plantar surface of the foot is stimulated. Pinching the dorsal surface of the foot elicits a definite conscious response when stimulated, and the flexor reflex is present even though the toes are not flexed.

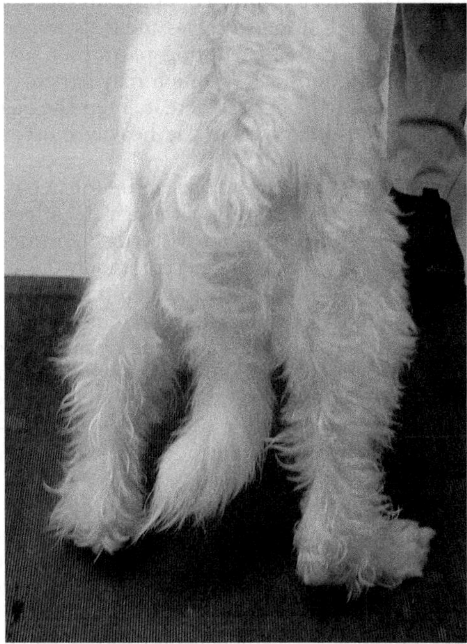

Figure 5-6 Bilateral tibial nerve paralysis in a dog resulting from improper immobilization of the pelvic limbs during a castration procedure. Note the dropped hocks in both pelvic limbs, a result of distal nerve injury of the tibial nerves.

Isolated tibial nerve injury may follow injections into the thigh muscles. Large so-called trophic ulcers may develop in the digital pads of small animals because of decreased circulation over bony prominences.[21,22] Affected animals apparently do not move their limbs to the degree necessary to relieve soft tissue compression.[23] In those animals unsuccessfully treated conservatively, surgical correction necessitates grafting of skin from normally innervated cutaneous regions.[24]

Femoral Nerve. The femoral nerve arises from the L3-6 spinal cord segments and supplies the extensor muscles of the stifle. The major motor component is from L5.[25] The saphenous branch of the femoral nerve is the sensory pathway from the skin on the medial surface of the foot, limb, stifle, and thigh. Peripheral injuries to this nerve are not common because of its short and well-protected course before innervating the quadriceps muscle. Rarely, unilateral damage restricted to the ventral gray matter of the L4-6 segments results in a neuropathy involving the femoral nerve. Bilateral femoral nerve injury has been seen in dogs after extreme extension of the hips. With femoral nerve lesions, the stifle cannot be fixed (extended) for weight bearing and the animal usually carries the affected limb. Lesions involving the peripheral femoral nerve cause anesthesia in areas innervated by the saphenous nerve. Selective lesions involving the gray matter of the spinal cord produce motor dysfunction only. The patellar reflex is absent or diminished; however, the flexor reflex is normal, except for decreased flexion of the hip. The hopping reaction is greatly decreased in the affected limb because weight bearing is inhibited. However, if the animal's weight is supported, proprioceptive placement should be normal when only the femoral nerve is affected.

Femoral neuropathy can be associated with iliopsoas muscle pathology. The injury can be secondary to bleeding disorders, neoplasia, or to primary injury of the iliopsoas muscle.[26,27] The muscle pathology can be detected using ultrasonography or computed tomography (CT), but magnetic resonance imaging (MRI) may provide better visualization.[28] Tenectomy of the muscle insertion can relieve signs of hip pain.

In large animals, femoral nerve paralysis results in severe monoparesis. The affected limb is poorly advanced and collapses during weight bearing. In calves and foals, femoral nerve paralysis results from trauma during parturition.[7,29] Forced extraction from the "hip-lock" position may hyperextend the hip and overstretches the nerve where it enters the quadriceps muscle. Incidence is increased in the heavily muscled cattle breeds.

Obturator Nerve. Injuries to the obturator nerve in dogs or cats do not cause monoparesis, although the affected limb may slide laterally when the animal stands on a smooth surface. Obturator paralysis occurs most commonly during parturition in cows. The obturator nerve lies on the medial surface of the ilium and innervates the adductor muscles of the limb. Injuries cause marked pelvic limb weakness, especially on slick surfaces. The limbs may be placed in a wide-based stance that is exaggerated as the animal runs. The gait abnormality is less pronounced with unilateral lesions. Most dystocia-related injuries in cows also damage branches of the sciatic nerve.[7]

Spinal Cord Diseases

Unilateral spinal cord lesions caudal to the T2 spinal cord segment result in monoparesis. Lesions at L4-S2 cause LMN deficits, whereas those at T3-L3 spinal cord segments cause GP/UMN signs. Sensory deficits usually also occur. In most cases, several spinal cord segments are involved, and dysfunction affects multiple nerves (polyneuropathy). The most common cause is infarction caused by fibrocartilaginous embolism and other vascular-related diseases. Occasionally, spinal cord trauma, neoplasia, or, more rarely, inflammation has a unilateral distribution and produces monoparesis. In horses, protozoal encephalomyelitis can produce selective gray matter lesions causing ipsilateral paresis. Pertinent disorders that produce unilateral spinal cord lesions are discussed in the chapters on pelvic limb paresis (see Chapter 6) and tetraparesis (see Chapter 7).

Acute Nonprogressive Diseases, Monoparesis of the Thoracic Limbs

Peripheral Nerve Injuries

Nerves that innervate the muscles of the thoracic limbs and clinical signs associated with injuries of these nerves are listed in Table 5-1. Proximal radial nerve injuries cause paralysis of the triceps brachii muscle, and extensor muscles of the carpus and digits. Because the animal is unable to extend the elbow and carpus, it cannot bear weight or properly place the foot. The elbow also is dropped. Injury to the musculocutaneous nerve causes paralysis of biceps brachii and brachialis muscles and the animal cannot flex the elbow. Paralysis of the carpal flexor muscles as a result of median and ulnar nerve injury is more subtle, causing overextension of the carpus during weight bearing.

Evaluation of spinal reflexes helps to identify which muscle groups are functional. The flexor reflex is useful in assessing muscle strength and identifying partial lesions. Sensory evaluation is essential to mapping the cutaneous areas of decreased sensation (see Chapter 1). This section discusses injuries to the brachial plexus, and radial and suprascapular nerves because injuries to these nerves are more common in clinical practice.

Trauma to the Brachial Plexus. The nerves of the brachial plexus originate from the C6-T2 spinal cord segments (see Table 5-1). In addition, the sympathetic nerves that innervate the eye originate from neurons in the first three thoracic segments and travel along the roots of the brachial plexus as they exit the vertebral canal. Trauma that abducts and caudally displaces the thoracic limb may damage the dorsal and ventral roots of the brachial plexus.[30-34] Typically, the trauma occurs intradurally at the point where the nerve roots arise from the spinal cord (Figure 5-7). Injuries that place severe traction on the spinal cord also may damage GP/UMN spinal pathways involving the ipsilateral pelvic limb. Rarely, the plexus is damaged by a direct blow to the shoulder, thus causing contusion or hemorrhage. This lesion is usually not complete.

The myotomal distribution of the ventral spinal nerve roots varies to some extent from one dog to the next so that the degree of dysfunction induced by any single root

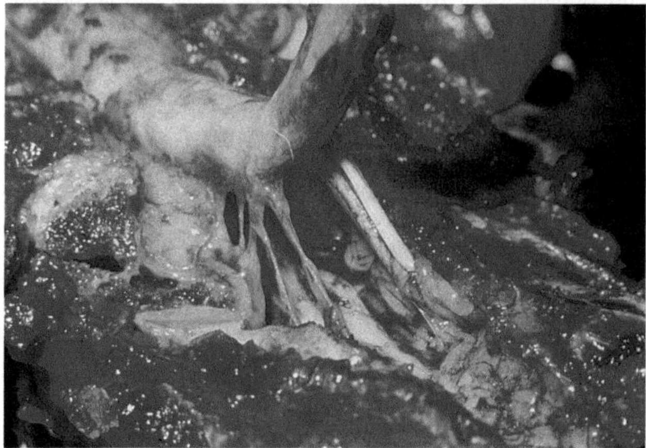

Figure 5-7 The cervical spinal cord from a 3-year-old Labrador retriever euthanized for brachial plexus avulsion after falling out of a pickup truck. Note the avulsion of the nerve roots from the spinal cord.

injury cannot be fully predicted. Injuries have been broadly categorized as complete, cranial, and caudal, depending on the extent of nerve root avulsion.[31,32] Complete brachial plexus injuries involve the entire plexus. In Griffiths' original classification, caudal brachial plexus injuries involve the C8 and T1 nerve roots, whereas cranial avulsions involve the C6 and C7 roots.[31,32] Complete and caudal brachial plexus injuries cause paralysis of the triceps brachii muscle so that affected dogs cannot extend the elbow or bear weight on the limb. Postural reactions and the flexor, extensor carpi radialis, and triceps brachii reflexes are weak or absent. The paw is knuckled over and dragged (Figure 5-8), potentially causing severe abrasion and ulceration of the dorsal surface. Dogs with caudal avulsions walk with the elbow and shoulder flexed. Elbow extensors are spared with cranial avulsions so that the dog can still bear weight on the limb but cannot flex the elbow or protract the limb. The supraspinatus and infraspinatus muscles are atrophied. With each form of brachial plexus injuries, neurogenic muscle atrophy begins in the distribution of the denervation in about 1 week (Video 5-1).

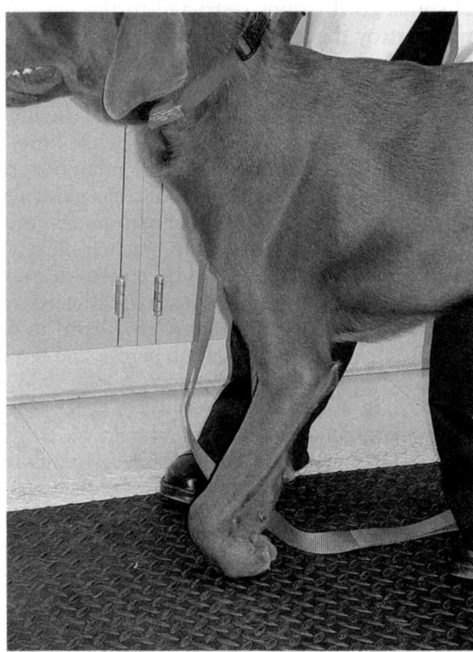

Figure 5-8 Left brachial plexus injury in a 2-year-old Labrador retriever, a result of a car accident. Note the knuckled paw and the inability to support weight on the limb. Atrophy is present in the scapular and triceps muscles.

The pattern of sensory loss allows more critical clinical definition of the nature of the injury (Figure 5-9).[30-32] With complete brachial plexus injuries, pain perception is essentially lost distal to the elbow. Bailey[30] has provided a detailed description of sensory deficits in selected incomplete lesions. A cranial brachial plexus injury involving the C6-8 roots caused a loss of cutaneous sensation over the cranial antebrachium distal to the elbow (radial nerve), the lateral and cranial brachium overlying the humerus (axillary and brachiocephalicus nerves), and an area over the cranial aspect of the dorsal spine of the scapula (dorsal cutaneous branch of C6). Sensory distribution over the caudal antebrachium, provided through cutaneous branches of the ulnar nerve, and a portion of the median antebrachium (musculocutaneous nerve) were spared. A caudal brachial plexus injury involving the C8 and T1 roots and the T2 communicating branch to T1 caused loss of sensation cranially and caudally over both the lateral and medial antebrachium (radial and ulnar nerves). Although sensation was lost over the lateral antebrachium, a sizeable medial portion retained sensation (musculocutaneous nerve). Areas innervated by cutaneous branches of the axillary and brachiocephalicus nerves over the cranial and lateral brachium also were spared.

Injury of the T1 ventral spinal nerve root affects the preganglionic sympathetic nerve fibers, resulting in miosis of the ipsilateral pupil (partial Horner's syndrome).[31,35] Other features of Horner's syndrome, such as ptosis, enophthalmos, and protrusion of the membrana nictitans, occur rarely unless the spinal roots for T1 and T2 or cranial sympathetic trunk also are involved. Another feature of brachial plexus injury is loss of the cutaneous trunci reflex ipsilateral to the lesion. This loss occurs with either complete or caudal injury resulting from injury of the C8 and T1 ventral spinal nerve roots, thus interrupting lateral thoracic nerve innervation of the cutaneous trunci (panniculus carnosus) muscle. The reflex is present on the side of the body contralateral to the lesion such that stimulation on either side of the trunk elicits a motor response only on the side opposite the brachial plexus injury. Injuries that place severe traction on the spinal cord also may cause damage to GP/UMN pathways. This damage causes pelvic limb deficits, particularly on the ipsilateral side.

Some limb function may return relatively quickly when intact axons recover from temporary conduction block. The prognosis for recovery of function, however, is generally poor, particularly when elbow extensors are denervated.[36] The best prognostic indicator predictive for return of function after brachial plexus injury is presence of pain perception.[36] Corrective orthopedic procedures such as carpal arthrodesis or tendon transplantation are not indicated in these cases but may be helpful in selected cases in which the proximal branches of the radial and the musculocutaneous nerves are spared. If such surgery is contemplated, EMG should be done

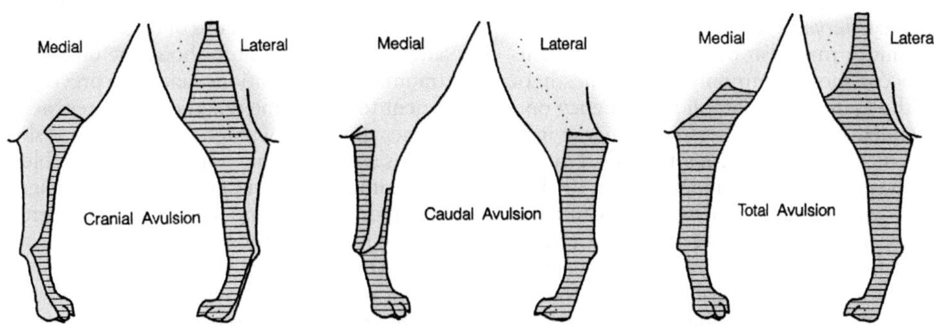

Figure 5-9 Maps of sensory loss in cranial, caudal, and total brachial plexus avulsions. (Data from Bailey CS: Patterns of cutaneous anesthesia associated with brachial plexus avulsions in the dog, J Am Vet Med Assoc 185:889, 1984.)

to ensure that the elbow extensors and muscles to be transplanted are not denervated.[37] Affected animals often develop severe limb contractures and may mutilate the limb, necessitating amputation.

Bilateral brachial plexus injury occurs in some animals, particularly when they have fallen from great heights and landed in a sternal position, severely abducting both thoracic limbs. Bilateral injury of the C5-7 nerve roots may cause diaphragmatic paralysis due to phrenic nerve involvement. Affected animals have dyspnea in addition to bilateral thoracic limb paralysis.

Suprascapular Nerve. Suprascapular paralysis occurs most frequently in large animals secondary to trauma or fractures involving the cranial and distal border of the scapula.[5,38] Severe supraspinatus and infraspinatus muscle atrophy occurs, resulting in a condition termed *sweeney*. Weight bearing is usually unaffected; however, in the acute stage of injury, the stride may be shortened and the shoulder may luxate laterally when weight is borne on the limb. Cattle may have this injury due to malfunctioning chutes or from striking the head gate with the shoulders. Working draft horses may be injured from poorly fitting collars. Electromyography is useful to ensure that other nerves are not affected. Surgical decompression of the nerve as it passes around the cranial surface of the scapula is recommended if spontaneous improvement does not occur.[39] Recommendations vary with early versus delayed surgery.[5] Results are probably best with exploration after about 1 month. Waiting for 3 months to ensure that spontaneous recovery does not occur is an alternative.

Contracture of the infraspinatus muscle occurs in dogs and results in thoracic limb lameness. The cause is presumed to be trauma to the muscle and possibly to the vasculature or the suprascapular nerve supplying the muscle.[40] Affected dogs tend to be working hunting breeds of dog. An understanding the normal function of the infraspinatus muscle helps appreciate the gait disturbance that occurs with contracture. The normal action of the muscle is to externally rotate and abduct the humerus and flex or extend the shoulder depending on the position of the joint when the muscle is stimulated. With contracture of the muscle, the humerus remains fixed in a slightly externally rotated and abducted position. In addition, the shoulder is fixed in flexion. During the swing phase of the gait, the stride of the limb may be slightly shortened. To compensate for the inability to extend the shoulder, there is excessive flexion of the elbow and a characteristic "flip" to the carpus. Additionally, the limb is abducted during the swing phase (Video 5-2). Transecting the insertion of the infraspinatus muscle is beneficial.[40]

Radial Nerve. The entire radial nerve may be injured by fractures of the first rib. Fractures of the humerus may injure the nerve distal to the branches that supply the triceps brachii muscle. Similarly, application of tourniquets proximal to the elbow during declaw or to assist with hemostasis for surgeries involving the antebrachium or foot, may result in compression or ischemia to the radial nerve. Typically, the lesion is transient but permanent injury may also occur. In large animals, radial nerve injuries occur most commonly during anesthetic procedures or when the animal is in lateral recumbency on a hard surface for extended periods.[5] Distal radial nerve injuries produce less severe gait abnormalities than do brachial plexus injuries. The elbow can be extended; however, the foot tends to knuckle over when the animal walks because the extensors of the carpus and the digits are paralyzed (Figure 5-10). Sensation is lost from the dorsal and cranial aspects of the limb distal to the elbow. Surgical exploration of the injured nerve with neurolysis or anastomosis is indicated, especially in distal radial nerve injuries.[41,42] Carpal arthrodesis or transposition of a flexor tendon may be helpful.[43] Paresthesia may lead to self-mutilation, however.

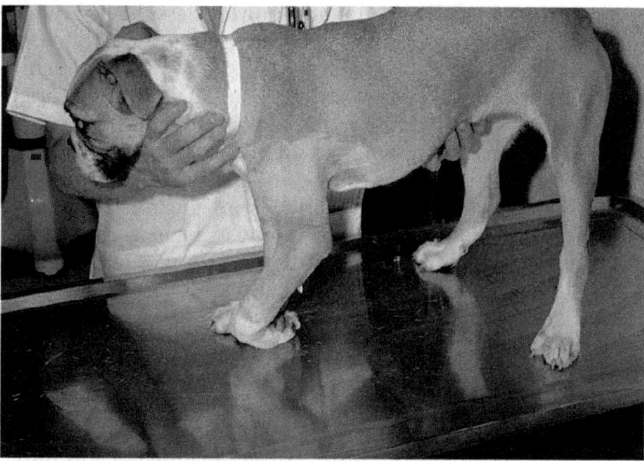

Figure 5-10 A mixed-breed dog with a distal fracture of the left humerus and suspected radial nerve paralysis.

Spinal Cord Diseases

Unilateral spinal cord lesions restricted to the gray matter at C6-T2 may destroy the motor neurons of the brachial plexus, resulting in LMN monoparesis while sparing sensory perception, depending on the degree of involvement of the dorsal horn sensory relay neurons. Lesions at this level usually involve the GP/UMN pathways of the ipsilateral pelvic limb, causing hemiparesis. The most common cause is infarction resulting from fibrocartilaginous embolism and other vascular-based diseases. Trauma, neoplasia, and inflammation also may cause focal spinal cord disease. Injury to the brachial plexus may be associated with paresis or paralysis of the ipsilateral pelvic limb if the spinal cord is compressed, contused, tethered, or otherwise damaged at the time of trauma. Spinal cord diseases are discussed in the chapters on pelvic limb paresis and tetraparesis.

Treatment of Nerve Injury

Animals with peripheral nerve injury should be treated with short-term antiinflammatory dosages of corticosteroids to relieve inflammation and swelling. The limb is immobilized to prevent further trauma. Nerve decompression or anastomosis is indicated if the site of injury is surgically accessible. Long-term management includes physiotherapy to maintain range-of-motion and minimize muscle atrophy of the remaining functional muscle groups, and prevention of further trauma to the affected limb.[44] Tendon transplantation and joint arthrodesis are performed primarily for distal radial nerve and common peroneal nerve injuries in small animals.[20] The most important aspect of long-term management is probably prevention of trauma to the distal extremity. Commercially available boots and orthotics that help protect the foot are easily applied by the owner and are well tolerated by the dog. Owners frequently request amputation of the affected limb because of distal extremity trauma. Generally, amputation of the limb should be delayed for 6 months unless traumatic complications cannot be prevented. This period is sufficient to determine whether nerve regeneration will occur. The owner should be warned that recovery is slow and that amputation is an irreversible solution to the problem.

Animals with cutaneous areas of anesthesia or hypesthesia (reduced sensory perception) frequently self-mutilate the affected area. In most instances in which there is anesthesia, concurrent paralysis precludes return of limb function. As a result, amputation should be strongly advocated. In animals that maintain sensory perception and self-mutilate the denervated region of the limb, the possible presence of neuropathic pain can be empirically treated with gabapentin at 2 to 10 mg/kg orally three times daily.

Many peripheral nerve injuries in large animals can be avoided by proper management when placed in lateral recumbency.[5] Adequate padding must be provided at all times, and recumbent animals should be turned at least three times daily. Excessive traction on limbs should be avoided during anesthesia, animal restraint and movement, or during fetal extraction. Injured limbs should be protected by bandages, splints, or casts. Cattle with obturator nerve paralysis must be kept on a nonslick surface. Hobbles on the pelvic limbs may be helpful. Recumbent animals should be supported with slings whenever possible.

Prognosis

The prognosis of peripheral nerve injuries depends on the type of damage and the severity of neurologic dysfunction. Nerve fibers that have been contused, compressed, or stretched may regain function slowly. Nerves that have been lacerated or avulsed from their spinal cord attachments, however, seldom regain function. Unfortunately, in routine practice, establishing which of these situations has occurred is sometimes difficult at the initial examination. For nerve fibers to regenerate, the nerve sheath must remain intact. Compressive lesions may cause demyelination without disrupting the axon. Recovery begins in about 3 to 4 weeks and continues for 1 to 2 months. Axonal regeneration occurs slowly, at a rate of approximately 1 mm per day (1 inch a month); however, the nerve sheath must be intact to guide the axon to the denervated muscle. The affected muscles may be reinnervated by axonal sprouting from adjacent intact neurons. Regardless of the repair process involved, return to function may take several months and may never be complete. As a general rule, reinnervation must occur in 12 months or less to be effective. Regeneration for distances greater than 12 inches is therefore unlikely.

In general, the prognosis for functional recovery of animals with severe motor dysfunction and complete anesthesia is poor. These lesions are usually severe and may involve complete disruption of nerve fibers. Some animals regain function; however, the outcome is often unsatisfactory. The prognosis is better for animals with partial loss of motor or sensory function because damage to the axons may be transitory and reinnervation from adjacent, intact nerve fibers is more predictable. In addition, animals with partial dysfunction may learn to compensate by using other, uninvolved muscle groups. In most cases, the distribution and the severity of sensory loss are the most important factors in establishing a prognosis.

If available, an EMG examination that includes nerve conduction studies and evoked potentials is useful for formulating a prognosis and assessing the recovery of peripheral nerve injuries.[37,45] This technique helps the clinician establish the severity and distribution of nerve injury. A total lack of voluntary motor potentials, an absence of response to nerve stimulation, and evidence of diffuse denervation are highly correlated with a poor prognosis. The presence of some motor unit activity and patchy denervation suggests that the lesion is not complete and that a better chance for nerve regeneration exists.[46] The EMG examination can be repeated periodically over several months to determine whether reinnervation is occurring. If tendon transplant surgery is contemplated before surgery, the muscle to be transplanted should be examined with EMG to ensure that denervation potentials are absent.

Acute Progressive Diseases and Monoparesis

Plexus Neuritis

Monoparesis can rarely be caused by inflammatory disorders, especially when the inflammation is localized to the plexuses or in the intumescences with myelitis. Reported cases have been described as an acute onset of thoracic limb paresis. When isolated to the brachial plexus, the involvement can be complete or incomplete and occur bilaterally. The pathogenesis is assumed to have an immunologic basis. The cases described in dogs and cats have been related to an all-horsemeat diet or associated with modified-live vaccines.[47-50] Definitive causality has not been established in other cases.

The weakness manifests as lower motor neuron signs to the thoracic limbs. Pain may or may not be manifested upon limb manipulation. The proximal limb muscles are more commonly affected. Electromyography and nerve conduction reveal changes consistent with denervation atrophy. Importantly, abnormalities are not identified in the pelvic limbs eliminating diffuse LMN disease from consideration. MRI reveals nerve swelling associated with an increase in signal intensity on T2 weighted images.[50] Cerebrospinal fluid (CSF) analysis is usually normal or may have elevated protein if the intradural nerve roots are affected. Nerve biopsy shows Wallerian degeneration and necropsy reveals inflammation isolated to the nerve roots and ventral branches of the spinal nerve.[47,49] Some affected animals respond to corticosteroid administration (along with diet change to a novel source of protein in cases in which an unusual diet is fed) and others resolve spontaneously. Recovery has been reported as slow or static.

Chronic Progressive Diseases and Monoparesis

Peripheral Nerve Sheath Tumors

Pathophysiology. Peripheral nerves may be affected primarily or secondarily by neoplasia. Nerve sheath tumors arise from Schwann cells (schwannoma) or connective tissue surrounding the nerves (neurofibroma, neurinoma, neurilemmoma). These two tumor tissue types are distinguished in part because the schwannoma is encapsulated and distinct from the nerve, whereas the neurofibroma is not encapsulated and indistinct from the nerve. However, the distinction is often difficult to make. Consequently, they are considered collectively under the term *nerve sheath tumor*.[51] Recently, the diagnostic classification of benign nerve sheath tumors has been reported.[52] The malignant counterparts are malignant schwannoma and neurofibrosarcoma and more generally termed, malignant peripheral nerve sheath tumor. In dogs, nerve sheath tumors have been reported in various anatomic sites but spinal nerves in the caudal cervical and cranial thoracic region, and cranial nerves (in particular cranial nerve V; see Chapter 9) are affected with greater frequency.[53] Most nerve sheath tumors originate peripherally and then slowly extend proximally to involve the spinal cord (Figure 5-11).[51,54] As tumors grow proximally, other nerves in the plexus become involved and by the time the dog has clinical signs multiple nerves often are affected. Nerve sheath tumors in the thoracolumbar spinal cord more commonly arise intradurally and compress the spinal cord initially.[54]

Other tumor types may secondarily involve peripheral nerves and nerve roots.[34] Meningiomas originating at the outfoldings of meninges around the nerve roots may compress or invade the root. Bony and soft tissue tumors also may compress nerve roots or peripheral nerves. Lymphoma, particularly in cats, may involve peripheral nerves and roots, especially at the cervical intumescence and in the brachial plexus.[55]

Clinical Signs. Some nerve sheath tumors affect peripheral nerves in the skin and cause only disfigurement, particularly true in cattle.[56] Other tumors can involve major peripheral nerves or roots and cause monoparesis. Those originating in the brachial plexus typically cause initial thoracic limb lameness (nerve root signature). Dogs are reluctant to bear weight on the involved limb and show pain during palpation. Affected dogs are frequently thought to have orthopedic disease given similar clinical presentations and the greater prevalence with which orthopedic disease is observed in small

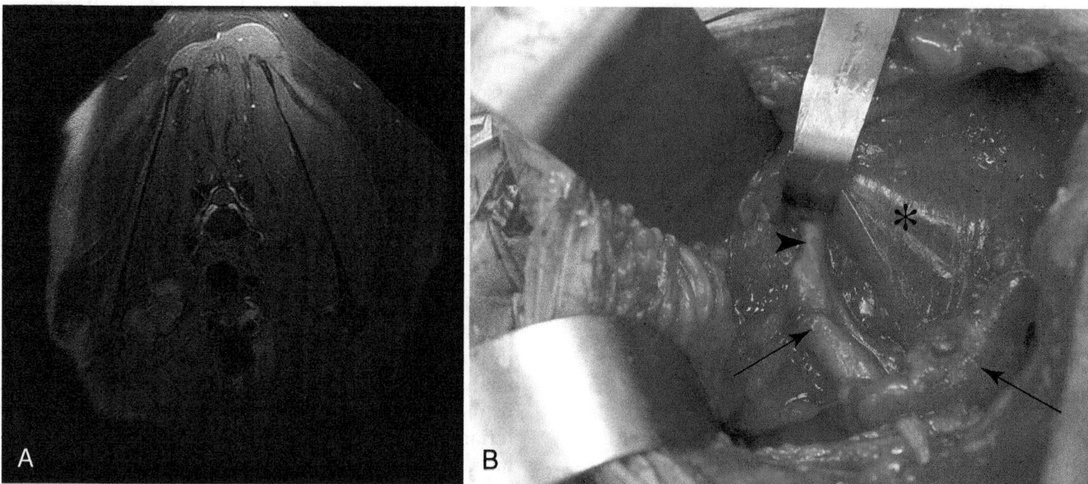

Figure 5-11 Intraoperative picture of the C7 spinal nerve in a 10-year-old Weimaraner dog that was evaluated for left thoracic lameness and chronic atrophy of the infraspinatus and supraspinatus muscles. EMG identified evidence of denervation only in the infraspinatus and supraspinatus muscles. On MRI (T1W imaging), the suprascapular nerve appeared enlarged, had an irregular course, and displayed contrast enhancement *(arrow)* **(A)**. During exploratory surgery via a lateral approach to the brachial plexus, the suprascapular nerve was markedly thickened, irregular shaped, and discolored **(B)**. The nerve was contiguous with the C7 spinal nerve *(large arrows)*. At the level of the intervertebral foramen, the C7 spinal nerve appeared grossly normal *(arrowhead)*. The lesion was resected 1 cm proximal to the lesion just deep to the scalenus muscle *(asterisk)*. A malignant nerve sheath tumor was diagnosed histologically. Microscopic evaluation of the proximal resected edge of the nerve was normal. Immediately postoperatively, the dog had a mild weight-bearing lameness. After 1 month, the lameness resolved. The dog's gait remained normal for 1½ years postoperatively. (Copyright 2010 University of Georgia Research Foundation, Inc.)

animals. Eventually, neurologic deficits such as neurogenic muscle atrophy become more pronounced. Tumors generally are not palpable, but large masses can be identified in the axillary region in some dogs.[34] Tumors involving the brachial plexus often extend proximally to compress the spinal cord and cause deficits in the opposite thoracic limb and pelvic limbs. Spinal nerve or nerve root involvement of the caudal cervical and cranial thoracic regions causes ipsilateral loss of the cutaneous trunci reflex and Horner's syndrome.

Diagnosis. Nerve root neoplasia should be suspected in animals with chronic progressive monoparesis associated with neurogenic muscle atrophy and signs of nerve root signature. Average time from development of signs to diagnosis ranges from 4 to 6 months.[53] Orthopedic disease can be excluded by careful examination and radiography of the thoracic limb. Thoracic radiography and abdominal ultrasonography are recommended to evaluate for metastatic disease. EMG evidence of denervation suggests neural involvement in animals with subtle neurologic deficits that otherwise might be thought to have orthopedic disease. Tumors that reach the vertebral canal may cause resorption of the bone and enlargement of the intervertebral foramen on survey radiographs. Compression of the spinal cord causes a characteristic intradural-extramedullary pattern on myelography (see Chapter 4).[54] The contrast material in the subarachnoid space splits at the tumor, resulting in a so-called golf-tee pattern in which the tumor is the golf ball and the enlarged contrast columns cranial and caudal to the mass are the golf tee. Tumors affecting the brachial and lumbosacral plexuses and paravertebral area may be detected by CT and MRI but visualization can be difficult early in the disease course. CT reveals masses that contrast enhanced to varying degrees with ring enhancement and hypoattenuation in areas indicating possible necrosis.[57] MRI reveals a multilobulated mass that is hyperintense on T2W and isointense on T1W images with varying intensities of contrast enhancement.[58,59] With multiplanar imaging, MRI best allows for delineation of proximal and distal tumor extent.[59]

Treatment. Local resection, limb amputation, laminectomy, or combinations of these are recommended surgical procedures. Tumors within the brachial plexus can be treated with local resection.[60] Tumors extending into the vertebral canal are explored with a laminectomy and durotomy. Nerve sheath tumors often are invasive and cannot be resected without injuring or removing portions of the involved nerve and causing substantial neurologic dysfunction. As tumors arising in the brachial plexus often have extended to other nerves by the time the diagnosis is made, incomplete resection is common. Amputation is often the best option. It is imperative that the proximal extent of the nerve resection (whether with amputation or with local tumor resection) be marked for microscopic examination at the margin(s) of the resection. Neoplastic involvement at the margin of the resection may necessitate re-resection or adjunctive therapy. Palliative pain management can be instituted using a combination of nonsteroidal antiinflammatory drugs (NSAIDs) and opioids. Gabapentin also can be empirically administered for neuropathic pain. Corticosteroids can reduce spinal cord edema.

Prognosis. Nerve sheath tumors have a high rate of recurrence, and overall long-term prognosis is considered poor.[53] Median survival time of dogs with root and peripheral nerve involvement is 5 and 12 months, respectively.[53] The median relapse free interval of root and plexus-associated tumors were 1 month and 7.5 months, respectively.[53] Early and aggressive surgical management may extend survival. Efficacy of radiation and chemotherapy is unknown in animals but may be beneficial in animals with incomplete resection.

CASE STUDIES

Key: *0*, Absent; *+1*, decreased; *+2*, normal; *+3*, exaggerated; *+4*, very exaggerated or clonus: *PL*, pelvic limb; *TL*, thoracic limb; *NE*, not evaluated.

CASE STUDY 5-1 *OLIVER*

 veterinaryneurologycases.com

▪ Signalment
Canine, Weimaraner, male, 6 years old.

▪ History
The dog was hit by a car 20 days ago. Since that day, he has been unable to use the right thoracic limb (TL). He has been dragging the foot and is unable to advance the limb or bear weight. Open sores have developed on the dorsum of the paw.

▪ Physical Examination
No abnormalities were found other than the neurologic problems described in the next section. Palpation reveals atrophy of the triceps, supraspinatus, infraspinatus, biceps brachii, and flexor carpi radialis muscles of the right thoracic limb.

▪ Neurologic Examination
Mental status
Alert

Gait and posture
Posture was normal with exception of the right TL. Gait showed severe paresis of the right thoracic limb. The dog drags the limb and the foot with the paw knuckling over. The dog can bear little weight on the limb.

Postural reactions
Absent proprioceptive positioning and hopping in the right thoracic limb.

Spinal reflexes
The triceps, extensor carpi radialis, and flexor reflexes were absent in the right thoracic limb. The cutaneous trunci reflex was absent on the right side.

Cranial nerves
The right pupil was constricted but responsive to a light stimulus

Sensory evaluation
Superficial pain perception—absent in the right TL.
Deep pain perception—markedly diminished in the right TL.

▪ Lesion Localization
The dog has monoparesis affecting the right thoracic limb and partial Horner's syndrome of the right eye. Lower motor neuron signs with sensory deficits in several nerves affecting only the right TL suggest a lesion of the right brachial plexus or spinal nerve or roots contributing to the plexus. A C6-T2 spinal cord lesion is discounted because the right pelvic limb is normal.

▪ Differential Diagnosis
1. Trauma
   a. Brachial plexus injury
   b. Caudal cervical vertebral column injury
   c. Injury to the nerve roots of the T1-3 causing Horner's syndrome
2. Vascular

▪ Diagnostic Plan
1. Evaluate the caudal cervical vertebral column with radiography or cross-sectional imaging
2. Electromyography can be used to evaluate muscle groups for evidence of denervation.

▪ Results
Spinal radiographs were within normal limits. Electromyography showed fibrillation potentials and sharp waves in several muscle groups of the thoracic limb.

▪ Diagnosis
Brachial plexus injury of the right thoracic limb

Treatment
Protect the foot with a boot. Perform physical rehabilitation to include range of motion and hydrotherapy. The owners were informed that the prognosis is very poor for functional use of the limb because the nerves, spinal nerves, or roots have been severely injured. Amputation may be needed in the future. The dog regained partial use of the limb in 6 months; however, he had to wear a boot continually to protect the foot. A persistent mild pupil constriction was present in the right eye.

CASE STUDY 5-2 *MURRAY*

 veterinaryneurologycases.com

▪ Signalment
Canine, boxer, male, 1 year old.

▪ History
The dog was hit by a car 10 months ago and was treated for shock and multiple pelvic fractures. The dog was referred 2 days after the initial injury because of severe dyspnea. Massive pleural effusion was treated with chest drains. The examination disclosed moderate paresis in the right pelvic limb (PL) and hypalgesia distal to the stifle. No treatment was given, and the dog was discharged 4 days later. He returned 10 months after the initial injury for follow-up examination, at which time no improvement in the right PL was noted.

▪ Physical Examination
Negative except for the neurologic problems. Deep ulcers are present in the plantar surfaces of the middle two digital pads; these toes are swollen.

Continued

CASE STUDY 5-2 *MURRAY—cont'd*

▪ Neurologic Examination

Mental status

Alert

Gait and posture

Posture was normal with the exception of the right PL. Moderate paresis of the right PL, with hyperflexion of the stifle; the paw knuckles over and the hock sinks during weight bearing; all other limbs are normal.

Palpation

Atrophy of the cranial tibialis and gastrocnemius muscle

Postural reactions

Proprioceptive positioning and hopping are absent in the right PL.

Spinal reflexes

The patellar reflex is increased in the right pelvic limb. On testing tap flexor muscle of the right pelvic limb, the hip and stifle joints flex but no flexion is observed in the hock joint. All other spinal reflexes are intact.

Cranial nerves

Normal

Sensory evaluation

Hyperesthesia—none
Superficial pain perception—blunted distal to stifle in right PL
Deep pain perception—absent in the two middle toes in the right PL

▪ Lesion Localization

The dog has monoparesis of the right pelvic limb. The presence of LMN signs with sensory deficits distal to the stifle localizes the lesion to the distal sciatic nerve involving the peroneal and tibial nerves.

▪ Differential Diagnosis

1. Trauma—fracture, injection injury
2. Vascular—thromboembolism

▪ Diagnostic Plan

1. Radiography is used to detect presence of fractures
2. Electromyography (EMG) can evaluate for evidence of denervation in muscles.

▪ Diagnostic Results

Pelvic radiographs revealed multiple pelvic fractures that are now healed but are displaced. Radiographs of the foot revealed bony lysis and proliferation involving the distal phalanges of the middle digits. EMG revealed diffuse denervation activity involving the muscles distal to the stifle; few fibrillation potentials and positive sharp waves in the gastrocnemius, the semitendinosus, and the semimembranosus muscles combined with nerve conduction studies, there was evidence of reinnervation in some muscles.

▪ Diagnosis

A distal sciatic nerve (peroneal and tibial nerves) injury is a result of a pelvic fracture. One may debate the cause of the nerve injury, that is, a pelvic fracture versus a needle (injection) injury. The neurologic examination is more consistent with the diagnosis of a needle (injection) injury because nerve damage usually occurs at the origin of the peroneal and the tibial nerves in the area caudal to the femur. The EMG, however, provides evidence that the lesion also is more proximal. Denervation of the semitendinosus and semimembranosus muscles probably is a result of the pelvic fractures because these muscles are rarely affected by injections in the thigh muscles.

▪ Treatment

Physical rehabilitation including range-of-motion exercises was to be performed. The middle two digits are infected, which requires antibiotic therapy. A boot was fitted on the dog to prevent further trauma. Because the sciatic nerve injury is partial and evidence of reinnervation is present, the dog may regain functional use of the limb. The dog regained good use of the limb and the boot eventually was removed.

CASE STUDY 5-3 *TUTU*

 veterinaryneurologycases.com

▪ Signalment

Feline, domestic, female, 7 years old.

▪ History

Mild lameness was noted in the right thoracic limb 6 to 8 weeks ago. The condition has slowly worsened, and the cat is unable to bear weight on the limb. She holds the limb extended with the paw flexed and is knuckling occasionally on the right pelvic limb.

▪ Physical Examination

Normal except for the neurologic problem. Palpation revealed mild atrophy of the scapular muscles in the right TL.

▪ Neurologic Examination

Mental status

Alert

Gait and posture

Posture is normal. Gait shows severe paresis of the right TL. The cat occasionally drags and knuckles the paw of the right PL.

Postural reactions

Proprioceptive positioning was absent in the right TL and decreased in the right PL. Hopping was absent in the right TL and decreased in the right PL. Extensor postural thrust was decreased in the right PL. Visual and tactile placing were absent in the right TL. The cutaneous trunci reflex was absent on the right side.

Spinal reflexes

The patellar reflex was +3 in the right PL. The right extensor carpi radialis and triceps reflexes were 0 to +1; the right flexor withdrawal reflex was absent in the right TL.

CASE STUDY 5-3 *TUTU—cont'd*

Cranial nerves
Mild pupillary constriction was present in the right eye. PLRs are normal.

Sensory evaluation
Hyperesthesia—present in right axillary space
Superficial pain perception—normal
Deep pain perception—normal

▪ Lesion Localization
Lower motor neuron signs are present in the right thoracic limb, and UMN signs are present in the right pelvic limb. In addition, mild Horner's syndrome is present in the right eye. A unilateral right C6-T2 spinal cord lesion would explain these signs. The history suggests that the lesion may have begun in the brachial plexus and progressed proximally.

▪ Differential Diagnosis
1. Neoplasia
2. Inflammation

▪ Diagnostic Plan
Radiography of the cervical spine and right thoracic limb may detect bony abnormalities or neoplasia.

MRI or CT/Myelography would evaluate for spinal cord compression.

CSF analysis would rule out inflammation.

▪ Diagnostic Results
Radiographs of the cervical vertebral column and right thoracic limb did not reveal any abnormalities. Myelography revealed an intradural-extramedullary mass at the right side of the cord over the C7 and T1 vertebrae. CSF analysis was normal (0 cells, 20 mg/dL protein).

▪ Diagnosis
A nerve sheath tumor of the right brachial plexus is the most likely diagnosis causing spinal cord compression of C6, C7, C8, and T1. The history is typical for a primary nerve sheath tumor or secondary tumor such as lymphoma involving the brachial plexus.

▪ Treatment
Dexamethasone can be administered to lessen the spinal cord edema and pain. Surgical removal may be possible but extension into the dura makes complete resection difficult and will likely cause permanent nerve and spinal cord. The right TL was amputated. A hemilaminectomy was performed at C7 for partial mass resection and decompression of the spinal cord.

REFERENCES

1. Bailey CS, Kitchell RL: Clinical evaluation of the cutaneous innervation of the canine thoracic limb, J Am Anim Hosp Assoc 20(11):939–950, 1984.
2. Haghighi SS, Kitchell RL, Johnson RD: Electrophysiologic studies of the cutaneous innervation of the pelvic limb of male dogs, Am J Vet Res 52(2):352–362, 1991.
3. Bailey CS, Kitchell RL: Cutaneous sensory testing in the dog, J Vet Intern Med 1(3):128–135, 1987.
4. Bennett GJ: An animal model of neuropathic pain: a review, Muscle Nerve 16:1040–1048, 1993.
5. Mayhew IG: Large animal neurology, ed 2, Ames, Iowa, 2009, Wiley-Blackwell.
6. Chambers JN, Hardie EM: Localization and management of sciatic nerve injury due to ischial or acetabular fracture, J Am Anim Hosp Assoc 22:539–544, 1986.
7. Cox VS, Breazile JE, Hoover TR: Surgical and anatomic study of calving paralysis, Am J Vet Res 36:427–430, 1975.
8. Walker TL: Ischiadic nerve entrapment, J Am Vet Med Assoc 178(12):1284–1288, 1981.
9. Jacobson A, Schrader SC: Peripheral nerve injury associated with fracture or fracture-dislocation of the pelvis in dogs and cats: 34 cases (1978-1982), J Am Vet Med Assoc 190(5):569–572, 1987.
10. Forterre F, Tomek A, Rytz U: Iatrogenic sciatic nerve injury in eighteen dogs and nine cats (1977-2006), Vet Surg 36:464–471, 2007.
11. Palmer RH, Aron DN, Purinton PT: Relationship of femoral intramedullary pins to the sciatic nerve and gluteal muscles after retrograde and normograde insertion, Vet Surg 17(2):65–70, 1988.
12. Fanton JW, Blass CE, Withrow SJ: Sciatic nerve injury as a complication of intramedullary pin fixation of femoral fractures, J Am Anim Hosp Assoc 19(5):687–694, 1983.
13. Cockshutt JR, Smith-Maxie LL: Delayed onset sciatic impairment following triple pelvic osteotomy, Prog Vet Neurol 4(2):60–63, 1993.
14. Stanton ME, Weigel JP, Henry RE: Ischiatic nerve paralysis associated with the biceps femoris muscle sling: case report and anatomical study, J Am Anim Hosp Assoc 24(4):429–432, 1988.
15. Sorjonen DC, Milton JL, Steiss JE: Hip dysplasia with bilateral ischiatic nerve entrapment in a dog, J Am Vet Med Assoc 197(4):495–497, 1990.
16. Andrews CM, Liska WD, Roberts DJ: Sciatic neurapraxia as a complication in 1000 consecutive canine total hip replacements, Vet Surg 37:254–262, 2008.
17. Autefage A, Fayolle P, Toutain PL: Distribution of material injected intramuscularly in dogs, Am J Vet Res 51(6): 901–904, 1990.
18. Levine JM, Fitch RB: Use of an ankle-foot orthotic in a dog with traumatic sciatic neuropathy, J Small Anim Pract 44:236–238, 2003.
19. Granger N, Moissonnier P, Fanchon L: Cutaneous saphenous nerve graft for the treatment of sciatic neurotmesis in a dog, J Am Vet Med Assoc 229:82–86, 2006.
20. Bennett D, Vaughan LC: The use of muscle relocation techniques in the treatment of peripheral nerve injuries in dogs and cats, J Small Anim Pract 17:99–108, 1976.
21. Read RA: Probable trophic pad ulceration following traumatic denervation. Report of two cases in dogs, Vet Surg 15(1):40–44, 1986.
22. Gibbons SE, McKee WM: Spontaneous healing of a trophic ulcer of the metatarsal pad in a dog, J Small Anim Pract 45:623–625, 2004.
23. Swaim SF, Hanson RR, Coates JR: Pressure wounds in animals, Compend Contin Educ Pract Vet 18(3): 203–219, 1996.

24. Danielson KS, Kent M, Cornell K: Successful treatment of a metacarpal trophic ulcer utilizing a neurovascular island flap, J Am Anim Hosp Assoc 45:176–180, 2009.
25. Wilson J: Relationship of the patellar tendon reflex to the ventral branch of the fifth lumbar spinal nerve in the dog, Am J Vet Res 39:1774–1779, 1978.
26. Breur GJ, Blevins WE: Traumatic injury of the iliopsoas muscle in three dogs, J Am Vet Med Assoc 210(11):1631–1634, 1997.
27. Rossmeisl JH, Rohleder J, Hancock R: Computed tomographic features of suspected traumatic injury to the iliopsoas and pelvic limb musculature of a dog, Vet Radiol Ultrasound 45:388–392, 2004.
28. Stephnick M, Olby NJ, Thompson RR: Femoral neuropathy in a dog with iliopsoas muscle injury, Vet Surg 35:186–190, 2006.
29. Tryphonas L, Hamilton GF, Rhodes GS: Perinatal femoral nerve degeneration and neurogenic atrophy of quadriceps femoris muscles in calves, J Am Vet Med Assoc 154:801–807, 1974.
30. Bailey CS: Patterns of cutaneous anesthesia associated with brachial plexus avulsions in the dog, J Am Vet Med Assoc 185(8):889–899, 1984.
31. Griffiths IR: Avulsion of the brachial plexus-1. Neuropathology of the spinal cord and peripheral nerves, J Small Anim Pract 15:165–176, 1974.
32. Griffiths IR, Duncan ID, Lawson DD: Avulsion of the brachial plexus-2. Clinical aspects, J Small Anim Pract 15:177–182, 1974.
33. Steinberg HS: Brachial plexus injuries and dysfunctions, Vet Clin North Am Small Anim Pract 18(3):565–580, 1988.
34. Wheeler SJ, Jones C, Wright JA: The diagnosis of brachial plexus disorders in dogs: a review of twenty-two cases, J Small Anim Pract 27:147–157, 1986.
35. Kern TJ, Aromando MC, Erb HN: Horner's syndrome in dogs and cats: 100 cases (1975-1985), J Am Vet Med Assoc 195(3):369–373, 1989.
36. Faissler D, Cizinauskas S, Jaggy A: Prognostic factors for functional recovery in dogs with suspected brachial plexus avulsion, J Vet Intern Med 16:370, 2002.
37. Steinberg HS: The use of electrodiagnostic techniques in evaluating traumatic brachial plexus root injuries, J Am Anim Hosp Assoc 15:621–626, 1979.
38. Schneider RK, Bramlage LR: Suprascapular nerve injury in horses, Compend Contin Educ Pract Vet 12:1783–1789, 1990.
39. Schneider JE, Adams OR, Easley KJ: Scapular notch resection for suprascapular nerve decompression, J Am Vet Med Assoc 187:1019–1020, 1985.
40. Bennett RA: Contracture of the infraspinatus muscle in dogs: a review of 12 cases, J Am Anim Hosp Assoc 22(4):481–487, 1986.
41. Knecht CD: The radial-brachial paralysis syndrome in the dog, J Am Vet Med Assoc 154(6):653–656, 1969.
42. Swaim SF: Peripheral nerve surgery in the dog, J Am Vet Med Assoc 161(8):905–911, 1972.
43. Okin R: Carpal arthrodesis in a cat with radial nerve damage, Feline Pract 12(4):18–20, 1982.
44. Sherman J, Olby NJ: Nursing and rehabilitation of the neurological patient. In Platt SR, Olby NJ, editors: BSAVA manual of canine and feline neurology, ed 3, Gloucester, UK, 2004, BSAVA.
45. Cuddon PA, Delauche AJ, Hutchison JM: Assessment of dorsal nerve root and spinal cord dorsal horn function in clinically normal dogs by determination of cord dorsum potentials, Am J Vet Res 60(2):222–226, 1999.
46. Griffiths IR, Duncan ID: Some studies of the clinical neurophysiology of denervation in the dog, Res Vet Sci 17(3):377–383, 1974.
47. Alexander JW, de Lahunta A, Scott DW: A case of brachial plexus neuropathy in a dog, J Am Anim Hosp Assoc 10(9):515–517, 1974.
48. Bright RM, Crabtree BJ, Knecht CD: Brachial plexus neuropathy in the cat: a case report, J Am Anim Hosp Assoc 14:612–615, 1978.
49. Cummings JF, Lorenz MD, deLahunta A: Canine brachial plexus neuritis: a syndrome resembling serum neuritis in man, Cornell Vet 63:589–617, 1973.
50. Garosi L, deLahunta A, Summer BA: Hypertrophic neuritis of the brachial plexus in a cat: magnetic resonance imaging and pathologic findings, J Feline Med Surg 8:63–68, 2006.
51. Braund KG: Neoplasia. In Oliver JE, Hoerlein BF, Mayhew IG, editors: Veterinary neurology, Philadelphia, 1987, WB Saunders.
52. Schoniger S, Summer BA: Localized, plexiform, diffuse, and other variants of neurofibroma in 12 dogs, 2 horses and a chicken, Vet Pathol 46:904–915, 2009.
53. Brehm DM, Vite CH, Steinberg HS: A retrospective evaluation of 51 cases of peripheral nerve sheath tumors in the dog, J Am Anim Hosp Assoc 31(4):349–359, 1995.
54. Bradley RL, Withrow SJ, Snyder SP: Nerve sheath tumors in the dog, J Am Anim Hosp Assoc 18:915–921, 1982.
55. Lane SB, Kornegay JN, Duncan JR: Feline spinal lymphosarcoma: a retrospective evaluation of 23 cats, J Vet Intern Med 8(2):99–104, 1994.
56. de Lahunta A, Glass E: Veterinary neuroanatomy and clinical neurology, St Louis, 2009, Saunders Elsevier.
57. McCarthy RJ, Feeney DA, Lipowitz AJ: Preoperative diagnosis of tumors of the brachial plexus by use of computed tomography in three dogs, J Am Vet Med Assoc 202(2):291–294, 1993.
58. Platt SR, Graham J, Chrisman CL: Magnetic resonance imaging and ultrasonography in the diagnosis of a malignant peripheral nerve sheath tumor in a dog, Vet Radiol Ultrasound 40(4):367–371, 1999.
59. Kraft SL, Ehrhart EJ, Gall D: Magnetic resonance imaging characteristics of peripheral nerve sheath tumors of the canine brachial plexus in 18 dogs, Vet Radiol Ultrasound 48:1–7, 2007.
60. Bailey CS: Long-term survival after surgical excision of a schwannoma of the sixth cervical spinal nerve in a dog. J Am Vet Med Assoc 196:754-756.

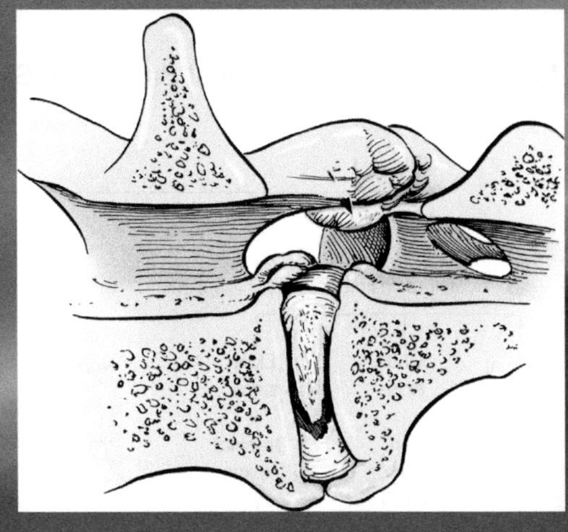

CHAPTER 6

Pelvic Limb Paresis, Paralysis, or Ataxia

Bilateral motor dysfunction of the pelvic limbs is termed *paraparesis or paraplegia*, depending on the severity of the motor loss. Loss of proprioception from the pelvic limbs results in general proprioceptive (GP) ataxia. In addition, loss of pain perception from the pelvic limbs may accompany the motor dysfunction. Lesion localization has been discussed in Chapter 2 and is summarized in Figure 6-1. A brief review follows.

LESION LOCALIZATION

Animals with pure pelvic limb paresis and GP ataxia have neurologic disease caudal to the second thoracic spinal cord segment. Lesions in the region of T3-L3 produce GP ataxia and upper motor neuron (UMN) paraparesis. The pelvic limb lower motor neurons (LMNs), located in segments L4-S3, remain intact and are capable of reflex motor activity; however, voluntary motor control from the brain is lost because the motor pathways in the spinal cord are damaged. The spinal reflexes are normal or exaggerated. Exaggerated reflexes result when UMN inhibitory influence on the LMNs is lost. Similarly, extensor hypertonus or spasticity also may develop. Ataxia results from damage to the spinal cord GP pathways, which transmit position sense signals from receptors in the pelvic limbs to the brain. Hypalgesia or analgesia caudal to the lesion results from disruption of sensory pathways from the pelvic limbs to the brain. Pain perception (nociception) is lost only if the lesion is bilateral and severe. Voluntary visceral functions (see Chapter 3), such as micturition, may be lost when UMN or sensory pathways in the spinal cord are damaged. Muscle atrophy from disuse may develop with time.

In summary, spinal cord lesions in the region of T3-L3 segments result in paresis, GP ataxia, decreased or absent postural reactions, normal reflexes or hyperreflexia, impaired micturition, and variable degrees of sensory loss caudal to the lesion. Examination of the thoracolumbar dermatomes may be helpful in the localization of lesions to spinal segments within this spinal cord region (see Chapter 1).

Lesions in the area of L4-S3 or those that involve the cauda equina (the L7 and S1-2 spinal nerve roots and spinal nerves) produce pelvic limb paresis of the LMN type. Lesions involving spinal cord segments of L4-S3 injure the motor neurons within the lumbosacral intumescence that form the lumbosacral plexus. Abnormalities related to femoral, sciatic, pudendal, and pelvic nerves are encountered in these patients. Pelvic limb reflexes are depressed or absent, and the muscles may be hypotonic. Neurogenic muscle atrophy develops. Sensory dysfunction (hypalgesia, analgesia) results from an injury to the sensory neurons and nerve fibers located in this region of the spinal cord. Abnormalities of visceral function result from an injury to the motor and sensory neurons that innervate the bladder and the anus. Lesions involving the caudal segments of the spinal cord and the cauda equina damage nerve fibers that form the sciatic, pudendal, pelvic, and caudal nerves. Because the femoral nerve is spared, the animal is able to support weight on the pelvic limbs but will have a plantigrade posture or stance. The patellar reflex is normal, and pain perception is perceived from the medial aspect of the first digit and the thigh. The clinical signs are related to motor and sensory dysfunction of the involved nerves. Figure 6-2 summarizes lesion localization for the problem of pelvic limb paresis based on motor signs.

DISEASES

The disorders or diseases that affect the spinal cord segments T3-L3 are classified in Tables 6-1 through 6-3. Disorders that affect spinal cord segments L4-S3 and the cauda equina are presented in Tables 6-4 through 6-6. Although many of the diseases are discussed in relationship to specific anatomic regions of the vertebral column and spinal cord (e.g., T3-L3 spinal cord segments), many can occur in any location. However, their inclusion in specific regions is based on their most common presentations. These tables are organized according to the logic used in the formulation of a neurologic diagnosis, discussed in Chapter 1. After the lesion has been localized to a region or segment of the spinal cord, nerve root, spinal nerve, or peripheral nerve, consideration is given to the possible etiologic categories that could produce the lesion. The etiologic categories are listed in the left-hand column of these tables and follow the DAMNITV classification scheme described in

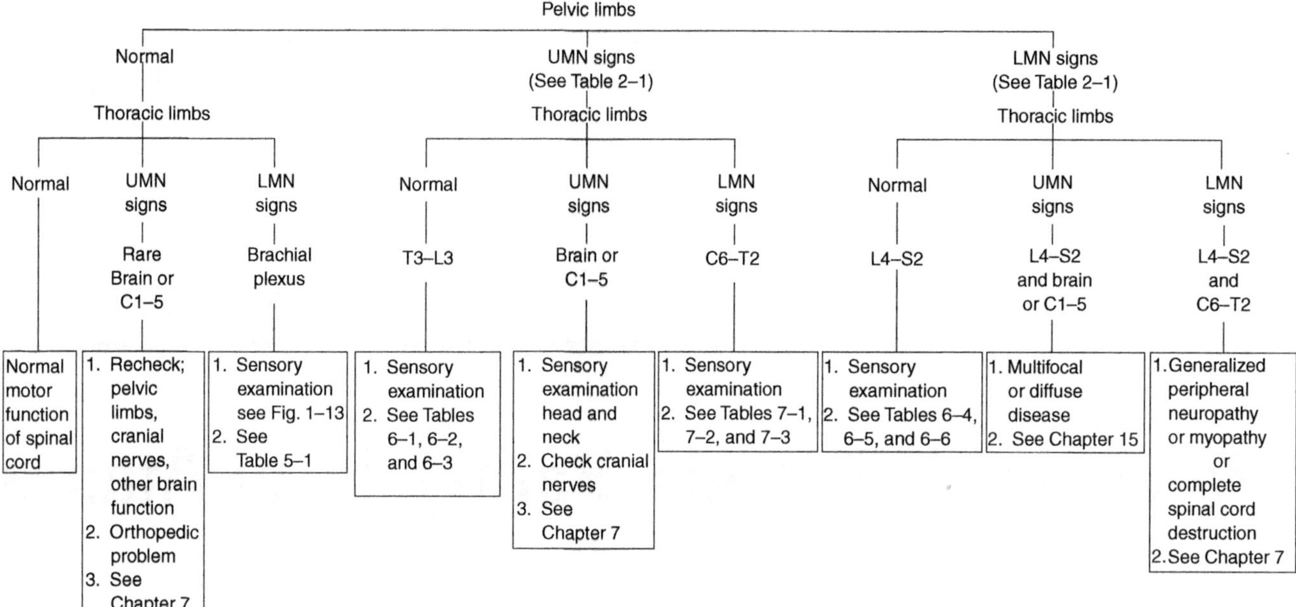

Figure 6-1 Localization of lesions based on motor function. *UMN,* Upper motor neuron; *LMN,* lower motor neuron; C, cervical; *T,* thoracic; *L,* lumbar; *S,* sacral. (From Hoerlein BF: Canine neurology: diagnosis and treatment, ed 3, Philadelphia, 1978, WB Saunders.)

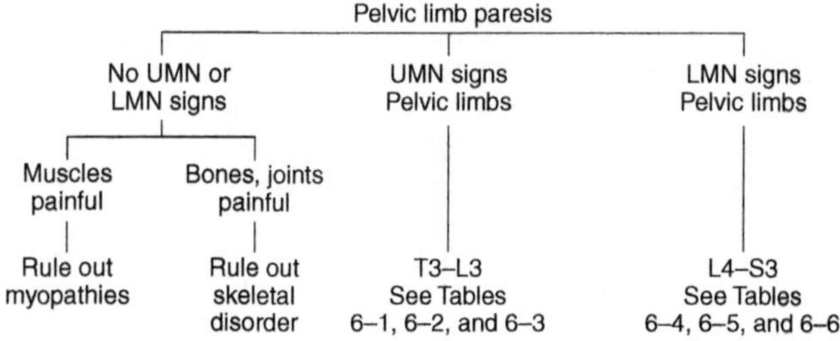

Figure 6-2 Algorithm for the localization of lesions causing pelvic limb paresis. *UMN,* Upper motor neuron; *LMN,* lower motor neuron.

Table 1-2. The diseases are further divided into acute progressive, acute nonprogressive, and chronic progressive categories based on historical information or on the clinical course of the illness. Most diseases have been included in the tables. The most important disorders are described in subsequent sections of this chapter. They are reviewed briefly with an emphasis on diagnosis and treatment. Some diseases are discussed in other chapters, as noted in the tables.

Acute Progressive Diseases, T3-L3

Degenerative

Thoracolumbar Intervertebral Disk Disease

Pathophysiology. The intervertebral disk (IVD) permits stable motion of the spine while supporting and distributing loads under movement. The annulus fibrosus is a multilayered ligament that makes up the periphery of the disk and attaches to the hyaline cartilage of the vertebral end plates. Its outer collagen layers blend with the ventral and dorsal longitudinal ligaments while the inner layers blend with the nucleus pulposus. The nucleus pulposus, an embryologic remnant of the notochord is the highly hydrated central portion of the disk.

The major molecular components of the disk are collagenous and noncollagenous proteins, proteoglycan aggregates, and glycoproteins. Glycosaminoglycans (GAG) are proteoglycans composed of repeating units of hexosamines: chondroitin sulfate (CS), dermatan sulfate, keratan sulfate (KS), and hyaluronic acid. One of the functions of GAGs is to bind water; thus concentrations of these proteoglycans are highest in the nucleus pulposus. Age-related or pathologic change is associated with a progressive decrease in the proteoglycans, resulting in a decrease in water content within the nucleus and annulus. The proportion of GAG also change with age: the structure of the aggregate changes, the core protein and GAG chains shorten, and there is an increase in the ratio of KS to CS. This common aging process is known as fibroid metaplasia. In chondrodystrophic breeds, these degenerative changes are accelerated causing early intervertebral disk degeneration. The process of premature disk degeneration is basically a chondroid metaplasia of the nucleus pulposus with degeneration and weakening of the annulus fibrosus.

Degenerative intervertebral disk disease (IVDD) is one of the most common disorders that produces paraparesis in the dog. Disk disease occurs in about 2% of canine patients seen at teaching hospitals.[1,2] It is rarely a problem in cats, horses, or food animals. Degenerative changes within the disk can result in IVD herniation. Intervertebral disk herniation may result in *protrusion* of the annulus fibrosus or *extrusion* of the nucleus pulposus into the vertebral canal. Basically, two types of disk degeneration (Hansen types I and II) that result in different clinical syndromes have been described by Hansen (Figure 6-3).[3,4] Hansen type I IVDD occurs primarily in the chondrodystrophic (hypochondroplastic) breeds (e.g., miniature poodle, dachshund, beagle, cocker spaniel, Pekingese, or mixed chondrodystrophic breeds). Type I IVD degeneration in chondrodystrophic breeds develops when the animal is young (i.e., 2 to 9 months of age); in affected dogs, clinical signs develop by the time the animal is 3 to 6 years of age.[2,5] Calcification of the degenerative disk commonly occurs and is radiographically apparent in affected dachshunds at 6 to 18 months of age.[6-8] Large nonchondrodystrophic breeds of dog (e.g., Doberman pinscher, German shepherd dog, and Labrador retriever) also can be affected with Hansen type I IVDD.

The process of Hansen type I IVDD leads to a weakened annulus that cannot restrain the degenerative nucleus, and normal movements of the vertebral column are sufficient to

TABLE 6-1

Small Animal Thoracolumbar Spinal Cord Diseases: Differential Diagnosis of T3-L3 Spinal Cord Disease Based on Clinical Course and Etiologic Categories*

Etiologic Category	Acute Nonprogressive	Acute Progressive	Chronic Progressive
Degenerative	None	Hansen type I IVDD (6) Hemorrhagic myelomalacia (6) Afghan hound myelinopathy (6)	Hansen type II IVDD (6) Degenerative myelopathy (6) Spondylosis deformans (6) Spinal dural ossification (6) Multiple cartilaginous exostoses (6) Spinal arachnoid cysts (6) Disseminated idiopathic skeletal hyperostosis (6) Spinal synovial cysts (6,7) Axonopathies (7) Demyelinating diseases (7) Neuronopathies (7)
Anomalous	None	None	Spinal cord malformation (6) Vertebral malformation (6) Spinal stenosis (6)
Metabolic	None	None	Endocrine neuropathies (8)
Neoplastic (6)	None	Metastatic Primary Vertebral Hematopoietic	Metastatic Primary Vertebral Hematopoietic
Nutritional	None	None	Hypervitaminosis A (cats) (15) Methionine deficiency (6)
Inflammatory	None	Rickettsial myelitis (15) Bacterial myelitis (15) Distemper virus myelitis (15) Protozoal myelitis (15) Mycotic myelitis (15) Discospondylitis (6) Vertebral abscess (6) Epidural empyema (6) Vertebral physitis	Feline infectious peritonitis (15) Granulomatous meningoencephalomyelitis (15) Necrotizing meningoencephalomyelitis (15)
Toxic	None	None	Various toxic neuropathies (7, 15)
Traumatic	Fractures (6) Luxations (6) Contusions (6) Intervertebral disk extrusion (6)	Hemorrhagic myelomalacia (6) Intervertebral disk extrusion (6)	None
Vascular	Fibrocartilaginous embolism (6) Aortic thromboembolism (6)	None	None

*Numbers in parentheses refer to chapters in which the entities are discussed.

initiate acute disk extrusion. The extrusion of nucleus pulposus results primarily in an acute, focal compressive myelopathy. In some cases a severe progressive myelopathy, known as ascending-descending myelomalacia (see later discussion), follows an acute and severe extrusion of the nucleus pulposus.[9]

Hansen type II IVD degeneration occurs in nonchondrodystrophic breeds, such as German shepherd dogs and Labrador retrievers.[1,2] Type II IVD develops at a slower rate, and clinical signs occur when the animal is 5 to 12 years of age. Fibroid metaplasia can lead to gradual disk protrusion. True extrusion of nucleus pulposus into the extradural space does not occur but rather a protrusion or bulge of the annulus fibrosus occurs. Both the annulus fibrosus and nucleus pulposus may protrude but the nucleus pulposus is contained within an intact, but degenerate annulus. Acute onset of clinical signs with Hansen type II IVDD is less common and compression from this protrusion results in a slowly progressive focal myelopathy. This syndrome is discussed in the section on chronic progressive spinal cord disorders.

Acute noncompressive nucleus pulposus extrusion is a less common phenomenon but has been better documented with the use of magnetic resonance imaging (MRI).[10] This type of IVD injury usually occurs during heavy exertional activity associated with peracute compressive types of injuries to

TABLE 6-2

Equine Thoracolumbar Spinal Cord Diseases: Differential Diagnosis of T3-L3 Spinal Cord Disease Based on Clinical Course and Etiologic Categories*

Etiologic Category	Acute Nonprogressive	Acute Progressive	Chronic Progressive
Degenerative	None	Degenerative myeloencephalopathy (7)	Spondylosis deformans (6) Neuronopathies (7) Demyelinating diseases (7) Axonopathies (7)
Anomalous	None	None	Vertebral malformation (6) Spinal cord malformation (6)
Neoplastic (6)	None	Metastatic Primary Skeletal Hematopoietic	Primary Skeletal Hematopoietic
Nutritional	None	None	Vitamin E deficiency (equine motor neuron disease) (7)
Inflammatory	None	Herpesvirus 1 (6) Protozoal myelitis (6) West Nile virus (6) Verminous migration (6) Mycotic myelitis (6) Rabies virus (15) Vertebral osteomyelitis (6)	See acute progressive
Toxic	None	None	Various neuropathies (7, 15)
Traumatic	Fractures (6) Luxations (6)	None	None
Vascular	Embolic myelopathy (6) Fibrocartilaginous emboli (6) Postanesthetic myelopathy	None	None

*Numbers in parentheses refer to chapters in which the entities are discussed.

the spine. Excessive forces placed on the intervertebral disk may result in expulsion of the nucleus pulposus toward the spinal cord through a rent in the annulus fibrosus. The gelatinous nucleus likely disperses along the floor of the spinal canal without causing spinal cord compression.

Spinal cord damage caused by compressive or concussive myelopathy primarily has been attributed to the mechanical derangement of neural tissue and hypoxic changes resulting from alterations to the vascular supply. Vascular embarrassment that results in ischemia and edema undoubtedly plays a role in the development of more severe spinal cord degeneration and the syndrome of ascending-descending myelomalacia. The severity of the spinal cord lesion is influenced by the amount of compression and its rate of development. The inflammatory reaction induced by the extruded nucleus pulposus and the diameter of the vertebral canal in comparison to the diameter of the spinal cord also are related to the severity of the clinical signs. Acute extrusions produce more severe spinal cord lesions than do chronic progressive extrusions/protrusions. Less severe lesions occur in areas where the vertebral canal is large in relation to the diameter of the spinal cord (e.g., the cervical vertebral column). Histopathologic changes progress from edema, demyelination, and necrosis of myelin and axons to the gross finding of myelomalacia.

Clinical Signs. In addition to the signs of paresis or paralysis that characterize spinal cord lesions, IVD herniation may compress the nerve roots and the meninges, resulting in severe pain and hyperesthesia when the vertebral column is manipulated. Hyperesthesia is an exaggerated cerebral response to a nonnoxious stimulus. An animal may arch its back (kyphotic posture) and tense its abdominal muscles that can mimic acute abdominal pain in disorders such as pancreatitis (Figure 6-4). Dogs with back pain alone or minimal neurologic deficits actually can have substantial spinal cord compression.[11] Such cases typically have a protracted history of pain. Lateralization of the IVD herniation and spinal cord compression often will cause asymmetry of neurologic deficits. Clinical signs of back pain only can progress in order of functional loss: (1) loss of general proprioception, (2) loss of voluntary motor function, and (3) lastly, loss of pain perception. Loss of bladder function usually occurs with paraplegia. Sensory examinations, such as pinching the skin and palpating the vertebrae, are important because they may allow the clinician to localize the lesion to within two or three spinal cord segments. Lesions that affect the pain (nociception) pathways abolish the cutaneous trunci reflex caudal to the lesion. This reflex is normally most apparent when the skin over the thoracolumbar junction is stimulated. Students may incorrectly believe that this apparent exaggeration of the skin twitch represents hyperesthesia and thus correlates with lesion location. Cooperative animals that cry out or try to bite when an area is palpated or pinched may be experiencing hyperesthesia, and the lesion is usually one or two segments cranial to the point at which the response was induced. In animals that are analgesic in the pelvic limbs, a point or line across the vertebral column, caudal to which the animal is analgesic, should be determined. Likewise, the lesion is usually one or two segments cranial to the point at which the animal first feels noxious stimuli (e.g., pinching the skin with a hemostat).

TABLE 6-3

Food Animal Thoracolumbar Spinal Cord Diseases: Differential Diagnosis of T3-L3 Spinal Cord Disease Based on Clinical Course and Etiologic Categories*

Etiologic Category	Acute Nonprogressive	Acute Progressive	Chronic Progressive
Degenerative	None	None	Progressive ataxia of Charolais cattle—B (7) Degenerative myeloencephalopathy—B, CA (7) Spondylosis deformans—All (6) Arthrogryposis—All (7) Demyelinating diseases—B (7) Neuronopathies—B, O (7)
Anomalous	None	None	Spinal cord malformation—All (6) Vertebral malformation—All (6) Vertebral canal stenosis—B (6)
Neoplastic (6)	None	Metastatic Primary Vertebral Hematopoietic	Metastatic Primary Vertebral Hematopoietic
Nutritional	None	None	Enzootic ataxia, copper deficiency—C, O (15) Hypervitaminosis A (15)
Inflammatory	None	Caprine arthritis-encephalomyelitis—C (6) Rabies myelitis—All (15) West Nile virus—CA (6) Equine herpesvirus 1—CA (6) Bacterial myelitis—All (15) Verminous migration—All (6) Protozoal myelitis (15) Mycotic myelitis (15) Vertebral osteomyelitis—All (6)	Maedi-visna—O (6) Verminous migration—All (6) Rabies myelitis—All (15)
Toxic	None	None	Various neuropathies (7, 15)
Traumatic	Fractures (6) Luxations (6) Contusions (6)	None	None
Vascular	Fibrocartilaginous embolism—B, P (6) Aortic thromboembolism—B (6) Embolic myelopathy	None	None

B, Bovine; *C*, caprine; *O*, ovine; *P*, porcine; *CA*, camelids.
*Numbers in parentheses refer to chapters in which the entities are discussed.

Dogs having peracute or acute thoracolumbar IVD herniations may manifest initial clinical signs consistent with "spinal shock" or Schiff-Sherrington postures. These phenomena are further discussed in the section on spinal trauma. It is important to recognize these clinical manifestations to avoid mistakes on localization. Hansen type I thoracolumbar IVD herniations may develop at IVD spaces T9-10 to L7-S1. The intercapital ligament usually prevents extrusion of the nucleus pulposus in the cranial and midthoracic IVDs. More than 65% of type I IVD herniations occur at sites T11-12, T12-13, T13-L1, and L1-2.[1,2,12] The most common site for type I IVD herniations in large breed dogs is the disk interspace between L1 and L2.[13] These areas should be evaluated carefully in dogs with suspected thoracolumbar IVDD. Less frequently, IVD herniations in dogs occur caudal to the L3-4 IVD space. Herniation at these sites produces LMN signs in the pelvic limbs because the compressive myelopathy directly affects the motor neurons of the lumbosacral intumescence that form the lumbosacral plexus.

A syndrome of ascending-descending ischemic necrosis of the spinal cord may occur with an incidence rate as high as 10% in dogs with acute thoracolumbar IVDD and complete sensory loss.[14,15] This syndrome is also known as ascending-descending *myelomalacia*. The syndrome of ascending-descending myelomalacia has an unknown pathogenesis, but vascular lesions leading to severe ischemia probably are important. This syndrome can follow severe acute spinal cord trauma of any cause and results in complete destruction of the nervous tissue of the spinal cord. The syndrome typically begins within the first several days after injury. The clinical signs result from necrosis of the motor neurons, descending motor fibers, and ascending sensory fibers. Clinical signs progress as the ischemic necrosis ascends and descends along the spinal cord. As the lesion ascends, there is a cranial migration

TABLE 6-4

Small Animal Lumbosacral and Cauda Equina Diseases: Differential Diagnosis of L4-S3 and Caudal Spinal Cord Disease Based on Clinical Courses and Etiologic Categories*

Etiologic Category	Acute Nonprogressive	Acute Progressive	Chronic Progressive
Degenerative	None	Hansen type I IVDD (6) Hemorrhagic myelomalacia (6)	Hansen type II IVDD (6) Degenerative myelopathy (6) Degenerative lumbosacral stenosis (6) Spondylosis deformans (6) Neuronopathies (7)
Anomalous	None	None	Spinal cord malformation (6) Vertebral malformation (6)
Metabolic	None	None	Endocrine neuropathies (7)
Neoplastic (6)	None	Metastatic Primary Vertebral Hematopoietic	Metastatic Primary Vertebral Hematopoietic
Inflammatory	None	Distemper virus myelitis (15) Bacterial myelitis (15) Rickettsial myelitis Protozoal myelitis (15) Mycotic myelitis (15) Discospondylitis (6) Vertebral abscess (6) Epidural empyema (6) Vertebral physitis (6)	Feline infectious peritonitis (15) Distemper virus myelitis (15) Granulomatous meningoencephalomyelitis (15) Necrotizing meningoencephalomyelitis (15) Postvaccinal rabies
Toxic	None	None	Various neuropathies (7, 15)
Traumatic	Fractures (6) Luxations (6) Contusions (6) Intervertebral disk extrusion (6)	Hemorrhagic myelomalacia (6) Intervertebral disk extrusion (6)	None
Vascular	Fibrocartilaginous embolism (6) Aortic thromboembolism (6) Embolic myelopathy	None	None

*Numbers in parentheses refer to chapters in which the entities are discussed.

of the line of analgesia and the cut-off of the cutaneous trunci reflex. This may be the first indications of the onset of this syndrome. Ascending signs of LMN paralysis include a loss of intercostal muscle function for respiration and an inability to remain sternal because of paralysis of the paraspinal muscles. The thoracic limbs may be rigidly extended, and hyperesthesia may develop in the limbs a few hours before the necrosis affects the caudal cervical spinal cord. As the lesion progresses cranially, the motor neurons involved in the innervation of the thoracic limb become affected. Ultimately, LMN paresis, hypotonia, and sensory loss involving the thoracic limbs develops. Finally, as the lesion ascends into the cervical spinal cord, there is a loss of the ability to ventilate. Respiratory failure occurs when the necrosis ascends to the level of the fifth and sixth cervical spinal cord segments and thus destroys the motor neurons of the phrenic nerves. Affected animals can die of respiratory failure within 2 to 4 days after the onset of clinical signs. As the lesion progresses caudally, there is a sequential loss of the patellar reflex and muscular tone of the pelvic limbs, followed by loss of the flexor reflex, and ultimately loss of anal and urethral sphincter tone. The anus may be dilated, and the perineal reflex is weak or absent. The bladder is usually distended (atonic) and easily expressed because of poor tone in the urethral sphincter. In addition, there is loss of tone of the abdominal wall musculature leading to a flaccid abdominal wall when palpated. This syndrome should be suspected in all animals that develop ascending analgesia or descending signs of LMN dysfunction after trauma and severe compression of the spinal cord. There is no treatment for this syndrome. Once the clinical signs develop, they usually continue to progress. This extent of myelomalacia is irreparable, and euthanasia should be performed on affected animals to prevent needless suffering. This syndrome apparently occurs with greatest frequency in dogs that develop acute paralysis and complete sensory loss. Owners of dogs with complete sensory loss should be warned of this possibility, particularly in cases in which surgical therapy is contemplated.

Importantly, these cases can be differentiated from those of a focal lesion affecting the L4-S2 spinal cord segments. In cases with ascending-descending myelomalacia, there is a more cranial location of hyperesthesia and a more cranial level of decreased sensation or point at which there is a loss of the cutaneous trunci reflex than would be expected for a lesion affecting the L4-S2 spinal segments.

Diagnosis. A tentative diagnosis of thoracolumbar IVDD is based on assessment of the clinical signs, breed signalment, and results of the neurologic evaluation. For example, an animal with asymmetric paresis and little to no hyperesthesia is

TABLE 6-5

Equine Lumbosacral and Cauda Equina Diseases: Differential Diagnosis of L4-S5 and Caudal Disease Based on Clinical Course and Etiologic Categories*

Etiologic Category	Acute Nonprogressive	Acute Progressive	Chronic Progressive
Degenerative	None	None	Spondylosis deformans (6) Neuronopathies (7) Demyelinating diseases (7) Axonopathies (7)
Anomalous	None	None	Vertebral malformation (6) Spinal cord malformation (6)
Neoplastic (6)	None	Metastatic Primary Skeletal Hematopoietic	Primary Skeletal Hematopoietic
Inflammatory	None	Herpesvirus 1 (6) Protozoal myelitis (6) Verminous migration (6) Vertebral osteomyelitis (6) Mycotic myelitis (6)	Neuritis of the cauda equina (6) (see also acute progressive)
Toxic	None	None	Various neuropathies (7, 15) Sorghum ataxia and cystitis (6)
Traumatic	Fractures (6) Luxations (6) Postfoaling paralyses (5)	None	None
Vascular	Embolic myelopathy (6) Fibrocartilaginous emboli (6) Postanesthetic myelopathy	None	None

*Numbers in parentheses refer to chapters in which the entities are discussed.

more likely to have a vascular infarct than a compressive lesion from IVD herniation. Of utmost importance is the fact that clinical signs related to IVD herniation are clinically indistinguishable from those of a focal spinal cord lesion related to another etiology. Consequently, formulating a presumptive diagnosis based on signalment, history, and clinical signs should be done with caution. Ultimately, definitive diagnosis relies on diagnostic tests such as imaging studies. The diagnosis can be suspected by a conventional radiography evaluating for evidence of degenerate disks, but myelography combined with computed tomography (CT) or MRI of the vertebral column and spinal cord provide the accurate presumptive diagnosis and importantly lesion localization required for surgical intervention.

Figure 6-5 demonstrates diagnostic lesions observed on survey radiographs of the vertebral column. General anesthesia or strong sedation provides the necessary relaxation needed for proper positioning of the dog to allow diagnostic radiographs of the vertebral column to be obtained. In our hospitals, radiographs are taken when surgical treatment is being considered. For cases treated by conservative medical procedures, radiographs are not routinely made unless another disease, such as discospondylitis, neoplasia, or trauma is to be excluded. Survey radiographic changes associated with IVD herniation include a narrowing or wedging of the IVD space, a narrowing of the space between the articular processes, and a smaller intervertebral foramen as compared with adjacent spaces. Importantly, the T10-T11 IVD space is normally narrow compared with other IVD spaces at the thoracolumbar junction of the spine. Sometimes mineralized disk material can be visualized in the vertebral canal or superimposed over the area of the intervertebral foramen. Survey radiography alone, however, lacks accuracy in identifying the exact location of the extruded disk material.

Myelography or cross-sectional imaging using CT or MRI of the spine is required to determine the active site of the compression. The diagnostic procedures requested by the surgeon are dependent upon ability to ascertain the lesion site, to increase the probability of identifying the side of the IVD herniation, and to rule out other diseases. Myelography has served as a standard for diagnosing spinal cord compression in dogs with IVDD (see Chapter 4). Attenuation of contrast medium within the subarachnoid space occurs at sites of compression and subarachnoid space occlusion; such patterns are described as extradural, intradural/extramedullary, and intramedullary (Figure 6-6). Lateral, ventrodorsal, and oblique views are useful for determining the circumferential and longitudinal location along the vertebral column and extent of the extradural compression. Longitudinal lesion localization by myelography in thoracolumbar IVDD has nearly 90% accuracy.[16,17] An intramedullary pattern associated with spinal cord edema or extensive hemorrhage is more common with acute extrusions and may obscure the site of extradural compression. The extent of spinal cord swelling seen with myelography may assist in establishing a prognosis. A study in dogs with loss of pain perception showed a significantly worse outcome if the extent of spinal cord swelling is greater than five times the length of L2.[18]

Cross-sectional imaging using MRI and CT has supplanted the use of myelography for the evaluation of animals with suspected IVDD. CT can be an adjunctive procedure to myelography to further delineate lateralization of the extruded IVD material or used as the sole technique for detecting IVD

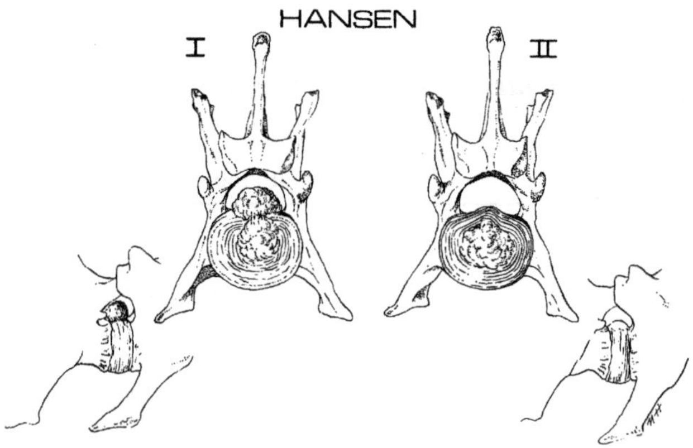

Figure 6-3 Drawings of Hansen type I and type II disk protrusions. (From Hoerlein BF: Canine neurology: diagnosis and treatment, ed 3, Philadelphia, 1978, WB Saunders.)

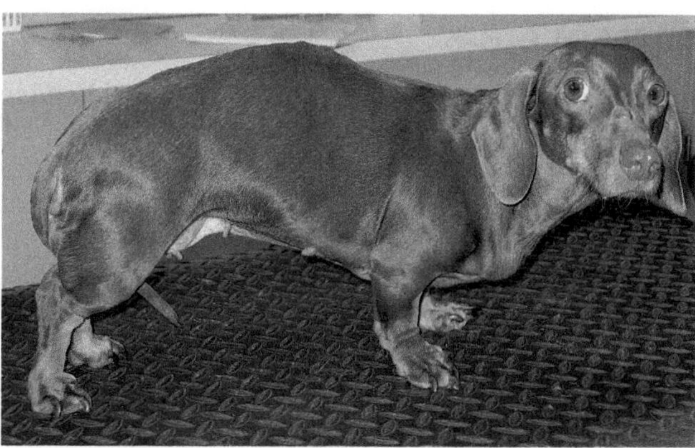

Figure 6-4 A 2-year-old female spayed dachshund showing a kyphotic posture that manifested paraspinal pain on palpation. Thoracolumbar intervertebral disk disease was confirmed with diagnostics and surgery.

TABLE 6-6

Food Animal Lumbosacral and Cauda Equina Diseases: Differential Diagnosis of L4-S3 and Caudal Disease Based on Clinical Course and Etiologic Categories*

Etiologic Category	Acute Nonprogressive	Acute Progressive	Chronic Progressive
Degenerative	None	None	Spondylosis deformans—All (6) Arthrogryposis—All (7) Neuronopathies—0, B (7)
Anomalous	None	None	Spinal cord malformation—All (6) Vertebral malformation—All (6)
Neoplastic (6)	None	Metastatic Primary Vertebral Hematopoietic	Metastatic Primary Vertebral Hematopoietic
Nutritional	None	None	Enzootic ataxia, copper deficiency—C, O (15)
Inflammatory	None	Bacterial myelitis—All (15) Vertebral osteomyelitis—All (7) Protozoal myelitis—All (15) Mycotic myelitis—All (15) Rabies virus—All (15)	Verminous migration—All (6) Vertebral osteomyelitis—All (7)
Toxic	None	None	Various neuropathies (7, 15) Sorghum ataxia and cystitis—B, O (6)
Traumatic	Fractures (6) Luxations (6) Contusions (6) Postcalving paralyses—B (5)	None	None
Vascular	Fibrocartilaginous embolism—B, P (6) Aortic thromboembolism—B (6) Embolic myelopathy	None	None

B, Bovine; C, caprine; O, ovine; *P*, porcine; *CA*, camelids.
*Numbers in parentheses refer to chapters in which the entities are discussed.

extrusion. Imaging the spine using CT alone is noninvasive and performed more quickly with fewer complications than myelography but experience is needed for accurate interpretation.[19] The lesion extent and lateralization of IVD material can be more distinct on CT than with myelography alone (Figure 6-7). Mineralized disk material and acute hemorrhage are identified in the vertebral canal using noncontrast-enhanced CT. The attenuation (brightness) of the disk material increases with the degree of mineralization. Acutely extruded IVD material typically is recognized as a heterogeneous and hyperattenuating extradural mass from a combination of disk material and hemorrhage.

MRI is superior in the recognition of intraparenchymal pathology and is the standard of care for assessment of acute

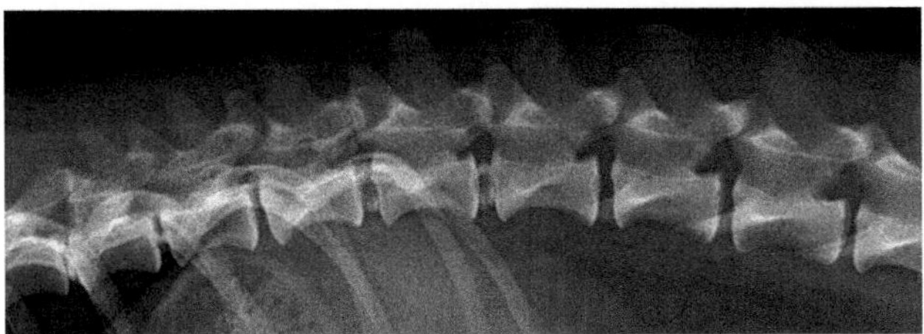

Figure 6-5 Lateral thoracolumbar radiograph showing wedging of the intervertebral space at T12-13. This is a radiographic lesion indicative of disk herniation. Mineralized disks are evident at T10-11, T13-L1, and L1-2. Mineralized disks in situ seldom cause active disease but are likely to herniate later.

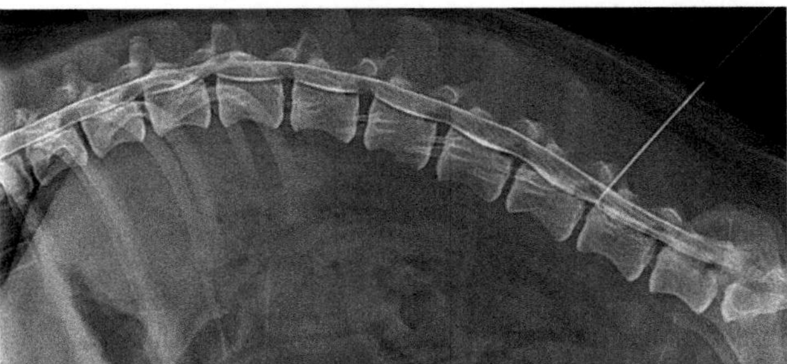

Figure 6-6 Lateral thoracolumbar radiograph and myelogram of a dog after injection of contrast into the subarachnoid space at L5-6. An extradural compression of the ventral contrast column and attenuation of the dorsal contrast column is visualized at T13-L1.

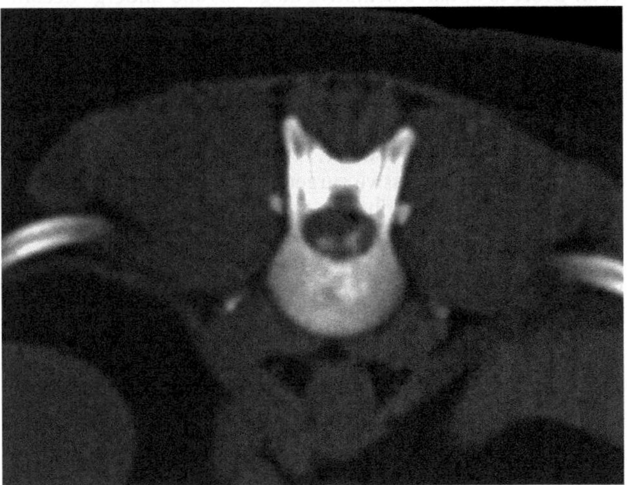

Figure 6-7 Transverse computed tomographic image of a Hansen type 1 intervertebral disk extrusion at T13-L1 demonstrating heterogeneous attenuation and opacity ventral to the spinal cord.

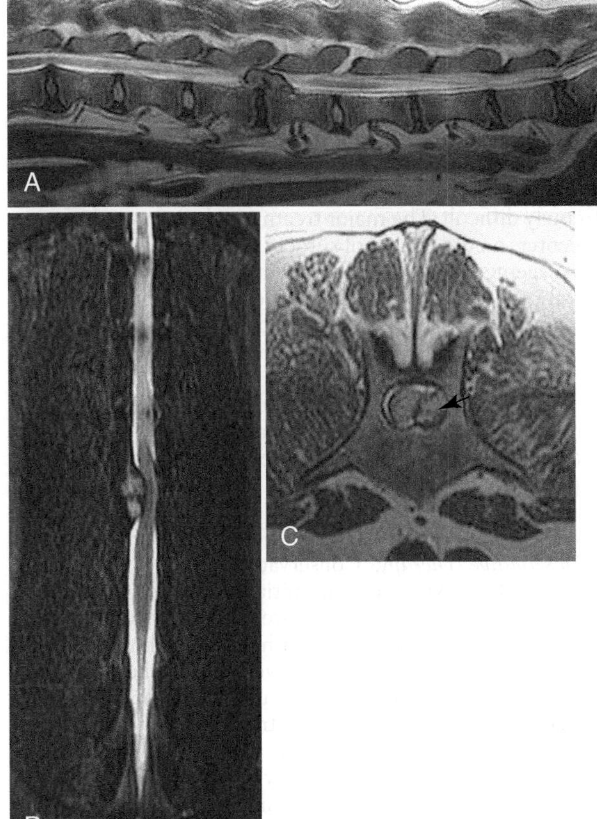

Figure 6-8 MRI from a 7-year-old German shepherd dog after L3-4 intervertebral disk extrusion of 2 weeks duration. **A,** Sagittal T2W image demonstrating heterogeneous intensity of a mass over the L3-4 disk interspace. Note the hyperintense normal nucleus pulposus at the L1-2, L2-3, and L4-5 disk interspaces and the hypointense to isointense degenerate nucleus pulposus at the T13-L1, L5-6, L6-7, and L7-S1 disk interspaces. **B,** Dorsal STIR image demonstrating left-sided lateralization of the extruded intervertebral disk causing displacement of the spinal cord to the right. **C,** Transverse image showing lateralization of the extruded disk material on the left side compressing the spinal cord to the right. Surgery confirmed a type I intervertebral disk herniation consisting of extruded nucleus pulposus with presence of old hemorrhage.

spinal cord injury (SCI) in animals (Figure 6-8). Standardized MRI protocols for intervertebral disk disease use T1- and T2-weighted sagittal and transverse imaging over areas of interest. MRI is also is ideal for early recognition of in situ disk degeneration based on a decrease in signal intensity (relative blackness) within the nucleus pulposus on T2-weighted images.[20] Focal signal void (blackness) within the IVD space or spinal canal may represent mineralization or extruded mineralized nucleus pulposus.[21,22] Acute pathologies of spinal cord tissue recognized as high-signal hypersensitivity on T2-weighted images (relative whiteness) include necrosis, inflammation, and edema. However, it is difficult to distinguish among these specific types of pathology. MRI may provide better clarity than other imaging techniques in detecting hemorrhage associated with IVD herniation. However, timing of MRI in relation to the onset of the lesion can confound interpretation of signal intensity since rapid changes can occur within areas of the hemorrhage in the early stages after injury.[23]

MRI has been used to predict prognosis in paraplegic dogs caused by IVD extrusion. Results of dogs undergoing MRI and surgery for IVDD suggest that an area of intramedullary spinal cord hyperintensity on sagittal T2-weighted MR images and at least the length of the L2 vertebral body have a poorer prognosis for functional recovery.[24] Success rate following surgery in dogs without hyperintensity of the spinal cord was 100% compared with 55% in those with areas of hyperintensity. Moreover, success rates reported for dogs with areas of hyperintensity and loss of pain perception was 31%, and the success rate in dogs with loss of pain perception and hyperintensity greater than three times the length of the L2 vertebral body was 10% (1/10 dogs).[24]

Levine et al[25] also found that intramedullary spinal cord hyperintensity on T2-weighted MR images was associated with the injury severity and also predictive of the recovery of the ability to walk long term.

Treatment. Many dogs with IVDD respond at least temporarily to attentive nursing care that promotes the spontaneous healing processes. Because of this finding, citing clear cut evidence of the superiority of one therapy over another is extremely difficult. The major treatment decision-making process centers on the benefit of surgery versus conservative medical management. In addition, the relative benefits of the various surgical procedures are still being debated. In comparing any treatment protocols, the severity and duration of the problem must be recognized as critical factors in recovery, regardless of treatment.[1] When those factors are constant, the literature is reasonably clear on appropriate treatment. Table 6-7 summarizes the indications for treatment and the forms of management currently recommended.

Special consideration for acute SCI is given to medical management and neuroprotection (see the Spinal Trauma section).

Conservative Therapy. Conservative therapy is indicated for animals that experience an initial episode of mild neurologic dysfunction (e.g., dogs that are ambulatory or have only mild GP ataxia) or pain alone, with owners who have financial constraints or for those that have other medical problems precluding general anesthesia and surgery. In general, management consists of pain control and strict confinement. Therapy should support the normal healing processes but not totally inhibit the beneficial inflammatory process induced by the extruded disk material. Analgesics and antiinflammatory drugs can be used but only if strict confinement is possible. Importantly, relief of pain may promote overactivity in affected dogs. Consequently, owners must be cautioned to remain vigilant in continuing to maintain strict exercise restriction despite clinical improvement. Overactivity may result in further IVD herniation and rapidly worsening clinical signs.

The most important aspect of conservative therapy is enforced cage rest, preferably under direct veterinary supervision. Animals should not be confined in baby cribs or playpens because to do so encourages the animal to jump in an attempt to get out. Confinement at home should be in a small pet crate placed in a quiet room where the animal will not be disturbed. The animal should be minimally exercised twice a day on a leash, away from other dogs or cats. Often strict cage confinement is recommended for a 4- to 6-week duration. If satisfactory progress is made, exercise is restricted to a leash for an additional 3 weeks. The most common mistake made by owners and veterinarians is to administer antiinflammatory drugs such as corticosteroids without exercise restriction. Predictably, these animals return in 36 to 48 hours with severe neurologic signs. Ideally, affected dogs should be hospitalized for observation for up to 1 week in facilities that have 24-hour monitoring.

Analgesics or other antiinflammatory drugs should be used at home only when the client agrees to cooperate fully with the instructions for strict cage rest. Prednisone, 0.25 to 0.5 mg/kg of body weight, is given every 12 hours for 72 hours and then the dosage is gradually tapered until discontinued. Nonsteroidal antiinflammatory drugs (NSAIDs) can then be administered as needed for pain management. However, NSAIDs and corticosteroids should not be concurrently administered because complications such as gastric ulceration and perforation occur frequently. If the medication is switched from corticosteroids to NSAIDs, a 72-hour "wash out" period is recommended. Furthermore, corticosteroids if continued longer than 5 to 7 days, can result in increased risk for gastrointestinal ulceration and urinary tract infection.[26] These dogs are already at risk for urinary tract infection with urine retention from a dysfunctional detrusor muscle. Gastrointestinal protection may be necessary during use of antiinflammatory drugs. Acupuncture and muscle relaxants also have been advocated as a treatment for pain management.

Dogs treated conservatively should be assessed twice daily for pain control, comfort, bladder emptying, evidence of decubital ulceration, and neurologic status. Cases with recurrent episodes of back pain uncontrolled by medication and/or worsening of neurologic status should undergo further diagnostics in an effort to obtain a definitive diagnosis and undergo decompressive surgery. Physical rehabilitation, weight control, and avoidance of jumping activities may reduce recurrence rates. If followed closely, these recommendations can result in considerable improvement; however, the owner must be aware that future episodes of clinical signs may occur and that the recurrence of deficits may be severe. If the animal's signs deteriorate at any time, decompressive surgery should be considered. Pain and its control are described in Chapter 14.

Success rates for conservative management of ambulatory dogs with thoracolumbar pain only and/or mild paresis range from 50% to 100%.[27-29] Predictably, recovery rates in nonambulatory dogs with intact pain perception are lower.[28,30]

TABLE 6-7

Outline of Recommendations for Management of Thoracolumbar Intervertebral Disk Disease*

Neurologic Classification	Initial Treatment Recommendations	Prognosis Medical Management	Prognosis Surgical Management
Paraplegia with no deep pain perception	<24-48 hr surgical decompression; >48 hr surgery not recommended	<12 hr >5%; >48 hr <5%	<12 hr 45%-76%; >48 hr 6%-33%
Paraplegia with deep pain perception and no superficial pain perception	Surgical decompression	50%	86%-89%
Paraplegia with intact pain perception	Surgical decompression	51%	79%-96%
Nonambulatory paraparesis	Surgical decompression	55%-85%	83%-95%
Ambulatory paraparesis	Conservative management	55%-85%	83%-95%
Spinal hyperesthesia only	Conservative management	55%-85%	83%-95%

*Modified from Frankel System (Frankel HL, et al: Paraplegia, 7:179–192, 1969; Levine M, et al: Am J Vet Res 67:283–287, 2006.)
The value of postural reaction in the initial management of closed injuries of the spine with paraplagia and tetraplasia.

Furthermore, recurrence rates are higher in studies following conservative treatment. Retrospective studies of dogs managed conservatively for presumptive thoracolumbar disk disease documented 30% to 50% recurrence rates in dogs with minimal clinical signs (e.g., maintained the ability to walk).[29,31] Dogs with thoracolumbar IVDD that were medically managed had recurrence within 6 months to 1 year from onset of the initial clinical signs.[31]

The absence of pain perception represents a severe, usually irreparable SCI. Paralyzed animals that have a loss of pain perception for 48 hours or longer have a grave prognosis (less than a 5% chance for recovering the ability to walk) with or without surgery.[14,28] Unless the owner definitely wants to try surgery in the face of these odds, the animal should be treated conservatively. Even with intensive therapy, the prognosis is grave.

Surgical Therapy. Indications for surgical management of thoracolumbar IVDD include spinal hyperesthesia or paresis refractory to conservative therapy, recurrence or progression of neurologic deficits, paraplegia with intact pain perception, and paraplegia with loss of pain perception for less than 24 to 48 hours. Ideally, dogs with acute paralysis and lack of pain perception should have immediate decompressive surgery. However, prolonged loss of pain perception (>48 hours) carries a poorer prognosis and owners should be made aware of this before surgery since surgery may not improve the recovery rate in such cases. Surgery can be performed in dogs with absence of pain perception for up to 48 hours; however, the rate and quality of recovery are much less predictable. As long as owners understand this, surgery should be performed with the hope that decompressive surgery may improve the potential for recovery in ambulatory status. If a paralyzed dog is to be referred for surgical decompression, principles of medical management of acute SCI are followed.

The various forms of surgical therapy have been reviewed extensively by Hoerlein and in other surgical textbooks.[1] The type of decompressive procedure may not affect outcome; however, the ability to retrieve the herniated disk material depends on the decompressive procedure. Decompressive procedures for thoracolumbar IVDD include dorsal laminectomy, hemilaminectomy, and pediculectomy. Hemilaminectomy significantly improves retrieval of extruded IVD material with minimal spinal cord manipulation (Figure 6-9). Hemilaminectomy provides the same degree of decompression as dorsal laminectomy and is less frequently associated with a postsurgical constrictive laminectomy membrane. Pediculectomy, in which the pedicle of the vertebra is removed with preservation of the articular processes, is the least invasive technique and can be used as an adjunct technique in cases of a bilateral approach to the vertebral canal. Radical bilateral dorsal laminectomy (removal of pedicles and dorsal laminae) has an increased risk of constrictive laminectomy membrane formation.[32] Studies have reported retrieval of disk material in 93% of dogs that had hemilaminectomy compared with 40% of dogs that had dorsal laminectomy, but initial neurologic recovery after hemilaminectomy was not significantly different compared with dorsal laminectomy.[33] Biomechanical studies have shown that unilateral hemilaminectomy and fenestration do not significantly destabilize a vertebral column with regards to the application of lateral bending forces.[34] Surgical complications include seroma formation, excessive hemorrhage, incomplete removal of IVD material, constrictive fibrosis, and rarely instability.

If the patient has loss of pain perception before surgery, a *durotomy* may be considered to allow visualization of the spinal cord. A longitudinal incision in the meninges allows for visualization of the spinal cord parenchyma to determine extent of swelling and presence of myelomalacia. Presence of diffuse myelomalacia indicates a grave prognosis. The owners should be informed of the care involved with a dog in a cart and warned of ascending/descending myelomalacia. Ideally, this discussion should be had with the owners before surgical intervention given the prognosis for regaining the ability to walk in dogs without pain perception. Moreover, absence of visual evidence of myelomalacia does not guarantee functional recovery; conversely, functional recovery may still occur in the presence of focal myelomalacia. A study reported that durotomy is ineffective as a therapy in improving the prognosis for dogs without pain perception that underwent decompressive surgery caused by IVD extrusion.[35]

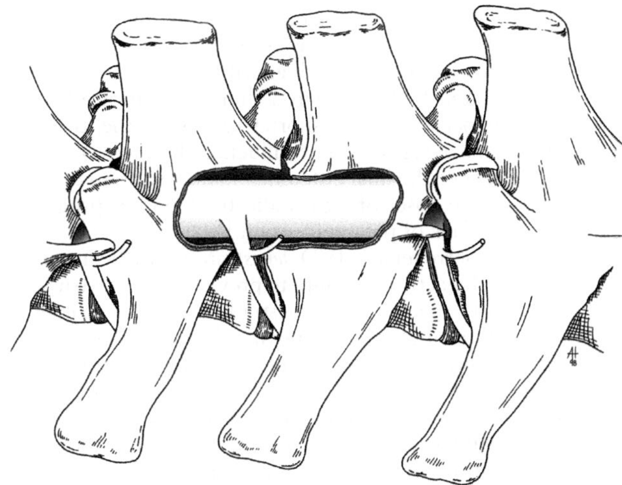

Figure 6-9 A depiction of a hemilaminectomy at L1-2. Note the removal of the articular processes, pedicles, lamina of L1 and L2. (From Coates JR, Hoffman A, Dewey CW: Surgical approaches to the spine. In Slatter D, editor: Textbook of small animal surgery, ed 3, Philadelphia, 2003, WB Saunders.)

In dogs that are nonambulatory paraparetic or paraplegic, decompressive surgery should be performed immediately. This recommendation is supported by several clinical and experimental studies that compared the time of onset (acute vs. chronic) and duration of spinal cord compression with the rate of recovery. Experimental studies by Tarlov et al is demonstrated that acute spinal cord compression with a force sufficient to produce complete sensorimotor paralysis can completely recover from the injury if the compression is less than 2 hours in duration.[36,37] Furthermore, the rate of recovery in Tarlov's study correlated directly with the duration of compression. Gradual compression of the spinal cord was better tolerated, and irreversible changes developed at a slower rate in these animals. Thus early decompressive surgery may have a positive influence on both the quality of restored function and the rate of recovery. Knecht also compared the outcome of dogs after hemilaminectomy and duration of clinical signs and showed that a delay before surgery does not influence outcome in dogs with mild neurologic dysfunction but does affect better functional recovery in paraplegic dogs when performed within 12 hours.[38] When indicated, spinal cord decompression should be performed without delay. Dogs treated conservatively with moderate to severe paresis or paraplegia for 24 to 48 hours and then performing surgery if no improvement occurs is not recommended. Doing so discounts the experimental data regarding the effects of spinal compression over variable periods and the clinical experience of many veterinary surgeons.[1]

Other clinically based studies in dogs with thoracolumbar disk extrusions have shown that those with a shorter duration and the gradual onset of neurologic dysfunction (less than 48 hours) before surgery have a faster recovery.[15,39,40] However, a study of 71 paraplegic dogs with intact pain perception demonstrated that although a shorter duration of signs was indeed associated with a shorter recovery time, the rate of onset of clinical signs did not influence the recovery time, but it did influence the final outcome.[41] This relates to the fact that the peracute onset of signs indicates a poorer prognosis for dogs with a lack of pain perception.[15]

Although controversial, IVD *fenestration* has been advocated as a prophylactic procedure to prevent future extrusions at adjacent IVD spaces. Disk fenestration involves making a "window" in the annulus and removing the accessible nucleus pulposus. This procedure often is performed at the site of the IVD herniation at the time of spinal decompression and is recommended to prevent continued extrusion of remaining in situ nucleus pulposus. Prophylactic fenestration of other IVD spaces at the time of decompression typically is performed from T11-12 to L3-4.

General agreement exists that IVD fenestration alone may benefit some animals by preventing further extrusion at other IVD spaces. Fenestration may also produce an acute inflammatory process that stimulates phagocytosis (the resorption of necrotic disk material) and the formation of fibrosis, which helps to stabilize the disk.[42] Percutaneous laser disk ablation has been successfully used as a replacement for surgical disk fenestration.[43] It is indicated for dogs that have multiple episodes of pain and no evidence of spinal cord compression. Using fluoroscopy, hypodermic needles are placed in the nucleus pulposus and a holmium-yttrium-aluminum-garnet laser is guided through the needle into the IVD. Bartels and colleagues[44] reported on the outcome and complications associated with prophylactic percutaneous laser disk ablation in dogs. Of 277 dogs treated, only 5 developed complications in the perioperative period. These researchers contacted 262 owners 1 to 85 months after the procedure; 76% of these owners indicated that their dogs were immediately improved, 22% indicated their dogs were the same, 2% indicated their dogs were worse, and 81% reported their dogs had not had any recurrence of thoracolumbar IVDD.

Published studies suggest recurrence rates of IVD herniation following surgery to range from 0%[45] to 24%[46] with prophylactic fenestration and from 2.7%[39] to 42%[47] without prophylactic fenestration. Dogs undergoing prophylactic fenestration tend to have lower recurrence rates. Brisson et al determined a 4.7% recurrence rate after multiple IVD fenestrations in 265 dogs but commented that prophylactic fenestration could promote IVD herniation at an adjacent nonfenestrated IVD.[48]

Prognosis. Prognosis in dogs with thoracolumbar IVDD after surgical decompression is summarized in Table 6-7. Overall success rates after decompressive surgery for thoracolumbar IVDD range from 58.8%[39] to 95%.[49] Specifically, prognosis is better than 95% in dogs that are ambulatory.[11,39,49,50] In dogs that are paraplegic with intact pain perception, the prognosis ranges from 79% to 96%.[40,41,47-51]

However, the success of decompressive surgery may depend on what criteria are used to define it, length of time after the surgery the patient is assessed, and the outcome that the pet owners are willing to accept. Surgical success may consist of improvement in the patient's neurologic status but still may not recover to complete normality. It has been reported that in dogs with loss of pain perception, approximately 40% of dogs that recovered continued to have fecal incontinence.[14] Residual signs such as fecal and urinary incontinence may not be acceptable to some pet owners.

As stated above, the rate of return to ambulation and for functional micturition is highly correlated with the duration and rate of the spinal cord compression. Reported mean time from postsurgery to ambulatory status varied from 10 days for dogs experiencing pain alone as a clinical sign or showing paraparesis to 52 days for paraplegic dogs.[39] Other long-term studies reported recovery times of 2 to 14 days for dogs that were either ambulatory or nonambulatory paraparetic and up to 4 weeks for dogs that were paraplegic.[52,53] Ruddle et al reported that 42% of dogs were ambulatory by 2 weeks and 79% were ambulatory by 4 weeks following decompression in 218 nonambulatory dogs with intact pain perception.[51] Patient age and weight also may impact the time required for ability to ambulate.[14] Generally in a paraplegic dog, if pain perception remains intact or returns shortly after surgery, good voluntary motor activity should return within 4 to 5 weeks, and the unassisted ability to support weight usually is restored within 6 to 8 weeks. Proprioception is the last function to return. Early decompression hastens the return of neurologic function. The quality of recovery depends on the severity of secondary injury to the spinal cord. Animals decompressed in the first 24 hours may be walking in the next 24 hours.

Pain perception (nociception) is considered the most important prognostic indicator for functional recovery. In general, the majority of dogs with intact pain perception, have an excellent prognosis, particularly if treated surgically. In general, dogs with loss of pain perception for longer than 24 to 48 hours before surgery have a poorer prognosis for return of function. Recovery rates for dogs with thoracolumbar IVDD and absent pain perception range from 0% to 76%.[54] Specifically, the prognosis ranges from 47% to 76% in dogs that lack pain perception and have surgical decompression within 12 to 24 hours.[14,15,35,39,51,54] If decompressive surgery is delayed by longer than 48 hours after losing pain perception, the prognosis diminishes to less than 5%.[14,15,35]

Recovery of pain perception within 2 weeks after surgery has been associated with a successful outcome to ambulatory status. In a study of 87 dogs with loss of pain perception, 58% regained pain perception and the ability to walk.[14] In summary, dogs with absent pain perception that have surgery within 24 hours have a better chance of more rapid and complete recovery than those with delay of surgery. Prognosis is considered poor if pain perception does not return within 4 weeks after surgery.

Supportive Care of the Paraplegic. Supportive care of the nonambulatory dog is directed at preventing the development of decubital ulcers, urinary tract infection, and muscle atrophy. Dogs that undergo physical rehabilitation may have shorter recovery times for return of ambulation.[51] Physical rehabilitation is briefly described in Chapter 14.

Dogs with thoracolumbar IVDD that are unable to ambulate often will have concomitant upper motor neuron urinary bladder dysfunction. These dogs will require manual bladder expression, or intermittent or indwelling urinary bladder catheterization. Incomplete bladder evacuation and use of urinary catheters may predispose dogs to urinary tract infection (UTI).[26] A prospective study in dogs with thoracolumbar IVDD determined that the prevalence of UTIs was 30% with higher incidence in dogs that were female and had lower intraoperative body temperatures.[26] Bladder care is further described in Chapter 3.

Inflammatory

Inflammatory infectious diseases can cause myelitis and meningitis or result in infection of the vertebral body and in the spinal canal. Inflammatory diseases often will cause multifocal signs (see Chapter 15). In this section, we will emphasize diseases that primarily manifest as paraparesis.

Equine Herpesvirus 1 Myeloencephalopathy/Pathogenesis. Equine herpesvirus (EHV) myeloencephalopathy is an acute progressive neurologic disease that usually affects adult horses and, less frequently, foals.[55-57] The neuropathic strain of EHV-1 can produce myeloencephalopathy and rarely, EHV-4. The virus is laterally transmitted by direct contact through inhalation and less frequently by direct contact with fetal and placental tissues. The EHV-1 infection occurs within groups of horses, usually in the winter and spring and most commonly causes respiratory disease, abortion, and stillbirths. Latency and reactivation are critical features of the epidemiology of EHV-1 infection.[57] Immunity to the virus is poor, so the virus usually persists in latent form and can recrudesce as myeloencephalopathy.[58] The virus infects the mononuclear cells, which disseminate the virus into other tissues including the central nervous system (CNS), rather than by direct infection of the neural tissues. Through cell-associated contact, the virus enters the CNS via the endothelial cells. Lesions are multifocal caused by vasculitis following infection of endothelial cells in the CNS with severe vasculitis followed by thrombosis/infarction and ischemia.[56] Histopathologic examination reveals diffuse to multifocal lymphocytic perivascular cuffing, edema, infarction, and necrosis throughout the spinal cord white matter and brain, but clinical signs usually reflect the spinal cord lesions.

Clinical Signs. Usually EHV-1 myeloencephalopathy occurs within 1 to 2 weeks after outbreaks of upper respiratory tract infections or abortions. Pregnant mares may be more susceptible to the development of severe spinal cord lesions and may abort if infected in the last trimester of pregnancy. Fever is an important physical examination finding. Neurologic signs develop acutely. In most cases, the clinical signs are those of thoracolumbar spinal cord dysfunction. The classic neurologic signs are those of a symmetric paresis with the pelvic limbs more severely affected than the thoracic limbs.[59] Common signs include pelvic limb ataxia, dysuria, flaccid anus and tail, and loss of sensation around the perineal area. A dog-sitting posture is not unusual. Tetraparesis may be severe if cervical spinal cord lesions are extensive. Disease progression is variable, depending on the severity of the initial spinal cord lesions. Affected horses may recover in 24 to 48 hours, or they may progress rapidly to severe tetraplegia or paraplegia. In a few cases, seizures occur with involvement of the cerebral cortex or cranial nerve dysfunction and vestibular signs with involvement of the brainstem. Both UMN and LMN signs may be noted relative to the site of vascular lesions in the spinal cord.

Diagnosis. Definitive antemortem diagnosis is difficult. Whenever neurologic disease appears to follow outbreaks of respiratory tract infection or abortion, EHV-1 myeloencephalopathy, a sporadic disease of horses, must be suspected. Analysis of the cerebrospinal fluid (CSF) reveals xanthochromia and significant elevations in protein levels (150 mg/dL or greater) with normal or slightly elevated cell counts. Virus culture and isolation is considered the gold standard test for making a laboratory diagnosis of EHV-1.[57] Presumptive diagnosis is based on serologic test interpretations in conjunction with the presenting clinical signs. Polymerase chain reaction (PCR) has become the diagnostic test of choice because of its high sensitivity and specificity.[57] Presence of the virus can be detected using PCR for the neuropathic strain in the nasal mucosa and blood, virus isolation, and seroconversion studies. Rising serum antibody titers may be observed in horses with neurologic disease; however, a sharp rise in antibody titers occurs during the respiratory phase of the disease some 1 to 3 weeks before the onset of neurologic signs, which complicates interpretation of serology.[60] Techniques using PCR may help to differentiate pathogenicity of strains and EHV-1 deoxyribonucleic acid (DNA) in tissues.[61] The definitive diagnosis coupled with presence of vasculitis is made by isolation of the virus from nervous tissue.

Treatment. No definitive treatment for this disease exists. Because an immune mechanism may be responsible for progression of clinical signs, some have suggested the use of anti-inflammatory drugs in the acute phase.[57] Administration of antiviral drugs may be effective early in the disease course. Many animals recover if given supportive nursing care, including catheterization of the urinary bladder and use of a sling in recumbent horses. Priorities for management include early diagnosis, prevention of further spread, and management of clinical cases.[62] As the disease is laterally transmitted, management practices for containing an outbreak should include closing down the hospital, disinfection procedures, and isolation of affected horses. An affected horse should remain in isolation for 21 days after resolution of clinical signs.[63] There is no evidence that current vaccines can prevent naturally occurring cases of EHV myeloencephalomyelitis.[57] A killed intramuscular (IM) vaccine is available that probably provides immunity to the respiratory disease but not to infection of the placenta or CNS. Therefore vaccinated animals may still have abortions or neurologic disease. Environmental stressors associated with transport, management practices, breeding, foaling, weaning, and castration can result in reactivation of the latent virus.[58]

Equine Protozoal Myeloencephalitis

Pathogenesis. Equine protozoal myeloencephalitis (EPM) is the most common neurologic disease in horses with multifocal or asymmetric neurologic deficits.[56,64] The disease is commonly characterized by either *sudden* or *gradual* onset of pelvic limb paresis and ataxia. Because lesions may be multifocal in the spinal cord or brain, neurologic signs may indicate involvement of any part of the CNS. EPM is most commonly caused by the apicomplexan, resembling *Sarcocystis neurona.*[65] A small number of EPM cases have been attributed to infection by *Neospora hughesi*. The opossum is the definitive host for *S. neurona* and harbors the sexual stages of the protozoa within its gastrointestinal tract.[66,67] Infective sporocysts are shed in the feces. After ingestion of the sporocysts by a natural intermediate host, the released merozoites travel in the bloodstream to skeletal or cardiac muscle tissue to undergo several cycles of asexual reproduction and re-form as sarcocysts. Natural intermediate hosts for *S. neurona* that have been identified include the skunk, raccoon, cat, Pacific harbor seal, and nine-banded armadillo. The horse is an aberrant dead-end host (the parasite cannot complete its life cycle in horses). The life cycle is completed when opossums eat sarcocyst-infected tissue from an intermediate host. Horses are infected after they ingest sporocysts shed in opossum feces. Following ingestion by horses, sporozoites emerge by exiting from sporocysts in the small intestine and enter the circulation. Sporozoites may replicate in endothelial cells and release tachyzoites. Tachyzoites may enter the CNS and provoke an inflammatory response. Moreover, tachyzoites are able to replicate (asexually) in neurons and microglial cells. Slowly growing *S. neurona* tachyzoites cause progressive loss of neurons and supporting cells, and along with resulting inflammation causes signs of neurologic dysfunction that refer to a specific neuroanatomic location. The organism invades and multiplies in the CNS rather than encysting in muscle.

Early reports suggested that the disease was most common in the eastern United States, but it has been reported in many other locations and may occur anywhere in North America with geographic distribution of the opossum.[68-70] There is a bimodal age distribution of 1 to 5 years and older than 13 years, which is associated with other risk factors: exposure to opossums, heavy exercise, breeding, transportation, and herd environment.[56,71] All breeds are susceptible to EPM. A higher frequency of EPM has been seen in the light breeds that race, show, and compete and also in farm and pleasure horses. Older horses are also at risk for EPM because they develop age-associated immunocompromise. It also appears that specific immunologic abnormalities may predispose to EPM, allowing the parasite to evade the host's immune response and gain entry into the CNS. Although a majority of horses in a geographic location that is endemic for *S. neurona* are infected by the protozoan, neurologic disease only develops in a minority (<1%) of infected horses.

Lesions within the CNS are focal or multifocal and usually are asymmetric. The lesion severity of myeloencephalomeningitis associated with EPM will vary. The histopathologic lesion is a nonsuppurative inflammation with a perivascular distribution affecting both gray and white matter. Organisms are seen in only half the cases. The identification of *S. neurona* at histopathology is significantly facilitated using immunohistochemical techniques.

Clinical Signs. No typical presentation or characteristic set of neurologic signs have been established for EPM, and symmetric neurologic disease does not preclude its diagnosis.[72] Frequently, the clinical manifestation of EPM begins with signs of subtle lameness that are difficult to localize using routine diagnostic tests (such as nerve anesthesia and radiography). Gradually, over the course of several weeks, the clinical signs become more prominent and a neurologic component becomes more readily apparent. Clinical signs may develop suddenly and progress slowly over days to weeks. Rapid progression sometimes also occurs. Asymmetric GP ataxia and paresis of the pelvic limbs are the most common manifestations. Because lesions may be multifocal, however, a mixture of UMN and LMN signs may be present in the pelvic and thoracic limbs, and brainstem signs may also be present. Lesions may be selective to involve only one nucleus or tract in the CNS. If the lesion occurs in the cervical spinal intumescence, the thoracic limb signs may be worse than the pelvic limb signs. These animals move with the thoracic limbs extended forward and the head held low. Asymmetry of clinical signs is a hallmark of the disease. The clinical signs may resemble those observed in the equine wobbler syndrome and EHV-1 myeloencephalitis; however, the asymmetry that is seen helps in the clinical differentiation of protozoal myelitis-encephalitis from the other two diseases. Three cardinal neurologic manifestations that are highly implicative for EPM include asymmetric signs; multifocal signs; and evidence of LMN lesion (focal muscle atrophy) (Figure 6-10).[73]

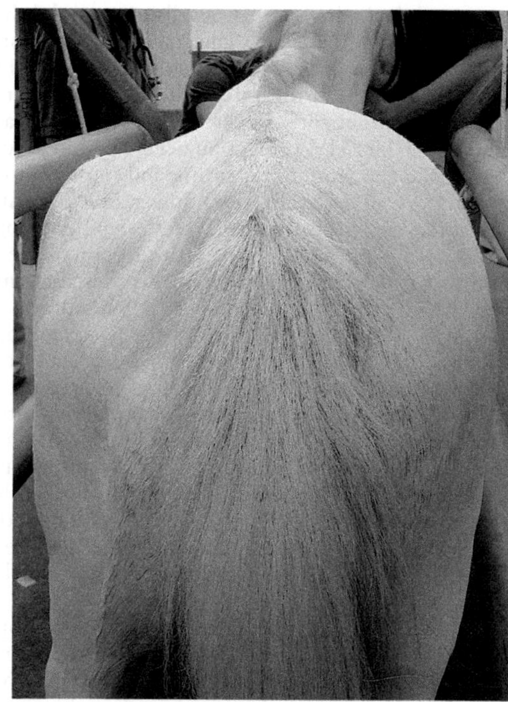

Figure 6-10 A photo of a horse presumptively diagnosed with equine protozoal myelitis. Note the severe atrophy of the left gluteal musculature. (Copyright 2010 University of Georgia Research Foundation, Inc.)

Diagnosis. Clinical diagnosis of EPM is a challenge and requires careful interpretation of clinicopathologic findings.[56,64] Diagnostic imaging procedures assist in ruling out other diseases (such as cervical vertebral trauma or cervical stenotic myelopathy) from the differential diagnosis. In EPM, unlike EHV-1 encephalomyelitis, few CSF abnormalities occur. Mildly increased concentrations of mononuclear cells and protein occasionally are found. Cervical spinal radiographs are normal, differentiating this disease from cervical stenotic myelopathy. Electromyography (EMG) can help to identify multifocal LMN damage, which is more common in this disease than in the others with similar clinical signs.

Postmortem evaluation is the gold standard for diagnosis of EPM. A presumptive diagnosis of EPM is supported by demonstrating antibodies against *S. neurona* in blood and/or in CSF. It should be emphasized that interpretation of these serodiagnostic tests in both blood and CSF are complicated by both false positive and false negative results. In those geographic locations in which *S. neurona* is endemic, positive antibody titers can be demonstrated in a majority of healthy horses, in the absence of neurologic signs. These positive antibody test results are attributed to the widespread extent to which horses are exposed to *S. neurona* in their natural environment: both the plasma and the CSF may contain antibodies in the absence of EPM. Therefore, caution must be exercised when interpreting results of serodiagnostic tests for *S. neurona* antibodies in equine patients. As a general rule, a positive *S. neurona* antibodies test result performed on CSF is regarded as being more likely implicative for an EPM diagnosis (in horses that are exhibiting neurologic signs) when compared with test results on plasma. However, it should be noted that antigen-specific antibody can be detected in the CSF of normal horses in which antigen has not been administered intrathecally.[74] Finally, serum and CSF from normal foals born to seropositive mares will test positive for EPM for up to days after birth.[75] Blood contamination often will confuse the interpretation of presence of antibody in the CSF.

There are presently four commercially available serodiagnostic tests for *S. neurona* antibodies (and some labs offer similar tests for *N. hughesi*): immunofluorescent antibody test (IFAT); enzyme-linked immunoabsorbent assay (ELISA) test; and the western immunoblot (WB). Currently, the generally recommended serodiagnostic test to support a diagnosis of EPM is the IFAT performed on either serum or CSF.[76] Results suggest that a sufficiently high titer is very strongly correlated with and predictive for a diagnosis of EPM. Another test evaluates for antibodies directed specifically against the SAG-1 epitope of *S. neurona*.[77] Testing for antibodies against SAG-1 may yield false-negative results because it has been shown that some strains of the parasite lack this epitope. Although analysis of serum or CSF using Western blot technology for the presence of antibody to *S. neurona* used to be the recommended method for determining a presumptive diagnosis, controversy exists regarding its specificity.[64,78] Its low specificity indicates that false-positive test results are likely[78]; however, its high sensitivity indicates that a negative test result is useful in ruling out EPM. Identification of *S. neurona* DNA in CSF via PCR is available, but the clinical sensitivity of this test is poor (usually fails to identify the protozoan in the CSF). PCR testing for *S. neurona* in the CSF is not currently recommended but it may be helpful for diagnosis of EPM based on tissue analysis postmortem.[64] Diagnosis of EPM is also supported by a positive response following institution of antiprotozoal treatment.[56,64] In many cases, it is not possible to make a definitive diagnosis of EPM while the patient is living, and a presumptive diagnosis is given with knowledge of the diagnostic testing results. Diagnosis of EPM can only be proven with demonstrable lesions in the CNS at necropsy. Making a necropsy diagnosis is also challenging because the size of the examined tissues is substantial in this large animal species.

Treatment. Treatment of EPM usually includes four strategies: antiprotozoal drugs; antiinflammatory drugs; immunomodulation; and minimization of stress factors that might have facilitated protozoal infection of the CNS.[56,64] Three antiprotozoal drug strategies have been developed, approved for use in EPM-affected horses, and marketed. The three approved drug products are pyrimethamine/sulfadiazine combination, nitazoxanide, and ponazuril. Presently, only the ponazuril product is commercially available to veterinarians. Diclazuril has also been developed and approved for use in EPM-affected horses, but has not been marketed. Where applicable, the pyrimethamine/sulfadiazine combination and nitazoxanide may be available from compounding pharmacies. Nonsteroidal antiinflammatory drugs are sometimes administered to EPM-affected horses for a few days to minimize debilitating inflammatory reactions to protozoal death that are sometimes reported at the outset of an antiprotozoal treatment period. Immunomodulators, such as levamisole, are sometimes advocated for purposes of "stimulating" the host's immune responsiveness to *S. neurona*. There was a vaccine produced for prevention of *S. neurona* infection but it is no longer available. Preventive management practices include removal of dead animals, carrion, and spilled foods around the premises, which attract opossums.

West Nile Virus

Pathogenesis. West Nile virus (WNV) is an ribonucleic acid (RNA) virus of the *Flavivirus* genus within the family Flaviviridae. WNV occurs worldwide and an outbreak of WNV occurred in the late 1990s in the northeastern United States with reports of infection in birds, horses, and people.[79-81] The persistent environment reservoir for this virus is in avian species that are not killed by infection. When active, mosquitoes serve as a vector to transmit the virus from the reservoir avian species to susceptible mammalian species (e.g., humans, horses, and others). Horses, humans, and other species are considered to be dead-end hosts. Dogs and ruminant species are less susceptible to infection.[80]

Clinical Signs. The disease can cause severe neurologic signs and mortality in horses but most infections are subclinical and go unrecognized. Horses that develop neurologic signs show multifocal signs that may predominate as spinal cord or brain dysfunction.[81,82] Signs of spinal cord dysfunction usually are asymmetric motor and proprioceptive deficits. Intracranial signs consist of cranial nerve deficits, seizures, and abnormal mentation. Other clinical signs include pyrexia and muscle fasciculation. Horses may be found acutely recumbent or dead.

Diagnosis. Diagnosis is based on clinical signs and time of year, CSF analysis, and ruling out other differentials. Exposure can be detected by use of serum neutralization assay using early and convalescent serum samples. CSF analysis reveals a marked increase in protein concentration and an increase in mononuclear cells.[83] CSF abnormalities are found in about 70% of affected horses. Encephalomyelitis is evident on histopathology and more definitive diagnosis is made with virus isolation. A presumptive diagnosis is mainly based on serum IgM ELISA and whole blood RT-PCR.[84,85]

Treatment. Treatment of animals with suspected WNV infection is supportive.[81] Empirical antiinflammatory therapies are used to lessen the CNS inflammation but treatment efficacy for specific therapies is unproven. Nursing care should include proper bedding and nutrition. Preventive management practices include vaccination in horses and mosquito control.

Verminous Migration

Clinical Signs. Onset of parasitic invasion into the neural tissue is acute and progressive with waxing and waning periods of improvement.[56] Neurologic signs are usually asymmetric and may show focal or multifocal distributions and reflect the area affected. The pathologies from migration include inflammatory, necrotic, and hemorrhagic processes.

Equine. The migration of several parasites through the spinal cord of horses has been described.[56,86] The most important of these organisms includes *Halicephalobus deletrix*, *Strongylus vulgaris*, *Draschia megastoma*, and *Hypoderma lineatum*. *S. vulgaris Paralaphostrongylus tenius* is the most common organism to cause verminous myelitis in the horse and the one most likely to affect the spinal cord.[86] Larvae of *Hypoderma*. spp. (warble fly or heel fly) can also cause verminous meningoencephalitis, but it usually affects the brain and not the spinal cord with asymmetric brainstem disease as the most common clinical manifestation. Both *Draschia* spp. and *Hypoderma* spp. tend to infect the brain. The clinical signs depend on the location of the parasite and may be asymmetric, focal, or multifocal. Embolization of *S. vulgaris* larvae into spinal or cerebral arteries may produce severe acute progressive or nonprogressive clinical signs.

Bovine. The larvae of *Hypoderma bovis* migrate through the epidural space of cattle.[87] Infestation usually occurs during the months of July through October. If the larvae die or are killed while in the epidural space, a severe immunologic reaction occurs, resulting in SCI. The clinical signs usually appear in cattle treated with organophosphate insecticides during the period of epidural larva migration. Clinical signs develop acutely hours to days after treatment and usually are caused by thoracolumbar spinal cord injury. Prominent signs include GP ataxia and paresis of pelvic limbs. If the lumbosacral cord is involved, LMN signs may be detected in the pelvic limbs. The signs are usually asymmetric.

The diagnosis is based on the history and the clinical signs.[87] The CSF changes reflect signs of degeneration (moderate increases in protein and cell concentrations). Eosinophils may not be present in the CSF. Affected animals should be treated with antiinflammatory drugs approved for use in food producing animals to reduce the secondary inflammatory reaction. If signs develop several days to weeks after organophosphate application, the possibility of organophosphate intoxication should be considered.

Ovine, Caprine, Camelids. Cerebrospinal nematodiasis caused by the migrating larvae of *Parelaphostrongylus tenuis* has been reported in sheep, goats, camelids, and other domestic livestock.[87] Cattle appear resistant to infection but llamas seem to be the most sensitive to development of disease. The disease is endemic in North America where white-tailed deer are common. In its natural life cycle, the adult parasite resides in the subarachnoid space of the white-tailed deer. The eggs are removed from the CNS through the venous circulation and enter the lungs. They are coughed up, swallowed, and passed in the feces. The larvae are ingested by snails or slugs and develop into third-stage larva. When the snail or slug is ingested by the aberrant hosts, the larvae are released from the digestive tract and migrate into the CNS. In species other than the white-tailed deer, the parasite enters the spinal cord and migrates. The aberrant hosts are not equally susceptible to disease produced by *P. tenuis*.[87]

Migration of this parasite through the CNS produces a variety of clinical signs that include pelvic limb paresis and ataxia. The clinical course is variable and may include progression, stasis, or improvement in clinical signs. Affected animals have a history of grazing in pastures that have been exposed to white-tailed deer. Antemortem diagnosis is based on clinical signs and CSF analysis. The CSF of these animals usually contains increased concentrations of protein and cells. A mononuclear and eosinophilic pleocytosis is usually encountered. Successful treatment of clinical CNS parelaphostrongylosis requires early diagnosis and institution of treatment.[87] Treatment with diethylcarbamazine, ivermectin, levamisole, or thiabendazole is recommended. The prognosis is guarded. Minimizing contact with white-tailed deer decreases the larval load on the premises. It has been recommended to administer an avermectin dewormer to camelids on a monthly basis after the last hard frost.[87]

Porcine. The kidney worm of swine, *Stephanurus dentatus*, may migrate through the lumbar spinal cord, producing pelvic limb paresis and GP ataxia. This organism must be considered in individual swine that develop acute paraparesis, particularly swine residing on farms in the southeastern United States.

Diagnosis. Confirmation of parasitic encephalomyelitis is difficult to make. The CSF may contain increased concentrations of eosinophils, neutrophils, macrophages, and red blood cells.[56] It may be mildly to moderately xanthochromic. Definitive diagnosis of parasitic encephalomyelitis is made by demonstrating the parasitic organism and characteristic lesions at necropsy.

Treatment. In suspected cases of verminous migration, broad spectrum anthelmintics have been recommended. Empiric therapies with antiinflammatory drugs can be used to decrease the inflammatory response to the dying worms and larvae. Recoveries are possible if animals are treated early in the disease course. Many animals will have permanent disability. Recumbency indicates a poorer prognosis. Prophylactic therapy is warranted for some parasites.

Ovine and Caprine Lentiviral Encephalomyelitis [Maedi-visna and Ovine Progressive Pneumonia (MVV/OPPV) and Caprine Arthritis-Encephalitis Virus (CAE)]

Pathogenesis. Lentiviral infections in sheep and goats share many clinical similarities and are characterized by insidious onset and slow progression.[88] Ovine and caprine lentiviruses belong to the family Retroviridae. These infections occur worldwide. The terms *maedi* (shortness of breath) and *visna* (shrinkage or wasting) arise from the original Icelandic descriptions of MVV/OPPV caused by lentiviral infection in sheep. The lentiviral infection in goats causes the disease syndrome of CAE, which manifests as respiratory disease, mastitis, arthritis, and encephalomyelitis. Respiratory signs are more common in adult sheep, whereas arthritis in adult goats is more common with CAE virus. The primary mode of transmission is through infected milk and colostrum consumed by neonates.[89,90]

Clinical Signs. Only a few infected animals will manifest clinical disease. In sheep with MVV/OPPV, neurologic signs of leukoencephalomyelitis rarely occurs and is characterized by an ascending paralysis.[90] In contrast to sheep, neurologic signs more commonly occur in the younger goat.[89] More than one kid is affected in most cases. Caprine leukoencephalomyelitis is characterized by symmetric or asymmetric paraparesis and GP ataxia. Cranial nerve signs may be observed. Neurologic signs in both species reflect multifocal disease, including involvement of the brain. Histopathology in both ovine/caprine lentiviral encephalomyelitis includes a periventricular encephalitis and widespread demyelination. As in other viral diseases, lesions may develop anywhere in the spinal cord, producing focal or multifocal asymmetric neurologic signs. Weight loss, arthritis, pneumonitis, and palpation of a firm udder may be present in one or more animals.

Diagnosis. The CSF usually contains markedly increased concentrations of mononuclear cells and modestly increased concentrations of protein. Electromyography may indicate evidence of LMN dysfunction. Serologic tests (ELISA and agar gel immunodiffusion) can be helpful if positive but does not confirm the virus. Many affected animals, however, have negative results. Combination of ELISA and PCR testing is now thought to be more useful for detection of lentivirus infections.[91]

Treatment. The neurologic syndrome is progressive and signs are permanent. There is no treatment. Prevention is directed toward identifying infected animals and minimizing transmission between infected dams and offspring and minimizing direct contact with infected animals.[88] Thus withholding calostrom is effective prevention. Serologic testing and cull programs can decrease prevalence within a flock or herd.

Discospondylitis and Vertebral Abscess. Several terms are used to describe vertebral infections.[92] Discospondylitis is an infection of the IVD and the adjacent vertebral bodies. Infection confined to the vertebra is called vertebral osteomyelitis or spondylitis. Infection when confined only within the IVD is called infectious diskitis. Vertebral physitis is inflammation confined to the physeal zones of the end plate.[93] All regions of the spine are prone to develop infections of the IVD or vertebrae.

Pathogenesis. Discospondylitis is an IVD infection with concurrent osteomyelitis of contiguous vertebrae.[92,94-96] Direct infection can occur from spinal surgery, penetrating wound, regional abscessation or migration of foreign material (e.g., plant awn).[94,96-98] In cats, bite wound abscesses can induce discospondylitis by direct inoculation of bacterial organisms.[99] In dogs, the most common bacterial causes are *Staphylococcus pseudintermedius* and, occasionally, *Streptococcus* spp., gram negatives, and *Brucella canis*.[92,95] Because of its zoonotic importance, *B. canis* is an important infectious agent to always consider in discospondylitis.[100-102] *Actinomyces* spp., a filamentous bacteria, often occurs with grass awn migration.[98] Some spinal infections in dogs are caused by fungal organisms, including *Aspergillus* spp., *Paecilomyces* spp., and *Coccidioides immitis*.[92] The most common route of infection is hematogenous spread of organisms from the genitourinary system, oral cavity, heart valves, or skin. Infection of the IVD and the vertebrae usually occurs secondary to infection of one of these primary foci. Discospondylitis in dogs often is associated with a urinary tract infection and bacteremia. With the exception of directly penetrating wounds and foreign object migration, discospondylitis infections usually start in the end plate of a vertebra, with subsequent spread into the IVD. The blood supply within the vertebral end plates consists of capillary beds, with reduced blood flow velocity.[103,104] The pores in the end plate allow for diffusion of nutrients into the IVD but also provides a route for organisms to enter the IVD. The minimal vascular supply of the IVD further perpetuates infection within the disk. The infection may involve cervical or thoracolumbar vertebrae; however, it most frequently develops in the lumbosacral, thoracolumbar, cervicothoracic, and midthoracic IVD spaces (Figure 6-11).[95,96] The most common site for discospondylitis in dogs is L7-S1 IVD space.[95,105] Lesions often are multifocal.

Vertebral abscesses are formed primarily in young or debilitated large animals.[56] An association is often present with omphalophlebitis (navel ill) in calves and foals, tail docking in lambs, erysipelas arthritis in swine, pneumonia in cattle, and enteric *Salmonella* spp. infections in horses.[106-108] The bacteria-producing vertebral abscesses in foals include *Salmonella* spp., *Streptococcus* spp., *Actinobacillus equuli*, *Eikenella corrodens*, and *Rhodococcus equi*.[56] In adult horses, *Staphylococcus* spp., *Brucella abortus*, and *Mycobacterium tuberculosis* are reported.[56] In cattle, *Bacteroides* spp. *Pasturella* spp., *Salmonella* spp., *Arcanobacterium pyogenes*, *Fusobacterium* spp., and

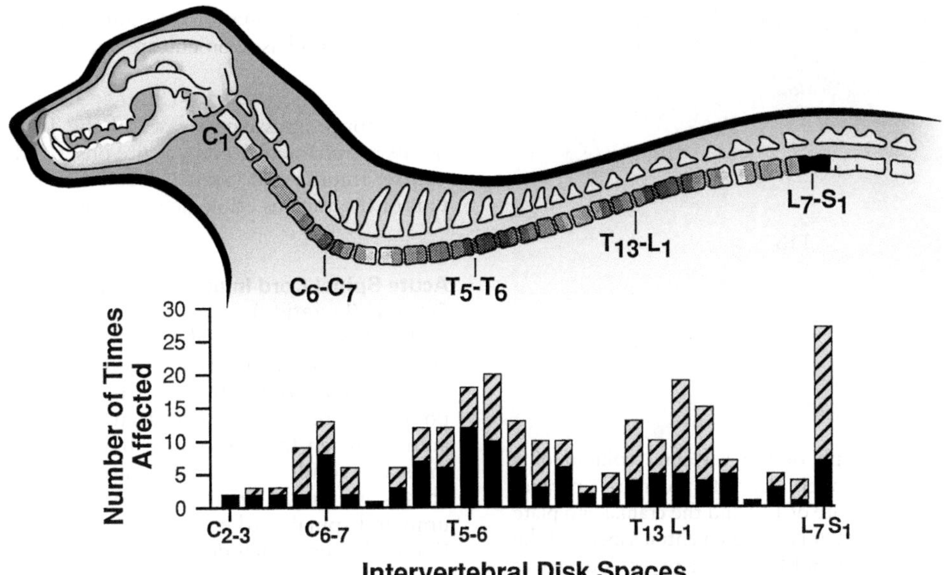

Figure 6-11 Histogram and schematic of frequency of intervertebral disk space involvement in 56 dogs with discospondylitis evaluated at the University of Georgia, College of Veterinary Medicine between 1976 and 1981 *(solid bars)* and 75 affected dogs evaluated at the North Carolina State University, College of Veterinary Medicine between 1983 and 1990 *(hatched bars)*. Some dogs had multiple infected sites. Combined data are expressed in the schematic of the vertebral column, with darker regions identifying areas affected most frequently. (From Kornegay JN: Discospondylitis. In Slatter DH, editor: Textbook of small animal surgery, ed 2, Philadelphia, 1993, WB Saunders.)

Staphylococcus spp. are the most common bacteria isolated and the fungus *Aspergillus* spp.[107,108] In pigs, *Staphylococcus* spp., *Streptococcus* spp., *Arcanobacterium pyogenes*, and *Erysipelothrix rhusiopathiae* are common.[106]

Neurologic signs develop from encroachment on the spinal cord or nerve roots by the expanding tissues, causing severe pain and, eventually, paresis. Destruction of the vertebrae may cause spinal instability with secondary compression of the spinal cord. Paresis or paralysis and ataxia caudal to the lesion results from spinal cord compression. The most common finding in large animals is suppurative osteomyelitis and epidural empyema.[56]

Clinical Signs. Discospondylitis and vertebral abscesses always are suspected in animals with fever, depression, anorexia, vertebral pain, and pelvic limb ataxia or paresis. Discospondylitis can affect animals of any age. It is more common in adult dogs with the mean age reported to be 5.1 years.[95] In dogs, discospondylitis more frequently occurs in males than in females (2:1 ratio).[94,95] In all animals, the usual course of clinical signs is chronic and progressive; however, in some affected animals signs may develop acutely and progress rapidly. Most animals have systemic signs including anorexia, depression, and pyrexia. Signs of urinary tract infection or endocarditis-myocarditis occasionally are detected. Dogs with brucellosis may have signs suggesting this disease (orchitis, epididymitis, abortion, infertility, and so forth).[100-102] Systemic signs, however, usually are not localizing to any organ system.

Frequently encountered clinical signs are directly referable to the musculoskeletal and nervous systems.[95,109] The most common presenting sign is pain localized to vertebral column.[94,95] Other signs include hyperesthesia in the area of vertebral involvement, stiff gait, and paresis or paralysis if spinal cord compression occurs. The syndrome is quite similar to intervertebral disk disease except animals with discospondylitis frequently are systemically ill and have a more chronic disease course. Large-breed dogs with type II IVDD rarely are in as much pain as those with discospondylitis. Specific neurologic signs are related to the site of involvement. Cervical vertebral column lesions may cause tetraparesis along with severe neck pain. Thoracolumbar lesions cause back pain and pelvic limb paresis and general proprioceptive ataxia.

Diagnosis. A definitive diagnosis is made with conventional radiography of the spine.[56,92,95,96,109] It is important to radiograph the entire spine to evaluate for multiple lesions. Typical radiographic findings include concentric lysis of adjacent vertebral end plates and various degrees of vertebral lysis surrounded by bone proliferation (Figure 6-12). Vertebral bodies may be shortened, and intervertebral disk spaces may be narrowed. Severely destructive lesions may cause vertebral luxation and spinal cord compression.[110] Occasionally, radiographic abnormalities are not detected in early lesions. Although typical clinical signs are present, radiographic evidence of infection may lag behind the onset of clinical signs for 2 to 3 weeks.[92] Radionuclide scintigraphy or CT and MR imaging may be useful if discospondylitis is strongly suspected and no vertebral lesions are seen on survey radiographs.[111]

Affected dogs occasionally have a leukocytosis composed of neutrophilia and monocytosis on CBC and evidence of pyuria. Leukocytosis is more common in dogs with associated endocarditis. The CSF analysis is usually normal, although elevations in protein concentration and mononuclear cells are occasionally encountered. Blood cultures in dogs yield positive results in about 45% to 75% of dogs with discospondylitis, and urine cultures are positive in about 25% to 50%.[95,112] *Staphylococcus pseudintermedius* is the most common bacterium isolated.[94,95] Results of blood cultures for brucella in dogs are less likely to yield a positive culture.[101] The tube agglutination test is usually positive in dogs affected with *B. canis*. Confirmation of brucellosis should be performed with IFA or PCR testing. Aspiration of lesions may be

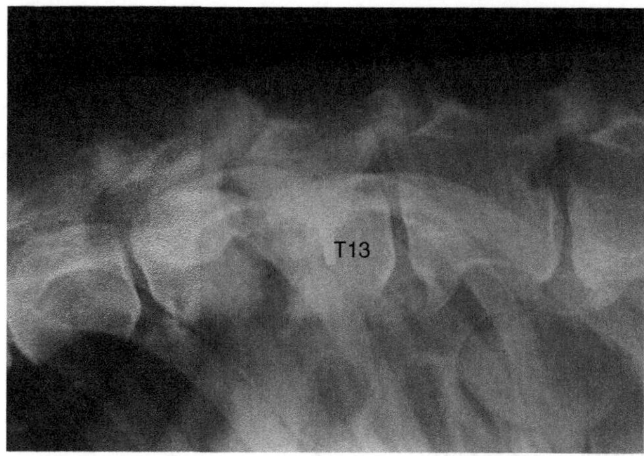

Figure 6-12 Lateral radiograph of the vertebral column of a 5-year-old female German shepherd dog with progressive paraparesis. Lysis of the caudal end plate of T12 and the cranial end plate of T13 is seen. Osteophytes extend from the ventral aspects of the vertebral bodies at the T13-L1 and L1-2 interspaces. A diagnosis of discospondylitis at T12-13 and spondylosis deformans at T13-L1 and L1-2 was made. (From Kornegay JN: Vertebral diseases of large breed dogs. In Kornegay JN, editor: Neurologic disorders: contemporary issues in small animal practice, vol 5, New York, 1986, Churchill Livingstone.)

accomplished with fluoroscopic guidance in small animals and by direct needle placement in large animals.[112] Specimens (blood, urine, or material aspirated from the affected IVD space) should be obtained for culture and sensitivity testing before antimicrobial therapy is initiated.

Treatment. Antibiotic therapy is based on susceptibility testing of bacteria isolated from urine or blood or from infected tissues (see Chapter 15).[113] Antibiotic therapy alone is suggested unless severe spinal cord compression is present or if after 5 days no response to therapy occurs. Prolonged therapy should be continued for at least 8 weeks. Cage rest and pain management using NSAIDs are also recommended. It is important to avoid use of corticosteroids. Compressive lesions require decompression, curettage, and stabilization in addition to long-term antibiotic therapy.[95,110] Discospondylitis of fungal origin or due to brucellosis is difficult to resolve and warrants a guarded prognosis.[95,101] Owners should be advised of its zoonotic potential with *B. canis* infection. Dogs with brucellosis should be neutered.

Spinal Epidural Empyema

Spinal epidural empyema is a suppurative and septic process within the epidural space. Infection results from hematogenous spread of bacteria or by direct local extension.[114] Empyema in dogs and cats has been associated with discospondylitis,[115,116] osteomyelitis,[117] and paraspinal abscessation.[114,118] Cardinal clinical signs are lethargy, fever, anorexia, profound paraspinal pain, and rapidly progressive myelopathy. Common clinicopathologic findings are a neutrophilic leukocytosis on a CBC and a neutrophilic pleocytosis in the CSF.[116] Diagnosis can be aided by myelography, CT, or MRI with identification of an extradural compression extending over multiple spinal cord segments.[114,115,119,120] Spinal radiography is not a reliable technique. MR imaging permits more accurate visualization of the severity and extent of changes within the spinal canal and paraspinal regions.[114] Surgery is the treatment of choice for spinal empyema because it allows decompression of the spinal cord, drainage of the infected material, and direct culture of the organism. Dogs with spinal empyema may have a good outcome when treated by surgical decompression and appropriate long-term (minimum of 8 weeks) antibiotic administration based on culture and sensitivity.[115,116]

Acute Nonprogressive Diseases, T3-L3

Acute nonprogressive diseases of the T3-L3 spinal cord segments are characterized by acute onset and with static clinical course. Trauma and vascular (see L4-S3) are the most important of the various etiologic categories.

Trauma

Acute Spinal Cord Injury (Thoracolumbar Vertebral Column Fracture/Luxation)

Pathophysiology. Spinal cord trauma, usually the result of automobile accidents, is a common neurologic injury.[121,122] The incidence is much greater in areas where leash laws are poorly enforced. Spinal cord trauma is more frequent in large animals when they are young but may occur in mature animals as a result of falls, trailer accidents, or overcrowding in chutes and holding pens. Primary injury to the vertebral column and spinal cord occurs from external or internal causes. External causes include automobile-related injury, falls, falling objects, and projectile missile damage; internal causes include IVDD, pathologic fractures, and vascular.[123,124] Mechanisms of the primary injury are the direct result of compression, shear, laceration, bending, and distraction.[125] The thoracolumbar vertebral column is the most commonly injured in the dog and cat. Fractures occur between T11 and L6 in 50% to 60% of patients after blunt trauma.[122,126] Fractures in the thoracic vertebral column may have little displacement because of the additional support provided by the ribs, ligamentous support, and epaxial musculature. Fracture or luxation of the thoracolumbar vertebral column are often associated with other systemic injuries: pneumothorax, pulmonary contusions, orthopedic injuries, urogenital injuries, and diaphragmatic hernia. Approximately 20% of patients with thoracolumbar vertebral column fractures have a second fracture-luxation.[121,126] The amount of neural tissue injury is related to the rapidity and severity of insult, and the amount and duration of compression.

Primary mechanical injury to the neural tissue can subsequently lead to secondary biochemical injury *(secondary injury theory)*.[124,127-129] Acute SCI causes both systemic and local vascular abnormalities. Primary injury can lead to progressive decrease in perfusion, edema, and necrosis of the injured area of the spinal cord. Secondary metabolic injury that results from ischemia includes abnormal release of excitatory neurotransmitters, abnormal accumulation of intracellular calcium, and activation of membrane phospholipases, and production of free radicals. Similar pathophysiologic mechanisms underlie primary and secondary brain injury (see Chapter 12). *Vascular mechanisms* include ischemia, impaired autoregulation, neurogenic shock, hemorrhage, microcirculatory disruption, vasospasm, and thrombosis. *Ionic derangements* include increased intracellular calcium and sodium, and increased extracellular potassium. *Alterations in neurotransmitters concentrations* include serotonin, catecholamines, and extracellular glutamate, which can potentiate neurotoxicity. The severity of the pathologic changes and the degree of recovery are related to the duration of acute compression as demonstrated in studies of animal models. New treatments are aimed at limiting the secondary injury spinal and those that promote regeneration of the injured spinal cord (oscillating field stimulators, polyethylene glycol, 4-aminopyridine).[127]

This section provides a concise review. The management of spinal cord trauma has been discussed extensively by others.[130-132] Veterinarians have two primary obligations in these cases. First, they must diagnose and treat systemic shock, major abdominal or thoracic hemorrhage, visceral rupture, or ventilation abnormalities. Second, they must be able to give owners accurate prognoses for the animal's recovery of neurologic function.

First Aid and Emergency Medical Treatment. During the period of early evaluation and treatment, the animal must be restrained to prevent further SCI.[131] If a spinal fracture is suspected, the animal should be secured and immobilized to a back board or rigid stretcher to prevent further injury. Movement should be discouraged, especially if vertebral fractures or luxations are suspected. Sedation may be necessary if the animal is struggling. Since some sedatives cause hypotension, before administering sedative drugs, animals must have the cardiovascular system stabilized. The animal should be evaluated in the position that it is presented, usually in lateral or sternal recumbency.

An injury of sufficient force to produce spinal cord trauma may result in another life-threatening injury.[121,133,134] Maintenance of a patent airway is of the utmost importance. Unconscious animals may require endotracheal intubation. Adequate ventilation and oxygenation are of great importance because hypoxia aggravates CNS edema. Spontaneous respiration or evidence of respiratory compromise is closely monitored, especially in patients with cervical SCI. Systemic shock, if present, must be treated. Intravenous isotonic fluids are given to restore vascular volume. Fluid therapy must be carefully monitored to prevent overhydration, but the patient must have fluid volume restored and maintained.

After providing initial treatment aimed at supporting cardiovascular and pulmonary functions, the veterinarian must perform a thorough physical examination. Exogenous spinal injury frequently is associated with multiple organ trauma. Abdominal or thoracic trauma may be difficult to appreciate immediately after an injury; therefore, visceral function must be monitored for several days. Little benefit exists in successfully repairing the spinal fracture only to have the animal die several days later from a diaphragmatic hernia or a ruptured urinary bladder; however, spinal cord trauma must be treated without delay to improve the odds of recovery.

Neurologic Examination. Most spinal cord injuries are the result of vertebral fracture, vertebral luxation, or traumatic IVD herniation, which may produce severe, irreversible neurologic deficits, especially if early treatment has not been provided. The functional status is determined by the neurologic examination. Somatosensory-evoked potentials may be of benefit to define spinal cord integrity more precisely (see Chapter 4). Localization of the spinal cord lesion and the prognosis based on the severity of the injury are determined by the neurologic examination. It is important to perform the neurologic examination with care to prevent further injury and displacement of the vertebral column. Cranial nerves, spinal reflexes, spinal palpation (for obvious deformity and areas of hyperesthesia), cutaneous trunci reflex, and assessment of pain perception can be performed with minimal manipulation of the animal. The vertebral column should be gently palpated for alterations in vertebral conformation because these changes have good localizing value. The principles of lesion localization were reviewed earlier. Table 6-8 summarizes the signs of complete spinal cord transection at various levels of the spinal cord.

It is important to recognize specific neurologic examination findings associated with acute SCI. *Schiff-Sherrington posture* is seen as increased extensor tone in the thoracic limbs and flaccidity in the pelvic limbs. This phenomenon is associated with lesions affecting the T2 to L4 spinal cord segments. The "border" cells located in the dorsal aspect of the ventral horn of segments L1-4(5) project an inhibitory innervation cranially within the fasciculus proprius to the alpha-motor neurons in the cervicothoracic intumescence that provide innervation to the extensor muscles of the thoracic limbs; thus these muscles are disinhibited. *Spinal shock* is usually manifested as flaccidity caudal to the lesion. Likewise, the spinal reflexes are depressed to absent and the bladder may be flaccid with urine retention and sphincter hypotonia.[135] The cause of spinal shock is unclear. A transient decrease in limb tone may be due to loss of descending supraspinal input on the alpha-motor neurons and interneurons along with an increase in segmental inhibition. The duration of spinal shock is proportional to the degree of species encephalization. Spinal shock is important to recognize to prevent improper lesion localization. In some cases, this may be difficult. Spinal shock should be considered in animals with LMN paraplegia in which other clinical findings (such as hyperesthesia, the point at which the cutaneous trunci reflex and line of analgesia are observed) are present cranial to lumbosacral intumescence. *Neurogenic shock* is the systemic complication associated with severe cervical or thoracic spinal cord injury. This syndrome results from sympathetic loss (decreased blood pressure and heart rate resulting from unopposed vagal tone) and continual vagal tone. Consequence of this phenomenon results in loss of spinal cord blood flow regulation and subsequent ischemia. Neurogenic shock should be treated with fluid therapy and pressor agents in an effort to maintain normal systemic blood pressure. These transient phenomena indicate acute and severe SCI but do not determine prognosis. The presence of these signs does not indicate that the lesion is irreversible. These signs may occur in animals that maintain pain perception. *Traction injury* often is traumatic in origin; common in cats following tail injury and with brachial plexus injury. This type of injury commonly affects the sacral and coccygeal or spinal nerves of the cervicothoracic spinal cord segments, respectively.

Assuming that the skeletal lesion can be stabilized, injured animals are categorized as shown in Table 6-7. The prognosis for reversibility of a spinal cord injury depends on severity and duration of the compressive force and extent of secondary vascular responses to the injury.[127] The spinal cord may be anatomically or physiologically transected. Physiologic or functional transection refers to instances in which all functional integrity of the spinal cord is lost (paralysis and absence of pain perception), yet the spinal cord remains structurally intact. In most cases, physiologic transection is the most common cause of irreversibility. Acute compression of the spinal cord is far worse than gradual compression. Acute experimental compression of the spinal cord with a force sufficient to produce paralysis, and loss of pain perception results in irreversible spinal cord injury if the duration of compression exceeds 4 hours. Most experimental studies documenting effective medical therapy of spinal cord trauma indicate that treatment must be given in the first hour.

Presence or absence of pain perception is the most important prognostic indicator. The key to prognosis is the *perceptual response* to noxious stimuli applied caudally to the lesion. Most often this is done by squeezing the digits or nailbed with a hemostat. In the absence of pain perception, the duration of the injury becomes the critical factor related to prognosis (see Table 6-7). The absence of pain perception is a very unfavorable sign, especially in cases of fracture-related trauma. The prognosis for animals with spinal fractures that lack pain perception caudal to the lesion is very poor to hopeless.[14]

Imaging Studies. Radiographs of the vertebral column are necessary if surgical treatment is contemplated. Survey radiography can determine precise lesion location(s) and extent, demonstrate multiple lesions, and help determine an appropriate surgical procedure (Figure 6-13). These findings dictate the surgical procedure needed to decompress and stabilize

TABLE 6-8

Signs of Complete Spinal Cord Transection

Spinal Cord Segments	SIGNS CAUDAL TO LESION		
	Motor	Sensory	Autonomic
C1-4	Tetraplegia (UMN)	Anesthesia	Apnea, no micturition
C5-6	Tetraplegia (UMN), LMN suprascapular nerve	Anesthesia, hyperesthesia—midcervical	Apnea—phrenic nerve, LMN, no micturition
C7-T2	Tetraplegia or paraplegia (UMN), LMN brachial plexus, Horner syndrome	Anesthesia, hyperesthesia—brachial plexus	Diaphragmatic breathing only, no micturition
T3-L3	Paraplegia (UMN), Schiff-Sherrington syndrome	Anesthesia, hyperesthesia—segmental	Diaphragmatic, some intercostal and abdominal respiration depending on level of lesion, no micturition
L4-S1	Paraplegia with LMN lumbosacral plexus S1 = anal sphincter; may be atonic	Anesthesia, hyperesthesia—segmental	No micturition
S1-3	Knuckling of hind foot, paralysis of tail; anal sphincter atonic	Anesthesia, hyperesthesia—segmental	No micturition, extenal sphincter atonic
Cd1-5	Paralysis of tail	Anesthesia, hyperesthesia—segmental	Traction injury may secondarily damage S1-3

C, Cervical; *T,* thoracic; *L,* lumbar; *S,* sacral; *Cd,* caudal; *LMN,* lower motor neuron; *UMN,* upper motor neuron.

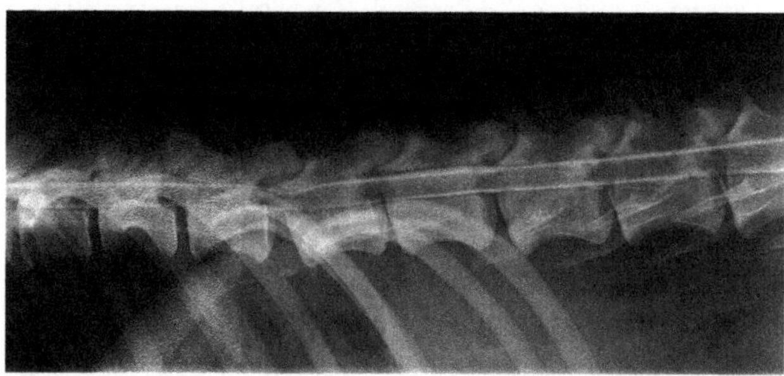

Figure 6-13 Myelogram of a dog with a subluxation at T12-13. The compression of the spinal cord and instability of the vertebral column were not apparent on survey films.

the injury. The initial views are performed over the region in question, with subsequent evaluation of the entire vertebral column. Radiography is performed with the animal in lateral recumbency. Two views should be obtained. To minimize patient movement, the ventrodorsal view may be acquired using a horizontal beam technique. When questionable, fluoroscopy may be used for assessing spinal stability during cautious spinal manipulation. This should be done with extreme caution because the spinal cord can easily be injured.

Myelography or cross-sectional imaging (CT and MRI) is used to provide greater three-dimensional evaluation of the injury, when the radiographic findings do not correlate with neurologic examination, to evaluate spinal cord swelling in concussive injuries, and to further assess severity of spinal cord compression. CT and MRI is useful for further evaluating bone and spinal cord tissues, respectively. CT with sagittal reconstruction of images or MR images are obtained through areas of suspicion based on conventional radiography. CT provides better definition of spinal canal encroachment by bone fragments and for fractures through laminae and pedicles. MRI of the appropriate spinal region will more definitively rule out intramedullary spinal cord lesion and extramedullary compression caused by traumatic IVD herniation or epidural hematoma, and bony fractures. It is important to keep in mind that imaging provides a static representation of displacement at the time of evaluation and not the actual displacement, which occurs at the time of injury.

Spinal stability is assessed using the three-compartment concept (Figure 6-14).[124] The vertebral column is divided into three compartments defined by anatomic structures. The dorsal compartment contains the articular processes, laminae, pedicles, spinous processes, and interarcuate and interspinous ligaments. The middle compartment contains the dorsal longitudinal ligament, dorsal annulus, and dorsal vertebral body. The ventral compartment contains the remainder of the vertebral body, lateral and ventral aspects of the annulus fibrosus, nucleus pulposus, and ventral longitudinal ligament. When two or three compartments are affected or displaced, the fracture is considered unstable. Disruption of the ventral compartment by itself can cause spinal instability.[136]

Specific Treatment of Acute Spinal Cord Injury. The pathophysiology of acute SCI has led to relevant neuroprotective approaches to attenuate the effects of secondary injury. Fluid therapy to maintain spinal cord perfusion is most important in management of animals with severe SCI. General medical management of patients with spinal trauma should include restoring normal blood pressure, enhancing intravascular volume, preventing hypoxemia, and preventing hyperthermia/hypothermia in an effort to enhance spinal cord perfusion. Hypotension will often follow SCI due to multiple factors: interruption to preganglionic neurons of the sympathetic nervous system resulting in unopposed parasympathetic influence and bradycardia; spinal shock causing loss of muscle tone and secondary hypovolemia from venous pooling; and blood loss from other associated injuries. Integrity of the circulatory system is monitored with assessment of the heart rate, capillary refill time, packed cell volume, total protein, and blood pressure.

Neuroprotection. Administration of high-dose corticosteroids is controversial from the standpoint of countering

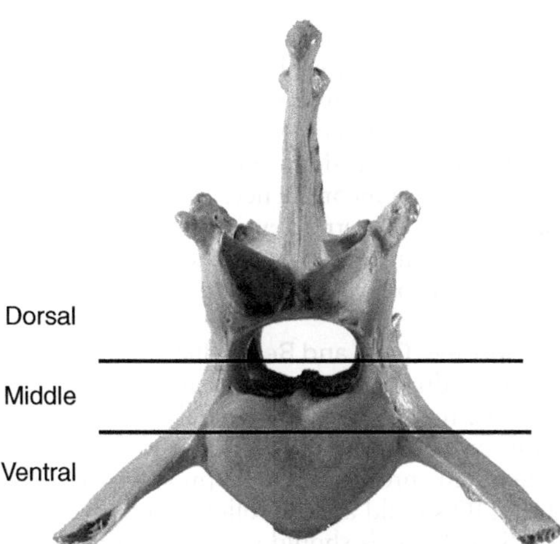

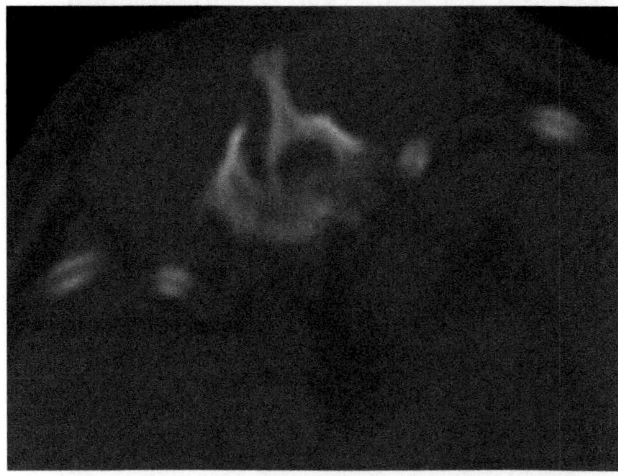

Figure 6-14 **A,** Depiction of the three-compartment model (dorsal, middle, and ventral) for assessing spinal instability. **B,** Disruption of more than one compartment or the ventral compartment alone compromises stability of the vertebral column as shown in the CT transverse image of a three-compartment T13 fracture.

pathophysiologic mechanisms associated with secondary injury processes and efficacy still remains to be proven. The only drug shown to be of benefit in randomized human and laboratory animal clinical trials is methylprednisolone sodium succinate (MPSS).[137,138] Neuroprotective effects of MPSS include inhibition of lipid peroxidation, calcium influx into the neuron, ischemia, axonal dieback, and cytoskeletal degradation, and possession of free-radical scavenging and antiinflammatory effects.[139,140] In the setting of acute SCI resulting in lack of pain perception due to traumatic fractures or luxations of the vertebral column, the administration MPSS should be considered. MPSS, 30 mg/kg, is given intravenously (IV) on presentation, followed by 15 mg/kg IV 4 and 6 hours later and then continuous infusion of 5 mg/kg per hour for 24 hours.[141] Initiation of the MPSS regimen should not be administered after 8 hours from time of onset because of lack of beneficial effects. Although MPSS remains the standard of care in humans with acute SCI, the therapeutic efficacy of MPSS has been questioned. Additionally, in humans the use of MPSS is associated with an increased rate of sepsis and pneumonia. No scientific randomized controlled clinical trials exist for the use of MPSS in animals. Complications of corticosteroid therapy in dogs include diarrhea, melena, vomiting, hematochezia, hematemesis, and anorexia.[142,143] Patients administered corticosteroids also are at higher risk for urinary tract infection. Dimethyl sulfoxide (DMSO) is often recommended, especially for large animals.[56] Most controlled studies do not indicate efficacy, but the literature is controversial.[144] In large animals, it is used at an IV dose of 1 g/kg, 10% DMSO in 5% dextrose.

Conservative Management. Conservative management of spinal fractures consists of strict cage confinement for 6 to 8 weeks. Indications include minimal neurologic deficits, minimal vertebral displacement, involvement of a single compartment of the vertebral canal (with the exception of the ventral compartment), and lack of significant spinal cord compression. Using external coaptation with a splint will depend upon the animal's demeanor, size, and age. Goal of external support is to provide immobilization of the vertebral segments cranial and caudal to the injured area.[131] External coaptation may not resist axial compression and is not ideal when there is failure of the ventral compartment. It is important to follow principles of bandage care when using methods of external support. The patient will need to be turned regularly and kept clean and dry to prevent urine scalding.

Surgical Stabilization. Although some vertebral fractures can be managed conservatively, surgery is indicated for fractures or luxations that are unstable (>1 compartment) (Figure 6-14, *B*). Goals for spinal fractures/luxation repair are decompression, realignment of the vertebrae, and fixation of involved vertebral segments until physiologic/structural fusion occurs. Surgical management often provides a more rapid rate and a more complete neurologic recovery. Indications for surgical stabilization include rapidity of neurologic progression, vertebral column instability, severe compressive injury, hypoventilation, and intractable pain. If decompression is warranted, selection of the decompressive procedure should be conservative so as to not further disrupt the integrity of the vertebrae or further compromise stability, but large enough to relieve compression. Hemilaminectomy is the favored approach for decompression because any method of fixation can be used with this procedure and because it creates less instability. Dorsal laminectomy often is used in the lumbosacral region (Figure 6-15).

There are many methods of internal fixation that are commonly used to stabilize spinal fractures and the reader is referred to other texts and references for in-depth descriptions of the various surgical techniques.[131,145,146] The method is dependent upon the size of the patient, fracture type, and surgeon preference. The decision as to the method of stabilization is based on imaging findings and on observations made during the surgery. Common techniques used for internal stabilization include securing flexible plates to the dorsal spinous processes, vertebral body plating, pins/screws and polymethylmethacrylate (PMMA) (Figure 6-16), articular process stabilizing, and segmental spinal instrumentation. It also is important to consider incorporating bone grafting into the procedure to enhance healing. Compression fractures of the vertebral body and fractures of the transverse processes without displacement may still be stable. Fractures of the vertebral body with luxation or fractures involving the articular processes require reduction and stabilization. Successful outcome after surgical fixation depends not only on the severity of the SCI but also on the type and strength of fixation, the surgeon's skill and knowledge of the spinal anatomy, and accuracy of vertebral column alignment.

Prognosis. Prognosis for animals with acute thoracolumbar injury is dependent upon the neurologic examination. The prognosis for recovery from a spinal fracture or luxation that results in paraplegia with loss of pain perception is considered

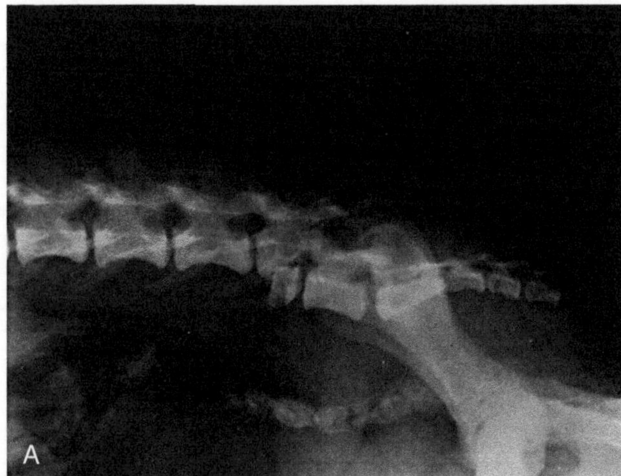

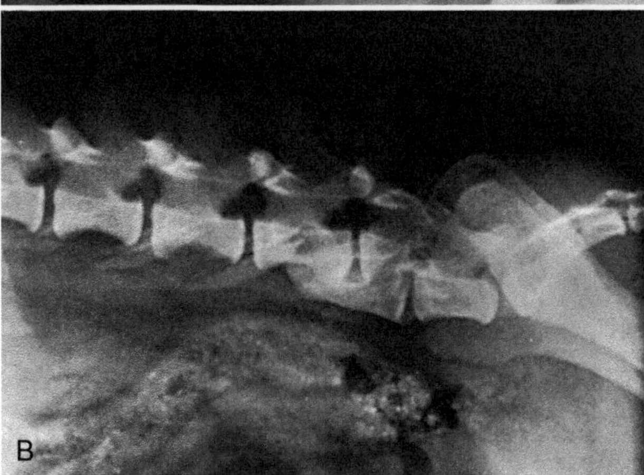

Figure 6-15 **A,** Lumbosacral lateral radiograph demonstrating a fracture of L6. These injuries entrap the spinal nerve roots that form the sciatic, pelvic, pudendal, and caudal nerves. **B,** Follow-up postsurgical radiograph of the same dog. The fracture site was decompressed, and the nerves in the vertebral canal were freed from compression. A callus had bridged the fracture site, although no internal stabilization had been provided.

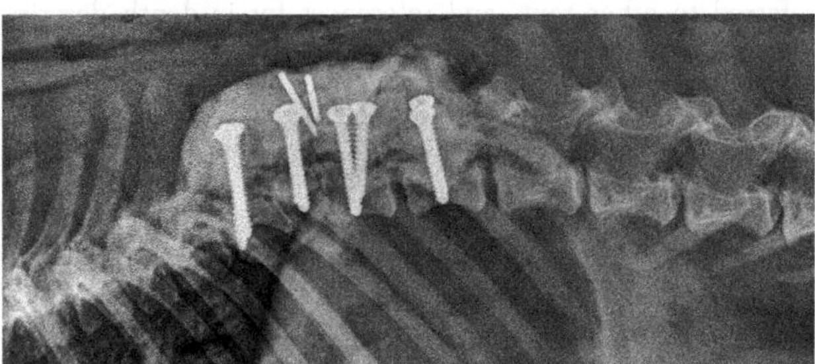

Figure 6-16 Survey lateral thoracolumbar radiograph demonstrating use of polymethylmethacrylate and screws for stabilizing a three-compartment T12 compression fracture in a young bull- dog.

poor.[14] One study of 211 dogs and cats with vertebral fractures found minimal difference between medical and surgical management.[122] Other studies summarize a 70% to 95% recovery rate for conservative management on selective cases.[147-149] Dogs with cervical vertebral column injury may respond well to external coaptation techniques.[150] Although considerable displacement may occur, results of spinal stabilization tend to be good if pain perception is intact in the tail and digits of the pelvic limbs, and perineal sensation is present (as an indicator of injury severity to the sacral segments).[148,149,151] Patients that maintain pain perception may still require months to recover and have residual neurologic deficits including urinary and/or fecal incontinence. Traction injury of sacral nerves usually results in permanent fecal and urinary incontinence. Unfortunately, in veterinary medicine, the outcome of the case often depends on the dedication and financial cooperation of the owner.

Supportive Care and Rehabilitation. Few animals become ambulatory during the first week after surgery following severe SCI. Most remain paretic or paralyzed and require attentive nursing care and physical therapy and a rehabilitation period. In general, the procedures for supportive care of the paraplegic with IVDD should also be followed up after surgery for traumatic SCI. Animals should improve within 2 to 3 weeks, and significant improvement should be seen in a month. Failure to show improvement during this time is strongly correlated with permanent spinal cord damage; however, every clinician encounters a few dogs that regain functional use of the pelvic limbs when the initial outlook has seemed hopeless. Surprisingly, some cats and dogs regain the ability to walk without regaining pain perception, a phenomenon known as *"spinal walking or spinal locomotion"* based on intact reflex pathways associated with the central pattern generators of the spinal cord.[152] Spinal locomotion is dependent on the development and preparation of the spinal locomotor pattern generators, afferent stimulation (of cutaneous receptors), changes in neurochemistry within the spinal cord, and midlumbar spinal cord input.[153]

Chronic Progressive Diseases, T3-L3

Chronic progressive diseases of the T3-L3 region are characterized by insidious onset and slow progression of the neurologic signs. Degenerative, anomalous/malformation (see L4-S3), and neoplastic diseases are the most important of the various etiologic categories. Although the diseases listed in the right-hand column of Tables 6-1 through 6-3 may start in the T3-L3 spinal cord segments, progression into other regions may occur. With long-standing disease, cervical spinal cord involvement predominates, causing tetraparesis or hemiparesis. These problems are discussed in Chapter 7.

Degenerative

Canine Degenerative Myelopathy

Pathogenesis. Canine degenerative myelopathy (DM) was first described in 1973 by Averill as an insidious, progressive, GP ataxia and UMN spastic paresis of the pelvic limbs beginning in late adulthood, ultimately leading to paraplegia and necessitating euthanasia.[154] The disease was termed *degenerative myelopathy* because of its histopathologic nature as a nonspecific degeneration of spinal cord tissue of undetermined cause. In 1975, Griffiths and Duncan published a series of cases with signs of hyporeflexia and nerve root involvement, and they termed the condition *chronic degenerative radiculomyelopathy*.[155] Though most of the dogs in these initial reports were German shepherd dogs (GSDs), other breeds were represented. Nonetheless, for many years, DM was considered a UMN and GP disease in the GSD.[156]

In general, the pathology of DM is consistent with a noninflammatory axonal degeneration.[154-156] Regional axonal loss in the spinal cord is severe in many DM-affected dogs with complete loss of axonal and myelin profiles and replacement by large areas of astrogliosis.[154-158] Lesion distribution involves the spinal cord myelin and axons in all funiculi but affects the midthoracic to caudal thoracic region most extensively.[154-156,158] There is a tendency for increased lesion severity

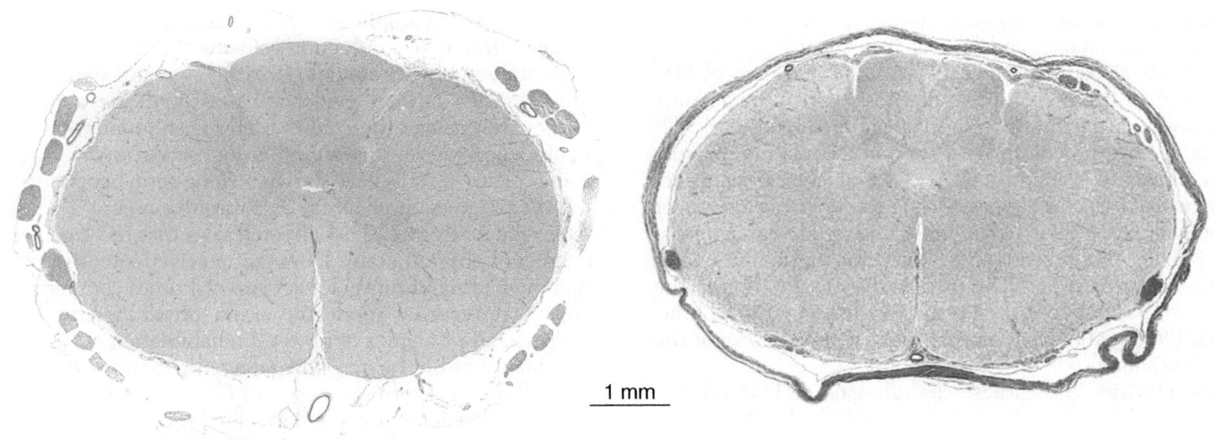

Figure 6-17 Histopathology using Luxol fast blue with periodic acid-Schiff counter-staining of the thoracic spinal cord from a normal and degenerative myelopathy (DM)–affected dog. Note the severity of pallor in the white matter of the DM-affected dog. (Courtesy PA March Cummings School of Veterinary Medicine at Tufts University.)

within the dorsal portion of the lateral funiculus involving the peripheral and deeper white matter tracts[154-156,158] and in the dorsal funiculus in some dogs (Figure 6-17).[154,158] The transverse and longitudinal extent of spinal cord lesions also parallel the severity of the neurologic deficits.[158] The more severely affected dogs show significantly greater axonal degeneration and loss in the thoracic spinal cord segments and progression to the cervical and lumbar spinal cord.[158] Characterization of the brain pathology of DM-affected dogs has been limited. Johnston et al[157] described abnormalities in the red nucleus and lateral vestibular nucleus of the brainstem, and in the lateral (dentate) and fastigial nucleus of the cerebellum. Despite these findings, clinical signs related to intracranial lesions are uncommon.

Historically, DM has been considered a disease that results solely in GP/UMN deficits. Recently, affected dogs have been indentified in which late in the natural progression of the disease, generalized LMN signs develop. With DM, the nerve pathology and LMN signs do not become evident until later in the disease progression. When examined in earlier reported cases, nerves have been described as normal or exhibiting sporadic axonal loss.[154,158] A recent study documented neuromuscular pathology in DM-affected dogs manifesting LMN signs.[159] Nerve specimens showed nerve fiber loss resulting from axonal degeneration, endoneurial fibrosis, numerous inappropriately thinly myelinated fibers, and secondary demyelination. Muscle specimens from dogs with advanced DM show excessive variability in myofiber size, with large and small groups of atrophic fibers typical of denervation. Canine DM may now be most accurately classified as a *multisystem central and peripheral axonopathy*.

Immunologic,[160-162] metabolic or nutritional,[163-167] oxidative stress,[168] excitotoxic,[169] and genetic mechanisms have been explored as underlying the pathogenesis of DM. The uniformity of clinical signs, histopathology, age, and breed predilections suggest an inherited basis for DM; however, the late onset of disease has made it difficult to collect data from parents and siblings to substantiate this theory. Segregation of DM in families has been reported in the Siberian husky,[170] Pembroke Welsh corgi,[168] and Chesapeake Bay retriever.[171] Familial DM also occurs in the Rhodesian ridgeback and boxer. Clemmons et al reported a point mutation in hypervariable region 2 of *DLA-DRB1* in GSDs with DM and offers a DNA test for DM based on this allele.[171a] Others were unable to confirm a correlation between this mutation and DM in GSDs.[172] Awano et al[159] used a genome-wide association and determined a missense mutation in the superoxide dismutase 1 (*SOD1*) gene. Mutations in the *SOD1* gene are known to cause amyotrophic lateral sclerosis (ALS) in humans, which is also known as Lou Gehrig disease. The disease derives its name from the combined degeneration of UMNs and LMNs motor neurons projecting from the brain and spinal cord. The Greek derivation of amyotrophy means "muscles without nourishment." Lateral is the location within the spinal cord of axonal disease and sclerosis refers to diseased axons being replaced by sclerosis or "scar" tissue. Equine motor neuron disease also resembles human ALS and is further discussed in Chapter 7. Dogs testing homozygous for the mutation are *at risk* for developing DM. Some dogs are homozygous for the mutation, but remain free of clinical signs, which suggests age-related incomplete penetrance.

Although the clinical signs, disease progression, and genetic analysis are provocative for considering DM as a canine model of ALS, there remain significant pathologic and clinical differences. These include the absence of any evidence of neuronal cell body degeneration or loss in the ventral horn of the spinal cord and the diffuse nature of the axonopathy that involves sensory tracts and UMN tracts. Studies are underway to further describe the neuronal cell body, nerve root, and spinal nerve pathology associated with DM.

Signalment. There is no sex predilection. Age of onset of neurologic signs is usually 5 years or older with a mean age of 9 years in large dog breeds with DM.[154,155,157,173] A study in Pembroke Welsh corgis (PWCs) reported a mean age of onset of 11 years.[168] Histopathologically confirmed cases of DM have been reported in the following dog breeds: GSD,[154-157,159] Siberian husky,[170] miniature poodle,[174] boxer,[159,175] PWC,[158,168] Chesapeake Bay retriever,[159,171] Rhodesian ridgeback,[159] and mixed breed.[154] Other previously reported breeds presumptively diagnosed without histopathologic confirmation include the Irish terrier,[155] Kerry blue terrier,[155] Labrador retriever,[173] Bernese mountain dog,[173] Hovawart,[173] Kuvasz,[173] collie,[173] Belgian shepherd,[173] giant schnauzer,[173] soft-coated wheaten terrier,[173] mastiff,[173] borzoi,[173]and Great Dane.[176] Recently, we have been able to histopathologically confirm DM in the Bernese mountain dog, standard poodle, Kerry blue terrier, Cardigan Welsh corgi, golden retriever, wire fox terrier, American Eskimo dog, soft-coated wheaten terrier, and pug (Zeng—publication pending).

Clinical Signs. Progressive, asymmetric UMN paraparesis, pelvic limb GP ataxia, and lack of paraspinal hyperesthesia are key clinical features of DM. The clinical course of DM can vary after the presumptive diagnosis with a mean time for disease duration of 6 months in larger dog breeds.[154,156,157] Most large dog breeds progress to nonambulatory paraparesis within 6 to 9 months from onset of clinical signs. Pet owners usually elect euthanasia when the dogs can no longer support weight in their pelvic limbs and need walking assistance. Smaller dog breeds can be cared for by the pet owner over a longer time.[168,174] The median disease duration in the PWC was 19 months.[168] As a result of a longer survival time, affected PWCs often have signs of thoracic limb paresis at the time of euthanasia.

Early Disease. The earliest clinical signs of DM are GP ataxia and mild spastic paresis in the pelvic limbs. Worn nails and asymmetric pelvic limb weakness are apparent upon physical examination. Asymmetry of signs at disease onset is frequently reported.[154,168,173,174] At disease onset, spinal reflex abnormalities are consistent with UMN paresis localized in the T3 to L3 spinal cord segments.[154] Patellar reflexes may be normal or exaggerated to clonic; however, hyporeflexia of the patellar reflex has also been described in dogs at similar disease stage.[155] Flexor (withdrawal) reflexes may also be normal or show crossed extension (suggestive of chronic UMN dysfunction). Often dogs progress to nonambulatory paraparesis and are euthanized during this disease stage.

Late Disease. If the dog is not euthanized early, clinical signs will progress to LMN paraplegia and ascend to affect the thoracic limbs.[154,168,173,174] Flaccid tetraplegia occurs in dogs with advanced disease.[159,168,174] The paresis becomes more symmetric as the disease progresses. LMN signs emerge as hyporeflexia of the patellar and withdrawal reflexes, flaccid paralysis, and widespread muscle atrophy beginning in the pelvic limbs as the dogs become nonambulatory.[159,174] Widespread and severe loss of muscle mass occurs in the appendicular muscles in the late stage of DM. Most reports attributed loss of muscle mass to disuse[154,155,168,170,174] but flaccidity in dogs with protracted disease suggests denervation.[159,174] Cranial nerve signs include swallowing difficulties and inability to bark.[159,168,174] Urinary and fecal continence usually are spared also until the latter disease stage with paraplegia.[154,168,170,173]

Diagnosis. Accurate antemortem diagnosis is based on pattern recognition of the progression of clinical signs followed by a series of diagnostic steps to exclude other disorders.[177,178] Neurodiagnostic techniques for evaluation of spinal cord disease include CSF analysis, electrodiagnostic testing, and spinal cord imaging procedures. A presumptive diagnosis of DM often is made based on lack of clinically relevant compressive myelopathy as determined by MRI. If MRI is unavailable, CT/myelography can also be used. MRI is especially useful for identifying early intramedullary spinal cord neoplasia and evidence of extradural compressive myelopathy. Unfortunately, imaging often reveals IVD herniation, which can confound a diagnosis of DM. The clinician must be guided by clinical experience to evaluate for rapidity of disease progression, presence of paraspinal hyperesthesia, and amount of spinal cord compression to account for the severity of the myelopathy.

CSF analysis can help rule out meningitis. Abnormalities in electrodiagnostic testing have been reported.[155,159,168,173] Early in the progression of DM, no abnormal spontaneous activity is detected by electromyography (EMG) and nerve conduction velocities are within normal limits.[159] Later in the disease course, EMG reveals multifocal spontaneous activity in the distal appendicular musculature. Recordings of compound muscle action potentials (M waves) from stimulation of the tibial and ulnar nerves have shown temporal dispersion and decreases in amplitudes. A reduction in the proximal and distal motor nerve conduction velocities has been observed.[159]

Management Strategies. Treatment regimens have been empiric with lack of evidence-based medicine approaches. Although it is hypothesized that DM is an immune-mediated neurodegenerative disease, immunosuppressive therapies using corticosteroids have shown no long-term benefits in halting the progression of DM.[176,179] Kathmann et al[173] reported survival data from 22 DM-affected dogs that received varying degrees of physiotherapy. Dogs that received intensive physiotherapy had significantly longer survival times compared with dogs that received moderate or no physiotherapy. Physiotherapy and principles of physical rehabilitation may improve the quality of life for the DM-affected pet and pet owner.[180] Overall the long-term prognosis of DM is poor.

Other Specific Axonal and Myelin Degenerative Disorders. Myelinopathies, axonopathies, and neuronopathies can present initially with progressive signs of paraparesis that eventually affect the thoracic limbs. Many of these disorders are breed-specific and inherited. Summaries of these degenerative conditions are further described in Chapter 7. Primary myelin degenerative disorders can be classified as hypomyelination and dysmyelination (leukodystrophy or myelinolytic diseases) and clinical signs are manifested in the pelvic limbs most severely. Disorders of hypomyelination often have tremor and are discussed in Chapter 10. Dysmyelination refers to when myelin synthesis or function is defective and cannot be maintained. Myelinolysis is a degeneration and destruction or necrosis of the spinal cord myelin. Clinical signs often are acute and rapidly progressive, causing paraplegia and eventually affect the thoracic limbs.

In 1973, Cockrell et al[181] described a demyelinating spinal cord disease in related, young Afghan hounds. The age at onset varied from 3 to 13 months, and the clinical course was 2 to 6 weeks. Affected dogs progressed rapidly from pelvic limb ataxia and spastic paresis to paraplegia within 7 to 10 days. Spinal reflexes were usually normal or exaggerated. In some dogs, mild thoracic limb deficits were detected. The disorder progressed to tetraplegia and death from respiratory failure in 2 to 6 weeks. Severe destruction of myelin and necrosis with relative sparing of axons was found in the ventral, lateral, and sometimes dorsal funiculi. The lesions were prominent in spinal cord segments C5-L3 and can extend into the brainstem. The most severe changes were found in the cranial thoracic spinal cord. The pathogenesis is unknown and the disease is thought to have an autosomal recessive inheritance patten. There is no effective treatment. Similar disorders, which vary in onset, have been reported in Leonbergers,[182] miniature poodle,[183] and Dutch kooiker dog.[184] Degenerative myeloencephalopathies that are inherited or caused by toxins and nutritional-related disorders occur in other species (see Chapter 7).[185]

Type II Intervertebral Disk Disease

Pathogenesis. Hansen type II disk disease occurs primarily in older (5 to 12 years of age), large-breed, nonchondrodystrophic dogs. Similar IVD protrusions are sometimes seen in smaller dogs and in cats.[1,2,186] The pathologic change within the intervertebral disk is a fibroid degeneration and a weakening of the dorsal annulus (see Figure 6-3).[4] Recurrent partial IVD protrusion produces a dome-shaped mass that eventually becomes large enough to compress the spinal cord or to irritate meninges and nerve roots. The neurologic signs and spinal cord lesions are those of a compressive myelopathy.

Clinical Signs. As with type I IVD herniation, clinical signs relate to the region of the spinal cord affected. Intervertebral disk herniation involving spinal cord segments T3-L3 result in UMN signs, whereas IVD herniations involving segments caudal to L3 can produce LMN signs to the pelvic limbs. The cutaneous trunci reflex may be decreased caudal to the level of the lesion. The presence of hyperesthesia on spinal palpation has great localizing value. Importantly, the clinical signs are similar to other common spinal cord disorders that result in chronic progressive clinical signs. Other common conditions include degenerative myelopathy and spinal neoplasia. Consequently, definitive diagnosis or exclusion of other conditions cannot be made solely based on clinical signs. Despite this, several findings may increase the index of suspicion for type II IVD herniation. With type II IVD protrusions, hyperesthesia in the area of the IVD herniation may be present, in contrast to the lack of hyperesthesia in degenerative myelopathy. However, many dogs with type II IVDD are not painful presumably because of the slow progression of the syndrome. Likewise, voluntary micturition may be affected by the compressive myelopathy, whereas micturition usually remains normal in the early stages of degenerative myelopathy.

Diagnosis. Conventional radiography cannot provide a definitive diagnosis, although suggestive changes may be seen. Increased opacity in the interverterbral foramen and narrowing of the disk space are not consistently present in type II IVD protrusions. Myelography, CT, or MRI is usually necessary to demonstrate the compressive nature of the disk in question. It is not uncommon to find multiple disk spaces affected. Dogs may also have concurrent disease such as degenerative myelopathy or degenerative lumbosacral stenosis.

Treatment. Patients with early and mild signs may respond temporarily to antiinflammatory drugs such as corticosteroids or NSAIDs; however, the signs may recur and progressively worsen. Dogs with pain as the only clinical sign can be treated medically, but decompressive surgery with removal of the IVD protrusion is more satisfactory in most cases. Decompressive surgery may be indicated for dogs with paresis. Surgery should be performed early to prevent further neurologic deterioration. The prognosis with surgery is fair to good in that most dogs regain normal neurologic function. There is a greater risk with dogs with chronic disk disease being transiently worse after surgery. All owners should be cautioned that concurrent degenerative myelopathy is always a risk.

Spinal Dural Ossification. Dural ossification, also known as ossifying pachymeningitis, is a common radiographic or necropsy finding in middle-aged or older large-breed dogs (Figure 6-18).[187] Plaques of bone develop on the inner dural surface in response to an unidentified factor and are often identified in association with vertebral spondylosis. The disease usually affects the cervical and lumbar areas. The bony plaques are of little clinical importance except in rare cases in which they entrap a nerve root or cause pain. Rarely, large dural plaques cause local spinal cord edema, necrosis, or fibrosis. Radiographs are useful for establishing the diagnosis. Myelographic, CT, or MRI evidence of compression warrants exploratory decompression of the lesion. Medical treatment is usually directed toward pain management. Clinicians should make every attempt to find other causes for the neurologic signs before assuming that dural ossification is the cause.

Spondylosis Deformans (Hypertrophic Spondylosis). This noninfectious, nonseptic condition is a common finding during routine radiographic or necropsy examinations. Spondylosis deformans is characterized by the formation of new bone and bony bridges at the intervertebral disk spaces (see Figure 6-18).[188-190] The term *spondylitis* originally was used to describe this condition because investigators believed that inflammation produced the bony reaction. Further work suggested that the condition was a noninflammatory process associated with degeneration of the annulus fibrosus of the intervertebral disk.[191] The term *spondylosis deformans* is therefore preferred. Spondylosis occurs in most species but is most frequent in dogs, bulls, and pigs.[56,190,192] Spondylosis

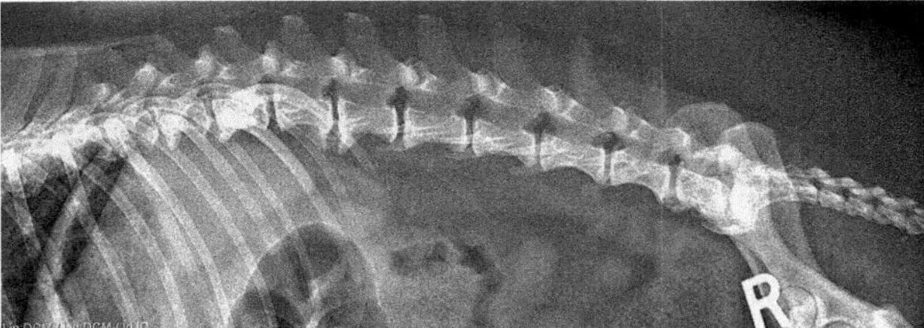

Figure 6-18 Spondylosis of the lumbar vertebrae was an incidental finding in this dog. These changes seldom cause neurologic signs.

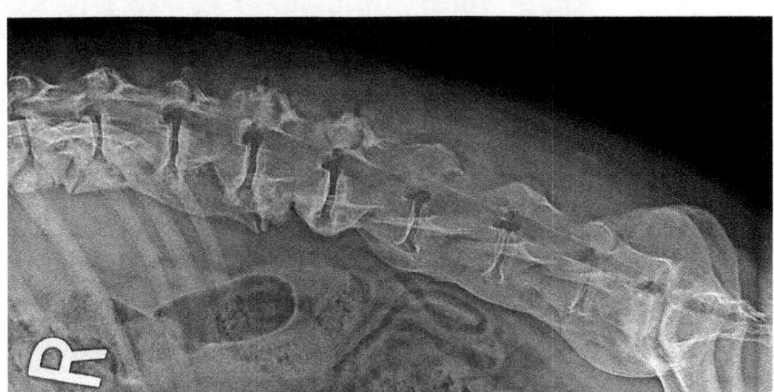

Figure 6-19 A lateral radiograph of the thoracolumbar spine from a 6-year-old male boxer demonstrating disseminated idiopathic spinal hyperostosis (DISH), which consists of contiguous bridging spondylosis and bony proliferation of the articular processes. The neurologic examination was normal.

deformans has higher prevalence and heritability in the boxer breed.[193]

The lesions often are incidental findings on radiography and do not compress the associated neural tissues. Osteophyte formation within the vertebral canal in dogs is very rare and seldom, if ever, results in spinal cord or nerve root compression.[191,194] The condition in dogs may be present anywhere in the spine but is most common in the caudal thoracic and caudal lumbar vertebrae.[191] As with dural ossification, clinicians must search for other causes of the neurologic signs before assuming that spondylosis is the cause. Spondylosis occasionally causes spinal and nerve root pain, especially after exercise. An association may exist between radiographically apparent spondylosis and type II IVDD.[195] However, the presence of spondylosis at a disk space is not proof of disk protrusion. It also is frequently seen at the L7-S1 disk space in dogs and may be associated with stenosis of the vertebral canal or intervertebral foramina that produce pain and LMN signs (see the degenerative lumbosacral stenosis section).[194,196,197]

In large animals (bulls, pigs, and horses), spondylosis deformans is more often associated with clinical signs of limited vertebral movement, neck and back pain, and ataxia.[56,192,198,199] Spondylosis occurs at low prevalence in horses with back pain.[198] Bulls with spondylosis may have an acute onset of paraplegia or paraparesis.[192]

Other Vertebral Lesions Causing Compressive Myelopathy

Disseminated Idiopathic Skeletal Hyperostosis (DISH). DISH refers to extensive ossification through the axial and appendicular skeleton, including the vertebrae in dogs and cats.[200,201] This disorder is characterized by a proliferative bony response to minor stresses. The cause is unknown. Radiographic signs are characterized by a flowing ossification primarily located at the ventrolateral aspect of the spine, extending for at least four contiguous vertebrae (Figure 6-19). The interspinous ligaments also may be ossified as well as extraspinal ligamentous attachments. Clinical signs of gait

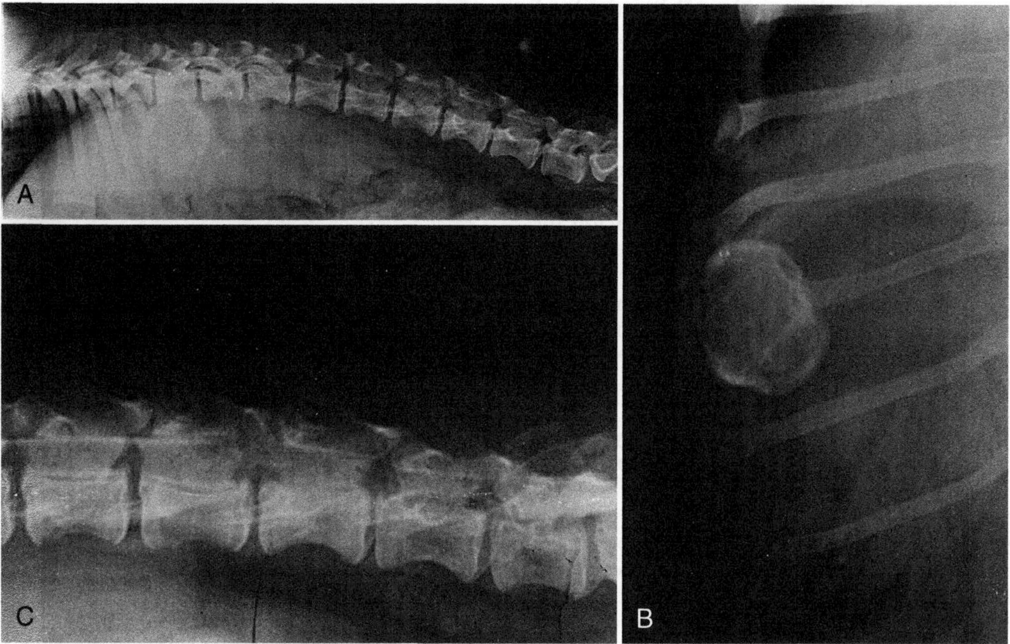

Figure 6-20 **A,** Multiple cartilaginous exostoses affecting the vertebrae of a young dog. Note the cystlike structures within the vertebrae. **B,** Radiograph of a cystlike bone lesion in the rib of the same dog. These bony, bullae-like structures are diagnostic of multiple cartilaginous exostoses. **C,** Myelogram demonstrating severe spinal cord compression from L4 to L6. Occasionally, these lesions undergo malignant transformation to chondrosarcoma.

abnormalities reflect the effects of periarticular involvement of the axial and appendicular skeleton. Decompressive surgery may be indicated in severe cases of spinal cord compression.

Solitary or Multiple Cartilaginous Exostoses. Multiple cartilaginous exostoses, also known as osteochondromatoses, osteocartilaginous exostoses, and multiple osteochondromas, are conditions that occur in dogs, cats, and horses.[202-205] The disease is a benign proliferation of cartilage and bone that affects the bones formed by endochondral ossification. Lesions may be found as a single (solitary) lesion or as multiple lesions. In addition to the appendicular skeleton, lesions may develop in the vertebral bodies or the spinous processes (Figure 6-20, *A*). The ribs are also commonly affected (see Figure 6-20, *B*). A small percentage of cartilaginous exostoses may undergo malignant transformation into chondrosarcomas or osteosarcomas.[206] Clinical evidence indicates that the condition may be inherited in the dog and horse.[204,207]

Clinical signs in dogs appear during the period of active bone growth and thoracolumbar vertebral involvement is frequent. Pain or loss of neurologic function develops when adjacent structures are compressed or distorted by the boney lesions. Spinal cord compression with neurologic deficits caudal to the lesion is common (see Figure 6-20, C) in dogs. Compressive lesions in the cervical spine may produce progressive tetraparesis.[205] Radiographically, the bony exostoses are characterized as variably sized radiopaque lesions with large radiolucent areas.[204,205] Vertebral lesions tend to be circular. Radiography provides strong supportive evidence of the diagnosis. CT or MRI can aid in further characterization of the lesion extent.[208] However, a definitive diagnosis of solitary or multiple cartilaginous exostoses is based on microscopic examination to differentiate the condition from vertebral neoplasia. In dogs, the exostoses apparently stop growing after physeal closure.

Although microscopically identical, the disease in cats differs from that in dogs. In cats, lesions occur after skeletal maturity is reached and continue to progress. Solitary lesions typically affect older cats and are more commonly associated with joints of the appendicular skeleton. Multiple cartilaginous exostoses affects young adult cats.[209] The disease is associated with feline leukemia virus. A type C viral particles, suggestive of FeLV or feline sarcoma virus, have been identified in bony lesions.[210] In both dogs and cats, treatment involves surgical decompression.

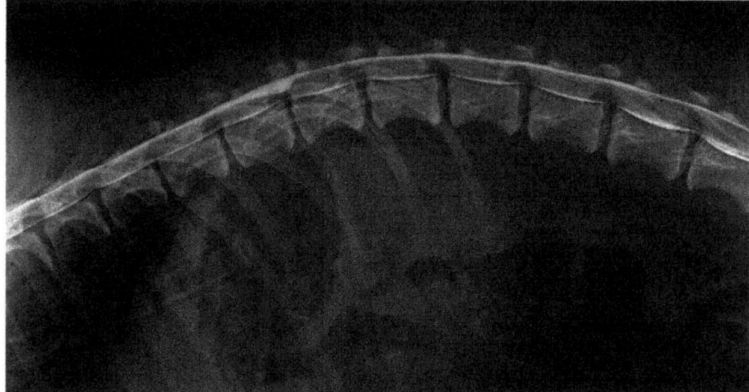

Figure 6-21 Myelogram from a 5-year-old dachshund with progressive paraparesis demonstrating a contrast-filled diverticulum in the dorsal subarachnoid space at the level of the T12-13 intervertebral disk space.

Spinal Arachnoid Cysts. Spinal arachnoid cysts or diverticula consist of accumulations of CSF within a focal area of the subarachnoid space (Figure 6-21).[211,212] Arachnoid cysts involving the spinal cord can cause a progressive compressive myelopathy. Arachnoid cysts occur in the cervical and thoracolumbar spinal cord. Large-breed dogs appear to develop cervical lesions more frequently, whereas small-breed dogs develop lesions more frequently in the thoracolumbar region.[212] This disorder has been more commonly reported in rottweilers.[211]

Spinal arachnoid cysts also occur in cats.[213,214] The neurologic signs reflect the region of spinal cord affected. In the thoracolumbar region, clinical signs and course may be protracted over weeks to years. Most dogs develop UMN paraparesis and urinary incontinence. In the cervical region, neurologic signs include GP ataxia and tetraparesis. The lesions can be delineated with myelography, CT/myelography, and MRI.[211,212,215] MRI is more sensitive in detecting associated spinal cord syringomyelia.[215] Various surgical procedures involve spinal cord decompression and removal or draining the cyst with fenestration or marsupialization of the dura mater.[211,212] Prognosis is good for young dogs and for dogs treated soon after the onset of clinical signs.[211,212]

Spinal Synovial Cysts. Spinal synovial cysts tend to occur in young, large-breed dogs in the cervical vertebral column[216-218] but involve the thoracolumbar vertebral column in older, large-breed dogs.[219,220] These extradural synovial cysts or ganglion cysts arise from the articular facets. Pathogenesis is thought to be a result of excessive motion placing biomechanical stress on the vertebral articulations, which predisposes the joint to osteoarthritis and synovial cyst formation. Histopathology consists of fibrous connective tissue with a synovial cell lining. Diagnosis is based on evidence of degenerative joint disease of the articular processes. Spinal cord compression is detected using myelography, CT/myelography, and MRI. Attenuation of subarachnoid contrast is recognized medial to the articular processes (hourglass appearance). Surgical decompression is indicated when neurologic function is progressive and in cases of refractory pain. Laminectomy and removal of the proliferative tissue alleviates spinal compression. The prognosis is good depending on the severity and duration of neurologic signs.

Compressive Myelopathy in Shiloh Shepherd Dogs. An unusual degenerative joint disease that affects the articular processes of the thoracolumbar spinal cord has been described in Shiloh shepherd dogs.[221] Clinical signs develop from 9 weeks to 16 months of age and include GP ataxia and UMN paraparesis. Proliferative lesions involving the articular processes from T11 to L2 were observed radiographically and were responsible for a dorsal compressive myelopathy. Surgery was beneficial in two cases and not beneficial in one case. One dog partially responded to medical treatment consisting of exercise restriction and a reduced protein diet. The disease may be inherited.

Neoplasia of the Spine and Spinal Cord

General Description

Pathogenesis. Tumors affecting the vertebrae, meninges, nerve roots, or spinal cord may result in neurologic signs. Collectively, these tumors are often referred to as spinal tumors. Tumors are classified according to anatomic location and histologic tumor type as primary, secondary (metastatic), or those that arise from adjacent structures and secondarily invade the vertebral column (e.g., prostatic tumors, hematopoietic, or skeletal). Anatomic location with respect to the spinal cord includes extradural, intradural-extramedullary, or intramedullary (Table 6-9). In general, the most common tumors are extradural that secondarily compress or invade the spinal

TABLE 6-9

Characteristics of Vertebral and Spinal Cord Tumors

	TUMOR LOCATION		
Characteristic	**Extradural**	**Intradural/Extramedullary**	**Intramedullary**
Frequency	50%	35%	15%
Tumor types	Bone tumors Metastatic tumors Lymphoma	Neurofibromas Meningiomas Lymphoma Nephroblastomas	Gliomas Ependymomas Astrocytoma Metastatic
Rate of growth	Rapid	Slow	Usually slow
Clinical signs			
Pain	Early severe	Early, variable	Unusual, late
Paresis	Early, rapidly progressive, usually bilateral	Late, slowly progressive, may be unilateral	Early asymmetric; late, rapidly progressive, usually bilateral
Sensory evaluation	Usually intact until late	Usually intact until late	Usually intact until late
Course	Acute onset, rapid progression	Very slow progression	Insidious onset, rapid progression
Diagnosis			
CSF	Increased protein, normal cells	Increased protein, normal cells	Increased protein, normal cells, may be xanthochromic
Radiography	Skeletal lesions if bone	Possibly large intervertebral foramen (neurofibroma)	Possible widened vertebral canal
Myelography	Extradural compression	Variable, may be cupping of contrast column	Widened spinal cord, attenuated contrast column
MRI	Extradural compression Hyperintensity in spinal cord from edema	Variable Hyperintensity in spinal cord from edema, mass in intradural space	Widened spinal cord Hyperintensity in spinal cord from edema and mass

Modified with permission from Prata RG: Diagnosis of spinal cord tumors in the dog, Vet Clin North Am 7:165–185, 1977.

TABLE 6-10

Differential Diagnosis for Progressive Spinal Cord Disorders in Dogs

			INFLAMMATION		
Characteristic	**Spinal Cord Tumor**	**Degenerative Myelopathy**	**Meningitis and Myelitis**	**Discospondylitis**	**Hansen Type II Intervertebral Disk Disease**
Age	Adult too old	>8 yr	Any	Any	Middle age—older
Progression	Usually slow	Slow	Variable	Variable	Slow
Focal signs	Yes, unless metastatic; may be painful	T3-L3, not painful; L4-S3 and TL with LMN signs later in disease	Sometimes early, later progresses to other areas; frequently painful	Yes, may be multifocal; usually painful	Yes, may or may not be painful
Imaging survey radiography	Sometimes vertebral changes	Normal, frequently have spondylosis because of age and breed	Normal	Characteristic, osteomyelitis	May be normal, frequently have spondylosis because of age and breed
Myelography, CT, MRI	Defines extent: extradural, intradural, intramedullary	Normal	Normal spinal cord tissue hyperintensity on MRI	May demonstrate extradural compression, hyperintensity in bone on MRI, bony lysis on CT	Extradural compression at disk space
CSF	Increased protein, normal cells	Normal protein (variable), normal cells	Increased protein, increased cells	Variable, may be normal	Increased protein (variable), normal cells

cord, spinal nerve roots, or spinal nerves. Most tumors slowly compress the spinal cord, producing signs similar to those of degenerative myelopathy and type II disk disease (Table 6-10). Despite this, many affected animals have an acute onset of neurologic signs. Extradural tumors frequently cause signs of paraspinal pain, often before significant paresis occurs.[222,223] Intradural-extramedullary tumors are usually meningiomas or nerve sheath tumors and may be painful. Paraspinal pain usually is not a clinical feature of intramedullary spinal cord tumors. Sudden onset of neurologic dysfunction may be seen with intramedullary neoplasms affecting the spinal cord, presumably when blood vessels are compromised. Some tumors such as lymphoma may embolize arteries of the spinal cord. Certain tumors occur more commonly in specific regions of the vertebral column and spinal cord. Meningiomas[224,225] and nerve sheath tumors[226] commonly occur in the cervical region, whereas lymphoma in cats[227,228] and spinal nephroblastoma (neuroepitheliomas)[229] occur in the thoracolumbar region. In dogs, meningiomas are the most common primary spinal cord tumor. Although secondary in origin, lymphoma is the most common tumor to affect the spinal cord in cats.[227,230]

Diagnosis. Conventional radiography detects vertebral tumors that are lytic. Sometimes an enlarged vertebral canal or intervertebral foramina as a result of osteonecrosis form slow expansile tumors within the vertebral canal or intervertebral foramen, respectively. Myelography or CT/myelography is useful for delineating extradural, intradural extramedullary, and intramedullary involvement. MRI is the gold standard imaging modality for evaluation and characterization of vertebral and spinal cord tumors.[231] Analysis of CSF for spinal cord tumors often is nonspecific and reveals albuminocytologic dissociation.[232]

Treatment. In general, treatment involves surgery, radiation therapy, and chemotherapy, alone or in variation combinations depending on anatomic location, extent of disease, and histologic tumor type. A decompressive laminectomy procedure by itself will relieve clinical signs associated with compression. However, complete excision is often not feasible. Surgical resection is a viable option for some extradural and intradural extramedullary tumors.[222,224,225,233] Rarely, intramedullary tumors also can be resected using a myelotomy procedure. More often, surgical resection is used to provide decompression. Radiation therapy may be used for tumors not surgically accessible or as an adjunct to partial surgical resection.[234,235] Chemotherapy is used for hematopoietic tumors.[236] Corticosteroids are used as palliative therapy to reduce peritumoral edema and are also used with definitive therapies (e.g., in conjunction with surgery).

Primary Spinal Cord Tumors. Tumors affecting the spinal cord may be primary or secondary. Anatomically, these tumors can occur as intramedullary or intradural/extramedullary masses.[222,237-239] Intradural/extramedullary tumors may arise from nerve roots (nerve sheath tumors) or from meninges (meningiomas). Nerve sheath tumors, including schwannomas and neurofibromas, arise from nerve roots or peripheral nerves. As these tumors grow, they follow the nerve proximally to invade or compress the spinal cord, resulting in asymmetric neurologic signs caudal to the lesion. These tumors are further described in Chapter 5.

Meningioma. Meningiomas usually grow slowly and cause progressive compression of the spinal cord. The average age in dogs with meningiomas is 9 years (range, 5 to 14 years).[224] Although affected dogs tend to be large-breed dogs, no breed predilection exists.[240] Spinal meningiomas are the most common primary spinal cord tumors in cats older than 8 years of age.[227] The clinical signs reflect the spinal cord region involved. Paraspinal pain or signs of radicular pain may be evident. The clinical course usually resembles that of type II disk disease or degenerative myelopathy. Myelography or MRI is necessary for detection of extramedullary spinal cord compression.[224,241] With MRI, these tumors are isointense to hypointense on T1-weighted (T1W) images, hyperintense on T2-weighted (T2W) images, and demonstrate strong, uniform contrast enhancement.[230] These lesions should be surgically explored because many meningiomas can be completely or partially removed and therefore may be associated with prolonged survival after surgery.[224,225,233] Postoperative radiation therapy may be used adjunctively to prolong survival in dogs with incompletely excised tumors. Treatment with surgery and radiation therapy can result in a fair to excellent prognosis.[224] Surgical results are guarded when meningiomas are associated with intumescence involvement and tumors with ventral location and invasion of the spinal cord.[241]

Nephroblastoma. Spinal nephroblastoma (neuroepithelioma) is a unique intradural-extramedullary tumor that affects the T10-L2 spinal cord segments and has been reported in young dogs 6 months to 3 years of age.[242,243] GSDs may be predisposed.[243] Myelography shows an intradural extramedullary patten but MRI may be more sensitive for determining the extent of intramedullary involvement (Figure 6-22).[244] In most instances, spinal nephroblastoma occurs as a solitary lesion without renal involvement. Primary renal involvement is assessed by abdominal radiography and ultrasound.[245] Early detection is important for surgical resection. Prognosis is considered guarded if the tumor has invaded the spinal cord tissue. In some cases, gross resection is possible and can be associated with long-term remission of clinical signs.

Intramedullary Tumors. Primary intramedullary tumors originate from within the spinal cord tissue and include astrocytoma,[246,247] oligodendroglioma,[248] and ependymoma.[249,250] Metastatic tumors can metastasize to the spinal cord.[251] Initial signs may be unilateral; however, as the tumor grows, bilateral signs develop. Myelography can detect presence of these tumors based on a focal intramedullary pattern (Figure 6-23).

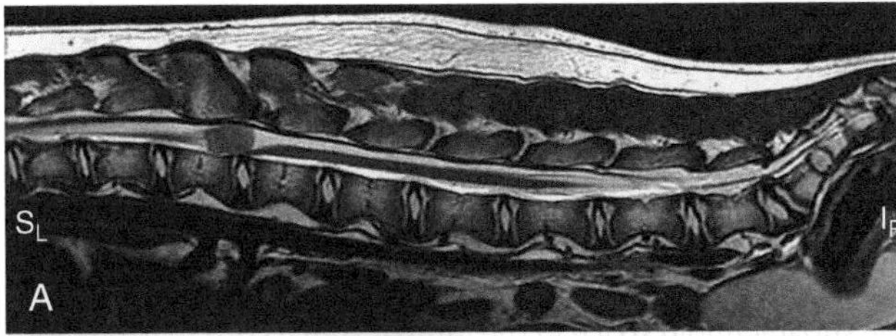

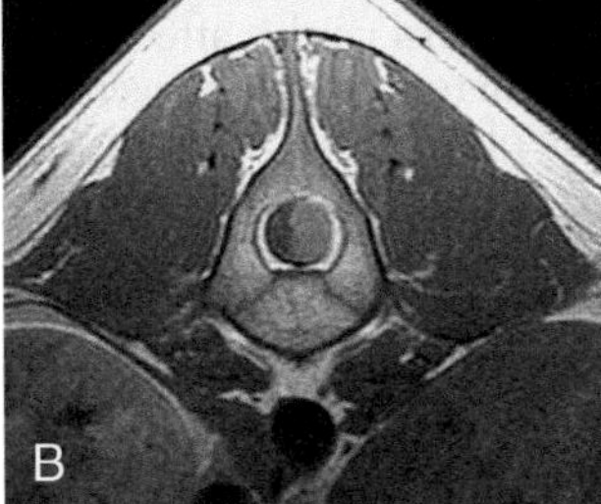

Figure 6-22 **A,** Sagittal T2W MRI from a 1-year-old Great Dane with progressive paraparesis demonstrating an intradural isodense mass over the L1 and L2 vertebrae. **B,** Transverse T1W postcontrast image demonstrating homogeneous contrast enhancement of the mass and compressing the spinal cord to the right. The mass was histopathologically confirmed as a nephroblastoma after surgical resection. (Copyright 2010 University of Georgia Research Foundation, Inc.)

However, MRI is much more sensitive in determining presence and lesion extent. The prognosis is poor because these tumors are generally inoperable, although newer microsurgical techniques may allow resection in some cases.[252]

Skeletal (Vertebral) Tumors. Vertebral tumors may be primary or may arise from metastases or invasion from adjacent structures.[253] Generally, as the tumors grow into the vertebral canal, the spinal cord is compressed slowly, producing signs of a slowly progressive myelopathy. Occasionally, the tumor causes considerable vertebral destruction without spinal cord compression. With severe vertebral involvement, the vertebrae may fracture, resulting in acute spinal cord compression and therefore an acute presentation. Vertebral tumors are usually painful because of periosteal and, perhaps, meningeal and nerve root irritation. Primary vertebral tumors include osteomas, osteosarcomas, fibrosarcomas, hemangiosarcomas, chondromas, chondrosarcomas (Figure 6-24), and hematopoietic tumors, such as plasma cell tumors (Figure 6-25) and lymphoma.[223,235] In small-breed dogs, osteosarcomas will commonly metastasize to the axial skeleton.[253] Conventional radiography of the spine is usually diagnostic for vertebral involvement but cytologic or histologic confirmation is necessary for definitive diagnosis. Other imaging modalities, such as CT or MRI, may provide more information on lesion location and extent.[223,231] Treatment is usually palliative, although total vertebra removal with vertebral column fixation has been advocated for certain primary vertebral tumors.[254] Malignant tumors may be surgically debulked and then treated with radiation therapy; this approach is also usually palliative.[235]

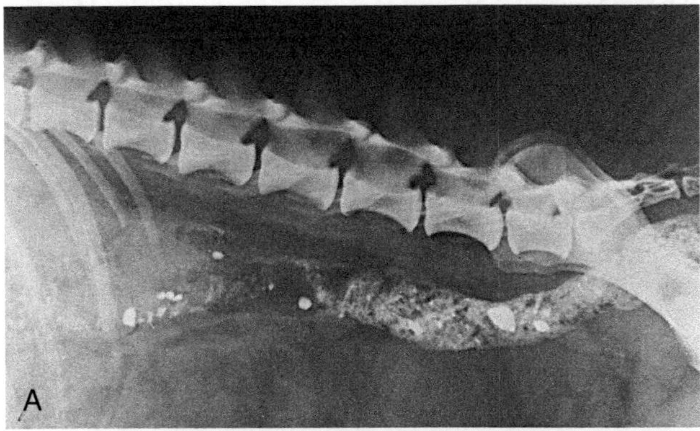

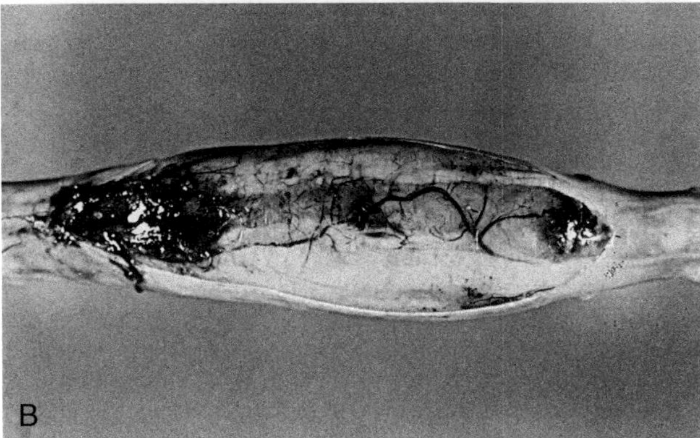

Figure 6-23 **A,** Lateral radiograph of a dog with progressive lower motor neuron paraparesis, constipation, and urinary incontinence. Note the enlarged vertebral canal of L4 and L5. These changes are characteristic of expanding intramedullary tumors. **B,** Spinal cord section from the same dog, which was affected with an intramedullary tumor. The expanding tumor produced the radiographic changes in **A.**

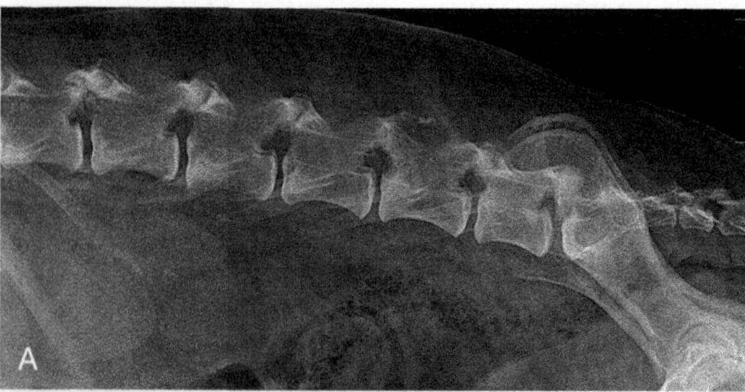

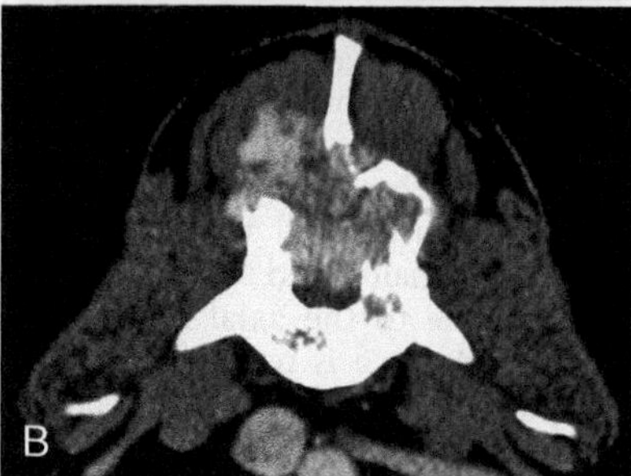

Figure 6-24 **A,** Lateral radiograph of a 10-year-old golden retriever with progressive lower motor neuron paraparesis and urinary retention. Note the lysis of the lamina extending into the dorsal spinous process of L6. **B,** Transverse CT image demonstrating the extensive osseous mass in the vertebral canal. A CT-guided biopsy confirmed chondrosarcoma.

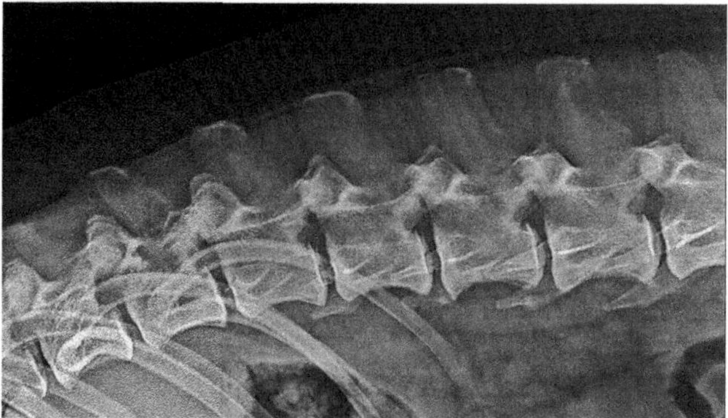

Figure 6-25 Lateral thoracolumbar radiograph of a 9-year-old rottweiler with paraspinal pain at the thoracolumbar junction demonstrating multiple areas of bone lysis in the T13 vertebra. These changes are characteristic for a plasma cell tumor.

Metastatic Tumors. Malignant tumors can metastasize or arise in adjacent anatomic structures and secondarily invade the vertebrae and spinal cord. A variety of carcinomas and sarcomas have been reported to metastasize to the vertebrae.[223,235] In dogs, mammary tumors, prostatic adenocarcinomas, thyroid carcinomas, and hemangiosarcomas are the tumors that most frequently metastasize to the vertebrae. Vertebral plasma cell tumors also may involve one or more vertebrae, sometimes producing multifocal signs.[236] Lymphoma and hemangiosarcoma are common tumors that frequently will metastasize to the spinal cord.[251] Spinal cord tumors can also be a result of spread in the CSF (drop metastasis) from other CNS locations, such as choroid plexus tumors, histiocytic tumors, and glioma that are in close proximity to the ventricular system. In general, neurologic signs related to vertebral tumors result from spinal cord compression secondary to vertebral instability

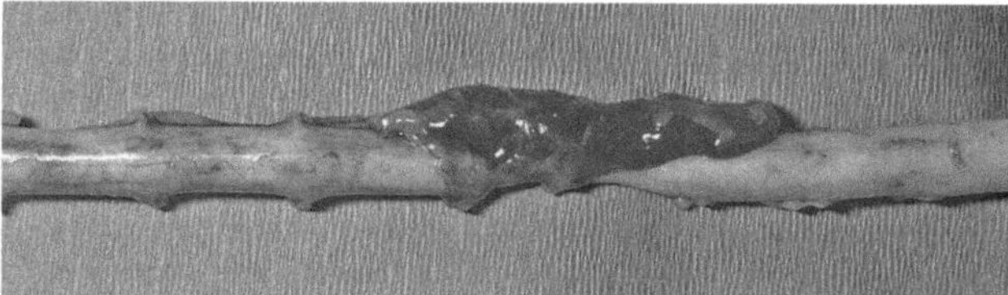

Figure 6-26 An extradural mass confirmed causing severe compression of the thoracolumbar spinal cord from a young cat with progressive paraparesis. Histopathology confirmed the mass to be lymphoma.

and pathologic fracture or direct compression by the neoplastic mass. Spinal radiography, CT/myelography, and MRI assist with determining a suspected diagnosis, localization, and lesion extent. These tumor types are confirmed by cytology or histopathology. Treatment usually is palliative.

Lymphoma. Lymphoma involving the vertebral canal and spinal cord is frequently encountered in cats[228,255] and cattle[256] but is uncommon in dogs[257] and horses.[258] Spinal lymphoma of cattle is caused by the bovine leukosis virus. Spinal lymphoma is the most common spinal tumor in cats.[227] Young male cats that test positive for FeLV may be at risk for spinal lymphoma.[228,255] Median age for cats with spinal lymphoma has been reported to be less than 2 years and 4.5 years by others.[227,228] The reason for the higher median age of cats with spinal lymphoma in later studies could be due to increased testing for FeLV and reduced incidence.

These secondary tumors grow in the vertebral canal and are often located in the epidural space. Tumor growth within the vertebral canal produces a compressive myelopathy. Several segments of the spinal cord may be involved, but lesions in the cat and cattle are most common in thoracolumbar segments (Figure 6-26). Spinal lymphoma must be considered in any cat or in older cows with a history of progressive neurologic dysfunction of the pelvic limbs.[256] However, lymphoma must be differentiated from other spinal tumors, IVDD, and the neurologic form of feline infectious peritonitis in cats with paraparesis.

In addition to pelvic limb GP ataxia and paresis, regional hyperesthesia may be present. Clinical signs of spinal lymphoma can be acute in onset. Radiographs are usually normal. Myelography, CT, and MRI may reveal extensive compression because the tumor may fill the vertebral canals of several vertebrae. Analysis of the CSF yields variable results. The CSF is normal when the tumor is outside the meninges. In some animals, the CSF may contain malignant lymphocytes and may have increased protein concentrations. Samples taken from the subarachnoid space in the lumbar spinal cord may be more diagnostic when the thoracolumbar spinal cord is affected.[232] In addition, PCR for analysis of antigen receptor rearrangement can be used to detect the presence of neoplastic lymphocytes in CSF.[259]

Lymphoma that is multicentric in origin requires full systemic examination to include CBC, biochemistry screening, radiography, abdominal ultrasound, retroviral screening, and lymph node and bone marrow aspirate.[257] The safest and most reliable method of obtaining a diagnosis of multicentric lymphoma in cats that involves the CNS is extraneural confirmation of lymphoma in another visceral organ.[227,260] Primary renal lymphoma in cats can relapse to the CNS.[261] Histopathology/cytology of tissue collected by fluoroscopically guided percutaneous fine-needle aspiration of epidural masses or surgical biopsy will establish a definitive diagnosis of the spinal involvement.[262] Combination therapy involving chemotherapy, radiation therapy, and surgical excision may result in remission in some cats.[228,255,260] Corticosteroids may temporarily alleviate some of the clinical signs caused by edema and spinal cord compression and induce a temporary remission. In general, prognosis for spinal lymphoma in cats is poor.

Acute Progressive Diseases, L4-S3

The acute progressive diseases that affect the caudal lumbar and sacral spinal cord segments are listed by etiologic category in Tables 6-4 through 6-6. Most of these diseases have been discussed in the previous sections that considered T3-L3 disorders. Remember that some of these degenerative diseases of the axons and myelin initially occur as pelvic limb paresis but may progress to involve the cervical spinal cord. Tetraparesis (tetraplegia) may develop as the disease progresses (see Chapter 7).

Acute Nonprogressive Diseases, L4-S3

Trauma and vascular are the most important of the various etiologic categories. In this section, diseases described are fractures involving the lumbosacral, sacral, and sacrococcygeal vertebral column, fibrocartilaginous embolism, and aortic thromboembolism.

Trauma

Fracture/Luxation of the Pelvis, and Caudal Lumbar, Lumbosacral, and Sacrococcygeal Vertebral Column. Pelvic fractures, caudal lumbar fractures, and lumbosacral subluxations are very common skeletal injuries in animals. Traumatic lesions in this area may involve the termination of the spinal cord or the cauda equina. These injuries may compress or entrap the roots of the sciatic, pelvic, and pudendal nerves, resulting in severe neurologic dysfunction of the pelvic limbs, urinary bladder, and anal sphincter (Figure 6-27). The diagnosis and management of sciatic nerve injury are discussed in Chapter 5.

Sacral and Pelvic Fractures. The assessment of sacral and pelvic fractures or lumbosacral subluxations must include a neurologic evaluation of the pelvic limbs, the external anal sphincter, and the urinary bladder and urethral sphincter function. The prognosis for recovery is much better in animals with normal neurologic function. Fractures medial to the sacral foramina (axial) frequently result in urinary or fecal incontinence, or both, loss of perineal sensation, and tail analgesia.[263] Fractures lateral to the sacral foramina (abaxial fractures) more frequently result in pelvic limb deficits.

Caudal Lumbar Fractures. Fractures of the L6 and L7 vertebrae are common where the vertebral column caudal to the fracture/luxation is displaced cranioventrally.[121] The spinal cord terminates cranially, so only spinal nerve roots and spinal nerves (cauda equina) occupy this region. Neurologic signs reflect damage to the sciatic, sacral, pelvic, and caudal nerves. Diagnosis is based on radiographic findings. Myelography or CT/MRI may be necessary to further establish spinal cord, spinal nerve root, or spinal nerve compression or damage. Spinal instability is assessed based upon the degree of vertebral damage.[136]

Treatment can involve conservative management or surgical stabilization. Conservative treatment can be successful if neurologic deficits are mild and there is little to no instability present.[147,264] Several surgical techniques of internal spinal fixation involving pins or screws and polymethylmethacrylate for management of caudal lumbar vertebral fractures have been reported.[131,146,151,265-267] External spinal fixation has been used successfully to facilitate stability and healing.[268] A dorsal laminectomy can evaluate for compression and spinal nerve root or spinal nerve integrity. Although considerable displacement may occur, the results of stabilization tend to be good if pain perception and micturition are intact.

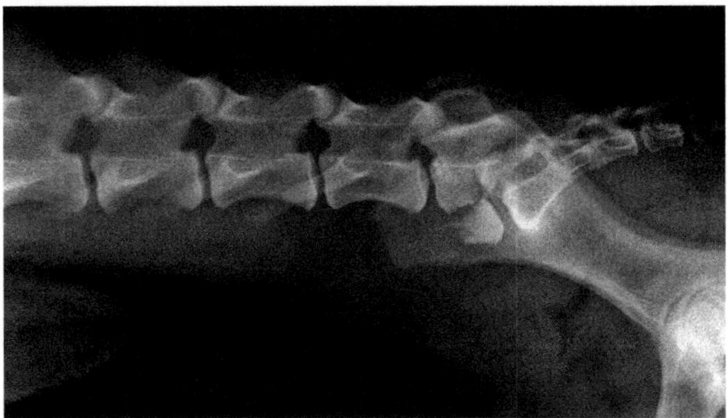

Figure 6-27 Vertebral body fracture and luxation of L7 in this 3-year-old mixed-breed dog produced sciatic nerve injury, tail anesthesia, and bladder atony. Prognosis is poor with the severity of neurologic signs.

Sacrocaudal (Coccygeal) Vertebral Fracture/Luxation. Sacral and caudal (coccygeal) fractures are common, especially in cats, but they also occur in dogs, horses, and cattle.[56,269] Sacrocaudal vertebral luxation can occur with tail restraint in horses and cattle. The syndrome in cats is usually caused by a traction injury at the sacrocaudal junction. Injury to the cauda equina and the sacral spinal cord results in loss of innervation to the tail, perineum, anal sphincter, and urinary bladder. Functional assessment of the anal sphincter affords a good indirect assessment of bladder function; however, some animals have normal anal sphincter function with no bladder function. The mechanism is not clear but may indicate intrapelvic injury to the pelvic nerves. Diagnosis is made by clinical signs and radiography. Tail amputation is recommended to prevent further traction injury to the lumbosacral spinal cord. Animals with absent pain perception (complete denervation) to the perineum with lack of anal sphincter, bladder, and urethral function have a grave prognosis. Cats that do not become continent within 1 month have a poor prognosis for regaining urinary function (see Chapter 3 for management of neurogenic bladder).[269]

Vascular

Fibrocartilaginous Embolic Myelopathy and Spinal Cord Infarction. Although fibrocartilaginous embolism can affect any spinal cord segment, it occurs most frequently in the caudal lumbar area and less frequently in the midcervical to caudal cervical spinal cord. For this reason, we have elected to discuss it with the other L4-S3 disorders. Fibrocartilaginous embolism has a brief progressive course (a few hours) and then becomes nonprogressive. We have therefore classified it as a nonprogressive disease.

Pathogenesis. Although emboli to the CNS can develop from a variety of sources such as endocarditis, sepsis, and fat, the most common form causing spinal cord infarction is a fibrocartilaginous material that histochemically stains in a manner similar to nucleus pulposus. The cause of this disease is unknown. Fibrocartilaginous embolic myelopathy occurs most frequently in dogs but also in horses, cats, pigs, sheep, and humans.[270-276] Fibrocartilaginous material found in arterioles and veins of the meninges and spinal cord results in an ischemic necrotizing myelopathy (Figure 6-28). Exactly how this material is distributed into the circulation of the spinal cord is not known, but several theories have been proposed. Most of these are based on the belief that fibrocartilaginous emboli originate from the intervertebral disks. The most probable mechanism is herniation of the nucleus pulposus into the body of the vertebrae, followed by entrance into an internal

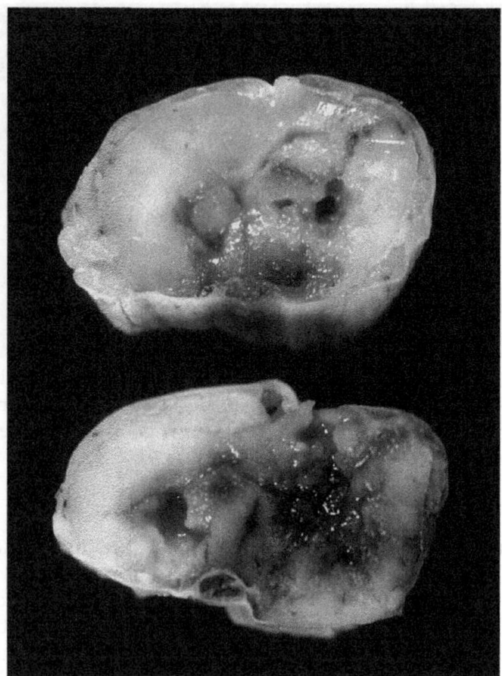

Figure 6-28 Adjacent sections of spinal cord from the lumbar intumescence from a Great Dane with acute asymmetric paraplegia resulting from histologically confirmed fibrocartilaginous embolism. Note the right side of the spinal cord is markedly necrotic and contains hemorrhage.

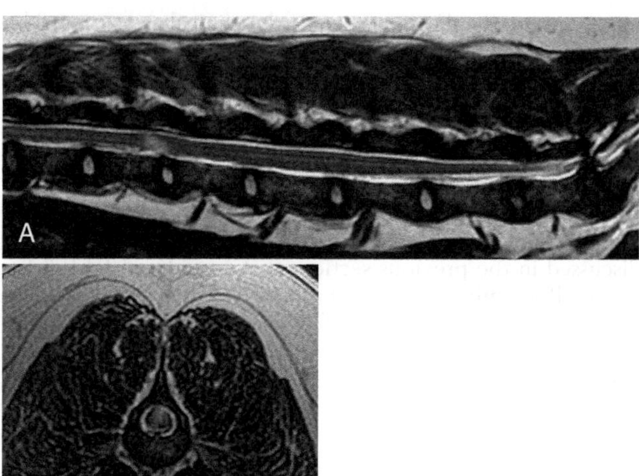

Figure 6-29 **A,** Sagittal T2W MRI of the lumbar spine from a young dog with acute onset paraplegia demonstrating hyperintensity in the spinal cord at the level of the L1-2 intervertebral disk space. **B,** Transverse T2W MRI at the same level demonstrating asymmetric hyperintensity in the spinal cord. A presumptive diagnosis of fibrocartilaginous embolism was made. (Copyright 2010 University of Georgia Research Foundation, Inc.)

vertebral venous plexus and then into an arteriovenous anastomosis. The material could then enter the spinal cord in arteries, veins, or both.[270,273]

Larger-breed dogs have been studied most intensely, but spinal cord infarction occurs in smaller-breed dogs as well. A breed predisposition may exist for miniature schnauzers, GSDs, and Irish wolfhounds.[277-280] Fibrocartilaginous embolism occurs more frequently in nonchondrodystrophic breeds. Interestingly, chondrodystrophic breeds with a predisposition for Hansen type I disk disease are affected infrequently.[281]

Clinical Signs. The key clinical features of fibrocartilaginous embolism are acute onset, nonprogressive course (except for the first few hours), and nonpainful, asymmetric paresis.[272,282] The clinical signs develop acutely and progress rapidly within 1 to 2 hours from initial pain to unilateral or bilateral paralysis. Spinal hyperesthesia may be present at onset of signs but is absent after the clinical signs stabilize. Trauma is not in the history, but dogs are frequently reported to be exercising at the time of onset. Asymmetry is not found in every case but is a valuable sign when present. Asymmetry is explained by the frequency of unilateral branches of the central branch of the ventral spinal artery. Lateralization of signs is very suggestive of fibrocartilaginous embolism because spinal cord compression generally causes bilateral signs. Although asymmetry may be present in disease processes that result in compression (e.g., IVD herniation), the asymmetry rarely is strikingly disparate as is often the case in a fibrocartilaginous embolism. With a fibrocartilaginous embolism, it is not uncommon to have one pelvic limb lack voluntary motor ability while the contralateral limb displays minimal deficits. Despite this presentation, bilateral signs also occur in a fibrocartilaginous embolism. The degree and character of the neurologic deficit correspond to the site and the extent of the spinal cord infarction. Infarction of gray matter of an intumescence may cause LMN signs in affected limbs. Absence of spinal hyperesthesia distinguishes embolic myelopathy diseases in which there is compression, such as Hansen type I IVDD, neoplasia, or vertebral fractures and disease processes in which there is inflammation such as meningomyelitis.

Diagnosis. Diagnosis is based on history, clinical findings, and exclusion of other causes. No definitive antemortem diagnostic procedure exists for fibrocartilaginous embolic myelopathy. The diagnosis is supported by evidence that rules out the presence of spinal cord compression. Survey radiography and myelography findings are usually within normal limits. The myelogram may show a slight swelling of the spinal cord for the first few days. The CSF may contain a slight increase in protein. MRI has become the imaging modality of choice for a presumptive diagnosis while excluding other causes. The MRI findings are characterized by focal, intramedullary, hyperintense lesions on T2W images with varying degrees of contrast enhancement (Figure 6-29).[283,284] Lesions are often present in a segment of the spinal cord overlying an IVD in which the nucleus pulposus has undergone degenerative changes resulting in a loss of signal intensity on T2W images. The severity of clinical signs is associated with the presence and extent of the lesion on MRI.[283,284] Animals should be evaluated for conditions such as hypertension and hypothyroidism that might predispose to CNS vascular occlusion and infarction.

Treatment. Corticosteroid therapy for fibrocartilaginous embolism is considered controversial. Corticosteroids such as methylprednisolone sodium succinate are aimed largely at reducing spinal cord edema and inflammation. However, a study revealed lack of significant association with corticosteroid administration and outcome.[284] Neurologic improvement may be noted within a few days, but functional recovery may require several weeks. Although rest is advocated, physical rehabilitation may have a positive role during the recovery phase.[272]

Prognosis. The clinical signs of complete paralysis, loss of pain perception, or LMN involvement have been associated with a poor prognosis.[272,282] If motor neurons are destroyed in an infarcted area of the spinal cord that innervates the limbs or bladder, the deficit is likely to be permanent. Because recovery from white matter damage is more likely to occur, animals with UMN deficits have better prognoses. Animals with functional recovery in 2 weeks seem to have a better prognosis.[282] Severity of neurologic signs and lesion extent on MRI are associated with outcome in dogs with ischemic myelopathy.[284] Many dogs, especially smaller dogs, make satisfactory recoveries, so early euthanasia is discouraged.

Aortic Thromboembolism (Ischemic Neuromyopathy). Thromboembolism of the aorta or iliac arteries occurs with moderate frequency in cats and occasionally in dogs and horses. In cats it is associated with cardiomyopathy.[285,286] Thrombi extend from the aorta into the iliac arteries. Vasoactive substances are believed to be involved in the pathogenesis of the ischemic changes. Clinically the syndrome is characterized by an acute onset with little progression. Pelvic limb pain and paralysis are common. The femoral pulses are weak or absent and the distal limbs are cool. Distal limb muscles are affected more than proximal muscles. Pain perception may be absent as a consequence of the ischemic neuromyopathy. Creatine kinase is markedly elevated early on after the embolic episode. Although functional recovery may be possible, recurrences are common, and cardiomyopathy must be considered.[286] In cats that survive, the average length for long-term survival is 11 months.[286] Surgical removal of the thrombus may improve recovery, but its efficacy is controversial. In dogs, the aortic thromboembolism may occur secondary to a hypercoagulable state associated with protein-losing nephropathies or hyperadrenocorticism. A similar syndrome is seen in performance horses. Associations with *Strongylus vulgaris* arteritis, thrombotic diseases, and cardiomyopathy have not been conclusively demonstrated.[56]

Chronic Progressive Diseases, L4-S3

Degenerative

Degenerative Lumbosacral Stenosis (Cauda Equina Syndrome). Compression of the cauda equina at the lumbosacral articulation is relatively common and has been reported in dogs of various ages and breeds.[287] Degenerative lumbosacral stenosis (DLSS) is also being recognized with increasing frequency in the cat.[288] In several studies, middle-aged to older large-breed dogs, such as GSDs, Labrador retrievers, border collies, or crossbreeds were affected more frequently.[289-293] The male:female ratio in GSDs is 2:1.[290,291] Sometimes DLSS in dogs is not recognized because of occurrence of other musculoskeletal problems in these breeds.[294-296]

Pathogenesis. Stenosis of the lumbosacral canal is caused by a combination of anatomic factors causing compression of the cauda equina.[287,294,297,298] Stresses on the annulus fibrosus lead to proliferative changes and IVD protrusion. This is a Hansen type II IVD degeneration with additional changes in the articulations and vertebral end plates. Narrowing of the IVD space causes the intervertebral foramen to be smaller. When osteophytes are around the foramen, the L7 spinal nerve is entrapped (Figure 6-30). In some cases ventral displacement of the sacrum occurs relative to L7, further narrowing the vertebral canal. Proliferation of the soft tissues of the joints, annulus fibrosus, and interarcuate ligament further contributes to the compression. Extension of the joint causes additional folding of these tissues, thereby increasing pressure on the nerve roots (Figure 6-31).[197]

Predisposing factors for DLSS include congenital vertebral abnormalities.[299] The high incidence in GSDs suggests a developmental predisposition, even though the clinical signs tend to occur in older dogs. Lumbosacral transitional vertebrae are congenital abnormalities of the spine with the vertebrae having characteristics of both spinal segments and can be symmetric or asymmetric. In dogs, lumbosacral transitional vertebrae have been associated with both hip dysplasia and

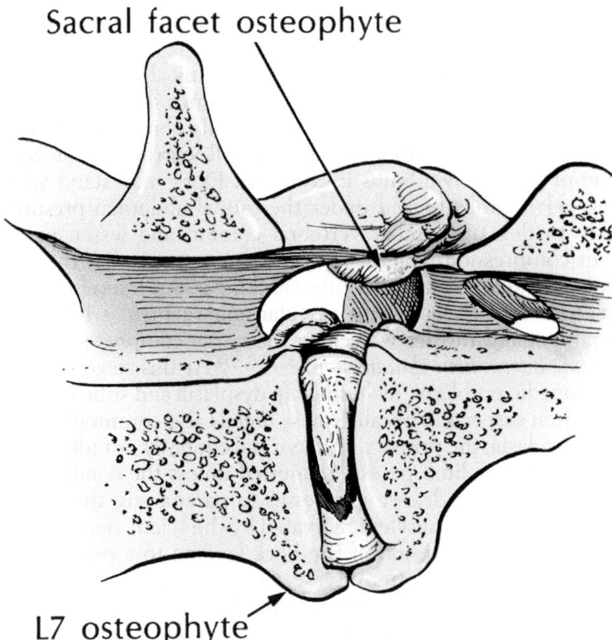

Figure 6-30 Degenerative lumbosacral stenosis. Compromise of intervertebral foramen by articular osteophytes that have formed on facet and vertebral body. (From Chambers JN: Degenerative lumbosacral stenosis in dogs, Vet Med Rep 1:166–180, 1989.)

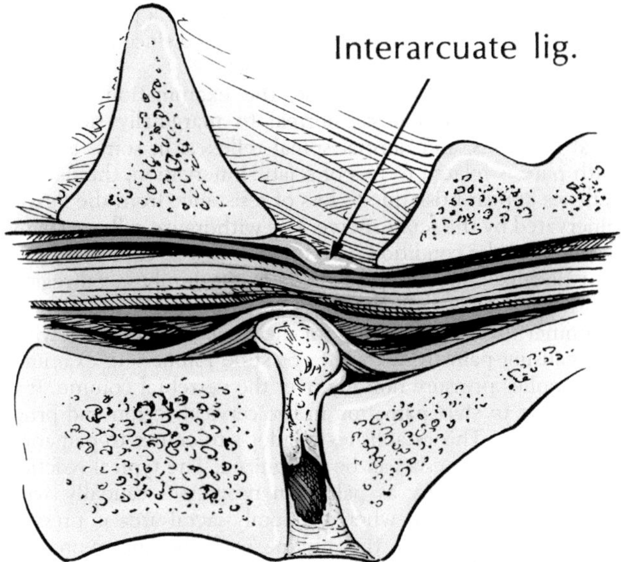

Figure 6-31 Degenerative lumbosacral stenosis. Compression of the cauda equina in a sagittal plane by the combined effects of disk herniation and ventral folding of the interarcuate ligament. Note how extension would increase the compression. (From Chambers JN: Degenerative lumbosacral stenosis in dogs, Vet Med Rep 1:166-180, 1989.)

DLSS.[300,301] Additionally, smaller facet angles of the joints of the lumbosacral articular processes may be a predisposing factor.[292] A related common initiating factor for the degenerative changes is probably abnormal motion at the lumbosacral articulations.[302,303] The biomechanical abnormality causes cumulative microtrauma, resulting in proliferation of fibrous connective tissue and osteophytes. A few animals appear to have a narrow canal with shortened pedicles, suggesting a developmental stenosis.[303]

Clinical Signs. The most common clinical sign of DLSS is caudal lumbar pain. Dogs may experience difficulty rising, and at this stage the clinical signs are easily confused with hip dysplasia or other orthopedic disorders. Recurring lameness of one or both pelvic limbs is common. Dogs may stand with the pelvic limbs tucked under the caudal abdomen presumably to flex the lumbar vertebral column and lessen nerve root compression. The owner frequently reports that the dog does not jump or has difficulty climbing stairs. Exercise often exacerbates the signs with vascular engorgement within the foramen, and further worsening the nerve compression, *neurogenic intermittent claudication*.[287,295,304] At this stage, various orthopedic problems, including hip dysplasia and stifle disease, are often suspected. Because these breeds also commonly have hip dysplasia, the primary problem is frequently not identified initially. Pelvic limb paresis is unusual unless the condition is advanced. If the disease progresses to paraparesis, the weakness involves the muscles innervated by the sciatic nerve, causing decreased extension of the hock leading to a plantigrade stance. Only in the latter disease stage are significant postural reaction deficits present. A few animals appear to have paresthesia in the tail or perineal region and may lick or chew the affected area. Frequently the owner may notice an altered tail carriage.

Abnormalities in urination and fecal incontinence are commonly associated with clinical signs attributed to compression of the sacral nerves.[305] The anal sphincter may be atonic, and the perineal reflex may be weak or absent. The urinary incontinence is of the LMN type with overflow incontinence. The bladder is flaccid and distended as a result of a poor detrusor reflex. The sphincter tone is still maintained since innervation by the hypogastric nerve remains intact.

Early in the disease course, the examination indicates lameness without paresis, normal to marginally slow postural reactions, and normal spinal reflexes. In some animals with paresis related to loss of sciatic innervation, the patellar reflexes appear brisk due to loss of resistance from the flexors innervated by the sciatic nerve. The withdrawal reflex remains intact until the condition is severe. The key to clinical diagnosis is localization of hyperesthesia in the lumbosacral region. More than 90% of affected dogs are in pain.[289-291,297,306] The examiner must elicit pain from the lumbosacral region without causing pain from the hip or stifle joints. The examiner first applies pressure dorsally over the vertebral column. It is preferable to start palpation in the cervical region and progress caudally. This establishes the dog's tolerance to palpation so that hyperesthesia can be recognized. The typical reaction is increasing anxiety as palpation progresses caudally, with a significant reaction when the lumbosacral area is pressed. Placing the thumbs on the midline, with the fingers on each ilium, allows the examiner direct pressure at the correct location without stressing the dog's hips.[294] If this fails to elicit a reaction, the tail is elevated with continued pressure on the lumbosacral region. Each pelvic limb can also be extended caudally to stress the lumbosacral articulation even further. Remember, extension of the lumbosacral articulation causes maximal compression and pain. Extension of the hips also may cause pain if hip dysplasia is present; however, abduction and rotation of the hips should also cause pain in hip dysplasia but not stress the lumbosacral junction. The animal can be placed in a laterally recumbent position to minimize stress placed on the hip and stifle joints and the palpation procedure is repeated. By rectal palpation, pressure can be applied to the ventral aspect of the lumbosacral IVD space. Motor dysfunction varies with severity of neural tissue compression. These techniques enable comparison between the dog's response to lumbosacral extension and response to hip manipulation and enable the examiner to distinguish degenerative lumbosacral stenosis from hip dysplasia.

Diagnosis. Degenerative lumbosacral stenosis must be differentiated from disease syndromes with similar clinical signs. These disorders include various causes of compression, such as trauma and neoplasia; inflammatory diseases such as discospondylitis and spinal empyema (abscesses); orthopedic diseases, such as arthritis, hip dysplasia, and cranial cruciate disease; and spinal cord diseases, such as degenerative myelopathy and IVDD. Correct localization is a critical first step in establishing a diagnosis as it rules out most of these diseases. Those that affect the cauda equina require additional diagnostic tests. Electromyography can be a valuable tool for mapping the distribution of denervation and localizing the lesion to specific nerve roots.[306,307]

Survey radiography is useful to rule out other causes of DLSS (e.g., discospondylitis and vertebral neoplasms). Abnormal findings that have been evaluated in dogs with DLSS include osteochondrosis of the sacral end plate,[194,298,308] transitional vertebrae,[309] spondylosis,[196] subluxation, sclerosis of the end plates, and bony proliferation of the articular processes. Stress radiography (extension and flexion) has been used to identify underlying instability of the LS junction. Controversy still exists as to the significance of these radiographic signs. A recent retrospective study of spondylosis deformans found higher rates of spondylosis at sites with type II IVD protrusions.[195] However, other studies have shown that spondylosis deformans is not consistently associated with clinical signs of DLSS.[310] Dogs with evidence of transitional vertebrae[301,309] or osteochondrosis[298] on survey radiographs have increased risk for development of DLSS. However, results of a recent study suggested that specific radiographic abnormalities may be of limited use to identifying working dogs that may be *at risk* for developing DLSS.[310] Myelography is a contrast procedure mainly used to rule out other causes of compressive myelopathies cranial to L4. Discography and epidurography are other contrast procedures that have been used in the past before cross-sectional imaging become available to evaluate for dynamic and compressive lesions within the epidural space of the LS region.[307,311]

CT and MR imaging have the advantage of better bone and soft tissue resolution, respectively. Transverse, dorsal, and sagittal planes provide determination of lesion extent. Both flexed and extended views are used to accentuate any abnormal compression and help establish the presence of a dynamic lesion, which may impact surgical treatment (Figure 6-32). The articular processes, intervertebral disk, and foramina also can be evaluated. Abnormalities detected by CT include: loss of epidural fat, increased soft tissue opacity in the intervertebral foramen, bulging of the intervertebral disk, thecal sac displacement, spondylosis, narrowed vertebral canal, thickened articular processes, and osteophyte formation of articular processes in the intervertebral foramen.[312-314] MRI is superior to CT with regard to soft tissue definition of the associated neural and ligamentous tissues.[194,287,292,315] The spinal cord, cerebrospinal fluid, intervertebral disks, ligaments, and nerve roots can be directly visualized. MRI can provide early recognition of intervertebral disk degeneration. Importantly, imaging findings based on CT and MR may be disparate when compared with the severity of clinical signs and predicting the surgical outcome.[316] Consequently, imaging findings should not be used in formulating the prognosis. See Chapter 4 and the references for additional discussion and for imaging techniques.

Treatment. The management of DLSS is based on an evaluation of the severity and duration of the clinical signs. Indications for conservative management include the first episode of

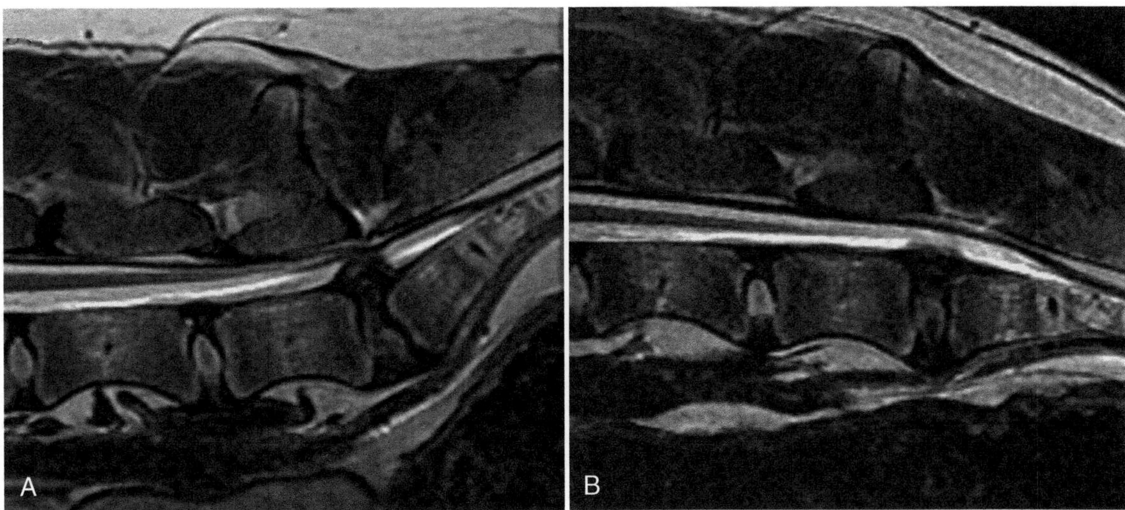

Figure 6-32 **A,** Sagittal T2W MR image of the caudal lumbar spine in extension of a German shepherd dog with hyperesthesia over the lumbosacral spine demonstrating dorsal and ventral compression of the cauda equina and loss of hyperintensity of CSF in the thecal sac. Note the IVD degeneration of the L6-L7 and L7-S1 disk. **B,** Sagittal T2W MR image from the same dog with the spine in flexion. This thereby demonstrates a dynamic lesion of the lumbosacral disk space. (Copyright 2010 University of Georgia Research Foundation, Inc.)

clinical signs or when the pain is intermittent. Confined rest for 4 to 8 weeks and pain management are recommended for dogs with an initial episode of only pain. The recovery rate with conservative management is between 24% and 50%.[291] Signs often recur when exercise is resumed. Injection of methylprednisolone sodium acetate injections into the lumbosacral epidural space results in clinical improvement in 79% and complete resolution of signs in 53% of affected dogs.[293]

Indications for surgical management include failure of conservative management, severe pain, and severe neurologic deficits (in particular incontinence). Choices of surgical procedures include dorsal decompression, discectomy, facetectomy, foraminotomy, and fixation-fusion.[287] The dorsal laminectomy procedure allows decompression and visualization of the cauda equina (Figure 6-33).[294,297,317] The nerve roots can be retracted laterally for visualization of the disk for annular fenestration. It is important to preserve the articular processes because sacrifice of these structures may destabilize the lumbosacral articulation. A lateral approach that minimizes bony removal of the processes has been developed for foraminotomy.[318] Dorsal laminectomy alone provides relief of pain in most dogs. Short-term outcome success using a decompressive laminectomy procedure ranges between 41% to 78%.[194,290,292,297,319] Recent attention also has been paid to biomechanical implications associated with decompressive procedures. Studies have shown that laminectomy alone does not cause instability of the lumbosacral articulation, but the addition of diskectomy reduces stiffness and the further addition of removal of the articular processes is likely to have devastating consequences to stability of the lumbosacral articulation. Dorsal stabilization procedures include distraction-fusion, fusion, lag screw articular processes, and Kirschner techniques.[320,321] The purpose of the distraction-fusion technique is to enlarge the collapsed disk space and intervertebral foramina (Figure 6-34). The lag screw technique has the potential to distract but may further weaken and fracture the articular process if not properly placed.

Postoperative care includes meticulous attention to the maintenance of bladder function if this is a problem (see Chapter 3). Exercise should be restricted for at least 6 weeks. Dogs that become active too early often have recurrent episodes of

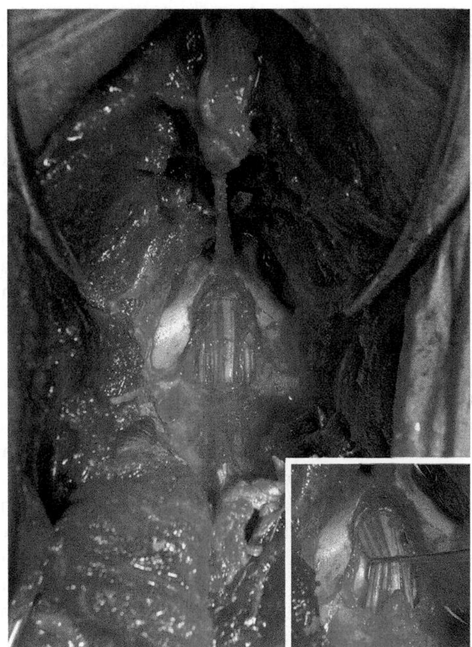

Figure 6-33 An intraoperative photograph after performing a dorsal laminectomy exposing the cauda equina. The inset demonstrates mild retraction of the nerve roots exposing annular protrusion of the L7-S1 disk. Note that the articular processes are preserved. (Copyright 2010 University of Georgia Research Foundation, Inc.)

pain. Nonsteroidal analgesics may be given to reduce pain during the postoperative period. Prognosis depends on the severity and duration of signs. Dogs with pain as the only sign have an excellent prognosis for complete recovery, although they may experience episodes of discomfort after vigorous exercise.

Prognosis. Prognosis is fair to good if clinical signs improve with surgery and with early surgical intervention. Recurrence rates for degenerative lumbosacral stenosis vary between 3% and 18% in the working dog.[290,319] Working dogs

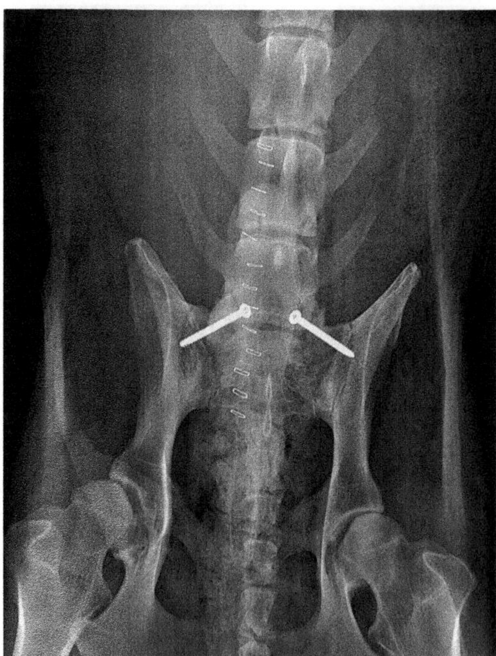

Figure 6-34 Ventrodorsal radiograph of the lumbosacral spine after a dorsal laminectomy and stabilization of the lumbosacral spine with screws placed in the articular processes along with a bone graft for fusion. (Copyright 2010 University of Georgia Research Foundation, Inc.)

that are younger at time of onset and have mild signs have a good prognosis with surgical decompression alone; however, recurrence still may be seen.[322] Dogs with severe neurologic deficits, and urinary and fecal incontinence for more than a few weeks before surgery have a guarded to poor prognosis.[319] Other reported recurrence rates have varied with relation of activity level of the dog, with the active working dog having a higher level of recurrence.

Anomalous

Vertebral Column and Spinal Cord Malformations. Spinal cord and vertebral anomalies are classified based on embryologic origin of the tissue.[323,324] Tissues of mesodermal origin are the vertebral body and intervertebral disk. Tissues originating from the ectoderm include the dorsal arch of the vertebra, spinal cord, and meninges. Mesodermal anomalies commonly involve failure of the vertebra to separate or fuse. Malformations involving the spinal cord are referred to as myelodysplasia. There are reviews of vertebral and spinal cord for dogs,[324] cats,[325] sheep,[326] pigs,[327] cattle,[328] camelids,[329] and horses.[330] [56,331] Vertebral/spinal cord anomalies are usually congenital, may have known or unknown inheritance, are acquired from in utero exposure to toxins or nutritional deficiencies or excesses, or occur sporadically. Also vertebral anomalies can result from perinatal trauma during the birth process. In large animals, arthrogryposis can occur secondary to spinal cord anomalies. Some anomalies are considered complex, involving developmental defects of both the vertebra and spinal cord that result in secondary abnormalities of the spinal cord and vertebral column. See Table 6-11 for a summary of abnormalities and classifications.

Vertebral Anomalies. Vertebral anomalies of the thoracolumbar vertebral column are common in dogs with a screw tail, such as the English and French bulldogs and the Boston terrier (Figure 6-35).[323] They are reported in other species, especially the cat.[325] Vertebral malformations have been recognized as a global problem in Holstein cattle.[332] Incomplete separation of the vertebral bodies, arches, or entire vertebra is called *block vertebrae*. *Hemivertebra* is potentially of clinical importance. Failure of ossification of one half of the vertebral body may cause the development of unilateral, dorsal, or ventral hemivertebra. Unilateral hemivertebra causes scoliosis, dorsal hemivertebra causes kyphosis, and ventral hemivertebra causes lordosis (Figure 6-36). A *butterfly vertebra* has a sagittal cleft in the vertebral body. These anomalies are most common in the thoracic vertebral column and rarely cause clinical signs. Dorsal displacement of a ventral hemivertebra may induce chronic progressive spinal cord compression. Vertebral intermediates of two adjacent segments of the vertebrae are called *transitional vertebrae*. Cervicothoracic transitional vertebrae have transverse processes that resemble ribs. Thoracolumbar transitional vertebrae may also have spinous processes resembling ribs, absence of a rib on one side, or fusion of the last rib like a transverse process. The major significance is in the location of the correct interspace in spinal surgery, where the T13-L1 interspace is identified as a landmark from which the affected site can be correctly identified. The last lumbar vertebra may fuse with the first sacral vertebra bilaterally or unilaterally. Unilateral sacralization may cause deviation of the pelvis and possibly nerve root entrapment. The appearance of transverse processes on the first sacral vertebra is called *lumbarization* and may lead to instability (see DLSS section).

Vertebral anomalies involving the cervical vertebral column such as atlantoaxial subluxation and occipitoatlantoaxial malformation are discussed in Chapter 7.

Spina Bifida. Spina bifida is the incomplete closure or fusion of the dorsal vertebral arches. Spina bifida may affect any vertebra but is most common in the caudal lumbar and sacral areas. In some cases it occurs in association with protrusion of the meninges (meningocele) or the spinal cord and meninges (meningomyelocele) through the vertebral defect (spina bifida cystica). These defects are forms of myelodysplasia also known as spinal dysraphism. Often these meningeal or spinal cord protrusions adhere to the skin where the neuroectoderm failed to separate from other ectodermal structures. The adhesions may produce a small depression or dimple in the skin at the site of attachment (Figure 6-37). In some cases this defect is open and spinal fluid leaks onto the skin, producing epidermal ulceration (spina bifida aperta). Because the meninges are exposed in this situation, meningitis may develop. In most cases that have been investigated, the caudal and some of the sacral nerves are either severely attenuated or incomplete. Spina bifida manifesta is termed when there are associated clinical signs. Other associated anomalies may include myeloschisis, tethering of the distal spinal cord, and hydrocephalus.[333] Spina bifida is most common in the Manx cat and the bulldog as a result of sacrocaudal dysplasia but can occur in all species.[334-337] Rachischisis occurs when the vertebral canal is open in its entire length and the spinal cord is exposed.

Clinical signs range from clinically silent (spina bifida occulta), to mild, to occasionally severe depending on the severity of the involvement of the spinal cord or the cauda equina. Some animals have signs similar to those of spinal dysraphism. In the bulldog with spina bifida of the sacrum, clinical signs often are related to dysfunction in the areas innervated by the cauda equina.[338] Mild to moderate pelvic limb ataxia and paresis may be present. Many animals have decreased innervation of the muscles supplied by the sciatic nerve. The limb may be fixed in extension owing to the unopposed contraction of the quadriceps muscle. Affected dogs consistently have fecal and urinary incontinence, and pelvic limb paresis is usually present. Pain perception may be decreased in the perineal area and from the distal regions of the pelvic limbs.

TABLE 6-11

Summary of Vertebral and Spinal Cord Malformations in Domestic Animals

Abnormality	Description	Imaging Characteristics	Clinical Significance
Vertebral Body (Mesodermal Origin)			
Block vertebra	Abnormal segmentation of somites	Fusion of adjacent vertebrae	Incidental finding
Butterfly vertebra	A cleft in the vertebral body causing an indentation	Appears like a butterfly on a ventrodorsal radiograph	Incidental finding
Hemivertebra	Ossification failure of the vertebral body or displacement of somites	Wedge shape of vertebra	Can lead to scoliosis, lordosis, and kyphosis with secondary instability and compressive myelopathy
Transitional	Characteristics of adjacent regions of the vertebral column, which occur at the cervicothoracic, thoracolumbar, lumbosacral, and sacrocaudal junctions	Lumbarization of T13 or S1, sacralization of L7	Incidental finding; lumbosacral transitional vertebrae may be predisposed to degenerative lumbosacral stenosis
Atlantoaxial subluxation	Hypoplasia or aplasia of the odontoid process (dens)	Absence or shortening of dens; displacement of the axis into the vertebral canal	Can lead to spinal instability and compressive myelopathy
Occipitoatlantoaxial malformation	Developmental defect in formation of atlanto-occipital joint	Fusion of atlas to occipital bones and shortening of axis with malformation of dens	Can lead to displacement of the axis into the foramen magnum and spinal instability and compressive myelopathy and secondary syrinx formation
Vertebral Arch and Spinal Cord			
Spina bifida occulta	Bony defect involving only incomplete closure of the vertebral arch; overlying skin is normal	Defect of fusion of spinous process	Incidental finding
Spina bifida cystica	Meningocele or meningomyelocele concurrent with bony defect	Herniation of the meninges from the vertebral canal through the bony defect; may see skin dimple or thin membrane	Meningomyelocele manifests signs of myelopathy
Spina bifida aperta	The above lesions communicate with the environment	Lack of skin over defect	Leakage of CSF and meningitis
Rachischisis	Vertebral canal is open over its entire length	Spinal cord is exposed and deformed	Not compatible with life
Sacrocaudal dysgenesis	Defect in formation of sacral and caudal vertebrae and spinal cord segments	Varying degrees of spina bifida occulta, cystica, aperta	Neurologic impairment involving sacral nerves
Syringomyelia	Syringomyelia—fluid-filled cavitation and no communication with central canal	Intramedullary fluid accumulation	Can be occult or clinical; associated with scoliosis and Chiari malformation
Hydromyelia	Dilation of the central canal	Intramedullary fluid accumulation	Can be occult or clinical
Other myelodysplasias	Duplication of spinal cord in vertebral column—diplomyelia Duplication of vertebral column—diastematomyelia Segmental hypoplasia or aplasia Absence of median fissure	Unknown	Varying degrees of myelopathy that may or may not be compatible with life

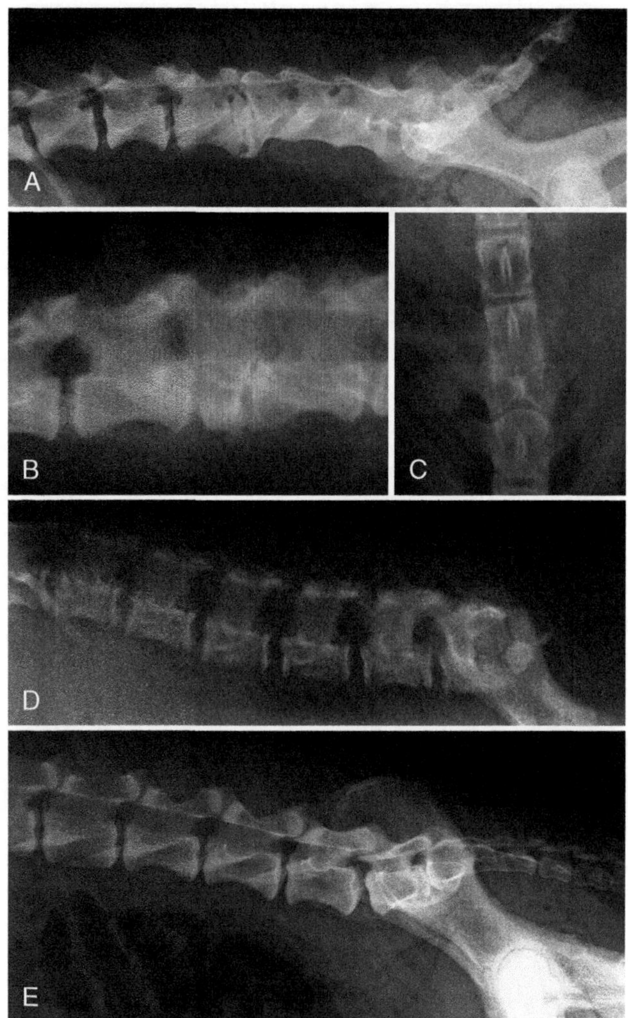

Figure 6-35 Composite of radiographic images demonstrating **A,** block vertebrae; **B,** hemivertebra; **C,** butterfly vertebra; **D,** sacral agenesis; **E,** transitional vertebra of S1.

Spina bifida without myelomeningocele is not associated with any neurologic deficits.

Spina bifida can be confirmed by radiography (Figure 6-38). The presence of meningocele and myelomeningocele can be determined myelographically or with MRI (Figure 6-39). MRI provides a more sensitive means of identifying the presence and extent of the lesion. No specific treatments are available for spina bifida. Surgical correction of the tethered spinal cord can be attempted in animals with intact urinary and fecal function (see Figure 6-37, *B*).[333] If there is extensive loss of normal nerve supply to the bladder and anus, recovery is unlikely in most of these animals. Meningoceles can be closed surgically to prevent the leakage of CSF and to prevent meningeal infection.

Spinal Dysraphism (Myelodysplasia). The dysraphic conditions are congenital defects that result from failure of normal closure of the neural tube. They may affect the brain or spinal cord, often with accompanying abnormalities in the surrounding bone and other tissues. Those affecting the vertebral column or the spinal cord in animals include spinal dysraphism, diplomyelia (duplicate spinal cord), diastematomyelia (duplicate vertebral canal), syringomyelia, spina bifida with or without meningocele, myelomeningocele, or myeloschisis and caudal vertebral hypoplasia (Figure 6-40).

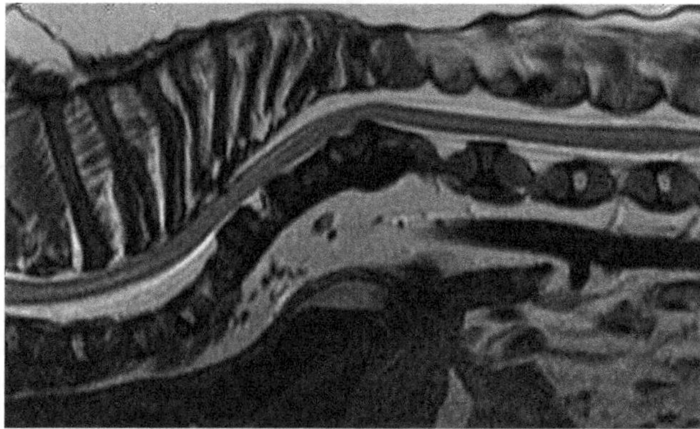

Figure 6-36 Sagittal T2W MRI from a young bulldog demonstrating kyphosis of the thoracic vertebral column and spinal cord. Note the spinal cord compression at T10-11.

Spinal dysraphism occurs in several breeds of dogs, cattle, and pigs but has been documented most frequently in the Weimaraner.[327,339,340] Changes within the spinal cord include absence, distention, or duplication of the central canal. Other changes include hydromyelia, syringomyelia, and anomalies of the ventral median fissure. Fluid-filled cavitations are commonly observed in dysraphic spinal cords, and spinal dysraphism, particularly in the Weimaraner, has been called *syringomyelia*. The fluid-filled cysts in the dysraphic spinal cords of Weimaraners probably result from abnormal vascularization that produces ischemia, degeneration, and cavitation. The thoracic spinal cord is most commonly affected. Because dysraphic lesions are the cause of the clinical signs, the term *spinal dysraphism* is preferred to the term *syringomyelia*.

Clinical signs become apparent at 6 to 8 weeks of age, although in mild cases the dog may not be presented for examination until it is several months old. The classic clinical signs include a symmetric hopping gait with the pelvic limbs (bunny hopping), a crouching posture, and a wide-based stance. Postural reactions in the pelvic limbs are abnormal, and the animal may occasionally knuckle over on the dorsum of the foot. The postural reactions are depressed. The spinal reflexes are usually normal, and exaggerated scratch reflexes may be present. Pain perception is usually intact. The neurologic signs are nonprogressive but become more obvious as the animal matures. Less common clinical signs include abnormal hair streams or hair whorls in the dorsal cervical area, kinking of the undocked tail, scoliosis, and depression of the sternum.

Diagnosis is based on typical clinical signs and the breed involved. Spinal radiographs and CSF analysis help eliminate the diagnosis of a treatable disease. Syringomyelia is detected by MRI. No effective treatment is available. Because the syndrome is probably inherited as a codominant lethal trait in the Weimaraner, owners are advised to cease breeding animals that have produced affected puppies.[341]

Syringohydromyelia in dogs often is associated with caudal occipital malformation syndrome (COMS—Chiari malformation) often will involve mainly the cervical spinal cord and is discussed in Chapter 7.

Sacrocaudal Dysplasia in Manx Cats. The Manx cat has been bred selectively to have a bobtail. These tail types have been classified as rumpy (no caudal vertebrae), rumpy-riser (fusion of several caudal vertebrae), stumpy (several caudal vertebrae that are mobile) and longie (normal tail).[334] Spinal cord anomalies include dysraphism, syringomyelia, meningocele, and myelomeningocele.[334,335,337] The Manx factor, or

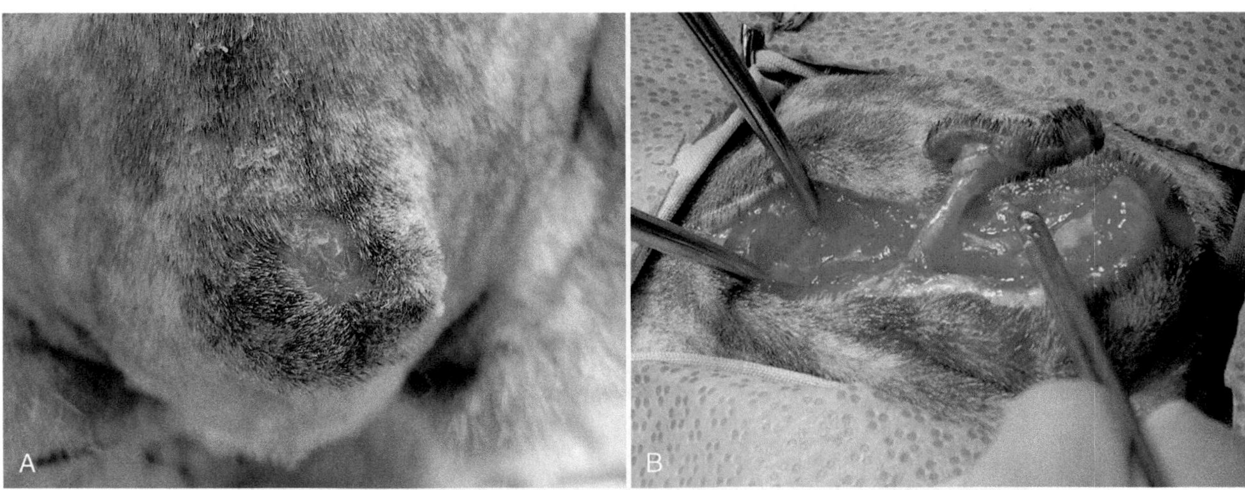

Figure 6-37 **A,** Photograph of a tail from a 12-week-old Manx kitten demonstrating a thin epithelial covering of a meningocele, which periodically leaked cerebrospinal fluid. **B,** An intraoperative photograph from the cat of a fistulous tract that extended from the skin lying over the caudal vertebrae into the thecal sac. The sacral nerves were unaffected.

taillessness, is apparently inherited as an autosomal dominant trait of incomplete penetrance.[335] In addition to caudal dysgenesis, sacral hypoplasia may occur. Spina bifida is also commonly encountered in this breed.

The neurologic signs are related to abnormal development and tethering of the nerves in the cauda equina as the cat grows. The clinical signs are present from birth and are nonprogressive. These signs include LMN deficits to the anus, the urinary bladder, and the pelvic limbs. Urinary and fecal incontinence and fecal retention are major problems. Undoubtedly a certain degree of spinal dysraphism is present in these so-called normal cats. Severely affected cats have pelvic limb paresis or paralysis. Primary uterine inertia has also been observed. The diagnosis is based on the breed, the clinical signs, and radiographic evidence of sacrocaudal abnormalities (see Figure 6-38). Therapy is directed at managing urinary and fecal retention. In some cases the filum terminale can be dissected free along with the fistulous tract (see Figure 6-37, *B*).[336,342]

Inflammatory

Although discussed in the section on acute progressive T3-L3 spinal cord disease, other inflammatory diseases of the vertebral column and spinal cord such as discospondylitis (Figure 6-41) can also affect the lumbosacral region of the vertebral column.

Neuritis of the Cauda Equina (Polyneuritis Equi)

Pathogenesis. Polyneuritis equi is a severe, slowly progressive granulomatous LMN disease that primarily affects adult horses. The neuritis of the cauda equina is usually restricted to the caudal spinal nerves and spinal nerve roots. The lesion is a demyelination with a granulomatous neuritis and meningitis involving the extradural components of the sacral and coccygeal nerve roots.[343,344] Cranial and peripheral nerve involvement may also occur in some cases, hence the term *polyneuritis equi*.[344-346] The lesion resembles allergic neuritis, and the evidence suggests that this is an autoimmune polyneuritis.[343] As in coonhound paralysis and Landry-Guillain-Barré syndromes, a factor such as a virus probably initiates the immune reaction. Although the cause is unknown, a history of vaccination or respiratory illness is reported in some cases.[347]

Clinical Signs. Early signs reflect a slowly progressive, symmetric deficit localized to the cauda equina. Clinical signs of hyperesthesia include tail rubbing and hypersensitivity to touch of the perineal area and are followed by urine scalding and constipation. Subsequent LMN signs include poor tail tone, paralysis of the tail, anus, rectum, and bladder. Thus animals often have fecal and urinary retention that subsequently cause colic and overflow urinary incontinence. Decreased sensory perception and anesthesia in the perineal area occur as the disease progresses. In male horses, pudendal nerve paralysis results in a dropped penis or the inability to retract the penis. Hypalgesia to the penis also may occur. Cranial nerves V, VII, and VIII are frequently affected. Thus signs such as head tilt, nystagmus, and facial paralysis may occur in some horses.

Diagnosis. If both the cauda equina and cranial nerves are affected, the diagnosis of polyneuritis is highly suspected. If only the cauda equina is involved, sacral fractures should be ruled out by rectal palpation and radiography. Abnormal findings on electromyography and evoked potentials may further support a localization to the cauda equina. Collection of spinal fluid at the lumbar cistern is often diagnostic of cauda equina neuritis. Cerebrospinal fluid analysis from the lumbosacral space is frequently xanthochromic and reveals moderately increased concentrations of protein (100 to 300 mg/dL) and cells (>100 cells/mm^3). The cytologic composition is mainly macrophages, neutrophils, and lymphocytes. High P_2 myelin antibody titers can be demonstrated by ELISA, but the test is not specific for polyneuritis equi.[348] Definitive diagnosis is based on histopathology.

Treatment. No specific treatment is known and the primary therapy is palliative. Evacuation of the bladder and bowel may allow the animal to live for prolonged periods; however, denervation of the genital tract precludes breeding stallions. The prognosis is usually poor.

Sorghum Cystitis and Ataxia

Pathogenesis. A syndrome of ataxia and bladder paralysis occurs more frequently in horses, and less often in cattle and sheep that ingest sorghum, Johnson, or Sudan grass. Lesions develop primarily in the lumbar, sacral, and caudal spinal cord segments. The histopathology is characterized by focal axonal degeneration and demyelination with associated lipid-laden macrophages. Neurotoxicity is suspected from chronic sublethal doses of hydrocyanic acid found in plants of the genus *Sorghum*. Production of a lathyrogenic principle (nitrile-related amino acid) has also been postulated.[349,350]

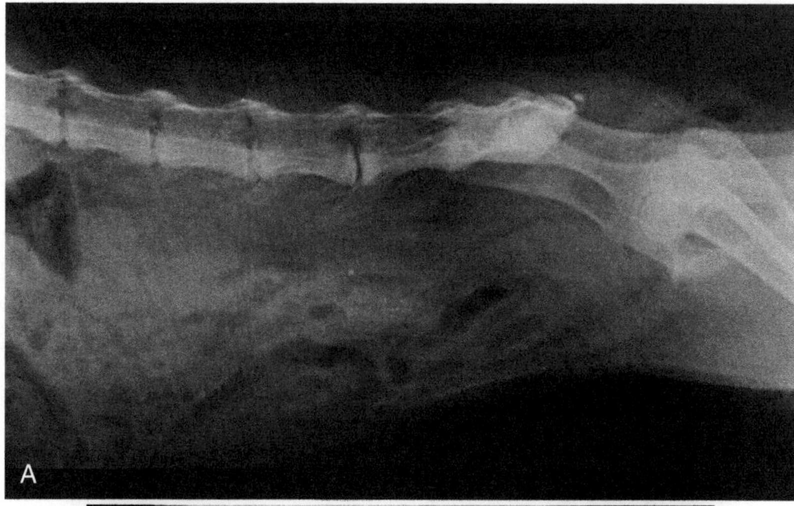

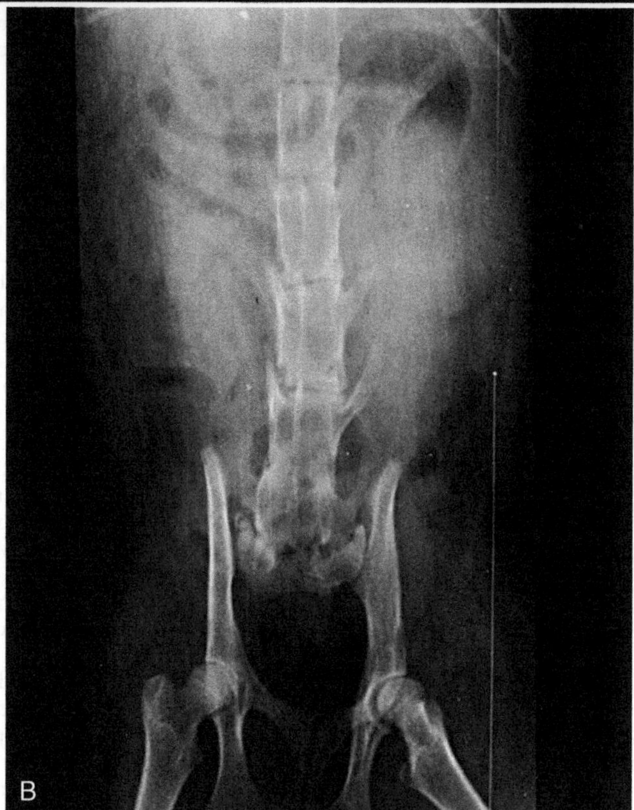

Figure 6-38 Lateral lumbosacral (A) and ventrodorsal (B) radiographs of a Manx cat with sacrocaudal abnormalities. Note the short, malformed sacrum and the absence of caudal vertebrae.

Enzootics of this disease occur in horses of all ages that graze in sorghum or Sudan grass pastures. The disease usually occurs when the plants are young and rapidly growing, but mature and second-growth plants also have been incriminated. Apparently the toxins do not persist in cured hay or silage.

Clinical Signs. Although the signs of urinary incontinence are most noticeable in many horses, neurologic signs involving the pelvic limbs and tail usually develop first. Signs include flaccidity of the anus and tail and pelvic limb ataxia. Occasionally, severe LMN paralysis of the pelvic limbs progressively develops over 24 hours from the first onset of weakness. In mares, clinical signs include continual opening and closing of the vulva and dribbling of urine. Urine scald and thick urine deposits occur on the buttocks, the thighs, and the hocks. Male horses drip urine from a relaxed and extended penis. Urinary incontinence is intensified when the animal is forced to move suddenly. Postural reaction deficits and hyporeflexia are detectable in the pelvic limbs. Clinical signs rarely extend to the thoracic limbs, even though brainstem and cerebral cortical lesions have been reported. Pregnant mares may abort, and these foals may have severe ankylosis (arthrogryposis). Arthrogryposis also may occur in full-term foals when the dam has grazed hybrid Sudan plants.

Diagnosis. The diagnosis is suspected from the history and the clinical signs. Affected horses have a severe fibrinopurulent cystitis secondary to neurogenic urine retention. Several

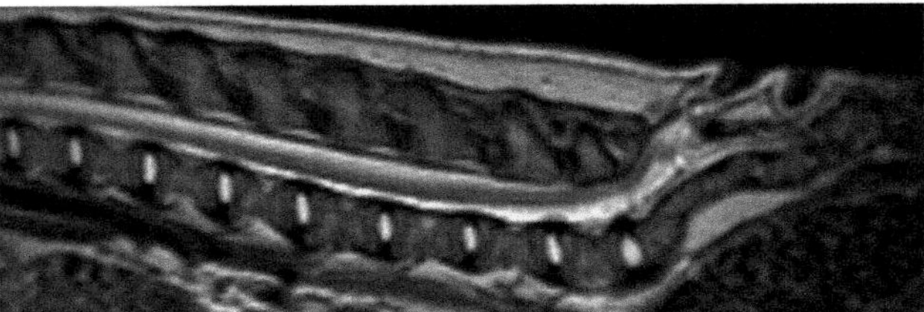

Figure 6-39 A sagittal TW2 MRI from a young bulldog demonstrating a meningocele over the sacral vertebrae.

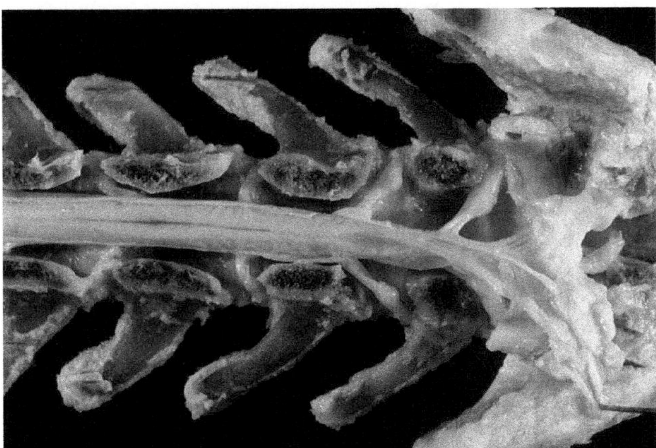

Figure 6-40 Caudal region of the vertebral column, spinal cord, and cauda equina from a 2-year-old female English bulldog with urinary-fecal incontinence since birth. Portions of the cauda equina extend dorsally into a meningeal sac, and a dorsal longitudinal spinal cleft is present. A diagnosis of meningomyelocele with associated myeloschisis was made. (From Kornegay JN: Lesions of the lumbosacral intumescence and cauda equina. In Slatter DH, editor: Textbook of small animal surgery, Philadelphia, 1985, WB Saunders.)

different bacteria have been isolated from the urine of affected horses. Some animals develop severe ascending pyelonephritis from the chronic cystitis. The sensory loss in the perineum is less than that from cauda equina neuritis or sacral fracture. Ancillary diagnostic tests are of little benefit. Mild changes in the CSF are found. Protein elevations are slight (60 to 80 mg/dL), and cell counts range from 5 to 10 mononuclear cells/μL. Urine or serum can be tested for high levels of thiocyanate, the major detoxification product of cyanide.

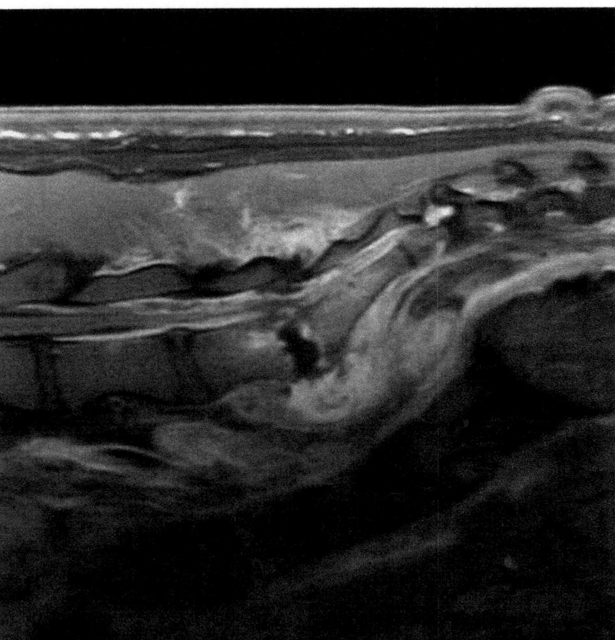

Figure 6-41 A sagittal postcontrast T1W MRI of the lumbosacral vertebral column demonstrating discospondylitis of the L7-S1 intervertebral disk space. Note the hyperintensity of the surrounding soft tissues. (Copyright 2010 University of Georgia Research Foundation, Inc.)

Treatment. Treatment involves removing the affected horses from pasture and supportive care. Improvement will occur slowly over several months. Bladder management includes catheterization and antibiotic therapy for the urinary tract infection. Horses should not be allowed to graze in sorghum pastures while the plants are rapidly growing or are stunted by drought. Plants are generally safe if they are yellow, are more than 2 feet tall, or have formed fruiting heads. Pastures can be checked periodically to determine the amount of cyanide present when toxic forage is suspected.

CASE STUDIES

CASE STUDY 6-1 *LUCY*

 veterinaryneurologycases.com

▪ Signalment
Canine, Labrador retriever, female, 6 years old.

▪ History
Two days ago, the dog suddenly cried out in pain and developed paresis in the pelvic limbs. Within 2 hours she became totally paralyzed in the pelvic limbs (PLs). No possibility of trauma was evident. The dog developed signs while under the owner's observation in the backyard.

▪ Physical Examination
No abnormalities were found other than the neurologic problem described in the next section. The bladder was full on palpation.

▪ Neurologic Examination
Mental status
Alert

Gait
Paraplegia; thoracic limbs normal

Continued

CASE STUDY 6-1 LUCY—cont'd

Posture
Normal, except gait

Postural reactions
Proprioceptive positioning absent in both PLs

Spinal reflexes
Left PL: patellar reflex decreased and withdrawal reflex decreased with decreased muscular tone of the limb. Muscle tone was increased in the right PL. Spinal reflexes were exaggerated in right PL. The perineal and cutaneous trunci reflexes were intact.

Cranial nerves
All normal

Sensory evaluation
Hyperesthesia—no pain elicited on spinal palpation
Superficial pain perception—intact
Deep pain perception—intact

▪ Lesion Location
This lesion localization is difficult to reconcile in one anatomic region. This dog has paraplegia characterized by (1) UMN paralysis in the right PL and (2) LMN paralysis in the left limb. There is no evidence of hyperesthesia. An asymmetric lesion best explains this localization. Signs in the left PL are consistent with L4-S1 spinal cord segments. However, one would expect that similar neurologic findings in the right PL. The lesion has spared spinal cord sensory pathways. Likewise, the lesion spared S2-3 as the perineal reflex was normal. Acute nonprogressive diseases should be considered.

▪ Differential Diagnosis
1. Fibrocartilaginous embolism
2. Intervertebral disk disease

▪ Diagnostic Plan
1. Spinal radiography to rule out bony lesion
2. Myelography/CT or MRI to rule out compressive myelopathy. MRI would be best to perform since an infarct is most likely based on lack of paraspinal hyperesthesia.
3. CSF analysis to substantiate infarction and rule out inflammatory disease processes

▪ Diagnostic Results
Spinal radiography was within normal limits. Sagittal T2W MRI sequences revealed intramedullary spinal cord hyperintensity extending from the L5 to L7 vertebrae; on axial T2W imaging, the hyperintensity was located in the area of the left gray matter of the spinal cord; there was no uptake of gadolinium contrast on T1W imaging.

▪ Diagnosis
Based on the history, neurologic examination, and MRI results, the most likely diagnosis is fibrocartilaginous embolism. This constellation of neurologic examination findings is common for dogs with fibrocartilaginous embolism. The UMN paralysis of the right pelvic limb remains unexplained by the anatomic location of the lesion.

▪ Treatment
Physical rehabilitation involving range of motion exercises and hydrotherapy was recommended. Bladder management required manual expression three times a day. The prognosis is guarded to fair based on deep pain perception. If the dog shows improvement in motor function within 2 weeks, the prognosis will be good. The dog started to regain movement in the PLs and voluntary micturition within 1 week.

CASE STUDY 6-2 GRETEL

 veterinaryneurologycases.com

▪ Signalment
Canine, dachshund, female, 7 years old.

▪ History
Two days ago the dog had a sudden onset of difficulty walking in the pelvic limbs and within 6 hours became paralyzed in both pelvic limbs (PLs). When the dog was examined initially, the PL reflexes were present, but pain perception was absent in both PLs. The thoracic limbs were normal.

▪ Physical Examination
Urinary incontinence, hematuria, and shallow abdominal respirations are present. The dog cries periodically as if it were in pain. Palpation revealed hypotonus in both PLs and a flaccid abdomen.

▪ Neurologic Examination
Mental Status
Apprehensive

Gait
No voluntary movements of PLs; short, choppy steps with thoracic limbs

Posture
Cannot maintain sternal recumbency

Postural reactions
Postural reactions were absent in both PLs. Postural reactions in the thoracic limbs were normal.

Spinal reflexes
Patellar reflex and flexor withdrawal reflex was absent in both PLs. The perineal reflex was absent. Anal sphincter tone was greatly reduced. The cutaneous trunci reflex was absent caudal to the T3 vertebra.

Cranial nerves
All normal

Sensory evaluation
Hyperesthesia—present at T2-T3 vertebrae
Superficial pain perception—absent caudal to the scapula
Deep pain perception—absent caudal to the scapula

CASE STUDY 6-2 GRETEL—cont'd

■ **Lesion Location**

Motor examination reveals severe bilateral LMN disease in both pelvic limbs and the pudendal nerve. The symmetry of the signs suggests severe disease in segments L4-S3. The sensory examination reveals complete analgesia caudal to the shoulders. This finding suggests a severe lesion extending cranial to the T3 vertebra. In addition, the LMN neurons to the abdominal and intercostal muscles are involved. Therefore, diffuse symmetric disease of the spinal cord caudal to T3 should be suspected. The history suggests lesion progression insofar as spinal reflexes in the pelvic limbs were present 2 days ago. The lesion involves both gray and white matter throughout the spinal cord caudal to T3 vertebra.

■ **Differential Diagnosis**

1. Ascending/descending myelomalacia secondary to spinal cord compression from type I IVDD

■ **Diagnostic Plan**

None—the history and neurologic examination findings essentially provide a definitive diagnosis. Given the prognosis, diagnostics are not pursued.

■ **Treatment**

The prognosis is hopeless and euthanasia is recommended. Necropsy revealed severe ascending/descending myelomalacia secondary to a herniated disk at T13-L1.

CASE STUDY 6-3 THOR

 veterinaryneurologycases.com

■ **Signalment**

Canine, German shepherd dog, female, 1.5 years old.

■ **History**

Six weeks ago, the dog became lame in the right pelvic limb (PL). Since then, paresis and GP ataxia have gradually developed in both PLs, more so on the right side than on the left. Three days ago the dog became completely paralyzed in both PLs.

■ **Physical Examination**

Findings are normal except for the neurologic problem.

■ **Neurologic Examination**

Mental status

Alert

Gait

Paraplegia; thoracic limbs normal

Posture

Paraplegia; but otherwise normal

Postural reactions

Postural reactions are absent in the PLs. Postural reactions in the thoracic limbs were normal.

Spinal reflexes

Patellar reflex is exaggerated; flexor reflexes present in both PLs. The cutaneous trunci reflex was absent caudal to L2.

Cranial nerves

All normal

Sensory evaluation

Hyperesthesia—paraspinal pain at L2-3
Superficial pain perception—absent caudal to L2
Deep pain perception—blunted caudal to L2-3

■ **Lesion Location**

The neurologic examination reveals bilateral UMN paralysis to both pelvic limbs, suggesting a lesion in spinal cord segment T3-L3. The clinical course suggests a progressive disease. Sensory evaluation suggests a lesion at segment L2-3.

■ **Differential Diagnosis**

1. Type II IVDD
2. Neoplasia
3. Meningomyelitis
4. Discospondylitis

■ **Diagnostic Plan**

1. Spinal radiography will determine presence of bony lesions, such as primary vertebral tumor or discospondylitis
2. Imaging with myelography/CT or MRI will identify compressive myelopathy; MRI is more sensitive for evaluating the spinal cord and lesion extent.
3. Cerebrospinal fluid will identify any evidence of meningomyelitis.

■ **Diagnostic Results**

Spinal radiography and myelography were normal. Myelography disclosed a pattern consistent with an intramedullary lesion at L1-2. CSF contained 1 WBC/mm^3, 33.5 mg/dL protein.

■ **Diagnosis**

Despite the dog's age, the lesion was consistent with a spinal cord neoplasm. Other differentials such as myelitis, intramedullary hematoma, and infarction were considered unlikely given the CSF analysis (myelitis and hematoma) and history (infarction). A presumptive diagnosis of spinal nephroblastoma was made based on signalment and lesion location. Depending on the invasiveness of these tumors, surgery may be performed. In most cases, gross excision of the tumor is not possible. However, the combination of surgery and radiation may provide long-term control in some cases. Before surgery, MRI may provide greater detail regarding the extent and invasiveness of the tumor. The prognosis is considered guarded.

■ **Treatment**

Corticosteroids were recommended for palliative treatment of edema and spinal pain. Euthanasia was eventually performed. A nephroblastoma at L1-2 was diagnosed on histopathology.

CASE STUDY 6-4 UGA

veterinaryneurologycases.com

▪ Signalment
Canine, bulldog, male, 7 weeks old

▪ History
Since he became ambulatory, the puppy has had a spastic, ataxic gait in the PLs. Urinary and fecal incontinence have been present for at least 2 weeks.

▪ Physical Examination
Urinary incontinence is present. No tone in anal sphincter. There was a small depression over the dorsal, midline area just cranial to sacrum.

▪ Neurologic Examination

Mental status
Alert, responsive

Gait
Ambulatory paraparesis with a bunny-hopping gait; normal in thoracic limbs

Posture
Wide-based stance in the PLs

Postural reactions
Proprioceptive positioning was absent in both PLs. Hopping and extensor postural thrust reactions were decreased in both PLs. Tactile placing was absent in both PLs,

Spinal reflexes
Patellar reflex was normal in both PLs. The flexor reflex was decreased to absent in both PLs. The perineal reflex was absent. The cutaneous trunci reflex was intact.

Cranial nerves
All normal

Sensory evaluation
Hyperesthesia—none
Superficial pain perception—absent in perineal area
Deep pain perception—present but decreased in tail

▪ Lesion Location
LMN signs with blunted pain perception suggest a bilateral lesion in the spinal cord segments L6-S2 or in the lumbosacral plexus. The urinary and fecal incontinence is explained by a lesion in this region. The age and the breed suggest an anomalous/congenital abnormality.

▪ Differential Diagnosis
1. Congenital/anomalous
   a. Spina bifida
   b. Spinal dysraphism
2. Trauma
3. Inflammatory (infectious)

▪ Diagnostic Plan
1. Radiography of the lumbosacral vertebrae to evaluation for vertebral anomalies
2. EMG of the perineal muscles
3. MRI of the lumbosacral vertebral column to detect spinal cord anomalies
4. CSF analysis to rule out inflammatory infectious diseases.

▪ Diagnostic Results
Radiographs revealed evidence of spina bifida involving the sacrum. MRI was performed and a meningomyelocele was demonstrated. EMG and CSF analysis were not performed.

▪ Diagnosis
The diagnosis was spina bifida with concurrent myelomeningocele.

▪ Treatment
None; the owners could not have a dog with urinary incontinence. The dog was euthanized.

CASE STUDY 6-5 TONTO

 veterinaryneurologycases.com

▪ Signalment
German shepherd dog, 7-year-old FS

▪ History
Five months before admission, the dog jumped off a retaining wall and was injured. She showed back pain and difficulty moving, which has progressively gotten worse. The dog was initially treated for a urinary tract infection after *E. coli* was isolated from the urine.

▪ Physical Examination
The dog is thin and vitals were within normal limits.

▪ Neurologic Examination

Mental status
Dull

Gait
General proprioceptive ataxia and paraparesis

Posture
Mild kyphosis

Postural reactions
Proprioceptive positioning is reduced in both PLs. Hopping reactions are decreased in both PLs. Thoracic limbs have no deficits.

Spinal reflexes
Patellar reflex was normal to increased in both PLs. The cutaneous trunci reflex was intact.

Cranial nerves
All normal

CASE STUDY 6-5 *TONTO*—cont'd

Sensory evaluation
Hyperesthesia—marked paraspinal pain in the cranial aspect of the lumbar vertebral column
Superficial pain perception—normal
Deep pain perception—not assessed

▪ Lesion Location

The neurologic examination reveals bilateral UMN paraparesis to both pelvic limbs, suggesting a lesion in spinal cord segment T3-L3. The clinical course suggests a progressive disease. The hyperesthesia suggests a lesion involving the cranial lumbar spinal cord segment(s). Structures that may be involved are those that are pain sensitive, such as the vertebra, meninges, nerve roots, and disk.

▪ Differential Diagnosis

1. Degenerative
   a. Hansen type II IVDD
2. Neoplasia
   a. Vertebral body—osteosarcoma, chondrosarcoma, fibrosarcoma
   b. Extradural—metastatic
   c. Intradural extramedullary—meningioma, nerve sheath tumor
3. Inflammatory (infectious/noninfectious)
   a. Discospondylitis
   b. Meningomyelitis—GME, bacterial, rickettsial, protozoal
4. Trauma

▪ Diagnostic Plan

1. A systemic workup due to the physical examination abnormalities.
2. Radiography of the vertebral column to evaluate for bony neoplasms and infection involving the bone and disk spaces.
3. MRI to further assess vertebral column lesions and lesions in the spinal cord.
4. CSF analysis to rule out inflammatory infectious diseases.

▪ Diagnostic Results

Ultrasonography of kidneys revealed pyelonephritis. Survey radiographs of spine revealed a discospondylitis lesion at L1-2 IVD space and multiple lesions in the thoracic spine. Serology for *Brucella canis* was negative. Urinalysis revealed presence of fungal hyphae. Urine and blood cultures specifically for bacteria yielded no growth. Urine was then specifically cultured for fungal agents and *Aspergillus terreus* was isolated.

▪ Diagnosis

A. terreus causes disseminated aspergillosis with discospondylitis being a common feature. The disease has been most commonly reported in German shepherd dogs from Western Australia but isolated cases are reported in the United States.

▪ Treatment

Treatment with antifungal agents may slow the disease progression but often long-term prognosis is poor. After diagnosis, the dog continued to deteriorate and the owner elected euthanasia.

REFERENCES

1. Hoerlein BF: Intervertebral disc disease. In Oliver JE, Hoerlein BF, Mayhew IG, editors: Veterinary neurology, Philadelphia, 1987, WB Saunders.
2. Hoerlein BF: Intervertebral disc disease. In Hoerlein BF, editor: Canine neurology: diagnosis and treatment, ed 3, Philadelphia, 1978, WB Saunders.
3. Hansen HJ: A pathologic-anatomical study on disc degeneration in dog, Acta Orthop Scand, Suppl 11:1–117, 1952.
4. Hansen HJ: A pathologic-anatomical interpretation of disc degeneration in dogs, Acta Orthop Scand 20:280–293, 1951.
5. Priester WA: Canine intervertebral disc disease–occurrence by age, breed, and sex among 8,117 cases, Theriogenology 6(2-3):293–303, 1976.
6. Stigen Ø: Calcification of intervertebral discs in the dachshund. A radiographic study of 327 young dogs, Acta Vet Scand 32(2):197–203, 1991.
7. Stigen Ø: Calcification of intervertebral discs in the dachshund: a radiographic study of 115 dogs at 1 and 5 years of age, Acta Vet Scand 37(3):229–237, 1996.
8. Jensen VF, Arnbjerg J: Development of intervertebral disk calcification in the dachshund: a prospective longitudinal radiographic study, J Am Anim Hosp Assoc 37:274–282, 2001.
9. Griffiths IR: The extensive myelopathy of intervertebral disc protrusions in dogs (ascending syndrome), J Small Anim Pract 13:425, 1972.
10. De Risio L, Adams V, Dennis R, et al: Association of clinical and magnetic resonance imaging findings with outcome in dogs with presumptive acute noncompressive nucleus pulposus extrusion: 42 cases (2000-2007), J Am Vet Med Assoc 234(4):495–504, 2009.
11. Sukhiani HR, Parent JM, Atilola MA, et al: Intervertebral disk disease in dogs with signs of back pain alone: 25 cases (1986-1993), J Am Vet Med Assoc 209(7):1275–1279, 1996.
12. Gage ED: Incidence of clinical disc disease in the dog, J Am Anim Hosp Assoc 11:135–138, 1975.
13. Cudia SP, Duval JM: Thoracolumbar intervertebral disk disease in large, nonchondrodystrophic dogs: a retrospective study, J Am Anim Hosp Assoc 33(5):456–460, 1997.
14. Olby N, Levine J, Harris T, et al: Long-term functional outcome of dogs with severe injuries of the thoracolumbar spinal cord: 87 cases (1996-2001), J Am Vet Med Assoc 22:2762–2769, 2003.
15. Scott HW, McKee WM: Laminectomy for 34 dogs with thoracolumbar intervertebral disc disease and loss of deep pain perception, J Small Anim Pract 40:417–422, 1999.
16. Kirberger RM: Recent developments in canine lumbar myelography, Compend Contin Educ Pract Vet 16(7):847–854, 1994.
17. Olby NJ, Dyce J, Houlton JEF: Correlation of plain radiographic and lumbar myelographic findings with surgical findings in thoracolumbar disc disease, J Small Anim Pract 35(7):345–350, 1994.

18. Duval J, Dewey C, Roberts R, et al: Spinal cord swelling as a myelographic indicator of prognosis: a retrospective study in dogs with intervertebral disc disease and loss of deep pain perception, Vet Surg 25(1):6–12, 1996.
19. Olby NJ, Muñana KR, Sharp NJ, et al: The computed tomographic appearance of acute thoracolumbar intervertebral disc herniations in dogs, Vet Radiol Ultrasound 41(5):396–402, 2000.
20. Naude SH, Lambrechts NE, Wagner WM, et al: Association of preoperative magnetic resonance imaging findings with surgical features in dachshunds with thoracolumbar intervertebral disk extrusion, J Am Vet Med Assoc 23:2702–2708, 2008.
21. Besalti O, Ozak A, Pekcan Z, et al: The role of extruded disk material in thoracolumbar intervertebral disk disease: a retrospective study in 40 dogs, Can Vet J 46:814–820, 2005.
22. Besalti O, Pekcan Z, Sirin S, et al: Magnetic resonance imaging findings in dogs with thoracolumbar intervertebral disk disease: 69 cases (1997-2005), J Am Vet Med Assoc 22:8902–8908, 2006.
23. Tidwell AS, Specht A, Blaeser L, et al: Magnetic resonance imaging features of extradural hematomas associated with intervertebral disc herniation in a dog, Vet Radiol Ultrasound 43:319–324, 2002.
24. Ito D, Matsunaga S, Jeffery ND, et al: Prognostic value of magnetic resonance imaging in dogs with paraplegia caused by thoracolumbar intervertebral disk extrusion: 77 cases (2000-2003), J Am Vet Med Assoc 227:1454–1460, 2005.
25. Levine JM, Fosgate GT, Chen A, et al: Magnetic resonance imaging in dogs with neurologic impairment due to acute thoracic and lumbar intervertebral disk herniation, J Vet Intern Med 23:1220–1226, 2009.
26. Stiffler KS, Stevenson MAM, Sanchez S: Prevalence and characterization of urinary tract infections in dogs with surgically treated type 1 intervertebral disc extrusion, Vet Surg 35:330–336, 2006.
27. Funkquist B: Investigations of the therapeutic and prophylactic effects of disc evacuation in cases of thoracolumbar herniated discs in dogs, Acta Vet Scand 19:441–457, 1978.
28. Davies JV, Sharp NJH: A comparison of conservative treatment and fenestration for thoracolumbar intervertebral disc disease in the dog, J Small Anim Pract 24:721–729, 1983.
29. Levine JM, Levine GJ, Johnson SI, et al: Evaluation of the success of medical management for presumptive thoracolumbar intervertebral disk herniation in dogs, Vet Surg 36:482–491, 2007.
30. Funkquist B: Thoraco-lumbar disk protrusion with severe cord compression in the dog II: clinical observations with special reference to the prognosis in conservative treatment, Acta Vet Scand 3:317–343, 1962.
31. Mann FA, Wagner-Mann CC, Dunphy ED, et al: Recurrence rate of presumed thoracolumbar intervertebral disc disease in ambulatory dogs with spinal hyperpathia treated with anti-inflammatory drugs: 78 (1997-2000), J Vet Emerg Crit Care 17:53–60, 2007.
32. Horne TRJ, Powers RD, Swaim SF: Dorsal laminectomy techniques in the dog, J Am Vet Med Assoc 171(8):742–749, 1977.
33. McKee WM: A comparison of hemilaminectomy (with concomitant disc fenestration) and dorsal laminectomy for the treatment of thoracolumbar disc protrusion in dogs, Vet Rec 130(14):296–300, 1992.
34. Schulz KS, Waldron DR, Grant JW, et al: Biomechanics of the thoracolumbar vertebral column of dogs during lateral bending, Am J Vet Res 57(8):1228–1232, 1996.
35. Loughin CA, Dewey CW, Ringwood PB, et al: Effect of durotomy on functional outcome of dogs with type I thoracolumbar disc extrusion and absent deep pain perception, Vet Comp Orthop Traumatol 18:141–146, 2005.
36. Tarlov I, Klinger H: Spinal cord compression studies II: time limits for recovery after acute compression in dogs, Arch Neurol Psychiatry 71:271–290, 1954.
37. Tarlov I, Klinger H, Vitale S: Spinal cord compression studies I: experimental techniques to produce acute and gradual compression, Arch Neurol Psychiatry 70:813–819, 1953.
38. Knecht CD: The effect of delayed hemilaminectomy in the treatment of intervertebral disc protrusion in dogs, J Am Anim Hosp Assoc 13:449, 1970.
39. Brown NO, Helphrey ML, Prata RG: Thoracolumbar disk disease in the dog: a retrospective analysis of 187 cases, J Am Anim Hosp Assoc 13:665–672, 1977.
40. Gambardella PC: Dorsal decompressive laminectomy for treatment of thoracolumbar disc disease in dogs: a retrospective study of 98 cases, Vet Surg 9(1):24–26, 1980.
41. Ferreira AJA, Correia JHD, Jaggy A: Thoracolumbar disc disease in 71 paraplegic dogs: influence of rate of onset and duration of clinical signs on treatment results, J Small Anim Pract 43:158–163, 2002.
42. Shores A, Cechner PE, Cantwell HD, et al: Structural changes in thoracolumbar disks following lateral fenestration. A study of the radiographic, histologic, and histochemical changes in the chondrodystrophoid dog, Vet Surg 14(2):117–123, 1985.
43. Dickey DT, Bartels KE, Henry GA, et al: Use of the holmium yttrium aluminum garnet laser for percutaneous thoracolumbar intervertebral disk ablation in dogs, J Am Vet Med Assoc 208(8):1263–1267, 1996.
44. Bartels KE, Higbee RG, Bahr RJ, et al: Outcome of and complications associated with prophylactic percutaneous laser disk ablation in dogs with thoracolumbar disk disease: 277 cases (1992-2001), J Am Vet Med Assoc 222(12):1733–1739, 2003.
45. Black AP: Lateral spinal decompression in the dog: a review of 39 cases, J Small Anim Pract 29(9):581–588, 1988.
46. Knapp DW, Pope ER, Hewett JE, et al: A retrospective study of thoracolumbar disk fenestration in dogs using a ventral approach: 160 cases (1976 to 1986), J Am Anim Hosp Assoc 26:543–549, 1990.
47. Funkquist B: Decompressive laminectomy in thoracolumbar disc protrusion with paraplegia in the dog, J Small Anim Pract 11:445–451, 1970.
48. Brisson BA, Moffatt SL, Swayne AL, et al: Recurrence of thoracolumbar intervertebral disk extrusion in chondrodystrophic dogs after surgical decompression with or without prophylactic fenestration: 265 cases (1995-1999), J Am Vet Med Assoc 224:1808–1814, 2004.
49. Schulman A, Lippincott CL: Dorsolateral hemilaminectomy in the treatment of thoracolumbar intervertebral disk disease in dogs, Compend Contin Educ Pract Vet 9(3):305–310, 1987.
50. Forterre F, Gorgas D, Dickomeit M, et al: Incidence of spinal compressive lesions in chondrodystrophic dogs with abnormal recovery after hemilaminectomy for treatment of thoracolumbar disc disease: a prospective magnetic resonance imaging study, Vet Surg 39(2):165–172, 2010.
51. Ruddle TL, Allen DA, Schertel ER, et al: Outcome and prognostic factors in nonambulatory Hansen type I intervertebral disc extrusions: 308 cases, Vet Comp Orthop Traumatol 19:29–34, 2006.

52. Yovich JC, Read R, Eger C, et al: Modified lateral spinal decompression in 61 dogs with thoracolumbar disc protrusion, J Small Anim Pract 35:351–356, 1994.
53. Scott HW: Hemilaminectomy for the treatment of thoracolumbar disc disease in the dog: a follow-up study of 40 cases, J Small Anim Pract 38(11):488–494, 1997.
54. Anderson SM, Lippincott CL, Gill PJ: Hemilaminectomy in dogs without deep pain perception. A retrospective study of 32 cases, Calif Vet: 45:24–28, 1991.
55. Pusterla N, David WW, Madigan JE, et al: Equine herpesvirus-1 myeloencephalopathy: a review of recent developments, Vet J 180(3):279–289, 2009:review.
56. Mayhew IG: Large animal neurology, ed 2, Ames, Iowa, 2009, Wiley-Blackwell.
57. Lunn DP, Davis-Poynter N, Flaminio MJBF, et al: Equine herpesvirus-1 consensus statement, J Vet Intern Med 23:450–461, 2009.
58. Allen GP, Bryans JT: Molecular epizootiology, pathogenesis and prophylaxis of equine herpesvirus-1 infection, Prog Vet Microbiol 2:78–144, 1986.
59. Jackson TA, Osburn BI, Cordy DR, et al: Equine herpesvirus 1 infection of horses: studies on the experimentally induced neurologic disease, Am J Vet Res 38(6):709–719, 1977.
60. Kydd JH, Townsend HG, Hannant D: The equine immune response to equine herpesvirus-1: the virus and its vaccines, Vet Immunol Immunopathol 11:115–130, 2006.
61. Allen GP: Development of a real-time polymerase chain reaction assay for rapid diagnosis of neuropathogenic strains of equine herpesvirus-1, J Vet Diagn Invest 19:69–72, 2007.
62. Allen GP: Epidemic disease caused by equine herpesvirus-1: recommendations for prevention and control, Equine Vet Educ 4:177–183, 2002.
63. Henninger RW, Reed SM, Saville WJ, et al: Outbreak of neurologic disease caused by equine herpesvirus-1 at a university equestrian center, J Vet Intern Med 21(1):157–165, 2007.
64. Sellon DC, Dubey JP: Equine protozoal myeloencephalitis. In Sellon DC, Long MT, editors: Equine infectious diseases, St Louis, 2007, Elsevier.
65. Dubey JP, Davis SW, Speer CA: *Sarcocystis neurona* n. sp. (Protozoa: *Apicomplexa*), the etiologic agent of equine protozoal myeloencephalitis, J Parasitol 77:212–218, 1991.
66. Dubey JP, Lindsay DS, Saville WJ, et al: A review of *Sarcocystis neurona* and equine protozoal myeloencephalitis (EPM), Vet Parasitol 95:89–131, 2001.
67. Fenger CK, Granstrom DE, Langemeier JL, et al: Identification of opossums *(Didelphis virginiana)* as the putative definitive host of, *Sarcocystis neurona.* J Parasitol 81(6):916–919, 1995.
68. Fayer R, Mayhew IG, Baird JD, et al: Epidemiology of equine protozoal myeloencephalitis in North America based on histologically confirmed cases. A report, J Vet Intern Med 4(2):54–57, 1990.
69. Clark EG, Townsend HGG, McKenzie NT: Equine protozoal myeloencephalitis: a report of two cases from Western Canada, Can Vet J 22(5):140–144, 1981.
70. Dorr TE, Higgins RJ, Dangler CA, et al: Protozoal myeloencephalitis in horses in California, J Am Vet Med Assoc 185(7):801–802, 1984.
71. Cohen ND, Mackay RJ, Toby E, et al: A multicenter case-control study of risk factors for equine protozoal myeloencephalitis, J Am Vet Med Assoc 231(12):1857–1863, 2007.
72. Mayhew IG: Measurements of the accuracy of clinical diagnoses of equine neurologic disease, J Vet Intern Med 5(6):332–334, 1991.
73. Furr M, MacKay R, Granstrom D: Clinical diagnosis of equine protozoal myeloencephalomyelitis, J Vet Intern Med 16:618–621, 2002.
74. Furr M: Antigen-specific antibodies in cerebrospinal fluid after intramuscular injection of ovalbumin in horses, J Vet Intern Med 16(5):588–592, 2002:Erratum appears in *J Vet Intern Med* 16(6):748, 2000.
75. Cook AG, Buechner-Maxwell V, Morrow JK, et al: Interpretation of the detection of *Sarcocystis neurona* antibodies in the serum of young horses, Vet Parasitol 95(2-4):187–195, 2001.
76. Duarte PC, Ebel ED, Traub-Dargatz J, et al: Indirect fluorescent antibody testing of cerebrospinal fluid for diagnosis of equine protozoal myeloencephalitis, Am J Vet Res 67:869–876, 2006.
77. Crowdus CA, Marsh AE, Saville WJ, et al: SnSAG5 is an alternative surface antigen of *Sarcocystis neurona* strains that is mutually exclusive to SnSAG1, Vet Parasitol 158(1-2):36–43, 2008.
78. Daft BM, Barr BC, Gardner IA, et al: Sensitivity and specificity of western blot testing of cerebrospinal fluid and serum for diagnosis of equine protozoal myeloencephalitis in horses with and without neurologic abnormalities, J Am Vet Med Assoc 221(7):1007–1013, 2002.
79. Ostlund EN, Crom RL, Pederson DD: Equine West Nile encephalitis, United States, Emerg Infect Dis 7:665–669, 2001.
80. McLean RG, Ubico SR, Bourne D, et al: West Nile virus in livestock and wildlife, Curr Top Microbiol Immunol 267:271–308, 2002.
81. Castillo-Olivares J, Wood J: West Nile virus infection of horses, Vet Res 35(4):467–483, 2004.
82. Porter MB, Long MT, Getman LM, et al: West Nile virus encephalomyelitis in horses: 46 cases (2001), J Am Vet Med Assoc 222(9):1241–1247, 2003.
83. Wamsley HL, Alleman AR, Porter MB, et al: Findings in cerebrospinal fluids of horses infected with West Nile virus: 30 cases (2001), J Am Vet Med Assoc 221(9):1303–1305, 2002.
84. Kleiboeker SB, Loiacono CM, Rottinghaus A, et al: Diagnosis of West Nile virus infection in horses, J Vet Diagn Invest 16(1):2–10, 2004.
85. Porter MB, Long M, Gosche DG, et al: Immunoglobulin M-capture enzyme-linked immunosorbent assay testing of cerebrospinal fluid and serum from horses exposed to West Nile virus by vaccination or natural infection, J Vet Intern Med 18(6):866–870, 2004.
86. Lester G: Parasitic encephalomyelitis in horses, Compend Contin Educ Pract Vet 14(12):1624–1631, 1992.
87. Nagy DW: *Parelaphostrongylus tenuis* and other parasitic diseases of the ruminant nervous system, Vet Clin Food Anim 20:393–412, 2004.
88. Callan RJ, Van Metre DC: Viral diseases of the ruminant nervous system, Vet Clin Food Anim 20:327–362, 2004.
89. Rowe JD, East NE: Risk factors for transmission and methods for control of caprine arthritis-encephalitis virus infection, Vet Clin North Am Food Anim Pract 13(1):35–53, 1997.
90. de la Concha-Bermejillo A: Maedi-visna and ovine progressive pneumonia, Vet Clin Food Anim 13:13–33, 1997.
91. de AD, Klein D, Watt NJ, et al: Diagnostic tests for small ruminant lentiviruses, Vet Microbiol 107(1-2):49–62, 2005:review.
92. Thomas WB: Diskospondylitis and other vertebral infections, Vet Clin North Am Small Anim Pract 30:169–182, 2000.

93. Jimenez MM, O'Callaghan MW: Vertebral physitis: a radiographic diagnosis to be separated from discospondylitis. A preliminary report, Vet Radiol Ultrasound 36(3):188–195, 1995.
94. Hurov L, Troy G, Turnwald G: Diskospondylitis in the dog: 27 cases, J Am Vet Med Assoc 173(3):275–281, 1978.
95. Kornegay JN, Barber DL: Diskospondylitis in dogs, J Am Vet Med Assoc 177(4):337–341, 1980.
96. Kornegay JN: Canine diskospondylitis, Compend Contin Educ Pract Vet 1(12):930–934, 1979.
97. Jacob F, Bagley RS, Moore MP, et al: Cervical intervertebral disk protrusion, diskospondylitis, and porcupine quill foreign body in a dog, Prog Vet Neurol 7(2):53–55, 1996.
98. Johnston DE, Summers BA: Osteomyelitis of the lumbar vertebrae in dogs caused by grass-seed foreign bodies, Vet J 47:289, 1971.
99. Malik R, Lattimer JC, Love W: Bacterial diskospondylitis in a cat, J Small Anim Pract 31:404–406, 1990.
100. Henderson RA, Hoerlein BF, Kramer TT, et al: Discospondylitis in three dogs infected with, Brucella canis, J Am Vet Med Assoc 165(5):451–455, 1974.
101. Kerwin SC, Lewis DD, Hribernik TN, et al: Diskospondylitis associated with *Brucella canis* infection in dogs: 14 cases (1980-1991), J Am Vet Med Assoc 201(8):1253–1257, 1992.
102. Turnwald GH, Shires PK, Turk MA, et al: Diskospondylitis in a kennel of dogs: clinicopathologic findings, J Am Vet Med Assoc 188(2):178–183, 1986.
103. Turnbull IM: Microvasculature of the human spinal cord, J Neurosurg 35(2):141–147, 1971.
104. Crock HV, Goldwass M: Anatomic studies of the circulation in the region of the vertebral end-plate in adult greyhound dogs, Spine 9:702, 1984.
105. Gilmore DR: Lumbosacral diskospondylitis in 21 dogs, J Am Anim Hosp Assoc 23:57–61, 1987.
106. Doige C: Discospondylitis in swine, Can J Comp Med 44:121–128, 1980.
107. Sherman DM, Ames TR: Vertebral body abscesses in cattle: a review of five cases, J Am Vet Med Assoc 188(6):608–611, 1986.
108. Finley GG: A survey of vertebral abscesses in domestic animals in Ontario, Can Vet J 16:114–117, 1975.
109. Divers TJ: Acquired spinal cord and peripheral nerve disease, Vet Clin Food Anim 20:231–242, 2004.
110. Davis MJ, Dewey CW, Walker MA, et al: Contrast radiographic finding in canine bacterial discospondylitis: a multicenter, retrospective study of 27 cases, J Am Anim Hosp Assoc 36:81–85, 2000.
111. Kraft SL, Mussman JM, Smith T, et al: Magnetic resonance imaging of presumptive lumbosacral discospondylitis in a dog, Vet Radiol Ultrasound 39(1):9–13, 1998.
112. Fischer A, Mahaffey MB, Oliver JE: Fluoroscopically guided percutaneous disk aspiration in 10 dogs with diskospondylitis, J Vet Intern Med 11(5):284–287, 1997.
113. Gage ED: Treatment of discospondylitis in the dog, J Am Vet Med Assoc 166(12):1164–1169, 1975.
114. Holloway A, Dennis R, McConnell F, et al: Magnetic resonance imaging features of paraspinal infection in the dog and cat, Vet Radiol Ultrasound 50:285–291, 2009.
115. Destefani A, Garosi LS, McConnell FJ, et al: Magnetic resonance imaging features of spinal epidural empyema in five dogs, Vet Radiol Ultrasound 49(2):135–140, 2008.
116. Lavely JA, Vernau KM, Vernau W, et al: Spinal epidural empyema in seven dogs, Vet Surg 35(2):176–185, 2006.
117. Jerram RM, Dewey CW: Suspected spinal epidural empyema and associated vertebral osteomyelitis (physitis) in a dog, J Vet Emerg Crit Care 8(2):103–108, 1998.
118. Cherrone KL, Eich CS, Bonzynski JJ: Suspected paraspinal abscess and spinal epidural empyema in a dog, J Am Anim Hosp Assoc 38(2):149–151, 2002:review.
119. Dewey CW, Kortz GD, Bailey CS: Spinal epidural empyema in two dogs, J Am Anim Hosp Assoc 34(4):305–308, 1998.
120. Nykamp SG, Steffey MA, Scrivani PV, et al: Computed tomographic appearance of epidural empyema in a dog, Can Vet J 44(9):729–731, 2003.
121. Turner WD: Fractures and fracture-luxations of the lumbar spine: retrospective study in the dog, J Am Anim Hosp Assoc 23(4):459–464, 1987.
122. Selcer RR, Bubb WJ, Walker TL: Management of vertebral column fractures in dogs and cats: 211 cases (1977-1985), J Am Vet Med Assoc 198(11):1965–1968, 1991.
123. Rucker NC: Management of spinal cord trauma, Prog Vet Neurol 1(4):397–412, 1990.
124. Shores A: Spinal trauma. Pathophysiology and management of traumatic spinal injuries, Vet Clin North Am Small Anim Pract 22(4):859–888, 1992.
125. Janssens LAA: Mechanical and pathophysiological aspects of acute spinal cord trauma, J Small Anim Pract 32(11):572–578, 1991.
126. Feeney DA, Oliver JE: Blunt spinal trauma in the dog and cat: neurologic, radiologic, and therapeutic correlations, J Am Anim Hosp Assoc 16:664–668, 1980.
127. Olby N: Current concepts in the management of acute spinal cord injury, J Vet Intern Med 13(5):399–407, 1999.
128. Coughlan AR: Secondary injury mechanisms in acute spinal cord trauma, J Small Anim Pract 34:117–122, 1993.
129. Griffiths IR: Spinal cord blood flow after acute experimental cord injury in dogs, J Neurol Sci 27(2):247–259, 1976.
130. Shores A, Braund KG, Brawner WR Jr: Management of acute spinal cord trauma, Vet Med 85(7):724–743, 1990.
131. Bagley RS: Spinal fracture or luxation, Vet Clin North Am Small Anim Pract 30:130–153, 2000.
132. Bagley RS, Silver GM, Connors RL, et al: Exogenous spinal trauma: surgical therapy and aftercare, Compend Contin Educ Pract Vet 22:218–230, 2000.
133. Braund KG, Shores A, Brawner WR Jr: The etiology, pathology, and pathophysiology of acute spinal cord trauma, Vet Med 85(7):684–691, 1990.
134. Bagley RS, Harrington ML, Silver GM, et al: Exogenous spinal trauma: clinical assessment and initial management, Compend Contin Educ Pract Vet 21(12):1138–1144, 1999.
135. Smith PM, Jeffery ND: Spinal shock—comparative aspects and clinical relevance, J Vet Intern Med 19(6):788–793, 2005.
136. Shires PK, Waldron DR, Hedlund CS: A biomechanical study of rotational instability in unaltered and surgically altered canine thoracolumbar vertebral motion units, Prog Vet Neurol 2:6–14, 1991.
137. Bracken MB, Shepard MJ, Collins WF, et al: A randomized, controlled trial of methylprednisolone or naloxone in the treatment of acute spinal-cord injury. Results of the second national acute spinal cord injury study, N Engl J Med 322(20):1405–1411, 1990.
138. Bracken MB, Shepard MJ, Holford TR, et al: Methylprednisolone or tirilazad mesylate administration after acute spinal cord injury: 1-year follow-up. Results of the third national acute spinal cord injury randomized controlled trial, J Neurosurg 89(5):699–706, 1998.

139. Hall ED, Wolf DL, Braughler JM: Effects of a single large dose of methylprednisolone sodium succinate on experimental posttraumatic spinal cord ischemia. Dose-response and time-action analysis, J Neurosurg 61(1):124–130, 1984.
140. Faden AI, Salzman S: Pharmacological strategies in CNS trauma, Trends Pharmacol Sci 13(1):29–35, 1992.
141. Braughler JM, Hall ED, Means ED, et al: Evaluation of an intensive methylprednisolone sodium succinate dosing regimen in experimental spinal cord injury, J Neurosurg 67(1):102–105, 1987.
142. Boag AK, Otto CM, Drobatz KJ: Complications of methylprednisolone sodium succinate therapy in dachshunds with surgically treated intervertebral disc disease, J Vet Emerg Crit Care 11:105–110, 2001.
143. Culbert LA, Marino DJ, Baule RM, et al: Complications associated with high-dose prednisolone sodium succinate therapy in dogs with neurological injury, J Am Anim Hosp Assoc 34(2):129–134, 1998.
144. Hoerlein BF, Redding RW, Hoff EJ, et al: Evaluation of dexamethasone, DMSO, mannitol, and Solcoseryl in acute spinal cord trauma, J Am Anim Hosp Assoc 19(2):216–226, 1983.
145. Bruecker KA: Principles of vertebral fracture management, Semin Vet Med Surg (Small Anim) 11(4):259–272, 1996.
146. Sturges BK, LeCouteur RA: Vertebral fractures and luxations. In Slatter D, editor: Textbook of small animal surgery, ed 3, Philadelphia, 2003, WB Saunders.
147. Carberry CA, Flanders JA, Dietze AE, et al: Nonsurgical management of thoracic and lumbar spinal fractures and fracture luxations in the dog and cat: a review of 17 cases, J Am Anim Hosp Assoc 25(1):43–54, 1989.
148. Sharp NJH, Wheeler SJ: Small animal spinal disorders: diagnosis and surgery, London, 2005, Elsevier.
149. Bruce CW, Brisson BA, Gyselinck K: Spinal fracture and luxation in dogs and cats: a retrospective evaluation of 95 cases, Vet Comp Orthop Traumatol 21:280–284, 2008.
150. Hawthorne JC, Blevins WE, Wallace LJ, et al: Cervical vertebral fractures in 56 dogs: a retrospective study, J Am Anim Hosp Assoc 35(2):135–146, 1999.
151. Blass CE, Seim HB III: Spinal fixation in dogs using Steinmann pins and methylmethacrylate, Vet Surg 13(4):203–210, 1984.
152. Blauch B: Spinal reflex walking in the dog, Vet Med Small Anim Clin 72(2):169–173, 1977.
153. Rossignol S, Bouyer L, Barthelemy D, et al: Determinants of locomotor recovery in the cat following spinal cord lesions, Prog Brain Res 143:163–172, 2004.
154. Averill DR Jr: Degenerative myelopathy in the aging German shepherd dog: clinical and pathologic findings, J Am Vet Med Assoc 162(12):1045–1051, 1973.
155. Griffiths IR, Duncan ID: Chronic degenerative radiculomyelopathy in the dog, J Small Anim Pract 16(8):461–471, 1975.
156. Braund KG, Vandevelde M: German shepherd dog myelopathy: a morphologic and morphometric study, Am J Vet Res 39(8):1309–1315, 1978.
157. Johnston PEJ, Barrie JA, McCulloch MC, et al: Central nervous system pathology in 25 dogs with chronic degenerative radiculomyelopathy, Vet Rec 146(22):629–633, 2000.
158. March PA, Coates JR, Abyad RJ, et al: Degenerative myelopathy in 18 Pembroke Welsh corgi dogs, Vet Pathol 46:241–250, 2009.
159. Awano T, Johnson GS, Wade CM, et al: Genome-wide association analysis reveals a *SOD1* mutation in canine degenerative myelopathy that resembles amyotrophic lateral sclerosis, Proc Natl Acad Sci U S A 106:2794–2799, 2009.
160. Waxman FJ, Clemmons RM, Johnson G, et al: Progressive myelopathy in older German shepherd dogs. I. Depressed response to thymus-dependent mitogens, J Immunol 124(3):1209–1215, 1980.
161. Waxman FJ, Clemmons RM, Hinrichs DJ: Progressive myelopathy in older German shepherd dogs. II. Presence of circulating suppressor cells, J Immunol 124(3):1216–1222, 1980.
162. Barclay KB, Haines DM: Immunohistochemical evidence for immunoglobulin and complement deposition in spinal cord lesions in degenerative myelopathy in German shepherd dogs, Can J Vet Res 58(1):20–24, 1994.
163. Williams DA, Sharp NJH, Batt RM: Enteropathy associated with degenerative myelopathy in German shepherd dogs, Proc 1st ACVIM Forum 40, 1983.
164. Williams DA, Batt RM, Sharp NJH: Degenerative myelopathy in German shepherd dogs: an association with mucosal biochemical changes and bacterial overgrowth in the small intestine, Clin Sci 66:25, 1984.
165. Fechner H, Johnston PE, Sharp NJH, et al: Molecular genetic and expression analysis of alpha-tocopherol transfer protein mRNA in German shepherd dogs with degenerative myelopathy, Berl Much Tierarztl Wochenschr 11:631–636, 2003.
166. Johnston PEJ, Knox K, Gettinby G, et al: Serum α–tocopherol concentrations in German shepherd dogs with chronic degenerative radiculomyelopathy, Vet Rec 148:403–407, 2001.
167. Sheahan BJ, Caffrey JF, Gunn HM, et al: Structural and biochemical changes in a spinal myelinopathy in twelve English foxhounds and two harriers, Vet Pathol 28(2):117–124, 1991.
168. Coates JR, March PA, Oglesbee M, et al: Clinical characterization of a familial degenerative myelopathy in Pembroke Welsh corgi dogs, J Vet Intern Med 21(6):1323–1331, 2007.
169. Olby NJ, Sharp NJH, Muñana KR, et al: Chronic and acute compressive spinal cord lesions in dogs are associated with increased lumbar CSF glutamate levels, J Vet Intern Med 13(3):240, 1999:abstract.
170. Bichsel P, Vandevelde M, Lang J, et al: Degenerative myelopathy in a family of Siberian husky dogs, J Am Vet Med Assoc 183(9):998–1000, 1983.
171. Long SN, Henthorn PS, Serpell J, et al: Degenerative myelopathy in Chesapeake Bay retrievers, J Vet Intern Med 23:401–402, 2009.
171a. Abstract—clemmons et al: FASEB 2006.
172. Clark LA, Tsai KL, Murphy KE: Alleles of DLA-DRB1 are not unique in German shepherd dogs having degenerative myelopathy, Anim Genet 39(3):332, 2008.
173. Kathmann I, Cizinauskas S, Doherr MG, et al: Daily controlled physiotherapy increases survival time in dogs with suspected degenerative myelopathy, J Vet Intern Med 20:927–932, 2006.
174. Matthews NS, de Lahunta A: Degenerative myelopathy in an adult miniature poodle, J Am Vet Med Assoc 186(11):1213–1215, 1985.
175. Miller AD, Barber R, Porter BF, et al: Degenerative myelopathy in two boxer dogs, Vet Pathol 46(4):684–687, 2009.
176. Polizopoulou ZS, Koutinas AF, Patsikas MN, et al: Evaluation of a proposed therapeutic protocol in 12 dogs with tentative degenerative myelopathy, Acta Vet Hung 56(3):293–301, 2008.
177. Kneller SK, Oliver JE, Lewis RE: Differential diagnosis of progressive caudal paresis in an aged German shepherd dog, J Am Anim Hosp Assoc 11:414–417, 1975.
178. Braund KG: Hip dysplasia and degenerative myelopathy: making the distinction in dogs, Vet Med 782–789, 1987.

179. Clemmons RM: Degenerative myelopathy. In Kirk RW, editor: Current veterinary therapy X: small animal practice, Philadelphia, 1989, WB Saunders.
180. Sherman J, Olby NJ: Nursing and rehabilitation of the neurological patient. In Platt SR, Olby NJ, editors: BSAVA manual of canine and feline neurology, ed 3, Gloucester, UK, 2004, BSAVA.
181. Cockrell BY, Herigstad RR, Flo GL, et al: Myelomalacia in Afghan hounds, J Am Vet Med Assoc 162:362–365, 1973.
182. Oevermann A, Bley T, Konar M, et al: A novel leukoencephalomyelopathy of Leonberger dogs, J Vet Intern Med 22:467–471, 2008.
183. Douglas SW, Palmer AC: Idiopathic demyelination of brain-stem and cord in a miniature poodle puppy, J Pathol Bacteriol 82:67–71, 1961.
184. Mandigers PJJ, van Nes JJ, Knol BW, et al: Hereditary kooiker dog ataxia, Res Vet Sci 54:118–123, 1993.
185. Toenniessen JG, Morin DE: Degenerative myelopathy: a comparative review, Compend Contin Educ Pract Vet 17(2):271–283, 1995.
186. Heavner JE: Intervertebral disc syndrome in the cat, J Am Vet Med Assoc 159(4):425–427, 1971.
187. Morgan JP: Spinal dural ossification in the dog: incidence and distribution based on a radiographic study, J Am Vet Radiol Soc 10:43–48, 1969.
188. Larsen JS, Selby LA: Spondylosis deformans in large dogs—relative risk by breed, age and sex, J Am Anim Hosp Assoc 17(4):623–625, 1981.
189. Kornegay JN: Vertebral diseases of large breed dogs. In Kornegay JN, editor: Neurologic disorders (contemporary issues in small animal practice), New York, 1986, Churchill Livingstone.
190. Romatowski J: Spondylosis deformans in the dog, Compend Contin Educ Pract Vet 8(8):531–536, 1986.
191. Morgan JP: Spondylosis deformans in the dog, Acta Orthop Scand Suppl 9:61–88, 1967.
192. Weisbrode SE, Monke DR, Dodaro ST, et al: Osteochondrosis, degenerative joint disease, and vertebral osteophytosis in middle-aged bulls, J Am Vet Med Assoc 181(7):700–705, 1982.
193. Langeland M, Lingaas F: Spondylosis deformans in the boxer: estimates of heritability, J Small Anim Pract 36(4):166–169, 1995.
194. Adams WH, Daniel GB, Pardo AD, et al: Magnetic resonance imaging of the caudal lumbar and lumbosacral spine in 13 dogs (1990-1993), Vet Radiol Ultrasound 36(1):3–13, 1995.
195. Levine GJ, Levine JM, Walker MA, et al: Evaluation of the association between spondylosis deformans and clinical signs of intervertebral disk disease in dogs: 172 cases (1999-2000), J Am Vet Med Assoc 228:96–100, 2006.
196. Wright JA: Spondylosis deformans of the lumbo-sacral joint in dogs, J Small Anim Pract 21(1):45–58, 1980.
197. Mattoon JS, Koblik PD: Quantitative survey radiographic evaluation of the lumbosacral spine of normal dogs and dogs with degenerative lumbosacral stenosis, Vet Radiol Ultrasound 34(3):194–206, 1993.
198. Meehan L, Dyson S, Murray R: Radiographic and scintigraphic evaluation of spondylosis in the equine thoracolumbar spine: a retrospective study, Equine Vet J 41:800–807, 2009.
199. Doige CE: Pathological changes in the lumbar spine in boars, Can J Comp Med 44:382–389, 1980.
200. Morgan JP, Stavenborn M: Disseminated idiopathic skeletal hyperostosis (DISH) in a dog, Vet Radiol Ultrasound 32(2):65–70, 1991.
201. LeCouteur RA: Disease of the spinal cord. In Ettinger SJ, Feldman EC, editors: Textbook of veterinary internal medicine, ed 5, Philadelphia, 2000, WB Saunders.
202. Finnie JW, Sinclair IR: Multiple cartilaginous exostoses in a dog, J Small Anim Pract 22(9):597–602, 1981.
203. Reidarson TH, Metz AL, Hardy RM: Thoracic vertebral osteochondroma in a cat, J Am Vet Med Assoc 192(8):1102–1104, 1988.
204. Doige CE: Multiple cartilaginous exostoses in dogs, Vet Pathol 24(3):276–278, 1987.
205. Jacobson LS, Kirberger RM: Canine multiple cartilaginous exostoses: unusual manifestations and a review of the literature, J Am Anim Hosp Assoc 32(1):45–51, 1996.
206. Green EM, Adams WM, Steinberg H: Malignant transformation of solitary spinal osteochondroma in two mature dogs, Vet Radiol Ultrasound 40(6):634–637, 1999.
207. Shupe JL, Leone NC, Gardner EJ, et al: Hereditary multiple exostoses. Hereditary multiple exostoses in horses, Am J Pathol 104(3):285–288, 1981.
208. Caporn TM, Read RA: Osteochondromatosis of the cervical spine causing compressive myelopathy in a dog, J Small Anim Pract 37(3):133–137, 1996.
209. Pool RR, Harris JM: Feline osteochondromatosis, Feline Pract 5(2):24–25, 1975:28.
210. Gradner A, Weissenböck H, Kneissl S, et al: Use of latissimus dorsi and abdominal external oblique muscle for reconstruction of a thoracic wall defect in a cat with feline osteochondromatosis, J Feline Med Surg 10(1):88–94, 2008.
211. Rylander H, Lipsitz D, Berry WL, et al: Retrospective analysis of spinal arachnoid cysts in 14 dogs, J Vet Intern Med 16(6):690–696, 2002.
212. Skeen TM, Olby NJ, Munana KR, et al: Spinal arachnoid cysts in 17 dogs, J Am Anim Hosp Assoc 39:271–282, 2003.
213. Shamir MH, Shahar R, Aizenberg I: Subarachnoid cyst in a cat, J Am Anim Hosp Assoc 33(2):123–125, 1997.
214. Vignoli M, Rossi F, Sarli G: Spinal subarachnoid cyst in a cat, Vet Radiol Ultrasound 40(2):116–119, 1999.
215. Galloway AM, Curtis NC, Sommerlad SF, et al: Correlative imaging findings in seven dogs and one cat with spinal arachnoid cysts, Vet Radiol Ultrasound 40(5):445–452, 1999.
216. Dickinson PJ, LeCouteur RA, Sturges BK, et al: Extradural spinal synovial cysts in two dogs: clinical and pathological features, J Vet Intern Med 13(3):241, 1999:abstract.
217. Levitski RE, Chauvet AE, Lipsitz D: Cervical myelopathy associated with extradural synovial cysts in 4 dogs, J Vet Intern Med 13(3):181–186, 1999.
218. Levitski RE, Lipsitz D, Chauvet AE: Magnetic resonance imaging of the cervical spine in 27 dogs, Vet Radiol Ultrasound 40(4):332–341, 1999.
219. Dickinson PJ, Sturges BK, Berry WL, et al: Extradural spinal synovial cysts in nine dogs, J Small Anim Pract 42:502–509, 2001.
220. Perez B, Rollan E, Ramiro, et al: Intraspinal synovial cyst in a dog, J Am Anim Hosp Assoc 36(3):235–238, 2000.
221. McDonnell JJ, Knowles KE, de Lahunta A, et al: Thoracolumbar spinal cord compression due to vertebral process degenerative joint disease in a family of Shiloh shepherd dogs, J Vet Intern Med 17:530–537, 2003.
222. Luttgen PJL: Neoplasms of the spine, Vet Clin North Am Small Anim Pract 22(4):973–984, 1992.
223. Morgan JP, Ackerman N, Bailey CS, et al: Vertebral tumors in the dog: a clinical, radiologic, and pathologic study of 61 primary and secondary lesions, Vet Radiol Ultrasound 21:197–212, 1980.

224. Petersen SA, Sturges BK, Dickinson PJ, et al: Canine intraspinal meningiomas: imaging features, histopathologic classification, and long-term outcome in 34 dogs, J Vet Intern Med 22(4):946–953, 2008.
225. Fingeroth JM, Prata RG, Patnaik AK: Spinal meningiomas in dogs: 13 cases (1972-1987), J Am Vet Med Assoc 191(6):720–726, 1987.
226. Brehm DM, Vite CH, Steinberg HS, et al: A retrospective evaluation of 51 cases of peripheral nerve sheath tumors in the dog, J Am Anim Hosp Assoc 31(4):349–359, 1995.
227. Marioni-henry K, Vite CH, Newton AL, et al: Prevalence of diseases of the spinal cord of cats, J Vet Intern Med 18:851–858, 2004.
228. Lane SB, Kornegay JN, Duncan JR, et al: Feline spinal lymphosarcoma: a retrospective evaluation of 23 cats, J Vet Intern Med 8(2):99–104, 1994.
229. Summers BA, de Lahunta A: Unusual intradural extramedullary spinal tumours in twelve dogs, J Neuropathol Exp Neurol 45:322, 1986.
230. Petersen SA, Sturges BK, Vernau KM, et al: Spinal cord disease in dogs with neoplasia arising from the central nervous system, J Vet Intern Med 20:735, 2006.
231. Kippenes H, Gavin PR, Bagley RS, et al: Magnetic resonance imaging features of tumors of the spine and spinal cord in dogs, Vet Radiol Ultrasound 40(6):627–633, 1999.
232. Thomson CE, Kornegay JN, Stevens JB: Analysis of cerebrospinal fluid from the cerebellomedullary and lumbar cisterns of dogs with focal neurologic disease: 145 cases (1985-1987), J Am Vet Med Assoc 196(11):1841–1844, 1990.
233. Levy MS, Kapatkin AS, Patnaik AK, et al: Spinal tumors in 37 dogs: clinical outcome and long-term survival (1987-1994), J Am Anim Hosp Assoc 33(4):307–312, 1997.
234. Siegel S, Kornegay JN, Thrall DE: Postoperative irradiation of spinal cord tumors in 9 dogs, Vet Radiol Ultrasound 37(2):150–153, 1996.
235. Dernell WS, Van VB, Straw RC, et al: Outcome following treatment of vertebral tumors in 20 dogs (1986-1995), J Am Anim Hosp Assoc 36(3):245–251, 2000.
236. Rusbridge C, Wheeler SJ, Lamb CR, et al: Vertebral plasma cell tumors in 8 dogs, J Vet Intern Med 13(2):126–133, 1999.
237. Gilmore DR: Intraspinal tumors in the dog, Compend Contin Educ Pract Vet 5(1):55–66, 1983.
238. Wright JA: The pathological features associated with spinal tumours in 29 dogs, J Comp Pathol 95(4):549–557, 1985.
239. Wright JA, Bell DA, Clayton-Jones DG: The clinical and radiological features associated with spinal tumours in thirty dogs, J Small Anim Pract 20:461–472, 1979.
240. Luttgen PJ, Braund KG, Brawner WR Jr, et al: A retrospective study of twenty-nine spinal tumours in the dog and cat, J Small Anim Pract 21:213–226, 1980.
241. McDonnell JJ, Tidwell AS, Faissler D, et al: Magnetic resonance imaging features of cervical spinal cord meningiomas, Vet Radiol Ultrasound 46:368–374, 2005.
242. Moissonnier P, Abbott DP: Canine neuroepithelioma: case report and literature review, J Am Anim Hosp Assoc 29(5):397–401, 1993.
243. Summers BA, deLahunta A, McEntee M, et al: A novel intradural extramedullary spinal cord tumor in young dogs, Acta Neuropathol 75(4):402–410, 1988.
244. McConnell JF, Garosi LS, Dennis R, et al: Imaging of a spinal nephroblastoma in a dog, Vet Radiol Ultrasound 44(5):537–541, 2003.
245. Gasser AM, Bush WW, Smith S, et al: Extradural spinal, bone marrow, and renal nephroblastoma, J Am Anim Hosp Assoc 39:80–85, 2003.
246. Neer TM, Kreeger JM: Cervical spinal cord astrocytoma in a dog, J Am Vet Med Assoc 191(1):84–86, 1987.
247. Stigen Ø, Ytrehus B, Eggertsdottir AV: Spinal cord astrocytoma in a cat, J Small Anim Pract 42:306–310, 2001.
248. Wilson RB, Beckman SL: Mucinous oligodendroglioma of the spinal cord in a dog, J Am Anim Hosp Assoc 31(1):26–28, 1995.
249. Chaffee VW: Spinal cord ependymoma in a dog, Vet Med Small Anim Clin 72(12):1854–1858, 1977.
250. Luttgen PJ, Bratton GR: Spinal cord ependymoma: a case report, J Am Anim Hosp Assoc 12:788–790, 1976.
251. Waters DJ, Hayden DW: Intramedullary spinal cord metastasis in the dog, J Vet Intern Med 4(4):207–215, 1990.
252. Jeffery ND, Phillips SM: Surgical treatment of intramedullary spinal cord neoplasia in two dogs, J Small Anim Pract 36(12):553–557, 1995.
253. Cooley DM, Waters DJ: Skeletal neoplasms of small dogs: a retrospective study and literature review, J Am Anim Hosp Assoc 33(1):11–23, 1997.
254. Chauvet AE, Hogge GS, Sandin JA, et al: Vertebrectomy, bone allograft fusion, and antitumor vaccination for the treatment of vertebral fibrosarcoma in a dog, Vet Surg 28(6):480–488, 1999.
255. Spodnick GJ, Berg J, Moore FM, et al: Spinal lymphoma in cats: 21 cases (1976-1989), J Am Vet Med Assoc 200(3):373–376, 1992.
256. Rebhun WC, de Lahunta A, Baum KH, et al: Compressive neoplasms affecting the bovine spinal cord, Compend Contin Educ Pract Vet 6:396–400, 1984.
257. Rosin A: Neurologic diseases associated with lymphosarcoma in ten dogs, J Am Vet Med Assoc 181(1):50–53, 1982.
258. Williams MA, Welles EG, Gailor RJ, et al: Lymphosarcoma associated with neurological signs and abnormal cerebrospinal fluid in two horses, Prog Vet Neurol 3(2):51–56, 1992.
259. Burnett RC, Vernau W, Modiano JF, et al: Diagnosis of canine lymphoid neoplasia using clonal rearrangements of antigen receptor genes, Vet Pathol 40(1):32–41, 2003.
260. Noonan M, Kline KL, Meleo K: Lymphoma of the central nervous system: a retrospective study of 18 cats, Compend Contin Educ Pract Vet 19(4):497–504, 1997.
261. Mooney SC, Hayes AA, Matus RE, et al: Renal lymphoma in cats: 28 cases (1977-1984), J Am Vet Med Assoc 191(11):1473–1477, 1987.
262. Irving G, McMillan MC: Fluoroscopically guided percutaneous fine-needle aspiration biopsy of thoracolumbar spinal lesions in cats, Prog Vet Neurol 1(4):473–475, 1990.
263. Kuntz CA, Waldron D, Martin RA, et al: Sacral fractures in dogs: a review of 32 cases, J Am Anim Hosp Assoc 31(2):142–150, 1995.
264. Slocum B, Rudy RL: Fractures of the seventh lumbar vertebra in the dog, J Am Anim Hosp Assoc 11(2):167–174, 1975.
265. Beaver DP, MacPherson GC, Muir P, et al: Methylmethacrylate and bone screw repair of seventh lumbar vertebral fracture-luxations in dogs, J Small Anim Pract 37(8):381–386, 1996.
266. Ullman SL, Boudrieau RJ: Internal skeletal fixation using a Kirschner apparatus for stabilization of fracture/luxations of the lumbosacral joint in six dogs. A modification of the transilial pin technique, Vet Surg 22(1):11–17, 1993.

267. Weh JM, Kraus KH: Use of a four pin and methylmethacrylate fixation in L7 and the iliac body to stabilize lumbosacral fracture-luxations: a clinical and anatomic study, Vet Surg 36:775–782, 2010.
268. Shores A, Nichols C, Rochat M, et al: Combined Kirschner-Ehmer device and dorsal spinal plate fixation technique for caudal lumbar vertebral fractures in dogs, J Am Vet Med Assoc 195(3):335–339, 1989.
269. Smeak DD, Olmstead ML: Fractures/luxations of the sacrococcygeal area in the cat: a retrospective study of 51 cases, Vet Surg 14:319–324, 1985.
270. Penwick RC: Fibrocartilaginous embolism and ischemic myelopathy, Compend Contin Educ Pract Vet 11(3):287–299, 1989.
271. Cauzinille L: Fibrocartilaginous embolism in dogs, Vet Clin North Am Small Anim Pract 30:155–167, 2000.
272. Gandini G, Cizinauskas S, Lang J, et al: Fibrocartilaginous embolism in 75 dogs: clinical findings and factors influencing the recovery rate, J Small Anim Pract 44:76–80, 2003.
273. Gilmore DR, de Lahunta A: Necrotizing myelopathy secondary to presumed or confirmed fibrocartilaginous embolism in 24 dogs, J Am Anim Hosp Assoc 23:373–376, 1987.
274. Mikszewski JS, Van Winkle TJ, Troxel MT: Fibrocartilaginous embolic myelopathy in five cats, J Am Anim Hosp Assoc 42:226–233, 2006.
275. Benson JE, Schwartz KJ: Ischemic myelomalacia associated with fibrocartilaginous embolism in multiple finishing swine, J Vet Diagn Invest 10(3):274–277, 1998.
276. Jackson W, de Lahunta A, Adaska J, et al: Fibrocartilaginous embolic myelopathy in an adult Belgian horse, Prog Vet Neurol 6(1):16–19, 1995.
277. Hawthorne JC, Wallace LJ, Fenner WR, et al: Fibrocartilaginous embolic myelopathy in miniature schnauzers, J Am Anim Hosp Assoc 37:374–383, 2001.
278. Junker K, van den Ingh TSGAM, Bossard MM, et al: Fibrocartilaginous embolism (FCE) of the spinal cord in juvenile Irish wolfhounds, Vet Q 22:154–156, 2001.
279. Schubert TA: Fibrocartilaginous infarct in a German shepherd dog, Vet Med Sm Anim Clin 75(5):839–842, 1980.
280. Zaki FA, Prata RG: Necrotizing myelopathy secondary to embolization of herniated intervertebral disk material in the dog, J Am Vet Med Assoc 169(2):222–228, 1976.
281. Grünenfelder FI, Weishaupt D, Green R, et al: Magnetic resonance imaging findings in spinal cord infarction in three small breed dogs, Vet Radiol Ultrasound 46:91–96, 2005.
282. Cauzinille L, Kornegay JN: Fibrocartilaginous embolism of the spinal cord in dogs: review of 36 histologically confirmed cases and retrospective study of 26 suspected cases, J Vet Intern Med 10(4):241–245, 1996.
283. De Risio L, Adams V, Dennis R, et al: Magnetic resonance imaging findings and clinical associations in 52 dogs with suspected ischemic myelopathy, J Vet Intern Med 21(6):1290–1298, 2007.
284. De Risio L, Adams V, Dennis R, et al: Association of clinical and magnetic resonance imaging findings with outcome in dogs suspected to have ischemic myelopathy: 50 cases (2000-2006), J Am Vet Med Assoc 233(1):129–135, 2008.
285. Flanders JA: Feline aortic thromboembolism, Compend Contin Educ Pract Vet 8(7):473–484, 1986.
286. Laste NJ, Harpster NK: A retrospective study of 100 cases of feline distal aortic thromboembolism: 1977-1993, J Am Anim Hosp Assoc 31(6):492–500, 1995.
287. De Risio L, Thomas WB, Sharp NJH: Degenerative lumbosacral stenosis, Vet Clin North Am 30:111–132, 2000.
288. Newitt ALM, German AJ, Barr FJ: Lumbosacral transitional vertebrae in cats and their effects on morphology of adjacent joints, J Feline Med Surg 11:941–947, 2009.
289. Watt PR: Degenerative lumbosacral stenosis in 18 dogs, J Small Anim Pract 32(3):125–134, 1991.
290. Danielsson F, Sjostrom L: Surgical treatment of degenerative lumbosacral stenosis in dogs, Vet Surg 28(2):91–98, 1999.
291. Ness MG: Degenerative lumbosacral stenosis in the dog: a review of 30 cases, J Small Anim Pract 35:185–190, 1994.
292. Suwankong N, Meij BP, Voorhout G, et al: Review and retrospective analysis of degenerative lumbosacral stenosis in 156 dogs treated by dorsal laminectomy, Vet Comp Orthop Traumatol 21(3):285–293, 2008.
293. Janssens L, Beosier Y, Daems R: Lumbosacral degenerative stenosis in the dog. The results of epidural infiltration with methylprednisolone acetate: a retrospective study, Vet Comp Orthop Traumatol 22(6):486–491, 2009.
294. Chambers JN: Degenerative lumbosacral stenosis in dogs, Vet Med Rep 1(2):166–180, 1989.
295. Palmer RH, Chambers JN: Canine lumbosacral diseases. Part I. Anatomy, pathophysiology, and clinical presentation, Compend Contin Educ Pract Vet 13(1):61–69, 1991.
296. Palmer RH, Chambers JN: Canine lumbosacral diseases. Part II. Definitive diagnosis, treatment, and prognosis, Compend Contin Educ Pract Vet 13(2):213–222, 1991.
297. Chambers JN, Selcer BA, Oliver JE Jr: Results of treatment of degenerative lumbosacral stenosis in dogs by exploration and excision, Vet Comp Orthop Traumatol 3:130–133, 1988.
298. Lang J, Häni H, Schawalder P: A sacral lesion resembling osteochondrosis in the German shepherd Dog, Vet Radiol Ultrasound 33(2):69–76, 1992.
299. Morgan JP, Bailey CS: Cauda equina syndrome in the dog: radiographic evaluation, J Small Anim Pract 31:69–77, 1990.
300. Damur-Djuric N, Steffen F, Hassig M, et al: Lumbosacral transitional vertebrae in dogs: classification, prevalence, and association with the sacroiliac morphology, Vet Radiol Ultrasound 47:32–38, 2006.
301. Fluckiger MA, Damur-Djuric N, Hassig M, et al: A lumbosacral transitional vertebra in the dog predisposes to cauda equina syndrome, Vet Radiol Ultrasound 47:39–44, 2006.
302. Schmid V, Lang J: Measurements on the lumbosacral junction in normal dogs and those with cauda equina compression, J Small Anim Pract 34(9):437–442, 1993.
303. Morgan JP: Transitional lumbosacral vertebral anomaly in the dog: a radiographic study, J Small Anim Pract 40(4):167–172, 1999.
304. Jones JC, Hudson JA, Sorjonen DC, et al: Effects of experimental nerve root compression on arterial blood flow velocity in the seventh lumbar spinal ganglion of the dog: measurement using intraoperative Doppler ultrasonography, Vet Radiol Ultrasound 37(2):133–140, 1996.
305. Coates JR: Urethral dyssynergia in lumbosacral syndrome, Proceed 17 ACVIM Forum, Chicago: 299–302, 1999.
306. Oliver JE Jr, Selcer RR, Simpson S: Cauda equina compression from lumbosacral malarticulation and malformation in the dog, J Am Vet Med Assoc 173(2):207–214, 1978.
307. Sisson AF, LeCouteur RA, Ingram JT, et al: Diagnosis of cauda equina abnormalities by using electromyography, discography, and epidurography in dogs, J Vet Intern Med 6(5):253–263, 1992.
308. Hanna FY: Lumbosacral osteochondrosis: radiological features and surgical management in 34 dogs, J Small Anim Pract 42:272–278, 2001.

309. Morgan JP, Bahr A, Franti CE, et al: Lumbosacral transitional vertebrae as a predisposing cause of cauda equina syndrome in German shepherd dogs: 161 cases (1987-1990), J Am Vet Med Assoc 202(11):1877–1882, 1993.
310. Steffen F, Hunold K, Scharf G, et al: A follow-up study of neurologic and radiographic findings in working German shepherd dogs with and without degenerative lumbosacral stenosis, J Am Vet Med Assoc 231(10):1529–1533, 2007.
311. Selcer BA, Chambers JN, Schwensen K, et al: Epidurography as a diagnostic aid in canine lumbosacral compressive disease: 47 cases (1981-1986), Vet Comp Orthop Traumatol 3:97–103, 1988.
312. Jones JC, Sorjonen DC, Simpson ST, et al: Comparison between computed tomographic and surgical findings in nine large-breed dogs with lumbosacral stenosis, Vet Radiol Ultrasound 37(4):247–256, 1996.
313. Jones JC, Cartee RE, Bartels JE: Computed tomographic anatomy of the canine lumbosacral spine, Vet Radiol Ultrasound 36(2):91–99, 1995.
314. Jones JC, Wright JC, Bartels JE: Computed tomographic morphometry of the lumbosacral spine of dogs, Am J Vet Res 56(9):1125–1132, 1995.
315. de Haan JJ, Shelton SB, Ackerman N: Magnetic resonance imaging in the diagnosis of degenerative lumbosacral stenosis in four dogs, Vet Surg 22(1):1–4, 1993.
316. Jones JC, Banfield CM, Ward DL: Association between postoperative outcome and results of magnetic resonance imaging and computed tomography in working dogs with degenerative lumbosacral stenosis, J Am Vet Med Assoc 216(11):1769–1774, 2000.
317. Cook JR Jr: Decompressive procedures. Indications and techniques, Vet Clin North Am Small Anim Pract 22(4):917–921, 1992.
318. Godde T, Steffen F: Surgical treatment of lumbosacral foraminal stenosis, Vet Surg 36:705–713, 2007.
319. De Risio L, Sharp NJH, Olby NJ, et al: Predictors of outcome after dorsal decompressive laminectomy for degenerative lumbosacral stenosis in dogs: 69 cases (1987-1997), J Am Vet Med Assoc 219:624–628, 2001.
320. Auger J, Dupuis J, Quesnel A, et al: Surgical treatment of lumbosacral instability caused by discospondylitis in four dogs, Vet Surg 29(1):70–80, 2000.
321. Slocum B, Devine T: Optimal treatment for degenerative lumbosacral stenosis. Traction, internal fixation, and fusion, Vet Med Rep 1(2):249–257, 1989.
322. Linn LL, Bartels KE, Rochat MC, et al: Lumbosacral stenosis in 29 military working dogs: epidemiologic findings and outcome after surgical intervention (1990-1999), Vet Surg 32:21–29, 2003.
323. Bailey CS: An embryological approach to the clinical significance of congenital vertebral and spinal cord abnormalities, J Am Anim Hosp Assoc 11(7):426–434, 1975.
324. Bailey CS, Morgan JP: Congenital spinal malformations, Vet Clin North Am Small Anim Pract 22(4):985–1015, 1992.
325. Kroll RA, Constantinescu GM: Congenital abnormalities of the spinal cord and vertebrae. In August JR, editor: Consultation in feline internal medicine, ed 2, Philadelphia, 1994, WB Saunders.
326. Dennis SM: Congenital defects of the nervous system of lambs, Aust Vet J 51(8):385–388, 1975.
327. Woollen NE: Congenital abnormalities of pigs, Vet Clin North Am Food Anim Pract 9:163–181, 1993.
328. Leipold HW, Cates WF, Radostits OM, et al: Arthrogryposis and associated defects in newborn calves, Am J Vet Res 31(8):1367–1374, 1970.
329. Leipold H, Hiraga T, Johnson LW: Congenital defects in the llama, Vet Clin North Am Food Anim Pract 10:410–420, 1994.
330. Denoix JM: Thoracolumbar malformations or injuries and neurological manifestations, Equine Vet Educ 17:191–194, 2005.
331. Washburn KE, Streeter RN: Congenital defects of the ruminant nervous system, Vet Clin North Am Food Anim Pract 20:413–434, 2004.
332. Agerholm JS, Bendixen C, Andersen O, et al: Complex vertebral malformation in Holstein calves, J Vet Diagn Invest 13:283–289, 2001.
333. Fingeroth JM, Johnson GC, Burt JK, et al: Neuroradiographic diagnosis and surgical repair of tethered cord syndrome in an English bulldog with spina bifida and myeloschisis, J Am Vet Med Assoc 194(9):1300–1302, 1989.
334. Davidson AP: Congenital disorders of the Manx cat, Southwest Vet 37(2):115–119, 1986.
335. Kitchen H, Murray RE, Cockrell BY: Animal model for human disease. Spina bifida, sacral dysgenesis and myelocele. Animal model: Manx cats, Am J Pathol 68(1):203–206, 1972.
336. Plummer SB, Bunch SE, Khoo LH, et al: Tethered spinal cord and an intradural lipoma associated with a meningocele in a Manx-type cat, J Am Vet Med Assoc 203(8):1159–1161, 1993.
337. Kroll RA: Feline spinal cord disease: congenital abnormalities Proceed 10th ACVIM Forum, 265–267, 1992.
338. Wilson JW, Kurtz HJ, Leipold HW, et al: Spina bifida in the dog, Vet Pathol 16(2):165–179, 1979.
339. Engel HN, Draper DD: Comparative prenatal development of the spinal cord in normal and dysraphic dogs: embryonic stage, Am J Vet Res 43(10):1729–1734, 1982.
340. van den Broek AHM, Else RW, Abercromby R, et al: Spinal dysraphism in the Weimaraner, J Small Anim Pract 32(5):258–260, 1991.
341. Shelton MC: A possible mode of inheritance for spinal dysraphism with a more complete description of the clinical syndrome, Ames, IA, 1977, Iowa State University (thesis/dissertation).
342. Dorn AS, Joiner RW: Surgical removal of a meningocoele from a Manx cat, Feline Pract 6:37–40, 1976.
343. Cummings J, de Lahunta A, Timoney J: Neuritis in the cauda equina, a chronic idiopathic polyradiculoneuritis in the horse, Acta Neuropathol 46:17–24, 1979.
344. Wright JA, Fordyce P, Edington N: Neuritis of the cauda equina in the horse, J Comp Pathol 97(6):667–675, 1987.
345. Rousseaux CG, Futcher KG, Clark EG, et al: Cauda equina neuritis: a chronic idiopathic polyneuritis in two horses, Can Vet J 25(5):214–218, 1984.
346. Vatistas NJ, Mayhew IG, Whitwell KE, et al: Polyneuritis equi: a clinical review incorporating a case report of a horse displaying unconventional signs, Prog Vet Neurol 2(1):67–72, 1991.
347. Edington N, Wright J, Patel J, et al: Equine adenovirus 1 isolated from cauda equina neuritis, Res Vet Sci 37:252–254, 1984.
348. Fordyce PS, Edington N, Bridges GC, et al: Use of an ELISA in the differential diagnosis of cauda equina neuritis and other equine neuropathies, Equine Vet J 19(1):55–59, 1987.
349. Morgan SE, Johnson B, Brewer B, et al: Sorghum and cystitis ataxia syndrome in horses, Vet Hum Toxicol 32:582, 1990.
350. Van Kampen KR: Sudan grass and sorghum poisoning of horses: a possible lathyrogenic disease, J Am Vet Med Assoc 156:629–630, 1970.

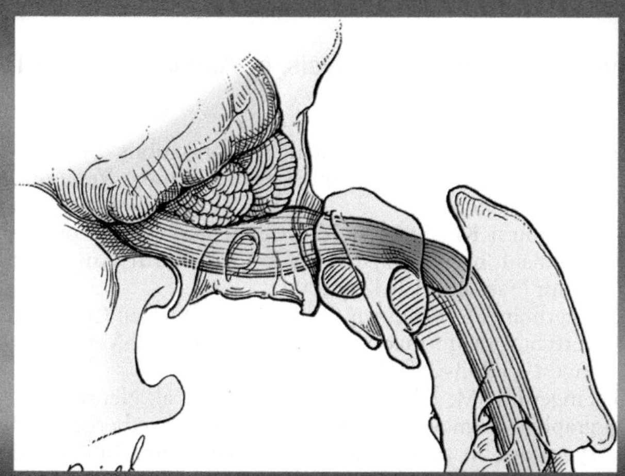

CHAPTER 7

Tetraparesis, Hemiparesis, and Ataxia

The term *tetraparesis* (-plegia) (quadriparesis, quadriplegia) refers to partial (-paresis) or complete (-plegia) loss of voluntary motor function in all limbs. Paresis may be manifested as an inability to support weight against gravity, gait abnormalities, or as postural reaction deficits. The term *hemiparesis* refers to motor dysfunction of two limbs on the same side. General proprioceptive (GP) ataxia is a frequently associated problem. Lesion localization is discussed in Chapter 2, summarized in Figure 7-1, and reviewed briefly in this chapter.

LESION LOCALIZATION

Animals with tetraparesis usually have neurologic disease. Diffuse muscle or skeletal diseases may result in weakness or gait abnormalities which at times are difficult to differentiate from a true neurologic lesion. Tetraparesis must be differentiated from generalized muscle weakness, orthopedic disease (e.g., polyarthritis), or obtundation associated with severe metabolic disease (e.g., adrenal insufficiency, hypoglycemia).

When initially presented with a tetraparetic animal, the clinician must decide which systems are involved (e.g., nervous, musculoskeletal, or general metabolic). Results of the history, physical examination, and laboratory tests usually provide sufficient evidence for the practitioner to make this differentiation. In this chapter, primary consideration is given to lesions involving the central and peripheral nervous systems (CNS and PNS).

Neurologic lesions that produce tetraparesis may involve the brainstem, cervical spinal cord, or lower motor neurons (LMNs). Lesion localization is based on the decisions outlined in Figure 7-1. Although the motor cortex is important for the performance of learned reactions and to help initiate gait (see Chapters 1 and 2), it does not maintain locomotion in domestic animals. Therefore, most animals with structural disease localized to the forebrain have a normal gait and do not display paresis. Importantly, the contralateral postural reaction deficits associated with unilateral forebrain lesions should not be misinterpreted as paresis. Instead, the postural reaction deficits with forebrain lesions represent dysfunction of the ascending GP pathways. Other signs of forebrain dysfunction, such as altered mental status, seizures, or blindness, may be present and may help in lesion localization. Furthermore, animals with diffuse forebrain disease often have little or no gait abnormality once the gait is initiated. Diffuse brainstem centers coordinate the gait with reinforcement from the forebrain. Consequently, lesions involving the midbrain or structures caudal to the midbrain are associated with paresis.

Cervical Spinal Cord

Clinical Signs of Brainstem or C1 to C5 Cervical Spinal Cord

Lesions involving the brainstem and cervical spinal cord result in an abnormal gait because motor pathways from brainstem centers to the LMNs of the spinal cord are disrupted. Tetraparesis develops if the lesion is bilateral, and hemiparesis (usually ipsilateral) develops if the lesion is unilateral. Ascending GP information is altered, resulting in GP ataxia. The GP ataxia frequently is associated with motor dysfunction (paresis) because of the close anatomic relationship between the ascending GP pathways and the descending upper motor neuron (UMN) pathways, in which a lesion involving one pathway will affect the other. In acute and severe spinal cord injuries, respiratory dysfunction may be a sequela, with disruption of the descending UMN pathways from the respiratory centers that lie in the medulla oblongata.

Lesions in the brainstem and C1-5 spinal cord segments result in UMN paresis of the limbs. As explained in Chapter 2, disruption of UMN signals that inhibit the segmental spinal reflexes results in "release," or disinhibition, of the LMNs. Exaggerated reflexes result when UMN inhibitory influence on the LMNs is lost. Similarly, extensor hypertonus or spasticity also may develop in all limbs. Brainstem and cranial cervical spinal cord lesions are differentiated by examination of the head, because lesions in either region can result in identical abnormalities in the limbs. The brainstem can be described as a cervical spinal cord that is modified by the presence of cranial nerve nuclei which are analogous to the LMN neurons that contribute to the innervations of the limbs. Evidence of dysfunction in these cranial nerve nuclei in conjunction with GP ataxia/UMN tetraparesis indicates brainstem disease.

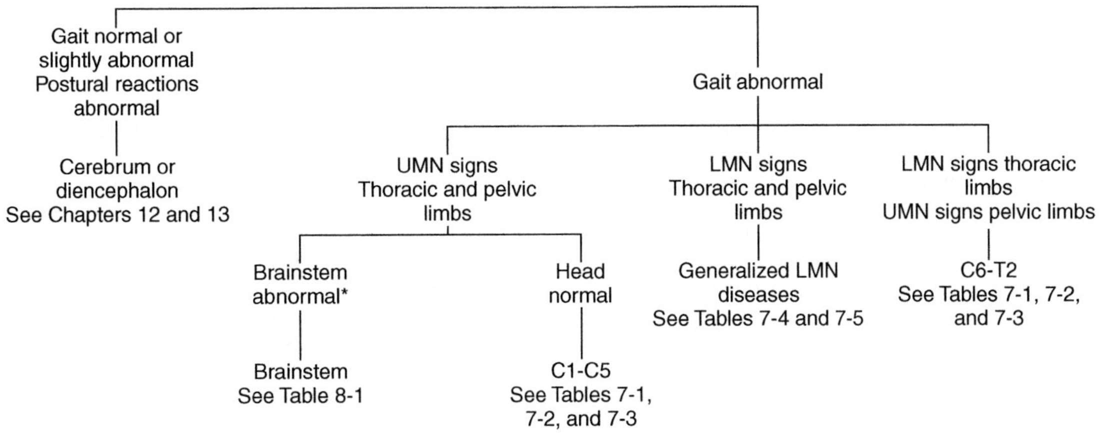

Gait normal or slightly abnormal Postural reactions abnormal
Cerebrum or diencephalon See Chapters 12 and 13
Gait abnormal
UMN signs Thoracic and pelvic limbs
Brainstem abnormal*
Brainstem See Table 8-1
Head normal
C1-C5 See Tables 7-1, 7-2, and 7-3
LMN signs Thoracic and pelvic limbs
Generalized LMN diseases See Tables 7-4 and 7-5
LMN signs thoracic limbs UMN signs pelvic limbs
C6-T2 See Tables 7-1, 7-2, and 7-3

*Brainstem involvement: one or more signs involving the head are present, e.g., head tilt, nystagmus, cranial nerve signs, seizures, and so forth.

Figure 7-1 Algorithm for the diagnosis of tetraparesis, hemiparesis, and ataxia.

Knowledge of the anatomic location of the cranial nerve nuclei allow localization of a lesion to a specific area of the brainstem (see Chapters 8 through 11). For example, paresis associated with vestibular signs, altered mental status, or other abnormal cranial nerve functions strongly suggest a lesion in the brainstem.

C6 to T2 Cervical Spinal Cord

Lesions involving the C6-T2 spinal cord segments result in tetraparesis and a distinct gait disturbance. In the thoracic limbs, LMN signs may be present as the motor neurons forming the brachial plexus are injured, whereas in the pelvic limbs, disruption of the GP and UMN pathways result in GP ataxia and UMN paresis. The thoracic limb gait is characteristic of LMN paresis (see later). Additional LMN signs in the thoracic limbs are related to dysfunction of the suprascapular, axillary, musculocutaneous, radial, median, and ulnar nerves. Thoracic limb reflexes may be depressed or absent, and the muscles may be hypotonic. Neurogenic muscle atrophy subsequently develops. In addition, Horner's syndrome may develop if the LMNs in T1-3 spinal cord segments that form the sympathetic nerve are injured. Sensory perception in the thoracic limbs also is invariably altered with significant lesions of the C6-T2 spinal cord segments. Moreover, UMN signs develop in the pelvic limbs because GP and UMN pathways are disrupted as they pass through the caudal cervical spinal cord.

Peripheral Nervous System (PNS)

Anatomy

Peripheral nervous system diseases result from pathology of the lower motor neuron or motor unit. A motor unit is composed of the neuronal cell body located within the CNS, its axon, the neuromuscular junction, and associated muscle fibers. A group of myofibers innervated by one neuron is considered the *motor unit.* An abnormality in any portion of the motor unit can result in clinical signs of neuromuscular disease—LMN signs. The functional component of the motor unit involves the *reflex arc.* The reflex arc consists of a sense organ, an afferent neuron (cell body in spinal ganglion), one or more synapses centrally, an efferent neuron (LMN), and an effector organ (muscle fiber). The classic example of a reflex arc is the patellar reflex. An all-or-none action potential is generated in the afferent nerve and modulated centrally to be generated again as an all-or-none potential in the efferent nerve. Transmission of the electrical impulse is conveyed by the axon and its myelin sheath. Myelin is formed by Schwann cells in the PNS and oligodendrocytes in the CNS. Processes from these cells wrap around an axon in a unique multilamellar structure analogized to a "Swiss roll" as it fuses with the inner axonal membrane. Schwann cells are aligned along the length of the axon and separated by a gap, the node of Ranvier. Myelin acts as an insulator by having high resistance and low capacitance within the internodal regions. This allows an electrical impulse to propagate rapidly down the axon, jumping from node to node, a process called *saltatory conduction.* The conduction velocity in myelinated fibers is much faster than in nonmyelinated fibers. The electrical impulse arriving at the axonal terminal (pre-synapse) results in influx of calcium and release of a transmitter (chemical transmission) that interacts with receptors within the postsynaptic membrane of the effector organ (muscle).

An individual peripheral nerve contains a variable mix of nerve fibers, myelinated and unmyelinated. Most nerves in the PNS contain both motor and sensory fibers. Motor axons of spinal nerves and cranial nerves originate from neuronal cell bodies that lie within the gray matter of the spinal cord (ventral horn) and brainstem, respectively. Cell bodies for sensory fibers are contained within the spinal ganglia or cranial ganglia. Afferent (sensory) fibers can be myelinated or nonmyelinated. Efferent (motor) fibers to skeletal muscle are always myelinated. Nonmyelinated fibers, however, comprise the postganglionic sympathetic fibers supplying smooth muscles and blood vessels.

Clinical Signs

Tetraparetic animals with LMN signs of the thoracic and pelvic limbs can have lesions involving the motor neuron cell bodies (neuronopathies) which are located in the spinal cord, axon (ventral spinal root, spinal nerve, nerve), neuromuscular junction (motor end plates), or muscle (see Tables 7-4 and 7-5). Neuropathies and neuromuscular junction and muscle disorders are commonly encountered in animals, whereas neuronopathies are rare. Lesions involving motor neurons, ventral nerve roots, or neuromuscular junctions do not produce altered sensory perception. Neuropathies may cause altered sensory perception, because most nerves contain both motor and sensory fibers. Animals with LMN signs in the limbs and normal sensory perception usually have a disease of the ventral nerve roots or the neuromuscular junction. Those with episodic neurologic signs (e.g., exacerbated by exercise) usually have neuromuscular junction disease involving the motor endplate. Occasionally, animals with diffuse muscle disease develop episodic LMN dysfunction. Careful muscle palpation, laboratory tests, electrophysiologic testing, and muscle/nerve biopsy are usually necessary to differentiate primary muscle disease from primary neuropathies or neuronopathies.

Diseases in which episodes of weakness are interspersed with periods of normalcy are perplexing because many different body systems may be involved. Episodic weakness can be a clinical sign of cardiovascular, metabolic, or neuromuscular disease. The neuromuscular disorders, myasthenia gravis, and several myopathies that may cause episodic weakness will be discussed. Other systemic and metabolic causes are discussed in Chapter 15.

DISEASES OF THE SPINAL CORD, C1-T2

The diseases discussed in this chapter include those that commonly affect the cervical spinal cord and those that diffusely affect the LMN system. Diseases that affect the forebrain and brainstem are discussed in Chapters 8 through 15. This section is organized according to the anatomic location of the lesion and the course of the disease (acute versus chronic, progressive versus nonprogressive). The disorders that affect spinal cord segments C1-T2 in small animals are presented in Table 7-1. Cervical spinal cord diseases of horses are presented in Table 7-2, and those of food animals are listed in Table 7-3. Diffuse LMN diseases involving neuropathies and myopathies are listed in Table 7-4 and Table 7-5.

Acute Progressive Diseases, C1-T2

The acute progressive disorders to involve degenerative diseases such as intervertebral disk disease and equine degenerative myelopathy (see Chapter 6), spinal cord and vertebral column neoplasia (see Chapter 6), and inflammatory noninfectious and infectious diseases (see Chapter 15) are discussed elsewhere.

Degenerative

Cervical Intervertebral Disk Disease

Pathophysiology. The pathophysiology of intervertebral disk disease (IVDD) is discussed in Chapter 6. Hansen type I IVDD in the cervical vertebral column occurs most frequently in the chondrodystrophic breeds (miniature poodle, dachshund, beagle, cocker spaniel) but can also occur in certain large-breed dogs such as the Doberman pinscher.[1] The incidence of cervical IVDD in dogs is lower than that of thoracolumbar IVDD. About 14% of all IVD herniations in the dog occur in the cervical vertebral column.[2] The most common sites for Hansen type I IVDD in the cervical vertebral column are C2-3 and C3-4 in small-breed dogs and C6-7 in larger-breed dogs.[1,3] Cervical IVD herniations rarely cause clinical signs in other species, primarily cats and horses.[2,4,5] In older cats, the cervical vertebral column has been reported as the most common site for IVD protrusion, followed by the mid- to caudal lumbar regions.[6,7] Older, nonchondrodystrophic large-breed dogs more commonly have Hansen type II IVDD of the caudal cervical vertebral column.[1,8]

Unlike thoracolumbar IVDD, cervical IVD herniations less commonly result in compressive myelopathy sufficient to cause paresis or paralysis. Although many factors may account for this finding, the larger diameter of the vertebral canal in the cervical vertebral column is probably the most logical explanation. Because of the greater space surrounding the cervical cord, IVD herniations in this area are less likely to result in focal compressive myelopathy. Likewise, the syndrome of ascending-descending myelomalacia rarely results from cervical IVDD or fracture of the cervical vertebral column.

Clinical Signs. Cervical spinal pain is the most common clinical sign of acute onset cervical IVDD. Low head and neck carriage, neck rigidity, and spasms of the cervical spinal muscles are common clinical manifestations of cervical spinal pain (Figure 7-2). Dogs may resist any attempt to move their head or neck. Pressure from herniated disk material on the nerve root can cause nerve root ischemia and severe pain. Dogs with pain alone as a clinical sign often have some evidence of spinal cord compression with diagnostic imaging.[9] Pain is often intermittent and manifests as thoracic limb lameness (root signature or radicular pain; see Chapter 5).[10] Forced movement of the thoracic limbs may cause considerable pain. Dogs that are in pain have a stiff, short-strided gait and may cry or whine if forced to change direction suddenly. Most dogs are reluctant or refuse to climb down stairs or jump. These clinical signs of cervical spinal pain are not pathognomonic for IVDD, but instead are similar to those associated with disease processes such as meningitis and polyarthritis (see Chapters 14 and 15).

The presence of neurologic signs other than pain strongly suggests spinal cord compression. Cervical IVD herniation can compress the cervical spinal cord causing tetra- or hemiparesis and GP ataxia of the thoracic and pelvic limbs. Rarely, a massive or acute IVD herniation produces tetraplegia or hemiplegia and development of the syndrome of ascending-descending myelomalacia.[11-13] Tetraplegia with loss of pain perception is not recognized, because respiratory arrest occurs with such a lesion. In a study in 32 dogs with cervical IVD herniation, fewer than one-third of dogs that were nonambulatory experienced loss of voluntary motor function; altered sensory perception was encountered even less frequently.[14]

In general, thoracic limb spinal reflexes are normal to hyperreflexic with a C1-5 spinal cord lesion and hyporeflexic with a C6-T2 lesion. However, spinal reflex evaluations may not be reliable for localization within the cervical spinal cord region. A decreased flexor reflex does not always indicate a lesion from C6-T2 and can also occur with lesions at C1-5 spinal cord level.[15] Intervertebral disk protrusions affecting the cervical spinal cord may also produce ipsilateral Horner's syndrome as a result of disruption of the descending lateral tectotegmental spinal tract that controls the sympathetic LMNs located in the T1-3 spinal cord segments. Other clinical signs associated with peracute cervical IVD extrusions are cardiac arrhythmia and respiratory dysfunction. Dysphonia or respiratory dysfunction can occur if edema and injury extends to the caudal brainstem or disrupts the descending respiratory pathways.[16]

Diagnosis. A presumptive diagnosis is based on clinical signs and signalment. Imaging studies of the spinal cord using myelography and/or computed tomography (CT) and magnetic resonance imaging (MRI) are necessary to confirm a diagnosis of IVDD and extent of the lesion (see Chapter 4 and 6). Radiography of the cervical vertebral column can provide evidence of in situ disk mineralization and may show narrowing of the IVD space (Figure 7-3) and rule out other bony lesions. Anesthesia is required for proper positioning of the cervical vertebral column in a patient. The use of survey radiography alone is an inaccurate means for identifying the site of IVD herniation.[17] Myelography can show attenuation and displacement of the contrast column (Figure 7-4).[9] Oblique views may further identify foraminal extrusions.[10]

CT and MRI (see Figure 7-3) more accurately access lesion extent and injury of the spinal cord.[18-20] MRI is the imaging modality of choice, as it allows assessment of the spinal cord. Cerebrospinal fluid (CSF) should be obtained to rule out meningomyelitis.

Treatment. As with thoracolumbar IVDD, dogs may be treated conservatively or surgically (see Chapter 6). Dogs with an initial episode of pain may be treated with conservative

TABLE 7-1

Small Animal C1-T2 Spinal Cord Diseases: Differential Diagnosis Based on Clinical Course and Etiologic Categories*

Etiologic Category	Acute Nonprogressive	Acute Progressive	Chronic Progressive
Degenerative	None	Hansen type I IVDD (6,7) Ascending descending myelomalacia (6) Myelinolysis (6)	Hansen type II IVDD (6,7) Cervical spondylomyelopathy (7) Spondylosis deformans (6) Neuronopathies (7) Myelinolysis (6) Dysmyelinating diseases (7) Axonopathies (7) Lysosomal storage diseases (8,15) Extradural synovial cysts (7)
Anomalous	None	None	Spinal cord malformation (6) Vertebral column malformation (6) Atlantoaxial subluxation (7) Atlantooccipital malformation (7) Chiari-like malformation (7) Intra-arachnoid cyst/diverticulum (6)
Neoplastic (6)	None	Primary Hematopoietic Skeletal Metastatic	Primary Hematopoietic Skeletal Metastatic
Nutritional	None	None	Hypervitaminosis A (cats) (15)
Inflammatory	None	Distemper myelitis (15) Bacterial myelitis (15) Rickettsial myelitis (15) Protozoal myelitis (15) Mycotic myelitis (15) Diskospondylitis (6) Epidural empyema (6) Vertebral physitis (6)	Feline infectious peritonitis (15) Granulomatous meningoencephalomyelitis (15) Steroid-responsive meningitis arteritis (15)
Traumatic	Fractures (6) Luxations (6) Contusions (6) Hansen type III disk extrusion (6)	Ascending descending myelomalacia (6)	None
Vascular	Fibrocartilaginous embolism (6,7) Vascular malformations (7) Embolic myelopathy (6)	None	None

*Numbers in parentheses refer to chapters in which the entities are discussed.

therapy. Many dogs with cervical IVDD respond at least temporarily to conservative therapy (see next section). Because of lower risk for severe, permanent neurologic dysfunction, cervical IVD extrusion is usually not considered a neurosurgical emergency, as is the case with thoracolumbar IVDD. Decisions regarding conservative or surgical therapy are based on the clinical signs and chronicity of the problem.

Conservative Therapy. Principles of conservative management are described in Chapter 6. Conservative therapy for cervical IVDD, as with thoracolumbar IVDD, should be restricted to dogs with an initial episode of neck pain. The most important element of the treatment is strict confinement to keep movement to a minimum. Conservative therapy is attempted while the dog is monitored for reduction of pain and improvement in neurologic status. Collars should be avoided and use of harnesses encouraged. If the animal is confined but still has considerable pain, opioid analgesics and corticosteroids or nonsteroidal antiinflammatory drugs may be used (see Chapter 14). Pain relief must be accompanied by strict confinement because otherwise, the animal may become too active. The owner is instructed to maintain confinement for at least 4 to 6 weeks, regardless of how much the dog improves. If signs worsen or paresis ensues within the early period of confinement, the dog should be reevaluated for surgery.

In dogs with cervical IVDD, conservative therapy alone often is ineffective and recurrence is common. A possible reason for lack of response to strict cage rest is that total immobility of the cervical vertebral column is difficult to maintain. It also has been shown in dogs with the presenting sign of cervical spinal pain alone that a significant amount of extruded IVD material is often present in the vertebral canal.[9] In the authors' experience, surgery is recommended when pain is

TABLE 7-2

Equine C1-T2 Spinal Cord Diseases: Differential Diagnosis Based on Clinical Course and Etiologic Categories*

Etiologic Category	Acute Nonprogressive	Acute Progressive	Chronic Progressive
Degenerative	None	Equine degenerative myeloencephalopathy (7)	Cervical spondylomyelopathy (7) Neuronopathies (7) Demyelinating diseases (7) Axonopathies (7)
Anomalous	None	None	Vertebral column malformation (6) Spinal cord malformation (6) Occipitoatlantoaxial malformation (7) Atlantoaxial luxation (7)
Neoplastic (6)	None	Metastatic Primary Skeletal Hematopoietic	Primary Skeletal Hematopoietic
Nutritional	None	Degenerative myeloencephalopathy (7)	
Inflammatory	None	Herpesvirus (6) Protozoal myelitis (6) Verminous migrations (6) Vertebral osteomyelitis (6) Mycotic myelitis (6)	See Acute Progressive
Traumatic	Fractures (6) Luxations (6) Brachial plexus injury (5)	None	None
Vascular	Embolic myelopathy (6) Fibrocartilaginous emboli (6) Postanesthetic myelopathy	None	None

*Numbers in parentheses refer to chapters in which the entities are discussed.

refractory to pain management for longer than 1 to 2 weeks or when progression of neurologic deficits occurs. There has been limited information on the success of conservative therapy for cervical IVDD in dogs. The recurrence rate has been reported as 36% in dogs treated conservatively for cervical IVDD.[21] More recently, Levine et al. reported that dogs with a presumptive diagnosis of cervical IVDD had a success rate of 48.9%, with 33% having recurrence of clinical signs and 18% having therapeutic failure.[22] Owners must be cautioned that clinical signs often recur after conservative therapy.

Surgical. Evidence of severe intractable pain, progression of paresis, or paresis at the onset of clinical signs are an indication for decompressive surgery. The various forms of surgical therapy have been reviewed extensively by Hoerlein.[2] In cervical IVDD, decompressive procedures by ventral or dorsal approaches are techniques of choice for removal of an extruded disk. Selection of the decompressive procedure is usually determined by the location of the herniated IVD material. The ventral slot technique is commonly performed for IVD material displaced ventral to the spinal cord (Figure 7-5).[23] Using identifying landmarks, the ventral tubercle of the C1 and the transverse processes of C6 vertebrae, to identify the IVD space of the herniation, a midline "slot" is created into the ventral aspect of the affected IVD and the adjacent cranial and caudal vertebral endplates/bodies of the vertebrae using a pneumatic drill. Advantages of the ventral decompressive technique include minimal muscle dissection, limited need for manipulation of the spinal cord to remove herniated disk material, and exposure for prophylactic fenestration of adjacent cervical disks.

Dorsal laminectomy involves dissection of the epaxial musculature and removal of the spinous process and the laminae.[24,25] Dorsal procedures provide spinal cord decompression and access for laterally extruded IVD material, but access is limited to extruded IVD material located ventral to the spinal cord. A lateral approach has been described for lateral or intraforaminal IVD extrusions at the C4-5 and C5-6 interspaces.[26,27] Prophylactic disk fenestration can be performed at the time of ventral decompression. Fenestration alone as a surgical treatment should not be performed, because the IVD material in the vertebral canal is not removed.[28-30]

Complications associated with cervical spinal surgery include excessive hemorrhage from damage to the internal vertebral venous plexi or vertebral artery and incomplete removal of disk IVD material, leading to inadequate decompression. In the ventral slot procedure, if the width of the slot is too wide (>40% to 50%), dogs may suffer from instability or subluxation.[31] Dogs undergoing cervical spinal surgery also are at higher risk for postoperative pneumonia.[32] Other related risk factors for pneumonia include tetraparesis, long anesthetic times (>1 hour), repeat anesthesias, and postrecovery vomiting.

The prognosis for functional recovery after decompression of most cervical IVD extrusions is excellent. Predictors for recovery outcomes in dogs with cervical IVDD are based on site of herniation, ambulatory status, and breed size. In a recent study of 190 dogs with cervical IVDD treated surgically, outcomes were no different for the ambulatory versus nonambulatory dogs with intact pain perception.[1] After surgery,

TABLE 7-3

*Food Animal C1-T2 Spinal Cord Diseases: Differential Diagnosis Based on Clinical Course and Etiologic Categories**

Etiologic Category	Acute Nonprogressive	Acute Progressive	Chronic Progressive
Degenerative	None	None	Myeloencephalopathies—B (7) Spondylosis deformans—all (6) Arthrogryposis—all (7) Neuronopathies—B, O (7) Axonopathies—B (7) Hypo-/demyelinating diseases—B, P, O (7)
Anomalous	None	None	Vertebral column malformations—all (6) Occipitoatlantoaxial malformations—B, O (6) Spinal cord malformations—all (6) Chiari-like malformation—B (7)
Neoplastic (6)	None	Primary Hematopoietic Skeletal Metastatic	Primary Hematopoietic Skeletal Metastatic
Nutritional	None	None	Enzootic ataxia, copper deficiency—C, O (15) Nicotinic acid deficiency—P
Inflammatory	None	Caprine arthritis-encephalomyelitis—C (6) Bacterial myelitis—all (15) Protozoal myelitis (6,15) Mycotic myelitis (15) Vertebral osteomyelitis—all (6)	Visna-Maedi—O (6,15) Verminous migration—all (6)
Toxic	None	Selenium—P (15)	
Traumatic	Fractures (6) Luxations (6) Contusions (6) Brachial plexus injury(5)	None	None
Vascular	Fibrocartilaginous embolism—P (6)	None	None

B, Bovine; *C*, caprine; *O*, ovine; *P*, porcine.
*Numbers in parentheses refer to chapters in which the entities are discussed.

99% of dogs had resolution of cervical spinal pain and were able to ambulate unassisted. In contrast, another study in 32 dogs with nonambulatory tetraparesis reported that only 62% had a complete recovery.[14] Predictors for recovery included higher likelihood of recovery in small-breed dogs and return of ambulatory function within 96 hours after surgery. However if given more time, many dogs still regained ambulatory function but had residual deficits. In contrast to some previous studies, site of IVD herniation was not a significant predictor of complete recovery.[14] In large-breed dogs with Hansen type II disk protrusions, recovery may be slow, which necessitates physical rehabilitation (see caudal cervical spondylomyelopathy). Previous studies have reported dogs with caudal cervical IVD extrusions respond less favorably and are more severely affected than dogs with cranial cervical IVD extrusions.[11,33,34] In large-breed dogs with Hansen type II IVDD and caudal cervical spondylomyelopathy, only a 66% success rate following ventral decompression has been reported.[35]

Recurrence of clinical signs after surgery in dogs with cervical IVDD ranges from 10%[1] to 33%.[33] The most common clinical sign of recurrence was cervical spinal pain. A second IVD extrusion at a site distinct from the initial lesion was the most common reason for recurrence.

Inflammatory

Cervical Meningomyelitis. Inflammation of the meninges caused by bacterial, viral, rickettsial, or fungal agents or subsequent to idiopathic diseases such as granulomatous meningoencephalomyelitis (GME), steroid responsive meningitis arteritis (SRMA), or the meningoencephalitides of unknown etiology (MUE), may produce clinical signs that are similar to those of cervical IVDD (see Chapter 15). Cervical spinal pain is common with meningitis. Involvement of the white or gray matter of the spinal cord results in GP ataxia, paresis, or paralysis. These diseases are sometimes characterized by polysystemic signs and multifocal neurologic lesions. In many cases, the course becomes chronic and progressive after the acute development of neurologic signs. Diagnosis is primarily based on clinical signs, imaging features, CSF abnormalities, and exclusion of other diseases. These disorders are discussed in Chapter 15.

Acute Nonprogressive Diseases, C1-T2

Traumatic

Cervical Spinal Cord Trauma

Pathogenesis. Traumatic compression of the cervical spinal cord, in contrast to that in the thoracolumbar area, is more likely to cause pain with little motor dysfunction; however,

TABLE 7-4

Diffuse Neuropathic and Neuromuscular Junction Diseases of Domestic Animals: Differential Diagnosis Based on Clinical Course and Etiologic Categories*

Etiologic Category	Episodic	Acute Progressive	Chronic Progressive
Degenerative	None	None	Arthrogryposis—all (7) Neuronopathies—B, O (7) Axonopathies—B (7) Hypo-/demyelinating diseases—B, P, O (7) Some storage diseases (7,8,15)
Anomalous	Congenital myasthenia gravis (NMJ)—Ca, F, B	None	
Metabolic (7,15)	None	None	Diabetes mellitus—Ca, F Hypothyroidism—Ca Hyperthyroidism—F Hyperoxaluria—F Hyperchylomicronemia—F
Neoplastic	None	Paraneoplastic—Ca (7) Hematopoietic	None
Nutritional	None	None	Enzootic ataxia, copper deficiency—C, O (15) Tyrosine/phenylalanine deficiency—F Pantothenic acid deficiency—P
Idiopathic	None	None	Idiopathic polyneuropathy—Ca, F Stringhalt—E
Inflammatory/immune mediated (7)	Aquired myasthenia gravis—Ca, F	Polyradiculoneuritis Polyneuritis Protozoal polyradiculoneuritis Ganglioradiculoneuritis	Chronic inflammatory demyelinating polyneuropathy—Ca, F
Toxic (7,15)	None	Fulminant myasthesia gravis (NMJ)—Ca Tick paralysis (NMJ)—all Botulism (NMJ)—all Drugs—vincristine, cisplatin, salinomycin, aminoglycosides	Heavy metals—lead, mercury, thallium, antimony, zinc Insecticides—organophosphates—F, B Other—trichloroethylene, *N*-hexane, acrylamide
Traumatic (all)	None	None	None
Vascular	None	None	None

B, Bovine; *C*, caprine; *Ca*, canine; *E*, equine; *F*, feline; *NMJ*, neuromusucular junction; O, ovine; *P*, porcine.
*Numbers in parentheses refer to chapters in which the entities are discussed.

extensive compression can result in severe motor and sensory dysfunction. Owing to an increased ratio of vertebral canal to spinal cord diameter in the cervical region, clinical signs in dogs with cervical vertebral column trauma more often manifest with cervical spinal pain and postural reaction deficits.[36] Approximately 70% of cervical vertebral fractures involve the C1 and C2 vertebrae, 10% to 15% are between C3 and C7, and multiple fractures are not uncommon (Figure 7-6).[36,37] A fracture between C1 and C5 spinal cord segments results in tetraparesis/plegia or ipsilateral hemiparesis/plegia. Spinal reflexes are normal or exaggerated. Horner's syndrome is possible with severe lesions. Severe lesions can also cause respiratory paresis or apnea from disruption of descending reticulospinal pathways that control muscles for respiration. Dogs with cervical spinal cord injury may require peri- and postoperative ventilatory support. A fracture between C6 and T2 spinal cord segments results in tetraparesis/plegia or ipsilateral hemiparesis/plegia. Thoracic limb spinal reflexes may be decreased or absent with hypotonia. An ipsilateral Horner's syndrome may follow damage of the T1-3 spinal cord segments, spinal roots, or nerves. Animals with monoparesis and LMN signs should be suspected to have a brachial plexus injury or avulsion. Injuries cranial to the C5 spinal cord segment may cause sudden death through disruption of the respiratory pathways to the phrenic and intercostal motor neurons. Tetraplegia with loss of pain perception caudal to the lesion, therefore, is rare because affected animals die of respiratory failure.

Diagnosis and Treatment. Diagnosis and management of spinal cord trauma are discussed in Chapter 6.

Prognosis. Prognosis is variable with cervical vertebral fractures in dogs, especially for large breeds and those receiving surgical management. Conservative treatment with neck

TABLE 7-5

Diffuse Myopathic Diseases of Domestic Animals: Differential Diagnosis Based on Clinical Course and Etiologic Categories*

Etiologic Category	Episodic	Acute Progressive	Chronic Progressive
Degenerative	Exercise-induced collapse in Labrador retrievers†	None	Muscular dystrophies—Ca, F, O Myopathy of Pietrain pigs Other breed-related myopathies—Ca, F Some storage diseases
Anomalous	None	None	
Metabolic (7,15)	Hypokalemia—all Hyperkalemia—all Hypocalcemia—all Hypercalcemia—all Periodic paralysis—E, Ca, F Adrenal insufficiency—all Malignant hyperthermia syndrome—Ca, P Recurrent exertional rhabdomyolysis	None	Hypothyroidism—Ca Hyperthyroidism—F Steroid myopathy—Ca, E Glycogen storage myopathies—Ca, E Polysaccharide storage myopathy—E Mitochondrial, lipid storage myopathy—Ca, E Myotonic myopathy/dystrophy—Ca, F, E, B (10)
Neoplastic (6)	None	Paraneoplastic	Paraneoplastic
Nutritional	None	Vitamin E, Se deficiency White muscle disease—E, B	Vitamin E, Se deficiency
Inflammatory	None	Bacterial myositis—all Protozoal myositis—Ca, F, E Masticatory muscle myositis—Ca Immune-mediated polymyositis—Ca, F Dermatomyositis—Ca Extraocular myositis—Ca	Chronic polymyositis—Ca, F
Toxic (all)	None	Drugs—trimethoprim sulfa Snakes, spider, tetanus Monensin	None
Traumatic (all)	Limber tail—Ca (7) Compartment syndrome (7) Contusions (6)	None	None
Vascular	Ischemic neuromyopathy—Ca, F (6,7)	None	None

B, Bovine; *C*, caprine; *Ca*, canine; *E*, equine; *F*, feline; *O*, ovine; *P*, porcine.
*Numbers in parentheses refer to chapters in which the entities are discussed.
†Now considered synaptic vesicle release abnormality in CNS.

immobilization (external coaptation) is a viable approach for many dogs with cervical fractures. Hawthorne et al. reported functional recovery in 25 of 28 dogs treated conservatively.[37] Surgical treatment was associated with higher mortality (56%). Overall, severity of neurologic deficits (nonambulatory) and prolonged interval to referral was associated with poorer outcome. Early neck immobilization and prompt referral are recommended.

Vascular

Fibrocartilaginous Embolism. This syndrome is described in Chapter 6. The disease can occur in the cervical spinal cord and seems to occur more commonly in small-breed dogs and cats (Figure 7-7).[38-42] The clinical signs develop acutely and progress rapidly in 1 to 2 hours from initial pain to tetraparesis or hemiparesis if only one side of the spinal cord is involved. Signs are compatible with acute cervical spinal cord compression, except affected dogs often have dramatic asymmetry and show lack of paraspinal hyperesthesia. Lesions at C6-T2 spinal cord segments frequently result in LMN signs in the thoracic limbs and GP/UMN signs in the pelvic limbs. Similar to involvement of the lumbosacral intumescence, a correlation between poor prognosis and involvement of intumescences, lesion symmetry, and absence of pain perception has been observed.[39] Diagnosis and management are discussed in Chapter 6.

Chronic Progressive Diseases, C1-T2

The chronic progressive diseases include anomalies and other degenerative diseases of the spinal cord. The degenerative spinal cord diseases often affect the pelvic limbs first but progress to also involve the thoracic limbs. Some degeneration diseases may also affect the brain, hence the term *degenerative myeloencephalopathy*. Malformations, with or without secondary spinal cord compression, affect the cervical vertebrae as elsewhere in the vertebral column (see Chapter 6 for a description of these anomalies). Malformations may be a component of "wobbler" syndrome, which we refer to as *cervical spondylomyelopathy*.

Primary Degenerative Spinal Cord Disorders

In general, these disorders are uncommon. Consideration should be given to these disorders based on clinical signs, typical young age of onset, and breed predilection that occur in many of these degenerative spinal cord diseases. The classification scheme for the degenerative spinal cord disorders of animals are further described in Table 7-6. Many of these degenerative spinal cord disorders have a breed predisposition which may suggest an inherited basis. Initial clinical signs often are worse in the pelvic limbs but then progress to involve the thoracic limbs and possibly the brainstem. Definitive diagnosis of these diseases is usually determined by histopathology of the CNS and PNS. Degenerative spinal cord disorders involving myelinopathy and axonopathy are classified based on their histopathologic features (Table 7-7).[149]

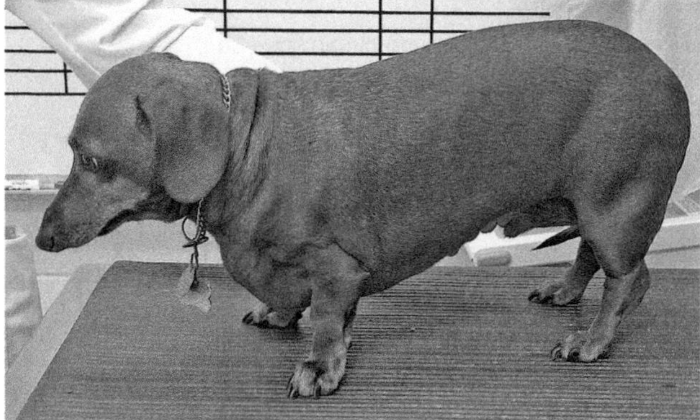

Figure 7-2 A 4-year-old male castrated dachshund shows horizontal neck placement. Dog was reluctant to move his neck and manifested paraspinal hyperesthesia on neck palpation. Hansen type I cervical intervertebral disk herniation was confirmed with diagnostics and surgery.

Central Myelinopathy. Primary myelin degenerative disorders can be classified as hypomyelination, dysmyelination (leukodystrophy), or myelinolytic diseases.[149,150] In hypomyelinogenesis, oligodendrocytes are decreased in numbers or unable to produce functional myelin. These disorders clinically manifest with whole body tremors (see Chapter 10). *Leukodystrophy* refers to inherited conditions of younger animals in which myelin synthesis or function is defective and cannot be maintained. Leukodystrophies have been reported in the dalmation,[151] Labrador retriever,[152] Scottish terrier,[153,154] bull mastiff,[155] and miniature poodle.[156] Onset is within 3 to 6 months of age. Clinical signs manifest as a GP/UMN paraparesis which progresses to tetraparesis. Signs of cerebellar involvement and seizures also may occur. Histopathology reveals myelin degeneration replaced by severe astrogliosis or Rosenthal fibers (astrocytic processes) that is widespread throughout the brain and spinal cord. Leukodystrophy has been described in Charolais cattle, with a progressive history of paraparesis leading to tetraparesis recumbency by 24 months of age.[157-159]

Myelinolysis is characterized by disintegration of initially normally formed myelin. These disorders have been described in the Leonberger,[160] Afghan hound,[161-163] and miniature poodle.[164] Onset of paraparesis is acute, and there is bilateral and symmetrical loss of myelin in all funiculi, with preservation of axons (see Chapter 6).

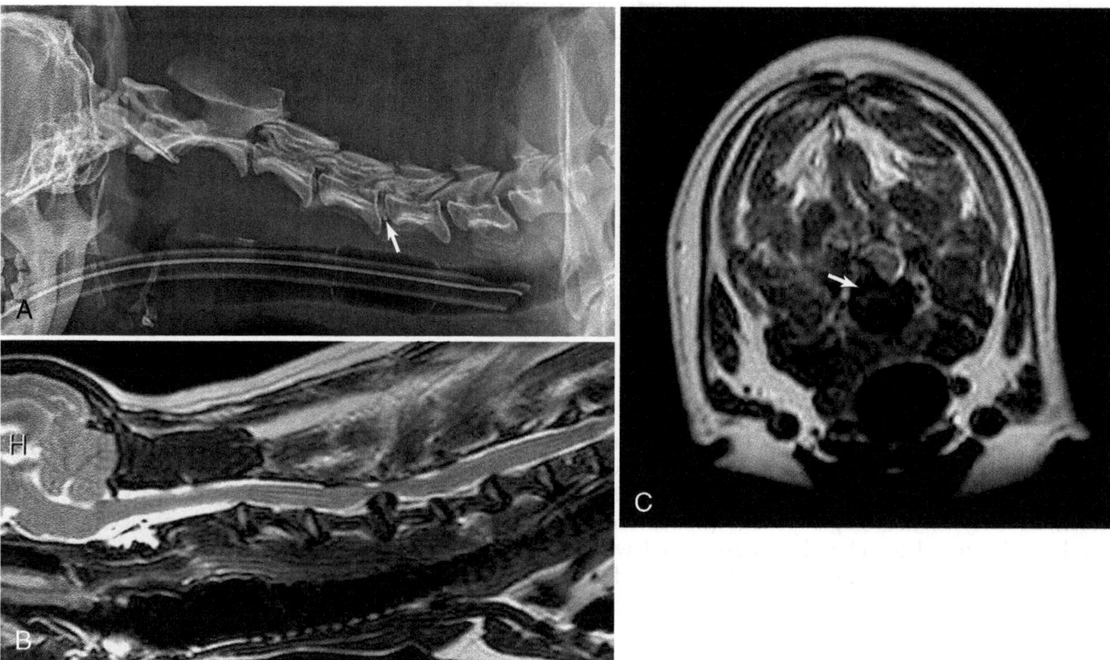

Figure 7-3 **A,** Lateral radiograph of cervical vertebral column in 5-year-old mixed-breed dog with cervical spinal pain. Note narrow intervertebral disk (IVD) space at C4-5 *(arrow)* and opacified nucleus pulposus and extrusion into vertebral canal. **B,** Sagittal T2-weighted image demontrating heterogeneous intensity of a mass at same IVD space. Mass is causing dorsal deviation of spinal cord and attenuation of dorsal subarachnoid space over C4 and C5 spinal cord segments. Degeneration of C4-5 IVD is evidenced by decreased intensity compared to other IVD spaces. **C,** Transverse imaging showing right-sided lateralization of extruded material displacing spinal cord dorsally and to the left. Dog responded well to a ventral slot and removal of extruded nucleus pulposus, typical for Hansen type I intervertebral disk disease.

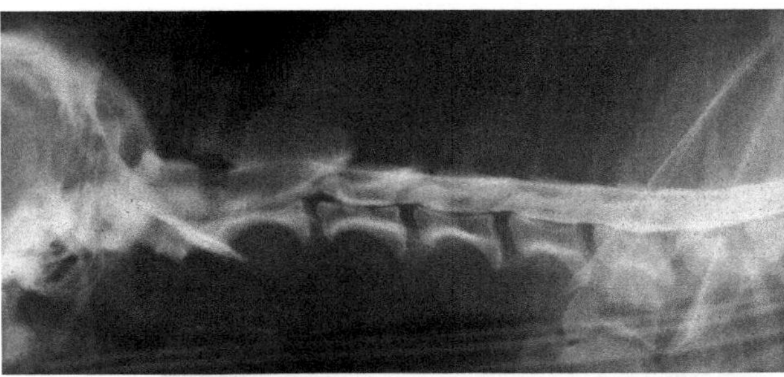

Figure 7-4 Cervical myelogram of dog, showing narrowing of C2-3 intervertebral disk (IVD) space and dorsal deviation of spinal cord over C2-3 IVD space. Lesion was not visualized on survey radiographs. Condition responded to a ventral slot and removal of extruded IVD material.

If the type of myelin degeneration cannot be determined, a more general term, *leukoencephalomyelopathy*, is used to classify these degenerative spinal cord disorders that may be inherited or acquired. Leukoencephalomyelopathies have been documented in the rottweiler[165,166] and Dutch Kooiker dog.[167] The age at onset of signs is within a few months to over 1 year. Progression is rapid in the Dutch Kooiker dog but slow and insidious in the rottweiler. The myelin is affected in all funiculi, with sparing of axons. *Spongy degeneration* is a nonspecific term used to denote that the affected tissue is vacuolated. Vacuolation can be seen in disorders that involve separation of the myelin sheath or that involve the neuronal cell body, as in the prion diseases. A spongiform leukoencephalomyelopathy has been reported in the Australian cattle dog,[168,169] Shetland sheepdog, and Labrador retriever.[170,171] Onset of signs occur within 2 to 9 months of age and are progressive. Clinical signs manifest as cerebellar ataxia, seizures, and opisthotonus. There is widespread vacuolation and myelin degeneration of the spinal cord, brainstem, and cerebellum, with involvement of the cerebral white matter in the Labrador retriever. A leukoencephalomyelopathy has been described in calves of the Murray Grey breed in Australia.[172] Calves manifest ataxia and paresis from birth. Histopathology reveals primarily myelin involvement in the brainstem and spinal cord.

Some lysosomal storage diseases such as globoid cell leukodystrophy cause demyelination by buildup of storage material and accumulation of psychosine.[173,174] Psychosine is a metabolite toxic to myelin-forming oligodendrocytes and Schwann cells. Other myelin disorders that affect primarily the peripheral nerves are discussed in the Lower Motor Neuron section of this chapter.

Central Axonopathy. Axonal degeneration results from disease within the neuronal cell body or within the axon itself. Lesion distributions are variable. Central axonopathy usually consists of bilateral and symmetric degeneration of the axon and myelin and affects both sensory and motor tracts of the spinal cord, with the longest fibers being the most vulnerable.[175] Breeds described include Jack Russell and smooth fox terriers,[176-178] Scottish terrier,[179] and Labrador retriever.[180] Lesions typify diffuse loss of myelinated fibers in the cerebellar white matter and/or in the dorsal funiculi and pyramidal tracts in the spinal cord. Swollen axons may show neurofilament accumulations. In Brown Swiss cattle, at 5 months of age affected calves develop paraparesis and ataxia, and signs insidiously progress over months. Histopathology reveals diffuse axonal degeneration in the spinal cord, with spheroids (axonal swellings) present in some brainstem nuclei and in the cerebellar granular layer.[181,182]

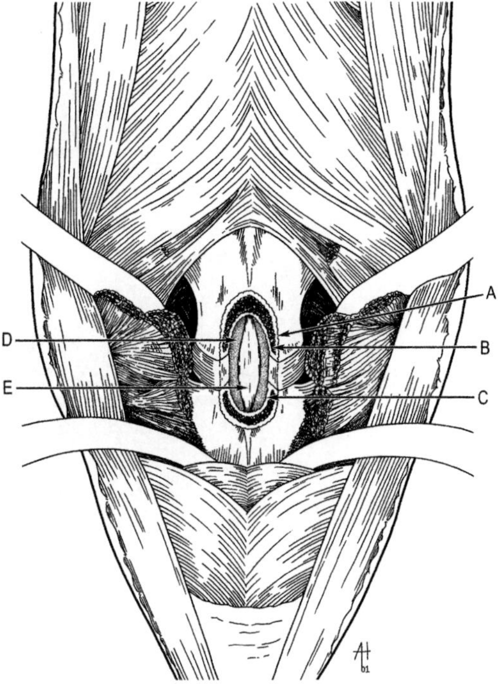

Figure 7-5 Depiction of a ventral slot procedure at C2-3 IVD space. Slot is more extensive in vertebra cranial to disk. Drilling depth is judged by recognition of **(A)** outer cortical bone, **(B)** cancellous bone, and **(C)** inner cortical bone. Other structures not easily seen are **(D)** paired venous sinuses, and **(E)** dorsal longitudinal ligaments. (From Coates JR, Hoffman A, Dewey CW: Surgical approaches to the spine. In Slatter D, editor: Textbook of small animal surgery, ed 3, Philadelphia, 2003, Saunders, pp 1148–1162.)

Those that selectively involve long-tract axons in the CNS and PNS are described as in central-peripheral distal axonopathy. Central-peripheral axonopathy of young dogs have been described in the Ibizan hound,[149] Alaskan husky,[183] boxer,[184-186] Pyrenean mountain dog,[187] and New Zealand Huntaway.[188] y is a central-peripheral axonopathy of older-aged dogs (see Chapter 6).

Those limited to the PNS are neuropathies.[149,189] Axonal degeneration or myelin degeneration may predominate. Sensorimotor neuropathy often shows degenerative changes in spinal ganglia or in the dorsal horn or ventral horn of the spinal cord.[189,190]

Multisystem neuronal degeneration involves axonopathy and neuronopathy throughout the CNS and may include neuropathy (see also Chapter 8). These have been described in the cairn terrier,[191-193] cocker spaniel,[194] golden retriever,[195] and rottweiler.[196]

Neuroaxonal Dystrophy. Neuroaxonal dystrophies (NADs) are primary disorders of axonal transport that occur in dogs, sheep, cats, and horses. They can be histopathologically distinguished from other diseases by the presence of spheroids that involve distal or preterminal parts of the axon and are found in gray matter with proximity to the neuronal cell bodies in the spinal cord and brainstem.[149] These disorders manifest as a progressive cerebellar ataxia and tetraparesis. In dogs, neuroaxonal dystrophy has been described in the rottweiler,[197-199] Chihuahua,[200] working collie sheepdog,[201] Jack Russell terrier,[202] German shepherd dog,[203] and papillon.[204,205] NAD has been sporadically described in cats.[206-208] A progressive ataxia and paraparesis which progressed to tetraparesis has been described in young Suffolk lambs with

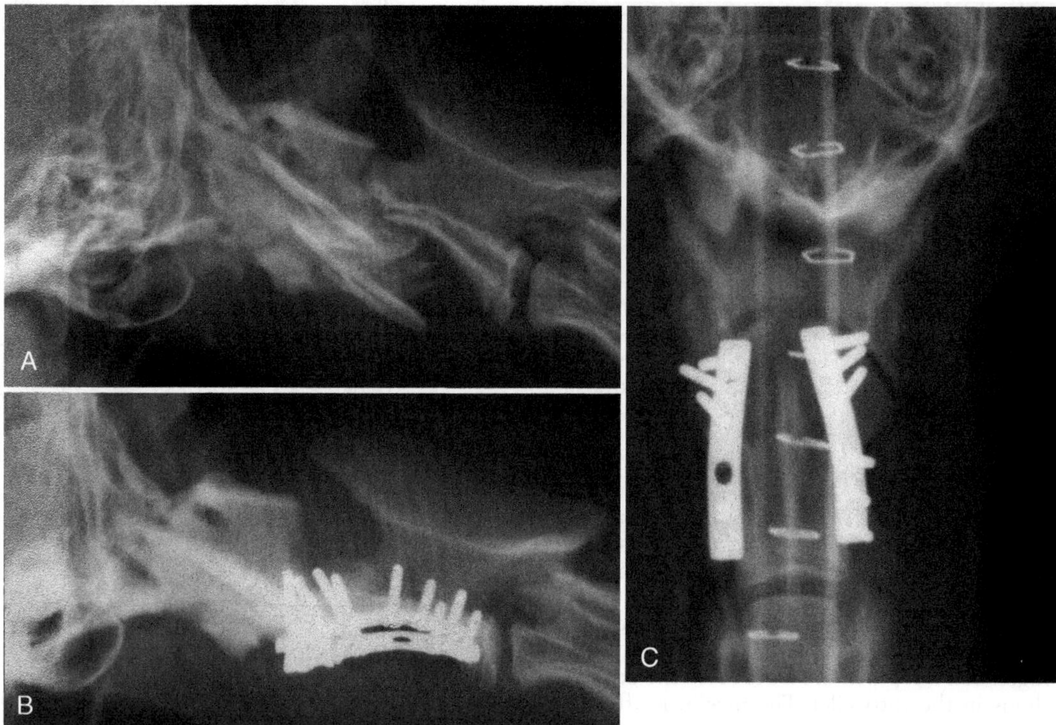

Figure 7-6 **A,** Lateral radiograph of cervical spine from 1-year-old Rottweiler with fracture of C2 vertebra, displaced craniodorsally. **B,** Lateral radiograph taken postoperatively demonstrating use of two plates realigning fracture. **C,** Ventrodorsal view.

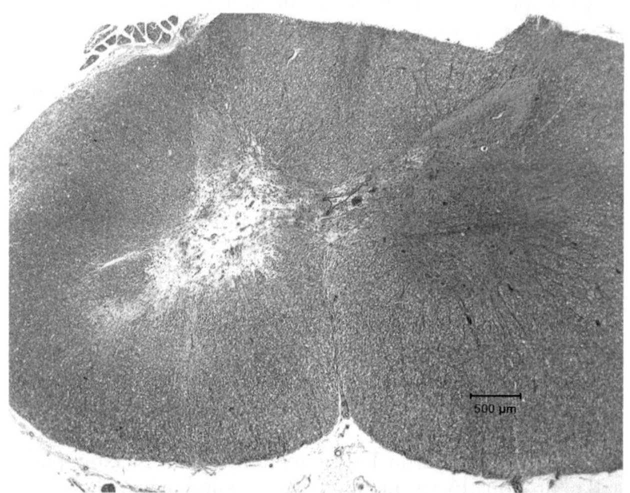

Figure 7-7 Histopathology using Luxol fast blue staining demonstrating malacia and tissue loss in ventral gray matter from a Pembroke Welsh Corgi presenting for acute-onset asymmetric hemiplegia. A presumptive diagnosis of fibrocartilaginous embolism was made. (Courtesy Dr. Gayle C. Johnson.)

neuroaxonal dystrophy.[209] Neuroaxonal dystrophy also has been described in other breeds of sheep in Australia and New Zealand.[210] A potentially familial form of neuroaxonal dystrophy is seen in Morgan horses.[211]

Equine Degenerative Myeloencephalopathy

Pathophysiology. Equine degenerative myeloencephalopathy occurs in light breeds of horses, captive Przewalski horses, zebras, and a few ruminant species.[212] The disease is characterized by acute, progressive, symmetric ataxia and paresis in young animals up to 24 months of age. Chronic progressive forms of the disease have been described. The disease has been diagnosed in Europe and North America, most commonly in the northeastern United States.[213,214] Histopathologically, the disease is characterized by diffuse myeloencephalopathy, with lesions in the spinal cord and brainstem of variable severity.[215] Degeneration of white matter occurs in all spinal cord funiculi and also involves the white matter in the sensory (proprioceptive) relay nuclei in the medulla oblongata, consisting of spheroid formation, astrogliosis, and axonal and myelin loss. Equine degenerative myeloencephalopathy is clinically indistinguishable from neuroaxonal dystrophy. Lesion distribution of NAD differs with its lesion confinement to the cuneate and gracilis nuclei in the brainstem.[216,217] A familial tendency to develop EDM has been observed in the Arabian, thoroughbred, Paso Fino, Appaloosa, and standardbred breeds and in some zebras.[218] A similar, potentially familial, form of neuroaxonal dystrophy is seen in Morgan horses.[211] The cause of degenerative myeloencephalopathy is unknown but may involve a complex interaction of many factors. In other species, degenerative myeloencephalopathies with similar histologic findings have been linked to etiologies such as vitamin E and copper deficiencies, genetics, and toxins. Risk factors associated with EDM include use of insecticides, exposure to wood preservatives, and frequency of time spent on dirt with limited exposure to forages containing adequate vitamin E content.[219] Some studies showed evidence of vitamin E deficiency,[218,220] but this finding has not been substantiated by others.[221] Consequently, the role of vitamin E and other related cofactors in the development of EDM remains unclear. The disease must be differentiated from NAD, cervical spondylomyelopathy, and protozoal myeloencephalitis.

Clinical Signs. Signs develop in horses that are younger than 2 years of age, with a mean age at onset of 0.4 years. Signs include symmetric GP ataxia and UMN paresis in all limbs, with signs disparately worse in the pelvic limbs.[215,217,222]

TABLE 7-6

Classification of Myelin, Axonal, and Neuronal Disorders of the CNS (Spinal Cord) and PNS

Neuroanatomic Pathology	Specific Description
CNS—Myelopathy/Encephalomyelopathy (see Table 7-7)	
Myelinopathy	Hypomyelination Dysmyelination: leukodystrophy; myelinolytic disorders Leukomyelopathy Leukoencephalomyelopathy
Spongy degeneration	Myelin vacuolation Neuronal vacuolation
Axonopathy—wallerian degeneration, distal axonopathy (dying-back neuropathy), segmental degeneration	Central axonopathy Central-peripheral axonopathy Central-peripheral distal axonopathy
Neuroaxonal dystrophy	Axonal transport disorder
Multisystem degeneration	Axonopathy, neuronopathy, and neuropathy
PNS—Neuropathy	
Neuronopathy—degeneration and loss of neurons, neurofibrillary accumulations in neurons	Motor neuronopathy (see Table 7-9) Sensory neuronopathy (see Table 7-10)
Myelinopathy (see Table 7-10)	Segmental demyelination Hypomyelination
Axonopathy (see Table 7-10)	Sensory-motor neuropathy: distal sensory motor; central-peripheral distal axonopathy Sensory neuropathy Metabolic neuropathy Autonomic neuropathy (see Chapters 3 and 15)

CNS, Central nervous system; *PNS,* peripheral nervous system.

Cutaneous trunci and other reflexes, such as with the slap test, may be decreased. Although the disease is progressive, tetraplegia is rare. The early onset of signs and the marked disparity in gait deficits between the thoracic and pelvic limbs raise the index of suspicion for degenerative myeloencephalopathy over other focal cervical myelopathies.

Diagnosis. Definitive diagnosis of EDM is only made based on histopathologic examination of the spinal cord and brainstem. Antemortem diagnosis is difficult. Radiography of the cervical vertebral column is useful in excluding cervical spondylomyelopathy from consideration if rigid criteria are followed (see Cervical Spondylomyelopathy: Diagnosis). Serum vitamin E concentrations should be greater than 1.5 mg/mL in normal horses. Levels in affected horses may be half that or less.[210] Analysis of CSF may disclose increased protein concentration, which lessens the likelihood of protozoal encephalomyelopathy.

Treatment. No specific treatment for EDM exists. Vitamin E supplementation in groups of horses with high prevalence of EDM has been associated with cessation of the development of new cases.[218,222] The recommended dose of vitamin E for horses at risk is 1000 to 2000 U daily. Higher dosing at 6000 U/day may provide beneficial effects in some affected horses.[210] Providing fresh green forage with an adequate vitamin E content may be better. The prognosis is poor for complete resolution of signs, although signs may stabilize.

Anomalies

Atlantoaxial Subluxation

Pathophysiology. Atlantoaxial (AA) subluxation (AA luxation, AA instability) usually results from congenital malformation or trauma to the associated bones, joint, and/or supporting ligamentous structures involved in the articulation of the atlas (C1) and axis (C2). Seven ossification centers exist during development of the axis and three for the atlas.[223,224] Specifically, the dens of the axis is composed of two ossification centers, of which the cranial bony element has its origin with the atlas.[224] All centers fuse by approximately 4 months postpartum.[223] A variety of lesions involving the atlas and axis have been reported.[225,226] The normal atlantoaxial articulation allows rotational and lateral movement. The dens projects from the body of the axis and is bound to the ventral arch of the atlas by a strong transverse ligament (Figure 7-8). This attachment prevents flexion between the atlas and the axis (Figure 7-9, *A*). Hypoplasia or aplasia of the dens causes failure of proper ligamentous development and support.[227-229] Dorsal angulation of the dens is common in affected dogs. Joint instability allows the axis to rotate caudodorsally. The spinal cord is then compressed between the axis and the dorsal arch of the atlas (see Figure 7-9, *B*). Cervical flexion accentuates the degree of spinal cord compression. Luxations caused by a fracture or congenital malformation of the dens tend to produce less severe neurologic signs, because less compression of the spinal cord occurs. Fractures of the body of the axis produce neurologic signs similar to those of acute traumatic luxation in other regions of the cervical vertebral column. Neurologic signs result from acute or chronic progressive compressive myelopathy. The congenital disorders are usually more chronic, with gradual progression of neurologic signs.

Atlantoaxial subluxation frequently affects young, small/toy breed dogs, but single case reports exist for older-aged and large-breed dogs.[230-233] It also has been reported in other species (e.g., horses, cattle, cats, deer).[234-237] Slowly progressive subluxation of the atlantoaxial articulation was originally described in 10 small-breed dogs.[238] These lesions include subluxations with either an intact or a congenitally malformed

Text continued on p.181.

TABLE 7-7

Summary of Degenerative Spinal Cord (SC) Disorders in Domestic Animals

Disease (Affected Breed or Breeds)	Age of Onset	Inheritance Pattern	Clinical Features	Histopathology	Reference
CNS Hypomyelinopathy					
Canine—dalmatian, springer spaniel, Samoyed, chow chow, Weimaraner, Lurcher, Bernese mountain dog	Birth	X-linked (springer spaniel); AR (Bernese mountain dog)	Bouncing gait; pendular nystagmus; tremor; cerebellar ataxia	Widespread CNS hypomyelination and myelin pallor; oligodendrocyte numbers are reduced or absent; astrogliosis in some	43-49
Siamese	Birth	Familial	Whole-body tremors	Hypomyelination of spinal cord	50
Swine—Type A I	Birth	Acquired from hog cholera	Rhythmic whole-body tremor; bouncing gait	CNS hypomyelinogenesis, cerebellar hypoplasia and dysplasia	51
Swine—Type A II	Birth	Acquired unknown viral agent	Same as above	CNS hypomyelinogenesis	51
Swine—Type A III in Landrace or Landrace cross	Birth	X-linked	Same as above	CNS hypomyelination; oligodendrocyte reduced in numbers	51, 52
Swine—Type A IV in Saddleback pigs	Birth	AR	Same as above	CNS hypomyelination; oligodendrocyte degeneration	51, 53
Swine—Type A V	Birth	Acquired from organophosphate	Same as above	CNS hypomyelination; cerebellar hypoplasia	54
Bovine—Angus shorthorn	Birth	Unknown	Unable to stand, tremor	Hypomyelination in medulla, cerebrum, cerebellum, SC	55
Jersey	Birth	Unknown	Same as above	Pallor in cerebellum and medulla; failure of axonal development in brainstem	56
Shorthorn and Hereford in Canada	Birth	Unknown	Same as above	Nonspecific changes in central WM	57
Lambs—hairy fleece	Birth	Unknown	Same as above	CNS hypomyelinogenesis	58
Dysmyelinopathy (Leukomyelopathy/Leukoencephalomyelopathy/Spongy Degeneration/Leukodystrophy)					
Myelinopathy Hound ataxia (foxhound, beagle, and harrier hounds)	2-7 yr	Acquired from methionine deficiency	Progressive GP ataxia and spastic paresis in PL	Myelin degeneration in all funiculi; mild in dorsal funiculi; thoracic SC most severely affected; degeneration tapers into brainstem	59-61

Myelinolytic disorder (Leonberger)	2-2.5 yr	Unknown	Slowly progressive paresis and ataxia, hypermetria of TL, increased extensor tone, postural reaction deficits all limbs, spinal reflexes intact	Bilateral symmetric demyelination in all funiculi, most severe in dorsal parts of lateral funiculus of cervical SC, extending cranially into brain and caudally into thoracic SC; lesion encroached in descending motor pathways; lesions in brain were most severe in cerebrospinal tract, tectospinal tract, pyramidal decussation, pyramids, medial lemniscus, and spinal tract of V; myelin loss replaced by gliosis; axons are preserved	62
Myelinolytic disorder (Afghan hound)	6 mos	AR?	Rapidly progressive symmetric spastic paraparesis and GP ataxia to paraplegia within 7-10 days; spastic TL involvement. Spinal reflexes increased.	Bilateral and symmetric loss of myelin in all funiculi in midthoracic SC; lesions extend cranially to midcervical SC that taper to only involve dorsal or ventral funiculus; fasciculus proprius is usually spared; few medullary lesions; tissue cavitation in rare cases; vacuolated myelin sheaths, gitter cells; axons are preserved	63-65
Myelinolytic disorder (miniature poodle)	9 wk	Unknown	Progressive spastic tetraparesis to tetraplegia	Extensive loss of myelinated fibers in SC and midbrain; bilateral symmetric loss of myelin in SC with sparing of fasciculus proprius; axonal integrity maintained	66
Leukomyelopathy (Dutch Kooiker dogs)	3-12 mo	AR	Rapidly progressive paraparesis and GP ataxia to tetraparesis; spinal reflexes increased	Diffuse leukomyelopathy affecting all funiculi in all regions; most severe in dorsal and ventral funiculi; myelin necrosis and cavitation; axon sparing unknown	67
Leukoencephalomyelopathy (rottweiler)	1.5 - 3.5 yr	Unknown, familial	Slowly progressive ataxia involving all limbs; UMN paresis with GP proprioceptive ataxia	Bilateral widespread primary demyelination; lesions most severe in dorsal funiculi of cervical SC and extend into thoracic SC; axons are preserved.	68, 69
Spongiform leukoencephalomyelopathy (Australian cattle dog and Shetland sheepdog)	2-9 mo	Maternal mitochondrial (missense mutation cytochrome B)	Progressive spastic paraparesis and cerebellar ataxia to tetraplegia; tremors; dysphagia; seizures	Widespread vacuolation of myelin in subcortical WM, brain, brainstem, spinal cord, and cerebellum; splitting of myelin sheaths	70, 71
Spongy degeneration (Labrador retriever)	4-9 mo	Familial	Cerebellar ataxia and dysmetria, paw placement normal, episodic limb extension and opisthotonos; spinal reflexes intact, generalized muscle atrophy	Vacuolation and myelin degeneration in central and peripheral nervous systems; lesions prominent in cerebellar peduncles and white matter, cerebral WM, and tracts in brainstem and SC; astrocytic proliferation in areas of vacuolation	72, 73
Leukoencephalomalacia (Labrador retriever)	4-18 mo	Familial	Central blindness; normal gait to dysmetria TL, ataxia in PL; cognitive dysfunction	Pallor in corona radiata of cerebrum; tissue necrosis; lesions not observed in cerebellar and brainstem WM; spinal cord not available	74
Birman cat leukoencephalomyelopathy	2-6 mo	Familial	Paraparesis; GP ataxia	Vacuolation affecting cerebral cortex, thalamus, caudal colliculus, medulla; wallerian degeneration in SC	75

Continued

TABLE 7-7

***Summary of Degenerative Spinal Cord (SC) Disorders in Domestic Animals*—cont'd**

Disease (Affected Breed or Breeds)	Age of Onset	Inheritance Pattern	Clinical Features	Histopathology	Reference
American Brown Swiss and Swiss Brown (Braunvieh)	Birth	AR	Recumbency, limb extension opisthotonos, tremor	Defective myelination, astrocytosis involving dorsal, dorsolateral SC funiculi	76-78
Progressive spinal myelinopathy in Murray Grey cattle and Limousin	Birth	AR	Paraparesis and GP ataxia	Diffuse myelopathy involving dorsal spinocerebellar and ventromedian tracts; myelin loss	79, 80
Leukodystrophies					
Globoid cell leukodystrophy (many breeds) (see Table 5-2)	3 mo	AR	Progressive ataxia and paraparesis; cerebellar signs; dull mentation; blindness reflexes may be depressed; euthanasia within 1 yr	Loss of myelin in brain, spinal cord, and nerves with perivascular accumulations of globoid macrophages	81, 82
Leukodystrophy (dalmatian dogs)	3-5 mo	AR	Progressive PL GP ataxia to TL; visual deficits; euthanized within 4 mo from onset	Bilateral cavitating lesions in cerebral WM also involving caudate nucleus and putamen; loss of myelin with preservation of axons; reactive astrocytosis; midbrain, cerebellum, medulla are normal; spinal roots and nerves are normal.	83
Leukodystrophy (Labrador retriever)	6 mo	Unknown	Progressive PL GP ataxia and paresis, wide-base stance; euthanized within 3-10 mo	Perivascular Rosenthal fibers and hypertrophic astrocytes in WM of cerebrum, basal nuclei and brainstem	84
Leukodystrophy (Scottish terrier)	6 mo	Unknown, familial	Progressive tetraparesis, ataxia, and head tilt; seizures; euthanasia within 3 mo	Widespread Rosenthal fibers and astrocytosis throughout brain and SC	85, 86
Leukodystrophy (bull mastiff)	6 mo	Unknown	Slow progressive spastic tetraparesis and ataxia; intermittent whole-body tremors; euthanized at 8 mo to 2 yr	Areas of myelin pallor throughout the major WM tracts with minimal astrocytosis; segmental demyelination; ultrastructural abnormalities in oligodendroglia	87
Leukodystrophy (miniature poodle)	3 mo	Unknown	Progressive tetraparesis and GP ataxia, tremors; euthanized at 6 mo of age	Widespread Rosenthal fibers and astrocytosis throughout brain and SC	88
Leukodystrophy (progressive ataxia in Charolais cattle)	1-2 yr	AR?	Spastic ataxia in PL and TL progressing to recumbency; head tremor	Primary oligodendrocyte dysplasia; eosinophilic plaques in WM of CNS involving cerebellum, internal capsule, corpus callosum, and SC	89-91

Axonopathy (Central Axonopathy, Central-Peripheral Axonopathy, Central-Peripheral Distal Axonopathy)					
Central-peripheral axonopathy *Canine degenerative myelopathy* (many breeds)	>8 yr	Autosomal recessive (*SOD1* mutation)	Slowly progressive general proprioceptive ataxia and spastic UMN PL paresis in early disease; ascending tetraparesis and GP ataxia to tetraplegia and LMN signs; euthanasia within 9 mo to 3 yr	Diffuse myelopathy in all funiculi most severe in dorsal portion of lateral funiculus and in fasciculus gracilis in thoracic SC; loss of axons, moderate astrocytosis; limited SC GM involvement; peripheral nerve involvement with axonal loss and secondary demyelination	92-101
Central axonopathy *Hereditary ataxia* (smooth fox terrier, Jack Russell terrier)	2-6 mo	AR	GP ataxia and paresis in PL; wide-base stance; hypermetria TL and PL; intention tremor; seizures in JRT	Bilaterally symmetric axon and myelin degeneration in dorsal part of lateral funiculus and in ventromedial part of ventral funiculus; myelin loss; degeneration of spinocerebellar tracts most severe in cervical SC; JRT also has changes in central auditory pathway, with presence of extensive spheroids	102-104
Central-peripheral axonopathy (Ibizan hound)	8 mo-2 yr	AR	Progressive GP and cerebellar ataxia; most severe in PL; signs progress to TL; hyporeflexia to absence of patellar reflex	Diffuse axonopathy of all funiculi of SC, worse in thoracic region; degeneration of ascending and descending tracts; many large spheroids in axons of auditory pathway in trapezoid body; spinal roots showed dilated myelin sheaths; many nerves contained excessive endoneurium; encephalopathy and neuropathy affecting axons	105
Central-peripheral axonopathy *Hereditary encephalomyelopathy* (Alaskan husky)	6-18 wk	AR	Generalized weakness progressing to recumbency; GP ataxia; LMN signs in TL; UMN and LMN signs PL; laryngeal paresis	Bilaterally symmetric axon and myelin of SC in all segments, with astrogliosis replacement; in cranial cervical region, areas of degeneration in dorsolateral and dorsal funiculi; midcervical to midthoracic areas of degeneration in caudal projecting pathways of ventral and lateral funiculi. Degeneration cranially extended into medulla and caudal cerebellar peduncle; brainstem and cerebellar nuclei lesions consisting of astrocytosis, spheroids, and no neuronal cell body abnormalities. Diffuse axonopathy and secondary demyelination in nerves.	106
Central-peripheral distal axonopathy *Progressive axonopathy* (boxer)	5-15 mo	Unknown	Progressive PL GP ataxia and paresis; loss of paw replacement; progress to TL; decreased spinal reflexes	Symmetric and bilateral axon and myelin degeneration in lateral and ventral funiculi of SC; spheroids more common in WM and cuneate, gracilic, olivary nuclei; cerebellum and cerebral cortex spared; nerves show axonal degeneration and demyelination.	107-109

Continued

TABLE 7-7

***Summary of Degenerative Spinal Cord (SC) Disorders in Domestic Animals*—cont'd**

Disease (Affected Breed or Breeds)	Age of Onset	Inheritance Pattern	Clinical Features	Histopathology	Reference
Central axonopathy (Labrador retriever)	3-5 mo	AR?	PL affected; initially short-strided and collapse; TL stiff; hypermetria all limbs; head tremors and dysmetria late in disease	Axonopathy of all funiculi; aplasia or hypoplasia of corpus callosum, spina bifida; bilaterally symmetric degeneration of SC WM in dorsal part of each lateral funiculus involving spinocerebellar tracts and in fasciculus gracilis and lesser in ventral funiculus; most extensive in thoracic SC and decreased in intensity in more caudal lumbar and sacral SC; degeneration cranially into medulla and cerebellar peduncles and cerebellum; partial loss of axons and myelin replaced by astrogliosis; more extensive loss of larger axons; presence of axonal spheroids; spheroids numerous in granular layer of neurons of cerebellar cortex; no cell body lesions in SC; in medulla, cell body degeneration was extensive in each olivary nucleus; neurofilament staining	110
Central axonopathy (Scottish terrier)	10-12 wk; 4 to 5 mo	Unknown	Tremors and ataxia	Diffuse degeneration of WM in SC, cerebral WM, cerebellum, brainstem; replaced by gliosis; some dystrophic axons and spheroids suggest axonal pathology; secondary demyelination	111
Central-peripheral axonopathy (Pyrenean mountain dog)	12 wk	Unknown	PL GP ataxia, postural reaction deficits, decreased spinal reflexes; nerve conduction slow	Diffuse axonal degeneration in dorsolateral, lateral and ventral WM from medulla to L5; axonal swelling, myelin degeneration in CNS and PNS	112
Central-peripheral axonopathy (New Zealand Huntaway)	8 wk	Familial	GP ataxia and spastic paresis in PL, hypermetria, postural reaction deficits, TL are normal; dogs euthanized at 20 mo of age	Severe degeneration of axons and myelin in SC; degeneration most severe in cranial cervical SC within dorsal funiculi, ventral medial part of ventral funiculi, lateral and dorsal part of lateral funiculus involving spinocerebellar tracts; fiber loss replaced by astrocytosis; nerve showed myelin and axonal degeneration; changes severe in tibial nerve.	113
Central-peripheral axonopathy; sensory ataxic neuropathy (golden retriever)	2 to 8 mo	Mitochondrial inheritance (*tRNA*^{Tyr} mutation)	GP ataxia, hyporeflexia; dogs euthanized by 3 yr of age	Mild to moderate WM degeneration in SC; degeneration most severe in fasciculus gracilis and dorsal part of lateral funiculus; peripheral nerve showed sensory fibers loss.	114, 115
Central-peripheral distal axonopathy (Birman cat)	8-10 wk	Sex limited?	Hypermetria, frequent falling, plantigrade stance, PL>TL	CNS shows loss of myelinated fibers and astrocytosis; PNS has degenerating nerve fibers with myelin debris and disrupted axons; selective loss of distal parts of CNS and PNS	116

Equine degenerative myeloencephalopathy (many pure breeds—Arabian, thoroughbred, Paso Fino, Appaloosa, standardbreds, Haflingers, clustering)	6 mo-2 yr	Unknown or familial; vitamin E deficiency	GP ataxia; progressive spastic paraparesis to tetraparesis	Loss of myelinated fibers in all funiculi but most severe in dorsal spinocerebellar tract; pronounced astrocytosis; neuroaxonal degeneration in nucleus thoracicus; spheroids inconsistently in brainstem nuclei	117, 118
Progressive degenerative myeloencephalopathy of Brown Swiss cattle *Weaver syndrome*	5-8 mo	Unknown	Slowly progressive GP ataxia and spastic pelvic limb paresis and dysmetria resulting in recumbency in 1-3 yr	Primary central axonopathy; spinal cord lesions with axonal swelling and degeneration; spongy degeneration; patchy loss of Purkinje cells	119
Encephalomyelopathy in Simmental and Limousin cattle	5-12 mo	Unknown	Progressive PL GP ataxia, wasting and recumbency in 6 mo; behavior change	Bilaterally symmetric, multifocal grayish areas of degeneration in internal capsule, caudate nucleus, putamen, brainstem, spinal cord GM	120-122
Congenital axonopathy in Holstein-Friesian calves (Australia)	1-7 days	Unknown	Recumbency; opisthotonic posture	Wallerian degeneration in all segments of spinal cord extending into brainstem	123
Degenerative thoracic myelopathy in Merino sheep	5 mo	Unknown	GP ataxia, tetraparesis	Degeneration of SC WM	124
Degenerative myeloencephalopathy in llamas	Adult	Unknown	GP ataxia, progressive paraparesis to tetraparesis	Myelopathy in all funiculi, most severe in dorsal portion of lateral funiculus and in fasciculus gracilis in thoracic SC; loss of axons moderate astrocytosis; limited SC GM involvement; few degenerate neurons in GM; degenerative neurons in brainstem	125
Neuroaxonal Dystrophy					
Rottweiler	1 yr	Familial	TL hypermetria; progress 1-2 yr to cerebellar ataxia	Brain shows mild cerebellar atrophy; numerous spheroids throughout GM, dorsal horn of SC, vestibular, gracilic, cuneate nuclei, lateral and medial geniculate nuclei, nucleus thoracicus	126-128
Chihuahua	7 wk	Familial	No description	Spheroids predominance in WM	129
Working collie sheepdog in New Zealand & Australia	2-4 mo	AR?	Hypermetria, wide-base, intention tremor, difficulty maintaining balance	Numerous spheroids; mild wallerian degeneration in central cerebellar WM and cerebellar and lateral vestibular nuclei	130
Jack Russell terrier	9 wk	Unknown	No description	Spheroids in brainstem nuclei and SC GM; absence of septum pellucidum; hypoplasia of corpus callosum; bilateral hydrocephalus	131
Giant axonal neuropathy in German shepherd dog	14-16 mo	Unknown	PL paresis and GP ataxia progressing to LMN signs; megaesophagus	Numerous swollen unmyelinated fibers containing neurofilament; SC distal portions of long tracts, fasciculus gracilis, dorsal spinocerebellar in cranial cervical cord; lateral funiculus involved caudal thoracic and lumbar; nuclei gracilis, cuneatus; spheroids in brainstem, cerebellar vermis; axonal swellings in tibial and recurrent laryngeal; central-peripheral distal axonopathy	132, 133

Continued

TABLE 7-7

Summary of Degenerative Spinal Cord (SC) Disorders in Domestic Animals—cont'd

Disease (Affected breed or breeds)	Age of Onset	Inheritance Pattern	Clinical Features	Histopathology	Reference
Papillon	13-16 wk	Unknown	Hypermetria, generalized tremors, absent proprioception	Spheroids in cerebral and cerebellar cortex; degeneration in axons and myelin in gray and white matter of brain and SC	134-136
Domestic shorthair	6- 9 mo	Unknown or familial	GP ataxia	Spheroids in brainstem, cerebellum, and SC	137, 138
Merino sheep—Australia	4 mo	Unknown	Tetraparesis, GP ataxia	Spheroids in midbrain, brainstem, cerebellum, and SC	139
Suffolk sheep	1.5-5 mo	Unknown	GP ataxia, tetraparesis	Spheroids in GM, SC, brainstem	140
Morgan horse	1 yr	Unknown or familial	GP ataxia, tetraparesis	Wallerian degeneration in SC, spheroids in lateral cuneate nucleus	141, 142
Multisystem Neuronal Degeneration					
Cairn terrier	<5 mo	Unknown	Progressive paresis, ataxia and brainstem signs, PL collapse patellar areflexia, tetraparesis, hypermetria, head tremor	Disease affects motor neurons in SC, brainstem, thalamic nuclei with degeneration in the SC WM and medulla	143-145
Cocker spaniel	10-14 mo	Unknown	Abnormal gait, tremors, thalamocortical dysfunction, vestibular signs, abnormal behavior	No SC lesions, pathology widespread in brain; neuronal cell body degeneration and loss with gliosis, axonal spheroids in cerebellum and axonal dystrophy	146
Golden retriever	3 mo	Familial	PL paresis that progressed to TL; fine resting muscle tremors; short-strided LMN tetraparesis with no proprioceptive ataxia; reflexes decreased; generalized LMN paresis	Severe axonopathy in lateral funiculi of SC; caudal medulla astrogliosis; motor nuclei of CNV had vacuoles; motor neuron loss in ventral GM; nerves had vacuolated myelin surrounding axons; macrophages, ventral root had wallerian degeneration; neurogenic muscle atrophy; axonopathy and neuronopathy	147
Rottweiler	6 wk-8 mo	Unknown	GP ataxia, tetraparesis worse in PL	Intracytoplasmic neuronal vacuolation prominent in deep cerebellar nuclei and nuclei of extrapyramidal system; vacuolation in dorsal root and autonomic ganglia; bilaterally symmetric axonal degeneration in dorsolateral and ventromedial SC WM	148

CNS, Central nervous system; *GM*, gray matter; *GP*, general proprioceptive; *LMN*, lower motor neuron; *PL*, pelvic limb; *PNS*, peripheral nervous system; *SC*, spinal cord; *TL*, thoracic limb; *UMN*, upper motor neuron; *WM*, white matter.

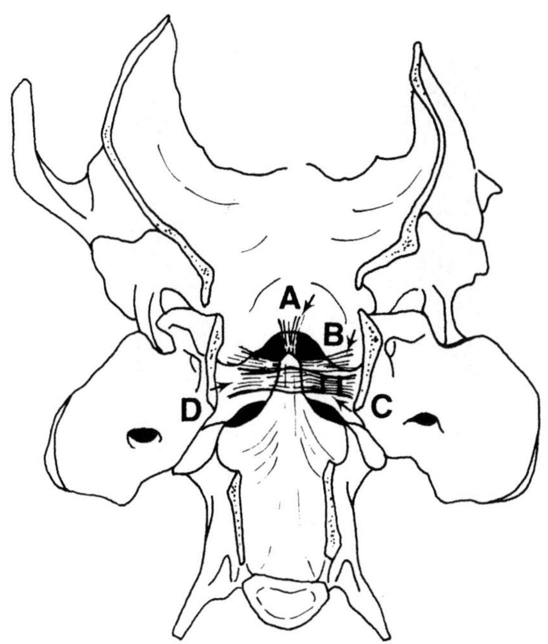

Figure 7-8 Ligamentous attachments of the dens. *A*, Apical. *B*, Alar. C, Lateral. *D*, Transverse atlantal. (From Oliver JE Jr, Lewis RE: Lesions of the atlas and axis in dogs, J Am Anim Hosp Assoc 9:307, 1973.)

dens and fractures of the axis or atlas. Some congenital malformations that involve the atlas, axis, and occipital bone are discussed in the next section.

Clinical Signs. Traumatic luxations or fractures involving the atlantoaxial articulation result in cervical spinal pain and GP ataxia/UMN tetraparesis. Neurologic signs may be asymmetric. The onset of clinical signs can be acute or chronic with a gradual progressive disease course. Temporal relation also may be associated with episodic bouts of cervical spinal pain or be static for years, with an acute exacerbation. Dogs with congenital lesions usually show signs during the first year of life; however, older dogs also may develop signs. Often the onset of clinical signs coincides with minor trauma such as jumping from furniture. Some dogs may not show clinical signs because adequate vertebral support by other fibrous and muscular structures prevents C1-2 subluxation. With age, these structures may weaken, allowing the axis to rotate caudodorsally and compress the spinal cord.

In the congenital form of the disorder, the initial clinical sign is usually cervical spinal pain. Neurologic signs can progress from pain alone to minor or severe motor dysfunction with GP ataxia/UMN tetraparesis or paralysis.[227,238] Neurologic examination findings are consistent with a lesion affecting the C1-5 spinal cord segments. Rarely, tetraplegia and respiratory compromise/failure may occur. Severe cervical spinal cord injury may disrupt descending reticulospinal pathways for control of respiration, thus necessitating perioperative ventilatory support.[239] Respiratory failure occurs when

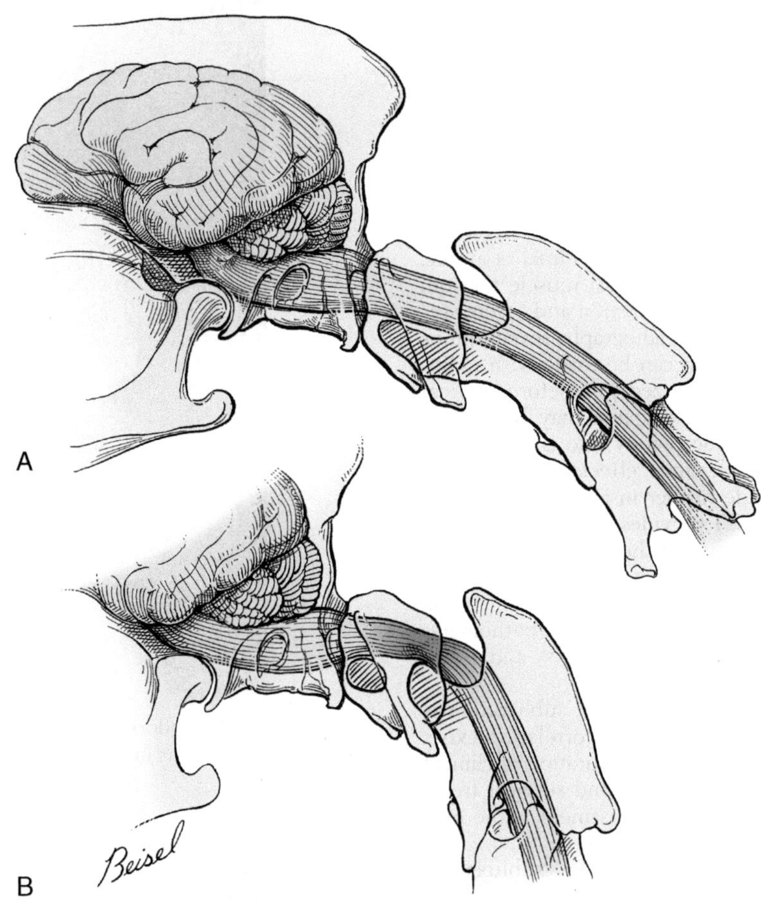

Figure 7-9 **A,** Drawing of normal atlantoaxial articulation. **B,** Drawing of atlantoaxial subluxation resulting from separation of dens from body of axis. Note dorsal displacement of axis, compressing spinal cord at this level.

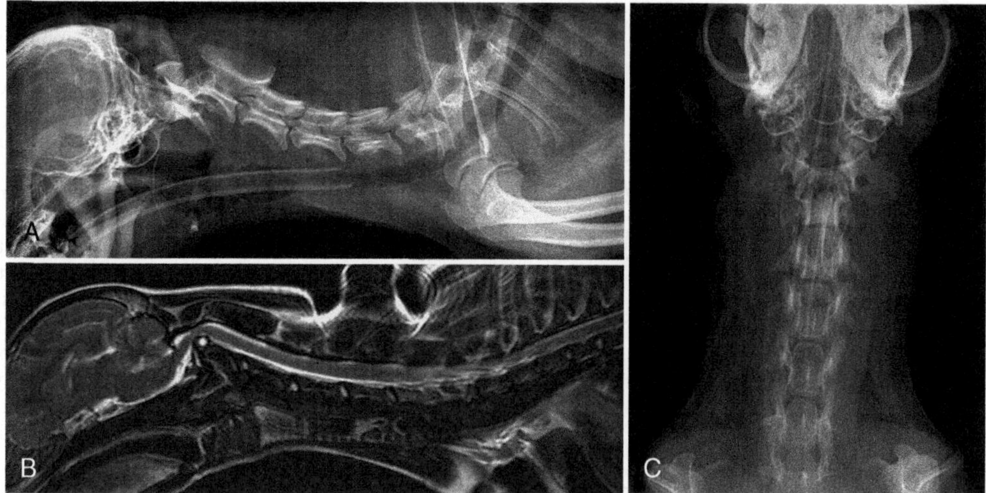

Figure 7-10 Lateral radiograph (A) and sagittal T2-weighted MRI (B) of cervical vertebral column of a 10-month-old Yorkshire terrier with cervical spinal hyperesthesia and atlantoaxial subluxation. Note marked dorsal luxation of axis relative to atlas, and severe spinal cord compression. C, Ventrodorsal view demonstrating presence of a hypoplastic dens.

these pathologic events compromise respiratory pathways. The displaced axis may be palpated as a firm swelling just caudal to the occiput.[225] Because flexing the neck causes severe pain and accentuates motor dysfunction, it should be avoided or done with extreme caution. When atlantoaxial luxation or fractures are suspected, extension of the neck must be maintained and flexion of the neck avoided.[225] This is especially important if the dog is to be sedated or undergo anesthesia, during which times muscle relaxation may further accentuate instability and lead to greater compression and worsening of clinical signs.

Diagnosis. Atlantoaxial subluxation must be suspected in all toy or miniature dogs with cranial cervical spinal pain, neck rigidity, and GP ataxia/UMN paresis or paralysis. Spinal radiography is useful for revealing the C1-2 malalignment (Figure 7-10). Survey radiographs should include lateral and ventrodorsal views and be taken while the animal is awake. Anesthetized dogs do not maintain cervical muscle tension, which increases the possibility of neck flexion and severe spinal cord compression. If the survey radiographs reveal minor displacement, a definitive diagnosis can be made with radiographs taken with the dog anesthetized just before surgical fixation.[225] Careful and gentle neck flexion may be needed to demonstrate the luxation. Fluoroscopy also is helpful for detecting instability and the dynamic effects of the lesion. Advanced imaging can provide further insight to other bony and soft-tissue abnormalities. CT provides more detailed bone resolution. Abnormal conformation of the dens can be seen in 70% of dogs with AA subluxation (Figure 7-11).[230,240] MRI gives excellent soft-tissue resolution of the neural parenchyma and provides identification of other spinal cord pathologies (e.g., syringo/hydromyelia and myelomalacia)[241] and intra-axial hemorrhage (see Figure 7-10).[242]

Treatment. The goal for treatment of AA subluxation is joint stabilization and fusion.[229] A positive correlation exists between neurologic recovery and decrease duration of clinical signs prior to admission for conservative and surgical treatments.[230,243] As a general rule, surgical treatment is the preferred method of therapy for AA subluxation.

Conservative. Conservative therapy of AA subluxation involves exercise restriction with cage rest, external coaptation of the cervical vertebral column and head, as well as pain control. Conservative therapy has been a plausible treatment option for dogs that show clinical signs of cervical spinal pain or minimal neurologic deficits, had minimal anatomic malalignment on radiography, or have owners with constraints that prevented surgical options.[243] Animals with immature bone that is not capable of withstanding implant placement also may benefit from temporary external coaptation.

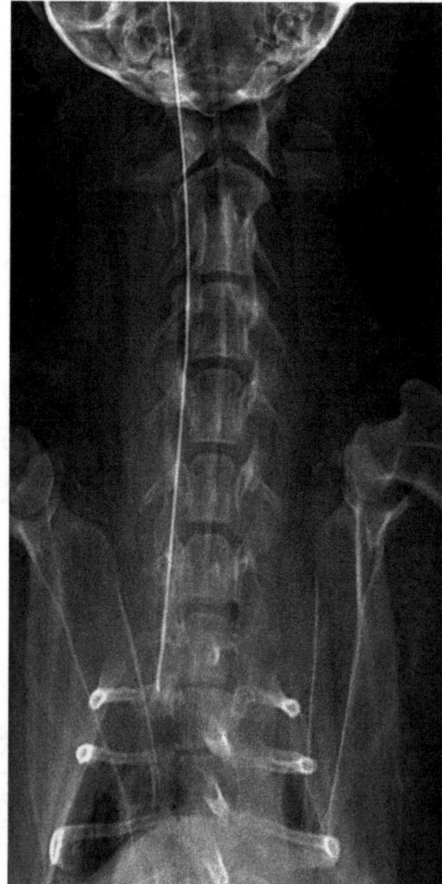

Figure 7-11 Ventrodorsal radiograph demonstrating almost complete absence of dens in dog with atlantoaxial subluxation.

External coaptation by use of cervical spinal splints is a noninvasive method to promote fibrous ankylosis of the AA joint. Methods of splint placement vary based on clinician preference. Types of splints include dorsal, ventral, circumferential, or soft padded bandage. To be effective, external coaptation must incorporate the head and thoracic limbs so as to eliminate flexion. External splints are usually maintained for 6 to 8 weeks, but the time required for adequate stabilization of the AA joint is unknown. Bandage changes are necessary every several days to ensure adequate immobilization. Necropsy and histopathologic confirmation of fusion of the AA joints after cervical spinal splinting has not been well described. It is suspected that fibrous tissue proliferation occurs at the articulations, thus providing some stability. Complications include inadequate joint stabilization, corneal ulceration, decubitus ulcers, dermatitis, and otitis externa secondary to bandage placement. Dogs with AA subluxation also can have pharyngeal and laryngeal weakness, predisposing them to aspiration pneumonia, dyspnea, and choking. Owners need to be well educated about bandage management and care and committed to frequent evaluations.

Most retrospective studies evaluating conservative therapy report good outcomes but lack adequate long-term follow-up.[37,244,245] A retrospective study evaluated long-term outcome in dogs treated by conservative therapy for 1 year or longer after removal of cervical spinal splint.[243] A good outcome was reported in 10 of 16 dogs that had placement of a cervical spinal splint. Neurologic grade upon admission, radiographic appearance of dens, and age at onset of clinical signs were not associated with outcome. This study suggested that use of a cervical spinal splint is a viable treatment option in young dogs with a first episode of acute onset of clinical signs, regardless of severity of their neurologic status.[243] Other studies report age as a predictor of outcome, with older dogs having poor neurologic recovery.[230]

Surgical Stabilization. Surgical techniques for stabilization include both ventral and dorsal techniques. *Ventral fusion* is the most common type of stabilization procedure for treatment of AA subluxation in dogs. Indications for ventral fusion techniques include chronic history of clinical signs, relapse of signs from conservative therapy, and bone maturity that is capable of withstanding implant placement.[246] Odontoidectomy may facilitate reduction and has been recommended if there is dorsal angulation of the dens but usually is not necessary to perform.[247,248] Techniques of fusion of the AA joint include transarticular fixation or multiple implants secured with polymethylmethacrylate. A ventral approach to the cranial cervical vertebral column allows adequate visualization of the AA joint. The articular cartilage is removed using a blade, pneumatic drill-burr, or bone curette. The joint is reduced and aligned, and screws or pins are placed across the C1-2 joint (Figure 7-12).[249] A cancellous bone autograft is placed to facilitate bony fusion. Polymethylmethacrylate may be place over the pins to prevent implant migration. Types of implants described include Kirschner wires, threaded pins, cortical screws, plates, and cannulated screws.[250] In recent years, several techniques using multiple implants have been described.[251-254] During the postoperative recovery period, an external splint may be applied to facilitate fusion and prevent implant breakage. It has been recommended that all forms of fixation be supplemented with external coaptation and combined with strict cage confinement for 8 weeks.

Main complications associated with ventral surgical stabilization are death or implant failure.[250,255,256] The incidence for repeat surgery ranges between 8.2% and 19% of cases.[240,255,256] Implant failures mainly are a result of migration, breakage, or loss of reduction. Postoperative complications for AA stabilization most commonly include respiratory-related complications: reflex gagging, laryngeal paralysis, tracheal collapse and necrosis, pulmonary edema, pneumonia, respiratory compromise, and death.[250] Other complications include permanent torticollis, worsening of neurologic status, and Horner's syndrome. Complications causing death have been reported to be as high as 30% with transarticular fixation.[255] Causes of death at time of surgery are usually associated with cardiac or respiratory arrest.[240] Risk factors that can affect the outcome of surgery for AA subluxation have been studied in dogs. Dogs younger than 24 months of age and those with signs of less than 10 months duration generally had better outcomes.[230] Severity of neurologic signs before surgery was only marginally predictive of a successful outcome. Residual neurologic signs were detected in a greater percentage of dogs following dorsal procedures, but the success rates of both procedures were nearly identical.[230]

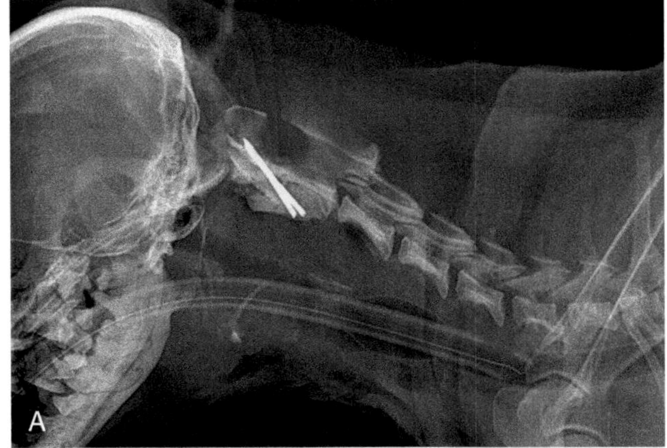

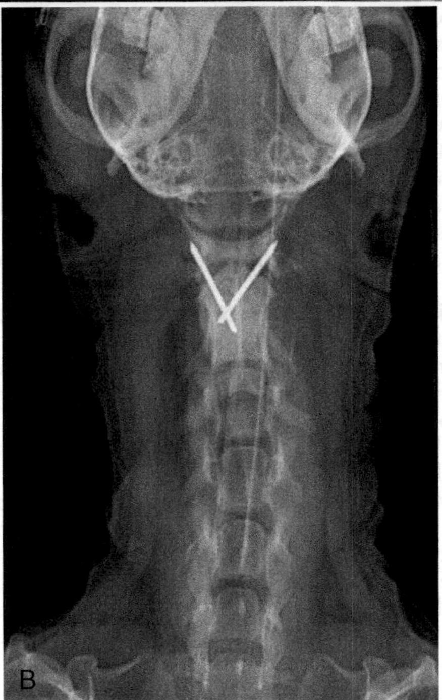

Figure 7-12 **A,** Lateral and **B,** ventrodorsal radiograph of 11-month-old Maltese after stabilization of atlantoaxial subluxation with two threaded pins and polymethylmethacrylate.

Dorsal wire fixation entails a loop of wire or suture passed beneath the dorsal arch of C1 and cut and tightened to provide adequate reduction of C1 and C2.[225,229,257] The nuchal ligament also can be used for dorsal stabilization of the AA joint.[258] Failure rate has been reported as high as 37%.[259]

Usually there is breakage of the wire or suture; the spinous process of C2 or the dorsal arch of C1 also may fracture. A metallic clip positioned around the cranial aspect of the laminae of the atlas and anchored to the axis has also been used to stabilize luxations.[260] Mortality rate has been reported as 16%.[250] Dorsal stabilization techniques do not eliminate rotation and shear forces acting across the joint and are more prone to failure.[261] Complications are usually respiratory failure or cardiac arrest from spinal cord compression during the surgical procedure or after breaking of the wire or suture.

Occipitoatlantoaxial Malformation. Occipitoatlantoaxial malformation is a congenital malformation that includes fusion of the atlas to the occipital bone; it is reported in horses, cattle, cats, and dogs.[262-264] Congenital asymmetric occipitoatlantoaxial malformations and asymmetric atlantooccipital fusion are presumed to be inherited in Arabian horses.[264,265] Ataxia, tetraparesis, and a stiff neck may be found in neonates or in weanling foals. The abnormal cervical articulations usually can be palpated. Diagnosis is based on radiography.

Occipitoatlantal Luxations. Traumatic luxations of the occipitoatlantal articulation are rare. They have been reported in dogs, a cat, and a goat.[266-270] The luxations can be managed with conservative therapy in which the luxation is manual reduced and a cast with the neck in flexion is applied or with surgical stabilization. This rare injury would be expected to cause death in most cases, but some animals have relatively minimal neurologic deficits.

Chiari-Like Malformation (Caudal Occipital Malformation Syndrome) and Syringomyelia

Pathogenesis. Syringomyelia is a condition characterized by gradual formation of a fluid-filled cavity (syrinx) within the spinal cord. In many cases, it is difficult to discern that the abnormal fluid-filled cavity is a syrinx rather than dilated central canal or a combination of both. In such cases, the term *syringohydromyelia* may be applied. In humans, syringomyelia may be caused by a several conditions, including abnormalities of the posterior fossa (Chiari malformation). In dogs, the observation of similar but not the same exact abnormalities has led to the term *Chiari-like malformation* (CM). Another term used is *caudal occipital malformation syndrome* (COMS). Chiari-like malformation is a hereditary condition, first described in the Cavalier King Charles spaniel (CKCS), that can lead to syringohydromyelia.[271] This condition is also named *occipital dysplasia* and *caudal occipital malformation*.[272] Occipital dysplasia is a malformation of the occipital bone consisting of a variation in the dorsal extent of the foramen magnum in normal dogs or associated with cranial cervical spinal cord anomaly.[273,274] This also has been described in the CKCS.[275] The anomaly of CM consists of an abnormally small caudal fossa, with secondary herniation of the cerebellar vermis through the foramen magnum and subsequent formation of syringohydromyelia (Figure 7-13). There appears to be a breed predilection for CM in CKCSs and the Griffon Bruxellois (Brussel Griffon), but other toy and small-breed dogs can be affected.[272,276-280] The incidence of CM and syringohydromyelia may be high even in the asymptomatic population of CKCS.[281,282] Imaging studies of CKCS with CM have identified a small caudal fossa in dogs with clinicals signs; however, there lacks correlation between a small caudal fossa and development of syringohydromyelia.[281,282] The incidence is high for other congenital diseases of the craniocervical junction in dogs with CM, especially the CKCS and Griffon Buxellois.[283]

Syringohydromyelia can be a debilitating neurologic condition with signs ranging from severe pain to neurologic deficits referable to the spinal cord. In a normal state, pulsatile flow of CSF occurs across the foramen magnum from the intracranial subarachnoid space to the cervical spinal subarachnoid space during systole and reverses flow direction during diastole. The pathophysiology of CM may be related to the overcrowding of the caudal fossa obstructing the normal flow of CSF across the foramen magnum, resulting in abnormal pressure dynamics and hydrocephalus.[284-286] The intramedullary pulse pressure theory is a plausible explanation for syrinx formation.[287] With each arterial pulse, the brain moves back and forth, and the herniated cerebellum is forced caudally. The CSF pressure increases, and CSF is redirected into the perivascular channels along the spinal cord, causing progressive fluid accumulation and syrinx formation.

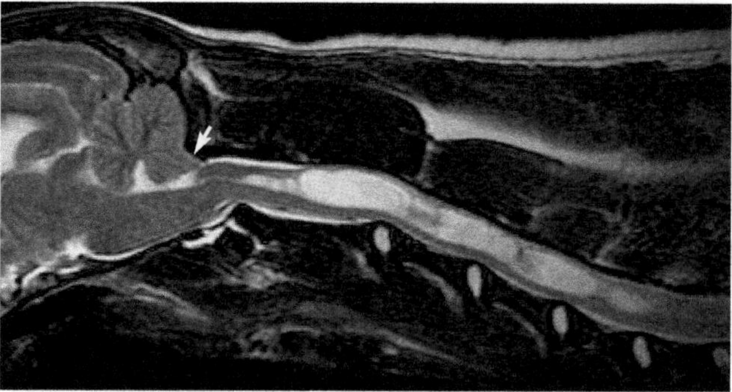

Figure 7-13 Sagittal T2-weighted MRI of a Griffon Buxellois that presented for persistent scratching of the neck region and cervical spinal pain. Note herniated cerebellar vermis *(arrow)* and extensive syringohydromyelia extending from C2 to C5 vertebrae. (Photograph by Marc Kent © 2010, University of Georgia Research Foundation Inc.)

The etiology for CM in CKCSs is suspected to have an inherited basis. In the early 1900s, the modern CKCS breed was established and line breeding was used extensively.[275] The onset of signs of syringohydromyelia occurs in younger dogs, and the signs are more severe in dogs from more highly inbred lines.[288] A DNA collection program is underway for future genetic studies of this complex genetic disease.[289]

Diagnosis. Chiari-like malformation is diagnosed by MRI.[277,279,290,291] The most useful view is a mid-sagittal image of the caudal aspect of the brain that includes the cervical spinal cord. Characteristic MRI findings in dogs include attenuation of the dorsal subarachnoid space at the cervicomedullary junction, rostral displacement of the caudal cerebellum by the occipital bone, varying degrees of syringohydromyelia in the cervical spinal cord, obstructive hydrocephalus, and herniation of the caudal cerebellar vermis.[279,292] A "kinked" appearance of the caudal medulla oblongata has been occasionally noted.[272] Ultrasonography of the craniocervical junction also can be used to identify cerebellar herniation and syringomyelia but lacks sensitivity.[281]

MRI has increased the recognition of CM in the CKCS as well as in other small and toy breed dogs. A study in which MRI was used to measure dimensions of the foramen magnum in CKCS with CM and syringomyelia showed no apparent correlation between neurologic signs, severity of cerebellar herniation, and extent of syringohydromyelia.[279] The severity of clinical signs correlates to the height and width of the syrinx in affected CKCS.[282,293] It has been shown that up to 40% of clinically normal CKCSs have syringomyelia evident on MRI.[282,293] These dogs, however, tend to have a smaller and less extensive syrinx. Thus, the major factor for dogs becoming symptomatic for CM is still unknown.

Clinical Signs. Chiari-like malformation can be responsible for clinical signs involving the forebrain, caudal brainstem, and cervical spinal cord.[287,294] The most devastating clinical sign of CM is severe cervical spinal pain. Excessive scratching of the ear, neck, or shoulder, vocalization, and facial rubbing also may be the prominent or sole features of CM.[271] These signs are a reflection of paresthesia or *neuropathic pain*. The enlarged syrinx is most likely associated with development of the neuropathic pain, owing to damage in the dorsal horn of the gray matter and alterations in neural processing of sensory information.[287] GP ataxia/UMN paresis consistent with signs of a C1-5 lesion or LMN paresis of the thoracic limbs and GP ataxia/UMN paresis of the pelvic limbs if the syrinx affects the C6-T2 spinal cord segments. Central vestibular and cerebellovestibular may occur with cerebellar and brainstem involvement. Seizures and other encephalopathic signs are referable to the secondary obstructive hydrocephalus. Scoliosis also can be a secondary phenomenon to syringohydromyelia.[295]

Treatment. The goals of medical management are pain control and decreasing CSF production. Combination analgesics are often required for pain management.[272,296] Acetazolamide and furosemide may be used to decrease CSF production.[297] Corticosteroids provide antiinflammatory effects and also decrease CSF production. Recently gabapentin or pregabalin have been used to treat neuropathic pain.[283] Although medical management may improve clinical signs, it does not prevent further disease progression.

Surgical management is indicated when analgesics are unable to control the discomfort or when neurologic deficits are present and are unacceptable or progressive. Surgery consists of decompressing the cerebellum by a suboccipital craniectomy, which enlarges the foramen magnum, and a dorsal laminectomy of the first or second cervical vertebra.[296,297] A durotomy is also performed at the level of the decompression sites and resecting any dural bands that constrict the neural tissue. Decompressive surgery can relieve the pain but may not result in resolution of the syringohydromyelia.[296,297] Even with surgery, the clinical signs may not completely resolve, and recurrence is possible. A recurrence of clinical signs of up to 47% can occur within months to years after surgery.[296,297] Cranioplasty techniques may provide some benefit for preventing recurrence of signs.[298]

Cervical Spondylomyelopathy in Dogs and Horses. The growing popularity of giant-breed dogs and performance horses during the past 20 years is probably responsible for the increased interest in this neurologic syndrome. The disorder appears with greater frequency in Great Danes, Doberman pinschers, and thoroughbred horses, but it has been recognized in several other breeds of dogs and horses. Controversy still exists regarding proper terminology for this syndrome. Currently, *cervical spondylopathy*, *cervical spondylomyelopathy*, *cervical vertebral malformation-malarticulation*, and *cervical vertebral stenotic myelopathy* appear to be the most useful names encompassing the forms of the disease in all affected animals. Some investigators prefer to group all breeds together, whereas others prefer to characterize each breed separately. Our objective is to describe similarities and differences in the pathologic lesions and management of cervical spondylomyelopathy in the dog and horse and emphasize breed variations.

Pathophysiology. The pathologic lesions responsible for the clinical signs in young Great Danes, Doberman pinschers, and thoroughbreds form the basic model with which the disease in other animals is compared. In affected animals, neurologic signs develop because of progressive spinal cord compression from surrounding vertebral bony and soft-tissue structures. Abnormalities of the midcervical to the caudal cervical vertebrae or their articulations (or both) are usually identified with imaging studies or at necropsy. Because the exact cause is unknown, the term *cervical spondylomyelopathy* is used broadly to encompass the various vertebral and soft-tissue abnormalities.

Early studies suggested that excessive mobility of the caudal cervical vertebrae was primarily responsible for spinal cord compression. Subsequent studies demonstrated that malformation of the cervical vertebrae of dogs and horses resulted in stenosis of the vertebral canal.[299-302] These changes are more consistently present in young Great Danes and include narrowing and dorsoventral flattening of the cranial vertebral foramina of C5, C6, and C7.[301,303,304] The sixth cervical vertebra is usually most severely affected. In young thoroughbred horses, rottweilers, and basset hounds, these findings are more common at C3 and C4.[303,305,306]

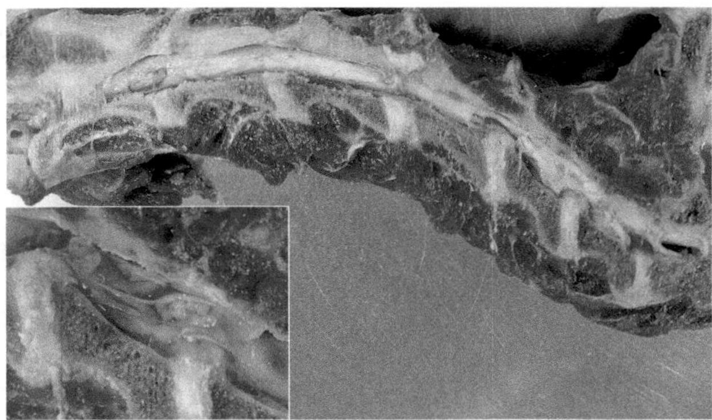

Figure 7-14 Parasagittal cut of cervical vertebral column from 7-year-old FS Doberman pinscher with progressive tetraparesis and severe general proprioceptive (GP) ataxia of pelvic limbs. Spinal cord is compressed ventrally at both C5-6 and C6-7 by proliferative dorsal annulus fibrosis and dorsal longitudinal ligament (see inset). Findings are consistent with caudal cervical spondylomyelopathy of C5-6 and C6-7 intervertebral disk spaces.

Dogs. Cervical spondylomyelopathy has been recognized as a disease in large and giant-breed dogs. The Doberman pinscher and Great Dane often are overrepresented, with other breeds reported sporadically. Recently the disease also has been thoroughly described in young to middle-aged Bernese mountain dogs.[307] In dogs, CSM has variable forms which differ between the Doberman pinscher and the giant breeds. Dobermans have a peak incidence between 4 and 8 years of age.[303,308,309] Common pathologic features in affected Doberman pinschers include hypertrophy of the interarcuate and dorsal longitudinal ligaments and Hansen type II disk protrusion involving the caudal cervical vertebrae (Figure 7-14).[149,246,310-312] Since Hansen type II IVDD is common, the term *disk-associated wobbler syndrome* (DAWS) has been proposed.[311,313] In some affected dogs, there is remodeling along with abnormal rotation of the body of the C6 vertebra. An MRI study of Doberman pinschers demonstrated that vertebral canal stenosis and wider IVD spaces distinguished CSM affected dogs from clinically normal dogs.[314] Still, clinically normal Doberman pinschers had a high incidence of disk degeneration, foraminal stenosis, and asymptomatic spinal cord compression. The vertebral malformation in Dobermans tends to lead to malarticulation and vertebral instability. Apparently as a consequence of the instability, soft tissues that support and strengthen the cervical articulations proliferate. In Dobermans, hypertrophy of the interarcuate ligament, dorsal longitudinal ligament, or dorsal annulus may compress the spinal cord at the vertebral articulations. These changes are identified using imaging procedures to visualize the *dynamic compressive lesions* (Figure 7-15, *A-D*).

Great Danes and other giant breeds typically present with clinical signs at 2 years of age. The pathology includes dorsal and dorsolateral compression secondary to osteoarthrosis of the articular processes and hypertrophy of the joint capsules and interarcuate ligament (Figure 7-16).[149,246,303] Any site can be affected, but the C5-6 and C6-7 sites are most common. Osteoarthrosis has been considered a form of osteochondrosis dissecans.[315]

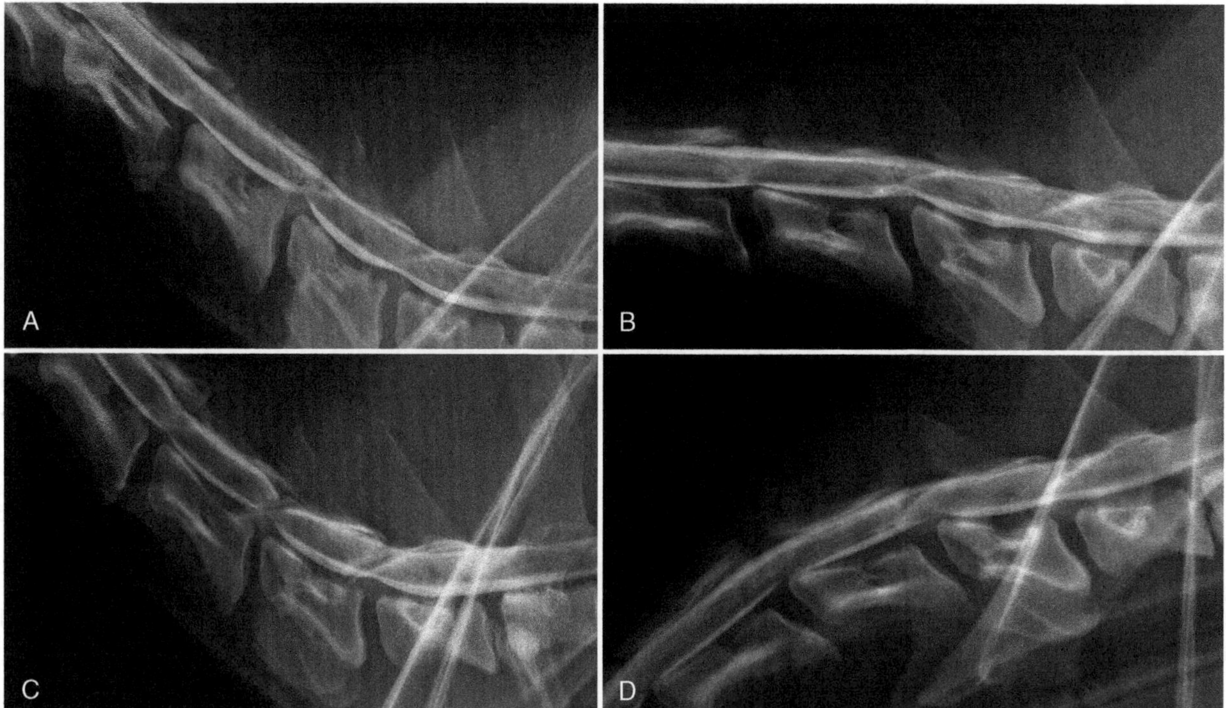

Figure 7-15 Lateral myelogram with dynamic positioning of caudal cervical spine from a Doberman with caudal cervical spondylomyelopathy that is severe at C5-6 and mild at C6-7. **A,** Neutral position showing spinal cord is severely compressed ventrally at C5-6 vertebrae and mildly compressed at C6-7. Compression is most likely caused by ligamentous proliferation in this area. **B,** Traction of cervical spine demonstrating improvement of compression and indicating a dynamic lesion. **C,** Extended positioning of cervical spine demonstrating that compression is more pronounced both dorsally and ventrally (recommended not to perform this view, owing to risk of worsening neurologic status). **D,** Flexed positioning of cervical spine, demonstrating improvement of ventral compression.

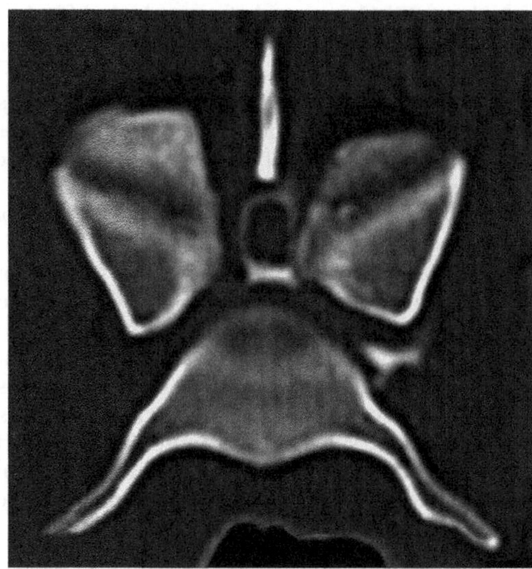

Figure 7-16 Transverse CT/myelogram image of C6 vertebra after myelography from a 1.5-year-old male Great Dane with severe pelvic limb general proprioceptive (GP) ataxia and tetraparesis. Note proliferative articular processes causing lateral spinal cord compression more severe on the left.

Although many, perhaps genetically controlled, factors may contribute to cervical spondylomyelopathy, the exact cause is unknown. Many of the large and giant breeds have been selected for their size and rapid growth. The disease occurs primarily in horses that are large for their age and breed. The very large head of certain breeds of dogs may exert an unusual force on the midcervical to caudal cervical vertebrae. Great Danes in particular have been selected for a prancing, high-stepping gait that some consider to be a mild form of hypermetria. Breeding for this gait actually may select for this disorder. One study of Great Danes established a relationship between excessive nutrition and several skeletal changes that also involved the cervical vertebrae.[316] The exact cause of the disorder awaits further classification.

Horses. Cervical spondylomyelopathy (cervical vertebral malformation [CVM]) occurs in horses of any age and breed but is most common in thoroughbreds of young age.[306] Neurologic signs are a result of progressive spinal cord compression involving structural changes to the vertebral canal and the surrounding soft tissues.[210,317] As a result of vertebral malformation, the vertebral canal stenosis may be static or dynamic with flexion or extension of the neck. Malformation of the articular processes associated with delayed ossification and osteochondrosis can potentiate vertebral canal stenosis. Likewise, proliferation of the joint capsules of the articular processes can result in cyst formation, adding to the soft-tissue structures compressing the spinal cord. Other malformations include angular deformity of the vertebral body and extensions of the vertebral arch.[317,318] Based on these pathologic abnormalities, CVM in horses is classified into two types.[210] Type I CVM tends to occur in younger animals, from unweaned foals up to 2 years of age. The pathologic changes include vertebral canal stenosis, angular deformity, osteochondrosis, and extension of the vertebral arch. The lesions tend to occur between C2 and C5. These horses are rapid growing, which supports a nutritional role. There may also be a familial influence. Type II

CVM tends to occur in older horses (mean age of 8.5 years) that are male, with warmbloods and the Tennessee Walking horse being predisposed.[319] There is evidence of osteoarthritis of the articular processes, with subsequent formation of synovial cysts and cranial extension of the vertebral arch involving the laminae and interarcuate ligament. Trauma also may be a predisposing factor. Dynamic vertebral canal stenosis between C5 and C7 occurs with neck flexion and extension.[319] The cause of CVM in horses appears to be multifactorial involving genetic and environmental influences.[320]

Clinical Signs. In most affected Great Danes and young horses and in some Doberman pinschers, clinical signs develop at 3 to 18 months of age. Clinical signs develop later in life at 3 to 8 years of age in most Doberman pinschers and in horses with osteoarthrosis of the articular processes. The disease in younger horses occurs earlier than 3 years of age and at 8 years of age in horses with osteoarthrosis of the articular processes.[210,319] In dogs, there is no sex predilection.

Although the cervical spinal cord is compressed, clinical signs usually remain more severe in the pelvic limbs in both dogs and horses. Dogs typically develop mild pelvic limb GP ataxia that progresses to tetraparesis. Compression of ascending proprioceptive pathways is responsible for these neurologic signs. With increasing compression, involvement of descending motor pathways causes UMN paresis or paralysis. Ataxia and paresis in the thoracic limbs may be pronounced in some cases but are sometimes detected only by careful neurologic examination in other cases. Forcing the dog to wheelbarrow with its head extended so that it cannot see the floor accentuates proprioceptive deficits in the thoracic limbs. Some tetraparetic dogs and horses may have LMN paresis in the thoracic limbs because of C6-T2 gray matter involvement of the spinal cord causing the stride length to be short and choppy. In horses, the abnormalities of the pelvic limbs are usually one grade worse than those of the thoracic limbs.[210,321] This also is often true in dogs.

Cervical spinal pain is usually absent unless the disorder is associated with cervical IVD protrusion. Extension of the neck may cause pain. Signs worsen progressively, and urinary incontinence may occur as a late manifestation in dogs. In some animals, trauma may precede the development of acute signs. Unlike most dogs, most horses have acute ataxia, paresis, and spasticity of all four limbs. After an initial period of progression, the equine disease usually stabilizes.

Diagnosis. The diagnosis of cervical spondylomyelopathy is made using various radiographic and cross-sectional imaging using CT and MRI.

Dogs. Changes observed on survey radiography in dogs include the following[246,310,322]:

1. Changes in shape or opacity, or both, of the intervertebral disk and/or disk space; this change is more common in the older Doberman pinscher.
2. Changes in shape or opacity, or both, of the articular facets to sclerosis and exostosis
3. Vertebral displacement (subluxation); however, diagnosis of subluxation based on survey radiographs is not definitive because of considerable variability in normal dogs.
4. Stenosis of the vertebral canal
5. Malformed or misshapen vertebral bodies (often involving C6 vertebra)
6. Misshapen spinous processes

Myelography can be used to identify minor changes in vertebral column architecture, compression by soft tissues (ligamentous structures and disk protrusions), and to define whether the lesion is associated with compression of one or multiple sites (see Figure 7-15). Myelograms made with the neck extended often reveal dynamic soft-tissue or bony

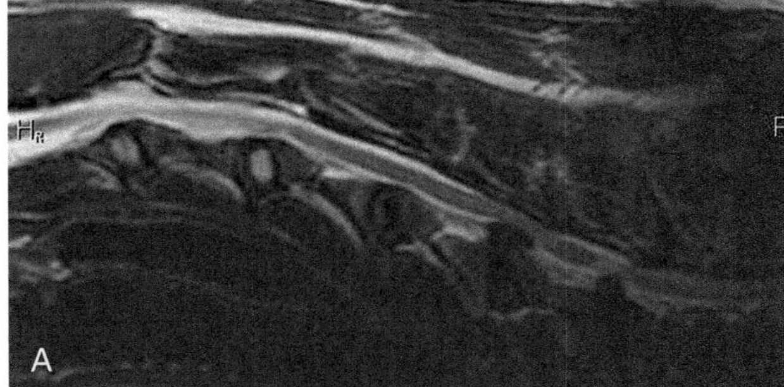

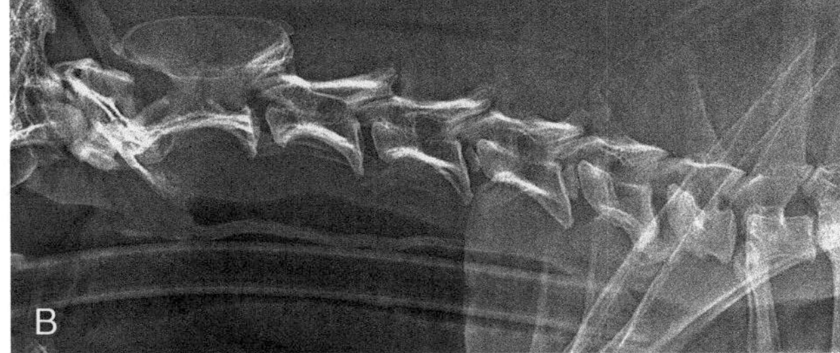

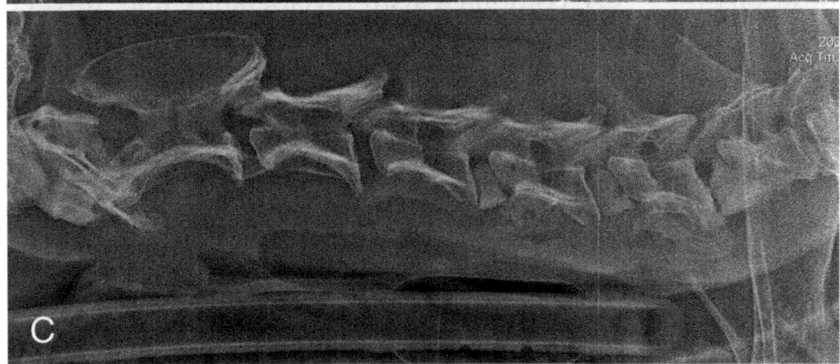

Figure 7-17 **A,** Sagittal T2-weighted MRI of cervical vertebral column from 8-year-old MC Doberman pinscher with a progressive tetraparesis and cervical spinal pain. Note degenerate intervertebral disks at C4-5, C5-6, and C6-7. Cervical spinal cord is severely compressed at C5-6 and C6-7 intervertebral disk interspaces. **B,** Lateral cervical radiograph demonstrating mineralized opacity of C4-5 and C5-6 intervertebral disks and ventral spondylosis at C6-7 intervertebral disk space. **C,** Lateral radiograph after placement of polymethylmethacrylate plugs in C4-5, C5-6, and C6-7 intervertebral disk spaces, with overlaying of autologous bone graft.

compression that may be missed if the neck is imaged only in normal (neutral) position. This dynamic compression often is alleviated by flexion or traction (see Figure 7-15, *B* and *D*). Based on the myelographic results, rational surgical therapy can be instituted. Dynamic (flexion, extension, and traction) views on myelography or cross-sectional imaging should be performed with caution. Dynamic imaging is mandatory in older Doberman pinschers to exclude disk disease as the primary cause of the neurologic signs. Myelography combined with CT or MRI alone may provide additional information, particularly on the degree of spinal cord atrophy.[323]

MRI provides more definitive information for soft-tissue structures causing spinal cord compression, as well as showing evidence of spinal cord pathology.[314,324] Spinal cord hyperintensity on T2-weighted images may suggest gliosis, edema, or syrinx formation. The finding of extensive hyperintensity in the grey matter of the spinal cord at the site of compression may portend a poorer prognosis for return of function following surgery. Intervertebral disk degeneration associated with CSM and other intervertebral disks causing compressive myelopathy also can be visualized more accurately on MRI (Figure 7-17, *A*).

Horses. In horses, cervical spondylomyelopathy must be differentiated from degenerative myeloencephalopathy, protozoal myeloencephalitis, and other disorders that affect the spinal cord. Radiography usually indicates combinations of vertebral canal stenosis and osteoarthrosis of the articular processes. Correct positioning is critical for accurate assessment in horses.[210] Minimal sagittal diameters have been used to presumptively diagnose CVM. Values lower than the control population indicates compression.[325,326] In one study, determination of the ratio of the minimum sagittal diameter of the vertebral canal to the sagittal width of the vertebral body had a sensitivity and specificity of ≥ 89% for diagnosis of cervical spondylomyelopathy.[325] This finding suggests that vertebral canal stenosis plays a critical role in affected horses. Radiography combined with myelography is required for a definitive diagnosis of spinal cord compression with CSM in horses.[327,328] Diagnosis is established by identifying a 50% or greater decrease in the sagittal diameter of the dorsal and ventral contrast columns between affected and unaffected sites.[320] Others report better diagnostic accuracy using a 20% reduction of the same measurement with the neck in either neutral or flexed positions.[210,329] CT combined with myelography may further delineate the compression in horses with osteoarthrosis.[319,330]

Therapy. Conservative therapy includes management of pain and strict exercise restriction similar to that involving conservative management of IVD herniation. Goals of surgery are to stabilize the vertebrae and decompress the spinal cord.

Dogs. No consensus exists on the best treatment for dogs with CSM. Some dogs improve with conservative therapy (cage rest, physiatry, and analgesics). Restriction of activity may reduce the dynamic component of spinal cord compression.[309,314] Short-term corticosteroid therapy may provide analgesic and antiinflammatory effects. However, there was no significant difference in outcome for dogs treated conservatively with or without corticosteroids.[309] Corticosteroids are contraindicated in young, growing animals. A study evaluating treatment of CSM in Dobermans and other breeds found no difference in outcome or survival time between dogs treated conservatively or surgically.[309]

Some clinicians feel the best long-term benefits are provided by surgical stabilization or decompression or both. Ventral[331-333] or dorsal[301,334-337] decompression may be indicated, depending on the sites of compression. Dorsal decompression techniques are used in dogs with dorsal or dorsolateral compression and multiple sites of involvement. Distraction-fusion procedures are used in dogs in which the spinal cord compression observed with imaging is relieved by traction of the cervical vertebral column (see Figure 7-17, C). Distraction techniques using interbody screws, bone grafts, metallic spacers, polymethylmethacrylate, or implants anchored by polymethylmethacrylate are used by many surgeons.[338-341] Newer techniques involve locking-plate fixation and interbody bone grafting.[312,342] Surgical treatment of dogs with multiple lesions is particularly problematic. Dorsal laminectomy extending over the entire area of involvement is associated with high morbidity immediately after surgery.[334,335,337] Distraction techniques can also be applied to span multiple adjacent disk spaces (see Figure 7-17, C).[339]

Surgical complications include implant failure and collapse of the intervertebral disk space, penetration of implants into the vertebral canal, failure of fusion and worsening of neurologic deficits. However, distraction techniques can put further stress on adjacent IVD spaces, risking a domino effect whereby the adjacent IVD space becomes affected as a consequence of the abnormal forces applied to it as a result of stabilization.[343-345] The plethora of surgical interventions establishes the importance of surgical planning that is tailored to each animal for the best possible surgical outcome.

Success rates for various surgical procedures in dogs with dynamic CSM have ranged from 70% to 80% to having a 33% success rate.[35,313,333] In general, the prognosis for full recovery is poor in tetraplegic dogs and guarded in others. Factors that contribute to poor recovery include (1) irreparable spinal cord damage, (2) failure to provide adequate decompression or stabilization, (3) development of compression at sites adjacent to the initial lesions, and (4) postsurgical complications caused by difficulty in rehabilitating large, recumbent dogs.[246] Studies of long-term outcome are lacking. One study comparing outcome in two different surgical techniques in Doberman pinschers with CSM found that 64% of the dogs were euthanized related to cervical spondylomyelopathy between 24 and 40 months after surgery.[345] Although dogs with dorsal compression or multiple-site involvement undergoing a dorsal laminectomy are transiently worse after surgery, long-term outcome and recurrence rates were comparable to other techniques.[337] Regardless of the procedure, surgical results largely depend on the degree of preexisting spinal cord damage.

Horses. Conservative therapy for equine cervical spondylomyelopathy is similar to that for dogs. Early in the course of the disease, young horses may improve when fed a balanced, minimal-growth diet, with a goal of retarding bone growth. This may allow the vertebral canal to enlarge while relieving spinal cord compression.[210,320] Stall rest and antiinflammatory agents may transiently improve clinical signs.

Cervical vertebral interbody fusion using a basket implant device provides intervertebral stability.[346] Ventral cervical fusion is indicated for horses with spinal cord compression caused by cervical vertebral instability. This technique results in improvement of neurologic status in 44% to 90% of horses, and up to 62% may return to athletic function.[346] Dorsal decompression is used to treat stenotic lesions that cause cord compression but is associated with higher risk of complication.[346,347] Dorsal laminectomy results in improvement of neurologic status in 40% to 75% of cases.[346,347] The results of ventral cervical fusion appear to be better than those with subtotal dorsal decompression.[347,348] Results of surgery depend to some degree on the severity, distribution, and duration of cervical cord compression.[320]

Extradural Synovial Cysts. Extradural synovial cysts associated with the articular processes of the cervical vertebral column have been reported in dogs and older horses and may cause a compressive myelopathy. Compressive cervical myelopathy has been reported in young Great Danes and mastiffs and other giant breeds.[349,350] Males may be more common. Age of onset can range from 4 to 36 months of age. Dogs will show progressive tetraparesis and GP ataxia before examination. The neurologic signs are suggestive of cervical myelopathy, and dogs often exhibit cervical spinal pain. Survey cervical spinal radiographs often reveal degenerative joint disease and proliferation of the articular processes from C2-3 to C6-7. Myelography is consistent with dorsolateral extradural spinal cord compression medial to the articular processes. Cross-sectional imaging using MRI or CT often will reveal extensive dorsolateral compression by fluid-filled structures that appear hyperintense on T2-weighted MRI. CSF analysis reveals albuminocytologic dissociation (increased protein concentrations with normal cell count). Dogs are treated by dorsal decompressive surgery and cyst removal. The diagnosis is confirmed with histopathologic analysis, with the synovial cysts constituting the major compressive lesion. Long-term recovery rates are favorable.[349,350]

Neoplastic

See Chapter 6.

DISEASES OF THE NERVES AND NEURONAL CELL BODY

These diseases often cause diffuse LMN signs. Diseases that affect one or more components of the LMNs (Figure 7-18) result in hyporeflexic or areflexic flaccid paresis or paralysis. Sensory perception may be normal or decreased. Hyperesthesia can be manifested with some diseases. The various diseases listed in Tables 7-4 and 7-5 can be classified as acute progressive, chronic progressive, or episodic. All are characterized by diffuse symmetric or asymmetric involvement of LMNs. The neurologic examination must be done carefully and thoroughly in these patients; in the early stages of more chronic diseases, LMN signs are subtle. Decreased strength of the flexor reflex may be the most prominent sign in the early stages of the disease course.

Peripheral neuropathies consist of disorders that affect the axon, axonopathies; the Schwann cells or myelin directly, myelinopathies (dysmyelinating diseases); or both the axons and Schwann cells, demyelinating diseases. Underlying pathologic processes of the nerve include wallerian degeneration, axonal degeneration, and segmental and diffuse myelin degeneration.[351] In most cases, these pathologies are not disease specific but occur in a variety of peripheral nerve diseases. Axonal degeneration and demyelination specify the underlying pathologic process and location to the peripheral nerve but rarely occur as separate disease entities. Motor neuron disorders occur when the disease process primarily affects the cell body, causing degeneration and loss.

Peripheral neuropathies are broadly classified as motor neuron disease, motor neuropathy/radiculopathy, sensory neuropathy, autonomic neuropathy, and mixed neuropathy. Most peripheral neuropathies or polyneuropathies involving spinal nerves are considered mixed neuropathies that affect motor, sensory, and autonomic nerves in varying degrees. Pathologic studies of peripheral neuropathy often show a combination of demyelination and axonal degeneration. The distal axon of the nerve is more sensitive to disease as a result of increased distance from the cell body and interruption of axonal transport. As a consequence, clinical signs such as weakness are worse in the distal musculature of the limbs. Some peripheral nerve diseases affecting the axons and myelin have involvement of both the CNS and PNS, but clinical signs may predominantly manifest as disease of the PNS, since the nerve itself is the final common pathway. Disease differentials for polyneuropathy or neuronopathy consist of a wide spectrum of diseases (see Table 7-4).

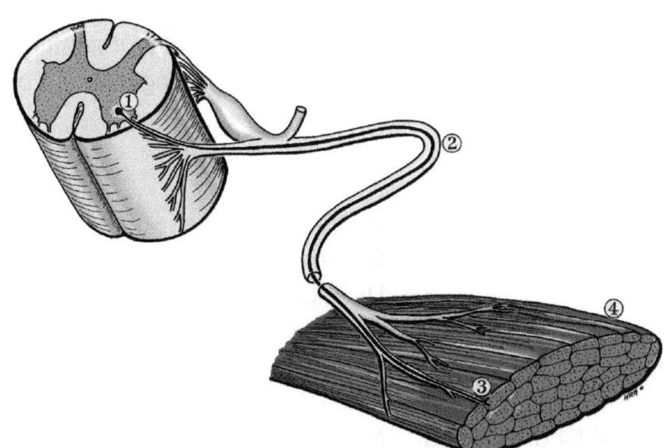

Figure 7-18 Schematic of anatomic sites of neuromuscular disease. *(1)* Neuronal cell bodies (neuronopathy), *(2)* peripheral nerves (neuropathy), *(3)* neuromuscular junction (junctionopathy), and *(4)* muscles (myopathy). (From Kornegay JN: Feline neurology [Problems in veterinary medicine series], Philadelphia, 1991, JB Lippincott.)

Peripheral neuropathies that involve the motor nerve and nerves roots often manifest hallmark signs of LMN disease with impairment of motor function. Motor neuropathies are characterized by a flaccid paresis or paralysis, postural reaction deficits, neurogenic muscle atrophy, and reduced to absent spinal reflexes.[352] Muscle fasciculations, spasms, and cramps also can occur. Neurogenic muscle atrophy is rapid and severe, occurring within 1 to 2 weeks from onset of clinical signs, and can progress to joint contracture in chronic cases.[352, 353] Neurogenic muscle atrophy results from a loss of the trophic influence of the axon on the muscle; denervation results in a loss of this trophism and consequently atrophy develops. As an aside, muscle atrophy is a clinical feature for wallerian degeneration and axonal degeneration but not for pure myelinopathies (axons still remain intact). Tremors also can be a clinical feature with some pure myelinopathies.[354,355]

Gait disturbances are a reflection of weakness and are not a result of incoordination. Often animals with lower motor neuron dysfunction will have a shortened stride and an inability to support weight, associated with the appendicular and axial musculature. Limb tone is reduced, and flaccidity often becomes more apparent in the distal limbs.[356] Limb posture will be crouched, with a tendency for joints to be flexed. Neck flexion also signifies generalized weakness. Dogs with just distal polyneuropathy often show a high-steppage or pseudohypermetric pelvic limb gait.[357] This represents a compensatory response to allow the carpi or tarsi to "flip" forward for limb placement. It is not uncommon for polyneuropathy to first manifest as paraparesis before tetraparesis because the longer (sciatic nerve) and more myelinated proprioceptive fibers usually are affected first.

Loss of tendon and flexor reflexes is a sign of peripheral nerve disease. Early in acute polyneuropathy, reflexes may be diminished but not absent, but they become more reduced over time. Reflexes can be diminished out of proportion to weakness because of greater involvement of the large afferent fibers of muscle spindles. Consequently, the loss of reflexes is a result of greater dysfunction of the afferent limb of the reflex arc.

Polyneuropathy can also present with multiple cranial nerve deficits. Cranial nerves V, VII, VIII, IX, X, and XI usually are involved. Affected animals may exhibit clinical signs of dysphagia, dysphonia, and dyspnea.[358] Dyspnea associated with upper respiratory tract signs suggests laryngeal paralysis.[359] The laryngeal abductor muscles are innervated by the recurrent laryngeal nerve, which is one of the longest peripheral nerves and thus susceptible to diseases causing neuropathy. Polyneuropathy needs to be considered as an underlying cause of laryngeal paralysis.[360,361] Diffuse motor neuropathies also cause respiratory compromise if the intercostal and phrenic nerves are involved.

Acute Progressive Diseases

Inflammatory

Acute Idiopathic Polyradiculoneuritis (Coonhound Paralysis). This acute neurologic syndrome has been recognized largely in hunting dogs that have been exposed to raccoons, but it also has been observed in dogs with no exposure to raccoons.[362,363] The disease is remarkably similar to acute polyneuritis in humans (Landry-Guillain-Barré syndrome). Other inflammatory neuropathies occasionally are reported in dogs and some other animals, including a cat[364,365] and a goat[366] (see discussion of chronic polyradiculoneuritis in cats). Polyneuritis equi (cauda equina neuritis) is relatively common in horses and is discussed in Chapter 6. Chronic polyneuropathies are discussed separately.

Pathophysiology. Immune-mediated segmental demyelination and degeneration of axons are found in dogs exposed to raccoons. Apparently, a transmissible substance in raccoon saliva produces the disease.[367] The Landry-Guillain-Barré syndrome in humans has been induced by several diseases, including respiratory infections and influenza vaccinations. Postvaccinal polyradiculoneuritis has also been seen in a dog.[368] The disease affects primarily the ventral roots and spinal nerves. Characteristic microscopic lesions include segmental demyelination, degeneration of both myelin and axons, leukocyte infiltration, secondary degeneration of the ventral horn neurons, and neurogenic muscle atrophy.[363,369] Neurologic signs develop because impulse transmission from the ventral horn of the spinal cord and motor nerve fibers to the myofibers is blocked.

Clinical Signs. Neurologic signs develop in some dogs 7 to 14 days after raccoon exposure. Early clinical signs include pelvic limb paresis and hyporeflexia. Ascending weakness or paralysis develops quickly. Affected dogs become tetraparetic within 24 to 48 hours after the neurologic signs first develop. Spinal reflexes are severely depressed or absent. Passive flexion and extension of the limbs reveal severe hypotonus of affected muscles. Cerebral responses to painful stimuli are normal or exaggerated. Diffuse hyperesthesia is occasionally seen in the paws and along the vertebral column upon palpation. Dogs with rapidly progressive disease may develop respiratory paralysis. Cranial nerve involvement is uncommon, although the dog's bark may be weak. Swallowing, gag reflex, and esophagus are normal. The patient remains alert, responsive, and afebrile. Defecation, urination, and tail mobility usually are normal because the sacral and caudal nerve roots are relatively spared. Muscle atrophy can be detected by direct palpation 10 to 14 days after the onset of paresis. Occasionally, the initial clinical signs are detected in the thoracic limbs and progress to the pelvic limbs. The thoracic limbs may remain preferentially involved in some acute forms of polyradiculoneuritis.[370,371] Complete respiratory paralysis can rarely occur.

Diagnosis. The diagnosis is suspected based on rapidity of clinical signs. The differential diagnosis should include tick paralysis, botulism, and fulminant myasthenia gravis, because these diseases produce clinical signs that are essentially identical to those of the early stages of polyradiculoneuritis (see the Neuromuscular Junction Diseases section). Table 7-8 compares the diagnostic features of polyradiculoneuritis, tick paralysis, and botulism. Polyradiculoneuritis is suspected when no ticks are found on physical examination, and exposure to botulinum toxin is not possible. Laboratory and radiographic studies are normal. Analysis of CSF collected from the lumbar subarachnoid space shows an increase in protein concentration, with a normal cell count.[369,372] A diagnosis of polyradiculoneuritis is supported by electrophysiologic evidence of diffuse denervation of affected muscles. These changes occur 5 to 7 days after injury of the motor axon. The electromyographic (EMG) abnormalities include increased insertion activity, fibrillation potentials, and positive sharp waves. Evoked potentials are slightly reduced in amplitude and may be polyphasic but are not as severely affected as with botulism or tick paralysis.[373] Nerve conduction velocities are reduced later in the course of the disease. F-waves are delayed and dispersed after paralysis has developed fully.[372] An enzyme-linked immunosorbent assay using raccoon saliva as the antigen shows some promise as a diagnostic test.[374]

Treatment. No specific treatment for polyradiculoneuritis exists. Controlled clinical trials using corticosteroids have not been reported. A study in humans did not show benefit of high-dose intravenous methylprednisolone early in Landry-Guillain-Barré syndrome.[375] Corticosteroids should not be used in dogs with polyradiculoneuritis, because they do not improve clinical signs or shorten the disease course.[376] Chronic corticosteroid therapy may cause urinary tract infection, further muscle wasting, and delayed healing of decubital ulcers. Plasmapheresis has been effective in human patients with Landry-Guillain-Barré syndrome,[377] has been used in other immune-mediated diseases of dogs[378] and could be beneficial in dogs with polyradiculoneuritis. Supportive care consists of attentive nursing that (1) prevents decubital ulcers, (2) minimizes muscle atrophy and contractures, (3) prevents urinary tract infection, (4) prevents pneumonia, and (5) supports respiratory function. Animals should be kept on padded bedding, turned frequently, and kept clean. Voluntary micturition usually is preserved; however, many dogs cannot produce

TABLE 7-8

Diagnostic Comparison of Acute Progressive Lower Motor Neuron Disorders

	Polyradiculoneuritis	Tick Paralysis	Botulism
History	Single case; previous exposure to raccoon in some cases	Single case—engorged tick	Multiple cases very suggestive; access to carrion or spoiled food
Pathophysiology	Nonsuppurative nerve root inflammation and demyelination	Interference with action potential or blocks release of acetylcholine	Toxin blocks release of acetylcholine by altering docking of synaptic vesicles
Esophageal motility	Normal	Normal	Reduced to absent
Hyperesthesia	Frequently present	Absent	Absent
Anal sphincter tone	Normal	Normal	Reduced to absent
Autonomic signs	Rare	Rare	Common
Cranial nerve involvement	Rare (sometimes CN VII)	Rare	Usually (often involving tongue and pharynx)
Electromyography	Fibrillation potentials and positive sharp waves	No denervation	Usually no denervation
Conduction velocity	Normal to decreased	Normal to slightly decreased	Normal
Evoked potentials	Reduced	Reduced	Reduced; decrement of amplitude on repetitive stimulation
Special tests	None	None	Toxin in feces and serum
Treatment	Supportive	Tick removal	Supportive
Recovery time	3-6 wk	24-48 hr	2-3 wk

a normal abdominal press and may fail to empty their bladders completely. Gentle manual expression of the bladder is helpful. Physical rehabilitation consisting of muscle massage and passive manipulation of the limbs is important.[379] Hydrotherapy is helpful for preventing muscle atrophy and contractures and for keeping the dog clean.

Prognosis. The prognosis for recovery is usually good. The clinical course is usually 3 to 6 weeks but may be prolonged up to 2 to 4 months or longer.[380,381] Improvement begins by the third week, and complete recovery may take 6 to 8 weeks. In patients that develop severe muscle atrophy, recovery will be prolonged and may not be complete. Neurologic signs usually abate in the reverse order of development. Relapses have been observed. Some dogs appear to be particularly susceptible to recurrences.

Protozoal Polyradiculoneuritis. *Neospora caninum* and *Toxoplasma gondii* can cause inflammation of the peripheral nerves, muscles, and/or CNS.[382-385] In the PNS, the spinal nerve roots are more severely affected. *Neospora caninum* and *T. gondii* infections can be distinguished using serologic, immunohistochemical, and morphologic criteria.[382] *Neospora caninum* is the likely causative agent in many cases originally thought to be toxoplasmosis.[385,423] Ingestion of raw or undercooked meat appears to be a risk factor for *N. caninum and T. gondii* infection.[424] Transplacental (vertical) mode of transmission underlies the congenital form of neosporosis.[423] In young puppies, pelvic limb extensor rigidity (genu recurvatum) is a classic feature of protozoal muscle and nerve infection.[383,384] Affected pups are normal at birth but then develop an asymmetric paraparesis and plantigrade stance. Ataxia and a bunny-hopping gait may develop along with hyporeflexia and severe muscle atrophy in the pelvic limbs. Because infections may be subclinical, evidence of seroconversion 2 or more weeks after the initial immunoglobulin G (IgG) antibody titer is required for a diagnosis (see Chapter 15). All dogs with clinical neosporosis have had serum titers greater than 1:200, but titers greater than 1:800 have been seen in clinically normal dogs.[425]

Diagnosis is based on clinical signs and serology or PCR testing. The creatine kinase (CK) is frequently elevated. Electrophysiologic testing supports evidence of neuropathy and myopathy. CSF analysis may show a mixed-cell pleocytosis and increased protein concentration. Muscle and nerve biopsies may show inflammation and presence of bradyzoites in muscle or tachyzoites within the CNS or nerve.

Treatment should include trimethoprim-sulfadiazine (15 mg/kg orally, every 12 hours) and pyrimethamine (1 mg/kg orally, every 24 hours) or clindamycin (15 to 20 mg/kg orally, every 12 hours). Treatment should continue for 4 to 6 weeks. Early treatment may be beneficial, but if muscle contracture is present, recovery is unlikely.

Chronic Progressive Diseases

Degenerative

Congenital and Inherited Motor Neuronopathies. Motor neuronopathies (Table 7-9) are disorders of the ventral horn neurons that cause generalized weakness. These chronic progressive diseases are characterized by progressive degeneration of motor neurons in the gray matter of the ventral horn of the spinal cord and nuclei of the brainstem. Progressive denervation of muscle fibers results in paresis, paralysis, and severe muscle atrophy. The diseases in dogs resemble the inherited spinal muscular atrophies of humans. A characteristic feature of motor neuron disease that differs from peripheral neuropathy is muscular weakness and fasciculations with muscle atrophy, but preservation of reflexes until the disease is advanced.[426] Other clinical signs include tremor, flexion of the neck, and dysphagia. Motor neuron diseases are rare and usually occur in young growing animals, with an insidious and progressive clinical disease course. These disorders have been mostly described in dogs and cats. Inherited forms have been described in the Brittany spaniel,[427] English pointer,[428] Swedish Lapland dogs,[429] and suspected for other breeds.[426] Motor neuron disease of young onset has been reported in the Maine coon and domestic shorthair cats.[430,431] An adult onset form of unknown cause has been reported in cats.[432] Bovine spinal muscular atrophy has been reported in Brown Swiss cattle and related breeds and has an autosomal recessive inheritance.[433-435] Motor neuron disease also has been reported in Romney lambs in New Zealand.[436]

Equine Motor Neuron Disease

Pathogenesis. Equine motor neuron disease is a spontaneous motor neuron disease which results from degeneration of motor neurons in the spinal cord and brainstem.[437,438] The disease primarily affects horses in the northeastern United States.[439] Various breeds and ages are affected, but most horses are older than 2 years of age. The exact cause is unknown, but vitamin E deficiency is a primary risk factor.[440] Vitamin E levels were significantly lower in affected horses.[441] Some horses have improved after being allowed on pasture and given supplemental vitamin E. Lesions are similar to those of the other spinal muscular atrophies.[442] Environmental risk factors include absence of grazing for more than 1 year and provision of poor-quality hay, dietary deficiency of vitamin E, and excessive dietary copper.[441] Hallmark pathologic findings include loss of ventral horn motor neurons supplying the highly oxidative type I muscle fibers. Approximately 30% of motor neurons are lost in horses with clinical signs.[443] Increased lipopigment in motor neurons and capillary endothelial cells suggest underlying oxidative damage.[437] Equine motor neuron disease has similarities to sporadic amyotrophic lateral sclerosis (ALS, or Lou Gehrig's disease).[444]

Clinical Signs. Characteristic initial signs include weight loss, muscle wasting, excessive recumbency, and trembling. Constant shifting of weight in the pelvic limbs, abnormally low head carriage, and muscle fasciculations reflect muscle weakness (Figure 7-19).[437] Black pigment deposits may be evident on the surface of the incisors in some affected horses. Funduscopic examination reveals brown streaking which represents abnormal ceroid lipofuscin in the retinal pigmented epithelium.[445,446]

Diagnosis. Diagnosis is based on clinical signs and by ruling out other diseases. Plasma vitamin E concentrations are less than 1 mcg/mL.[440] Vitamin A levels are usually low normal. Concentrations of muscle-derived enzymes such as CK are increased. Spontaneous activity is consistently seen on EMG, particularly in the proximal thoracic limbs.[447] A tentative antemortem diagnosis can be established by demonstrating degeneration of myelinated axons in biopsy samples of the ventral branch of the accessory nerve or denervation of the sacrocaudalis dorsalis medialis muscle.[448,449]

Treatment. Treatment consists of supplementing vitamin E by administering 5000 to 10,000 IU of alpha-tocopherol daily or grazing the horse on high-quality pasture.[449] Exercise should be limited during active disease for 2 to 3 months. Prevention of equine motor neuron disease requires maintaining adequate intake of vitamin E. Green forages are a major source of vitamin E.[450]

Peripheral Myelinopathies. Demyelination is caused by disease of the Schwann cell or myelin sheath (Table 7-10). Demyelination is loss of the myelin sheath along the length of the internode (segmental demyelination) or near the paranodal area (paranodal demyelination). Disease can occur continuously (diffuse demyelination) or randomly along the course of the nerve. In immune-mediated neuropathies, nerves are damaged by cellular or humoral mechanisms directed against various components of myelin. Repeated processes of demyelination and remyelination also occur with some disease

TABLE 7-9

Motor Neuron Disorders in Domestic Animals*

Breed and Species	Age of Onset	Inheritance	Clinical Signs	References
Canine				
Brittany spaniel (model of infantile SMA)	Homozygotes develop clinical signs 6-8 wk; heterozygotes develop signs 6 mo to 2 yr; euthanized at 7 yr	AD	Homozygotes rapidly progress to tetraplegia and dysphagia (SMA type I); heterozygotes have intermediate and chronic forms. Atrophy first in proximal muscles, with signs of PL weakness.	386-388
Collie	8 wk	Unknown	Exercise intolerance, weakness, decreased patellar reflexes	389
Doberman pinscher	4 wk	Unknown	Severe muscle atrophy; paraparesis progressing to tetraparesis	390
English pointer	4.5 to 6 mo	AR	Acute progressive tetraparesis with LMN signs; distal muscles more severe; tetraplegia; accumulation of lipids	391, 392
German shepherd dog	2 wk	Unknown	Angular limb deformities caused by muscle atrophy	393
Griffon Briquet Vendeen	6 wk	Unknown	Paraparesis first in extensor muscles then flexors	394
Rottweiler	4 wk	Unknown; familial	Regurgitation and megaesophagus; diminished growth, progressive PL ataxia; LMN signs	395
Saluki	9 wk	Unknown	Progressive tetraparesis; angular limb deformity in TL; muscle atrophy; neck ventroflexion; fine head tremor	396
Swedish Lapland dog	5 to 7 wk	AR?	Acute recumbency with severe muscle atrophy; distal limbs	397
New Zealand dogs—collies, pug, dachshund, fox terrier	3 to 9 mo of age	Unknown	Acute progressive paraparesis to flaccid tetraparesis; severe muscle atrophy	398
Stockard's paralysis—Great Dane x St. Bernard x bloodhound	8 to 12 wk	Unknown	Acute-onset paraparesis; distal appendicular muscles affected first, with sparing of paraspinal muscles; priapism	399
Canine degenerative myelopathy† many breeds	Older than 8 yr	AR (*SOD1* mutation)	Slowly progressive general proprioceptive ataxia and spastic UMN PL paresis in early disease; ascending tetraparesis and ataxia to tetraplegia and LMN signs; euthanasia within 9 mo to 3 years; pathology reflects central-peripheral axonopathy *without* motor neuron loss	400-409
Feline				
Maine coon	4 mo	AR (*LIX1-LNPEP* mutation)	Tremor; proximal muscle weakness and atrophy	410, 411
DSH	10 wk	Unknown	Acute progressive paraparesis to tetraplegia; appendicular muscle atrophy	412
Bovine				
Brown Swiss cattle (Bovine spinal muscular atrophy)	3 to 4 wk	AR	Progressive weakness in thoracic and pelvic limbs; neurogenic muscle atrophy	413-416
Red Danish dairy—related to Brown Swiss	Birth to 21 wk	Familial	Recumbent	417
German Braunvieh—related to Brown Swiss	3 wk	Familial	Ataxia, muscle atrophy, recumbency	418
Ovine				
Romney lambs	1 wk	Familial	Progressive weakness, hyporeflexia	419

Continued

TABLE 7-9

Motor Neuron Disorders in Domestic Animals*—cont'd

Breed and Species	Age of Onset	Inheritance	Clinical Signs	References
Equine				
Equine motor neuron disease (thoroughbreds, standardbreds, quarter horse, Appaloosas, Walking horses, Arabians, Welsh pony, Morgan)	15 mo to 25 yr	Familial, vitamin E deficiency	Progressive tetraparesis, muscle fasciculations, muscle atrophy, weight loss	420-422

*Disorders characterized by motor neuron loss.
†Mutations of the *SOD1* gene causing DM in dogs cause some forms of human ALS, which is characterized histopathologically with motor neuron loss.

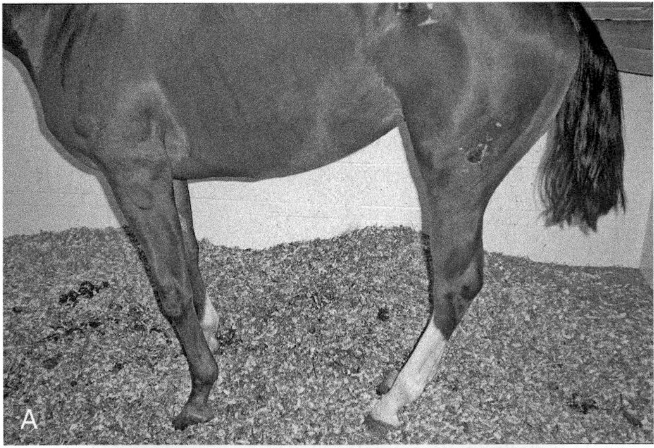

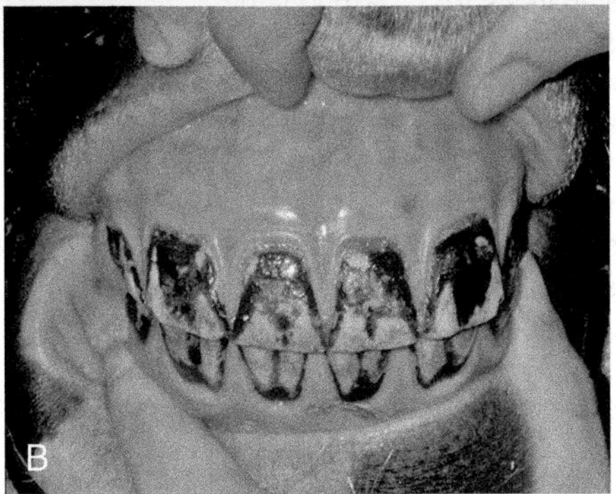

Figure 7-19 **A,** A 4-year-old horse with equine motor neuron disease, showing characteristic tucked placement of limbs beneath torso. Also note decubitus ulcers over bony prominences of pelvic limbs from prolonged recumbency. This horse also showed muscle fasciculations and shifting of weight between limbs. **B** shows black pigment on surface of incisors from same horse. (Courtesy Philip Johnson.)

processes, such as inflammatory demyelinating polyneuropathies. Remyelination can partially restore function. Disruption of the myelin sheath will cause the electric current of the action potential to dissipate through the internode as a result of increased capacitance and decreased resistance. This will result in a longer time to depolarize the next internode, thus prolonging the conduction time. Conduction failure occurs with severe demyelination. Diffuse myelinopathy occurs with inherited, metabolic, and toxic disorders. Most reported cases of canine hypomyelination primarily involve the CNS (see Chapter 10) and defects of the oligodendrocytes. Hypomyelination in the PNS is due to primary defects in Schwann cell function.

Schwann Cell Defects. Severe hypomyelination due to an underlying defect in Schwann cell function involving only the PNS has been reported in golden retriever puppies[552, 553] and Tibetan mastiffs.[554-557] Clinical signs are characterized by weakness, hypotonia, and hyporeflexia. Often there is a plantigrade stance in the pelvic limbs and a bunny-hopping gait. In the Tibetan mastiff, the disease is called *inherited hypertrophic neuropathy* because successive bouts of remyelination and demyelination result in gross hypertrophy of the nerve.[554] Autosomal recessive inheritance is suspected in the Tibetan mastiff,[558] and the disease is considered familial in the golden retriever. Clinicals signs will stabilize, and some affected dogs may recover the ability to walk with residual weakness.

Laminin-α_2 Deficient Muscular Dystrophy. This disorder due to deficiency of laminin α_2 has been reported in a domestic shorthair (DSH) and a Siamese cat.[559] Laminin α_2 is a large glycoprotein found in the basement membrane of muscle, Schwann cells, and in blood vessels within the brain and other tissues. Age of onset of clinical signs is 6 months. These cats develop progressive weakness of the spinal and head musculature, with the pelvic limbs first affected. The pelvic limbs develop marked atrophy and rigid contracture which eventually progress to involve the thoracic limbs. Limbs, spine, and tail are rigid. Moderate trismus also develops. Laminin α_2–deficient muscular dystrophy occurs sporadically in cats; a genetic predisposition is unknown at this time. The prognosis in cats with laminin-α_2 deficiency is considered poor because of its progressive nature.

Inherited Distal Sensorimotor Polyneuropathy

Pathogenesis. Axonal degeneration results from disease within the neuronal cell body or of the axon itself. These disorders often are inherited (see Table 7-10) and are distinguished from idiopathic or toxins based on the age of onset. The age of onset in dogs and cats usually is within a few months or young to middle age. Often the degeneration of the axon and its myelin sheath begins distally and extends proximally to the neuronal cell body. The neuron undergoes chromatolysis. This process has been termed *dying-back neuropathy*, *distal axonopathy*, or *distal sensorimotor neuropathy*. These processes preferentially affect long, large-caliber, myelinated nerve fibers. These inherited motor and sensory (mixed) neuropathies affect motor, sensory, and autonomic nerves in varying degrees. In mixed neuropathies, often the clinical signs reflect early motor

TABLE 7-10

Inherited and Breed-Associated Motor, Mixed, and Sensory Neuropathies of Domestic Animals

Disease (Breeds)	Age of Onset	Inheritance Pattern (Mutation)	Clinical Features	Predominant Neuropathy	Reference
Distal Sensorimotor Polyneuropathies					
Canine					
Alaskan Malamute polyneuropathy	10-18 mo	Suspect AR	Progressive tetraparesis PL>TL; distal limb muscle atrophy; paraspinal hyperesthesia; laryngeal mm. paresis	Distal sensorimotor polyneuropathy	451, 452
Dancing Doberman disease	6-7 yr	Suspect AR	Initial flexion of one PL progressing to opposite limb and flexion of both, causing preference of dog to sit; progresses to tetraparesis	Sensorimotor autonomic neuropathy	453
Familial German shepherd neuropathy	9-10 yr	Familial	Paraparesis progressing to tetraparesis, PL muscle atrophy; hyporeflexia; increased CK	Dying-back peripheral axonopathy	454
Distal symmetric polyneuropathy (Great Dane)	1.5-5 yr	Unknown	Paraparesis progressing to tetraparesis, atrophy of masticatory and distal limb muscles	Dying-back peripheral axonopathy	455, 456
Progressive axonopathy in boxer	5-15 mo	Unknown	Progressive PL ataxia and paresis; loss of paw replacement; progress to TL; decreased spinal reflexes	Central-peripheral distal axonopathy	457-459
Giant axonal neuropathy in German shepherd dogs	14-16 mo	Unknown	Plantigrade stance, progressive paraparesis to tetraparesis; decreased sensory perception; late—megaesophagus, fecal incontinence, laryngeal dysfunction	Central-peripheral axonopathy	454, 460-464
Bouvier des Flandres Laryngeal paralysis	4-6 mo	AD	Inspiratory distress, laryngeal paralysis unilateral or bilateral, dysphonia	Distal axonopathy; degeneration of motor neuronal cell bodies in brainstem	465-467
Laryngeal paralysis (Siberian husky, husky cross-breeds, bull terriers Leonberger, white German shepherd)	4-6 mo	Unknown	Inspiratory distress, laryngeal paralysis unilateral or bilateral, dysphonia	Distal axonopathy	468-470
Laryngeal paralysis polyneuropathy complex (dalmatian, rottweiler, Pyrenean mountain dog)	2-6 mo	Unknown	Laryngeal paralysis, megaesophagus, atrophy of laryngeal and appendicular muscles; tetraparesis	Dying-back distal axonopathy	187, 471-473
Inherited polyneuropathy in Leonberger dogs	1-3 yr	Suspect X-linked	Distal muscle atrophy, high-steppage gait, reduced flexion of distal joints, hyporeflexia, laryngeal paralysis	Distal polyneuropathy	474, 475

TABLE 7-10

***Inherited and Breed-Associated Motor, Mixed, and Sensory Neuropathies of Domestic Animals*—cont'd**

Disease (Breeds)	Age of Onset	Inheritance Pattern (Mutation)	Clinical Features	Predominant Neuropathy	Reference
Rottweiler distal sensorimotor polyneuropathy	1.5-4 yr	Unknown	Slowly progressive paraparesis to tetraparesis; hyporeflexia; appendicular muscle atrophy	Dying-back distal sensorimotor polyneuropathy	476
Italian Spinoni	8-10 yr	Suspect AR	Weakness, high-steppage gait in pelvic limbs, plantigrade stance, atrophy of distal limbs	Distal symmetric polyneuropathy	477
Feline					
Snowshoe cat	Young-2 yr	Unknown	Paraparesis	Distal axonopathy	478
Birman cat	8-10 wk	Sex limited?	Hypermetria, frequent falling, plantigrade stance, PL>TL	Central-peripheral distal axonopathy	479
Myelin-Associated Polyneuropathies					
Canine					
Congenital hypomyelination neuropathy in golden retriever	7 wk	Unknown	Bunny-hop gait, crouched PL, hyporeflexia	Hypomyelination Suspect Schwann cell defect	480, 481
Hypertrophic neuropathy (Tibetan mastiff)	7-10 wk	AR	Rapid onset of generalized weakness, hypotonia, dysphonia; recumbent by 3 mo of onset	Schwann cell defect	482-485
Hypertrophic polyneuropathy (DSH)	1 yr	Unknown	Tremor, hyporeflexia, sensory deficit	Peripheral myelin degeneration	486
Feline					
Laminin α_2-deficient muscular dystrophy (DSH, Siamese, Maine coon)	6-12 mo	Unknown	Paraparesis progressing to tetraparesis, trismus, severe extensor contracture, and muscle atrophy	Lack of laminin-α_2 in Schwann cell basement membrane	487, 488
Primary Sensory Neuropathies					
Long-haired dachshund	8-12 wk	Unknown	Mild ataxia, proprioceptive deficits, loss of nociception, urinary incontinence, self-mutilation	Distal central-peripheral axonopathy	489, 490
English pointer and German shorthaired pointer	2-12 mo	AR	Nociceptive loss in distal limbs, acral changes and self-mutilation	CNS and primary sensory neuropathy; loss of substance P	491-495
Jack Russell terrier	6 yr	Unknown	Proprioceptive deficits, loss of nociception, self-mutilation	Primary sensory neuropathy	496
French spaniel	3-12 mo	AR	Self-mutilation of distal extremities, loss of nociception	No light microscopic lesions	497
Golden retriever	Puppyhood	Mitochondrial (*tRNA^{Tyr}* mutation)	GP ataxia, postural reaction deficits, absent spinal reflexes	Central-peripheral sensory neuropathy	498, 499, 602
Breeds (single reports)—golden retriever, rough-coated collie, border collie, Doberman pinscher, Siberian husky, whippet, Scottish terrier					498, 500-504

Continued

TABLE 7-10

Inherited and Breed-Associated Motor, Mixed, and Sensory Neuropathies of Domestic Animals—cont'd

Disease (Breeds)	Age of Onset	Inheritance Pattern (Mutation)	Clinical Features	Predominant Neuropathy	Reference
Metabolic Neuropathies					
Hyperoxaluria (DSH)	5-9 mo	AR (*GRHPR* mutation)	Crouched stance, reluctant to walk, reduced postural reactions, areflexia	PNS changes include swollen axons in nerve root and ganglia secondary to neurofilament accumulation; deficient hepatic enzyme activity of D-glycerate dehydrogenase and glyoxylate reductase	505, 506
Hyperchylomicronemia (Siamese, Himalayan, Persian, European)	4 wk	AR (*LPL* mutation)	Clinical signs reflect asymmetric focal neuropathies affecting spinal and cranial nerves	Foraminal nerve compression by lipid granulomas; decreased activity of lipoprotein lipase	507-514
Familial neuropathy and glomerulopathy of Gelbvieh cattle	Young to 20 mo	Familial	Intermittent GP ataxia and paraparesis progressing to recumbency	Wallerian degeneration in dorsal and ventral nerve roots; minimal fiber degeneration in SC; multifocal myonecrosis	515, 516
Lysosomal Storage Disorders (see also Table 15-3)					
Fucosidosis (English springer spaniel)	6 mo-3 yr	AR (mutation *α-L-fucosidase*)	Slow learners, ataxia, hypermetria, progressive incoordination, hoarse bark, dysphagia, and hearing and visual deficits	Gross findings include enlargement of some nerves and nerve roots. Axonal spheroids and swollen neurons in CNS; vacuolated macrophages; deficiency of α-L-fucosidase	517-521
Globoid cell leukodystrophy (West Highland white terrier, cairn terrier, beagle, poodle, basset hound, bluetick hound, Pomeranian, Irish setter, DSH and DLH; Dorset sheep)	Ca-*West Highland white terrier* (2-5 mo), *cairn terrier* (2-5 mo), beagle (4 mo), poodle (2 yr), basset hound (1.5-2 yr), blue tick hound (4 mo), Pomeranian (1.5 yr), *Irish setter* (6 mo); F-DSH, DLH (5-6 wk); O-Dorset (4-18 mo)	AR or Unknown (mutation *galactosylceramidase* in West Highland white terrier and cairn terrier)	Reflect multifocal disease, progressive paraparesis to tetraparesis, cerebellar dysfunction, hyporeflexia, muscle atrophy	CNS lesions are confined to white matter in brain and spinal cord, with destruction of myelin and infiltration of PAS (+) macrophages (globoid cells); PNS lesions include segmental demyelination, axonal degeneration, and accumulation of macrophages containing globoid cells; deficiency of lysosomal enzyme galactosyl-ceramidase	522-532
Glycogenosis type IV (Norwegian forest cat, quarter horse, paint horse)	F-5 mo E-neonatal	AR (mutation in *glycogen branching enzyme 1*)	Generalized muscle tremors, bunny-hop gait, severe muscle atrophy, contracture, hyporeflexia	Abnormal accumulation of glycogen in PNS and CNS; loss of axons and myelin in peripheral nerves. Extensive storage in CNS; deficiency of glycogen branching enzyme α-1,4-D-glucan: α-1,4 glucan 6-glucosyl transferase	533-539

TABLE 7-10

***Inherited and Breed-Associated Motor, Mixed, and Sensory Neuropathies of Domestic Animals*—cont'd**

Disease (Breeds)	Age of Onset	Inheritance Pattern (Mutation)	Clinical Features	Predominant Neuropathy	Reference
Mannosidosis (DSH, DLH, Persian; Murray grey, Aberdeen Angus)	F-DSH (7 mo), DLH, *Persian* (8 wk); B-Galloway, Murray grey, Aberdeen Angus (birth)	AR (mutation *α-D-mannosidase* in Persians)	Cerebellar ataxia, tremor, corneal opacity, skeletal anomalies, neuropathy; B-cerebellar ataxia, aggressiveness	Vacuolated glia and neurons in CNS; vacuolated macrophages in peripheral nerves; defective myelin in CNS and PNS; hypomyelination in CNS and PNS; deficiency of α-D-mannosidase	540-546
Phenotypic variant of Niemann-Pick disease type A (miniature poodle, Balinese, Siamese, Hereford)	Ca-miniature poodle (2-4 mo); F-Balinese, Siamese (2-3 mo); B-Hereford (5 mo)	Unknown; AR Siamese	Absent postural reactions, hypo- to areflexia, hypotonia, fine tremors, plantigrade stance	Peripheral nerve changes include widespread demyelination, with many vacuolated macrophages; CNS also mildly affected; reduction in CNS and visceral lysosomal sphingomyelinase activity	547-551

AD, Autosomal dominant; *AR*, autosomal recessive; *B*, bovine; *C*, caprine; *Ca*, canine; *CK*, creatine kinase; *E*, equine; *F*, feline; *GP*, general proprioceptive; *O*, ovine; *P*, porcine; *PL*, pelvic limb; *SC*, spinal cord; *TL*, thoracic limb.

nerve dysfunction with less obvious signs of sensory nerve dysfunction. Both primary axonal degeneration and wallerian degeneration will cause neurogenic muscle atrophy later in the disease course. These diseases are progressive and relentless.

Clinical Signs. Clinical signs usually are recognized first in the distal limbs as a consequence of distance of the nerve from the cell body. The signs progress to nonambulatory paraparesis and tetraparesis. Hyporeflexia manifests first in the distal limbs. These disorders manifest as diffuse polyneuropathy that involve the distal appendicular musculature in the Alaskan Malamute,[560,561] Doberman pinscher (dancing Doberman disease),[562] German shepherd dog,[203,563,564] Great Dane,[565,566] Leonberger,[357,567] border collie,[568] and rottweiler.[569] In the border collie, there was initial sensory nerve dysfunction with progressive motor nerve dysfunction.

Some inherited distal neuropathies may be asymmetric at onset. A distal neuropathy has been reported in Doberman pinschers and is termed *dancing Doberman disease*.[562] Pelvic limb weakness is noted initially. Age of onset varies from 6 months to 7 years and slowly progresses over years. Typically, affected dogs flex one pelvic limb while standing. These dogs are unable to stand still, so that the dog alternately flexes each limb as if it is dancing. Patellar reflexes tend to be exaggerated. Weakness initially develops in the pelvic limbs and progress to involve the thoracic limbs. Muscle atrophy is especially prominent in the gastrocnemius muscle. Abnormalities are noted on EMG while nerve conduction velocities are within normal limits. Histopathology reveals both axonopathy and myopathy.

A distal axonopathy, with associated neurogenic muscle atrophy, has been identified in horses with Australian stringhalt.[570-572] Affected horses flex one or both pelvic limbs excessively during attempted movement. In contrast to classic stringhalt, this disease has a seasonal incidence, and affected horses may recover spontaneously (see Chapter 10).

Since the recurrent laryngeal is a long nerve, laryngeal paralysis is often a sequela to the acquired and inherited distal polyneuropathies.[361,573-575] For similar reasons, esophageal dysfunction also may occur.[576] Laryngeal paralysis is a predominant clinical manifestation in the Bouvier des Flandres and is inherited as an autosomal dominant trait.[577,578] Laryngeal paralysis occurs in a number of other breeds summarized in Chapter 9. A laryngeal paralysis polyneuropathy complex occurs in dalmatians,[579] rottweiler,[580] and Pyrenean mountain dog.[187] Male Leonberger dogs manifest a severe distal polyneuropathy and laryngeal paralysis that may be inherited as an X-linked trait.[357]

Diagnosis. Diagnosis is based on ruling out other acquired disorders. Electromyography is characterized by spontaneous activity which includes fibrillation potentials and sharp waves in the distal and proximal appendicular muscular with changes more severe in the distal musculature. Motor nerve conduction velocities may be slow as a result of the secondary demyelination. Nerve and muscle biopsy further assist with understanding the disease process and ruling out other acquired disorders.[581] On muscle biopsy, changes are characterized by excessive variability in myofiber size with atrophic fibers of both fiber types, large and small grouped atrophy, and hypertrophy. Fiber type grouping, an indicator of chronicity, may be evident if denervation is followed by reinnervation. Nerve biopsies show more severe changes in the distal nerve. Abnormal findings include axonal degeneration, loss of myelinated fibers of varying diameter, and axonal necrosis. If nerve regeneration is occurring, regenerating clusters and sprouts may be found. Teased fiber studies may further show axonal degeneration and evidence of demyelination and remyelination.

Treatment and Prognosis. Treatment is aimed toward supportive care. In dogs with laryngeal paralysis, "tie-back" procedures may lessen signs of upper airway obstruction. Physiotherapy can assist with maintaining range of motion. Prognosis is guarded to poor especially in the more rapidly progressive neuropathies

Central-Peripheral Distal Axonopathy. Central-peripheral distal axonopathy is characterized by the presence of axonal degeneration in selected pathways of the CNS and PNS (see Table 7-10). Clinical signs predominate as a peripheral neuropathy. These disorders have been well described in the Birman cat,[582] boxer (progressive axonopathy of boxer dogs),[184-186,583] and German shepherd dog (giant axonal neuropathy).[563,584] The CNS pathology involves the dorsal and lateral funiculi of the spinal cord. Swollen axons containing excessive neurofilaments are present in the spinal cord. Pathology of the nerve involves variable axonal loss and secondary demyelination. Motor and sensory fibers are affected. Onset of signs in Birman cats is between 8 and 10 weeks of age. These cats manifest a plantigrade stance and progressive GP ataxia and paresis in the pelvic limbs. The age at onset varies in boxers. These dogs manifest GP ataxia and paresis in the pelvic limbs that progress to involve the thoracic limbs. Myotatic reflexes are reduced, but flexor reflexes remain intact. Age at onset of signs in German shepherd dogs is between 1 and 2 years of age. Clinical signs in these dogs are manifested by a plantigrade stance, and GP ataxia and paresis in the pelvic limbs. Spinal reflexes are absent. Megaesophagus, laryngeal dysfunction, and fecal incontinence manifest late in the disease course.

Sensory Neuronopathy and Neuropathy. An animal with a *pure* sensory neuropathy may show decreased nociception, paresthesia, evidence of self-mutilation, and reduced to absent spinal reflexes *without* muscle atrophy.[356] Urinary incontinence may also develop. The absence of weakness and normal muscle tone and the ability to support weight provide evidence that the motor fibers are unaffected. In cases of acral mutilation, the location often involves the distal extremities and/or facial region. Affected dogs will undergo autoamputation of nail, digits, and footpads and walk on the mutilated paws without showing evidence of pain. Clinical signs are first noted within the first year of life. Clinical signs of self-mutilation have been reported in the long-haired dachshund,[585] English and short-haired pointer in North America,[586] English springer spaniel in Australia,[587] French spaniel[588] and in the Jack Russell terrier.[589]

Pure sensory nociceptive neuropathies are rare and often have an inherited cause (see Table 7-10).[189] Some acquired diseases also may show sensory disturbances in perception.[376] Unlike in humans, clinical signs of sensory loss (numbness, pain, temperature alterations) associated with polyneuropathy in animals often are impossible to recognize and go undetected. Individual cases have been documented in various breeds: Jack Russell terrier,[589] golden retriever,[590] rough-coated collie,[591] border collie,[592,593] Doberman pinscher, Siberian husky, whippet, and Scottish terrier.[594] Sensory neuronopathy of autosomal recessive inheritance has been well described in English pointer dogs in North America,[595] in short-haired pointers in Czech Republic,[586,596] and French spaniels.[588] Autosomal recessive inheritance is suspected in the long-haired dachshund.[597]

Diagnosis is based on clinical signs, electrophysiology, and biopsy. EMG and motor nerve conduction velocities are normal. Sensory nerve action potential cannot be elicited. Based on electrophysiologic abnormalities, one investigator suggested that dogs with acral lick dermatitis may have a mild sensory axonal polyneuropathy.[598] Histologic changes in sensory neuronopathy with nociceptive loss include decrease neuronal cell bodies in the spinal ganglia and paucity of myelinated axons in dorsal roots and peripheral nerves.[586] Severe depletion of both large myelinated and unmyelinated fibers occurs. Reduced density in the nociceptive pathways was observed. In affected English pointers, loss of the sensory neurons was associated with reduction of substance P immunoreactivity.[599] The lesion distribution in long-haired dachshunds and pointer dogs is characterized as a distal central-peripheral axonopathy, although the clinical signs predominate to involve the sensory nerve.[586,595,597] The lesion is confined to the nerve in the Jack Russell,[589] and minimal lesions in the nerve and ganglion were observed in the French spaniel.[588] Ganglioneuritis with involvement of spinal and cranial ganglia has been described.[594,600]

In cases of sensory neuropathy that involve acral mutilation, prognosis is considered poor. In the absence of a genetic test, the recommendation to prevent recurrence of a recessive disorder is to remove affected animals and their parents from the breeding program.

Hereditary neuropathies involving the central and peripheral sensory pathways without nociceptive involvement will manifest GP ataxia without acral automutilation.[590,601] Sensory ataxic neuropathy was recently identified in golden retrievers.[601] These dogs have GP ataxia, postural reaction deficits, and reduced to absent spinal reflexes. Onset of signs occurs during puppyhood and is slowly progressive. Dogs are often euthanized by 3 years of age. Histopathology revealed degeneration of the sensory pathways in both the central and peripheral nervous systems. Pedigree analysis revealed that all dogs belong to one maternal lineage, and statistical analysis showed that the disorder is of mitochondrial origin.[601] A deletion in the mitochondrial *tRNA*^{Tyr} gene was determined as the causative mutation for sensory ataxic neuropathy in golden retrievers.[602]

Metabolic

High metabolic demand of the peripheral nerve predisposes to effects associated with endocrine disorders. Storage disorders including sphingomyelinosis variant type A, mannosidosis, glycogen storage disease type IV, fucosidosis, and globoid cell leukodystrophy may also have peripheral nerve involvement, and therefore affected animals may display LMN weakness (see also Chapter 15).[189]

Hypothyroid Neuropathy. Hypothyroidism causes polyneuropathy and myopathy in dogs.[376,575,603-606] Nerve pathology involves both the axon and myelin.[575,604,607] Muscle biopsy will show neurogenic atrophy of both type I and II myofibers or type II myofiber atrophy, suggestive of primary myopathic disease.[606,607] Underlying pathophysiologic mechanisms for hypothyroid neuropathy include impaired energy metabolism of the motor neuron and alterations in microtubule assembly and axonal transport.[376,608] Myxedematous tissues may be associated with compressive neuropathy as the nerves exit through foramina of the cranium or the intervertebral foramina.[376]

Clinical Signs. Dogs may have signs of diffuse LMN dysfunction, peripheral or central vestibular dysfunction,[609,610] encephalopathy,[611,612] and cranial nerve dysfunction (VII, VIII, IX, X).[575,604] Peripheral neuropathy is the most common of the neurologic signs.[575] The paresis may vary in symmetry and involve one limb or all limbs.[575,604,613] Exercise intolerance may be evidence of myopathic involvement. Hyporeflexia may be evident with the polyneuropathy. Clinical signs of cranial nerve dysfunction include megaesophagus,[614] facial paralysis,[615] or laryngeal paralysis.[573,575]

Diagnosis. During the early stages when clinical signs are vague, the diagnosis is often overlooked. These vague presenting complaints include weakness, intermittent lameness, and signs of cranial nerve V, VII, VIII, IX, and X dysfunction (see Chapters 8 and 9). Many affected animals may or may not have the classical systemic signs of hypothyroidism such as lethargy, weight gain, alopecia, bradycardia, pyoderma, and seborrhea. Blood work abnormalities may include nonregenerative anemia, hypercholesterolemia, and increased CK and alkaline phosphatase activity.[575,605-607] The diagnosis is confirmed by reduced free and total serum thyroxine levels, with an elevation in thyroid-stimulating hormone levels. Electromyography and nerve-conduction studies can further characterize the neuropathic or myopathic disease and document evidence for both axonal degeneration and demyelination.[575,604,613] Degenerative changes may be seen in nerve and muscle biopsy specimens. Hypothyroidism also has been associated with acquired myasthenia gravis in dogs.[616] Diagnosis also is based on a positive clinical response to administration of levothyroxine.[613]

Treatment and Prognosis. The rate and degree of recovery subsequent to levothyroxine treatment depend on the severity of the denervation and myopathy. In hypothyroid myopathy, improvement of systemic signs and weakness after supplementation is noted within several days.[605] Actual improvement of motor function in hypothyroid neuropathy may take weeks to months. Animals with severe denervation have a more guarded prognosis for recovery.[605,617] Cranial nerve deficits associated with megaesophagus and laryngeal paralysis are less likely to improve.[575,605]

Diabetic Neuropathy

Pathophysiology. Peripheral neuropathy has been documented in association with diabetes mellitus in both cats and dogs.[618-621] Nerve biopsy studies in cats reveals that the distal axons are susceptible, and demyelination may predominate over the axonal pathology.[622,623] Moreover, the pelvic limbs are initially involved. Theories for underlying pathophysiologic mechanisms of diabetic neuropathy include metabolic alterations in the polyol pathway that results in sugar accumulations in the nerve, depletion of myoinositol, impaired sodium-potassium ATPase, growth factor deficiencies, impaired vascular supply to the nerve, and oxidative stress.[376,603]

Clinical Signs. Clinical signs include LMN paraparesis that may progress to tetraparesis. Hyporeflexia and distal muscle atrophy may occur. Affected cats characteristically have a plantigrade stance and show reluctance to jump (Figure 7-20).[624] Clinical signs of neuropathy may precede those more typically associated with diabetes mellitus. Although difficult to document, sensory nerve dysfunction may result in paresthesia and hyperesthesia.[624] Rarely, autonomic signs such as Horner's syndrome can occur.[625]

Diagnosis. Diagnosis is suspected based on demonstrating diabetes mellitus in the presence of signs of neuropathy. Electrodiagnostic testing may reveal patchy abnormalities on EMG and reduced motor and sensory nerve-conduction velocities. Abnormalities in the nerve can be detected both proximally and distally.[624] Subclinical electrophysiologic abnormalities may be present in diabetic animals.[620,626] Sensory nerves may be preferentially involved. Nerve biopsy documents the axonopathy and demyelination.[620,622,624]

Treatment and Prognosis. Therapy is directed toward control of the diabetes mellitus and other contributing disorders.[603,621] With improved glycemic control, clinical signs may reverse, but varying degrees of weakness may still persist. Other anecdotal therapies aimed at countering oxidative stress have been used.[627]

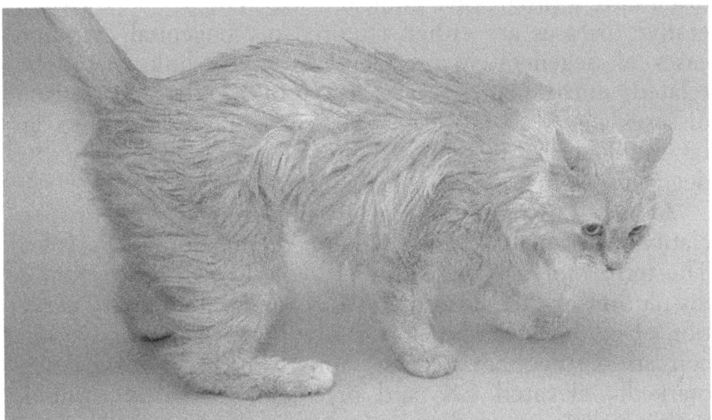

Figure 7-20 A 10-year-old domestic longhair cat diagnosed with diabetes mellitus. Note plantigrade and palmigrade stance suggestive for diabetic neuropathy. (Courtesy Dennis P. O'Brien.)

Hyperchylomicronemia in Cats. Jones described hyperchylomicronemia in two related male domestic shorthair cats.[628] The disease has been subsequently reported in other DSH cats[629,630] and Himalayan,[631] Persian,[632] European,[633] and Siamese cats.[634] Affected cats with chylomicronemia have a clinical phenotype similar to humans with lipoprotein lipase (LPL) deficiency. Hyperchylomicronemia is defined by increased concentrations of chylomicrons in plasma caused by a decrease in clearance of the lipoprotein from plasma.[635] Lipoprotein lipase regulates lipoprotein metabolism through the hydrolysis of triglycerides from chylomicrons and very low density lipoproteins (VLDL) which contribute to the formation of high density lipoproteins (HDL).[636]

Onset of clinical signs ranges between 4 and 8 weeks of age. Common clinical signs include fasting hyperlipidemia (increase chylomicrons and VLDL), lipemia retinalis, xanthomata, and various peripheral neuropathy.[628,635,637] Common sites for xanthomata formations include pressure points and sites where nerves exit the intervertebral or cranial foramina, causing compressive neuropathy affecting peripheral, cranial, and sympathetic nerves. A compressive peripheral neuropathy develops slowly over a course of months, and localization reflects multifocal disease in the area(s) of nerve compression. Horner's syndrome and tibial and radial nerve paralysis are most frequently detected.[638] Less commonly, systemic signs include anemia, splenomegaly, and lipid keratopathy.[628,638] Most affected cats have a fasting hyperchylomicronemia. Serum electrophoresis identifies an increase in chylomicrons and VLDL reflective of reduced LPL activity.[628,639]

Reduced LPL activities have been demonstrated in cats, using different biochemical methods.[628,629,631,638] Hyperchylomicronemia in cats has a familial incidence.[628,631,634,638] In New Zealand, related affected cats showed an autosomal recessive inheritance pattern.[639] The mutation for the lipoprotein lipase gene subsequently has been characterized.[639] A low-fat diet results in resolution of peripheral neuropathy.[629,632]

Hyperoxaluria in Cats. Domestic short-haired cats with D-glycerate dehydrogenase deficiency develop renal failure due to deposition of oxalate crystals in the renal tubules and LMN signs.[640] Axons of the ventral horn cells of the spinal cord, ventral roots, and intramuscular nerves are distended with neurofilaments. The cause of the axonal swellings is likely due to accumulation of neurofilaments. Clinical signs are apparent between 5 and 9 months of age. Onset is acute, with development of anorexia, dehydration, and weakness over a few days. Kidneys are painful on abdominal palpation. Neurologic examination demonstrates a crouched stance with adduction of the hock joints, tetraparesis, reduced myotatic and flexor reflexes, and decreased pain perception. Findings on serum biochemistry analysis reflect acute renal failure. Pedigree analysis was found to give a good fit, with an expected 3:1 ratio for a recessive gene.[640] A genetic mutation has been found in the feline glyoxylate reductase (*GRHPR*) gene.[641] Prognosis is poor.

Familial Neuropathy and Glomerulopathy of Gelbvieh Cattle. Gelbvieh calves clinically present with progressive GP ataxia and paresis in the pelvic limbs and progress over 20 months to recumbency.[642,643] Hypotonia develops, and spinal reflexes become hyporeflexic. Histopathology confirmed peripheral neuropathy and a proliferative glomerulopathy. The lesions are most severe in peripheral nerves, dorsal and ventral spinal nerve roots, and mild in the dorsal fasciculi of the spinal cord. Multifocal muscle necrosis may develop. Pedigree analysis of affected animals from one herd indicated a strong familial relationship.[642]

Neoplastic

Paraneoplastic Neuropathies. Neoplasia can affect peripheral nerves because of either direct involvement (see Chapter 5) or paraneoplastic ("remote") effects.[644] Paraneoplastic neuropathy has been mainly described in dogs[645,646] and rarely described in cats[647] with lymphoma. Effects on peripheral nerves may be difficult to distinguish from those caused by side effects of chemotherapy or irradiation.[648] Paraneoplastic effects are thought to be immune mediated due to antigen mimicry. An immune response is generated when antigens present within the neoplasm are shared with the peripheral nerve.[644] Subclinical pathologic evidence of peripheral neuropathy has been identified in dogs with distant neoplasia.[645] Braund[649] documented combinations of axonal necrosis, demyelination, and remyelination in dogs with malignant tumors including bronchogenic carcinoma, malignant melanoma, insulinoma, osteosarcoma, thyroid carcinoma, and mast cell tumors.

Many malignant tumor types have been associated with paraneoplastic neuropathy. Pancreatic β–islet cell tumors (insulinoma) has been the most completely documented example. Other tumor types implicated in paraneoplastic neuropathy include bronchogenic carcinoma,[650,651] gastric leiomyosarcoma,[652] hemangiosarcoma,[652] lymphoma,[653] and multiple myeloma.[654]

With β–islet cell tumors, neurologic signs in affected dogs are the result of profound hypoglycemia that affects the metabolism of the CNS, causing seizures, behavioral abnormalities, and other signs of forebrain disease (see Chapters 12, 13 and 15). Polyneuropathy can be profound in dogs with insulinoma.[655-658] Paraparesis that progresses to tetraparesis, with muscle atrophy and reduced spinal reflexes has been reported. The pathogenesis for β–islet cell tumor associated polyneuropathy is unclear. Insulin may have direct neurotoxic effects or indirect effects from the hypoglycemia or immune system. Dogs might benefit from corticosteroid therapy independent of insulin antagonism.[659]

Treatment of paraneoplastic polyneuropathy involves supportive care and addressing the underlying neoplasm. Immunomodulatory therapies including corticosteroids, immunosuppressants, plasmapheresis, and intravenous immunoglobulins have been utilized in human patients. Treatments directed toward the neoplasm can result in clinical improvement.[651,654,659]

Inflammatory

Chronic Idiopathic Polyneuritis (Chronic Inflammatory Demyelinating Polyneuropathy). This syndrome affects primarily mature dogs[670,671] and less frequently cats.[365,672] Early clinical signs involve the pelvic limbs and later over several months progress to involve the thoracic limbs. Signs of flaccid paresis, muscle atrophy, and hyporeflexia eventually result in paralysis in all limbs. The neurologic findings vary with the stage of the illness. Cranial nerve involvement may manifest with facial paralysis, dysphonia, megaesophagus, and laryngeal paralysis. Hypalgesia becomes evident as sensory nerves become involved. The clinical course varies from several months to years. Pathologic studies suggest that nonsuppurative inflammation, perhaps with an immune basis, is responsible for the disease.[670,671] If the spinal ganglia and cranial nerves are affected and causing sensory deficits, this condition has been called *ganglioradiculitis* or *sensory neuronopathy*.[600]

Electromyography may show spontaneous activity. Motor nerve conduction velocities are slow and show decreased amplitude of the compound motor action potential. Analysis of CSF may show nonspecific finding of increased protein concentration and cellularity. These changes are suggestive of axonal and myelin disease. The diagnosis is made by muscle and nerve biopsy which confirm denervation muscle atrophy and axonopathy with demyelination. Demyelination is the predominant pathologic finding. Some animals, especially cats, appear to benefit from corticosteroid therapy but then relapse and continue to worsen. Because of the disease's waxing-waning character, the benefit of corticosteroids is not proven.

Idiopathic

Idiopathic Polyneuropathy. These diseases are recognized more frequently in dogs now than a few years ago, but they are relatively uncommon in other species. The chronic neuropathies have an insidious onset and progress slowly over several months. Disease progression may be interrupted by periods of spontaneous improvement. Definition of the cause of chronic polyneuropathy is often elusive. Better diagnostic techniques, especially electrophysiologic tests and histopathologic assessment of muscle and nerve biopsy samples, have contributed to a greater understanding of this problem.

Toxicity

Toxic Neuropathies. Table 7-4 lists some toxins that may cause neuropathy. None of these are common. The potential for neurotoxicity varies among species. Drug-induced neuropathy has been reported in dogs with use of vincristine,[648] nitrofurantoin, and cistplatin.[376] Discontinuation of the drug results in regression of neurologic signs.

MYOPATHIC DISEASE

Skeletal muscle is composed of slow (type I) and fast (type II) twitch myofibers relatively resistant to fatigue. Cats also have fast-twitch fatigable myofibers. Myofibers utilize energy from glycogen in anaerobic conditions. Mitochondrial fatty acid oxidation is ideal for sustained exercise requiring endurance. The hallmark clinical sign of myopathy is weakness. Clinical signs can be persistent or episodic and exercise induced. Gait often is stiff and short strided. Cats will show an inability to jump. A unique clinical sign to cats is flexion of the neck. Generalized muscle atrophy can be a feature for some myopathies; alternatively, muscle hypertrophy develops in some conditions. Likewise, the distribution can be focal or generalized. Muscle pain (myalgia), failure of muscles to relax (myotonia), and sudden muscle contraction (cramp) also suggest muscle disease (see also Chapter 10).[673] Proprioception and spinal reflexes are normal unless the disorder is severe and diffuse.

In general, myopathies may be a result of inflammation (myositis) or degeneration. Inflammatory muscle diseases may be infectious or immune mediated and are acute in onset and often have a progressive clinical disease course.[674,675] Degenerative diseases are either acquired or congenital. Acquired cases of degenerative muscle disorders include metabolic-related, nutritional, neoplastic, trauma, toxic, and vascular diseases.[617,676-678] Most of the congenital myopathies are inherited (see Table 7-11). The most common of the inherited degenerative myopathies are the muscular dystrophies.[801,802]

Acquired myopathies may also be classified based on association with exercise and evidence of rhabdomyolysis.[678,803] The term *rhabdomyolysis* is represented by disintegration or dissolution of skeletal muscle associated with urinary excretion of myoglobin. The clinical syndrome of rhabdomyolysis consists of myofiber necrosis, muscle pain, limb weakness, markedly elevated CK, and myoglobinuria.[678] A common pathophysiologic mechanism relates to injury of the sarcolemmal membrane or failure of energy utilization causing an increase of intracellular calcium and ultimately destruction of myofibrils and myonecrosis.[678] Muscle disorders associated with rhabdomyolysis include some degenerative and storage myopathies, exercise-related disorders, nutritional, metabolic, toxic, trauma, and inflammatory diseases. In horses, diseases such as "tying up," Monday morning disease, azoturia, equine rhabdomyolysis, and equine myoglobinuria—once thought to be a distinct disease syndrome—are now considered common clinical manifestations for different muscle disorders of different causes.[803] Early recognition of rhabdomyolysis is important because myoglobinuria can cause renal failure and myonecrosis will cause severe electrolyte disturbances.

The signs of diffuse muscle disease are very similar to those of polyneuropathies. Because of ambiguities in establishing the diagnosis of myopathy through clinical signs alone, increasing attention should be given to evaluation of serum CK levels, serology, EMG, metabolic urine and plasma screening, molecular genetic testing, and muscle biopsy.[581,627,804] When a metabolic myopathy is suspected, screening tests should be performed at rest and after exercise. Often more than one diagnostic modality is required to confirm the cause of an inflammatory myopathy.[805] Muscle biopsy is necessary to determine presence and characterization of the inflammatory cell infiltrate, myonecrosis, and abnormal accumulations. Molecular genetic testing is becoming a valuable resource for disease when the causative mutation has been defined.[806] Myopathies of domestic animals are classified in Table 7-5. These disorders are discussed in subsequent sections of this chapter and further categorized as acute progressive (noninfectious and infectious inflammatory, metabolic), chronic progressive (degenerative, metabolic, nutritional), and episodic (metabolic).

Acute Progressive Myopathies

Inflammatory myopathies are a group of disorders characterized by inflammatory infiltrate of skeletal muscle. These disorders usually are acute in onset and progressive. Inflammatory myopathy can be classified focal or generalized, and noninfectious or infectious. Focal inflammatory myopathies include disorders such as masticatory muscle myositis and extraocular myositis. Infectious myositis can be focal or multifocal in distribution. Causes of generalized inflammatory myopathies encompass disorders that are noninfectious (e.g., immune mediated [polymyositis], idiopathic, toxic, paraneoplastic) or infectious.[805]

Inflammatory: Noninfectious

Immune-Mediated Polymyositis. Polymyositis is classified as diffuse muscle inflammation of immune-mediated origin.[675,805] Polymyositis may occur in association with systemic lupus erythematosus, as a paraneoplastic syndrome, or with some drugs, notably trimethoprim-sulfadiazine in Doberman pinschers and D-penicillamine in humans.[674,807-810] These disorders have also been described as idiopathic in origin.[674,811] Dogs seem to be most commonly affected[675,812]; cats may also develop polymyositis.[813] Adult animals are usually affected, although one report described two 7-month-old German wirehaired pointer littermates as being affected.[814]

Clinical Signs. Common clinical signs include generalized weakness, stiff and stilted gait, generalized and progressive muscle atrophy, regurgitation from megaesophagus, dysphonia, and pharyngeal weakness. Muscle pain or myalgia is not a prominent clinical feature.[805] Dogs with polymyositis may be lethargic, pyrexic, and anorexic. Many of these signs mimic those of chronic polyneuritis or other neuromuscular (e.g., myasthenia gravis) disorders. Episodes that are acute and painful must be differentiated from meningitis and skeletal diseases. The clinical course can be acute or insidious or chronic, progressive, and followed by periods of spontaneous remission.

Diagnosis. Diagnostic suspicion is gained from elevated CK levels, abnormal EMG, and testing that excludes infectious disease.[674] Disease confirmation is based on muscle biopsy results revealing mononuclear infiltrates and necrosis in skeletal muscle. It is important to rule out paraneoplastic disease through screening procedures such as thoracic radiography and abdominal ultrasound. In a study of 200 dogs with inflammatory myopathy, 88 dogs were diagnosed with immune-mediated polymyositis, of which 12 dogs subsequently developed neoplasia.[805] Of those 12 dogs, 8 were boxers diagnosed with lymphoma. Thymoma has been associated with polymyositis in dogs and cats.[815,816] Likewise, polymyositis can also occur concurrently with other underlying immune-mediated diseases which need to be investigated using immunologic testing.[809,810] Sarcolemma-specific antibodies have been identified in boxers and Newfoundlands.[817] The Newfoundlands had a younger age of onset, with megaesophagus and dysphagia as the predominating clinical signs.

Treatment. It is essential to determine whether an underlying infectious etiology exists. In animals with polymyositis, immunosuppression forms the basis of treatment. Typically, immunosuppressive doses of corticosteroids are given until remission is achieved. Alternate-day therapy is then instituted to maintain remission. Commensurate with improvement in clinical signs, the dosage is gradually tapered.

Treatment can be discontinued in some dogs, without recurrence of signs. Adjunctive immunosuppressive therapy often is used in conjunction with corticosteroids when corticosteroids alone are unable to obtain a clinical response, to maintain remission, or when there are severe and intolerable side effects.[818] Dogs with megaesophagus may develop aspiration pneumonia. Management of these cases is difficult, and the prognosis for regaining normal esophageal function is guarded.

Masticatory Muscle Myositis

Pathophysiology. Inflammation affecting primarily the muscles of mastication is seen more commonly in dogs than is polymyositis.[819-821] Masticatory muscle myositis (MMM) is a focal, immune-mediated inflammatory myopathy that affects the muscles of mastication (temporalis, masseter, pterygoid and rostral portion of the digastricus).[822] Selective involvement of the masticatory muscles is due to differences in histochemical and biochemical properties of the masticatory muscles.[822] Antibodies are produced against a specific myosin isoform in type 2M fibers of the masticatory muscles.[823] The autoimmune reaction may be initiated by a bacterial antigen.[804] Cellular infiltrates are present in both acute and chronic MMM, whereas extensive muscle atrophy and myofiber replacement with fatty tissue are present in the chronic form of this disease.[820] German shepherd dogs may be predisposed, but other large breeds usually are affected at a young age.[805] Bilateral atrophy of the masticatory muscles also can be caused by cachexia and prolonged exposure to excessive corticosteroids.[804,805,824,825]

Clinical Signs. In the acute stages of masticatory muscle myositis, the temporal and masseter muscles are firm, swollen, and painful. The jaw movements may be restricted, termed *trismus*. In the chronic phase, marked masticatory muscle atrophy is seen, and trismus often is present (Figure 7-21). The muscle atrophy is usually, but not always, symmetric.

Diagnosis. Diagnosis of masticatory muscle myositis is based on clinical signs and diagnostic testing. The gold standard is histopathologic confirmation of inflammation, atrophy, fibrosis, and necrosis involving the muscles of mastication.[820] Testing for the presence of circulating antibodies against type 2M myofibers is a noninvasive and sensitive confirmatory test.[820] Serum CK levels may be normal or mildly elevated in the acute phase. Electrophysiology further localizes the disease to the masticatory muscle group. Imaging with MRI or CT also may assist with diagnosis of canine inflammatory

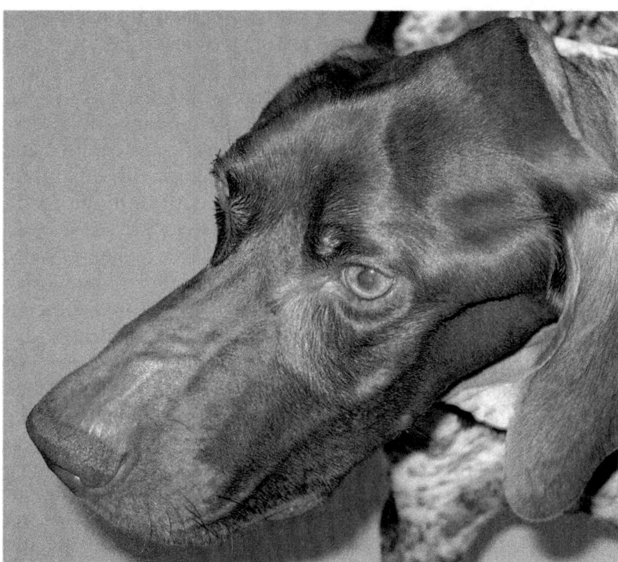

Figure 7-21 A 5-year-old German shorthair pointer with chronic masticatory muscle myositis. Note severe loss of muscle mass of temporalis and masseter muscles. Examiner was unable to open mouth owing to trismus from secondary muscle fibrosis.

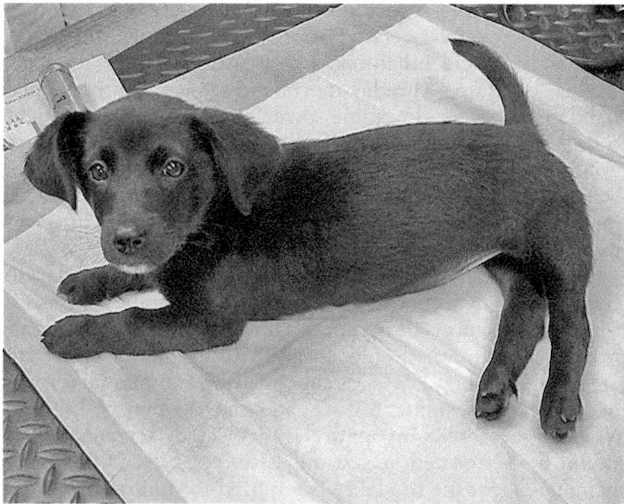

Figure 7-22 A 3-month-old mixed-breed puppy with extensor rigidity of pelvic limbs and presumptively diagnosed with protozoal myositis.

myopathies.[826-828] Overlap may exist between masticatory muscle myositis and polymyositis.[805]

Treatment. MMM is treated by immunosuppressive doses of corticosteroids for 3 to 4 weeks, and then the dosage is gradually tapered to every other day at the lowest dose until remission of clinical signs. Prognosis is good if the disease is treated aggressively in its early stage.[819] In chronic cases, other immunosuppressive agents may be necessary.

Extraocular Myositis. Myositis restricted to the extraocular muscles has been reported in two unrelated golden retrievers[829] but also reported in young dogs of other breeds.[830] In the acute phase, clinical signs are of bilateral exophthalmos. Fibrosis resulting in restrictive strabismus and enophthalmos occurs in the chronic phase. Other muscles groups of the head are unaffected. If treated during the acute phase, the disease responds well to corticosteroid treatment. Surgery may correct the restrictive strabismus.[830]

Dermatomyositis. Dermatomyositis is an inherited immune-mediated disease of the skin, vasculature, and muscle, reported most frequently in collies and Shetland sheepdogs.[831,832] A case report also exists in the Pembroke Welsh corgi.[833] The dermatitis that is most severe on the ears, face, tail, and distal extremities develops by 6 months of age. Myositis frequently involves the muscles of mastication and the distal appendicular muscles.[832] Clinical signs can include megaesophagus and dysphagia. Skin and muscle biopsies confirm the diagnosis. Histopathology of the muscle is characterized by perivascular to infiltrative mixed-cell inflammatory response. Therapy includes treatment of the skin lesions, vitamin E, and immunosuppression. Pentoxifylline, a methylxanthine derivative that increases the microvascular flow, may also be used.[834] Sunlight should be avoided. The prognosis for dogs that are less severely affected is good. An autosomal-dominant inheritance with incomplete penetrance and an immune-mediated pathogenesis is suspected.[832] Genetic studies have established linkage to the phenotype.[835]

Inflammatory: Infectious

Infectious Myositis. Clinical signs often are nonspecific and may include weakness, muscle atrophy, and myalgia. Increased serum CK and EMG abnormalities are nonspecific findings. A combination of clinical signs, serologic or PCR testing for infectious agents, and immunophenotyping on muscle tissue are required to identify a specific infectious etiology.[805] Definitive diagnosis is made by identification of the organism in a muscle biopsy. Serologic and PCR testing for infectious disease is part of the minimum database in any dog with generalized myositis.[805]

Protozoal Infection. Protozoal infections are common causes of infectious myositis, often without systemic signs of disease. The distribution in muscle is sporadic and multifocal with variation in severity of myopathic signs. Infection by *N. caninum* is more common than *T. gondii* and usually occurs in dogs younger than 1 year of age but also can occur in adult dogs.[382,836] Many dogs have concurrent polyradiculoneuritis and exhibit rigid pelvic limb extension and muscle atrophy (see also Protozoal Polyradiculoneuritis and Figure 7-22). Cats more commonly are infected with *T. gondii*. Myopathic signs are more related to weakness and possible muscle pain.[674] Along with the myopathy, presence of circulating antibodies to infectious agents such as *T. gondii* or *N. caninum* is suggestive of infectious myositis. The clinical response to antimicrobial therapy of some of these dogs alone supports this contention. Eosinophils are not uncommon in the muscle biopsy specimens from dogs with protozoal infection.[805] Antimicrobial treatment with clindamycin, 10 to 15 mg/kg every 8 to 12 hours, or a combination of trimethoprim-sulfadiazine and pyrimethamine is recommended. Prognosis is favorable if treatment is started early in the disease course.

Hepatozoon canis and *H. americanum* have been associated with infectious myositis. Clinical signs include severe muscle pain, muscle atrophy, cachexia, fever, periosteal bone proliferations and severe neurophilic and monocytic leukocytosis.[837,838] Diagnosis is based on identification of merozoites in muscle. PCR testing also is available. Therapy is based on halting the life cycle with combination therapy including trimethoprim-sulfadiazine, clindamycin, and pyrimethamine. An antiprotozoal agent, decoquinate, is administered indefinitely.[839] Prognosis is guarded, as relapse frequently occurs.

Trypanosoma cruzi usually infects the heart but can cause generalized myositis and other neurologic signs.[840,841] Infection with *Leishmania* spp. has been described in dogs with bilateral masticatory muscle pain and atrophy.[842]

Bacterial and Rickettsial Infection. Generalized infectious myositis has been associated with *Leptospira* spp.[843] Along with renal and hepatic involvement, clinical signs include myalgia, myoglobinuria, and fever. Clostridial myositis occurs following penetrating wounds or iatrogenic procedures.[844,845] Severe atrophy and limb rigidity occur. In horses, *Streptococcus equi* has been associated with a severe and rapidly progressive necrotizing myopathy.[846] Purpura hemorrhagica in horses is characterized by vasculitis as a sequela to infection or exposure to *Streptococcus* spp., *Rhodococcus* spp., and *Corynebacterium* spp.[847] Rarely will rickettsial and *Borrelia* spp. infection in dogs cause myositis.[805]

Trauma

Compartment Myopathy

Postanesthetic Myopathy. Heavy and larger animals have pain and swelling of groups of muscles and in some cases a compressive neuropathy after prolonged anesthesia.[210] The condition is caused, at least in part, by a compartment syndrome of affected muscles. Prolonged recumbency causes increased pressure in the muscle, with subsequent ischemia and necrosis. Treatment includes supporting the animal in a sling, administering IV fluids and electrolytes, and providing analgesics for pain relief. Massage and passive manipulation of the limbs help to increase blood flow and reduce the risk of decubital ulcers. The prognosis is good if the horse is standing. Recumbent animals may develop severe muscle atrophy. Preventative measures include careful padding, elevation of the uppermost limb, and avoidance of hypotension during anesthesia.

Limber Tail. This condition is known among people with hunting dogs as *limp tail*, *cold tail*, and *rudder tail*. Breeds primarily affected are English pointers and Labrador retrievers but also other hunting breeds.[848] Typically, dogs acutely manifest a flaccid tail. The tail is held out horizontally from base and then hangs down. Dogs show recovery within a few days to weeks. Major predisposing factors are prolonged cage transport, changes in climate, and overexertion.[849] Treatment usually consists of rest. The muscle damage is located to specific muscle groups within the tail, suggestive of compartment syndrome.[850]

Fibrotic Myopathy. Fibrotic myopathy has been documented most frequently in the German shepherd dog, especially those involved in strenuous training exercises.[851] The gracilis and semimembranosus/tendinosus muscles are usually involved. A tight band is palpated within these muscle groups. Affected dogs have a distinct lameness detected on gait. One or both pelvic limbs may be affected. The gait is characterized by a shortened stride with internal rotation of the foot, external rotation of the hock, and internal rotation of the stifle during the swing phase of the stride. History reveals an acute or insidious onset of lameness. The underlying cause remains unknown, but muscle strain is suspected. Surgical treatments that have been tried include excision of the gracilis muscle and semitendinosus tenectomy or tenotomy. Results have been disappointing, with temporary relief and recurrence of lameness within weeks to months.[851]

Toxic

Drug and Toxins. Acute onset of necrotizing myopathy may be a result of exposure to drugs or toxins (see also Chapter 15). These agents exert direct or indirect effects through a variety of mechanisms that include altered metabolism, instability of the muscle membrane, secondary hypokalemia, overexertion, and ischemia.[678] Often severe rhabdomyolysis and myoglobinuria may result from exposure to these toxins.

Vascular

Ischemic Neuromyopathy. Ischemic neuromyopathy is often secondary to thrombosis of the aorta or iliac arteries and occurs more frequently in cats with cardiomyopathy. Protein-losing nephropathy is a common cause in dogs. Loss of antithrombin secondary to glomerulopathy underlies the pathogenesis. Clinical signs are acute in onset. Asymmetric pelvic limb pain and paralysis are common. Femoral pulses are weak to absent. Distal limb muscles are more severely affected. The limb may be hypothermic and nail beds cyanotic. Limb muscles are painful and firm on palpation. The diagnosis is based on clinical signs and diagnostic tests. Creatine kinase activity is extremely high. Blood glucose measurements taken from the affected limb are approximately 25% or less than blood glucose measurements in unaffected limbs. Supportive care with vasodilators, fluid therapies, and thrombolytic drugs may assist with recovery. Anticoagulant therapy is used chronically. Recurrences are not uncommon.

Chronic Progressive Myopathies

Degenerative

Muscular Dystrophies. The muscular dystrophies are inherited primary degenerative myopathies (Table 7-11) characterized by progressive degeneration of skeletal muscle. These are a heterogeneous group of hereditary degenerative myopathies that are well described in humans, dogs, and cats.[801,802] In humans, one form of muscular dystrophy is known as *Duchenne muscular dystrophy* and has wide prevalence in young boys. Genetic mutations coding for the dystrophin protein or associated proteins lead to abnormal formation of the dystrophin-glycoprotein complex which lies in the sarcolemmal muscle membrane. Dystrophin is closely associated with other transmembrane proteins, an external protein known as *laminin-*α_2, sarcoglycan, and the actin myofilaments. Dystrophin deficiency is the most common cause of human, canine, and feline muscular dystrophies.[801] Dystrophin deficiencies are X-linked, so males manifest clinical signs. However, variations of phenotypic expression occurs among female carriers through a process called *lyonization*, in which the mutant or normal X chromosome is inactivated.[852-854]

Dystrophin-associated muscular dystrophy of dogs have been reported in golden retrievers (Figure 7-23),[855-857] Irish terriers,[858] Samoyeds,[859] rottweilers,[860] the Belgian Groenendaeler shepherd,[861] miniature schnauzer,[862]Alaskan malamute,[863] wire-haired fox terrier,[801] German shorthaired pointer,[864] rat terrier,[865] Pembroke Welsh corgi,[801] Japanese spitz dog,[866] Brittany spaniel,[867] Labrador retriever,[868] grand basset griffon,[869] and Cavalier King Charles spaniel.[870] X-linked dystrophin deficient muscular dystrophy has also been reported in domestic cats.[871-873] Dystrophin deficiency in dogs and cats is usually slowly progressive, causing generalized weakness and cardiomyopathy. Pathologic changes of dystrophic muscle include variation in size of myofibers, combination of degenerating and regenerating myofibers, fibrosis, and in some cases calcium deposits. Immunohistochemistry using antibodies against the muscle membrane proteins will determine if dystrophin or other dystrophy-associated proteins are absent or reduced.

X-linked Canine Dystrophinopathy. This form of muscular dystrophy is similar to Duchenne muscular dystrophy in humans and has been best characterized in the golden retriever.[856,874] The membrane-associated muscle protein, dystrophin, is decreased or absent in affected dogs (Figure 7-24) and humans. The myopathic phenotype is common in male dogs. Phenotypic variations occur among female carriers. Genetic mutations have been described in the golden retriever,[875] rottweiler[860] and German shorthaired pointer.[864] Female carriers of dystrophin mutations show little overt clinical evidence of the disease; however, the CK levels are often elevated. Still, carriers can manifest variations in histopathologic and expression of dystrophin.[852]

TABLE 7-11

Breed-Associated Inherited and Degenerative Myopathies and Junctionopathies of Domestic Animals

Disease (Breeds)	Age of Onset	Inheritance Pattern (Mutation)	Clinical Features	Predominant Pathology	Reference
Muscular Dystrophies					
X-linked canine dystrophinopathy (golden retriever, Irish terrier, Samoyed, rottweiler, Belgian Groenendaeler shepherds, miniature schnauzer, Alaskan Malamute, rat terrier, wired-haired fox terrier, German shorthaired pointer, Pembroke Welsh corgi, Japanese spitz dog, Brittany spaniel, Labrador retriever, Cavalier King Charles spaniel, Grand Basset Griffon)	Birth to few weeks; some later onset	X-linked (dystrophin gene: golden retriever, rottweiler, German shorthaired pointer); some carriers may manifest clinical signs—lyonization	Pelvic limb stiffness progressive to tetraparesis, dysphagia, tongue hypertrophy, neck flexion; spinal reflexes eventually become hyporeflexic, muscle atrophy, pseudohypertrophy, trismus, respiratory compromise; cardiomyopathy; elevated CK	Dystrophic changes—variability of myofiber size, degenerating and regenerating fibers, endomysial fibrosis; some show calcium deposits	679-697
X-linked feline dystrophinopathy (DSH)	3-6 mo	X-linked (dystrophin gene)	Neck and shoulder hypertrophy, tongue enlargement, lingual calcification, regurgitation, cardiomyopathy; hepatosplenomegaly	Dystrophic changes	698-700
Alpha-dystroglycan deficiency (Devon rex, Sphynx)	3-24 wk	AR (α-dystroglycan gene)	Neck flexion, high-steppage gate; dog-begging position, weakness in scapular musculature, dysphagia	Dystrophic changes	701-703
Sarcoglycanopathy (Boston terrier, cocker spaniel, Chihuahua	7-11 mo	AR	Failure to thrive, lethargic, exercise intolerance, CK elevations	Dystrophic changes	688, 704
Laminin-α_2 deficiency (Brittany springer spaniel mix; DSH, Siamese, Maine coon)	C-young; F- 2.5 mo	AR?	Paraparesis to rigid tetraparesis; CK elevations	Dystrophic changes; demyelination	705-707
Ovine muscular dystrophy (Merino sheep—Australia)	3 wk-6 mo	AR	Progressive stiffness in all limbs	Dystrophic degeneration of type I myofibers	708, 709
Nondystrophic Myopathies					
Centronuclear myopathy (Labrador retriever myopathy, type II fiber deficiency)	6 wk-7 mo	AR (*PTPLA* gene)	Stilted, bunny-hopping gait; atrophy in proximal limb and temporalis muscles; neck flexion; absence of myotatic reflexes; CK mild elevation	Variation in myofiber size, group atrophy; fiber angulation; type II myofibers involved; centralized nuclei	710-714
Bouvier des Flandres dysphagia-associated myopathy	2 yr	Unknown	Dysphagia involving pharyngeal, laryngeal, and esophageal muscles	Dystrophic changes in pharyngeal muscles	715, 716
Nemaline rod myopathy (C-border collie, vary; F-DSH; B-Braunvieh x American Brown Swiss)	C-10 mo-vary F-6-18 mo B-2 wk	Unknown	Progressive tetraparesis; muscle atrophy; decreased myotatic reflexes; increased CK	Myofiber size variation, centralization of nuclei, nemaline rods	717-720

Distal myopathy of rottweilers	6 wk	Unknown	Distal appendicular muscle weakness, plantigrade and palmigrade stance, hock flexion; mild increase CK	Myofiber atrophy, necrosis, fatty deposits	721
Inherited myopathy of Great Danes	6 mo	Unknown	Progressive muscle wasting, exercise intolerance, tremors, excitement-induced collapse; CK elevation	Dark-staining areas within myofibers	722
Glycogen Storage Diseases (GSDs)					
GSD type II (Pompe's disease; Swedish Lapland dog; beef shorthorn, Brahman; Corriedale sheep)	3-6 mo	AR	Progressive weakness, regurgitation, dysphonia	PAS-positive deposits in muscle; deficiency of alpha-glucosidase activity	723-728
GSD type III (Cori's disease; Akita, German shepherd dog, curly-coated retriever)	2 mo	AR (*AGL* gene)	Episodic muscular weakness, lethargy, exercise intolerance	PAS-positive deposits in muscle; deficiency in the glycogen branching enzyme	729-731
GSD type IV (Andersen's disease; Norwegian forest cat; quarter and paint horse)	F-4 mo E-neonatal	AR (*GBE1* gene)	Muscle tremors, weakness, contracture; progressive tetraparesis; cerebellar signs; seizures; CK elevation	PAS-positive deposits in muscle; glycogen branching enzyme deficiency	732-736
GSD type V (McArdle's disease; Charolais)	Young	AR (myophosphorylase gene)	Exercise intolerance, rhabdomyolysis, CK elevation	PAS-positive deposits in muscle; myophosphorylase deficiency	737-740
GSD type VII (Tarui's disease) (English springer spaniel, American cocker spaniel)	8 mo	AR (*PFK* gene)	Episodic progressive myopathy; CK elevated	PAS-positive deposits in muscle; phosphofructokinase deficiency	741-743
Other Metabolic Myopathies					
Polysaccharide storage myopathy (quarter horse, draft horses—Belgian Percheron, warmbloods—Arabians, Morgan, Tennessee Walking	5-8 yr	AD (*GYS1* gene)	Muscle stiffness, fasciculation, weakness; sweating; reluctance to move; rhabdomyolysis; CK elevation	PAS-positive deposits ± amylase resistance; glycogen synthase deficiency	744-748
Mitochondrial myopathy (Old English sheepdog, Jack Russell terrier, Sussex spaniel, Clumber spaniel, German shepherd dog; Arabian horse)	<1 yr	AR (cytochrome oxidase c gene)	Episodic weakness, exercise intolerance, cramping, myalgia, muscle atrophy, CK and lactate elevation	Histochemical evidence of "ragged red" fibers, myofiber necrosis; pyruvate dehydrogenase deficiency	749-755
Lipid storage myopathy (English pointer, cocker spaniel)	<1 yr	AR	Episodic weakness, exercise intolerance, cramping, myalgia, muscle atrophy, CK and lactate elevation	Lipid accumulations, "ragged red" fibers	756, 757
Pietrain creeper syndrome	3-12 wk	AR	Muscle weakness progressing to recumbency; crouched posture with creeping-type gait on flexed limbs	Atrophy of type I myofibers in proximal muscles	758, 759

Continued

TABLE 7-11

***Breed-Associated Inherited and Degenerative Myopathies and Junctionopathies of Domestic Animals*—cont'd**

Disease (Breeds)	Age of Onset	Inheritance Pattern (Mutation)	Clinical Features	Predominant Pathology	Reference
Myotonic Myopathies					
Myotonia congenita (Ca-miniature schnauzer, chow chow, Staffordshire terrier, Australian cattle dog, cocker spaniel, West Highland white terrier, Great Dane, Jack Russell terrier; F-Siamese, DSH, DLH; E-horse; O-Shropshire; caprine	Birth	Ca-AR (miniature schnauzer, chow chow, Staffordshire terrier, Australian cattle dog); unknown; C-AD or AR (mutation in chloride channel gene [*gCCl-1*], miniature schnauzer, Australian cattle dog; goat) O-AR	Signs begin soon after animals become ambulatory; muscle stiffness, hypertrophy; bunny-hopping gait, percussion myotonia, regurgitation, stridor; decreased range of motion in jaw	Myofiber hypertrophy, centrally located nuclei, increased sarcolemmal nuclei, myofiber degeneration	760-773 82-84
Myotonic dystrophy (Ca-boxer, Rhodesian ridgeback; E-foal	Adult	Unknown	Muscle hypertrophy and atrophy, stiff gait, percussion myotonia, excessive salivation; CK elevations	Myofiber size variation, centralization of nuclei, atrophy of type II myofibers; loss of type I myofibers	774-776
Myotonic myopathy in horses (quarter horse, thoroughbred, standardbred, Swedish halfbred, Appaloosa, Arabian, Welsh pony)	Birth or first mo	Unknown	Stiffness, hypertrophied and atrophic muscles; percussion myotonia	Myofiber size variation	776-778
Episodic Myopathies					
Episodic induced collapse in Labrador retrievers	7 mo-2 yr	AR (dynamin 1 [*DNM1*] gene)	During exercise, dogs hyperventilate, develop ataxia, collapse; loss of patellar reflex	No abnormalities Synaptic vesicle abnormality in CNS	779-781
Malignant hyperthermia syndrome (dogs, quarter horse, P-Pietrain, Poland China, Landrace)	Any age	P, C-AR E-AD (Ryanodine receptor [*RYR1*] gene)	Anesthesia, stress-induced rhabdomyolysis	Myonecrosis	777, 782-786
Hyperkalemic periodic paralysis (HyPP) (E-quarter horse, American paint, Appaloosa, cross-bred; Ca-pit bull)	Adult to 3 yr	E-AD (skeletal muscle sodium channel [*SCN4A*] gene)	Muscle fasciculation, tremors, recumbency, pharyngeal and laryngeal dysfunction	Myonecrosis	787-792
Congenital myasthenia gravis (Ca-English springer spaniels, dachshund, Jack Russell terrier, smooth fox terrier; F-DSH)	Birth	AR-Jack Russell, smooth fox terrier	Episodic exercise intolerance, megaesophagus	No abnormalities; absence of acetylcholine receptors	793-798
Congenital myasthenia syndrome (Ca-Gammel Dansk Honsehund; B-Red Brahman)	Birth	AR (B-epsilon subunit acetylcholine receptor *bovCHRNE* gene)	Progressive weakness and recumbency; episodic exercise intolerance	No abnormalities	799, 800

There is variation in disease severity even with the same mutation; some pups die near birth, while in others, the disease slowly progresses over months to years. Affected pups are weak at birth and may die before a diagnosis is made. Stilted gait, trismus, muscle atrophy, stunted growth, and drooling may be seen as early as 6 weeks of age. Affected dogs have flexion of the neck. Spinal reflexes, particularly the patellar reflex, are decreased to absent. Muscle atrophy, kyphosis, and debilitating muscle contractures subsequently develop (Figure 7-25). Pseudohypertrophy of some groups of muscles is attributed to deposition of adipose and connective tissues, whereas true hypertrophy occurs in the cranial sartorius muscle.[876] Muscles selectively involved include the tongue, masticatory, and truncal muscles. Muscle hypertrophy causes enlargement of the base of the tongue (see Figure 7-25). Trismus may occur and is caused by hypertrophy of the pharyngeal muscles and megaesophagus. Respiratory function also is compromised and contributes to exercise intolerance. Rhabdomyolysis can occur on rare occasions.[870,877] Signs often stabilize to some extent after 6 months of age in golden retrievers but ultimately progress to inability to ambulate and pharyngeal to esophageal dysfunction.

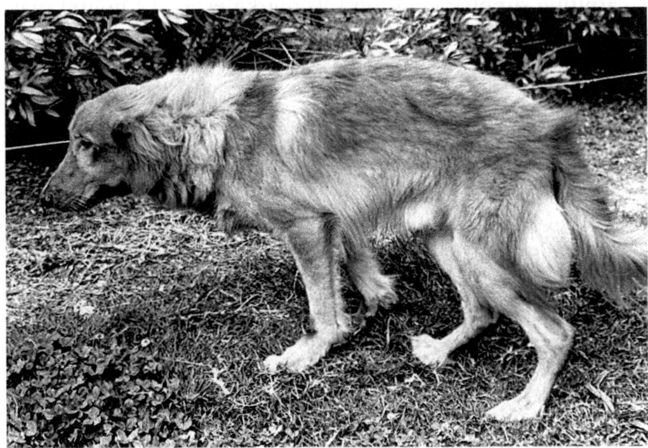

Figure 7-23 Dog with golden retriever muscular dystrophy at approximately 18 months of age. Note characteristic kyphosis, plantigrade stance, and temporalis muscle atrophy. (From Sharp NJH, Kornegay JN, Lane SB: The muscular dystrophies, Semin Vet Med Surg [Small Anim] 4:133–140, 1989.)

Genetic testing in golden retrievers confirms the disease[875] and may be used to identify carriers.[878] Thoracic radiography will reveal asymmetry and undulation of the diaphragm and gastroesophageal hiatal hernia.[879] Myocardial involvement is more severe in the golden retrievers compared to other breeds, and heart failure may occur in older dogs.[880] Serum muscle enzymes often are dramatically elevated in affected animals as a result of leakage through the defective muscle membrane; CK values greater than 20,000 U/L are seen as early as 1 day of age. Complex repetitive discharges are noted on EMG. Histopathologic changes include myofiber necrosis and phagocytosis, variation in myofiber size, and myofiber mineralization. Colonies of muscular dystrophy–affected golden retrievers and cats have been established. Molecular genetic therapies are currently being studied.

X-Linked Feline Muscular Dystrophy. Male cats with X-linked dystrophin deficiency are affected between 3 and 6 months of age.[871-873] Physical features of cats with muscular dystrophy are shoulder and neck muscle hypertrophy, enlargement of the tongue, and interestingly, lingual calcification. Regurgitation is a common clinical sign secondary to esophageal stenosis caused by hypertrophy of the diaphragm and megaesophagus.[872,881] During ambulation, cats have a bunny-hopping stride and develop exercise intolerance. Rhabdomyolysis has been associated with general anesthesia in these cats.[882] Gait evaluation often reveals a stiff gait with adduction of the hocks, bunny hopping, and inability to jump. Cats may also have hepato- and splenomegaly and dilated cardiomyopathy.[881,883] Biochemical and histopathologic findings are similar to those described in dystrophic dogs. Affected cats can live with this disease, but stress and inhalant anesthesia should be avoided. A genetic mutation has been characterized in the dystrophin gene.[884]

α-Dystroglycan Deficiency (Spasticity). Another muscular dystrophy in cats has been recognized in the Devon rex[885] and Sphynx[886] breeds, which manifest a slowly progressive myopathy. Age of onset is variable from 3 to 24 weeks of age. The inheritance pattern in the Devon rex is autosomal recessive.[887] Flexion of the neck is the most consistent clinical sign. These cats show a high-stepping gait of the thoracic limb and weakness of the scapular musculature. Cats often show exertion with exercise and will sit in a "dog begging" position. Cats have difficulty swallowing and prehending food, creating airway obstruction and choking. The CK levels are not elevated. Muscle biopsy show characteristic findings of muscular

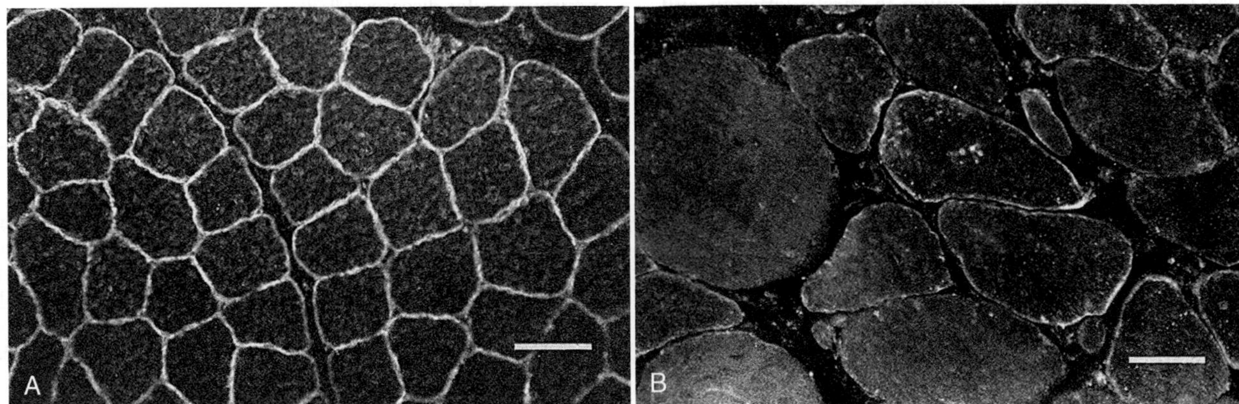

Figure 7-24 Characteristic subsarcolemmal staining pattern of dystrophin in a normal dog **(A)** and relative absence of staining in a littermate affected with golden retriever muscular dystrophy **(B)**. Several myofibers show focal peripheral staining in **B.** Marked variation in myofiber size is also noted in affected dog. Bar = 75 microns in **A** and 38 microns in **B.** Immunofluorescence: C-terminal domain antibody. (From Kornegay JN: The X-linked muscular dystrophies. In Kirk RW, Bonagura JD, editors: Current veterinary therapy XI, Philadelphia, 1992, Saunders.)

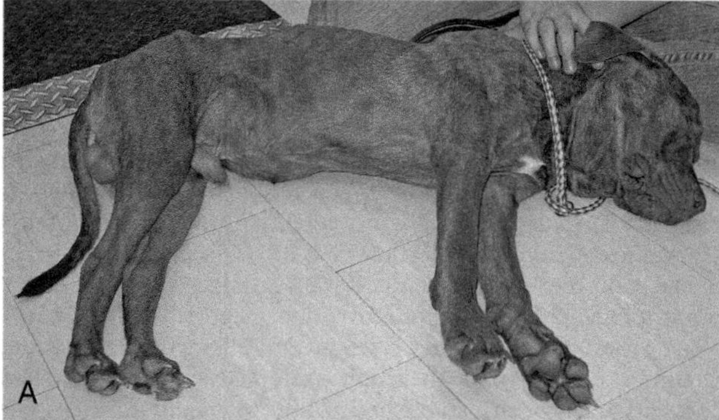

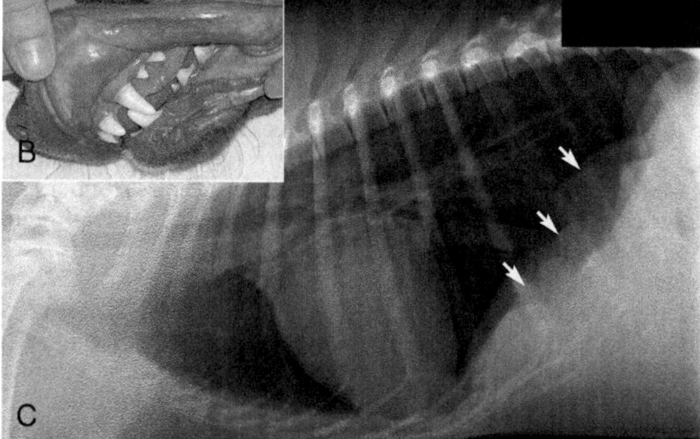

Figure 7-25 A 10-month-old male American Staffordshire terrier with muscular dystrophy and showing clinical signs of progressively stiff gait and weakness. Dog was having difficulty swallowing, and jaw had trismus. Muscle biopsy revealed histopathology consistent with muscular dystrophy. **A,** Dog in lateral recumbency, demonstrating muscle rigidity. **B,** Oral examination revealed hypertrophy of tongue. **C,** Lateral thoracic radiography demonstrates overinflation and undulating of diaphragm caused by muscle hypertrophy.

dystrophy. The muscular dystrophy is caused by a deficiency in α-dystroglycan protein.[886]

Sarcoglycanopathy. The protein sarcoglycan spans the sarcolemmal membrane while bridging dystrophin and the dystroglycan complex. Sarcoglycan deficiencies have been identified in the Boston terrier,[877] cocker spaniel, and Chihuahua.[801] Clinical signs include failure to thrive, lethargy, and exercise intolerance. The CK levels are elevated. Electromyography shows spontaneous activity in various muscle groups. Some dog have abnormalities on echocardiography. Muscle histopathology is typical for muscular dystrophy, and immunohistochemistry shows reduction to absence in the various sarcoglycan proteins.

Laminin α_2 Deficiency. Laminin-α_2 is a glycoprotein associated with the basal lamina of skeletal muscle and Schwann cells. This muscular dystrophy has been associated with absence of laminin α_2 in a young Brittany springer spaniel mixed breed[852] and in domestic shorthair, Siamese, and Maine coon cats.[559,888] In cats, pelvic limb weakness started at 2.5 months of age. Eventually, contracture of the extensor muscles develop. The CK levels are increased, and dystrophic changes are present in muscle biopsies of affected cats. Immunohistochemical stains revealed absence of laminin α_2. The prognosis is poor.

Muscular Dystrophy in Merino Sheep. This is an autosomal recessive inherited myopathy of Merino sheep in Australia.[889,890] Clinical signs develop between 3 weeks and 6 months as progressive stiffness in gait involving all limbs and neck. Disease progression can vary in flocks. The CK levels are within normal limits. The dystrophic degeneration is restricted to the oxidative type I myofibers.[891,892]

Other Nondystrophic Breed-Specific Myopathies

Centronuclear Myopathy (Labrador Retriever Myopathy, Type II Fiber Deficiency, Autosomal Recessive Muscular Dystrophy). This inherited myopathy in Labrador retrievers has been confirmed as centronuclear myopathy.[893] Signs develop between 6 weeks and 7 months of age and are generally much less severe than those in the X-linked dystrophy.[894-897] Affected dogs may have a stilted and bunny-hopping gait. These dog often show adduction of the hock and carpal joints. Muscle atrophy predominates in the proximal limb muscles and involves the temporalis muscles. Affected dogs have neck flexion. The myotatic or tendon reflexes, particularly the patellar, are depressed or absent. Signs generally stabilize by 6 to 12 months of age. Some dogs develop megaesophagus. The CK levels are usually only slightly elevated. Pathologic changes include variation in fiber size, myofiber group atrophy, and angular fibers. Central nuclei only become evident in muscle around 2 to 3 years of age. Type II myofibers may be preferentially involved in some muscles. Weakness often worsens with stress, exercise, and in cold weather; L-carnitine supplementation (50 mg/kg every 12 hours) may improve clinical signs. A mutation has been found in the *PTPLA* gene, a gene expressed during myogenesis; a genetic test is available.[893]

Bouvier des Flandres Myopathy. Degeneration of the pharyngeal, laryngeal, and esophageal muscles, with normal nerves, has been identified in Bouviers with dysphagia.[898,899] Regurgitation occurs beginning around 2 years of age. Muscle biopsy revealed dystrophic changes.[899]

Nemaline Rod Myopathy. This disorder has been reported in young cats, dogs, and calves. Cats developed weakness at 6 to 18 months of age.[900] Cats were reluctant to move and had hypermetria with jerky movements. The skin twitched vigorously when two of the cats were examined. Patellar reflexes were depressed. Flexor reflexes and sensory evaluation were normal. The scapular and gluteal muscle groups were atrophied. The CK levels were increased, but the EMG was normal. Muscle biopsy showed myofiber size variation, centralization of nuclei, and fibers contained nemaline rods. Affected cats eventually need to be euthanized. A nemaline rod myopathy has been reported as a congenital myopathy in neonatal Braunvieh X American Brown Swiss calves.[901] Nemaline rods also can be a pathologic finding in various other neuromuscular diseases.[606,902]

Distal Myopathy of Rottweilers. At time of ambulation, affected dogs have plantigrade and palmigrade stance, hock hyperflexion, and splayed forepaw digits.[903] Histopathologic changes of muscle include myofiber atrophy and necrosis, endomysial fibrosis, and fatty deposits. Plasma and muscle carnitine levels are decreased.

Inherited Myopathy of Great Danes (Previously Known as Central Core Myopathy). Disease onset is 6 months of age. Clinical signs include progressive weakness, exercise intolerance, muscle atrophy, and tremor.[904] Hyporeflexia may be observed. Other supportive finds of myopathy include elevated CK levels and abnormalities on EMG. Muscle biopsy will reveal presence of dark-staining centrally located cores. Many dogs are euthanized by 1 year of age.

Metabolic Myopathy

The metabolic myopathies include diseases in which either a primary biochemical defect involving skeletal muscle, or a generalized metabolic or endocrine disorder, causes muscle dysfunction. Major endocrine myopathies are discussed later in this chapter.

Disorders of Glycogen Metabolism. Given the metabolic demands necessary for normal function, muscle may be predominantly affected in some of the storage disorders. The glycogen storage myopathies result from deficiencies of specific enzymes involved in glycogen formation or metabolism. Abnormal glycogen accumulates intracellularly, and skeletal muscle often is affected. Clinical signs of muscle weakness predominate as exercise intolerance, tremor, and collapse. Other neurologic signs may manifest as cerebellar ataxia and seizures. Diagnosis is based on clinical signs, histopathology, enzymatic testing, and genetic testing is available for some disorders. Creatine kinase levels are often elevated. Findings of periodic acid–Schiff (PAS)-positive deposits in muscle indicate accumulation of glycogen or polysaccharide material. Several glycogen storage diseases exist in animals.

Glycogen Storage Disease Type II (Pompe's disease). This disorder is cause by a deficiency of α-glucosidase activity and has been reported in Swedish Lapland dogs.[905,906] By 6 months of age, affected dogs had progressive weakness, vomiting, regurgitation, and dysphonia. Dogs are euthanized before 18 months of age. Beef shorthorn and Brahman calves also have been affected with progressive muscle weakness within 3 months after birth.[907-909] Corriedale sheep develop ataxia and lethargy by 6 months of age and acute death within 10 months.[910]

Glycogen Storage Disease Type III (Cori's Disease). This is a disorder in the glycogen debranching enzyme, with an autosomal recessive inheritance pattern. Episodic muscular weakness was noted as early as 2 months of age in German shepherd dogs and Akitas.[911,912] Recently a milder form of the disorder has been identified in the curly-coated retriever observed to have exercise intolerance, collapse, and lethargy.[913] The genetic mutation in the *AGL* gene has been identified in the curly-coated retriever, and a DNA sequence-based carrier test has been developed.[913]

Glycogen Storage Diseases Type IV (Glycogen Branching Enzyme Deficiency [Andersen's Disease]). In deficiencies in glycogen branching enzyme, cardiac and skeletal muscles and the brain are unable to store and mobilize glycogen. Abnormal glycogen subsequently accumulates in skeletal and cardiac muscle, nerve, and the CNS. Norwegian forest cats with glycogen storage disease type IV developed clinical disease after 4 months of age.[914,915] Clinical signs progress from muscle tremors and weakness to nonambulatory tetraparesis with limb contracture. The inheritance pattern is autosomal recessive. A mutation in the glycogen branching enzyme 1 (*GBE1*) gene results in tissue deposition of an amylopectin-like substance.[916] Glycogen branching enzyme deficiency in quarter and paint horses also is an autosomal recessive trait caused by a mutation in the *GBE1* gene.[917] Stillbirths are common. Foals that survive are weak and develop limb contractures, cardiac abnormalities, and hypoglycemic seizures.[918] Most affected foals are euthanized by 8 weeks of age.

Glycogen Storage Disease Type V (McArdle's Disease). Glycogen storage disease type V results from deficiency of myophosphorylase and has been reported in Charolais calves in North America and New Zealand.[919,920] The inheritance pattern is autosomal recessive. Calves manifest with exercise intolerance and recumbency. A rhabdomyolysis and myoglobinuria develop with repeated attacks. A mutation has been found in the myophosphorylase gene, and a DNA test is available.[921,922]

Glycogen Storage Disease Type VII (Tarui's disease). Phosphofructokinase deficiency (PFK) (glycogen-storage disease type VII; Tarui's disease) is inherited as an autosomal recessive trait in English springer spaniels and American cocker spaniels.[923,924] Affected English springer spaniels at 8 months of age develop hemolytic anemia without overt muscle weakness. However, CK levels may be elevated. Older dogs may develop an episodic progressive myopathy.[925] A genetic test is available to identify PFK-deficient dogs and carriers.

Polysaccharide Storage Myopathy

Pathophysiology. Polysaccharide storage myopathy (PSSM), also described as "Monday morning disease" or "azoturia," was first discovered in quarter horses[926] but has since been recognized in draft horses (Belgian and Percheron), warmbloods, and other breeds such as Arabians, Morgans, and Tennessee Walking horses.[927,928] The incidence is lowest (27%) in thoroughbreds and highest (86%) in the draft-related horses.[928] Although the age at onset is variable, mean age is 5 years in quarter horses and 8 years in the draft horses and warmbloods. Risk factors include irregular exercise regimens, high-grain diets, and anesthesia. Histopathologic features in the original study included presence of vacuoles containing PAS-positive staining with amylase resistance for muscle glycogen.[926,929] An autosomal dominant mutation in the glycogen synthase 1 gene (*GYS1*) has been identified.[930] However, there is a subset of horses with similar clinical signs that lack the mutation. Thus, the disease is now referred to as *type 1 PSSM* for horses with abnormal glycogen storage and the *GYS1* mutation and *type 2 PSSM* for horses with abnormal glycogen storage and lacking the *GYS1* mutation. Overall, the prevalence of the *GYS1* mutation in PSSM horses is high in the draft (87%) and quarter (72%) horses and lower in warmbloods (18%) and other breeds (24%).[931]

Clinical Signs. The most common clinical signs in quarter horses include firm painful muscles, stiffness, fasciculations, weakness, sweating, and reluctance to move. Muscle pain occurs within 20 minutes and may last for a couple of hours. Signs are similar in warmbloods. The disease is subclinical in many draft horses. Some horses may have severe rhabdomyolysis and myoglobinuria.

Diagnosis. A presumptive diagnosis is based on clinical signs and signalment. Criteria for definitive diagnosis of type 1 PSSM is based on a muscle biopsy containing abnormal or increased accumulation of PAS-positive material and presence of the *GYS1* mutation. Other criteria used for diagnosis of PSSM are based on sensitivity to amylase on PAS staining: grade 1 (mild, amylase sensitive) and grade 2 (moderate, amylase resistant). The frequency of the *GYS1* mutation is higher in horses with grade 2 PSSM.[931] Muscle biopsy usually is taken from semimembranosus or semitendinosus muscle. Other supportive evidence for disease includes threefold elevations in CK and AST activities after exercise. Muscle enzyme activities may be persistently elevated in the quarter horse.

Treatment. Dietary modification and appropriate levels of exercise are crucial to management of PSSM.[932] Diets low in carbohydrates and at least 13% in fat may be the most effective way to reduce muscle glycogen.[933] Affected horses should be kept on pasture with little grain supplementation. When starting an exercise program in horses with PSSM, the owner should include dietary adaptation, restriction of exercise duration and intensity, and regular exercise that is gradually introduced and consistent while minimizing days without exercise.[934] In acute exacerbations, administration of dantrolene may reduce the severity of rhabdomyolysis. Additionally, horses should be confined for no longer than 48 hours and then allowed access to free pasture.

Mitochondrial and Lipid Storage Myopathies

Pathogenesis. Another subgroup of metabolic myopathies, the mitochondrial myopathies, has been reasonably well characterized in humans and to a lesser degree in animals. Inherited enzymatic defects within the mitochondrial electron-transport (respiratory) chain generally cause dysfunction in energy metabolism. Metabolism in fatty acids provides a primary energy source for skeletal and cardiac muscle. Carnitine plays a key role in cellular energy metabolism as a carrier for long-chain fatty acids from the cytosol into the mitochondria and as a buffer against organic acid accumulations. Most carnitine in the body is found in skeletal and cardiac muscle. Coenzyme Q_{10} plays a role in energy metabolism in the inner mitochondria as a carrier of electrons within the electron transport chain.

Mitochondrial myopathies associated with lactic acidemia have been reported in the Old English sheepdog,[935] Jack Russell terrier,[936] Sussex and Clumber spaniels,[937,938] and in a German shepherd dog.[939] A pyruvate dehydrogenase deficiency has been confirmed in the Clumber and Sussex spaniels.[938,940] The mutation has been identified in Clumber and Sussex spaniels in the pyruvate dehydrogenase phosphatase 1 gene, and a genetic test is available.[941] A mitochondrial myopathy with altered cytochrome C oxidase activity and reduced mitochondrial mRNA has been described in Old English sheepdog litter mates.[935,942] Mitochondrial myopathy also has been reported in a 3-year-old Arabian mare having muscle stiffness, myalgia, sweating, and exercise intolerance.[943]

Likely a form of mitochondrial dysfunction, lipid storage myopathy has been reported in the cocker spaniel and in a litter of English pointers with neurogenic muscular atrophy.[944,945] Dyserythropoiesis, cardiomegaly, and polymyopathy characterized by gross muscle atrophy and histologic evidence of myofiber size variation and poorly defined inclusions have been reported in English springer spaniels.[946] However, the underlying cause of this myopathy has not yet been defined.

Clinical Signs. Dogs with mitochondrial and lipid storage myopathies have onset of signs usually within the first year of life. Lipid storage myopathies, however, can have an adult onset. Episodic weakness, exercise intolerance, and cramping are typical signs of clinical presentation. Severe cases may have myalgia, muscle atrophy, and myoglobinuria. The serum CK and plasma lactate levels are elevated. Complex repetitive discharges are observed on EMG.

Diagnosis. Definitive diagnosis of mitochondrial and lipid storage myopathies is difficult and often requires microscopic evaluation of muscle specimens along with complete biochemical and molecular testing. It is important to consult with the laboratory performing the procedures in order to properly collect samples. Typical histopathologic changes include bizarre mitochondria on ultrastructural evaluation and histochemical evidence of "ragged red" fibers.[935,936] Intermediary metabolites, most often glycogen or lipid, typically also accumulate within some myofibers. Cytochrome oxidase deficiency has been identified in fibroblast cultures.[942]

Lactic acidemia has been associated with lipid storage and mitochondrial myopathies. Plasma lactate and pyruvate levels typically are elevated at rest and postexercise. Lactic acid is a byproduct of anaerobic metabolism of glucose. Thus, lactate levels will be increased even in normal animals after strenuous and prolonged exercise.[947] Lactic acidemia results from a defect in metabolism of pyruvate. Documentation of lactic acidosis with a normal lactate-to-pyruvate rate is consistent with a defect in pyruvate dehydrogenase or in one of the enzymes of gluconeogenesis. Lactic acidosis in association with a high lactate-to-pyruvate ratio is found in abnormalities within the mitochondrial electron transport chain, pyruvate decarboxylase deficiency, or the mitochondrial myopathies. Further investigation to determine a specific metabolic abnormality should also include evaluation of urinary organic acid quantification by gas chromatography/mass spectroscopy, plasma amino acid concentrations, and quantification of total, free, and esterified carnitine in plasma, urine, and muscle.[948-950] Lactic acidemia and lactic and pyruvic aciduria have been documented in dogs with lipid storage and mitochondrial myopathy.[951] Carnitine concentrations also were reduced in the plasma and muscle, and affected animals had evidence of increased urinary excretion.

Treatment. A therapeutic regimen for lipid storage and mitochondrial myopathies has included supplementation with L-carnitine, coenzyme Q_{10}, and B vitamins.[617,818] Some dogs have shown dramatic improvements following these supplementations[617]; L-carnitine is neuroprotective through its antioxidative and membrane stabilizing properties and typically administered at a dosage of 50 mg/kg PO twice daily. Coenzyme Q_{10} plays a role as an antioxidant and free radical scavenger. A dosage of 100 mg/day has been recommended.[818] For mitochondrial myopathy, a diet higher in fat (>50%) and lower in carbohydrates (<20%) will lead to a reduction in lactate and improvement of clinical signs.

Endocrine-Related Myopathies

Steroid-Induced Myopathy in Dogs. Dogs with endogenous and iatrogenic Cushing's disease resulting from corticosteroid excess develop muscle atrophy and weakness.[825,952] Affected dogs may have other characteristic signs of hyperadrenocorticism: polyuria and polydypsia, generalized muscle atrophy, abdominal distension, bilaterally symmetrical alopecia, and weakness. Clinical signs may be protracted for years before gait abnormalities become apparent; thus the muscle changes may be subclinical.[824] Some dogs develop an associated pseudomyotonic syndrome (see Chapter 10).[953] Pelvic limb stiffness may be unilateral or bilateral and eventually may involve the thoracic limbs (Figure 7-26). The proximal appendicular musculature may become hypertrophied. Severe pelvic limb rigidity develops in some dogs. The CK levels can be elevated.[952] Complex repetitive discharges that do not wax and wane are typical on EMG. The exact biochemical cause of steroid-induced myopathy is not known. Corticosteroid excess increases muscle protein catabolism and alters carbohydrate metabolism.[617] Type II myofiber atrophy is a consistent abnormality on muscle biopsy.[824,825,952] Other myopathic changes include myofiber necrosis, regeneration, and increased muscle fat and connective tissue. Nemaline rods and "ragged red fibers" have been found in type I fibers, suggesting

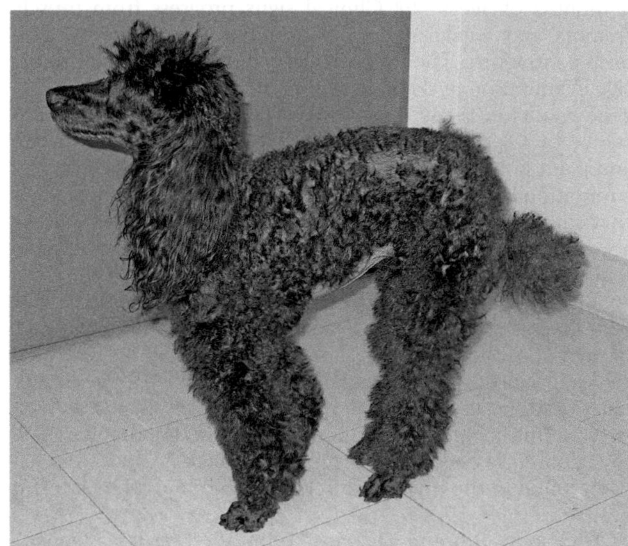

Figure 7-26 A 14-year-old FS standard poodle diagnosed with Cushing's disease and demonstrating Cushing's myopathy. Note rigid extension in both thoracic and pelvic limbs. Dog ambulated with very stilted gait in all limbs. Complex repetitive discharges were observed on EMG.

mitochondrial dysfunction.[824,902] The muscle weakness will improve in some dogs upon withdrawal of exogenous corticosteroids or suppression of endogenous corticosteroids.[952] Dogs with severe limb rigidity may not improve even after plasma steroid levels are decreased. Dogs that improve with appropriate therapy may have persistent complex repetitive discharges on EMG.[952]

Steroid Myopathy in Horses. Horses with pituitary pars intermedia dysfunction or equine Cushing's disease develop a myopathy. Morgans and ponies of middle-aged and geriatric horses appear to be at higher risk.[954] Common clinical signs include hirsutism, hyperhidrosis, polydipsia, polyuria, and muscle wasting with decreased strength.[954] Electromyography and CK levels are usually within normal limits.[955] A noninflammatory myopathy with atrophy of type II myofibers and myofiber size variation.[955]

Hypothyroid Myopathy. Weakness and muscle degeneration have been described in hypothyroid dogs.[604,607] These changes are less pronounced than those of the neuropathy previously described. Clinical signs suggestive of hypothyroid myopathy include weakness, stiffness, myalgia, and muscle wasting. The CK levels may or may not be elevated. Histopathology reveals atrophy of type II myofibers.[604,606,607] Other myopathic changes include predominance of type I myofibers with chronicity, presence of nemaline rod inclusions, and accumulations of abnormal mitochondria.[606] Electromyographic and muscle histopathologic changes have been described as being subclinical.[606,607] Myopathic changes are indicative of altered energy metabolism and depletion of skeletal muscle carnitine concentrations.[606] Prognosis for resolution of the myopathic signs of hypothyroidism is excellent with levothyroxine supplementation.

Foals that are hypothyroid have various neonatal musculoskeletal abnormalities that include ruptured tendons, angular limb deformities, forelimb contractures, and mandibular prognathism.[956]

Hyperthyroid Myopathy. Hyperthyroidism in cats is associated with muscle weakness in about 15% of cases.[957,958] These cats may show an inability to jump, flexion of the neck, and exercise-induced fatigue. Hyperthyroid cats that are hypokalemia can manifest severe muscle weakness.

Splayleg in Piglets. Splayleg, also known as *spreadleg*, is a weakness of the adductor muscle in newborn pigs and occurs more frequently in male piglets.[959] An underlying cause of corticosteroid excess from stress and hormonal imbalance in the sow may result in a myopathy.[960] However, another study determined a delay in spinal cord myelination and found no evidence of a myopathy.[961] Nutritional deficiencies of methionine and choline are suspected, since supplementation of these amino acids reduces the disease incidence.[961]

Pietrain Creeper Syndrome. This autosomal recessive inherited trait occurs in Pietrain pigs that are susceptible to stress.[962,963] Muscular weakness is noted at 3 weeks and progresses to recumbency by 12 weeks. These pigs have a crouched posture and a creeping-type gait using flexed limbs. Atrophy of type I myofibers is prominent in proximal muscles. No treatment exists.

Myotonic Myopathies. Contraction of muscle that persists after the cessation of voluntary effort or stimulation is called *myotonia* (if generalized) or *cramp* (if localized). Myotonia results from altered muscle membrane excitability from inherited abnormalities of ion conductance and acquired disorders associated with metabolic and toxin-induced diseases.[964] Myotonic myopathies are discussed in Chapter 10.

Nutritional

White Muscle Disease. White muscle disease, a degenerative myopathy of many species caused by dietary deficiency of vitamin E or selenium,[210] occurs most frequently in calves, foals, and lambs, less frequently in pigs, and rarely in other large animals, dogs, and cats.[965-969] Vitamin E and glutathione peroxidase function as biological antioxidants and play a protective role from lipid peroxidation. Selenium, a component of the enzyme glutathione peroxidase, functions to destroy peroxides and thus acts as a cell membrane protectant. Although selenium deficiency plays a major factor in development of muscle atrophy, not all selenium-deficient animals exhibit clinical signs.[968] Other risk factors include unacclimated exercise, inclement weather, and transport. Acute and chronic forms of the disease occur. The acute form in foals is characterized by sudden death that occurs during exertion and is due to cardiac muscle degeneration. Subacute disease in foals causes muscular weakness and dysphagia. Foals may have pain around the base of the tail and in tissues involving the area beneath the mane, tongue, and submandibular region. The chronic form is marked by a gradual onset of tetraparesis in calves 2 weeks of age or older. Lambs develop a stiff gait and tetraparesis at 10 days to 2 months of age. Muscles may be swollen and painful. Other diseases linked to selenium deficiency include mulberry heart disease in piglets, recurrent exertional rhabdomyolysis, and retained placenta in cattle. The diagnosis is based on clinical signs, histologic examination of biopsy samples from affected muscles, quantitation of glutathione peroxidase levels, and response to therapy.[968] The CK levels are markedly elevated. Foals can have life-threatening electrolyte abnormalities.[970] On necropsy, gross examination of skeletal muscle degeneration is characterized by symmetric grayish or white streaks that represent necrosis and edema. Histopathology reveals myonecrosis and regeneration, fibrosis, and calcification. Diets should be corrected if selenium deficiencies are found. Supplementation with selenium and vitamin E is beneficial if the signs are severe. In foals, supplementation of the food ration during gestation is paramount to disease prevention.[968] Response to therapy is always guarded in horses with steatitis and myodegeneration.[968,971]

Episodic Myopathies

Exercised-induced weakness often is characteristic of myopathic disease.

Metabolic

Exercise Intolerance and Collapse in Labrador Retrievers. This syndrome has been seen with increasing frequency in young Labrador retrievers, especially excitable, hard-driving dogs bred for field trial work.[972,973] Clinical signs develop between 7 months and 2 years of age. There is no sex or coat color predilection. After 5 to 15 minutes of strenuous exercise, dogs hyperventilate, become weak, ataxic, and then collapse. Prior to exercise, the patellar reflex is normal. However, loss of the patellar reflex during an episode of exercise-induced gait abnormalities or collapse is a consistent finding. Body temperatures are usually severely elevated during episodes but are normal at rest. Inability to regulate body temperature does not initiate the episodes.[947] At rest, no differences in phenotype (physical or neurologic examination findings) or biochemical testing are evident between affected and normal Labrador retrievers.[973] However, following 10 minutes of exercise, several affected dogs showed a significantly decreased $Paco_2$ and increased heart rate, Pao_2, and glucose compared to normal dogs.[973] Muscle biopsy on histopathology and pre- and postexercise lactate and pyruvate concentrations are within normal limits.

The diagnosis of exercise intolerance and collapse is made by ruling out other muscle disorders and cardiovascular diseases. There is no specific treatment, but most dogs respond well to avoiding strenuous exercise and excitement. The exercised-induced collapse has a familial pattern consistent with autosomal recessive inheritance.[972] Recently the genetic mutation was discovered, revealing a mutation in the dynamin 1 (*DNM1*) gene encoding for a protein involved in neurotransmission and synaptic vesicle endocytosis.[974] Understanding of the mutation explains the lack of abnormalities on muscle biopsy and that there is a reasonable likelihood for a CNS origin causing the collapse.

Malignant Hyperthermia Syndrome. Malignant hyperthermia is not a single disease but a clinical syndrome characterized by increases in $PaCO_2$, elevated body temperature, cardiac arrhythmias, hyperkalemia, and muscle necrosis.[677] This disease is seen more commonly in pigs and rarely in dogs, cats, or horses. A hypersensitive calcium-release mechanism that causes high levels of sarcoplasmic calcium levels apparently initiates the increased muscle activity and hyperthermia.[677] Muscle contraction is unopposed, leading to release of cations and enzymes into the circulation, increased heat production, and acidosis. Two types of calcium channels exist for coupling excitation and contraction of muscles. Depolarization first activates a voltage-gated channel and changes its conformation, which in turns opens a second calcium-release channel (ryanodine receptor). Calcium is subsequently released into the cytosol.

The disorder often is subclinical but becomes clinically evident in anesthetized animals, characterized by elevations in carbon dioxide and body temperature. Anesthetic agents known to trigger malignant hyperthermia include all the volatile anesthetics (e.g., halothane, isoflurane, sevoflurane) and depolarizing neuromuscular agents (e.g., succinylcholine). Dantrolene, a calcium-release channel antagonist has been shown to reverse clinical signs. Treatment of malignant hyperthermia includes discontinuing the triggering agent, dantrolene IV, fluid therapy, appropriate cooling regimens and diuresis.[677] Blood gases, CK, glucose and electrolytes should be monitored. Hyperkalemia can be treated with intravenous fluids (0.9% NaCl), insulin, and glucose. Mortality in anesthetized horses, dogs, and cats is high.

Pigs (Porcine Stress Syndrome). The trait is apparently inherited in Pietrain, Poland China, and Landrace pigs.[210] Clinical signs are exhibited after stressors such as anesthesia, administration of depolarizing muscle relaxants, hot weather, exercise, or restraint. Pigs exhibit stiffness, reluctance to move, and dyspnea. Sudden death may occur. Anesthetized pigs develop muscle rigidity, high body temperature, and tachycardia.[975] Laboratory findings include lactic acidemia, hyperkalemia, hypercarbia, and increased CK levels. On necropsy, muscles are pale, soft, and liquefied. In all pigs, malignant hyperthermia is inherited as an autosomal recessive trait. A mutation in the calcium-release channel gene (*RYR1*) has been identified. The condition is recessive in pigs, requiring two copies of the mutant allele for phenotypic expression.[976] Halothane may be used diagnostically to detect susceptible pigs. Reducing stress and selective breeding are recommended for prevention.

Horses. Malignant hyperthermia in horses is characterized by tachypnea, progressive increase in $PaCO_2$ even with controlled ventilation, and elevated body temperature. The onset of signs is slower and occurs after long periods of anesthesia. The hyperthermic episodes can be induced by halothane anesthesia or after succinylcholine administration.[977,978] Muscle biopsies reveal evidence of myonecrosis. Diagnosis for malignant hyperthermia is based on detecting lactic acidosis and hyperthermia. Treatment involves preventing these episodes by pretreatment with dantrolene before anesthesia. The prognosis is poor once a fulminant episode ensues. An autosomal dominant mutation in the *RYR1* gene was found in two quarter horses that developed hyperthermia and lactic acidosis while under anesthesia.[979] Both affected horses were homozygous for the mutation; the prevalence of the mutation is less than 1% in the quarter horse population.[979] The syndrome of malignant hyperthermia may overlap with hyperkalemic periodic paralysis and exertional rhabdomyolysis.

Dogs. Unlike affected pigs, affected dogs may not display lactic acidosis and extensor rigidity. The most consistent sign of malignant hyperthermia in dogs is a slow increase in $PaCO_2$ and body temperature. Elevations in $PaCO_2$ may precede elevations in body temperature. There is no specific breed sensitivity from previous reports.[677] A mutation in the calcium-release channel gene (*RYR1*) has been identified.[980] The inheritance pattern is autosomal dominant, and a single copy of the mutant *RYR1* is completely penetrant.

Recurrent Exertional Rhabdomyolysis. This disorder has been recognized in racing greyhounds and horses and known as *Monday morning disease*, *tying up*, and *paralytic myoglobinuria*. A similar syndrome in exotic animals is called *capture syndrome*. The specific cause is unknown. Studies suggest that the sustained muscle contraction is caused by abnormal regulation of intracellular calcium. Myoglobinuria is often seen. The muscles are painful and swollen on palpation. Serum muscle enzyme levels are elevated. Muscle atrophy may persist after recovery. The final events appear to be muscle swelling and necrosis.

Dogs. Gannon[981] has categorized the clinical signs in dogs as hyperacute, acute, and subacute. Predisposing factors include lack of physical fitness, excitement before racing, hot and humid conditions, and excessive frequency of running. In the more acute forms of the disease, clinical signs are observed during the race. The most severe signs include generalized muscle pain, tachypnea, and myoglobinuria. Death may occur within 48 hours. In the subacute (milder) form of the disease, muscle pain is confined to the longissimus thoracicus muscle and may not be apparent for 24 to 72 hours after the race. Myoglobinuria is rarely observed in subacute exertional rhabdomyolysis. The hyperacute and acute forms of the disease are treated similarly. Intravenous fluids are given to treat or prevent hypovolemic shock and to aid in renal excretion of myoglobin. Sodium bicarbonate is added to the fluid to combat muscle acidosis and to help prevent precipitation of myoglobin in renal tubules. The patient is cautiously cooled to remove excess heat. Precautionary measures to prevent recurrence may include installation of air conditioning in kennels, reduction of body temperature with cool-water baths before racing, administration of oral bicarbonate-glucose solutions before kenneling for racing, alkalinization of the urine with sodium bicarbonate or potassium citrate, administration of an oral potassium supplement, and reduction in the frequency of racing.[981]

Horses. This condition seems to be inherited as an autosomal dominant trait with variable phenotype in thoroughbred horses.[982] Horses develop exertional rhabdomyolysis during racing season, with recurrence in 17% of horses.[983,984] Horses clinically manifest signs of muscle stiffness, shifting hindlimb lameness, tachypnea, sweating, muscle pain in the hindquarters, and have reluctance to move. Lactic acidosis is not associated with the pathogenesis. Risk factors include horses that are fed a high-grain diet, female, young, anxious, irregular exercise, and have concurrent lameness.[984] Presumptive diagnosis is based on clinical signs, signalment, increased CK levels post exercise, and muscle biopsy. Histopathologic features include centrally located nuclei in type II myofibers, with variable amounts of necrosis and regeneration.[985]

In acute cases, goals are to minimize pain and restore fluid and electrolyte balances. Administration of dantrolene (2 to 4 mg/kg IV) may decrease muscle contracture and lessen myonecrosis. In severe cases, hyperkalemia should be managed with balanced electrolyte and fluid administration. Since lactic acidosis is no longer implicated, and horses are usually alkalotic, bicarbonate administration is not deemed appropriate. Additional support includes a few days of stall rest, with gradual return of exercise and hay diet. Long-term management includes modifying the environment, amount of exercise, and diet. A nutritionally balanced diet containing less than 20% supplied by starch and at least 15% in fat, along with adequate vitamins and minerals, are key to treating exertional rhabdomyolysis.[934]

Hyperkalemic Periodic Paralysis

Pathophysiology. This disease causes episodic muscle weakness and muscle trembling in quarter horses, American paint horses, Appaloosas, and cross-bred quarter horses. In horses, hyperkalemic periodic paralysis (HyPP) is an autosomal dominant inherited disease caused by a mutation in the alpha subunit of the skeletal muscle sodium channel, *SCN4A* gene.[986-990] The lineage of affected progeny stems from the founder sire, Impressive.[988] These horses are well muscled, as there is preferential selection of this trait. Homozygous animals are more severely affected than heterozygotes. Signs usually appear by 3 years of age. Severity of signs is variable, and episodes can last from minutes to hours; horses are normal between episodes. Exercise and rest and stressful events such as transport, weaning, and anesthesia may precipitate episodes.[991] A similar syndrome has been reported in one dog.[992]

Clinical Signs. Clinical signs range from mild muscle tremors to complete recumbency. Prolapse of the nictitans membrane may be the initial sign. The most frequent clinical sign is muscle fasciculation in the shoulders, flank, and neck.[993] Severe episodes may include tetany followed by a state of flaccidity and hyporeflexia. Pharyngeal and laryngeal dysfunction may occur alone, particularly in foals.[994,995] Acute death can occur from hyperkalemia-induced cardiac standstill.

Diagnosis. Suspicion for diagnosis is based on breed and clinical signs. Currently, the most accurate way to confirm a diagnosis of HyPP is by genetic testing through a licensed laboratory.[989] Before the development of a genetic test, other diagnostic testing procedures were performed. Blood samples taken during an episode may show hemoconcentration and hyperkalemia (5.0 to 11.7 mEq/L).[986] However, many affected horses are normokalemic. The CK level usually is within normal limits. Evidence of complex repetitive discharges on EMG is suggestive. A diagnosis also is suggested by inducing signs through administration of potassium chloride (0.1 g/kg orally initially; increase in 0.025 g/kg increments every 48 hours to a total of 0.2 g/kg), but this can cause death.[993] Prior to genetic testing, EMG combined with induction of signs with KCl gave the most accurate diagnosis.

Treatment. Acute episodes should be treated by intravenous administration of sodium bicarbonate, dextrose, or calcium solutions. Diuretic therapy using acetazolamide, 2.2 mg/kg orally 2 to 3 times daily, may lessen the frequency and severity of attacks.[986] Diuretics will increase renal potassium excretion and stimulate insulin secretion. Readily absorbable sources of carbohydrates may be fed to promote insulin induced uptake of potassium. Stressors, diets high in potassium (e.g., alfalfa, brome and orchard grass hays, soybean meal, and molasses) and irregular feeding need to be avoided.

Hypokalemic Myopathy of Cats

Pathogenesis. Potassium depletion can occur in any species, causing muscle weakness (see also Chapter 15). A generalized polymyopathy associated with hypokalemia of cats has been well characterized.[676,996-998] Mechanisms to account for the weakness are not fully understood. Decreased extracellular potassium (<3.0 mEq/L) causes an increase in the resting membrane potential difference, which leads to the myofiber being refractory to depolarization.[999] Additionally, glycogen metabolism in muscle and blood flow during exercise become impaired.[998] Hypokalemia can occur secondary to underlying diseases such as hyperthyroidism and renal dysfunction.[996,1000] Hypokalemia itself can induce further renal dysfunction.

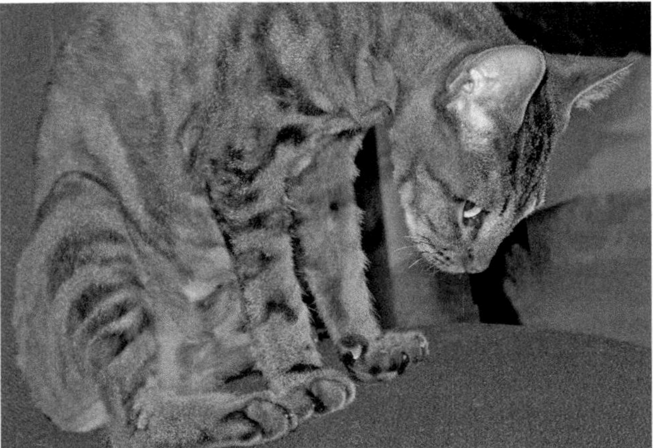

Figure 7-27 A 7-year-old MC domestic shorthair cat showing flexion of neck as a clinical sign of muscular weakness. Blood work revealed hypokalemia. Clinical signs resolved after potassium supplementation.

A similar syndrome involving hypokalemia and episodic weakness has been reported in Burmese cats between 2 and 6 months of age.[1001,1002] Clinical signs manifest as neck flexion.

Clinical Signs. Affected cats have signs of muscular weakness characterized by neck flexion, episodic weakness affecting the pelvic limbs, exercise intolerance, and a stiff gait (Figure 7-27). Muscle pain may be elicited on palpation. Tiring and lethargy may be observed before obvious weakness is noticed. Persistent flexion of the neck is a hallmark feature of this disease.

Diagnosis. Suspicion for the diagnosis is based on low serum potassium levels (<3.1 mEq/L).[998] Actual potassium concentrations in muscle are much lower than what serum values may reflect. Serum CK levels in these cats is moderately to severely elevated, with an average CK values of 2337 IU/L (normal, 0 to 156 IU/L).[996] Abnormal electromyography can further support myopathic disease. All affected cats should be assessed for underlying renal dysfunction.

Treatment. Clinical signs of myopathy associated with hypokalemia often resolve after potassium supplementation. Cats with muscle weakness are treated with oral potassium gluconate at an initial dosage of 2 to 5 mEq orally every 12 hours. Dilution of the potassium gluconate with water is helpful to avoid vomiting. Once the serum potassium normalizes, continued supplementation is necessary to prevent recurrence. It is important to avoid metabolic acidosis in chronic supplementation. Affected cats should be provided diets replete with potassium. Some diets can be low in potassium.[1003] Rapid correction of dehydration with fluids that are not supplemented with potassium may lead to exacerbation of hypokalemia. Severely affected cats that are moribund should be given potassium chloride (diluted in lactated Ringer's solution) at a rate of 0.5 to 1 mEq/kg/hr until 3.5 mEq/L is reached. Continuous ECG monitoring is recommended to avoid arrhythmias and asystole. Prognosis is good depending upon the underlying cause of the hypokalemia.

NEUROMUSCULAR JUNCTION DISEASES

Electrical transmission of impulses down the motor nerve is converted to chemical transmission as the nerve synapses with the muscle-neuromuscular junction. As the impulse travels to the end of the motor terminal, calcium is released into the presynaptic bouton. Increased Ca^{2+} concentration destabilizes the storage vesicles, which allows fusion of the vesicle to the presynaptic terminal membrane. The acetylcholine (ACh)-containing vesicles dock and fuse with the plasmalemma at the synaptic cleft region. The process results in exocytosis of ACh into the synaptic cleft. Nicotinic receptors are located in skeletal muscle. Once released from the presynaptic terminal, ACh diffuses to the postsynaptic membrane of the myofiber and binds to nicotinic ACh receptors (AChR). Binding of ACh to these receptors increases Na^+ and K^+ conductance of the membrane, and resultant influx of Na^+ produces a depolarizing potential called the *end plate potential* (EPP). The EPP causes depolarization of the adjacent muscle membrane. The muscle action potential subsequently initiates a muscle contraction. There is an overabundance of available ACh and AChR; this excess is referred to as the *safety margin* of neuromuscular transmission. The safety margin insures that there will be more than enough ACh available for neuromuscular transmission. At higher concentrations of ACh, the accumulation of ACh may result in fibrillation of muscle fibers. This is a result of sustained muscle membrane depolarization causing *neuromuscular junction blockade*.

Disorders affecting the neuromuscular junction are presynaptic or postsynaptic and sometimes both. These processes may increase or decrease the activity at the NMJ by the following: (1) increasing or decreasing presynaptic ACh release by altering ACh synthesis, transport, reuptake or presynaptic release; (2) altering the concentration or duration of ACh in the synaptic cleft by altering removal of ACh from the synaptic cleft; and (3) acting as an ACh agonist or antagonist at the NMJ by affecting the interaction between ACh and the postsynaptic receptor.[627,1004,1005]

Acute Progressive Diseases

Toxic

Botulism

Pathophysiology. For many years, this disease was suspected in dogs but was never documented. Carrion eaters and some carnivores, including dogs, were thought to be resistant to botulism toxin. In 1978 Barsanti and co-workers[1006] documented an outbreak of type C botulism in foxhounds in Georgia. Botulism also has been reported in dogs in Great Britain, the European continent, and Australia.[1007-1009] Before a detailed description of polyradiculoneuritis was published, many hunting dogs with acute progressive LMN disease were thought to have botulism. After the Cummings and Haas report[1010] on coonhound paralysis, most dogs were believed to have this disorder. Both conditions are now known to exist in dogs, but it can be difficult to make a differential diagnosis.

In large animals, botulism results from ingestion of toxin or from the contamination of an ulcerated gastrointestinal tract with proliferating *Clostridium botulinum* spores. Outbreaks in horses occur as a result of the ingestion of hay, silage, or water that has been contaminated by dead rodents.[1011] The shaker foal syndrome occurs most frequently in foals 2 to 5 weeks of age. Foals that are given highly nutritious feed develop gastrointestinal ulcers. These ulcers are colonized by *C. botulinum*, which then produces the offending toxin.[1012-1014] Botulism can also occur from wound infection.[1015]

Clinical signs develop when the preformed *C. botulinum* toxin is ingested. Several different strains of exotoxin-producing organisms have been identified. Types A, B, and E are most commonly associated with human disease. Types C and D, found in carrion, cause most cases of botulism in birds and mammals other than humans. Most cases reported in dogs and horses are caused by type C. Type B also has been reported in large animals.[1016] The toxin has been shown to bind to selective presynaptic receptors and is then translocated into the presynaptic terminus of the axon. Botulinum toxin produces generalized neuromuscular blockade by inhibiting the release of ACh from the terminals of cholinergic nerve fibers.[1017] Part of the toxin alters a docking and fusion protein of synaptic vesicles with the presynaptic membrane, thus preventing release of ACh.[1018]

Clinical Signs. The incubation period is less than 6 days. Clinical signs are those of a progressive, symmetric, generalized LMN disorder. Severity varies with the amount of toxin ingested and ranges from mild generalized weakness to tetraplegia with respiratory failure. Both cranial and spinal nerves are affected.[1006,1007] Cranial nerve signs include mydriasis with decreased pupillary light reflexes, decreased jaw tone, decreased gag reflex, decreased tongue movements, decreased palpebral reflexes, and change in bark and vocalization. Megaesophagus and intestinal ileus also can occur in dogs with botulism. Decreased anal sphincter tone and urinary bladder function also occur. In dogs, the usual clinical course is less than 14 days.

Diagnosis. Botulism must be suspected in animals with acute progressive LMN disease. Botulism is especially likely when multiple animals are affected. Given the clinical similarities to other acute LMN diseases such as tick paralysis and polyradiculoneuritis, a definitive diagnosis of botulism is difficult to make (see Table 7-8). Tick paralysis and polyradiculoneuritis are sporadic diseases that involve individual animals. EMG studies may help to differentiate botulism from polyradiculoneuritis, but some similarity exists, depending on the stage of disease. Electrophysiologic findings in affected humans include normal motor nerve conduction velocity, decreased M-wave amplitude, decrement/increment of the M wave with slow/rapid repetitive nerve stimulation, respectively, and increased "jitter" with single fiber EMG.[1019] Electrophysiologic evidence of peripheral nerve involvement also has been collected from affected dogs.[1020] Identification of toxin in the food, carrion, serum, feces, or vomitus of an affected animal confirms the diagnosis. The organism can be isolated from the viscera and feces of clinically normal animals.

Treatment. Treatment of botulism is largely supportive. To be effective, the specific antitoxin must be administered before the botulinum toxin binds to receptors at the neuromuscular junction. This approach is rarely possible because signs usually are present before the animal is treated. Polyvalent products that contain type C antitoxin generally are not available. The efficacy of antibiotic therapy has not been proven. The prognosis for recovery is generally good unless the dog develops severe, rapidly progressive signs. Ventilatory support may be necessary in some dogs. Mildly affected animals recover without therapy.[1006]

Tick Paralysis

Pathophysiology. This disease has been recognized worldwide, but most in-depth reports have come from the United States and Australia.[1021] The clinical signs are similar to those of polyradiculoneuritis and botulism. The toxin probably comes from the salivary glands of the engorged feeding female ticks. The neurotoxin either inhibits depolarization in the terminal portions of motor nerves or blocks the release of ACh at the neuromuscular junction. The toxin may affect both motor and sensory nerve fibers by altering ionic fluxes that mediate action potential production. In the United States, *Dermacentor andersoni* and *D. variabilis* are the primary ticks involved. In Australia, the disease is produced by *Ixodes holocyclus*, although *Ixodes cornuatus* and *Ixodes hirsti* are also incriminated.[1021]

Clinical Signs. Clinical signs develop 7 to 9 days after attachment of the tick. The earliest clinical sign is marked ataxia with rapid progression to paresis, paralysis, areflexia, and hypotonus. In the United States, cranial nerve involvement is rare. Nystagmus is occasionally observed. Death can occur from respiratory failure if the ticks are not removed. Painful stimuli normally are perceived. In Australia, affected dogs or cats develop more severe signs.[1022-1024] Asymmetric signs are not uncommon with *I. holocyclus*.[1025] Respiratory failure and autonomic signs occur with greater frequency in these animals than in those from the United States. In the Australian syndrome, clinical signs may progressively worsen even though the ticks have been removed.[1021,1024] In the U.S. syndrome, dramatic improvement follows tick removal.

Diagnosis. Tick paralysis is diagnosed by rapid improvement after tick removal. In unusual cases, EMG can be used to differentiate this disease from acute polyradiculoneuritis.[373] In tick paralysis, no EMG evidence of denervation exists, but the amplitude of evoked motor potentials is markedly reduced. Repetitive stimulation does not cause further decrement in the amplitude. Nerve conduction velocities may be slightly slower than normal, and terminal conduction times may be prolonged.[1026]

Treatment. In the United States syndrome, removal of the tick results in marked improvement within 24 hours and complete recovery within 72 hours. Animals must be examined thoroughly for ticks. The areas evaluated should include the ear canals and interdigital spaces. Ticks are removed carefully so that the head is not left embedded in the animal's skin. Since the toxin is secreted from the salivary glands, failure to remove the head may cause worsening of the clinical signs. Given the lack of side effects associated with treatment, all dogs with an acute onset of diffuse LMN signs should be treated with a commercially available ectoparasiticide therapy. The prognosis for complete recovery is good. In Australian tick paralysis, tick removal does not prevent further progression of the disease. Hyperimmune dog serum has been advocated to prevent death from respiratory failure.[1021]

Snake Envenomation. Envenomation by one of three species of coral snake, *Micruroides fulvius fulvius* (eastern coral snake), *M. fulvius tenere* (Texas coral snake), and *M. fulvius barbouri* (South Florida coral snake) is associated with diffuse LMN disease.[1027] The coral snake is recognized by its distinct color pattern of a black nose and a repeating pattern of black, yellow, followed by red circumferential bands. Envenomation has been reported in the dog and cat.[1028,1029] Affected animals develop acute onset of LMN signs within hours of envenomation, but signs may be delayed up to 7 days.[1028,1029] Tissue reaction at the site of envenomation varies from mild to severe. Death due to respiratory paralysis can occur. Clinicopathologic changes include hemolysis and increased CK levels.[1027] Electrophysiology is consistent with neuromuscular blockade.[1028] Treatment is directed at supportive care, broad-spectrum antibiotics, and monitoring of ventilatory capacity. Severely affected animals may need mechanical ventilation.[1029] With aggressive supportive care, the prognosis for recovery is good. The effects of the venom decline over 18 hours but may last for 7 to 10 days. [1028,1029] There is currently no approved antivenin.

Drug-Induced Neuromuscular Blockade. Several drugs have been shown to block neuromuscular transmission.[1004] These include aminoglycosides, antiarrhythmic agents, phenothiazine, penicillins, and magnesium. It is important to be aware of drug side effects, especially when treating myasthenia gravis. We observed one animal after aminoglycoside administration develop severe muscle weakness and hyporeflexia after 5 days of gentamicin therapy for deep pyoderma. The clinical signs resolved within 48 hours after the drug was discontinued.

Organophosphate and Carbamate Toxicity

Pathogenesis. Animal poisoning from organophosphate (chlorpyrifos, diazinon, dichlorvos) and carbamate (aldicarb, methomyl, carbofuran, carbaryl) insecticides commonly results from overapplication or accidental ingestion.[1030,1031] Organophosphates inhibit the action of acetylcholinesterase, resulting in an accumulation of ACh in the synaptic cleft. This leads to activation of nicotinic, muscarinic, and CNS cholinergic synapses. Carbamates are reversible cholinesterase inhibitors with reactivation of cholinesterase activity when the carbamate insecticide and enzyme separate. Some organophosphate insecticides bind covalently to the enzyme (aging), resulting in irreversible inhibition. Recovery depends upon resynthesis of acetylcholinesterase. Cats are especially sensitive to these agents and can develop delayed-onset neuropathy.[1032-1034]

Clinical Signs. Clinical signs of acute organophosphate toxicity include the effects of muscarinic, nicotinic stimulation on the CNS and PNS. These signs develop within minutes to hours depending upon dose and route of the intoxication. Muscarinic signs reflect the parasympathomimetic effects and include hypersalivation, lacrimation, urination, increased gastrointestinal motility, miosis, cyanosis, and incontinence. Signs of nicotinic stimulation of the PNS involve fasciculation, tremor, and muscle weakness which usually is generalized. Acetylcholine accumulation increases at the neuromuscular junction, causing a depolarization block. CNS signs include hyperactivity, anorexia, and seizures.

Diagnosis. Reduced cholinesterase activity (<50%) in blood is supportive of exposure in dogs. Evaluation of cholinesterase activity cannot be performed in cats because feline blood contain pseudocholinesterase that is very sensitive to inhibition by organophosphate.

Treatment. Atropine blocks the effects of accumulated ACh at the muscarinic receptors and is the first-line drug of choice. The dose for acute organophosphate toxicity ranges from 0.2 to 2 mg/kg. Dramatic cessation of parasympathetic signs usually is observed within a few minutes after administration.

Diphenhydramine has some antinicotinic effects and blocks nicotinic receptor overstimulation. The dose recommended ranges from 1 to 4 mg/kg PO every 8 hours.[1035] Muscle tremors should abolish over time. Pralidoxime chloride (2-PAM), an enzyme reactivator, acts specifically on the organophosphate-enzyme complex and frees the enzyme.[1033] The recommended dose is 10 to 15 mg/kg IM every 8 to 12 hours and is used to relieve tremors and other nicotinic signs. Therapy should be continued until signs are abolished.

Episodic Diseases

Degenerative/Immune Mediated

Acquired Myasthenia Gravis

Pathophysiology. Myasthenia gravis (MG) (grave muscle disease) is a disease of the motor end plate and results in progressive loss of muscle strength with exercise. Myasthenia gravis can be acquired or congenital. Acquired MG is an immune-mediated disorder in which autoantibodies against nicotinic AChR of skeletal muscle result in impairment of neuromuscular transmission.[1036] Acetylcholine receptors of the post synaptic membrane of the neuromuscular junction are decreased. The decreased number of functional AChR reduces the probability that ACh molecules will react with AChRs on the postsynaptic membrane and increases the chance of failure of neuromuscular transmission, the safety margin is reduced. With repetitive firing of a motor nerve ending, stores of ACh are depleted; the few available AChR are soon bound with ACh molecules and desensitized to further stimulation. Severe muscle weakness and fatigue results.

In acquired MG, the α_1 subunit of the nicotinic AChR is targeted by an autoimmune response.[1036,1037] The autoimmunity involves both the antibody response of B cells and the helper T cells with destruction of the neuromuscular junction and complement mediated destruction and simplification of the postsynaptic membrane. It has been suggested that molecular mimicry of the ACh receptor could initiate the immune response. The thymus is suspected to be the site of initiation of the autoimmune response to AChR in MG. Moreover, thymic neoplasms also have been associated with MG.[816,1038-1040]

Acquired MG is one of the most commonly treated neuromuscular diseases in dogs but is less common in cats.[1004] A bimodal age of onset (<5 years and >7 years) has been reported in dogs. Female dogs are at greater risk. Breeds predisposed include German shepherd dog, golden retriever, and Labrador retriever. A report evaluating relative risk in breeds of dogs found the Akita to have the highest risk.[1041] Newfoundlands and Great Danes may have an inherited predisposition.[1042,1043] The breeds in cats at higher risk include the Somalis, Abyssinians, and domestic shorthair.[1044] A cranial mediastinal mass also was commonly associated with acquired MG in cats. Cats treated with methimazole for hyperthyroidism may also develop acquired MG.[1044]

Clinical Signs. The hallmark clinical feature of MG is episodic muscle weakness. The neurologic examination can be normal when the animal is rested. With exercise, muscle weakness becomes progressively worse. This phenomenon is most apparent in the appendicular muscles of the pelvic limbs. Animals become fatigued, develop a shortened stride, and then lie down to rest. Strength returns after rest. The spinal and cranial nerve reflexes may at first be intact but with repetitive testing can show fatigue. The most sensitive reflex to evaluate for fatigue is the palpebral reflex.

There are 3 forms of MG that have been described in dogs and cats: (1) the focal form which consists of megaesophagus alone or facial and pharyngeal weakness; signs include ptosis of the upper eyelids, sialosis, regurgitation of food, and dysphagia[1045]; (2) the generalized form which presents as tetraparesis with the pelvic limbs most severely affected; megaesophagus, facial and pharyngeal weakness also may be present; and (3) the acute fulminating form presents as acute, rapidly progressive, profound generalized muscle weakness, megaesophagus, frequent episodes of regurgitation, and respiratory distress.[1046,1047] In dogs, generalized weakness with megaesophagus and megaesophagus alone are the most common clinical signs of MG.[1041] Moreover, some dogs with presumed idiopathic megaesophagus or laryngeal paralysis without generalized muscle weakness have MG.[1045]

In cats, clinicals signs are more variable and include generalized weakness, megaesophagus and dysphagia.[1044] About 15% of cats with acquired MG had only focal disease as opposed to 36% of dogs with acquired MG.[1046,1048] Megaesophagus is not as common in cats because of the increased proportion of smooth muscle in the esophagus as compared with the canine esophagus, which is composed predominantly of skeletal muscle. Other common signs of MG in cats include vomiting/regurgitation, exercise intolerance, dysphagia, change in voice, and dropped jaw.[1048] Cat may manifest with flexion of the neck as a sign of weakness.

Aspiration pneumonia often is a sequela of megaesophagus and is a complicating factor when managing treatment for MG. Third-degree atrioventricular block has been reported in dogs with acquired MG, although a cause-and-effect relationship was not proved.[1049] Other immune-mediated disease may occur concurrently with MG. Polymyositis or immune-mediated endocrinopathies have been reported in dogs with MG.[616,1050]

As MG may develop as part of the paraneoplastic syndrome, affected animals may display clinical signs related to a primary neoplasm. Thymoma is the most common neoplasm associated with MG in dogs and cats.[816,1038,1051] The incidence of thymoma associated with MG is higher in cats than in dogs.[1041,1044] Myasthenia gravis may also be a paraneoplastic effect of other tumors such as osteogenic sarcoma, cholangiocellular carcinoma, anal sac adenocarcinoma, and lymphoma.[644,1004,1052,1053]

Diagnosis. Standard of care for definitive diagnosis of MG is based on testing for serum autoantibodies to AChR by immunoprecipitation radioimmunoassay.[1004,1036,1054] A titer result of above 0.6 nmol/L in dogs and above 0.3 nmol/L in cats is compatible with a diagnosis of acquired MG.[1004] This test should be performed before administering corticosteroids to prevent false-negative results. About 90% of dogs with acquired MG have AChR antibodies, and approximately 2% with generalized MG are seronegative.[1004,1041] Dogs that are seronegative may have antibodies against other endplate components, lack production of antibodies, or the antibodies are lost during the testing procedure.[1004] Diagnosis is aided by the exclusion of cardiovascular and metabolic diseases with appropriate laboratory or electrophysiologic tests. Exercise-induced weakness, a decremental response to repetitive nerve stimulation, and a positive response to anticholinesterase drugs support a presumptive diagnosis of MG.

Testing with intravenous edrophonium chloride (Tensilon test) may aid in establishing a presumptive diagnosis of acquired MG with signs of appendicular muscle weakness.[1004] Edrophonium chloride is an ultra-short-acting anticholinesterase agent. In theory, the drug enables more ACh molecules to be available and interact with the remaining functional ACh receptors. A presumptive diagnosis of acquired MG may be made if a patient responds positively to IV injection of 0.1 to 0.2 mg/kg of edrophonium after inducing weakness with exercise. A patient that demonstrates obvious improvement in muscle strength shortly after edrophonium is considered to have a positive response. Due to the short half-life, improvement will only last for a few minutes. Care must be exercised in both test performance and interpretation of test results. A lack of improvement in muscle strength does not eliminate a diagnosis of MG.[1004] Moreover, dogs with other neuromuscular diseases such as polymyositis may have a partial response to edrophonium chloride. Anticholinesterase drugs are nonspecific-acting cholinergics and stimulate both nicotinic and muscarinic receptors. Overstimulation of these receptors may induce a cholinergic crisis: severe muscle weakness, vomiting, salivation, and defecation. Accordingly, atropine should be given before edrophonium to block muscarinic receptors only and thereby limit the muscarinic cholinergic effects. Nicotinic receptors are not affected by atropine, and therefore affected animals can still display a positive response.

Electrophysiologic testing may also provide a presumptive diagnosis of MG. The EMG is usually normal in MG, although variability in amplitude of motor units and occasional fibrillation potentials may be seen. Analogous to the observation of fatiguing the palpebral reflex with repeated testing, repetitive nerve stimulation is an electrophysiologic test in which repeated stimulation of a nerve and the measurement of the amplitude of resultant muscle action potential is performed. In normal animals, repetitive nerve stimulation at 5 Hz does not cause any decrement in the amplitude or area of the evoked muscle action potential.[1055,1056] In animals with MG, the amplitudes of the evoked nerve stimulation will decreases by at least 10% to 20% in the first 10 responses. Definitive studies on large numbers of myasthenic dogs, however, have not been reported. Any decrement on stimulation is suspect for neuromuscular junction disease. If a decrement is demonstrated, administration of edrophonium chloride intravenously should cause a normal response for a few minutes. Although the decremental response is abnormal in most myasthenic animals, both false-positive and false-negative results may occur. Single-fiber EMG analysis is reported to be the most definitive electrodiagnostic test for establishing a diagnosis of MG in humans and has been studied in normal dogs.[1057] Single-fiber

EMG measures uniformity of latency times (time from stimulus to response) of the compound motor unit action potential after repeat stimulation over the motor point. In MG, there is variability in latency times which is called *jitter* (see Chapter 4). Often these studies require lengthy anesthesia, which should be avoided in dogs with MG.

Other supportive diagnostics include thoracic radiography to evaluate for aspiration pneumonia, presence of megaesophagus, and evaluation for a cranial mediastinal mass. Abdominal ultrasound is performed to screen for neoplasia; likewise the thorax is screened for metastasis.

Treatment. In acquired MG, there are three major modalities of therapeutic intervention: anticholinesterase therapy, immunomodulatory therapy, and thymectomy. Once the diagnosis has been confirmed, initial therapy should include anticholinesterase agents (pyridostigmine bromide, 0.5 to 3 mg/kg, 2 or 3 times daily, orally).[1004,1054,1058] Long-acting anticholinesterase drugs prolong the action of ACh at the neuromuscular junction by reversibly inhibiting acetylcholinesterase. There is improvement in muscle strength within the first few days of therapy. To avoid overstimulation of ACh receptors, patients are started at the low end of the dosage range, and the dose is gradually increased to effect. Some patients cannot tolerate the oral form of medication because of frequent regurgitation from megaesophagus. Instead, intramuscular neostigmine bromide can be administered at 0.4 mg/kg. It is important that the dosages are titrated to an optimal level based on changes in muscle strength.

Excessive amounts of acetylcholinesterase inhibitors result in the accumulation of ACh and cause fibrillation of muscle fibers. Paradoxical muscle weakness may occur as a result of this neuromuscular blockage of the motor endplate. Additionally, excessive stimulation of muscarinic receptors also will cause SLUDD (cholinergic crisis). This may be difficult to distinguish from worsening of the MG (*myasthenic crisis*), which also will reflect as profound muscle weakness. Edrophonium can be used to differentiate between these conditions. If the patient shows no relief or worsens with edrophonium, most likely excessive acetylcholinesterase inhibitor is the cause. The anticholinesterase drug should be temporarily discontinued or dosage amount and frequency lowered.

The pathophysiology of acquired MG as an autoimmune disorder implies that immunosuppression may be necessary to resolve the underlying disease. However, the use of immunosuppressive therapy for acquired MG has been controversial. Immunosuppression may be contraindicated in patients that are at risk for developing or have already developed aspiration pneumonia. Corticosteroid administration also has been associated with muscular weakness in several species and could further accentuate weakening of a MG patient. The dosage of prednisone should be started at a low antiinflammatory dosage of 0.25 mg/kg once daily and then gradually increased to an immunosuppressive dose. DO NOT start the dose at immunosuppressive levels, because this could send a patient into a myasthenic crisis. Immunosuppressive doses of prednisone, 1 to 2 mg/kg PO twice daily, are administered for 2 to 4 weeks, and the titers are reevaluated. If the titers are within the normal reference range, the dose is gradually reduced or tapered very slowly every 4 weeks. The ultimate goal is alternate-day therapy at the lowest dose as clinical signs stabilize. High-dose corticosteroid therapy also can lead to undesirable side effects such as gastric ulceration, hepatic dysfunction, and iatrogenic hyperadrenocorticism. Other immunosuppressive agents (cyclosporine, mycophenolate mofetil, azathioprine) that modulate T-cell function have been administered alone or in combination with corticosteroids, with varying success.[1059-1061] Plasmapheresis has been attempted in dogs and is used in human medicine.[1062]

Thymectomy should be considered for dogs with thymoma or those that respond poorly to medical therapy.[1040,1051,1063] AChR antibody levels may persist despite clinical improvement after thymectomy. Careful consideration is recommended before a thymectomy because of the stress of anesthesia and risks associated with thoracotomy.

The ACh receptor antibody titers should be monitored until remission is achieved. The dosage of anticholinesterase drugs and corticosteroids is gradually decreased and, if possible, discontinued. Drastic changes in the therapy should be avoided. There is excellent correlation between resolution of clinical signs and return of AChR antibody titers to less than 0.6 nmol/L.[1004]

It is important to use supportive treatments when other complicating factors occur: managing the megaesophagus, treatment of aspiration pneumonia, fluid therapy, nutritional support (elevated feedings, gastrostomy tube), respiratory support, GI motility modifiers, and increasing lower esophageal sphincter tone. Drugs that may affect the neuromuscular junction transmission should be avoided. Acquired drug-induced MG should be considered in hyperthyroid cats after initiation of treatment with methimazole.[1044,1064] Intact females should be spayed, although the anesthesia may exacerbate the MG.

Prognosis. The prognosis in the early stages is guarded. In one study, up to 50% of dogs diagnosed with MG were euthanized within 2 weeks.[1046] The mortality rate within 1 year from time of diagnosis was 40%. A recent study documented the natural disease course in dogs with MG and treated with anticholinesterase drugs alone.[1065] Many of these dogs went into spontaneous remission, suggesting caution with use of immunosuppression because of its higher mortality risks. Cats appear to have a better prognosis for focal or generalized MG than that which has been reported in dogs.[1048] It also has been noted that cats may respond better to immunosuppressive therapy than to anticholinesterase therapy.[1004]

Anomalies

Congenital Myasthenia Gravis. Congenital MG, a rare disease, has been mainly documented in young dogs including English springer spaniels,[1066] dachshunds,[1067] Jack Russell terriers,[1068] and smooth fox terriers.[1069] Congenital MG has been described in few cats.[1070,1071] The congenital form is caused by a deficiency of AChR at the postsynaptic membrane, without evidence of autoimmunity. Myasthenic syndrome, in which there is a presynaptic defect in the release of ACh, has been described in the Gammel Dansk honsehund dog.[1072] Autosomal recessive inheritance has been determined for the Jack Russell and smooth fox terriers and the Gammel Dansk honsehund.[1068,1072,1073] Congenital myasthenia syndrome due to a mutation in the gene encoding the epsilon subunit (*bovCHRNE*) of the AChR has been documented as an autosomal recessive trait in Red Brahman cattle in South Africa.[1074]

Diagnosis is based on signalment and clinical signs of fatigue during ambulation. Puppies may have megaesophagus. There may not be a response to the edrophonium chloride test if there is complete absence of receptors. A biopsy of the external intercostal muscle collected origin to insertion can be used to quantify a reduced number or lack of AChRs at the neuromuscular junction. Since an immune response is not involved in congenital MG, serologic testing for AChR antibody is negative and should not be performed.

Treatment response depends upon the underlying cause of congenital MG. If there is a deficiency of AChRs and not complete absence, anticholinesterase therapy may be effective. However, desensitization to the drug occurs over time. The weakness may be progressive, and presence of megaesophagus will predispose to aspiration pneumonia. There is a congenital syndrome in the miniature dachshund, which resolves with age.[1004]

CASE STUDIES

CASE STUDY 7-1 ASTRO

 veterinaryneurologycases.com

▪ Signalment
Canine, mixed breed, male, 6 months old

▪ History
An acute onset of tetraparesis progressing rapidly to complete paralysis. The dog has been paralyzed for 24 hours prior to examination.

▪ Physical Examination
No abnormalities were found on physical examination.

▪ Neurologic Examination

Mental Status
Alert

Gait
Tetraplegic

Posture
Unable to support weight or maintain sternal recumbency. The tail could still wag.

Postural Reactions
Postural reaction absent in all limbs

Spinal Reflexes
The patellar and extensor carpi reflexes were absent. The flexor withdrawal reflexes were severely reduced in all limbs. All limbs had reduced muscular tone. No muscle atrophy was appreciated. The perineal and cutaneous trunci reflexes were normal.

Cranial Nerves
All normal

Sensory Evaluation
Hyperesthesia—no pain elicited on spinal palpation
Superficial pain perception—intact
Deep pain perception—intact

▪ Lesion Location
Based on reduced to absent spinal reflexes without obvious sensory deficits, the lesion is localized to the lower motor neuron system–neuromuscular. All limbs are affected, indicating a diffuse disease process. Generalized neuropathy, myopathy, or neuromuscular junction disease should be suspected. Although rare, neuronopathy should be considered.

▪ Differential Diagnosis
1. Tick paralysis
2. Polyradiculoneuritis
3. Botulism
4. Fulminant myasthenia gravis
5. Polyneuropathy (metabolic, endocrine, toxic)

▪ Diagnostic Plan
1. Closely examine the entire body for ticks. The ear canal should not be overlooked.
2. History of exposure to carrion and trash would be important in ruling out botulism.
3. Electromyography would be a procedure to perform 5 to 7 days after hospital admission. This is the time frame during which denervation would be evident in cases of polyradiculoneuritis.
4. CSF analysis may reveal increased protein concentration and a mild inflammatory response in polyradiculoneuritis.

▪ Diagnostic Results
After close inspection, a tick was found embedded in the inner pinna. An engorged female *Dermacentor* spp. tick was carefully removed, and the dog was also treated with an insecticide.

▪ Diagnosis
Tick paralysis

▪ Treatment
Within 12 hours, the dog was able to become sternal; by 24 hours, the dog was ambulatory and regaining muscle strength. This is the typical time frame for recovery from tick paralysis. Topical insecticide treatment should be performed in all dogs with similar presentation to this case, as ticks may be difficult to identify, especially in long-haired dogs.

CASE STUDY 7-2 MILO

 veterinaryneurologycases.com

Signalment

Canine, Shetland sheepdog, male, 3 years old

History

Seven days prior, the dog had an acute onset of falling to the right, with paresis of both pelvic limbs and paralysis of the right thoracic limb. There was no history of trauma. The clinical signs have not progressed.

Physical Examination

Normal

Neurologic Examination

Mental Status

Alert

Gait

With assistance, the dog can support weight. Minimal voluntary motor function was present in the right thoracic and pelvic limbs. Voluntary motor function appears almost normal in the left pelvic limb. The left thoracic limb appears to have normal strength and voluntary motor function. The paw of right thoracic limb remains knuckled over.

Posture

Lateral recumbency

Postural Reactions

Proprioceptive positioning is normal in the left thoracic and pelvic limbs, decreased in the right pelvic limb, and absent in the right thoracic limb. Hopping in the right thoracic and pelvic limbs was decreased to absent. Hopping in the left pelvic limb was mildly decreased. Hopping in the left thoracic limb was normal.

Spinal Reflexes

In the pelvic limbs, the patellar reflex is exaggerated (+3) on the right and normal on the left (+2). The flexor withdrawal reflexes are normal in both pelvic limbs. Muscle tone and muscle mass are normal in the pelvic limbs. In the right thoracic limb, the extensor carpi radialis reflex and the flexor withdrawal reflex are decreased. There is decreased muscular tone in the right thoracic limb. Palpation reveals atrophy of the right supraspinatus, biceps brachii, and triceps muscles. The flexor withdrawal reflex, muscle tone, and muscle mass are normal in the left thoracic limb.

Cranial Nerves

All normal

Sensory Evaluation

Hyperesthesia—none
Superficial pain perception—normal
Deep pain perception—not evaluated

Lesion Location

There are abnormal postural reactions and paresis in all of the limbs except the left thoracic limb, indicating neurologic dysfunction of these limbs. Despite this, the dog is significantly worse on the right side; right hemiparesis. The right hemiparesis is characterized by LMN paresis in the thoracic limb and UMN paresis in the pelvic limb. The lesion is most likely affecting the C6-T2 spinal cord segments. This dog did not manifest any evidence of paraspinal hyperesthesia, which may suggest that compressive or inflammatory diseases affecting pain-sensitive structures (meninges, spinal nerves, or spinal ganglia) are less likely.

Differential Diagnosis

1. Fibrocartilaginous embolism
2. Cervical intervertebral disk disease
3. Myelitis
4. Trauma
5. Neoplasia

Diagnostic Plan

1. Spinal radiography may be helpful in excluding an obvious vertebral fracture or luxation. May also provide evidence of intervertebral disc disease.
2. Imaging with myelography/CT or MRI will identify compressive myelopathy; MRI is more sensitive for evaluating the spinal cord and identifying the extent of the lesion.
3. Cerebrospinal fluid will identify any evidence of meningomyelitis

Diagnostic Results

Spinal radiography was within normal limits. Sagittal T2-weighted MRI disclosed an intraaxial hyperintensity extending from C5 to C7 spinal cord segment. The lesion was primarily located on the right side of the spinal cord on axial plane T2-weighted images. Analysis of cerebrospinal fluid obtained from the cerebellomedullary cistern contained 1 WBC/μL and 25 mg/dL protein (reference range < 24 mg/dL).

Diagnosis

Based on the findings of the MRI, spinal cord infarction presumably caused by a fibrocartilaginous embolism (FCE). Other supportive evidence includes history of an acute onset. Additionally asymmetric neurologic deficits and lack of paraspinal support FCE as the etiology.

Treatment

Based on the presence of voluntary motor function and normal pain perception, the prognosis is favorable for return of function. Treatment for FCE is supportive care and physical rehabilitation. Corticosteroids have not been shown to be of benefit. Rehabilitation included daily exercise in an underwater treadmill. The dog was placed in an underwater treadmill on a daily basis and began to show improved limb movements in the right pelvic limb within 3 days; within 7 days, the right thoracic limb began to show minimal movements. One month after the onset, the dog was ambulating on its own in all limbs but still had residual weakness in the right thoracic limb. The right thoracic limb may always be weak because there may be permanent ischemic injury that resulted in loss of motor neurons.

CASE STUDY 7-3 *ARIZONA*

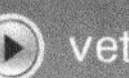 veterinaryneurologycases.com

▪ Signalment
Canine, miniature poodle, male, 11 years old

▪ History
One month ago, lameness developed in the left thoracic limb, progressing to both thoracic limbs within 7 days. Two weeks later, the dog developed general proprioceptive ataxia of both pelvic limbs, and 1 week prior to admission, the dog progressed to nonambulatory tetraparesis. The dog does not wag his tail.

▪ Physical Examination
Grade IV/VI holosystolic murmur with loudest intensity over the cardiac apex suggestive of mitral valve regurgitation. Lung auscultation revealed crackles.

▪ Neurologic Examination
Mental Status
Alert

Gait
Nonambulatory tetraparesis

Posture
Sternal recumbency

Postural Reactions
Absent in all limbs

Spinal Reflexes
Patellar reflex and extensor carpi radialis reflexes were exaggerated (+3) on the right side; flexor withdrawal reflexes were intact in all limbs.

Cranial Nerves
All normal

Sensory Evaluation
Hyperesthesia—paraspinal pain on palpation of the cervical vertebral column
Superficial pain perception—normal
Deep pain perception—not evaluated

▪ Lesion Location
The neurologic examination reveals UMN tetraparesis. There is no evidence of intracranial disease (i.e., abnormal mental status or cranial nerve dysfunction). Consequently, the lesion localization is between the C1 and C5 spinal cord segments. Other important clinical findings include paraspinal hyperesthesia and the progressive clinical signs.

▪ Differential Diagnosis
1. Cervical intervertebral disk disease
2. Neoplasia
3. Meningomyelitis
4. Discospondylitis

▪ Diagnostic Plan
1. Spinal radiography will determine presence of bony lesions such as a primary vertebral tumor or discospondylitis. Findings suggestive of intervertebral disk disease may also be identified.
2. Imaging with myelography/CT or MRI will identify compressive myelopathy; MRI is more sensitive for evaluating the spinal cord and identifying the extent of the lesion.
3. Cerebrospinal fluid will identify any evidence of meningomyelitis

▪ Diagnostic Results
Spinal radiography revealed in situ mineralization at the nucleus pulposus of the C2-3 intervertebral disk. Myelography disclosed a pattern consistent with an extradural compressive lesion at C2-3. Prior to injection of iodinated contrast medium, analysis of CSF contained 10 WBC/μL (reference range <5 cells/μL, 40 mg/dL protein (reference range <24 mg/dL). Cellular differential was 30% neutrophils, 40% mononuclear cells, and 30% macrophages.

▪ Diagnosis
Although this dog had other medical problems, diagnostics and surgery were recommended because of the severity of clinical signs. Had the clinical signs been less severe, evaluation of the heart murmur and crackles would have been pursued. Imaging findings are suggestive of Hansen type I IVDD. The findings on CSF analysis are typical of a mild inflammatory response associated with a compressive myelopathy.

▪ Treatment
A ventral slot procedure was performed at the C2-3 IVD space. A large amount of "chalky" material typical of degenerative IVD material was removed from the vertebral canal. Final diagnosis was a Hansen type I IVD extrusion. After surgery, the dog recovered well and was ambulatory with support at discharge. Other concurrent medical conditions were treated.

CASE STUDY 7-4 *LUKE*

 veterinaryneurologycases.com

▪ Signalment
Canine, toy poodle, male, 1 year old

▪ History
Five weeks prior, the dog experienced severe neck pain and could not walk up or down the stairs. The dog held the head slightly flexed, and the neck was stiff. One week prior, the dog bumped his head, cried out in pain, fell down, and became stiff in all limbs. The dog cries out when the head or neck is moved.

▪ Physical Examination
The dog was 5% dehydrated. Cranial palpation revealed a fontanelle.

▪ Neurologic Examination
Mental Status
Alert, anticipates pain when neck is touched

Gait
Nonambulatory tetraparesis

CASE STUDY 7-4 *LUKE*—cont'd

Posture
Extensor rigidity/spasticity in all limbs, and neck is extended.

Postural Reactions
Symmetrical abnormalities were observed. Proprioceptive positioning was reduced in the thoracic limbs and absent in the pelvic limbs. Hopping was reduced in the thoracic limbs and absent in the pelvic limbs.

Spinal Reflexes
Patellar and extensor carpi radialis reflexes were exaggerated (+3). The flexor withdrawal reflexes were intact in all limbs. Muscle tone was increased. No muscle atrophy was observed.

Cranial Nerves
All normal

Sensory Evaluation
Hyperesthesia—present in the cranial cervical vertebral column. There was resistance of the neck on lateral manipulation.
Superficial pain perception—normal
Deep pain perception—not assessed

▪ Lesion Location
The neurologic examination reveals UMN tetraparesis with no evidence of intracranial disease. The clinical course suggests a progressive disease. Taking into account the area of paraspinal hyperesthesia and spinal reflexes, lesion location is between the C1 and C5 spinal cord segments. The signalment highly suggests an anomalous condition such as atlantoaxial (A/A) subluxation. With this differential, the neck should not be further manipulated, and neck flexion should be avoided at all times.

▪ Differential Diagnosis
1. Congenital/anomalous
   a. Atlantoaxial subluxation
   b. Caudal occipital malformation syndrome
2. Trauma
3. Meningomyelitis

▪ Diagnostic Plan
1. Radiography of the cervical vertebrae to evaluate for vertebral anomalies
2. MRI of the cervical vertebral column to detect spinal cord anomalies
3. CSF analysis should not be performed from the cerebellomedullary cistern until an atlantoaxial subluxation is ruled out.

▪ Diagnostic Results
Spinal radiography revealed caudal and dorsal displacement of the spinous process of C2 from the dorsal arch of C1, indicative of AA subluxation. An MRI was performed to rule out concurrent or secondary pathology as well as other congenital cervical malformations. Aside from spinal cord compression at the AA articulation, there was no evidence of additional spinal cord pathology on MRI. Collection of CSF was not performed.

▪ Diagnosis
The diagnosis was AA subluxation.

▪ Treatment
Surgical stabilization was recommended. A ventral approach to the C1-2 vertebrae was made to perform transarticular stabilization. A bone graft was placed between the ventral AA articulation. The dog recovered well from the surgery. A soft-padded bandage was applied for 6 weeks in order to minimize neck movement until the joint arthrodesis was complete. Upon recheck examination 6 weeks after the surgery, the dog was ambulating well, and radiography showed evidence of bony fusion.

CASE STUDY 7-5 *BORIS*

 veterinaryneurologycases.com

▪ Signalment
Canine, Labrador retriever, mixed-breed, 6-year-old FS

▪ History
Four weeks prior to admission, the dog began to walk with a stiff gait in all limbs. The owner also noticed muscle atrophy. One week prior to admission, the dog appeared painful during eating and drinking. There was a copious amount of saliva in the water bowl.

▪ Physical Examination
Normal with the exception that the dog is thin.

▪ Neurologic Examination
Mental Status
Alert

Gait
Stiff, short strided in all limbs, and the dog could only ambulate a short distance before sitting down.

Posture
Mild kyphosis at the thoracolumbar junction

Postural Reactions
Postural reactions were normal in all limbs.

Spinal Reflexes
Spinal reflexes were normal in all limbs. Generalized muscle atrophy of the appendicular and epaxial muscles. The temporalis and masseter muscles were also severely atrophied. There was asymmetry in loss of muscle mass in various muscle groups. There was severe loss of muscle mass of the head involving those of mastication.

CASE STUDY 7-5 *BORIS*—cont'd

Cranial Nerves
Gag reflex was decreased.

Sensory Evaluation
Hyperesthesia—none
Superficial pain perception—normal
Deep pain perception—not assessed

▪ Lesion Location

The neurologic examination is suspicious for a diffuse disorder affecting the lower motor neuron unit–neuromuscular system. A key historical finding in this dog is exercise intolerance, which may suggest myopathy or disease of the neuromuscular junction. There appeared to be no fatigue of the reflexes (e.g., palpebral), which makes a disorder of the neuromuscular junction such as myasthenia gravis less likely than myopathy. Generalized myopathy can affect any muscle group, including the pharyngeal muscles and esophagus.

▪ Differential Diagnosis

1. Infectious myositis
2. Immune-mediated polymyositis
3. Neuromuscular diseases such as myasthenia gravis; however the atrophy is not typical for MG.
4. Metabolic, endocrine, toxic
5. Neoplasia—paraneoplastic syndrome
6. Degenerative

▪ Diagnostic Plan

1. A minimum database (complete blood count, biochemical profile, and urinalysis) is performed to identify metabolic disease or to provide evidence for specialized testing to confirm endocrine or toxic disorders. Creatine kinase levels should be performed to identify myopathic disorders.
2. Radiography of the chest and abdominal ultrasound were performed to rule out paraneoplastic myopathy/neuropathy.
3. Electromyography and direct nerve stimulation tests may help differentiate myopathy from neuropathy and define which muscles or nerves are affected; rarely provide definitive diagnosis. Repetitive nerve stimulation may provide evidence of myasthenia gravis.
4. PCR testing for hepatozoonosis (if suggestive based on minimum database)
5. Edrophonium hydrochloride (Tensilon) testing; provocative testing for myasthenia gravis (if suggestive based on minimum database and electrophysiology)
6. Muscle and/or nerve biopsy will further assist defining the character of the disease process (i.e., inflammatory, degenerative, endocrine related).

▪ Diagnostic Results

CBC, chemistry profile, and urinalysis were within normal limits. The CK levels were 8000 IU/L (normal 51 to 519 IU/L). Thoracic radiographs and abdominal ultrasound were within normal limits. The EMG revealed complex repetitive discharges in multiple muscle groups of all the limbs, spine, and epaxial muscles. Nerve conduction studies were within normal limits. A muscle biopsy was performed. A joint tap and CSF analysis were still performed to rule out evidence of inflammatory disease elsewhere. Histopathology of the muscle revealed variation in myofiber size and inflammation within the endomysium. Serology for *Toxoplasma* spp. and *Neospora caninum* were negative.

▪ Diagnosis

Immune-mediated polymyositis was suspected. Other differentials for infectious disease and paraneoplastic disease have been ruled out.

▪ Treatment

Pending serology, the dog was initially placed on clindamycin, 15 mg/kg every 12 hours per os, for presumed protozoal myositis. Once serologic tests were negative, treatment would include immunosuppressive therapy. Prednisone at 2 mg/kg every 12 hours per os was added. The dog began to show improvement in muscle strength within 2 weeks; however, the side effects were unacceptable to the owner. Consequently, azathioprine, 1 mg/kg every 24 hours, was added so the prednisone dose could be reduced to 1 mg/kg every other day. This regimen was maintained for 1 month, and then the therapies were slowly decreased over 6 months. The dog continued to improve.

CASE STUDY 7-6 *LILA*

 veterinaryneurologycases.com

▪ Signalment

Pit bull, female, spayed, 6 years old

▪ History

Four weeks prior to admission, the dog began to walk with a stiff gait in the pelvic limbs. One week prior to admission, the dog appeared to have difficulty walking in all limbs and could not make it to the door the morning of admission. The owner noted undigested food in the yard.

▪ Physical Examination

During physical examination, the dog demonstrated at wet cough.

▪ Neurologic Examination

Mental Status
Alert

Gait
Unable to ambulate

Posture
Sternal recumbency

Postural Reactions
Proprioceptive positioning was normal when the dog was supported.

Spinal Reflexes
Spinal reflexes were intact, but the patellar reflex was difficult to assess at times.

Cranial Nerves
Gag reflex was decreased. The palpebral reflex was reduced after tapping on the lateral canthi a couple of times.

CASE STUDY 7-6 *LILA*—cont'd

Sensory Evaluation

Hyperesthesia—none
Superficial pain perception—normal
Deep pain perception—not assessed

▪ Lesion Location

The neurologic examination suggests a neuromuscular problem. The exercise intolerance may suggest muscle or neuromuscular junction disease. Fatiguing of the reflexes suggest neuromuscular weakness.

▪ Differential Diagnosis

1. Degenerative
2. Myasthenia gravis
3. Myopathy

▪ Diagnostic Plan

1. A systemic workup because of the physical examination abnormalities. Creatine kinase levels were requested.
2. Radiography of the chest and abdominal ultrasound were performed to rule out neoplasia and investigate for megaesophagus and aspiration pneumonia.
3. Tensilon test
4. Acetylcholine receptor antibody titer
5. Serology for infectious disease (e.g., *Toxoplasma* spp., *Neospora caninum*)

▪ Diagnostic Results

CBC, chemistry profile, and urinalysis were within normal limits. The CK levels were normal. Thoracic radiographs revealed evidence of megaesophagus but no evidence of aspiration pneumonia. A Tensilon test was performed by injecting 0.1 mg/kg edrophonium chloride IV. An IV catheter was placed prior to the injection, and atropine 0.02 mg/kg was administered to limit the muscarinic side effects. One minute after administration, the dog was able to get up on all limbs and ambulate a short distance.

▪ Diagnosis

Acquired myasthenia gravis. Confirmation of the diagnosis can only be performed by evaluating for antibodies against the acetylcholine receptor. The titer results were above the normal reference range. This dog had the generalized form of MG evidenced by appendicular limb weakness and megaesophagus. Chest radiographs did not reveal presence of thymoma, which can be an underlying cause of MG.

▪ Treatment

In acquired MG, there are three major modalities of therapeutic intervention: anticholinesterase therapy, immunomodulatory therapy, and thymectomy. In veterinary medicine, anticholinesterase therapy is most widely accepted. Long-acting anticholinesterase drugs prolong the action of ACh at the neuromuscular junction by reversibly inhibiting acetylcholinesterase. The agent most often used is pyridostigmine bromide (Mestinon, 0.5 to 3 mg/kg every 8 to 12 hours by mouth). To avoid overstimulation of ACh receptors, patients are started at the low end of the dosage range, and the dose is gradually increased to effect. Oral pyridostigmine is available in tablet and syrup form. Some patients cannot tolerate the oral form of medication because of frequent regurgitation from megaesophagus. In these dogs, intramuscular neostigmine bromide can be administered at 0.4 mg/kg. The dosages are titrated to an optimal level based on changes in muscle strength.

This dog responded well to the pyridostigmine bromide. Titers were reevaluated monthly and were within the normal reference range after 2 months. Spontaneous remission including resolution of the megaesophagus should be considered. Aspiration pneumonia can be a fatal complication of megaesophagus.

REFERENCES

1. Cherrone KL, Dewey CW, Coates JR, et al: A retrospective comparison of cervical intervertebral disk disease in nonchondrodystrophic large dogs versus small dogs, J Am Anim Hosp Assoc 40(4):316–320, 2004.
2. Hoerlein BF: Intervertebral Disc Disease. In Oliver JE, Hoerlein BF, Mayhew IG, editors: Veterinary Neurology, Philadelphia, 1987, W.B. Saunders, pp 321–341.
3. Dallman MJ, Palettas P, Bojrab MJ: Characteristics of dogs admitted for treatment of cervical intervertebral disk disease: 105 cases (1972-1982), J Am Vet Med Assoc 200(12):2009–2011, 1992.
4. Foss RR, Genetzky RM, Riedesel EA, et al: Cervical intervertebral disc protrusion in two horses, Can Vet J 24:188–191, 1983.
5. Nixon AJ, Stashak TS, Ingram JT, et al: Cervical intervertebral disk protrusion in a horse, Vet Surg 13(3):154–158, 1984.
6. King AS, Smith RN: Disc protrusions in the cat: Distribution of dorsal protrusions along the vertebral column, Vet Rec 72:335–337, 1960.
7. King AS, Smith RN: Disc protrusions in the cat: Age incidence of dorsal protrusions, Vet Rec 72:381–383, 1960.
8. Gage ED: Disc syndrome in the large breed of dog, J Am Anim Hosp Assoc 5:93–98, 1969.
9. Morgan PW, Parent J, Holmberg DL: Cervical pain secondary to intervertebral disc disease in dogs; radiographic findings and surgical implications, Prog Vet Neurol 4(3):76–80, 1993.
10. Felts JF, Prata RG: Cervical disk disease in the dog: intraforaminal and lateral extrusions, J Am Anim Hosp Assoc 19:755–760, 1983.
11. Waters DJ: Nonambulatory tetraparesis secondary to cervical disk disease in the dog, J Am Anim Hosp Assoc 25:647–653, 1989.
12. Olsson SE: The dynamic factor in spinal cord compression: A study on dogs with special reference to cervical disc protrusions, J Neurosurg 15:308–312, 1958.
13. Griffiths IR: A syndrome produce by dorsolateral "explosions" of the cervical intervertebral discs, Vet Rec 87:737–741, 1970.
14. Hillman RB, Kengeri SS, Waters DJ: Reevaluation of predictive factors for complete recovery in dogs with nonambulatory tetraparesis secondary to cervical disk herniation, J Am Anim Hosp Assoc 45(4):155–163, 2009.

15. Forterre F, Konar M, Tomek A, et al: Accuracy of the withdrawal reflex for localization of the site of cervical disk herniation in dogs: 35 cases (2004-2007), J Am Vet Med Assoc 232(4):559–563, 2008.
16. Bagley RS, Stefanacci JD, Hansen B, et al: Dysphonia in two dogs with cranial cervical intervertebral disk extrusion, J Am Anim Hosp Assoc 29(6):557–559, 1993.
17. Somerville ME, Anderson SM, Gill PJ, et al: Accuracy of localization of cervical intervertebral disk extrusion or protrusion using survey radiography in dogs, J Am Anim Hosp Assoc 37(6):563–572, 2001.
18. Drees R, Dennison SE, Keuler NS, et al: Computed tomographic imaging protocol for the canine cervical and lumbar spine, Vet Radiol Ultrasound 50(1):74–79, 2009.
19. Ryan TM, Platt SR, Llabres-Diaz FJ, et al: Detection of spinal cord compression in dogs with cervical intervertebral disc disease by magnetic resonance imaging, Vet Rec 163(1):11–15, 2008.
20. Levitski RE, Lipsitz D, Chauvet AE: Magnetic resonance imaging of the cervical spine in 27 dogs, Vet Radiol Ultrasound 40(4):332–341, 1999.
21. Russell SW, Griffiths RC: Recurrence of cervical disc syndrome in surgically and conservatively treated dogs, J Am Vet Med Assoc 153:1412–1416, 1968.
22. Levine JM, Levine GJ, Johnson SI, et al: Evaluation of the success of medical management for presumptive cervical intervertebral disk herniation in dogs, Vet Surg 36(5):492–499, 2007.
23. Swaim SF: Ventral decompression of the cervical spinal cord in the dog, J Am Vet Med Assoc 164(5):491–495, 1974.
24. Funkquist B: Decompressive laminectomy for cervical disk protrusion in the dog, Acta Vet Scand 3:88–101, 1962.
25. Gill PJ, Lippincott CL, Anderson SM: Dorsal laminectomy in the treatment of cervical intervertebral disk disease in small dogs: a retrospective study of 30 cases, J Am Anim Hosp Assoc 32(1):77–80, 1996.
26. Lipsitz D, Bailey CS: Lateral approach for cervical spinal cord decompression, Prog Vet Neurol 3(1):39–44, 1992.
27. Lipsitz D, Bailey CS: Clinical use of the lateral cervical approach for cervical spinal cord and nerve root disease: eight cases, Prog Vet Neurol 6(2):60–65, 1995.
28. Tomlinson J: Tetraparesis following cervical disk fenestration in two dogs, J Am Vet Med Assoc 187(1):76–77, 1985.
29. Denny HR: The surgical treatment of cervical disc protrusions in the dog: a review of 40 cases, J Small Anim Pract 19:251–257, 1978.
30. Lincoln JD, Pettit GD: Evaluation of fenestration for treatment of degenerative disc disease in the caudal cervical region of large dogs, Vet Surg 14(3):240–246, 1985.
31. Lemarié RJ, Kerwin SC, Partington BP, Hosgood G: Vertebral subluxation following ventral cervical decompression in the dog, J Am Anim Hosp Assoc 36(4):348–358, 2000.
32. Java MA, Drobatz KJ, Gilley RS, et al: Incidence of and risk factors for postoperative pneumonia in dogs anesthetized for diagnosis or treatment of intervertebral disk disease, J Am Vet Med Assoc 235(3):281–287, 2009.
33. Toombs JP: Cervical intervertebral disk disease in dogs, Compend Contin Educ Pract Vet 14(11):1477–1487, 1992.
34. Fitch RB, Kerwin SC, Hosgood G: Caudal cervical intervertebral disk diseases in the small dog: role of distraction and stabilization in ventral slot decompression, J Am Anim Hosp Assoc 36:68–74, 2000.
35. Chambers JN, Oliver JE Jr, Bjorling DE: Update on ventral decompression for caudal cervical disk herniation in Dobermann pinschers, J Am Anim Hosp Assoc 22:775–778, 1986.
36. Stone EA, Betts CW, Chambers JN: Cervical fractures in the dog: a literature and case review, J Am Anim Hosp Assoc 14(4):463–471, 1979.
37. Hawthorne JC, Blevins WE, Wallace LJ, et al: Cervical vertebral fractures in 56 dogs: a retrospective study, J Am Anim Hosp Assoc 35(2):135–146, 1999.
38. Abramson CJ, Platt SR, Stedman NL: Tetraparesis in a cat with fibrocartilagenous emboli, J Am Anim Hosp Assoc 38:153–156, 2002.
39. Gandini G, Cizinauskas S, Lang J, et al: Fibrocartilaginous embolism in 75 dogs: clinical findings and factors influencing the recovery rate, J Small Anim Pract 44:76–80, 2003.
40. Cauzinille L, Kornegay JN: Fibrocartilaginous embolism of the spinal cord in dogs: review of 36 histologically confirmed cases and retrospective study of 26 suspected cases, J Vet Intern Med 10(4):241–245, 1996.
41. MacKay AD, Rusbridge C, Sparkes AH, et al: MRI characteristics of suspected acute spinal cord infarction in two cats, and a review of the literature, J Feline Med Surg 7(2):101–107, 2005.
42. De Risio L, Adams V, Dennis R, et al: Association of clinical and magnetic resonance imaging findings with outcome in dogs suspected to have ischemic myelopathy: 50 cases (2000-2006), J Am Vet Med Assoc 233(1):129–135, 2008.
43. Duncan ID: Abnormalities of myelination of the central nervous system associated with congenital tremor, J Vet Intern Med 1(1):10–23, 1987.
44. Duncan ID, Hammang JP, Jackson KF: Myelin mosaicism in female heterozygotes of the canine shaking pup and myelin-deficient rat mutants, Brain Res 402(1):168–172, 1987.
45. Palmer AC, Blakemore WF, Wallace ME, et al: Recognition of 'trembler', a hypomyelinating condition in the Bernese mountain dog, Vet Rec 120(26):609–612, 1987.
46. Kornegay JN, Goodwin MA, Spyridakis LK: Hypomyelination in Weimaraner dogs, Acta Neuropathol (Berl) 72(4):394–401, 1987.
47. Cummings JF, Summers BA, de Lahunta A, et al: Tremors in Samoyed pups with oligodendrocyte deficiencies and hypomyelination, Acta Neuropathol (Berl) 71(3-4):267–277, 1986.
48. Mayhew IG, Blakemore WF, Palmer AC, et al: Tremor syndrome and hypomyelination in Lurcher pups, J Small Anim Pract 25:551–559, 1984.
49. Greene CE, Vandevelde M, Hoff EJ: Congenital cerebrospinal hypomyelinogenesis in a pup, J Am Vet Med Assoc 171(6):534–536, 1977.
50. Stoffregen DA, Huxtable CR, Cummings JF, et al: Hypomyelination of the central nervous system of two Siamese kitten littermates, Vet Pathol 30(4):388–391, 1993.
51. Bradley R, Done JT: Nervous and muscular systems. In Leman AD, Straw B, Clock RD, editors: Diseases of Swine, Ames, 1986, Iowa State University Press, pp 73.
52. Blakemore WF, Harding JD, Done JT: Ultrastructural observations on the spinal cord of a Landrace pig with congenital tremor type AIII, Res Vet Sci 17(2):174–178, 1974.

53. Blakemore WF, Harding JD: Ultrastructural observations on the spinal cords of piglets affected with congenital tremor type AIV, Res Vet Sci 17(2):248–255, 1974.
54. Bolske G, Kronevi T, Lindgren NO: Congenital tremor in pigs in Sweden, Nord Vet Med 30:534–537, 1978.
55. Young S: Hypomyelinogenesis congenita (cerebellar ataxia) in Angus-Shorthorn calves, Cornell Vet 52(23):394, 1962.
56. Saunders LZ, Sweet JD, Martin SM, et al: Hereditary congenital ataxia in Jersey calves, Cornell Vet 42:559–591, 1952.
57. Hulland TJ: Cerebellar ataxia in calves, Can J Comp Med 2172–2176, 1957.
58. Physick-Sheard PW, Hopkins JB, O'Connor RD: A border disease-like syndrome in a southern Ontario sheep flock, Can Vet J 21:53–60, 1980.
59. Palmer AC, Medd RK, Wilkinson GT: Spinal cord degeneration in hound ataxia, J Small Anim Pract 25:139–148, 1984.
60. Palmer AC, Medd RK: Hound ataxia, Vet Rec 122(11):263, 1988.
61. Sheahan BJ, Caffrey JF, Gunn HM, et al: Structural and biochemical changes in a spinal myelinopathy in twelve English foxhounds and two harriers, Vet Pathol 28(2):117–124, 1991.
62. Oevermann A, Bley T, Konar M, et al: A novel leukoencephalomyelopathy of Leonberger dogs, J Vet Intern Med 22:467–471, 2008.
63. Cockrell BY, Herigstad RR, Flo GL, et al: Myelomalacia in Afghan hounds, J Am Vet Med Assoc 16(2):362–365, 1973.
64. Cummings JF, de Lahunta A: Hereditary myelopathy of Afghan hounds, a myelinolytic disease, Acta Neuropathol (Berl) 42(3):173–181, 1978.
65. Averill DR, Bronson RT: Inherited necrotizing myelopathy of Afghan hounds, J Neuropathol Exp Neurol 36:734–747, 1977.
66. Douglas SW, Palmer AC: Idiopathic demyelination of brainstem and cord in a miniature poodle puppy, J Pathol Bact 8:267–271, 1961.
67. Mandigers PJJ, van Nes JJ, Knol BW, et al: Hereditary Kooiker dog ataxia, Res Vet Sci 54:118–123, 1993.
68. Gamble DA, Chrisman CL: A leukoencephalomyelopathy of rottweiler dogs, Vet Pathol 21(3):274–280, 1984.
69. Wouda W, van Nes JJ: Progressive ataxia due to central demyelination in Rottweiler dogs, Vet Quart 8:89–97, 1986.
70. Wood SL, Patterson JS: Shetland Sheepdog Leukodystrophy, J Vet Intern Med 15:486–493, 2001.
71. Li FY, Cuddon PA, Song J, et al: Canine spongiform leukoencephalopathy is associated with a missense mutation in cytochrome b, Neurobiol Dis 2:135–142, 2006.
72. O'Brien DP, Zachary JF: Clinical features of spongy degeneration of the central nervous system in two Labrador retriever littermates, J Am Vet Med Assoc 186(11):1207–1210, 1985.
73. Zachary JF, O'Brien DP: Spongy degeneration of the central nervous system in two canine littermates, Vet Pathol 22:561–571, 1985.
74. Neer TM, Kornegay JN: Leucoencephalomalacia and cerebral white matter vacuolar degeneration in two related Labrador retriever puppies, J Vet Intern Med 9(2):100–104, 1995.
75. Jones BR, Alley MR, Shimada A, Lyon M: An encephalomyelopathy in related Birman kittens, N Z Vet J 40(4):160–163, 1992.
76. Hafner A, Dahme E, Obermaier G, et al: Spinal dysmyelination in new-born Brown Swiss X Braunvieh calves, Zentralbl Veterinarmed B 40:413–422, 1993.
77. Agerholm JS, Andersen O: Ineritance of spinal dysmyelination in calves, Zentralbl Veterinarmed A 42:9–12, 1995.
78. Nissen PH, Shukri NM, Agerholm JS: Genetic mapping of spinal dysmyelination in cross-bred American Brown Swiss cattle to Bovine chromosome 11, Mamm Genome 12:180–182, 2001.
79. Richards RB, Edwards JR: A progressive spinal myelinopathy in beef cattle, Vet Pathol 23(1):35–41, 1986.
80. Palmer AC, Jackson PGG: A primary demyelinating disorder of young cattle, Neuropathol Appl Neurobiol 17:457–467, 1991.
81. Fletcher TF, Lee DG, Hammer RF: Ultrastructural features of globoid-cell leukodystrophy in the dog, Am J Vet Res 32(1):177–181, 1971.
82. Fankhauser R, Luginbuhl H, Hartley WJ: Leukodystrophie vom typus Krabbe beim hund, Schweizer Archiv Fur Tierheilkunde 105:198–207, 1963.
83. Bjerkas I: Hereditary 'cavitating' leucodystrophy in Dalmatian dogs, Acta Neuropathol (Berl) 40:163–169, 1977.
84. McGrath JT: Fibrinoid leukodystrophy (Alexander's disease). In Andrews EJ, Ward BC, Altman NH, editors: Spontaneous animal models of human disease Vol. 2, New York, 1979, Academic Press.
85. Cox NR, Kwapien RP, Sorjonen DC, et al: Myeloencephalopathy resembling Alexander's disease in a Scottish terrier dog, Acta Neuropathol (Berl) 71 (1-2):163–166, 1986.
86. Sorjonen DC, Cox NR, Kwapien RP: Myeloencephalopathy with eosinophilic refractile bodies (Rosenthal fibers) in a Scottish terrier, J Am Vet Med Assoc 190(8):1004–1006, 1987.
87. Morrison JP, Schatzberg SJ, de Lahunta A, et al: Oligodendroglial dysplasia in two bullmastiff dogs, Vet Pathol 43(1):29–35, 2006.
88. Richardson JA, Tang K, Burns DK: Myeloencephalopathy with Rosenthal fiber formation in a miniature poodle, Vet Pathol 28(6):536–538, 1991.
89. Cordy DR: Progressive ataxia of Charolais cattle-an oligodendroglial dysplasia, Vet Pathol 23(1):78–80, 1986.
90. Palmer AC, Blakemore WF, Barlow RM, et al: Progressive ataxia of Charolais cattle associated with a myelin disorder, Vet Rec 91(24):592–594, 1972.
91. Blakemore WF, Palmer AC, Barlow RM: Progressive ataxia of Charolais cattle associated with disordered myelin, Acta Neuropathol 29(Fasc.2):127–139, 1974.
92. Averill DR Jr: Degenerative myelopathy in the aging German shepherd dog: clinical and pathologic findings, J Am Vet Med Assoc 162(12):1045–1051, 1973.
93. Griffiths IR, Duncan ID: Chronic degenerative radiculomyelopathy in the dog, J Small Anim Pract 16(8):461–471, 1975.
94. Braund KG, Vandevelde M: German shepherd dog myelopathy–a morphologic and morphometric study, Am J Vet Res 39(8):1309–1315, 1978.
95. Awano T, Johnson GS, Wade CM, et al: Genome-wide association analysis reveals a *SOD1* mutation in canine degenerative myelopathy that resembles amyotrophic lateral sclerosis, Proc Natl Acad Sci U S A 106:2794–2799, 2009.
96. Kathmann I, Cizinauskas S, Doherr MG, et al: Daily controlled physiotherapy increases survival time in dogs with suspected degenerative myelopathy, J Vet Intern Med 20:927–932, 2006.

97. Bichsel P, Vandevelde M, Lang J, et al: Degenerative myelopathy in a family of Siberian husky dogs, J Am Vet Med Assoc 183(9):998–1000, 1983.
98. Matthews NS, de Lahunta A: Degenerative myelopathy in an adult miniature poodle, J Am Vet Med Assoc 186(11):1213–1215, 1985.
99. Miller AD, Barber R, Porter BF, et al: Degenerative myelopathy in two boxer dogs, Vet Pathol 46(4):684–687, 2009.
100. Coates JR, March PA, Oglesbee M, et al: Clinical characterization of a familial degenerative myelopathy in Pembroke Welsh Corgi dogs, J Vet Intern Med 21(6):1323–1331, 2007.
101. Long SN, Henthorn PS, Serpell J, et al: Degenerative Myelopathy in Chesapeake Bay Retrievers, J Vet Intern Med 23:401–402, 2009.
102. Bjorck G, Mair W, Olsson S-E, et al: Hereditary ataxia in fox terriers, Acta Neuropathol (Berl) (Suppl 1):45–48, 1962.
103. Hartley WJ, Palmer AC: Ataxia in Jack Russell terriers, Acta Neuropathol (Berl) 26(1):71–74, 1973.
104. Wessman A, Goedde T, Fischer A, et al: Hereditary ataxia in the Jack Russell terrier - Clinical and genetic investigations, J Vet Intern Med 18:515–521, 2004.
105. Summers BA, Cummings JF, de Lahunta A: Degenerative diseases of the central nervous system. In Summers BA, Cummings JF, de Lahunta A, editors: Veterinary Neuropathology, St. Louis, 1995, Mosby, pp 208–350.
106. Wakshlag JJ, de Lahunta A: Hereditary encephalomyelopathy and polyneuropathy in an Alaskan husky, J Small Anim Pract 50:670–674, 2009.
107. Griffiths IR, McCulloch MC, Abrahams S: Progressive axonopathy: an inherited neuropathy of boxer dogs. 3. The peripheral axon lesion with special reference to the nerve roots, J Neurocytol 15(1):109–120, 1986.
108. Griffiths IR: Progressive axonopathy: an inherited neuropathy of Boxer dogs. I. Further studies of the clinical and electrophysiological features, J Small Anim Pract 26(7):381–392, 1985.
109. Griffiths IR, Duncan ID, Barker J: A progressive axonopathy of Boxer dogs affecting the central and peripheral nervous systems, J Small Anim Pract 21(1):29–43, 1980.
110. de Lahunta A, Ingram JT, Cummings JF, et al: Labrador Retriever central axonopathy, Prog Vet Neurol 5(3):117–122, 1994.
111. van Ham L, Vandevelde M, Desmidt M, et al: A tremor syndrome with a central axonopathy in Scottish terriers, J Vet Intern Med 8(4):290–292, 1994.
112. Wright JA, Brownlie S: Progressive ataxia in a Pyrenean mountain dog, Vet Rec 116(15):410–411, 1985.
113. Jolly RD, Burbidge HM, Alley MR, et al: Progressive myelopathy and neuropathy in New Zealand Huntaway dogs, N Z Vet J 48:188–191, 2000.
114. Baranowska I, Jaderlund KH, Nennesmo I, et al: Sensory ataxic neuropathy in golden retriever dogs is caused by a deletion in the mitochondrial *tRNA^{Tyr}* gene, PLoS Genet 5:1–9, 2009.
115. Jaderlund KH, Orvind E, Johnsson E, et al: A neurologic syndrome in golden reterievers presenting as a sensory ataxic neuropathy, J Vet Intern Med 211:307–1315, 2007.
116. Moreau PM, Vallat JM, Hugon J, et al: Peripheral and central distal axonopathy of suspected inherited origin in Birman cats, Acta Neuropathol (Berl) 82(2):143–146, 1991.
117. Mayhew IG, Brown CM, Stowe HD, et al: Equine degenerative myeloencephalopathy: a vitamin E deficiency that may be familial, J Vet Intern Med 1(1):45–50, 1987.
118. Mayhew IG, de Lahunta A, Whitlock RH, et al: Equine degenerative myeloencephalopathy, J Am Vet Med Assoc 170(2):195–201, 1977.
119. Stuart LD, Leipold HW: Lesions in bovine progressive degenerative myeloencephalopathy ("Weaver") of Brown Swiss cattle, Vet Pathol 22(1):13–23, 1985.
120. Harper PA, Hartley WJ, Coverdale OR, et al: Multifocal symmetrical encephalopathy in simmental calves, Vet Rec 124:122–123, 1989.
121. Harper PA, Hartley WJ, Fraser GC, et al: Multifocal encephalopathy in limousin calves, Aust Vet J 67:111–112, 1990.
122. Steffen DJ, Vestweber JG, Cash W, et al: Multifocal subacute necrotizing encephalomyelpathy in Semmental calves, J Vet Diagn Invest 6:466–472, 1994.
123. Harper PAW, Healy PJ: Neurological disease associated with degenerative axonopathy of neonatal Holtein-Friesian calves, Aust Vet J 66:143–146, 1989.
124. Harper PAW, Plant JW, Walker KH, et al: Progressive ataxia associated with degenerative thoracic myelopathy in Merino sheep, Aust Vet J 68(11):357–358, 1991.
125. Morin DE, Toenniessen JG, French RA, et al: Degenerative myeloencephalopathy in two llamas, J Am Vet Med Assoc 204(6):938–943, 1994.
126. Cork LC, Troncoso JC, Price DL, et al: Canine neuroaxonal dystrophy, J Neuropathol Exp Neurol 42(3):286–296, 1983.
127. Chrisman CL, Cork LC, Gamble DA: Neuroaxonal dystrophy of Rottweiler dogs, J Am Vet Med Assoc 184(4):464–467, 1984.
128. Evans MG, Mullaney TP, Lowrie CT: Neuroaxonal dystrophy in a Rottweiler pup, J Am Vet Med Assoc 192(11):1560–1562, 1988.
129. Blakemore WF, Palmer AC: Nervous disease in the chihuahua characterised by axonal swellings, Vet Rec 117(19):498–499, 1985.
130. Clark RG, Hartley WJ, Burgess GS, et al: Suspected inheirited cerebellar neuroaxonal dystrophy in collie sheep dogs, N Z Vet J 30(7):102–103, 1982.
131. Sacre BJ, Cummings JF, de Lahunta A: Neuroaxonal dystrophy in a Jack Russell terrier pup resembling human infantile neuroaxonal dystrophy, Cornell Vet 83(2):133–142, 1993.
132. Duncan ID, Griffiths IR, Carmichael S, et al: Inherited canine giant axonal neuropathy, Muscle Nerve 4(3):223–227, 1981.
133. Duncan ID, Griffiths IR: Canine giant axonal neuropathy, Vet Rec 10:1438–1441, 1977.
134. Diaz JD, Duque C, Geisel R: Neuroaxonal dystrophy in dogs: case report in 2 litters of Papillon puppies, J Vet Intern Med 21:531–534, 2007.
135. Franklin RJM, Jeffery ND, Ramsey IK: Neuroaxonal dystrophy in a litter of papillon pups, J Small Anim Pract 36(10):441–444, 1995.
136. Nibe K, Kita C, Morozumi M, et al: Clinicopathological features of canine neuroaxonal dystrophy and cerebellar cortical abiotrophy in Papillon and Papillon-related dogs, J Vet Med Sci 69(10):1047–1052, 2007.
137. Carmichael KP, Howerth EW, Oliver JE Jr, et al: Neuroaxonal dystrophy in a group of related cats, J Vet Diagn Invest 5(4):585–590, 1993.
138. Woodard JC, Collins GH, Hessler JR: Feline hereditary neuroaxonal dystrophy, Am J Pathol 74(3):551–566, 1974.
139. Hartley WJ, Loomis LN: Murrurundi disease: an encephalopathy of sheep, Aust Vet J 57:399–400, 1981.

140. Cordy DR, Richards WP, Bradford GE: Systemic neuroaxonal dystrophy in Suffolk sheep, Acta Neuropathol 8:133–140, 1967.
141. Beech J, Haskins M: Genetic studies of neuraxonal dystrophy in the Morgan, Am J Vet Res 48(1):109–113, 1987.
142. Beech J: Neuroaxonal dystrophy of the accessory cuneate nucleus in horses, Vet Pathol 21:384–393, 1984.
143. Cummings JF, de Lahunta A, Gasteiger EL: Multisystemic chromatolytic neuronal degeneration in Cairn terriers. A case with generalized cataplectic episodes, J Vet Intern Med 5(2):91–94, 1991.
144. Palmer AC, Blakemore WF: A progressive neuronopathy in the young Cairn Terrier, J Small Anim Pract 30(2):101–106, 1989.
145. Zaal MD, van dan Ingh TSGAM, Goedegebuure SA, et al: Progressive neuronopathy in two Cairn terrier litter mates, Vet Quart 19:34–36, 1997.
146. Jaggy A, Vandevelde M: Multisystem neuronal degeneration in cocker spaniels, J Vet Intern Med 2(3):117–120, 1988.
147. da Costa RC, Parent JM, Poma R, de Lahunta A: Multisystem axonopathy and neuronopathy in Golden Retriever dogs, J Vet Intern Med 23:935–939, 2009.
148. Kortz GD, Meier WA, Higgins RJ, et al: Neuronal vacuolation and spinocerebellar degeneration in young Rottweiler dogs, Vet Pathol 34(4):296–302, 1997.
149. Summers BA, Cummings JF, de Lahunta A: Veterinary Neuropathology, St. Louis, 1995, Mosby, 189-207.
150. Duncan ID: Abnormalities of myelination of the central nervous system associated with congenital tremor, J Vet Intern Med 1(1):10–23, 1987.
151. Bjerkas I: Hereditary 'cavitating' leucodystrophy in Dalmatian dogs, Acta Neuropath (Berl) 40:163–169, 1977.
152. McGrath JT: Fibrinoid leukodystrophy (Alexander's disease). In Andrews EJ, Ward BC, Altman NH, editors: Spontaneous animal models of human disease vol. 2, New York, 1979, Academic Press.
153. Cox NR, Kwapien RP, Sorjonen DC, et al: Myeloencephalopathy resembling Alexander's disease in a Scottish terrier dog, Acta Neuropathol (Berl) 71(1-2):163–166, 1986.
154. Sorjonen DC, Cox NR, Kwapien RP: Myeloencephalopathy with eosinophilic refractile bodies (Rosenthal fibers) in a Scottish terrier, J Am Vet Med Assoc 190(8):1004–1006, 1987.
155. Morrison JP, Schatzberg SJ, de Lahunta A, et al: Oligodendroglial dysplasia in two bullmastiff dogs, Vet Pathol 43(1):29–35, 2006.
156. Richardson JA, Tang K, Burns DK: Myeloencephalopathy with Rosenthal fiber formation in a miniature poodle, Vet Pathol 28(6):536–538, 1991.
157. Cordy DR: Progressive ataxia of Charolais cattle-an oligodendroglial dysplasia, Vet Pathol 23(1):78–80, 1986.
158. Millar M, Scholes S, Morris M: Progressive ataxia of Charolais cattle, Vet Rec 154(12):379, 2004.
159. Zicker SC, Kasari TR, Scruggs DW, et al: Progressive ataxia in a Charolais bull, J Am Vet Med Assoc 192(11):1590–1592, 1988.
160. Oevermann A, Bley T, Konar M, et al: A novel leukoencephalomyelopathy of Leonberger dogs, J Vet Intern Med 22:467–471, 2008.
161. Averill DR, Bronson RT: Inherited necrotizing myelopathy of Afghan hounds, J Neuropathol Exp Neurol 36:734–747, 1977.
162. Cockrell BY, Herigstad RR, Flo GL, et al: Myelomalacia in Afghan hounds, J Am Vet Med Assoc 162362–162365, 1973.
163. Cummings JF, de Lahunta A: Hereditary myelopathy of Afghan hounds, a myelinolytic disease, Acta Neuropathol (Berl) 42(3):173–181, 1978.
164. Douglas SW, Palmer AC: Idiopathic demyelination of brain-stem and cord in a miniature poodle puppy, J Pathol Bact 82:67–71, 1961.
165. Gamble DA, Chrisman CL: A leukoencephalomyelopathy of rottweiler dogs, Vet Pathol 21(3):274–280, 1984.
166. Wouda W, van Nes JJ: Progressive ataxia due to central demyelination in Rottweiler dogs, Vet Quart 8:89–97, 1986.
167. Mandigers PJJ, van Nes JJ, Knol BW, et al: Hereditary Kooiker dog ataxia, Res Vet Sci 54:118–123, 1993.
168. Wood SL, Patterson JS: Shetland Sheepdog Leukodystrophy, J Vet Intern Med 15:486–493, 2001.
169. Li FY, Cuddon PA, Song J, et al: Canine spongiform leukoencephalopathy is associated with a missense mutation in cytochrome b, Neurobiol Dis 2:135–142, 2006.
170. O'Brien DP, Zachary JF: Clinical features of spongy degeneration of the central nervous system in two Labrador retriever littermates, J Am Vet Med Assoc 186(11):1207–1210, 1985.
171. Zachary JF, O'Brien DP: Spongy degeneration of the central nervous system in two canine littermates, Vet Pathol 22:561–571, 1985.
172. Richards RB, Edwards JR: A progressive spinal myelinopathy in beef cattle, Vet Pathol 23(1):35–41, 1986.
173. Suzuki K, Suzuki Y: Globoid cell leucodystrophy (Krabbe's disease): deficiency of glactocerebroside beta-galactosidase, Proc Natl Acad Sci U S A 66:302–309, 1970.
174. Fankhauser R, Luginbuhl H, Hartley WJ: Leukodystrophie vom typus Krabbe beim hund, Schweizer Archiv Fur Tierheilkunde 105:198–207, 1963.
175. Cavanagh JB: The significance of the "dying back" process in experimental and human neurological disease, Int Rev Exp Pathol 3:219–267, 1964.
176. Hartley WJ, Palmer AC: Ataxia in Jack Russell terriers, Acta Neuropathol (Berl) 26(1):71–74, 1973.
177. Wessman A, Goedde T, Fischer A, et al: Hereditary ataxia in the Jack Russell terrier - Clinical and genetic investigations, J Vet Intern Med 18:515–521, 2004.
178. Bjorck G, Mair W, Olsson S-E, et al: Hereditary ataxia in fox terriers, Acta Neuropath (Berl) (Suppl 1):45–48, 1962.
179. van Ham L, Vandevelde M, Desmidt M, et al: A tremor syndrome with a central axonopathy in Scottish terriers, J Vet Intern Med 8(4):290–292, 1994.
180. de Lahunta A, Ingram JT, Cummings JF, et al: Labrador Retriever central axonopathy, Prog Vet Neurol 5(3):117–122, 1994.
181. Stuart LD, Leipold HW: Lesions in bovine progressive degenerative myeloencephalopathy ("Weaver") of Brown Swiss cattle, Vet Pathol 22(1):13–23, 1985.
182. Oyster R, Leipold HW, Troyer D, et al: Clinical studies of bovine progressive degenerative myeloencephaly of Brown Swiss cattle, Prog Vet Neurol 2(3):159–164, 1991.
183. Wakshlag JJ, de Lahunta A: Hereditary encephalomyelopathy and polyneuropathy in an Alaskan husky, J Small Anim Pract 50:670–674, 2009.
184. Griffiths IR, McCulloch MC, Abrahams S: Progressive axonopathy: an inherited neuropathy of boxer dogs. 3. The peripheral axon lesion with special reference to the nerve roots, J Neurocytol 15(1):109–120, 1986.

185. Griffiths IR, Duncan ID, Barker J: A progressive axonopathy of Boxer dogs affecting the central and peripheral nervous systems, J Small Anim Pract 21(1):29–43, 1980.
186. Griffiths IR, McCulloch MC, Abrahams S: Progressive axonopathy: an inherited neuropathy of Boxer dogs. 2. The nature and distribution of the pathological changes, Neuropathol Appl Neurobiol 11:431–446, 1985.
187. Wright JA, Brownlie S: Progressive ataxia in a Pyrenean mountain dog, Vet Rec 116(15):410–411, 1985.
188. Jolly RD, Burbidge HM, Alley MR, et al: Progressive myelopathy and neuropathy in New Zealand Huntaway dogs, N Z Vet J 48:188–191, 2000.
189. Coates JR, O'Brien DP: Inherited peripheral neuropathies in dogs and cats, Vet Clin North Am Small Anim Pract 34:1361–1401, 2004.
190. Summers BA, Cummings JF, de Lahunta A: Diseases of the peripheral nervous system. In Summers BA, Cummings JF, de Lahunta A, editors: Veterinary Neuropathology, St. Louis, 1995, Mosby, pp 402–501.
191. Cummings JF, de Lahunta A, Gasteiger EL: Multisystemic chromatolytic neuronal degeneration in Cairn terriers. A case with generalized cataplectic episodes, J Vet Intern Med 5(2):91–94, 1991.
192. Palmer AC, Blakemore WF: A progressive neuronopathy in the young Cairn Terrier, J Small Anim Pract 30(2):101–106, 1989.
193. Zaal MD, van dan Ingh TSGAM, Goedegebuure SA, et al: Progressive neuronopathy in two Cairn terrier litter mates, Vet Quart 19:34–36, 1997.
194. Jaggy A, Vandevelde M: Multisystem neuronal degeneration in cocker spaniels, J Vet Intern Med 2(3):117–120, 1988.
195. da Costa RC, Parent JM, Poma R, et al: Multisystem axonopathy and neuronopathy in Golden Retriever dogs, J Vet Intern Med 23:935–939, 2009.
196. Kortz GD, Meier WA, Higgins RJ, et al: Neuronal vacuolation and spinocerebellar degeneration in young Rottweiler dogs, Vet Pathol 34(4):296–302, 1997.
197. Cork LC, Troncoso JC, Price DL, et al: Canine neuroaxonal dystrophy, J Neuropathol Exp Neurol 42(3):286–296, 1983.
198. Chrisman CL, Cork LC, Gamble DA: Neuroaxonal dystrophy of Rottweiler dogs, J Am Vet Med Assoc 184(4):464–467, 1984.
199. Chrisman CL: Neurological diseases of Rottweilers: neuroaxonal dystrophy and leukoencephalomalacia, J Small Anim Pract 33(10):500–504, 1992.
200. Blakemore WF, Palmer AC: Nervous disease in the chihuahua characterised by axonal swellings, Vet Rec 117(19):498–499, 1985.
201. Clark RG, Hartley WJ, Burgess GS, et al: Suspected inheirited cerebellar neuroaxonal dystrophy in collie sheep dogs, N Z Vet J 30(7):102–103, 1982.
202. Sacre BJ, Cummings JF, de Lahunta A: Neuroaxonal dystrophy in a Jack Russell terrier pup resembling human infantile neuroaxonal dystrophy, Cornell Vet 83(2):133–142, 1993.
203. Duncan ID, Griffiths IR: Canine giant axonal neuropathy; some aspects of its clinical, pathological and comparative features, J Small Anim Pract 22(8):491–501, 1981.
204. Diaz JD, Duque C, Geisel R: Neuroaxonal dystrophy in dogs: case report in 2 litters of Papillon puppies, J Vet Intern Med 21:531–534, 2007.
205. Franklin RJM, Jeffery ND, Ramsey IK: Neuroaxonal dystrophy in a litter of papillon pups, J Small Anim Pract 36(10):441–444, 1995.
206. Carmichael KP, Howerth EW, Oliver JE Jr, et al: Neuroaxonal dystrophy in a group of related cats, J Vet Diagn Invest 5(4):585–590, 1993.
207. Rodriguez F, Espinosa de los Monteros A, Morales M, et al: Neuroaxonal dystrophy in two Siamese kitten littermates, Vet Res 138:548–549, 1996.
208. Woodard JC, Collins GH, Hessler JR: Feline hereditary neuroaxonal dystrophy, Am J Pathol 74(3):551–566, 1974.
209. Cordy DR, Richards WP, Bradford GE: Systemic neuroaxonal dystrophy in Suffolk sheep, Acta Neuropathol 8:133–140, 1967.
210. Mayhew IG: Large Animal Neurology, ed 2, Ames, 2009, Wiley-Blackwell.
211. Beech J, Haskins M: Genetic studies of neuraxonal dystrophy in the Morgan, Am J Vet Res 48(1):109–113, 1987.
212. Toenniessen JG, Morin DE: Degenerative myelopathy: a comparative review, Compend Contin Educ Pract Vet 17(2):271–283, 1995.
213. Miller MM, Collatos C: Equine degenerative myeloencephalopathy, Vet Clin North Am 13:43–52, 1997.
214. Mayhew IG: Measurements of the accuracy of clinical diagnoses of equine neurologic disease, J Vet Intern Med 5(6):332–334, 1991.
215. Mayhew IG, de Lahunta A, Whitlock RH, et al: Equine degenerative myeloencephalopathy, J Am Vet Med Assoc 170(2):195–201, 1977.
216. Adam A, Collatos C, Fuenteabla C, et al: Neuroaxonal dystrophy in a two-year-old quarter horse filly, Can Vet J :3743, 1996.
217. Blythe LL, Craig AM: Equine degenerative myeloencephalopathy. Part I. Clinical signs and pathogenesis, Compend Contin Educ Pract Vet 14(9):1215–1226, 1992.
218. Mayhew IG, Brown CM, Stowe HD, et al: Equine degenerative myeloencephalopathy: a vitamin E deficiency that may be familial, J Vet Intern Med 1(1):45–50, 1987.
219. Dill SG, Correa MT, Erb HN, et al: Factors associated with the development of equine degenerative myeloencephalopathy, Am J Vet Res 51(8):1300–1305, 1990.
220. Blythe LL, Craig AM, Lassen ED, et al: Serially determined plasma α-tocopherol concentrations and results of the oral vitamin E absorption test in clinically normal horses and in horses with degenerative myeloencephalopathy, Am J Vet Res 52(6):908–911, 1991.
221. Dill SG, Kallfelz FA, de Lahunta A, et al: Serum vitamin E and blood glutathione peroxidase values of horses with degenerative myeloencephalopathy, Am J Vet Res 50(1):166–168, 1989.
222. Blythe LL, Craig AM: Equine degenerative myeloencephalopathy. Part II. Diagnosis and treatment, Compend Contin Educ Pract Vet 14(12):1633–1637, 1992.
223. Evans HE: Prenatal Development. In Evans HE, editor: Miller's Anatomy of the Dog, ed 3, Philadelphia, 1993, W.B. Saunders Company, pp 32–97.
224. Watson AG, Stewart JS: Postnatal ossification centers of the atlas and axis in miniature schnauzers, Am J Vet Res 51(2):264–268, 1990.
225. Oliver JE Jr, Lewis RE: Lesions of the atlas and axis in dogs, J Am Anim Hosp Assoc 9(3):304–313, 1973.
226. Bailey CS: An embryological approach to the clinical significance of congenital vertebral and spinal cord abnormalities, J Am Anim Hosp Assoc 11(7):426–434, 1975.
227. Watson AG, de Lahunta A: Atlantoaxial subluxation and absence of transverse ligament of the atlas in a dog, J Am Vet Med Assoc 195(2):235–237, 1989.

228. Evans HE: Arthrology. In Evans HE, editor: Miller's Anatomy of the Dog, Philadelphia, 1993, W.B. Saunders Company, pp 219–257.
229. Cook JR Jr, Oliver JE Jr: Atlantoaxial luxation in the dog, Compend Contin Educ Pract Vet 3(3):242–252, 1981.
230. Beaver DP, Ellison GW, Lewis DD, et al: Risk factors affecting the outcome of surgery for atlantoaxial subluxation in dogs: 46 cases (1978-1998), J Am Vet Med Assoc 216(7):1104–1109, 2000.
231. Huibregtse BA, Smith CW, Fagin BD: Atlantoaxial luxation in a Doberman Pinscher, Canine Pract 17(5):7–10, 1992.
232. Hurov L: Congenital atlantoaxial malformation and acute subluxation in a mature Basset Hound - surgical treatment by wire stabilization, J Am Anim Hosp Assoc 15(2):177–180, 1979.
233. Wheeler SJ: Atlantoaxial subluxation with absence of the dens in a Rottweiler, J Small Anim Pract 33(2):90–93, 1992.
234. Shelton SB, Bellah J, Chrisman C, et al: Hypoplasia of the odontoid process and secondary atlantoaxial luxation in a Siamese cat, Prog Vet Neurol 2(3):209–211, 1991.
235. Slone DE, Bergfeld WA, Walker TL: Surgical decompression for traumatic atlantoaxial subluxation in a weanling filly, J Am Vet Med Assoc 174(11):1234–1236, 1979.
236. Blikslager AT, Wilson DA, Constantinescu GM, et al: Atlantoaxial malformation in a half-Arabian colt, Cornell Vet 81(1):67–75, 1991.
237. White ME, Pennock PW, Seiler RJ: Atlanto-axial subluxation in five young cattle, Can Vet J 19:79–82, 1978.
238. Geary JC, Oliver JE, Hoerlein BF: Atlanto axial subluxation in the canine, J Small Anim Pract 8:577–582, 1967.
239. Beal MW, Paglia DT, Griffin GM, et al: Ventilatory failure, ventilator management, and outcome in dogs with cervical spinal disorders: 14 cases (1991-1999), J Am Vet Med Assoc 218:1598–1602, 2001.
240. Denny HR, Gibbs C, Waterman A: Atlanto-axial subluxation in the dog: a review of thirty cases and an evaluation of treatment by lag screw fixation, J Small Anim Pract 26(1):37–47, 1988.
241. Sanders SG, Bagley RS, Silver GM: Complications associated with ventral screws, pins, and polymethylmethacrylate for the treatment of atlantoaxial instability of 8 dogs, J Vet Intern Med 14(3):339, 2000.
242. Kent M, Eagleson JS, Neravanda D, et al: Intraaxial spinal cord hemorrhage secondary to atlantoaxial subluxation in a dog, J Am Anim Hosp Assoc 46(2):132–137, 2010.
243. Havig ME, Cornell KK, Hawthorne JC, et al: Evaluation of nonsurgical treatment of atlantoaxial subluxation in dogs, J Am Vet Med Assoc 227:257–262, 2005.
244. Lorinson D, Bright RM, Thomas WB, et al: Atlanto-axial subluxation in dogs: the results of conservative and surgical therapy, Canine Pract 23(3):16–18, 1998.
245. Gilmore DR: Nonsurgical management of four cases of atlantoaxial subluxation in the dog, J Am Anim Hosp Assoc 20(1):93–96, 1984.
246. Sharp NJH, Wheeler SJ: Small Animal Spinal Disorders: Diagnosis and Surgery, London, 2005, Elsevier, 1–379.
247. Swaim SF, Greene CE: Odontoidectomy in a dog, J Am Anim Hosp Assoc 11(5):663–667, 1975.
248. Johnson SG, Hulse DA: Odontoid dysplasia with atlantoaxial instability in a dog, J Am Anim Hosp Assoc 25(4):400–408, 1989.
249. Sorjonen DC, Shires PK: Atlantoaxial instability: a ventral surgical technique for decompression, fixation, and fusion, Vet Surg 10(1):22–29, 1981.
250. Sharp NJH, Wheeler SJ: Atlantoaxial subluxation. In Sharp NJH, Wheeler SJ, editors: Small Animal Spinal Disorders: Diagnosis and Surgery, ed 2, Edinburgh, 2005, Elsevier, pp 161–180.
251. Knipe MF, Sturges BK, Vernau KM et al. Atlantoaxial instability in 17 dogs. In Proceedings of the 20th Annual ACVIM Forum Dallas, TX, May 29-June 1, 2002.
252. Sanders SG, Bagley RS, Silver GM, et al: Outcomes and complications associated with ventral screws, pins, and polymethylmethacrylate for atlantoaxial instability in 12 dogs, J Am Anim Hosp Assoc 40:204–210, 2004.
253. Platt SR, Chambers JN, Cross A: A modified ventral fixation for surgical management of atlantoaxial subluxation in 19 dogs, Vet Surg 33:349–354, 2004.
254. Schulz KS, Waldron DR, Fahie M: Application of ventral pins and polymethylmethacrylate for the management of atlantoaxial instability: results in nine dogs, Vet Surg 26(4):317–325, 1997.
255. Thomas WB, Sorjonen DC, Simpson ST: Surgical management of atlantoaxial subluxation in 23 dogs, Vet Surg 20(6):409–412, 1991.
256 Beaver DP, Ellison GW, Lewis DD, et al: Risk factors affecting the outcome of surgery for atlantoaxial subluxation in dogs: 46 cases (1978-1998), J Am Vet Med Assoc 216(7):1104–1109, 2000.
257. Chambers JN, Betts CW, Oliver JE: The use of nonmetallic suture mterial for stabilization of atlantoaxial subluxation, J Am Anim Hosp Assoc 13:602–604, 1977.
258. LeCouteur RA, McKeown D, Johnson J, Eger CE: Stabilization of atlantoaxial subluxation in the dog, using the nuchal ligament, J Am Vet Med Assoc 177(10):1011–1017, 1980.
259. McCarthy RJ, Lewis DD, Hosgood G: Atlantoaxial subluxation in dogs, Compend Contin Educ Pract Vet 17(2):215–227, 1995.
260. Kishigami M: Application of an atlantoaxial retractor for atlantoaxial subluxation in the cat and dog, J Am Anim Hosp Assoc 20(3):413–419, 1984.
261. van Ee RT, Pechman R, van Ee RM: Failure of the atlantoaxial tension band in two dogs, J Am Anim Hosp Assoc 25(6):707–712, 1989.
262. Jaggy A, Hutto VL, Roberts RE, et al: Occipitoatlantoaxial malformation with atlantoaxial subluxation in a cat, J Small Anim Pract 32(7):366–372, 1991.
263. Watson AG, Hall MA, de Lahunta A: Congenital occipitoatlantoaxial malformation in a cat, Compend Contin Educ Pract Vet 7(3):245–254, 1985.
264. Wilson WD, Hughes SJ, Ghoshal NG, et al: Occipitoatlantoaxial malformation in two non-Arabian horses, J Am Vet Med Assoc 187(1):36–40, 1985.
265. Watson AG, Mayhew IG: Familial congenital occipitoatlantoaxial malformation (OAAM) in the Arabian horse, Spine 11:334–339, 1986.
266. DeCamp CE, Schirmer RG, Stickle RL: Traumatic atlantooccipital subluxation in a dog, J Am Anim Hosp Assoc 27(4):415–418, 1991.
267. Crane SW: Surgical managment of traumatic atlanto-occipital instability in a dog, Vet Surg 7(2):39–42, 1978.
268. Lappin MR, Dow S: Traumatic atlanto-occipital luxation in a cat, Vet Surg 12(1):30–32, 1983.
269. Greenwood KM, Oliver JE Jr: Traumatic atlanto-occipital dislocation in two dogs, J Am Vet Med Assoc 173(10):1324–1327, 1978.

270. Sorjonen DC, Powe TA, West M, et al: Ventral surgical fixation and fusion for atlanto-occipital subluxation in a goat, Vet Surg 12(3):127–129, 1983.
271. Rusbridge C: Persistent scratching in Cavalier King Charles spaniels, Vet Rec 141(7):179, 1997.
272. Dewey CW, Berg JM, Stefanacci JD, et al: Caudal occipital malformation syndrome in dogs, Compend Contin Educ Pract Vet 26(11):886–895, 2004.
273. Parker A, Park RD: Occipital Dysplasia in the dog, J Am Anim Hosp Assoc 10:520–525, 1974.
274. Bagley RS, Harrington ML, Tucker RL, et al: Occipital dysplasia and associated cranial spinal cord abnormalities in two dogs, Vet Radiol Ultrasound 37(5):359–362, 1996.
275. Rusbridge C, Knowler SP: Hereditary aspects of occipital bone hypoplasia and syringomyelia (Chiari type I malformation) in Cavalier King Charles spaniels, Vet Rec 153:107–112, 2003.
276. Bynevelt M, Rusbridge C, Britton J: Dorsal dens angulation and a Chiari type malformation in a Cavalier King Charles spaniel, Vet Radiol Ultrasound 41(6):521–524, 2000.
277. Rusbridge C, MacSweeny JE, Davies JV, et al: Syringohydromyelia in Cavalier King Charles spaniels, J Am Anim Hosp Assoc 36(1):34–41, 2000.
278. Rusbridge C, Knowler SP: Hereditary aspects of occipital bone hypoplasia and syringomyelia (Chiari type I malformation) in Cavalier King Charles spaniels, Vet Rec 153(4):107–112, 2003.
279. Lu D, Lamb CR, Pfeiffer DU, et al: Neurological signs and results of magnetic resonance imaging in 40 Cavalier King Charles spaniels with Chiari type 1-like malformations, Vet Rec 153(9):260–263, 2003.
280. Rusbridge C, Knowler SP, Pieterse L, et al: Chiari-like malformation in the Griffon Bruxellois, J Small Anim Pract 50(8):386–393, 2009.
281. Couturier J, Rault D, Cauzinille L: Chiari-like malformation and syringomyelia in normal Cavalier King Charles spaniels: a multiple diagnostic imaging approach, J Small Anim Pract 49(9):438–443, 2008.
282. Cerda-Gonzalez S, Olby NJ, McCullough S, et al: Morphology of the caudal fossa in Cavalier King Charles spaniels, Vet Radiol Ultrasound 50(1):37–46, 2009.
283. Cerda-Gonzalez S, Dewey CW: Congenital diseases of the craniocervical junction in the dogs, Vet Clin North Am Small Anim Pract 40:121–141, 2010.
284. Oldfield EH, Muraszko K, Shawker TH, et al: Pathophysiology of syringomyelia associated with Chiari I malformation of the cerebellar tonsils. Implications for diagnosis and treatment, J Neurosurg 80:3–15, 1994.
285. Klekamp J: The pathophysiology of syringomyelia - historical overview and current concept, Acta Neurochir (Wien) 144(7):649–664, 2002.
286. Gardner WJ: Hydrodynamic mechanism of syringomyelia: its relationship to myelocele, J Neurol Neurosurg Psychiatry 28:247–259, 1965.
287. Rusbridge C, Greitz D, Iskandar BJ: Syringomyelia: current concepts in pathogenesis, diagnosis, and treatment, J Vet Intern Med 20(3):469–479, 2006.
288. Rusbridge C, Knowler SP: Inheritance of occipital bone hypoplasia (Chiari type I malformation) in Cavalier King Charles spaniels, J Vet Intern Med 18(5):673–678, 2004.
289. Rusbridge C, Knowler P, Rouleau GA, et al: Inherited occipital hypoplasia/syringomyelia in the Cavalier King Charles spaniel: experiences in setting up a worldwide DNA collection, J Hered 96(7):745–749, 2005.
290. Bagley RS, Silver GM, Kippenes H, et al: Syringomyelia and hydromyelia in dogs and cats, Compend Contin Educ Pract Vet 22:471–479, 2000.
291. Milhorat TH, Johnson RW, Milhorat RH, et al: Clinicopathological correlations in syringomyelia using axial magnetic resonance imaging, Neurosurgery 37(2):206–213, 1995.
292. Dewey CW, Berg JM, Stefanacci JD, et al: Caudal occipital malformation syndrome in dogs, Compend Contin Educ Pract Vet 26:886–896, 2004.
293. Rusbridge C, Carruthers H, Dubé MP, et al: Syringomyelia in Cavalier King Charles spaniels: the relationship between syrinx dimensions and pain, J Small Anim Pract 48(8):432–436, 2007.
294. Rusbridge C, MacSweeny JE, Davies JV, et al: Syringohydromyelia in Cavalier King Charles spaniels, J Am Anim Hosp Assoc 20:34–41, 2000.
295. Bagley RS, Silver GM, Seguin B, et al: Scoliosis and associated cystic spinal cord lesion in a dog, J Am Vet Med Assoc 211(5):573–575, 1997.
296. Rusbridge C: Chiari-like malformation with syringomyelia in the Cavalier King Charles spaniel: long-term outcome after surgical management, Vet Surg 36(5):396–405, 2007.
297. Dewey CW, Berg JM, Barone G, et al: Foramen magnum decompression for treatment of caudal occipital malformation syndrome in dogs, J Am Vet Med Assoc 227(8):1270–1275, 2005.
298. Dewey CW, Marino DJ, Bailey KS, et al: Foramen magnum decompression with cranioplasty for treatment of caudal occipital malformation syndrome in dogs, Vet Surg 36(5):406–415, 2007.
299. Powers BE, Stashak TS, Nixon AJ, et al: Pathology of the vertebral column of horses with cervical static stenosis, Vet Pathol 23(4):392–399, 1986.
300. Chambers JN: Caudal cervical spondylopathy in the dog: a review of 20 clinical cases and the literature, J Am Anim Hosp Assoc 13:571–576, 1977.
301. Trotter EJ, de Lahunta A, Geary JC, et al: Caudal cervical vertebral malformation-malarticulation in Great Danes and Doberman Pinschers, J Am Vet Med Assoc 168(10):917–930, 1976.
302. Selcer RR, Oliver JE Jr: Cervical spondylopathy–wobbler syndrome in dogs, J Am Anim Hosp Assoc 11:175–179, 1975.
303. Lewis DG: Cervical spondylomyelopathy ('wobbler' syndrome) in the dog: a study based on 224 cases, J Small Anim Pract 30(12):657–665, 1989.
304. Olsson SE, et al: Compression of the spinal cord in Great Danes, Vet Med Small Anim Clin 77(11):1587, 1982.
305. Baum F III, de Lahunta A, Trotter EJ: Cervical fibrotic stenosis in a young Rottweiler, J Am Vet Med Assoc 201(8):1222–1224, 1992.
306. Wright F, Rest JR, Palmer AC: Ataxia of the Great Dane caused by stenosis of the cervical vertebral canal: comparison with similar conditions in the basset hound, Doberman pinscher, ridgeback and the thoroughbred horse, Vet Rec 92(1):1–6, 1973.
307. Eagleson JS, Diaz J, Platt SR, et al: Cervical vertebral malformation-malarticulation syndrome in the Bernese mountain dog: clinical and magnetic resonance imaging features, J Small Anim Pract 50(4):186–193, 2009.
308. McKee WM, Butterworth SJ, Scott HW: Management of cervical spondylopathy-associated intervertebral disc protrusions using metal washers in 78 dogs, J Small Anim Pract 40(10):465–472, 1999.

309. Costa RC, Parent JM, Holmberg DL, et al: Outcome of medical and surgical treatment in dogs with cervical spondylomyelopathy: 104 cases (1988-2004), J Am Vet Med Assoc 233(8):1284–1290, 2008.
310. VanGundy T: Canine wobbler syndrome. Part I. Pathophysiology and diagnosis, Compend Contin Educ Pract Vet 11(2):144–158, 1989.
311. VanGundy TE: Disc-associated wobbler syndrome in the Doberman pinscher, Vet Clin North Am Small Anim Pract 18(3):667–696, 1988.
312. Trotter EJ: Cervical spine locking plate fixation for treatment of cervical spondylotic myelopathy in large breed gogs, Vet Surg 38(6):705–718, 2009.
313. Jeffery ND, McKee WM: Surgery for disc-associated wobbler syndrome in the dog - an examination of the controversy, J Small Anim Pract :42574–42581, 2001.
314. Costa RC, Parent JM, Partlow G, et al: Morphologic and morphometric magnetic resonance imaging features of Doberman pinschers with and without clinical signs of cervical spondylomyelopathy, Am J Vet Res 67(9):1601–1612, 2006.
315. Lincoln JD: Cervical vertebral malformation/malarticulation syndrome in large dogs, Vet Clin North Am Small Anim Pract 22(4):923–935, 1992.
316. Hedhammer A: Overnutrition and skeletal disease: An experimental study in growing Great Dane dogs, Cornell Vet Suppl 51–160, 1974.
317. Mayhew IG, Donawick WJ, Green SL, et al: Diagnosis and prediction of cervical vertebral malformation in thoroughbred foals based on semi-quantitative radiographic indicators, Equine Vet J 25(5):435–440, 1993.
318. Stewart RH, Reed SM, Weisbrode SE: Frequency and severity of osteochondrosis in horses with cervical stenotic myelopathy, Am J Vet Res 52(6):873–879, 1991.
319. Levine JM, Adam E, MacKay RJ, et al: Confirmed and presumptive cervical vertebral compressive myelopathy in older horses: a retrospective study (1992-2004), J Vet Intern Med 21(4):812–819, 2007.
320. Stewart RH, Rush BR: Cervical vertebral stenotic myelopathy. In Reed SM, Warwick MB, Sellon DC, editors: Equine Internal Medicine, ed 2, St. Louis, 2004, W.B. Saunders, pp 594–599.
321. Reed SM, Bayly WM, Traub JL, et al: Ataxia and paresis in horses. Part I. Differential diagnosis, Compend Contin Educ Pract Vet 3(3):S88–S99, 1981.
322. Sharp NJH, Wheeler SJ, Cofone M: Radiological evaluation of 'wobbler' syndrome–caudal cervical spondylomyelopathy, J Small Anim Pract 33:491–499, 1992.
323. Sharp NJH, Cofone M, Robertson ID, et al: Computed tomography in the evaluation of caudal cervical spondylomyelopathy of the Doberman pinscher, Vet Radiol Ultrasound 36(2):100–108, 1995.
324. Lipsitz D, Levitski RE, Chauvet AE, et al: Magnetc resonance imaging features of cervical stenotic myelopathy in 21 dogs, Vet Radiol Ultrasound 42:20–27, 2001.
325. Moore BR, Reed SM, Biller DS, et al: Assessment of vertebral canal diameter and bony malformations of the cervical part of the spine in horses with cervical stenotic myelopathy, Am J Vet Res 55(1):5–13, 1994.
326. Hahn CN, Handel I, Green SL, et al: Assessment of the utility of using intra- and intervertebral minimum sagittal diameter ratios in the diagnosis of cervical vertebral malformation in horses, Vet Radiol Ultrasound 49(1):1–6, 2008.
327. Neuwirth L: Equine myelography, Compend Contin Educ Pract Vet 14(1):72–79, 1992.
328. Papageorges M, Gavin PR, Sande RD, et al: Radiographic and myelographic examination of the cervical vertebral column in 306 ataxic horses, Vet Radiol 28(2):53–59, 1987.
329. Biervliet Jv, Scrivani PV, Divers TJ, et al: Evaluation of decision criteria for detection of spinal cord compression based on cervical myelography in horses: 38 cases (1981-2001), Equine Vet J 36(1):14–20, 2004.
330. Moore BR, Holbrook TC, Stefanacci JD, et al: Contrast-enhanced computed tomography and myelography in six horses with cervical stenotic myelopathy, Equine Vet J 24(3):197–202, 1992.
331. Bruecker KA, Seim HB, Withrow SJ: Clinical evaluation of three surgical methods for treatment of caudal cervical spondylomyelopathy of dogs, Vet Surg 18(3):197–203, 1989.
332. Goring RL, Beale BS, Faulkner RF: The inverted cone decompression technique: a surgical treatment for cervical vertebral instability "wobbler syndrome" in Doberman pinschers. Part I, J Am Anim Hosp Assoc 27(4):403–409, 1991.
333. Chambers JN, Oliver JE Jr, Kornegay JN, et al: Ventral decompression for caudal cervical disk herniation in large- and giant-breed dogs, J Am Vet Med Assoc 180(4):410–414, 1982.
334. Lyman R: Continuous dorsal laminectomy is the procedure of choice, Prog Vet Neurol 2(2):143–146, 1991.
335. Lyman R: Continuous dorsal laminectomy for the treatment of Doberman pinschers with caudal cervical vertebral instability and malformation, San Diego, 1987, Abstracts of the 5th Annual Meeting of the Veterinary Medical Forum, 303–5.
336. De Risio L, Sharp NJH, Olby NJ, et al: Predictors of outcome after dorsal decompressive laminectomy for degenerative lumbosacral stenosis in dogs: 69 cases (1987-1997), J Am Vet Med Assoc 219:624–628, 2001.
337. De Risio L, Munana K, Murray M, et al: Dorsal laminectomy for caudal cervical spondylomyelopathy: postoperative recovery and long-term follow-up in 20 dogs, Vet Surg 31(5):418–427, 2002.
338. McKee WM, Lavelle RB, Richardson JL, et al: Vertebral distraction-fusion for cervical spondylopathy using a screw and double washer technique, J Small Anim Pract 31(1):22–27, 1990.
339. Dixon BC, Tomlinson JL, Kraus KH: Modified distraction-stabilization technique using an interbody polymethyl methacrylate plug in dogs with caudal cervical spondylomyelopathy, J Am Vet Med Assoc 208(1):61–68, 1996.
340. Bruecker KA, Seim HB III, Blass CE: Caudal cervical spondylomyelopathy: decompression by linear traction and stabilization with Steinmann pins and polymethyl methacrylate, J Am Anim Hosp Assoc 25:677–683, 1989.
341. Ellison GW, Seim HB, Clemmons RM: Distracted cervical spinal fusion for management of caudal cervical spondylomyelopathy in large-breed dogs, J Am Vet Med Assoc 193(4):447–453, 1988.
342. Bergman RL, Levine JM, Coates JR, et al: Cervical spinal locking plate in combination with cortical ring allograft for a one level fusion in dogs with cervical spondylotic myelopathy, Vet Surg 37(6):530–536, 2008.
343. Wilson ER, Aron DN, Roberts RE: Observation of a secondary compressive lesion after treatment of caudal cervical spondylomyelopathy in a dog, J Am Vet Med Assoc 205(9):1297–1299, 1994.

344. Marchevsky AM, Richardson JL: Disc extrusion in a Rottweiler dog with caudal cervical spondylomyelopathy after failure of intervertebral distraction/stabilisation, Aust Vet J 77(5):295–297, 1999.
345. Rusbridge C, Wheeler SJ, Torrington AM, et al: Comparison of two surgical techniques for the management of cervical spondylomyelopathy in dobermanns, J Small Anim Pract 39(9):425–431, 1998.
346. Moore BR, Reed SM, Robertson JT: Surgical treatment of cervical stenotic myelopathy in horses: 73 cases (1983-1992), J Am Vet Med Assoc 203(1):108–112, 1993.
347. Nixon AJ: Surgical management of equine cervical vertebral malformation, Prog Vet Neurol 2(3):183–195, 1991.
348. Wagner PC, Grant BD, Gallina A, et al: Ataxia and paresis in horses. Part III. Surgical treatment of cervical spinal cord compression, Compend Contin Educ Pract Vet 3(5):S192–S202, 1981.
349. Levitski RE, Chauvet AE, Lipsitz D: Cervical myelopathy associated with extradural synovial cysts in 4 dogs, J Vet Intern Med 13(3):181–186, 1999.
350. Dickinson PJ, Sturges BK, Berry WL, et al: Extradural spinal synovial cysts in nine dogs, J Small Anim Pract 42:502–509, 2001.
351. Duncan ID: Peripheral neuropathy in the dog and cat, Prog Vet Neurol 2(2):111–128, 1991.
352 de Lahunta A, Glass E: Lower motor neuron-general somatic efferent system. In de Lahunta A, Glass E, editors: Veterinary neuroanatomy and clinical neurology, St Louis, 2009, Saunders Elsevier.
353. Braund KG: Neuropathic disorders. In Braund KG, editor: Clinical neurology in small animals—Localization, diagnosis and treatment, Ithaca, 2003, International Veterinary Information Service (www.ivis.org), 2003.
354. Bagley RS: Tremor syndromes in dogs: diagnosis and treatment, J Small Anim Pract 33(10):485–490, 1991.
355. Cuddon PA: Tremor Syndromes, Prog Vet Neurol 1:285–299, 1990.
356. Glass EN, Kent M: The clinical examination for neuromuscular disease, Vet Clin North Am Small Anim Pract 32(1):1–29, 2002.
357. Shelton GD, Podell M, Poncelet L, et al: Inherited polyneuropathy in Leonberger dogs: a mixed or intermediate form of Charcot-Marie-Tooth disease, Muscle Nerve 27:471–477, 2003.
358. Jeffery N: Neurological abnormalities of the head and face. In Platt SR, Olby NJ, editors: BSAVA Manual of Canine and Feline Neurology, ed 3, Gloucester, 2004, Woodrow House, pp 172–188.
359. Monnet E: Laryngeal paralysis and devocalization. In Slatter DH, editor: Textbook of Small Animal Surgery, ed 3, Philadelphia, 2003, Elsevier Science, pp 837–845.
360. Thieman KM, Krahwinkel DJ, Sims MH, et al: Histopathological confirmation of polyneuropathy in 11 dogs with laryngeal paralysis, J Am Anim Hosp Assoc 46:161–167, 2010.
361. Braund KG, Steinberg HS, Shores A, et al: Laryngeal paralysis in immature and mature dogs as one sign of a more diffuse polyneuropathy, J Am Vet Med Assoc 194(12):1735–1740, 1989.
362. Northington JW, Brown MJ, Farnbach GC, et al: Acute idiopathic polyneuropathy in the dog, J Am Vet Med Assoc 179(4):375–379, 1981.
363. Cummings JF, Haas C: Coonhound paralysis: An acute idiopathic polyradiculoneuritis in dogs resembling Landry Guillain Barre syndrome, J Neurol Sci 4:51–81, 1967.
364. Lane JR, de Lahunta A: Polyneuritis in a cat, J Am Anim Hosp Assoc 20:1006–1008, 1984.
365. Flecknell PA, Lucke VM: Chronic relapsing polyradiculoneuritis in a cat, Acta Neuropathol (Berl) 41(1):81–84, 1978.
366. MacLachlan NJ, Gribble DH, East NE: Polyradiculoneuritis in a goat, J Am Vet Med Assoc 180(2):166–167, 1982.
367. Holmes DF, Schultz RD, Cummings JF, et al: Experimental coonhound paralysis: animal model of Guillain-Barre syndrome, Neurology 29(8):1186–1187, 1979.
368. Schrauwen E, Van Ham LML: Postvaccinal acute polyradiculoneuritis in a young dog, Prog Vet Neurol 6(2):68–70, 1995.
369. Cummings JF, de Lahunta A, Holmes DF, et al: Coonhound paralysis. Further clinical studies and electron microscopic observations, Acta Neuropathol (Berl) 56(3):167–178, 1982.
370. Alexander JW, de Lahunta A, Scott DW: A case of brachial plexus neuropathy in a dog, J Am Anim Hosp Assoc 10(9):515–517, 1974.
371. Bright RM, Crabtree BJ, Knecht CD: Brachial plexus neuropathy in the cat: a case report, J Am Anim Hosp Assoc 14:612–615, 1978.
372. Cuddon PA: Electrophysiologic assessment of acute polyradiculoneuropathy in dogs: comparison with Guillain-Barré syndrome in people, J Vet Intern Med 12(4):294–303, 1998.
373. Chrisman CL: Differentiation of tick paralysis and acute idiopathic polyradiculoneuritis in the dog using electromyography, Compend Contin Educ Pract Vet 11:455–458, 1975.
374. Cuddon PA: Electrophysiology in neuromuscular disease, Vet Clin North Am Small Anim Pract 32(1):31–62, 2002.
375. Double-blind trial of intravenous methylprednisolone in Guillain-Barré syndrome. Guillain-Barré Syndrome Steroid Trial Group, Lancet 341(8845):586–590, 1993.
376. Cuddon PA: Acquired canine peripheral neuropathies, Vet Clin North Am Small Anim Pract 32(1):207–249, 2002.
377. Dyck PJ, Daube J, O'Brien P, et al: Plasma exchange in chronic inflammatory demyelinating polyradiculoneuropathy, N Engl J Med 314(8):461–465, 1986.
378. Bartges JW: Therapeutic plasmapheresis, Semin Vet Med Surg (Small Anim) 12(3):170–177, 1997.
379. Sherman J, Olby NJ: Nursing and rehabilitation of the neurological patient. In Platt SR, Olby NJ, editors: BSAVA Manual of Canine and Feline Neurology, ed 3, Gloucester, 2004, BSAVA, pp 394–407.
380. Duncan ID: Polyradiculoneuritis—Coonhound paralysis revisted Proceedings ACVIM Forum 334–337, 1987.
381. Blackmore JA, Schaer M: Idiopathic polyradiculoneuritis and impaired ventilation in a dog: a case report, J Am Anim Hosp Assoc 20(5):487–490, 1984.
382. Dubey JP, Carpenter JL, Speer CA, et al: Newly recognized fatal protozoan disease of dogs, J Am Vet Med Assoc 192(9):1269–1285, 1988.
383. Cuddon P, Lin DS, Bowman DD, et al: *Neospora caninum* infection in English Springer Spaniel littermates. Diagnostic evaluation and organism isolation, J Vet Intern Med 6(6):325–332, 1992.
384. Knowler C, Wheeler SJ: *Neospora caninum* infection in three dogs, J Small Anim Pract 36(4):172–177, 1995.
385. Ruehlmann D, Podell M, Oglesbee M, et al: Canine neosporosis: a case report and literature review, J Am Anim Hosp Assoc 31(2):174–183, 1995.
386. Cork LC, Griffin JW, Adams RJ, Price DL: Animal model of human disease: motor neuron disease - spinal muscular atrophy and amyotrophic lateral sclerosis, Am J Pathol 100:599–602, 1980.

387. Lorenz MD, Cork LC, Griffin JW, et al: Hereditary spinal muscular atrophy in Brittany Spaniels: clinical manifestations, J Am Vet Med Assoc 175(8):833–839, 1979.
388. Cork LC, Griffin JW, Munnell JF, et al: Hereditary canine spinal muscular atrophy, J Neuropathol Exp Neurol 38:209–221, 1979.
389 de Lahunta A, Shively JN: Neurofibrillary accumlation in a puppy, Cornell Vet 65:240–247, 1975.
390. Summers BA, Cummings JF, de Lahunta A: Veterinary Neuropathology, St. Louis, 1995, Mosby, 189-207.
391. Inada S, Yamauchi C, Igata A, et al: Canine storage disease characterized by hereditary progressive neurogenic muscular atrophy: breeding experiments and clinical manifestation, Am J Vet Res 47(10):2294–2299, 1986.
392. Inada S, Sakamoto H, Haruta K, et al: A clinical study on hereditary progressive neurogenic muscular atrophy in Pointer dogs, Nippon Juigaku Zasshi 40:539–547, 1978.
393. Cummings JF, George C, de Lahunta A, et al: Focal spinal muscular atrophy in two German shepherd pups, Acta Neuropathol (Berl) 79(1):113–116, 1989.
394. Mandara MT, Meo Ad: Lower motor neuron disease in the Griffon Briquet Venden dog, Vet Pathol 35(5):412–414, 1998.
395. Shell LG, Jortner BS, Leib MS: Familial motor neuron disease in Rottweiler dogs: neuropathologic studies, Vet Pathol 24(2):135–139, 1987.
396. Kent M, Knowles K, Glass E, et al: Motor neuron abiotrophy in a saluki, J Am Anim Hosp Assoc 35(5):436–439, 1999.
397. Sandefeldt E, Cummings JF, de Lahunta A: Animal model of human disease. Infantile spinal muscular atrophy, Werdnig-Hoffman diease. Animal model: hereditary neuronal abiotrophy in Swedish Lapland dogs, Am J Pathol 82:649–652, 1976.
398. Hartley WJ: Lower motor neuron disease in dogs, Acta Neuropathol 2:334–342, 1963.
399. Stockard CR: An hereditary lethal factor for localized motor and preganglionic neurons with a resulting paralysis in the dog, Am J Anat 59:1–53, 1936.
400. Averill DR Jr: Degenerative myelopathy in the aging German shepherd dog: clinical and pathologic findings, J Am Vet Med Assoc 162(12):1045–1051, 1973.
401. Griffiths IR, Duncan ID: Chronic degenerative radiculomyelopathy in the dog, J Small Anim Pract 16(8):461–471, 1975.
402. Braund KG, Vandevelde M: German shepherd dog myelopathy–a morphologic and morphometric study, Am J Vet Res 39(8):1309–1315, 1978.
403. Awano T, Johnson GS, Wade CM, et al: Genome-wide association analysis reveals a *SOD1* mutation in canine degenerative myelopathy that resembles amyotrophic lateral sclerosis, Proc Natl Acad Sci U S A 106:2794–2799, 2009.
404. Kathmann I, Cizinauskas S, Doherr MG, et al: Daily controlled physiotherapy increases survival time in dogs with suspected degenerative myelopathy, J Vet Intern Med 20:927–932, 2006.
405. Bichsel P, Vandevelde M, Lang J, et al: Degenerative myelopathy in a family of Siberian husky dogs, J Am Vet Med Assoc 183(9):998–1000, 1983.
406. Matthews NS, de Lahunta A: Degenerative myelopathy in an adult miniature poodle, J Am Vet Med Assoc 186(11):1213–1215, 1985.
407. Miller AD, Barber R, Porter BF, et al: Degenerative myelopathy in two boxer dogs, Vet Pathol 46(4):684–687, 2009.
408. Coates JR, March PA, Oglesbee M, et al: Clinical characterization of a familial degenerative myelopathy in Pembroke Welsh Corgi dogs, J Vet Intern Med 21(6):1323–1331, 2007.
409. Long SN, Henthorn PS, Serpell J, et al: Degenerative Myelopathy in Chesapeake Bay Retrievers, J Vet Intern Med 23:401–402, 2009.
410. He QC, Lowrie C, Shelton GD, et al: Inherited motor neuron disease in domestic cats: a model of spinal muscular atrophy, Pediatr Res 57(3):324–330, 2005.
411. Fyfe JC, Menotti-Raymond M, David VA, et al: An ~140-kb deletion associated with feline spinal muscular atrophy implies an essential LIX1 function for motor neuron survival, Genome Res 16(9):1084–1090, 2006.
412. Vandevelde M, Greene CE, Hoff EJ: Lower motor neuron disease with accumulation of neurofilaments in a cat, Vet Pathol 13(6):428–435, 1976.
413. Troyer D, Leipold HW, Cash W, et al: Upper motor neurone and descending tract pathology in bovine spinal muscular atrophy, J Comp Pathol 107(3):305–317, 1992.
414. Hiraga T, Leipold HW, Cash WC, et al: Reduced numbers and intense anti-ubiquitin immunostaining of bovine motor neurons affected with spinal muscular atrophy, J Neurol Sci 118(1):43–47, 1993.
415. Hiraga T, Leipold HW, Vestweber JGE, et al: Cytoskeletal proteins in affected motor neurons in bovine spinal muscular atrophy, Prog Vet Neurol 4(4):137–142, 1993.
416. Nielsen JS, Andresen E, Basse A, Christensen LG, et al: Inheritance of bovine spinal muscular atrophy, Acta Vet Scand 31(2):253–255, 1990.
417. Agerholm JS, Basse A: Spinal muscular atrophy in calves of the Red Danish dairy breed, Vet Rec 134(10):232–235, 1994.
418. Dahme E, Hafner A, Schmidt P: Spinal muscular atrophy in German Braunvieh calves - comparative neuropathological evaluation, Neuropathol Appl Neurobiol 17(6):517, 1991.
419. Anderson PD, Parton KH, Collett MG, et al: A lower motor neuron disease in newborn Romney lambs, N Z Vet J 47(3):112–114, 1999.
420. Cummings JF, deLahunta A, Fuhrer L, et al: Equine motor neuron disease: a preliminary report, Cornell Vet 80:357–379, 1990.
421. Divers TJ, Cummings JE, deLahunta A, et al: Evaluation of the risk of motor neuron disease in horses fed a diet low in vitamin E and high in copper and iron, Am J Vet Res 67(1):120–126, 2006.
422. Divers TJ, Mohammed HO, Cummings JF, et al: Equine motor neuron disease: findings in 28 horses and proposal of a pathophysiological mechanism for the disease, Equine Vet J 26(5):409–415, 1994.
423. Dubey JP, Koestner A, Piper RC: Repeated transplacental transmission of Neospora caninum in dogs, J Am Vet Med Assoc 197(7):857–860, 1990.
424. Dubey JP, Lappin MR: Toxoplasmosis and neosporosis. In Greene CE, editor: Infectious Diseases of the Dog and Cat, 3rd edition, Philadelphia, 2006, Elsevier Saunders, pp 754–775.
425. Barber JS, van Ham L, Polis I, et al: Seroprevalence of antibodies to *Neospora caninum* in Belgian dogs, J Small Anim Pract 38(1):15–16, 1997.
426. Olby N: Motor neuron disease: inherited and acquired, Vet Clin North Am Small Anim Pract 34:1403–1418, 2004.
427. Lorenz MD, Cork LC, Griffin JW, et al: Hereditary spinal muscular atrophy in Brittany Spaniels: clinical manifestations, J Am Vet Med Assoc 175(8):833–839, 1979.

428. Inada S, Sakamoto H, Haruta K, et al: A clinical study on hereditary progressive neurogenic muscular atrophy in Pointer dogs, Nippon Juigaku Zasshi 40:539–547, 1978.
429. Sandefeldt E, Cummings JF, de Lahunta A: Animal model of human disease. Infantile spinal muscular atrophy, Werdnig-Hoffman diease. Animal model: hereditary neuronal abiotrophy in Swedish Lapland dogs, Am J Pathol 82:649–652, 1976.
430. He QC, Lowrie C, Shelton GD, et al: Inherited motor neuron disease in domestic cats: a model of spinal muscular atrophy, Pediatr Res 57(3):324–330, 2005.
431. Vandevelde M, Greene CE, Hoff EJ: Lower motor neuron disease with accumulation of neurofilaments in a cat, Vet Pathol 13(6):428–435, 1976.
432. Shelton GD, Hopkins AL, Ginn PE, et al: Adult-onset motor neuron disease in three cats, J Am Vet Med Assoc 212(8):1271–1275, 1998.
433. Dahme E, Hafner A, Schmidt P: Spinal muscular atrophy in German Braunvieh calves - comparative neuropathological evaluation, Neuropathol Appl Neurobiol 17(6):517, 1991.
434. Nielsen JS, Andresen E, Basse A, et al: Inheritance of bovine spinal muscular atrophy, Acta Vet Scand 31(2):253–255, 1990.
435. Troyer D, Leipold HW, Cash W, et al: Upper motor neurone and descending tract pathology in bovine spinal muscular atrophy, J Comp Pathol 107(3):305–317, 1992.
436. Anderson PD, Parton KH, Collett MG, et al: A lower motor neuron disease in newborn Romney lambs, N Z Vet J 47(3):112–114, 1999.
437. Divers TJ, Mohammed HO, Cummings JF, et al: Equine motor neuron disease: findings in 28 horses and proposal of a pathophysiological mechanism for the disease, Equine Vet J 26(5):409–415, 1994.
438. Cummings JF, deLahunta A, Fuhrer L, et al: Equine motor neuron disease: a preliminary report, Cornell Vet 80:357–379, 1990.
439. de la Rua-Domenech R, Mohammed HO, Atwill ER, et al: Epidemiologic evidence for clustering of equine motor neuron disease in the United States, Am J Vet Res 56(11):1433–1439, 1995.
440. Mohammed HO, Divers TJ, Summers BA, et al: Vitamin E deficiency and risk of equine motor neuron disease, Acta Vet Scand 49:17, 2007.
441. Divers TJ, Cummings JE, deLahunta A, et al: Evaluation of the risk of motor neuron disease in horses fed a diet low in vitamin E and high in copper and iron, Am J Vet Res 67(1):120–126, 2006.
442. Cummings JF, de Lahunta A, Mohammed HO, et al: Equine motor neuron disease: a new neurologic disorder, Equine Pract 13(9):15–18, 1991.
443. Polack EW, King JM, Cummings JF, et al: Quantitative assessment of motor neuron loss in equine motor neuron disease (EMND), Equine Vet J 30(3):256–259, 1998.
444. Green SL, Tolwani RJ: Animal models for motor neuron disease, Lab Anim Sci 49(5):480–487, 1999.
445. Riis RC, Jackson C, Rebhun W, et al: Ocular manifestations of equine motor neuron disease, Equine Vet J 31(2):99–110, 1999.
446. Verhulst D, Barnett KC, Mayhew IG: Equine motor neuron disease and retinal degeneration, Equine Vet Educ 13(2):59–61, 2001.
447. Podell M, Valentine BA, Cummings JF, et al: Electromyography in acquired equine motor neuron disease, Prog Vet Neurol 6(4):128–134, 1995.
448. Jackson CA, de Lahunta A, Cummings JF, et al: Spinal accessory nerve biopsy as an *ante mortem* diagnostic test for equine motor neuron disease, Equine Vet J 28(3):215–219, 1996.
449. Divers TJ, de Lahunta A, Hintz HF, et al: Equine motor neuron disease, Equine Vet Educ 13(2):63–67, 2001.
450. de la Rua-Domenech R, Mohammed HO, Cummings JF, et al: Intrinsic, management, and nutritional factors associated with equine motor neuron disease, J Am Vet Med Assoc 211(10):1261–1267, 1997.
451. Moe L: Hereditary polyneuropathy of Alaskan malamutes. In Kirk RW, Bonagura JD, editors: Kirk's Current Veterinary Therapy, ed 11, Philadelphia, 1992, W.B. Saunders Co., pp 1038–1039.
452. Braund KG, Shores A, Lowrie CT, et al: Idiopathic polyneuropathy in Alaskan malamutes, J Vet Intern Med 11(4):243–249, 1997.
453. Chrisman CL: Dancing Doberman disease: clinical findings and prognosis, Prog Vet Neurol 1(1):83–90, 1990.
454. Duncan ID, Griffiths IR: Canine giant axonal neuropathy, Vet Rec 101:438–441, 1977.
455. Braund KG, Luttgen PJ, Redding RW, et al: Distal symmetrical polyneuropathy in a dog, Vet Pathol 17(4):422–435, 1980.
456. Henricks PM, Steiss J, Petterson JD: Distal peripheral polyneuropathy in a Great Dane, Can Vet J 28:165–167, 1987.
457. Griffiths IR, McCulloch MC, Abrahams S: Progressive axonopathy: an inherited neuropathy of boxer dogs. 3. The peripheral axon lesion with special reference to the nerve roots, J Neurocytol 15(1):109–120, 1986.
458. Griffiths IR: Progressive axonopathy: an inherited neuropathy of Boxer dogs. I. Further studies of the clinical and electrophysiological features, J Small Anim Pract 26(7):381–392, 1985.
459. Griffiths IR, Duncan ID, Barker J: A progressive axonopathy of Boxer dogs affecting the central and peripheral nervous systems, J Small Anim Pract 21(1):29–43, 1980.
460. Duncan ID, Griffiths IR, Carmichael S, et al: Inherited canine giant axonal neuropathy, Muscle Nerve 4(3):223–227, 1981.
461. Duncan ID, Griffiths IR: Canine giant axonal neuropathy; some aspects of its clinical, pathological and comparative features, J Small Anim Pract 22(8):491–501, 1981.
462. Duncan ID, Griffiths IR: Peripheral nervous system in a case of canine giant axonal neuropathy, Neuropathol Appl Neurobiol 5:25–39, 1979.
463. Griffiths IR, Duncan ID: The central nervous system in canine giant axonal neuropathy, Acta Neuropath (Berl) 46:169–172, 1979.
464. Griffiths IR, Duncan ID, McCulloch M, et al: Further studies of the central nervous system in canine giant axonal neuropathy, Neuropathol Appl Neurobiol 6:421–432, 1980.
465. Ubbink GJ, Knol BW, Bouw J: The relationship between homozygosity and the occurrence of specific diseases in Bouvier Belge des Flandres dogs in the Netherlands, Vet Quart 14:137–140, 1992.
466. Venker-van Haagen AJ, Bouw J, Hartman W: Hereditary transmission of laryngeal paralysis in Bouviers, J Am Anim Hosp Assoc 17(1):75–76, 1981.
467. Venker-van Haagen AJ, Hartman W, Goedegebuure SA: Spontaneous laryngeal paralysis in young Bouviers, J Am Anim Hosp Assoc 14:714–720, 1978.
468. O'Brien JA, Hendriks J: Inherited laryngeal paralysis. Analysis in the husky cross, Vet Quart 8:301–302, 1986.

469. Ridyard AE, Corcoran BM, Tasker S, et al: Spontaneous laryngeal paralysis in four white-coated German shepherd dogs, J Small Anim Pract 41:558–561, 2000.
470. Venker-van Haagen AJ: Laryngeal diseases of dogs and cats. In Kirk RW, editor: Current Veterinary Therapy IX Small Animal Practice, ed 7, Philadelphia, 1986, W.B. Saunders, pp 265–269.
471. Braund KG, Shores A, Di Pinto N, et al: Laryngeal paralysis in dalmatians, J Vet Intern Med 6(2):117, 1992.
472. Braund KG, Shores A, Cochrane S, et al: Laryngeal paralysis-polyneuropathy complex in young Dalmatians, Am J Vet Res 55(4):534–542, 1994.
473. Mahony OM, Knowles KE, Braund KG, et al: Laryngeal paralysis-polyneuropathy complex in young Rottweilers, J Vet Intern Med 12(5):330–337, 1998.
474. Shelton GD, Podell M, Sullivan S, et al: Distal, symmetrical polyneuropathy with laryngeal paralysis in young, related Leonberger dogs, J Vet Intern.Med 14(3):339, 2000.
475. Shelton GD, Podell M, Poncelet L, et al: Inherited polyneuropathy in Leonberger dogs: a mixed or intermediate form of Charcot-Marie-Tooth disease, Muscle Nerve 27:471–477, 2003.
476. Braund KG, Toivio-Kinnucan M, Vallat JM, et al: Distal sensorimotor polyneuropathy in mature Rottweiler dogs, Vet Pathol 31(3):316–326, 1994.
477. Schatzberg SJ, Shelton GD: Newly identified neuromuscular disorders, Vet Clin North Am Small Anim Pract 34(6):1497–1524, 2004.
478. Matiasek LA, Feliu-Pascual AL, Shelton DG, et al: Axonal neuropathy with unusual clinical course in young Snowshoe cats, J Feline Med Surg 11(12):1005–1010, 2009.
479. Moreau PM, Vallat JM, Hugon J, et al: Peripheral and central distal axonopathy of suspected inherited origin in Birman cats, Acta Neuropathol (Berl) 82(2):143–146, 1991.
480. Braund KG, Mehta JR, Toivio-Kinnucan M, et al: Congenital hypomyelinating polyneuropathy in two golden retriever littermates, Vet Pathol 26(3):202–208, 1989.
481. Matz ME, Shell L, Braund K: Peripheral hypomyelinization in two golden retriever littermates, J Am Vet Med Assoc 197(2):228–230, 1990.
482. Cummings JF, Cooper BJ, de Lahunta A, et al: Canine inherited hypertrophic neuropathy, Acta Neuropathol (Berl) 53(2):137–143, 1981.
483. Cooper BJ, de Lahunta A, Cummings JF, et al: Canine inherited hypertrophic neuropathy: clinical and electrodiagnostic studies, Am J Vet Res 45(6):1172–1177, 1984.
484. Cooper BJ, Duncan I, Cummings J, et al: Defective Schwann cell function in canine inherited hypertrophic neuropathy, Acta Neuropathol (Berl) 63(1):51–56, 1984.
485. Sponenberg DP, de Lahunta A: Hereditary hypertrophic neuropathy in Tibetan Mastiff dogs, J Hered 72:287, 1981.
486. Dahme E, Kraft W, Scabell J: Hypertrophische polyneuropathie bei der Katze, J Vet Med 34:271–288, 1987.
487. Poncelet L, Resibois A, Engvall E, et al: Laminin alpha2 deficiency-associated muscular dystrophy in a Maine coon cat. [Review] [19 refs], J Small Anim Pract 44(12):550–552, 2003.
488. O'Brien DP, Johnson GC, Liu LA, et al: Laminin α2 (merosin) -deficient muscular dystrophy and demyelinating neuropathy in two cats, J Neurol Sci 18:937–943, 2001.
489. Duncan ID, Griffiths IR: A sensory neuropathy affecting long-haired dachshund dogs, J Small Anim Pract 23:381–390, 1982.
490. Duncan ID, Griffiths IR, Munz M: The pathology of a sensory neuropathy affecting longhaired dachshund dogs, Acta Neuropathol (Berl) 58(2):141–151, 1982.
491. Cummings JF, de Lahunta A, Simpson ST, McDonald JM: Reduced substance P-like immunoreactivity in hereditary sensory neuropathy of pointer dogs, Acta Neuropathol (Berl) 63(1):33–40, 1984.
492. Cummings JF, de Lahunta A, Braund KG, Mitchell WJ Jr: Hereditary sensory neuropathy. Nociceptive loss and acral mutilation in pointer dogs: canine hereditary sensory neuropathy, Am J Pathol 112(1):136–138, 1983.
493. Cummings JF, de Lahunta A, Winn SS: Acral mutilation and nociceptive loss in English pointer dogs. A canine sensory neuropathy, Acta Neuropathol (Berl) 53(2):119–127, 1981.
494. Sanda A, Pivnik L: Die Zehenneckrose bei kurzhaarigen Vorstehhunden, Kleintierpraxis 9:76–83, 1964.
495. Pivnik L: Zur vergleichenden problematik einiger akrodystrophischer neuropathien bei menschen und hund, Neurol Neurochir Psychiatr 112:365–371, 1973.
496. Franklin RJM, Olby NJ, Targett MP, et al: Sensory neuropathy in a Jack Russell terrier, J Small Anim Pract 33:402–404, 1992.
497. Paradis M, Jaham Cd, Page N, et al: Acral mutilation and analgesia in 13 French spaniels, Vet Dermatol 16(2):87–93, 2005.
498. Steiss JE, Pook HA, Clark EG, et al: Sensory neuronopathy in a dog, J Am Vet Med Assoc 190(2):205–208, 1987.
499. Jaderlund KH, Orvind E, Johnsson E, et al: A neurologic syndrome in golden reterievers presenting as a sensory ataxic neuropathy, J Vet Intern Med 211:307–1315, 2007.
500. Carmichael S, Griffiths IR: Case of isolated sensory trigeminal neuropathy in a dog, Vet Rec 109(13):280–282, 1981.
501. Vermeersch K, Ham LV, Braund KG, et al: Sensory neuropathy in two border collie puppies, J Small Anim Pract 46(6):295–299, 2005.
502. Wheeler SJ: Sensory neuropathy in a border collie puppy, J Small Anim Pract 28:281–289, 1987.
503. Wouda W, Vandevelde M, Oettli P, et al: Sensory neuronopathy in dogs: a study of four cases, J Comp Pathol 93(3):437–450, 1983.
504. van Nes JJ: Electrophysiological evidence of sensory nerve dysfunction in 10 dogs with acral lick dermatitis, J Am Anim Hosp Assoc 22(2):157–160, 1986.
505. McKerrell RE, Blakemore WF, Heath MF, et al: Primary hyperoxaluria (L-glyceric aciduria) in the cat: a newly recognised inherited disease, Vet Rec 125(2):31–34, 1989.
506. Goldstein RE, Narala S, Sabet N, et al: Primary hyperoxaluria in cats is caused by a mutation in the feline GRHPR gene, J Hered 100:S2–S7, 2009.
507. Jones BR, Johnstone AC, Cahill JI, et al: Peripheral neuropathy in cats with inherited primary hyperchylomicronaemia, Vet Rec 119(11):268–272, 1986.
508. Jones BR: Inherited hyperchylomicronaemia in the cat, J Small Anim Pract 34:493–499, 1993.
509. Jones BR: Hyperchlomicronemia in the cat. In Bonagura JD, Kirk RW, editors: Kirk's Current Veterinary Theraphy XII Small Animal Practice, ed 12, Philadelphia, 1995, W.B. Saunders Co., pp 1163–1166.
510. Jones BR, Wallace A, Harding DRK, et al: Occurence of idiopathic, familial hyperchylomicronaemia in a cat, Vet Rec 112(543):547, 1983.

511. Grieshaber TL, McKeever PJ, McKeever PJ, et al: Spontaneous cutaneous (eruptive) xanthomatosis in two cats, J Am Anim Hosp Assoc 27:509–512, 1991.
512. Bauer JE, Verlander JW: Congenital lipoprotein lipase deficiency in hyperlipemic kitten siblings, Vet Clin Pathol 13:7–11, 1984.
513. Brooks KD: Idiopathic hyperlipoproteinemia in a cat, Companion Anim Pract 19:5–9, 1989.
514. Sottiaux J: Cas clinique: hyperchylomicronémie primaire chez un chat, Le Point Vétérinaire 18:117–119, 1986.
515. Moisan PG, Steffen DJ, Sanderson MW, et al: A familial degenerative neuromuscular disease of Gelbvieh cattle, J Vet Diagn Invest 14(2):140–149, 2002.
516. Panciera RJ, Washburn KE, Streeter RN, et al: A familial peripheral neuropathy and glomerulopathy in Gelbvieh calves, Veterinary Pathology 40(1):63–70, 2003.
517. Herrtage ME: Canine fucosidosis, Vet Ann 28:223–227, 1988.
518. Barker CG, Herrtage ME, Shanahan F, et al: Fucosidosis in English springer spaniels: results of a trial screening programme, J Small Anim Pract 29(10):623–630, 1988.
519. Littlewood JD, Herrtage ME, Palmer AC: Neuronal storage disease in English springer spaniels, Vet Rec 112(4):86–87, 1983.
520. Skelly BJ, Sargan DR, Winchester BG, et al: Genomic screening for fucosidosis in English Springer Spaniels, Am J Vet Res 60(6):726–729, 1999.
521. Smith MO, Wenger DA, Hill SL, et al: Fucosidosis in a family of American-bred English springer spaniels, J Am Vet Med Assoc 209(12):2088–2090, 1996.
522. Selcer ES, Selcer RR: Globoid cell leukodystrophy in two West Highland white terriers and one Pomeranian, Compend Contin Educ Pract Vet 6(7):621–624, 1984.
523. Victoria T, Rafi MA, Wenger DA: Cloning of the canine GALC cDNA and identification of the mutation causing globoid cell leukodystrophy in West Highland White and Cairn terriers, Genomics (San Diego) 33(3):457–462, 1996.
524. Wenger DA, Victoria T, Rafi MA, et al: Globoid cell leukodystrophy in Cairn and West Highland White terriers 90(1):138–142, 1999.
525. Johnson GR, Oliver JE Jr, Selcer R: Globoid cell leukodystrophy in a Beagle, J Am Vet Med Assoc 167(5):380–384, 1975.
526. Zaki FA, Kay WJ: Globoid cell leukodystrophy in a miniature poodle, J Am Vet Med Assoc 163(3):248–250, 1973.
527. Luttgen PJ, Braund KG, Storts RW: Globoid cell leucodystrophy in a Basset hound, J Small Anim Pract 24:153–160, 1983.
528. McDonnell JJ, Carmichael KP, McGraw RA, et al: Preliminary characterization of globoid cell leukodystrophy in Irish Setters, J Vet Intern Med 14(3):339, 2000.
529. McGraw RA, Carmichael KP: Molecular basis of globoid cell leukodystrophy in Irish setters, Vet J 171(2):370–372, 2006.
530. Johnson KH: Globoid leukodystrophy in the cat, J Am Vet Med Assoc 157(12):2057–2064, 1970.
531. Pritchard DH, Naphtine DV, Sinclair AJ: Globoid cell leukodystrophy in polled Dorset sheep, Vet Pathol 17:399–405, 1980.
532. Sigurdson CJ, Basaraba RJ, Mazzaferro EM, et al: Globoid cell-like leukodystrophy in a domestic longhaired cat, Vet Pathol 39:494–496, 2002.
533. Coates JR, Paxton R, Cox NR, et al: A case presentation and discussion of type IV glycogen storage disease in a Norwegian Forest cat, Prog Vet Neurol 7(1):5–11, 1996.
534. Fyfe JC, Giger U, Van Winkle TJ, et al: Glycogen storage disease type IV: inherited deficiency of branching enzyme activity in cats, Pediatr Res 32(6):719–725, 1992.
535. Fyfe JC, Giger U, Van Winkle TJ, et al: Familial glycogen storage disease type IV (GSD IV) in Norwegian forest cats, Proceed 8th ACVIM Forum 1129, 1990.
536. Sponseller BT, Valberg SJ, Ward TL, et al: Muscular weakness and recumbency in a Quarter Horse colt due to glycogen branching enzyme deficiency, Equine Vet Educ 15(4):182–187, 2003.
537. Valberg SJ, Ward TL, Rush B, et al: Glycogen branching enzyme deficiency in Quarter Horse foals, J Vet Intern Med 15(6):572–580, 2001.
538. Wagner ML, Valberg SJ, Ames EG, et al: Allele frequency and likely impact of the glycogen branching enzyme deficiency gene in Quarter horse and Paint horse populations, J Vet Intern Med 20(5):1207–1211, 2006.
539. Ward TL, Valberg SJ, Adelson DL, et al: Glycogen branching enzyme (GBE1) mutation causing equine glycogen storage disease IV, Mamm Genome 15(7):570–577, 2004.
540. Berg T, Tollersrud OK, Walkley SU, et al: Purification of feline lysosomal alpha-mannosidase, determination of its cDNA sequence and identification of a mutation causing alpha-mannosidosis in Persian cats, Biochem J 328(3):863–870, 1997.
541. Blakemore WF: A case of mannosidosis in the cat: clinical and histopathological findings, J Small Anim Pract 27(7):447–455, 1986.
542. Cummings JF, Wood PA, de Lahunta A, et al: The clinical and pathologic heterogeneity of feline a-mannosidosis, J Vet Intern Med 2(4):163–170, 1988.
543. Healy PJ, Harper PA, Dennis JA: Phenotypic variation in bovine a-mannosidosis, Res Vet Sci 49(1):82–84, 1990.
544. Maenhout T, Kint JA, Dacremont G, et al: Mannosidosis in a litter of Persian cats, Vet Rec 122(15):351–354, 1988.
545. Vandevelde M, Fankhauser R, Bichsel P, et al: Hereditary neurovisceral mannosidosis associated with a-mannosidase deficiency in a family of Persian cats, Acta Neuropathol (Berl) 58(1):64–68, 1982.
546. Embury DH, Jerrett IV: Mannosidosis in Galloway calves, Vet Pathol 22(6):548–551, 1985.
547. Wenger DA, Sattler M, Kudoh T, et al: Niemann-Pick disease: A genetic model in Siamese cats, Science 208:1471–1473, 1980.
548. Yamagami T, Umeda M, Kamiya S, et al: Neurovisceral sphingomyelinosis in a Siamese cat, Acta Neuropathol (Berl) 79(3):330–332, 1989.
549. Baker HJ, Wood PA, Wenger DA, et al: Sphingomyelin lipidosis in a cat, Veterinary Pathology 24(5):386–391, 1987.
550. Somers KL, Royals MA, Carstea ED, et al: Mutation analysis of feline Niemann-Pick C1 disease, Mol Genet Metab 79(2):99–103, 2003.
551. Saunders GK, Wenger DA: Sphingomyelinase deficiency (Niemann-Pick disease) in a Hereford calf, Vet Pathol 45(2):201–202, 2008.
552. Braund KG, Mehta JR, Toivio-Kinnucan M, et al: Congenital hypomyelinating polyneuropathy in two golden retriever littermates, Vet Pathol 26(3):202–208, 1989.
553. Matz ME, Shell L, Braund K: Peripheral hypomyelinization in two golden retriever littermates, J Am Vet Med Assoc 197(2):228–230, 1990.

554. Cummings JF, Cooper BJ, de Lahunta A, et al: Canine inherited hypertrophic neuropathy, Acta Neuropathol (Berl) 53(2):137–143, 1981.
555. Dahme E, Kraft W, Scabell J: Hypertrophische polyneuropathie bei der Katze, J Vet Med 34:271–288, 1987.
556. Cooper BJ, de Lahunta A, Cummings JF, et al: Canine inherited hypertrophic neuropathy: clinical and electrodiagnostic studies, Am J Vet Res 45(6):1172–1177, 1984.
557. Cooper BJ, Duncan I, Cummings J, et al: Defective Schwann cell function in canine inherited hypertrophic neuropathy, Acta Neuropathol (Berl) 63(1):51–56, 1984.
558. Sponenberg DP, de Lahunta A: Hereditary hypertrophic neuropathy in Tibetan Mastiff dogs, J Hered 72:287, 1981.
559. O'Brien DP, Johnson GC, Liu LA, et al: Laminin α2 (merosin) -deficient muscular dystrophy and demyelinating neuropathy in two cats, J Neurol Sci 18:937–943, 2001.
560. Braund KG, Shores A, Lowrie CT, et al: Idiopathic polyneuropathy in Alaskan malamutes, J Vet Intern Med 11(4):243–249, 1997.
561. Moe L: Hereditary polyneuropathy of Alaskan malamutes. In Kirk RW, Bonagura JD, editors: Kirk's Current Veterinary Therapy, ed 11, Philadelphia, 1992, W.B. Saunders Co., pp 1038–1039.
562. Chrisman CL: Dancing Doberman disease: clinical findings and prognosis, Prog Vet Neurol 1(1):83–90, 1990.
563. Duncan ID, Griffiths IR: Peripheral nervous system in a case of canine giant axonal neuropathy, Neuropathol Appl Neurobiol 5:25–39, 1979.
564. Duncan ID, Griffiths IR, Carmichael S, et al: Inherited canine giant axonal neuropathy, Muscle Nerve 4(3):223–227, 1981.
565. Braund KG, Luttgen PJ, Redding RW, et al: Distal symmetrical polyneuropathy in a dog, Vet Pathol 17(4):422–435, 1980.
566. Henricks PM, Steiss J, Petterson JD: Distal peripheral polyneuropathy in a Great Dane, Can Vet J 28:165–167, 1987.
567. Shelton GD, Podell M, Sullivan S, et al: Distal, symmetrical polyneuropathy with laryngeal paralysis in young, related Leonberger dogs, J Vet Intern.Med 14(3):339, 2000.
568. Harkin KR, Cash WC, Shelton GD: Sensory and motor neuropathy in a border collie, J Am Vet Med Assoc 227(8):1263–1265, 2005.
569. Braund KG, Toivio-Kinnucan M, Vallat JM, et al: Distal sensorimotor polyneuropathy in mature Rottweiler dogs, Vet Pathol 31(3):316–326, 1994.
570. Armengou L, Climent F, Shelton GD, et al: Antemortem diagnosis of a distal axonopathy causing severe stringhalt in a horse, J Vet Intern Med 24(1):220–223, 2010.
571. Huntington PJ, Jeffcott LB, Friend SCE, et al: Australian stringhalt - epidemiological, clinical and neurological investigations, Equine Vet J 21(4):266–273, 1989.
572. Slocombe RF, Huntington PJ, Friend SCE, et al: Pathological aspects of Australian stringhalt, Equine Vet J 24(3):174–183, 1992.
573. Gaber CE, Amis TC, LeCouteur RA: Laryngeal paralysis in dogs: a review of 23 cases, J Am Vet Med Assoc 186(4):377–380, 1985.
574. MacPhail CM, Monnet E: Outcome of and postoperative complications in dogs undergoing surgical treatment of laryngeal paralysis: 140 cases (1985-1998), J Am Vet Med Assoc 218(12):1949–1956, 2001.
575. Jaggy A, Oliver JE, Ferguson DC, et al: Neurological manifestations of hypothyroidism: a retrospective study of 29 dogs, J Vet Intern Med 8(5):328–336, 1994.
576. Stanley BJ, Hauptman JG, Fritz MC, et al: Esophageal dysfunction in dogs with idiopathic laryngeal paralysis: a controlled cohort study, Vet Surg 39(2):139–149, 2010.
577. Venker-van Haagen AJ, Hartman W, Goedegebuure SA: Spontaneous laryngeal paralysis in young Bouviers, J Am Anim Hosp Assoc 14:714–720, 1978.
578. Venker-van Haagen AJ, Bouw J, Hartman W: Hereditary transmission of laryngeal paralysis in Bouviers, J Am Anim Hosp Assoc 17(1):75–76, 1981.
579. Braund KG, Shores A, Cochrane S, et al: Laryngeal paralysis-polyneuropathy complex in young Dalmatians, Am J Vet Res 55(4):534–542, 1994.
580. Mahony OM, Knowles KE, Braund KG, et al: Laryngeal paralysis-polyneuropathy complex in young Rottweilers, J Vet Intern Med 12(5):330–337, 1998.
581. Dickinson PJ, LeCouteur RA: Muscle and nerve biopsy, Vet Clin North Am Small Anim Pract 32(1):63–102, 2002.
582. Moreau PM, Vallat JM, Hugon J, et al: Peripheral and central distal axonopathy of suspected inherited origin in Birman cats, Acta Neuropathol (Berl) 82(2):143–146, 1991.
583. Griffiths IR: Progressive axonopathy: an inherited neuropathy of Boxer dogs. 1. Further studies of the clinical and electrophysiological features, J Small Anim Pract 26:381–392, 1985.
584. Duncan ID, Griffiths IR: Canine giant axonal neuropathy, Vet Rec 101:438–441, 1977.
585. Duncan ID, Griffiths IR: A sensory neuropathy affecting long-haired dachshund dogs, J Small Anim Pract 23:381–390, 1982.
586. Cummings JF, de Lahunta A, Braund KG, et al: Hereditary sensory neuropathy. Nociceptive loss and acral mutilation in pointer dogs: canine hereditary sensory neuropathy, Am J Pathol 112(1):136–138, 1983.
587. Mason LT: The occurrence and pedigree analysis of a hereditary sensory neuropathy in the English springer spaniel, Proceed Ann Am College Vet Dermatology 1523–1524, 1999.
588. Paradis M, Cd Jaham, Page N, et al: Acral mutilation and analgesia in 13 French spaniels, Vet Dermatol 16(2):87–93, 2005.
589. Franklin RJM, Olby NJ, Targett MP, et al: Sensory neuropathy in a Jack Russell terrier, J Small Anim Pract 33:402–404, 1992.
590. Steiss JE, Pook HA, Clark EG, et al: Sensory neuronopathy in a dog, J Am Vet Med Assoc 190(2):205–208, 1987.
591. Carmichael S, Griffiths IR: Case of isolated sensory trigeminal neuropathy in a dog, Vet Rec 109(13):280–282, 1981.
592. Wheeler SJ: Sensory neuropathy in a border collie puppy, J Small Anim Pract :28281–28289, 1987.
593. Vermeersch K, Ham LV, Braund KG, et al: Sensory neuropathy in two border collie puppies, J Small Anim Pract 46(6):295–299, 2005.
594. Wouda W, Vandevelde M, Oettli P, et al: Sensory neuronopathy in dogs: a study of four cases, J Comp Pathol 93(3):437–450, 1983.
595. Cummings JF, de Lahunta A, Winn SS: Acral mutilation and nociceptive loss in English pointer dogs. A canine sensory neuropathy, Acta Neuropathol (Berl) 53(2):119–127, 1981.
596. Sanda A, Pivnik L: Die Zehenneckrose bei kurzhaarigen Vorstehhunden, Kleintierpraxis 9:76–83, 1964.

597. Duncan ID, Griffiths IR, Munz M: The pathology of a sensory neuropathy affecting longhaired Dachshund dogs, Acta Neuropathol (Berl) 58(2):141–151, 1982.
598. van Nes JJ: Electrophysiological evidence of sensory nerve dysfunction in 10 dogs with acral lick dermatitis, J Am Anim Hosp Assoc 22(2):157–160, 1986.
599. Cummings JF, de Lahunta A, Simpson ST, et al: Reduced substance P-like immunoreactivity in hereditary sensory neuropathy of pointer dogs, Acta Neuropathol (Berl) 63(1):33–40, 1984.
600. Cummings JF, de Lahunta A, Mitchell WJ Jr: Ganglioradiculitis in the dog. A clinical, light- and electron- microscopic study, Acta Neuropathol (Berl) 60(1-2):29–39, 1983.
601. Jaderlund KH, Orvind E, Johnsson E, et al: A neurologic syndrome in golden reterievers presenting as a sensory ataxic neuropathy, J Vet Intern Med 21:1307–1315, 2007.
602. Baranowska I, Jaderlund KH, Nennesmo I, et al: Sensory ataxic neuropathy in golden retriever dogs is caused by a deletion in the mitochondrial *tRNA^Tyr* gene, PLoS Genet :51–59, 2009.
603. Towell TL, Shell LC: Endocrinopathies that affect peripheral nerves of cats and dogs, Compend Contin Educ Pract Vet 16(2):157–161, 1994:196.
604. Indrieri RJ, Whalen LR, Cardinet GH, et al: Neuromuscular abnormalities associated with hypothyroidism and lymphocytic thyroiditis in three dogs, J Am Vet Med Assoc 190(5):544–548, 1987.
605. Panciera DL: Hypothyroidism in dogs: 66 cases (1987-1992), J Am Vet Med Assoc 204(5):761–767, 1994.
606. Rossmeisl JH Jr, Duncan RB, Inzana KD, et al: Longitudinal study of the effects of chronic hypothyroidism on skeletal muscle in dogs, Am J Vet Res 70(7):879–889, 2009.
607. Braund KG, Dillon AR, August JR, et al: Hypothyroid myopathy in two dogs, Vet Pathol 18(5):589–598, 1981.
608. Coates JR: Neurologic manifestations of hypothyroidism, Canine Pract 22(1):27–28, 1997.
609. Higgins MA, Rossmeisl JH, Panciera DL: Hypothyroid-associated central vestibular disease in 10 dogs: 1999-2005, J Vet Intern Med :201363–201369, 2006.
610. Bichsel P, Jacobs G, Oliver JE Jr: Neurologic manifestations associated with hypothyroidism in four dogs, J Am Vet Med Assoc 192(12):1745–1747, 1988.
611. Chastain CB, Graham CL, Riley MG: Myxedema coma in two dogs, Canine Pract 9(4):20–34, 1982.
612. Vitale CL, Olby NJ: Neurologic dysfunction in hypothyroid, hyperlipidemic Labrador Retrievers, J Vet Intern Med 21(6):1316–1322, 2007.
613. Budsberg SC, Moore GE, Klappenbach K: Thyroxine-responsive unilateral forelimb lameness and generalized neuromuscular disease in four hypothyroid dogs, J Am Vet Med Assoc 202(11):1859–1860, 1993.
614. Plotnick AN: Megaesophagus and hypothyroidism in an english springer spaniel and response to thyroxine supplementation, Canine Pract 2414–2417, 1999.
615. Kern TJ, Erb HN: Facial neuropathy in dogs and cats: 95 cases (1975-1985), J Am Vet Med Assoc 191(12):1604–1609, 1987.
616. Dewey CW, Shelton GD, Bailey CS, et al: Neuromuscular dysfunction in five dogs with acquired myasthenia gravis and presumptive hypothyroidism, Prog Vet Neurol 6(4):117–123, 1995.
617. Platt SR: Neuromuscular complications in endocrine and metabolic disorders, Vet Clin North Am Small Anim Pract 32(1):125–146, 2002.
618. Wolf AM: Management of geriatric diabetic cats, Compend Contin Educ Pract Vet 11(9):1088–1093, 1989.
619. Johnson CA, Kittleson MD, Indrieri RJ: Peripheral neuropathy and hypotension in a diabetic dog, J Am Vet Med Assoc 183(9):1007–1009, 1983.
620. Braund KG, Steiss JE: Distal neuropathy in spontaneous diabetes mellitus in the dog, Acta Neuropathol (Berl) 57(4):263–269, 1982.
621. Kramek BA, Moise NS, Cooper B, et al: Neuropathy associated with diabetes mellitus in the cat, J Am Vet Med Assoc 184(1):42–45, 1984.
622. Mizisin AP, Shelton GD, Wagner S, et al: Myelin splitting, Schwann cell injury and demyelination in feline diabetic neuropathy, Acta Neuropathol (Berl) 95(2):171–174, 1998.
623. Mizisin AP, Nelson RW, Sturges BK, et al: Comparable myelinated nerve pathology in feline and human diabetes mellitus, Acta Neuropathol :113431–113442, 2007.
624. Mizisin AP, Shelton GD, Burgers ML, et al: Neurological complications associated with spontaneously occurring feline diabetes mellitus, J Neuropathol Exp Neurol 61:872–884, 2002.
625. Holland CT: Bilateral Horner's syndrome in a dog with diabetes mellitus, Vet Rec 160(19):662–664, 2007.
626. Steiss JE, Orsher AN, Bowen JM: Electrodiagnostic analysis of peripheral neuropathy in dogs with diabetes mellitus, Am J Vet Res 42(12):2061–2064, 1981.
627. Platt SR, Garosi LS: Neuromuscular weakness and collapse, Vet Clin North Am Small Anim Pract :341281–341305, 2004.
628. Jones BR, Wallace A, Harding DRK, et al: Occurence of idiopathic, familial hyperchylomicronaemia in a cat, Vet Rec 112(543):547, 1983.
629. Jones BR, Johnstone AC, Cahill JI, et al: Peripheral neuropathy in cats with inherited primary hyperchylomicronaemia, Vet Rec 119(11):268–272, 1986.
630. Grieshaber TL, McKeever PJ, McKeever PJ, et al: Spontaneous cutaneous (eruptive) xanthomatosis in two cats, J Am Anim Hosp Assoc 27:509–512, 1991.
631. Bauer JE, Verlander JW: Congenital lipoprotein lipase deficiency in hyperlipemic kitten siblings, Vet Clin Pathol, 137–11, 1984.
632. Brooks KD: Idiopathic hyperlipoproteinemia in a cat, Companion Anim Pract :195–199, 1989.
633. Sottiaux J: Cas clinique: hyperchylomicronémie primaire chez un chat, Le Point Vétérinaire 18:117–119, 1986.
634. Smerdon T: Hyperchylomicronaemia in a litter of Siamese kittens, Bulletin of the Feline Advisory Bureau 51–53, 1990.
635. Jones BR: Hyperchlomicronemia in the cat. In Bonagura JD, Kirk RW, editors: Kirk's Current Veterinary Theraphy XII Small Animal Practice, ed 12, Philadelphia, 1995, W.B. Saunders Co., pp 1163–1166.
636. Mayes PA: Lipid transport and storage. In Murray RK, Granner DK, Mayes PA, Rodwell VW, editors: Harper's Biochemistry ed 12, Norwalk, 1990, Appleton & Lange, pp 234–248.
637. Jones BR: Inherited hyperchylomicronaemia in the cat, J Small Anim Pract 34:493–499, 1993.
638. Watson TDG, Gaffney D, Mooney CT, et al: Inherited hyperchylomicronaemia in the cat: lipoprotein lipase function and gene structure, J Small Anim Pract 33:207–212, 1992.
639. Ginzinger DG, Lewis MES, Ma Y, et al: A mutation in the lipoprotein lipase gene is the molecular basis of chylomicronemia in a colony of domestic cats, J Clin Invest 97(5):1257–1266, 1996.
640. McKerrell RE, Blakemore WF, Heath MF, et al: Primary hyperoxaluria (L-glyceric aciduria) in the cat: a newly recognised inherited disease, Vet Rec 125(2):31–34, 1989.

641. Goldstein RE, Narala S, Sabet N, Goldstein O, et al: Primary hyperoxaluria in cats is caused by a mutation in the feline GRHPR gene, J Hered 100:S2–S7, 2009.
642. Panciera RJ, Washburn KE, Streeter RN, et al: A familial peripheral neuropathy and glomerulopathy in Gelbvieh calves, Vet Pathol 40(1):63–70, 2003.
643. Moisan PG, Steffen DJ, Sanderson MW, et al: A familial degenerative neuromuscular disease of Gelbvieh cattle, J Vet Diagn Invest 14(2):140–149, 2002.
644. Inzana KD: Paraneoplastic neuromuscular disorders, Vet Clin North Am Small Anim Pract 34:1453–1467, 2004.
645. Braund KG: Remote effects of cancer on the nervous system, Semin Vet Med Surg (Small Anim) 5(4):262–270, 1990.
646. Brown NO: Paraneoplastic syndromes of humans, dogs and cats, J Am Anim Hosp Assoc 17(6):911–916, 1981.
647. Cavana P, Sammartano F, Capucchio MT, et al: Peripheral neuropathy in a cat with renal lymphoma, J Feline Med Surg 11(10):869–872, 2009.
648. Hamilton TA, Cook JRJ, Braund KG, et al: Vincristine-induced peripheral neuropathy in a dog, J Am Vet Med Assoc 198(4):635–638, 1991.
649. Braund KG, McGuire JA, Amling KA, et al: Peripheral neuropathy associated with malignant neoplasms in dogs, Vet Pathol 24(1):16–21, 1987.
650. Sorjonen DC, Braund KG, Hoff EJ: Paraplegia and subclinical neuromyopathy associated with a primary lung tumor in a dog, J Am Vet Med Assoc 180(10):1209–1211, 1982.
651. Mariani CL, Shelton SB, Alsup JC: Paraneoplastic polyneuropathy and subsequent recovery following tumor removal in a dog, J Am Anim Hosp Assoc 35(4):302–305, 1999.
652. Dyer KR, Duncan ID, Hammang JP, et al: Peripheral neuropathy in two dogs: correlation between clinical, electrophysiological and pathological findings, J Small Anim Pract 27:133–146, 1986.
653. Hobbs SL, Cobb MA: A cranial neuropathy associated with multicentric lymphosarcoma in a dog, Vet Rec 127:525–526, 1990.
654. Villiers E, Dobson J: Multiple myeloma with associated polyneuropathy in a German shepherd dog, J Small Anim Pract 39(5):249–251, 1998.
655. Bergman PJ, Bruyette DS, Coyne BE, et al: Canine clinical peripheral neuropathy associated with pancreatic islet cell carcinoma, Prog Vet Neurol 5(2):57–62, 1994.
656. Braund KG, Steiss JE, Amling KA, et al: Insulinoma and subclinical peripheral neuropathy in two dogs, J Vet Intern Med 1(2):86–90, 1987.
657. Schrauwen E, Van Ham LML, Desmidt M, et al: Peripheral polyneuropathy associated with insulinoma in the dog: clinical, pathological, and electrodiagnostic features, Prog Vet Neurol 7(1):16–19, 1996.
658. Shahar R, Rousseaux C, Steiss J: Peripheral polyneuropathy in a dog with functional islet B-cell tumor and widespread metastasis, J Am Vet Med Assoc 187(2):175–177, 1985.
659. van Ham L, Braund KG, Roels S, et al: Treatment of a dog with an insulinoma-related peripheral polyneurpathy with corticosteroids, Vet Rec 141:98–100, 1997.
670. Bichsel P, Oliver JE Jr, Tyler DE, et al: Chronic polyneuritis in a Rottweiler, J Am Vet Med Assoc 191(8):991–994, 1987.
671. Cummings J, de Lahunta A: Chronic relapsing polyradiculoneuritis in a dogs: A clinical, light and electron-microscopic study, Acta Neuropath (Berl) 28:191–204, 1974.
672. Shores A, Braund KG, McDonald RK: Chronic relapsing polyneuropathy in a cat, J Am Anim Hosp Assoc 23:569–573, 1987.
673. Shelton GD: Muscle pain, cramps and hypertonicity, Vet Clin North Am Small Anim Pract 34:1483–1496, 2004.
674. Podell M: Inflammatory myopathies, Vet Clin North Am Small Anim Pract 32:147–167, 2002.
675. Shelton GD: From dog to man: the broad spectrum of inflammatory myopathies. [Review] [56 refs], Neuromuscul Disord 17(9-10):663–670, 2007.
676. LeCouteur RA, Dow SW, Sisson AF: Metabolic and endocrine myopathies of dogs and cats, Semin Vet Med Surg (Small Anim) 4(2):146–155, 1989.
677. Brunson DB, Hogan KJ: Malignant hyperthermia: a syndrome not a disease, Vet Clin North Am Small Anim Pract 34:1419–1433, 2004.
678. Shelton GD: Rhabdomyolysis, myoglobinuria, and necrotizing myopathies, Vet Clin North Am Small Anim Pract 34:1469–1482, 2004.
679. Kornegay JN, Sharp NJH, Camp SD, et al: Early pathologic features of golden retriever muscular dystrophy: a model of Duchenne muscular dystrophy 48(3):348, 1989.
680. Kornegay JN, Tuler S, Miller D, et al: Muscular dystorphy in a litter of golden retriever dogs, Muscle Nerve 11:1056–1064, 1988.
681. Valentine BA, Cooper BJ, Cummings JF, et al: Progressive muscular dystrophy in a golden retriever dog: light microscope and ultrastructural features at 4 and 8 months, Acta Neuropathologica 71(3/4):301–310, 1986.
682. Wentink GH, Meijer AEFH, Linde-Sipman JS, et al: Myopathy iin an Irish terrier with a metabolic defect of the isolated mitochondria, Zentralblatt fur Veterinarmedizin 21A(Heft 1):62–74, 1974.
683. Presthus J, Nordstoga K: Congenital myopathy in a litter of Samoyed dogs, Prog Vet Neurol 4(2):37–40, 1993.
684. Winand N, Pradham D, Cooper B: Molecular characterization of severe Duchenne-type muscular dystrophy in a family of rottweiler dogs. Molecular mechanisms of neuromuscular disease, Tucson (AZ), 1994, Muscular Dystrophy Association.
685. Ham LML, Desmidt M, Tshamala M, et al: Canine X-linked muscular dystrophy in Belgian Groenendaeler Shepherds, Vlaams Diergeneeskundig Tijdschrift 64(3):102–106, 1995.
686. Paola JP, Podell M, Shelton GD: Muscular dystrophy in a miniature schnauzer, Prog Vet Neurol 4(1):14–18, 1993.
687. Cardinet GH III, Holliday TA: Neuromuscular diseases of domestic animals: a summary of muscle biopsies from 159 cases, Ann N Y Acad Sci 317:290–313, 1979.
688. Schatzberg SJ, Shelton GD: Newly identified neuromuscular disorders, Vet Clin North Am Small Anim Pract 34(6):1497–1524, 2004.
689. Schatzberg SJ, Olby NJ, Breen M, Anderson LV, et al: Molecular analysis of a spontaneous dystrophin 'knockout' dog, Neuromuscul Disord 9(5):289–295, 1999.
690. Wetterman CA, Harkin KR, Cash WC, et al: Hypertrophic muscular dystrophy in a young dog, J Am Vet Med Assoc 216(6):878–881, 2000.
691. Jones BR, Brennan S, Mooney CT, et al: Muscular dystrophy with truncated dystrophin in a family of Japanese Spitz dogs, J Neurol Sci 217(2):143–149, 2004.
692. Van Ham LML, Roels SLMF, Hoorens JK: Congenital dystrophy-like myopathy in a Brittany Spaniel puppy, Prog Vet Neurol 6(4):135–138, 1995.

693. Bergman RL, Inzana KD, Monroe WE, et al: Dystrophin-deficient muscular dystrophy in a Labrador retriever, J Am Anim Hosp Assoc 38(3):255–261, 2002.
694. Piercy RJ, Walmsley G: Muscular dystrophy in Cavalier King Charles spaniels, Vet Rec 165(2):62, 2009.
695. Klarenbeek S, Gerritzen-Bruning MJ, Rozemuller AJM, et al: Canine X-linked muscular dystrophy in a family of Grand Basset Griffon Venden dogs, J Comp Pathol 137(4):249–252, 2007.
696. Sharp NJH, Kornegay JN, Camp SD, et al: An error in dystrophin mRNA processing in golden retriever muscular dystrophy, an animal homologue of Duchenne muscular dystrophy, Genomics (San Diego) 13(1):115–121, 1992.
697. Schatzberg S, Olby N, Steingold S, et al: A polymerase chain reaction screening strategy for the promoter of the canine dystrophin gene, Am J Vet Res 60(9):1040–1046, 1999.
698. Gaschen F, Gaschen L, Burgunder JM: Clinical study of a breeding colony affected with hypertrophic feline muscular dystrophy, J Vet Intern Med 9(3):207, 1995.
699. Carpenter JL, Hoffman EP, Ramanul FC, et al: Feline muscular dystrophy with dystrophin deficiency, Am J Pathol 135:909–919, 1989.
700. Vos JH, van der Linde-Sipman JS, Goedegebuure SA: Dystrophy-like myopathy in the cat, J Comp Pathol 96(3):335–341, 1986.
701. Malik R, Mepstead K, Yang F, et al: Hereditary myopathy of Devon rex cats, J Small Anim Pract :34539–34546, 1993.
702. Martin PT, Shelton GD, Dickinson PJ, et al: Muscular dystrophy associated with alpha-dystroglycan deficiency in Sphynx and Devon Rex cats, Neuromuscul Disord 18(12):942–952, 2008.
703. Robinson R: Spasticity in the Devon Rex cat, Vet Rec 130:302, 1992.
704. Deitz K, Morrison JA, Kline K, et al: Sarcoglycan-deficient muscular dystrophy in a Boston terrier, J Vet Med 22(2):476–480, 2008.
705. Shelton GD, Ling LA, Guo LT, et al: Muscular dystrophy in female dogs, J Vet Intern Med 15:240–244, 2001.
706. O'Brien DP, Johnson GC, Liu LA, et al: Laminin a2 (merosin) -deficient muscular dystrophy and demyelinating neuropathy in two cats, J Neurol Sci 18:937–943, 2001.
707. Poncelet L, Resibois A, Engvall E, et al: Laminin alpha2 deficiency-associated muscular dystrophy in a Maine coon cat. [Review] [19 refs], J Small Anim Pract 44(12):550–552, 2003.
708. Richards RB, Passmore IK, Bretag AH, et al: Ovine congenital progressive muscular dystrophy: clinical syndrome and distribution of lesions, Australian Veterinary Journal 63(12):396–401, 1986.
709. Richards RB, Lewer RP, Passmore IK, McQuade NC: Ovine congenital progressive muscular dystrophy: mode of inheritance, Aust Vet J 65(3):93–94, 1988.
710. Kramer JW, Hegreberg GA, Hamilton MJ: Inheritance of a neuromuscular disorder of Labrador retriever dogs, J Am Vet Med Assoc 179(4):380–381, 1981.
711. Kramer JW, Hegreberg GA, Bryan GM, et al: A muscle disorder of Labrador retrievers characterized by deficiency of type II muscle fibers, J Am Vet Med Assoc 169(8):817–820, 1976.
712. McKerrell RE, Braund KG: Hereditary myopathy in Labrador retrievers: clinical variations, J Small Anim Pract 28:479–489, 1987.
713. McKerrell RE, Braund KG: Hereditary myopathies in Labrador retrievers: a morphologic study, J Small Anim Pract 23:411–417, 1986.
714. Pele M, Tiret L, Kessler JL, Blot S, et al: SINE exonic insertion in the PTPLA gene leads to multiple splicing defects and segregates with the autosomal recessive centronuclear myopathy in dogs. [Erratum appears in Hum Mol Genet. 2005 Jul 1;14(13):1905-6], Hum Mol Genet 14(11):1417–1427, 2005.
715. Peeters ME, Ubbink GJ: Dysphagia-associated muscular dystrophy, Prog Vet Neurol 5(3):124, 1994.
716. Peeters ME, Ubbink GJ: Dysphagia-associated muscular dystrophy: a familial trait in the bouvier des Flandres, Vet Rec 134(17):444–446, 1994.
717. Cooper BJ, de Lahunta A, Gallagher EA: Nemalin myopathy of cats, Muscle Nerve 9:618–625, 1986.
718. Hafner A, Dahme E, Obermaier G, et al: Congenital myopathy in Braunvieh Brown Swiss calves, J Comp Pathol 115(1):23–34, 1996.
719. Delauche AJ, Cuddon PA, Podell M, et al: Nemaline rods in canine myopathies: 4 case reports and literature review, J Vet Intern Med 12(6):424–430, 1998.
720. Rossmeisl JH Jr, Duncan RB, Inzana KD, et al: Longitudinal study of the effects of chronic hypothyroidism on skeletal muscle in dogs, Am J Vet Res 70(7):879–889, 2009.
721. Hanson SM, Smith MO, Walker TL, et al: Juvenile-onset distal myopathy in Rottweiler dogs, J Vet Intern Med 12(2):103–108, 1998.
722. Targett MP, Franklin RJM, Olby NJ, et al: Central core myopathy in a Great Dane, J Small Anim Pract 35(2):100–103, 1994.
723. Walvoort HC, van Nes JJ, Stokhof A, et al: Canine glycogen storage disease type II: a clinical study of four affected Lapland dogs, J Am Anim Hosp Assoc 20:279–286, 1984.
724. Walvoort HC, Slee RG, Koster JF: Canine glycogen storage disease type II. A biochemical study of an acid alpha -glucosidase-deficient Lapland dog, Biochim Biophys Acta 715(1):63–69, 1982.
725. Dennis JA, Healy PJ: Genotyping shorthorn cattle for generalised glycogenosis, Aust Vet J 79(11):773–775, 2001.
726. Dennis JA, Healy PJ, Reichmann KG: Genotyping Brahman cattle for generalised glycogenosis, Aust Vet J 80(5):286–291, 2002.
727. Reichmann KG, Twist JO, Thistlethwaite EJ: Clinical, diagnostic and biochemical features of generalised glycogenosis type II and Brahman cattle, Aust Vet J 70(11):405–408, 1993.
728. Manktelow BW, Hartley WJ: Generalized glycogen storage disease in sheep, J Comp Pathol 85(1):139–145, 1975.
729. Ceh L, Hauge JG, Svenkerud R, et al: Glycogenosis type III in the dog, Acta Vet Scand 17(2):210–222, 1976.
730. Rafiquzzaman M, Svenkerud R, et al: Glycogenosis in the dog, Acta Vet Scand 17(2):196–209, 1976.
731. Gregory BL, Shelton GD, Bali DS, et al: Glycogen storage disease type IIIa in Curly-Coated Retrievers, J Vet Intern Med 21(1):40–46, 2007.
732. Fyfe JC, Giger U, Van Winkle TJ, et al: Glycogen storage disease type IV: inherited deficiency of branching enzyme activity in cats, Pediatr Res 32(6):719–725, 1992.
733. Coates JR, Paxton R, Cox NR, et al: A case presentation and discussion of Type IV glycogen storage disease in a Norwegian Forest cat, Prog Vet Neurol 7(1):5–11, 1996.
734. Fyfe JC, Kurzhals RL, Patterson DF: Feline glycogensosis type IV is caused by a complex rearrangement deleting 6 kb of the branching enzyme gene and eliminating a exon, Am J Hum Genet 61A251, 1997.
735. Ward TL, Valberg SJ, Adelson DL, et al: Glycogen branching enzyme (GBE1) mutation causing equine glycogen storage disease IV, Mamm Genome 15(7):570–577, 2004.

736. Valberg SJ, Ward TL, Rush B, et al: Glycogen branching enzyme deficiency in Quarter Horse foals, J Vet Intern Med 15(6):572–580, 2001.
737. Johnstone AC, McSporran KD, Kenny JE, et al: Myophosphorylase deficiency (glycogen storage disease Type V) in a herd of Charolais cattle in New Zealand: confirmation by PCR-RFLP testing, N Z Vet J 52(6):404–408, 2004.
738. Angelos S, Valberg SJ, Smith BP, et al: Myophosphorylase deficiency associated with rhabdomyolysis and exercise intolerance in 6 related Charolais cattle, Muscle Nerve 18(7):736–740, 1995.
739. Bilstrom JA, Valberg SJ, Bernoco D, et al: Genetic test for myophosphorylase deficiency in Charolais cattle, Am J Vet Res 59(3):267–270, 1998.
740. Soethout EC, Verkaar ELC, Jansen GH, et al: A direct StyI polymerase chain reaction-restriction fragment length polymorphism (PCR-RFLP) test for the myophosphorylase mutation in cattle, J Vet Med 49(6):289–290, 2002.
741. Giger U, Argov Z, Schnall M, et al: Metabolic myopathy in canine muscle-type phosphofructokinase deficiency, Muscle Nerve 11(12):1260–1265, 1988.
742. Giger U, Smith BF, Woods CB, et al: Inherited phosphofructokinase deficiency in an American cocker spaniel, J Am Vet Med Assoc 201(10):1569–1571, 1992.
743. Harvey JW, Calderwood MM, Gropp KE, et al: Polysaccharide storage myopathy in canine phosphofructokinase deficiency (type VII glycogen storage disease), Vet Pathol 27(1):1–8, 1990.
744. Valberg SJ, Cardinet GH, Carlson GP, et al: Polysaccharide storage myopathy associated with recurrent exertional rhabdomyolysis in horses, Neuromuscul Disord 2:351–359, 1992.
745. Valentine BA, Credille KM, Lavoie JP, et al: Severe polysaccharide storage myopathy in Belgian and Percheron draught horses, Equine Vet J 29220–29225, 1997.
746. Valentine BA, Cooper BJ: Incidence of polysaccharide storage myopathy, Vet Pathol 42:823–827, 2005.
747. McCue ME, Valberg SJ, Miller MB, et al: Glycogen synthase (GYS1) mutation causes a novel skeletal muscle glycogenosis, Genomics 91:458–466, 2008.
748. McCue ME, Valberg SJ, Lucio M, et al: Glycogen synthase 1 (GYS1) mutation in diverse breeds with polysaccharide storage myopathy, J Vet Intern Med 22:1228–1233, 2008.
749. Breitschwerdt EB, Kornegay JN, Wheeler SJ, et al: Episodic weakness associated with exertional lactic acidosis and myopathy in Old English sheepdog littermates, J Am Vet Med Assoc 201(5):731–736, 1992.
750. Olby NJ, Chan KK, Targett MP, et al: Suspected mitochondrial myopathy in a Jack Russell terrier, J Small Anim Pract 38(5):213–216, 1997.
751. Houlton JE, Herrtage ME: Mitochondrial myopathy in the Sussex spaniel, Vet Rec 106(9):206, 1980.
752. Herrtage ME, Houlton JEF: Collapsing Clumber spaniels 105(14):334, 1979.
753. Paciello O, Maiolino P, Fatone G, Papparella S: Mitochondrial myopathy in a German shepherd dog, Vet Pathol 40(5):507–511, 2003.
754. Valberg SJ, Carlson GP, Cardinet GH, et al: Skeletal muscle mitochondrial myopathy as a cause of exercise intolerance in a horse, Muscle Nerve 17305–17312, 1994.
755. Cameron JM, Maj MC, Levandovskiy V, et al: Identification of a canine model of pyruvate dehydrogenase phosphatase 1 deficiency, Mol Genet Metab 90(1):15–23, 2007.
756. Platt SR, Chrisman CL, Shelton GD: Lipid storage myopathy in a cocker spaniel, J Small Anim Pract 40:31–34, 1999.
757. Inada S, Yamauchi C, Igata A, et al: Canine storage disease characterized by hereditary progressive neurogenic muscular atrophy: breeding experiments and clinical manifestation, Am J Vet Res 47(10):2294–2299, 1986.
758. Wells GAH, Bradley R: Pietrain creeper syndrome: a primary myopathy of the pig? Neuropathol Appl Neurobiol 4(3):237–238, 1978.
759. Wells GAH, Pinsent PJN, Todd JN: A progressive, familial myopathy of the Pietrain pig: the clinical syndrome, Vet Rec 106(26):556–558, 1980.
760. Beck CL, Fahlke C, George AL: Molecular basis for decreased muscle chloride conductance in the myotonic goat, Proc Natl Acad Sci U S A 93:11248–11252, 1996.
761. Finnigan DF, Hanna WJB, Poma R, et al: A novel mutation of the CLCN1 gene associated with myotonia hereditaria in an Australian cattle dog, J Vet Intern Med 21(3):458–463, 2007.
762. Rhodes TH, Vite CH, Giger U, et al: A missense mutation in canine ClC-1 causes recessive myotonia congenita in the dog, FEBS Lett 45654–45658, 1999.
763. Farrow BRH, Malik R: Hereditary myotonia in the Chow Chow, J Small Anim Pract 22:451–465, 1981.
764. Shores A, Redding RW, Braund KG, Simpson ST: Myotonia congenita in a Chow Chow pup, J Am Vet Med Assoc 188(5):532–533, 1986.
765. Vite CH, Cozzi F, Rich M, et al: Myotonic myopathy in Miniature Schnauzers, J Vet Intern Med 12(3):208, 1998.
766. Shires PK, Nafe LA, Hulse DA: Myotonia in a Staffordshire terrier, J Am Vet Med Assoc 183(2):229–232, 1983.
767. Hill SL, Shelton GD, Lenehan TM: Myotonia in a cocker spaniel, J Am Anim Hosp Assoc 31(6):506–509, 1995.
768. Lobetti RG: Myotonia congenita in a Jack Russell terrier, J South African Vet Assoc 80(2):106–107, 2009.
769. Honhold N, Smith DA: Myotonia in the Great Dane, Vet Rec 119(7):162, 1986.
770. Steinberg SA, Botelho S: Myotonia in a horse, Science 137979–137980, 1962.
771. Hickford FH, Jones BR, Gething MA, et al: Congenital myotonia in related kittens, J Small Anim Pract 39(6):281–285, 1998.
772. Toll J, Cooper B, Altschul M: Congenital myotonia in 2 domestic cats, J Vet Intern Med 12(2):116–119, 1998.
773. Moore GA, Dyer KR, Dyer RM, et al: Autosomal recessive myotonia congenita in sheep, Genet Select Evolution 29(3):291–294, 1997.
774. Simpson ST, Braund KG: Myotonic dystrophy-like disease in a dog, J Am Vet Med Assoc 186(5):495–498, 1985.
775. Smith BF, Braund KG, Steiss JE, et al: Possible adult onset myotonic dystrophy in a boxer, J Vet Intern Med 12(2):120, 1998.
776. Reed SM, Hegreber GA, Bayly WM: Progressive myotonia in foals resembling human dystrophia myotonica, Muscle Nerve 11:291–296, 1988.
777. Mayhew IG: Large Animal Neurology, ed 2, Ames, 2009, Wiley-Blackwell.
778. Sarli G, Della Salda L, Marcato PS: Dystrophy-like myopathy in a foal, Vet Rec 135(7):156–160, 1994.
779. Taylor SM, Shmon CL, Shelton GD, et al: Exercise-induced collapse of Labrador retrievers: survey results and preliminary investigation of heritability, J Am Anim Hosp Assoc 44(6):295–301, 2008.

780. Taylor SM, Shmon CL, Adams VJ, et al: Evaluations of Labrador retrievers with exercise-induced collapse, including response to a standardized strenuous exercise protocol, J Am Anim Hosp Assoc 45(1):3–13, 2009.
781. Patterson EE, Minor KM, Tchernatynskaia AV, et al: A canine DNM1 mutation is highly associated with the syndrome of exercise-induced collapse, Nat Genet 40(10):1235–1239, 2008.
782. Berman MC, Harrison GG, Bull AB, et al: Changes underlying halothane induced malignant hyperpyrexia in Landrace pigs, Nature 225:653–655, 1970.
783. Riedesel DH, Hildebrand SV: Unusual response following use of succinylcholine in a horse anesthetized with halothane, J Am Vet Med Assoc 187(5):507–508, 1985.
784. Aleman M, Brosnan RJ, Williams DC, et al: Malignant hyperthermia in a horse anesthetized with halothane, J Vet Intern Med 19(3):363–366, 2005.
785. Brunson DB, Hogan KJ: Malignant hyperthermia: a syndrome not a disease, Vet Clin North Am Small Anim Pract 34:1419–1433, 2004.
786. Roberts MC, Mickelson JR, Patterson EE, et al: Autosomal dominant canine malignant hyperthermia is caused by a mutation in the gene encoding the skeletal muscle calcium release channel (RYR1), Anesthesiology 95(3):716–725, 2001.
787. Spier SJ, Carlson GP, Holliday TA, et al: Hyperkalemic periodic paralysis in horses, J Am Vet Med Assoc 197(8):1009–1017, 1990.
788. Spier SJ, Carlson GP, Harrold D, et al: Genetic study of hyperkalemic periodic paralysis in horses, J Am Vet Med Assoc 202(6):933–937, 1993.
789. Naylor JM, Robinson JA, Bertone J: Familial incidence of hyperkalemic periodic paralysis in quarter horses, J Am Vet Med Assoc 200(3):340–343, 1992.
790. Rudolph JA, Spier SJ, Byrns G, et al: Periodic paralysis in quarter horses: a sodium channel mutation disseminated by selective breeding, Nat Genet 2(2):144–147, 1992.
791. Cannon SC, Hayward LJ, Beech J, et al: Sodium channel inactivation is impaired in equine hyperkalemic periodic paralysis, J Neurophysiol 73(5):1892–1899, 1995.
792. Jezyk PF: Hyperkalemic periodic paralysis in a dog, J Am Anim Hosp Assoc 18:977–980, 1982.
793. Johnson RP, Watson ADJ, Smith J, et al: Myasthenia in springer spaniel littermates, J Small Anim Pract 16(10):641–647, 1975.
794. Dickinson PJ, Sturges BK, Shelton GD, et al: Congenital myasthenia gravis in smooth-haired miniature dachshund dogs, J Vet Intern Med 19(6):920–923, 2005.
795. Wallace ME, Palmer AC: Recessive mode of inheritance in myasthenia gravis in the Jack Russell terrier, Vet Rec 114(14):350, 1984.
796. Miller LM, Lennon VA, Lambert EH, et al: Congenital myasthenia gravis in 13 smooth fox terriers, J Am Vet Med Assoc 182(7):694–697, 1983.
797. Indrieri RJ, Creighton SR, Lambert EH, et al: Myasthenia gravis in two cats, J Am Vet Med Assoc 182(1):57–60, 1983.
798. Joseph RJ, Carrillo JM, Lennon VA: Myasthenia gravis in the cat, J Vet Intern Med 2(2):75–79, 1988.
799. Flagstad A, Trojaborg W, Gammeltoft S: Congenital myasthenic syndrome in the dog breed Gammel Dansk Honsehund: clinical, electrophysiological, pharmacological and immunological comparison with acquired myasthenia gravis, Acta Vet Scand 30(1):89–102, 1989.
800. Thompson PN, Steinlein OK, Harper CK, et al: Congenital myasthenic syndrome of Brahman cattle in South Africa, Vet Rec 153(25):779–781, 2003.
801. Schatzberg SJ, Shelton GD: Newly identified neuromuscular disorders, Vet Clin North Am Small Anim Pract 34(6):1497–1524, 2004.
802. Shelton GD, Engvall E: Canine and feline models of human inherited muscle diseases, Neuromuscul Disord 15:127–138, 2005.
803. Aleman M: A review of equine muscle disorders, Neuromuscul Disord 18:277–287, 2008.
804. Shelton GD, Cardinet GH III: Pathophysiologic basis of canine muscle disorders, J Vet Intern Med 1(1):36–44, 1987.
805. Evans J, Levesque D, Shelton GD: Canine inflammatory myopathies: a clinicopathologic review of 200 cases, J Vet Intern Med 18(5):679–691, 2004.
806. Fyfe JC: Molecular diagnosis of inherited neuromuscular disease, Vet Clin North Am Small Anim Pract 32:287–299, 2002.
807. Werner LL, Bright JM: Drug-induced immune hypersensitivity disorders in two dogs treated with trimethoprim sulfadiazine: case reports and drug challenge studies, J Am Anim Hosp Assoc 19:783–790, 1983.
808. Giger U, Werner LL, Millichamp NJ, et al: Sulfadiazine-induced allergy in six Doberman Pinschers, J Am Vet Med Assoc 186(5):479–484, 1985.
809. Krum SH, Cardinet GH, Anderson BC, et al: Polymyositis and polyarthritis associated with systemic lupus erythematosus in a dog, J Am Vet Med Assoc 170(1):61–64, 1977.
810. Grindem CB, Johnson KH: Systemic lupus erythematosus: literature review and report of 42 new canine cases, J Am Anim Hosp Assoc 19(4):489–503, 1983.
811. Smith MO: Idiopathic myositides in dogs, Semin Vet Med Surg (Small Anim) 4(2):156–160, 1989.
812. Kornegay JN, Gorgacz EJ, Dawe DL, et al: Polymyositis in dogs, J Am Vet Med Assoc 176(5):431–438, 1980.
813. Ginman AA, Kline KL, Shelton GD: Severe polymyositis and neuritis in a cat, J Am Vet Med Assoc 235(2):172–175, 2009.
814. Presthus J, Lindboe CF: Polymyositis in two German wirehaired pointer littermates, J Small Anim Pract 29(4):239–248, 1988.
815. Aronsohn MG, Schunk KL, Carpenter JL, et al: Clinical and pathologic features of thymoma in 15 dogs, J Am Vet Med Assoc 184(11):1355–1362, 1984.
816. Carpenter JL, Holzworth J: Thymoma in 11 cats, J Am Vet Med Assoc 181(3):248–251, 1982.
817. Hankel S, Shelton GD, Engvall E: Sarcolemma-specific autoantibodies in canine inflammatory myopathy, Vet Immunol Immunopathol 113(1/2):1–10, 2006.
818. Kent M: Therapeutic options for neuromuscular diseases, Vet Clin North Am Small Anim Pract 34:1525–1551, 2004.
819. Gilmour MA, Morgan RV, Moore FM: Masticatory myopathy in the dog: a retrospective study of 18 cases, J Am Anim Hosp Assoc 28:300–306, 1992.
820. Shelton GD, Cardinet GH III, Bandman E: Canine masticatory muscle disorders: a study of 29 cases, Muscle Nerve 10(8):753–766, 1987.
821. Melmed C, Shelton GD, Bergman R, et al: Masticatory muscle myositis: pathogenesis, diagnosis, and treatment, Compend Contin Educ Pract Vet 26(8):590–604, 2004.
822. Orvis JS, Cardinet GH: Canine muscle fiber types and susceptibility of masticatory muscles to myositis, Muscle Nerve 4(4):354–359, 1981.

823. Shelton GD, Bandman E, Cardinet GH: Electrophoretic comparison of myosins from masticatory muscles and selected limb muscles in the dog, Am J Vet Res 46(2):493–498, 1985.
824. Braund KG, Dillon AR, Mikeal RL, et al: Subclinical myopathy associated with hyperadrenocorticism in the dog, Vet Pathol 17(2):134–148, 1980.
825. Braund KG, Dillon AR, Mikeal RL: Experimental investigation of glucocorticoid-induced myopathy in the dog, Exp Neurol 68(1):50–71, 1980.
826. Platt SR, McConnell JF, Garosi LS, et al: Magnetic resonance imaging in the diagnosis of canine inflammatory myopathies in three dogs, Vet Radiol Ultrasound 47(6):532–537, 2006.
827. Bishop TM, Glass EN, Lahunta Ad, et al: Imaging diagnosis-masticatory muscle myositis in a young dog, Vet Radiol Ultrasound 49(3):270–272, 2008.
828. Reiter AM, Schwarz T: Computed tomographic appearance of masticatory myositis in dogs: 7 cases (1999-2006), J Am Vet Med Assoc 231(6):924–930, 2007.
829. Carpenter JL, Schmidt GM, Moore FM, et al: Canine bilateral extraocular polymyositis, Vet Pathol 26(6):510–512, 1989.
830. Allgoewer I, Blair M, Basher T, et al: Extraocular muscle myositis and restrictive strabismus in 10 dogs, Vet Ophthalmol 3(1):21–26, 2000.
831. Hargis AM, Haupt KH, Prieur DJ, et al: A skin disorder in three Shetland sheepdogs: comparison with familial canine dermatomyositis in collies, Compend Contin Educ Pract Vet 7(4):306–315, 1985.
832. Haupt KH, Prieur DJ, Moore MP, et al: Familial canine dermatomyositis: clinical, electrodiagnostic, and genetic studies, Am J Vet Res 46(9):1861–1869, 1985.
833. White SD, Shelton GD, Sisson A, et al: Dermatomyositis in an adult Pembroke Welsh Corgi, J Am Anim Hosp Assoc 28(5):398–401, 1992.
834. Rees CA, Boothe DM: Therapeutic response to pentoxifylline and its active metabolites in dogs with familial canine dermatomyositis, Vet Therap 4(3):234–241, 2003.
835. Clark LA, Credille KM, Murphy KE, et al: Linkage of dermatomyositis in the Shetland sheepdog to chromosome 35, Vet Dermatol 16(6):392–394, 2005.
836. Braund KG, Blagburn BL, Toivio-Kinnucan M, et al: *Toxoplasma* polymyositis/polyneuropathy–a new clinical variant in two mature dogs, J Am Anim Hosp Assoc 24:93–97, 1988.
837. Macintire DK, Vincent-Johnson N, Dillon AR, et al: Hepatozoonosis in dogs: 22 cases (1989-1994), J Am Vet Med Assoc 210(7):916–922, 1997.
838. Vincent-Johnson N, Macintire DK, Baneth G: Canine hepatozoonois: pathophysiology, diagnosis, and treatment, Compend Contin Educ Pract Vet 19(1):51, 1997.
839. Macintire DK, Vincent-Johnson NA, Kane CW, et al: Treatment of dogs infected with *Hepatozoon americanum*: 53 cases (1989-1998), J Am Vet Med Assoc 218(1):77–82, 2001.
840. Barr SC, Simpson RM, Schmidt SP, et al: Chronic dilatative myocarditis caused by *Trypanosoma cruzi* in two dogs, J Am Vet Med Assoc 195(9):1237–1241, 1989.
841. Berger SL, Palmer RH, Hodges CC, et al: Neurologic manifestations of trypanosomiasis in a dog, J Am Vet Med Assoc 198(1):132–134, 1991.
842. Vamvakidis CD, Koutinas AF, Kanakoudis G, et al: Masticatory and skeletal muscle myositis in canine leishmaniasis (*Leishmania infantum*), Vet Rec 146(24):698–703, 2000.
843. Poncelet L, Fontaine M, Balligand M: Polymyositis associated with *Leptospira australis* infection in a dog, Vet Rec 129(2):40, 1991.
844. Poonacha KB, Donahue JM, Nightengale JR: Clostridial myositis in a dog, J Am Vet Med Assoc 194(1):69–70, 1989.
845. Peek SF, Semrad SD, Perkins GA: Clostridial myonecrosis in horses (37 cases 1985-2000), Equine Vet J 35:86–92, 2003.
846. Sponseller BT, Valberg SJ, Tennent-Brown BS, et al: Severe acute rhabdomyolysis associated with *Streptococcus equi* infection in four horses, J Am Vet Med Assoc 227:1800–1807, 2005.
847. Pusterla N, Watson JL, Affolter VK, et al: Purpura haemorrhagica in 53 horses, Vet Res 153:118–121, 2003.
848. Hewison C: Frozen tail or limber tail in working dogs, Vet Rec 140:536, 1997.
849. Steiss JE: What is limber tail syndrome? Canine Pract 22(5-6):1, 1997.
850. Steiss J, Braund K, Wright J, et al: Coccygeal muscle injury in English pointers (limber tail), J Vet Intern Med 13(6):540–548, 1999.
851. Lewis DD, Shelton GD, Piras A, et al: Gracilis or semitendinosus myopathy in 18 dogs, J Am Anim Hosp Assoc 33(2):177–188, 1997.
852. Shelton GD, Ling LA, Guo LT, et al: Muscular dystrophy in female dogs, J Vet Intern Med 15:240–244, 2001.
853. Valentine BA, Kornegay JN, Cooper BJ: Clinical electromyographic studies of canine X-linked muscular dystrophy, Am J Vet Res 50(12):2145–2147, 1989.
854. Lyon M: Sex chromatin and gene action in mammalian X-chromosomes, Am J Hum Genet 14:135–148, 1962.
855. Kornegay JN, Sharp NJH, Camp SD, et al: Early pathologic features of golden retriever muscular dystrophy: a model of Duchenne muscular dystrophy 48(3):348, 1989.
856. Kornegay JN, Tuler S, Miller D, Levesque D: Muscular dystorphy in a litter of golden retriever dogs, Muscle Nerve 11:1056–1064, 1988.
857. Valentine BA, Cooper BJ, Cummings JF, et al: Progressive muscular dystrophy in a golden retriever dog: light microscope and ultrastructural features at 4 and 8 months, Acta Neuropathol 71(3/4):301–310, 1986.
858. Wentink GH, Meijer AEFH, Linde-Sipman JS, et al: Myopathy in an Irish terrier with a metabolic defect of the isolated mitochondria, Zentralblatt fur Veterinarmedizin 21A(Heft 1):62–74, 1974.
859. Presthus J, Nordstoga K: Congenital myopathy in a litter of Samoyed dogs, Prog Vet Neurol 4(2):37–40, 1993.
860. Winand N, Pradham D, Cooper B: Molecular characterization of severe Duchenne-type muscular dystrophy in a family of rottweiler dogs. Molecular mechanisms of neuromuscular disease, Tucson (AZ), 1994, Muscular Dystrophy Association.
861. Ham LML, Desmidt M, Tshamala M, et al: Canine X-linked muscular dystrophy in Belgian Groenendaeler shepherds, Vlaams Diergeneeskundig Tijdschrift 64(3):102–106, 1995.
862. Paola JP, Podell M, Shelton GD: Muscular dystrophy in a miniature schnauzer, Prog Vet Neurol 4(1):14–18, 1993.
863. Cardinet GH III, Holliday TA: Neuromuscular diseases of domestic animals: a summary of muscle biopsies from 159 cases, Ann N Y Acad Sci 317:290–313, 1979.
864. Schatzberg SJ, Olby NJ, Breen M, et al: Molecular analysis of a spontaneous dystrophin 'knockout' dog, Neuromuscul Disord 9(5):289–295, 1999.
865. Wetterman CA, Harkin KR, Cash WC, Nietfield JC, Shelton GD: Hypertrophic muscular dystrophy in a young dog, J Am Vet Med Assoc 216(6):878–881, 2000.

866. Jones BR, Brennan S, Mooney CT, et al: Muscular dystrophy with truncated dystrophin in a family of Japanese Spitz dogs, J Neurol Sci 217(2):143–149, 2004.
867. Van Ham LML, Roels SLMF, Hoorens JK: Congenital dystrophy-like myopathy in a Brittany Spaniel puppy, Prog Vet Neurol 6(4):135–138, 1995.
868. Bergman RL, Inzana KD, Monroe WE, et al: Dystrophin-deficient muscular dystrophy in a Labrador retriever, J Am Anim Hosp Assoc 38(3):255–261, 2002.
869. Klarenbeek S, Gerritzen-Bruning MJ, Rozemuller AJM, et al: Canine X-linked muscular dystrophy in a family of Grand Basset Griffon Venden dogs, J Comp Pathol 137(4):249–252, 2007.
870. Piercy RJ, Walmsley G: Muscular dystrophy in Cavalier King Charles spaniels, Vet Rec 165(2):62, 2009.
871. Gaschen F, Gaschen L, Burgunder JM: Clinical study of a breeding colony affected with hypertrophic feline muscular dystrophy, J Vet Intern.Med 9(3):207, 1995.
872. Carpenter JL, Hoffman EP, Ramanul FC, et al: Feline muscular dystrophy with dystrophin deficiency, Am J Pathol 135:909–919, 1989.
873. Vos JH, van der Linde-Sipman JS, Goedegebuure SA: Dystrophy-like myopathy in the cat, J Comp Pathol 96(3):335–341, 1986.
874. Meier H: Myopathies in the dog, Cornell Vet 48:313–330, 1958.
875. Sharp NJH, Kornegay JN, Camp SD, et al: An error in dystrophin mRNA processing in golden retriever muscular dystrophy, an animal homologue of Duchenne muscular dystrophy, Genomics (San Diego) 13(1):115–121, 1992.
876. Kornegay JN, Cundiff DD, Bogan DJ, et al: The cranial sartorius muscle undergoes true hypertrophy in dogs with golden retriever muscular dystrophy, Neuromuscul Disord 13(6):493–500, 2003.
877. Deitz K, Morrison JA, Kline K, et al: Sarcoglycan-deficient muscular dystrophy in a Boston terrier, J Vet Intern Med 22(2):476–480, 2008.
878. Bartlett RJ, Winand NJ, Secore SL, Singer JT, Fletcher S, Wilton S, et al: Mutation segregation and rapid carrier detection of X-linked muscular dystrophy in dogs, Am J Vet Res 57(5):650–654, 1996.
879. Brumitt JW, Essman SC, Kornegay JN, et al: Radiographic features of golden retriever muscular dystrophy, Vet Radiol Ultrasound 47(6):574–580, 2006.
880. Moise NS, Valentine BA, Brown CA, et al: Duchenne's cardiomyopathy in a canine model: electrocardiograhic and echocardiographic studies, J Am Coll Cardiol 17:812–820, 1991.
881. Gaschen FP, Hoffman EP, Gorospe JRM, et al: Dystrophin deficiency causes lethal muscle hypertrophy in cats, J Neurol Sci 110(1,2):149–159, 1992.
882. Gaschen F, Gaschen L, Seiler G, et al: Lethal peracute rhabdomyolysis associated with stress and general anesthesia in three dystrophin-deficient cats, Vet Pathol 35(2):117–123, 1998.
883. Berry CR, Gaschen FP, Ackerman N: Radiographic and ultrasonographic features of hypertrophic feline muscular dystrophy in two cats, Vet Radiol Ultrasound 33(6):357–364, 1992.
884. Winand NJ, Edwards M, Pradhan D, et al: Deletion of the dystrophin muscle promoter in feline muscular dystrophy, Neuromuscul Disord 4(5-6):433–445, 1994.
885. Malik R, Mepstead K, Yang F, et al: Hereditary myopathy of Devon rex cats, J Small Anim Pract 34:539–546, 1993.
886. Martin PT, Shelton GD, Dickinson PJ, et al: Muscular dystrophy associated with alpha-dystroglycan deficiency in Sphynx and Devon Rex cats, Neuromuscul Disord 18(12):942–952, 2008.
887. Robinson R: Spasticity in the Devon Rex cat, Vet Rec 130:302, 1992.
888. Poncelet L, Resibois A, Engvall E, et al: Laminin alpha2 deficiency-associated muscular dystrophy in a Maine coon cat, J Small Anim Pract 44(12):550–552, 2003.
889. Richards RB, Passmore IK, Bretag AH, et al: Ovine congenital progressive muscular dystrophy: clinical syndrome and distribution of lesions, Aust Vet J 63(12):396–401, 1986.
890. Richards RB, Lewer RP, Passmore IK, et al: Ovine congenital progressive muscular dystrophy: mode of inheritance, Aust Vet J 65(3):93–94, 1988.
891. Richards RB, Passmore IK, Dempsey EF: Skeletal muscle pathology in ovine congenital progressive muscular dystrophy. 1. Histopathology and histochemistry, Acta Neuropathol 77(2):161–167, 1988.
892. Richards RB, Passmore IK, Dempsey EF: Skeletal muscle pathology in ovine congenital progressive muscular dystrophy. 2. Myofiber morphometry, Acta Neuropathol 77(1):95–99, 1988.
893. Pele M, Tiret L, Kessler JL, et al: SINE exonic insertion in the PTPLA gene leads to multiple splicing defects and segregates with the autosomal recessive centronuclear myopathy in dogs, Human Mol Genet 14(11):1417–1427, 2005, [Erratum appears in Hum Mol Genet 2005;14(13):1905-1906].
894. Kramer JW, Hegreberg GA, Hamilton MJ: Inheritance of a neuromuscular disorder of Labrador retriever dogs, J Am Vet Med Assoc 179(4):380–381, 1981.
895. Kramer JW, Hegreberg GA, Bryan GM, et al: A muscle disorder of Labrador retrievers characterized by deficiency of type II muscle fibers, J Am Vet Med Assoc 169(8):817–820, 1976.
896. McKerrell RE, Braund KG: Hereditary myopathy in Labrador retrievers: clinical variations, J Small Anim Pract 28:479–489, 1987.
897. McKerrell RE, Braund KG: Hereditary myopathies in Labrador retrievers: a morphologic study, J Small Anim Pract 23:411–417, 1986.
898. Peeters ME, Ubbink GJ: Dysphagia-associated muscular dystrophy, Prog Vet Neurol 5(3):124, 1994.
899. Peeters ME, Ubbink GJ: Dysphagia-associated muscular dystrophy: a familial trait in the bouvier des Flandres, Vet Rec 134(17):444–446, 1994.
900. Cooper BJ, de Lahunta A, Gallagher EA: Nemalin myopathy of cats, Muscle Nerve 9:618–625, 1986.
901. Hafner A, Dahme E, Obermaier G, et al: Congenital myopathy in Braunvieh Brown Swiss calves, J Comp Pathol 115(1):23–34, 1996.
902. Delauche AJ, Cuddon PA, Podell M, et al: Nemaline rods in canine myopathies: 4 case reports and literature review, J Vet Intern Med 12(6):424–430, 1998.
903. Hanson SM, Smith MO, Walker TL, et al: Juvenile-onset distal myopathy in Rottweiler dogs, J Vet Intern Med 12(2):103–108, 1998.
904. Targett MP, Franklin RJM, Olby NJ, et al: Central core myopathy in a Great Dane, J Small Anim Pract 35(2):100–103, 1994.
905. Walvoort HC, van Nes JJ, Stokhof A, et al: Canine glycogen storage disease type II: a clinical study of four affected Lapland dogs, J Am Anim Hosp Assoc 20:279–286, 1984.
906. Walvoort HC, Slee RG, Koster JF: Canine glycogen storage disease type II. A biochemical study of an acid alpha -glucosidase-deficient Lapland dog, Biochim Biophys Acta 715(1):63–69, 1982.

907. Dennis JA, Healy PJ: Genotyping shorthorn cattle for generalised glycogenosis, Aust Vet Jl 79(11):773–775, 2001.
908. Dennis JA, Healy PJ, Reichmann KG: Genotyping Brahman cattle for generalised glycogenosis, Aust Vet J 80(5):286–291, 2002.
909. Reichmann KG, Twist JO, Thistlethwaite EJ: Clinical, diagnostic and biochemical features of generalised glycogenosis type II and Brahman cattle, Aust Vet J 70(11):405–408, 1993.
910. Manktelow BW, Hartley WJ: Generalized glycogen storage disease in sheep, J Comp Pathol 85(1):139–145, 1975.
911. Ceh L, Hauge JG, Svenkerud R, et al: Glycogenosis type III in the dog, Acta Vet Scand 17(2):210–222, 1976.
912. Rafiquzzaman M, Svenkerud R, Strande A, et al: Glycogenosis in the dog, Acta Vet Scand 17(2):196–209, 1976.
913. Gregory BL, Shelton GD, Bali DS, et al: Glycogen storage disease type IIIa in Curly-Coated Retrievers, J Vet Intern Med 21(1):40–46, 2007.
914. Fyfe JC, Giger U, Van Winkle TJ, et al: Glycogen storage disease type IV: inherited deficiency of branching enzyme activity in cats, Pediatr Res 32(6):719–725, 1992.
915. Coates JR, Paxton R, Cox NR, et al: A case presentation and discussion of Type IV glycogen storage disease in a Norwegian Forest cat, Prog Vet Neurol 7(1):5–11, 1996.
916. Fyfe JC, Kurzhals RL, Patterson DF: Feline glycogensosis type IV is caused by a complex rearrangement deleting 6 kb of the branching enzyme gene and eliminating a exon, Am J Hum Genet , 1997:61A251.
917. Ward TL, Valberg SJ, Adelson DL, et al: Glycogen branching enzyme (GBE1) mutation causing equine glycogen storage disease IV, Mamm Genome 15(7):570–577, 2004.
918. Valberg SJ, Ward TL, Rush B, et al: Glycogen branching enzyme deficiency in Quarter Horse foals, J Vet Intern Med 15(6):572–580, 2001.
919. Johnstone AC, McSporran KD, Kenny JE, et al: Myophosphorylase deficiency (glycogen storage disease Type V) in a herd of Charolais cattle in New Zealand: confirmation by PCR-RFLP testing, N Z Vet J 52(6):404–408, 2004.
920. Angelos S, Valberg SJ, Smith BP, et al: Myophosphorylase deficiency associated with rhabdomyolysis and exercise intolerance in 6 related Charolais cattle, Muscle Nerve 18(7):736–740, 1995.
921. Bilstrom JA, Valberg SJ, Bernoco D, et al: Genetic test for myophosphorylase deficiency in Charolais cattle, Am J Vet Res 59(3):267–270, 1998.
922. Soethout EC, Verkaar ELC, Jansen GH, et al: A direct StyI polymerase chain reaction-restriction fragment length polymorphism (PCR-RFLP) test for the myophosphorylase mutation in cattle, J Vet Med 49(6):289–290, 2002.
923. Giger U, Argov Z, Schnall M, et al: Metabolic myopathy in canine muscle-type phosphofructokinase deficiency, Muscle Nerve 11(12):1260–1265, 1988.
924. Giger U, Smith BF, Woods CB, et al: Inherited phosphofructokinase deficiency in an American cocker spaniel, J Am Vet Med Assoc 201(10):1569–1571, 1992.
925. Harvey JW, Calderwood MM, Gropp KE, et al: Polysaccharide storage myopathy in canine phosphofructokinase deficiency (type VII glycogen storage disease), Vet Pathol 27(1):1–8, 1990.
926. Valberg SJ, Cardinet GH, Carlson GP, et al: Polysaccharide storage myopathy associated with recurrent exertional rhabdomyolysis in horses, Neuromuscul Disord 2:351–359, 1992.
927. Valentine BA, Credille KM, Lavoie JP, et al: Severe polysaccharide storage myopathy in Belgian and Percheron draught horses, Equine Vet J 29:220–225, 1997.
928. Valentine BA, Cooper BJ: Incidence of polysaccharide storage myopathy, Vet Pathol 42:823–827, 2005.
929. Firshman AM, Valberg SJ, Bender JB, et al: Comparison of histopathologic criteria and skeletal muscle fixation techniques for the diagnosis of polysaccharide storage myopathy in horses, Vet Pathol 43:257–269, 2006.
930. McCue ME, Valberg SJ, Miller MB, et al: Glycogen synthase (GYS1) mutation causes a novel skeletal muscle glycogenosis, Genomics 91:458–466, 2008.
931. McCue ME, Valberg SJ, Lucio M, et al: Glycogen synthase 1 (GYS1) mutation in diverse breeds with polysaccharide storage myopathy, J Vet Intern Med 22:1228–1233, 2008.
932. De La Corte FD, Valberg SJ: Update of equine therapeutics: Treatment of polysaccharide storage myopathy, Compend Contin Educ Pract Vet 22(8):782–788, 2000.
933. De La Corte FD, Valberg SJ, MacLeay JM, et al: Glucose uptake in horses with polysaccharide storage myopathy, Am J Vet Res 60(4):458–462, 1999.
934. Valberg SJ: Heritable muscle diseases. In Robinson NE, Sprayberry KA, editors: Current Therapy in Equine Medicine, ed 6, St. Louis, 2009, Saunder/Elsevier, pp 461–468.
935. Breitschwerdt EB, Kornegay JN, Wheeler SJ, et al: Episodic weakness associated with exertional lactic acidosis and myopathy in Old English sheepdog littermates, J Am Vet Med Assoc 201(5):731–736, 1992.
936. Olby NJ, Chan KK, Targett MP, et al: Suspected mitochondrial myopathy in a Jack Russell terrier, J Small Anim Pract 38(5):213–216, 1997.
937. Houlton JE, Herrtage ME: Mitochondrial myopathy in the Sussex spaniel, Vet Rec 106(9):206, 1980.
938. Herrtage ME, Houlton JEF: Collapsing Clumber spaniels 105(14):334, 1979.
939. Paciello O, Maiolino P, Fatone G, Papparella S: Mitochondrial myopathy in a German shepherd dog, Vet Pathol 40(5):507–511, 2003.
940. Shelton GD, van Ham L, Bhatti S, et al: Pyruvate dehydrogenase deficiency in Clumber and Sussex spaniels in the United States and Belgium, J Vet Intern.Med 14(3):342, 2000.
941. Cameron JM, Maj MC, Levandovskiy V, et al: Identification of a canine model of pyruvate dehydrogenase phosphatase 1 deficiency, Mol Genet Metab 90(1):15–23, 2007.
942. Vijayasarathy C, Giger U, Prociuk U, et al: Canine mitochondrial myopathy associated with reduced mitochondrial mRNA and altered cytochrome c oxidase activities in fibroblasts and skeletal muscle, Comp Biochem Physiol Comp Physiol 109(4):887–894, 1994.
943. Valberg SJ, Carlson GP, Cardinet GH, et al: Skeletal muscle mitochondrial myopathy as a cause of exercise intolerance in a horse, Muscle Nerve 17:305–312, 1994.
944. Platt SR, Chrisman CL, Shelton GD: Lipid storage myopathy in a cocker spaniel, J Small Anim Pract 40:31–34, 1999.
945. Inada S, Yamauchi C, Igata A, et al: Canine storage disease characterized by hereditary progressive neurogenic muscular atrophy: breeding experiments and clinical manifestation, Am J Vet Res 47(10):2294–2299, 1986.

946. Holland CT, Canfield PJ, Watson ADJ, et al: Dyserythropoiesis, polymyopathy, and cardiac disease in three related English Springer Spaniels, J Vet Intern Med 5(3):151–159, 1991.
947. Matwichuk CL, Taylor SM, Shmon CL, Kass PH, et al: Changes in rectal temperature and hematologic, biochemical, blood gas, and acid-base values in healthy Labrador Retrievers before and after strenuous exercise, Am J Vet Res 60(1):88–92, 1999.
948. Hoffmann G, Aramaki S, Blum-Hoffmann E, et al: Quantitative analysis for organic acids in biological samples: batch isolation followed by gas chromatographic-mass spectrometric analysis, Clin Chem 35(4):587–595, 1989.
949. Ozand PT, Gascon GG: Organic acidurias: a review. Part 1, J Child Neurol 6(3):196–219, 1991.
950. Ozand PT, Gascon GG: Organic acidurias: a review. Part 2, J Child Neurol 6(4):288–303, 1991.
951. Shelton GD, Nyhan WL, Kass PH, et al: Analysis of organic acids, amino acids, and carnitine in dogs with lipid storage myopathy, Muscle Nerve 21:1202–1205, 1998.
952. Greene CE, Lorenz MD, Munnell JF, et al: Myopathy associated with hyperadrenocorticism in the dog, J Am Vet Med Assoc 174(12):1310–1315, 1979.
953. Duncan ID, Griffiths IR, Nash AS: Myotonia in canine Cushing's disease, Vet Rec 100:30–31, 1977.
954. Schott HC: Pituitary pars intermedia dysfunction: equine Cushing's disease, Vet Clin North Am Equine Pract 18:237–270, 2002.
955. Aleman M, Watson JL, Williams DC, et al: Myopathy in horses with pituitary pars intermedia dysfunction (Cushing's disease), Neuromuscul Disord 16:737–744, 2006.
956. McLaughlin BG, Doige CE, McLaughlin PS: Thyroid hormone levels in foals with congenital musculoskeletal lesions, Can Vet J 27(7):264–267, 1986.
957. Peterson ME, Kintzer PP, Cavanagh PG: Feline hyperthyroidism: pretreatment, clinical and laboratory evaluation of 131 cases, J Am Vet Med Assoc 183:103–110, 1983.
958. Joseph RJ, Peterson ME: Review and comparison of neuromuscular and central nervous manifestations of hyperthyroidism in cats and humans, Prog Vet Neurol 3114–3119, 1992.
959. Vogt DW, Gipson TA, Akremi B, et al: Associations of sire, breed, birth weight, and sex in pigs with congenital splayleg, Am J Vet Res 45(11):2408–2409, 1984.
960. Jirmanova I: The splayleg disease: a form of congenital glucocorticoid myopathy? Vet Res Commun 6(2):91–101, 1983.
961. Szalay F, Zsarnovszky A, Fekete S, et al: Retarded myelination in the lumbar spinal cord of piglets born with spread-leg syndrome, Anat Embryol 203(1):53–59, 2001.
962. Wells GAH, Bradley R: Pietrain creeper syndrome: a primary myopathy of the pig? Neuropathol Appl Neurobiol 4(3):237–238, 1978.
963. Wells GAH, Pinsent PJN, Todd JN: A progressive, familial myopathy of the Pietrain pig: the clinical syndrome, Vet Rec 106(26):556–558, 1980.
964. Vite CH: Myotonia and disorders of altered muscle cell membrane excitability, Vet Clin North Am Small Anim Pract 32:169–187, 2002.
965. Anderson PH, Bradley R, Berrett S, et al: The sequence of myodegeneration in nutritional myopathy of the older calf, Br Vet J 133:160–165, 1977.
966. Maas J, Bulgin MS, Anderson BC, et al: Nutritional myodegeneration associated with vitamin E deficiency and normal selenium status in lambs, J Am Vet Med Assoc 184:201–204, 1984.
967. Ross AD, Gee CG, Jackson ARB, et al: Nutritional myopathy in goats, Aust Vet J 66(11):361–363, 1989.
968. Lofstedt J: White muscle disease of foals, Vet Clin North Am Equine Pract 13(1):169–185, 1997.
969. Rensburg IBJV, Venning WJA: Nutritional myopathy in a dog, J South African Vet Assoc 50(2):119–121, 1979.
970. Perkins G, Valberg SJ, Madigan JM, et al: Electrolyte disturbances in foals with severe rhabdomyolysis, J Vet Intern Med 12:173–177, 1998.
971. Foreman JH, Potter KA, Bayly WM, et al: Generalized steatitis associated with selenium deficiency and normal vitamin E status in a foal, J Am Vet Med Assoc 189(1):83–86, 1986.
972. Taylor SM, Shmon CL, Shelton GD, et al: Exercise-induced collapse of Labrador retrievers: survey results and preliminary investigation of heritability, J Am Anim Hosp Assoc 44(6):295–301, 2008.
973. Taylor SM, Shmon CL, Adams VJ, et al: Evaluations of Labrador retrievers with exercise-induced collapse, including response to a standardized strenuous exercise protocol, J Am Anim Hosp Assoc 45(1):3–13, 2009.
974. Patterson EE, Minor KM, Tchernatynskaia AV, et al: A canine DNM1 mutation is highly associated with the syndrome of exercise-induced collapse, Nat Genet 40(10):1235–1239, 2008.
975. Berman MC, Harrison GG, Bull AB, et al: Changes underlying halothane induced malignant hyperpyrexia in Landrace pigs, Nature 225:653–655, 1970.
976. Fujii J, Otsu K, Zorzato F, et al: Identification of a mutation in porcine ryanodine receptor associated with malignant hyperthermia, Science 253(5018):448–451, 1991.
977. Riedesel DH, Hildebrand SV: Unusual response following use of succinylcholine in a horse anesthetized with halothane, J Am Anim Hosp Assoc 187(5):507–508, 1985.
978. Aleman M, Brosnan RJ, Williams DC, et al: Malignant hyperthermia in a horse anesthetized with halothane, J Vet Intern Med 19(3):363–366, 2005.
979. Aleman M, Nieto JE, Magdesian KG: Malignant hyperthermia associated with ryanodine receptor 1 (C7360G) mutation in Quarter Horses, J Vet Intern Med 23(2):329–334, 2009.
980. Roberts MC, Mickelson JR, Patterson EE, et al: Autosomal dominant canine malignant hyperthermia is caused by a mutation in the gene encoding the skeletal muscle calcium release channel (RYR1), Anesthesiology 95(3):716–725, 2001.
981. Gannon JR: Exertional rhabdomyolysis (myoglobinuria) in the racing Greyhound. In Kirk RW, editor: Current Veterinary Therapy VII, ed 7, St. Louis, 1980, WB Saunders, pp 783–787.
982. Dranchak PK, Valberg SJ, Onan GW, et al: Inheritance of recurrent exertional rhabdomyolysis in Thoroughbreds, J Am Vet Med Assoc 227:762–767, 2005.
983. Valberg SJ, MacLeay JM, Mickelson JR: Exertional rhabdomyolysis and polysaccharide storage myopathy in horses, Compend Contin Educ Pract Vet 19(9):1077–1086, 1997.
984. MacLeay JM, Sorum SA, Valberg SJ, et al: Epidemiologic analysis of factors influencing exertional rhabdomyolysis in Thoroughbreds, Am J Vet Res 60:1562–1566, 1999.
985. Valberg SJ, Mickelson JR, Gallant EM, et al: Exertional rhabdomyolysis in Quarter horses and Thoroughbreds: one syndrome, multiple aetiologies, Equine Vet J Suppl 30:533–538, 1999.

986. Spier SJ, Carlson GP, Holliday TA, et al: Hyperkalemic periodic paralysis in horses, J Am Vet Med Assoc 197(8):1009–1017, 1990.
987. Spier SJ, Carlson GP, Harrold D, et al: Genetic study of hyperkalemic periodic paralysis in horses, J Am Vet Med Assoc 202(6):933–937, 1993.
988. Naylor JM, Robinson JA, Bertone J: Familial incidence of hyperkalemic periodic paralysis in quarter horses, J Am Vet Med Assoc 200(3):340–343, 1992.
989. Rudolph JA, Spier SJ, Byrns G, et al: Periodic paralysis in quarter horses: a sodium channel mutation disseminated by selective breeding, Nat Genet 2(2):144–147, 1992.
990. Cannon SC, Hayward LJ, Beech J, et al: Sodium channel inactivation is impaired in equine hyperkalemic periodic paralysis, J Neurophysiol 73(5):1892–1899, 1995.
991. Robertson SA, Green SL, Carter SW, et al: Postanesthetic recumbency associated with hyperkalemic periodic paralysis in a quarter horse, J Am Vet Med Assoc 201(8):1209–1212, 1992.
992. Jezyk PF: Hyperkalemic periodic paralysis in a dog, J Am Anim Hosp Assoc 18:977–980, 1982.
993. Naylor JM, Jones V, Berry SL: Clinical syndrome and diagnosis of hyperkalaemic periodic paralysis in quarter horses, Equine Vet J 25(3):227–232, 1993.
994. Traub-Dargatz JL, Ingram JT, Stashak TS, et al: Respiratory stridor associated with polymyopathy suspected to be hyperkalemic periodic paralysis in four quarter horse foals, J Am Vet Med Assoc 201(1):85–89, 1992.
995. Guglick MA, MacAllister CG, Breazile JE: Laryngospasm, dysphagia, and emaciation associated with hyperkalemic periodic paralysis in a horse, J Am Vet Med Assoc 209(1):115–117, 1996.
996. Dow SW, Fettman MJ, Curtis CR, et al: Hypokalemia in cats: 186 cases (1984-1987), J Am Vet Med Assoc 194(11):1604–1608, 1989.
997. Dow SW, Fettman MJ, LeCouteur RA, et al: Potassium depletion in cats: renal and dietary influences, J Am Vet Med Assoc 191(12):1569–1575, 1987.
998. Dow SW, LeCouteur RA, Fettman MJ, et al: Potassium depletion in cats: hypokalemic polymyopathy, J Am Vet Med Assoc 191(12):1563–1568, 1987.
999. Shelton GD: Disorders of neuromuscular transmission, Semin Vet Med Surg (Small Anim) 4(2):126–132, 1989.
1000. Nemzek JA, Kruger JM, Walshaw R, et al: Acute onset of hypokalemia and muscular weakness in four hyperthyroid cats, J Am Vet Med Assoc 205(1):65–68, 1994.
1001. Mason K: A hereditary disease in Burmese cats manifested as an episodic weakness with head nodding and neck ventroflexion, J Am Anim Hosp Assoc 24:147–151, 1988.
1002. Jones BR, Swinny GW, Alley MR: Hypokalemic myopathy in Burmese kittens, N Z Vet J 36:150–151, 1988.
1003. Leon A, Bain SAF, Levick WR: Hypokalaemic episodic polymyopathy in cats fed a vegetarian diet, Aust Vet J 69:249–254, 1992.
1004. Shelton GD: Myasthenia gravis and disorders of neuromuscular transmission, Vet Clin North Am Small Anim Pract 32:189–206, 2002.
1005. Dewey CW: Acquired myasthenia gravis in dogs–Part I, Compend Contin Educ Pract Vet 19(12):1340–1353, 1997.
1006. Barsanti JA, Walser M, Hatheway CL, et al: Type C botulism in American Foxhounds, J Am Vet Med Assoc 172(7):809–813, 1978.
1007. Cornelissen JMM, Haagsma J, van Nes JJ: Type C botulism in five dogs, J Am Anim Hosp Assoc 21:401–404, 1985.
1008. Darke PG, Roberts TA, Smart JL, et al: Suspected botulism in foxhounds, Vet Rec 99(6):98–99, 1976.
1009. Marlow GR, Smart JL: Botulism in foxhounds, Vet Rec 111(11):242, 1982.
1010. Cummings JF, Haas DC: Coonhound paralysis. An acute idiopathic polyradiculoneuritis in dogs resembling the Landry-Guillain-Barré syndrome, J Neurol Sci 4(1):51–81, 1967.
1011. Ricketts SW, Greet TR, Glyn PJ, et al: Thirteen cases of botulism in horses fed big bale silage, Equine Vet J 16(6):515–518, 1984.
1012. Swerczek TW: Toxicoinfectious botulism in foals and adult horses, J Am Vet Med Assoc 176(3):217–220, 1980.
1013. Swerczek TW: Experimentally induced toxicoinfectious botulism in horses and foals, Am J Vet Res 41(3):348–350, 1980.
1014. Kelly AP, Jones RT, Gillick JC, et al: Outbreak of botulism in horses, Equine Vet J 16(6):519–521, 1984.
1015. Bernard W, Divers TJ, Whitlock RH, et al: Botulism as a sequel to open castration in a horse, J Am Vet Med Assoc 191(1):73–74, 1987.
1016. Divers TJ, Bartholomew RC, Messick JB, et al: *Clostridium botulinum* type B toxicosis in a herd of cattle and a group of mules, J Am Vet Med Assoc 188(4):382–386, 1986.
1017. Kao I, Drachman D, Price D: Botulinum toxin: Mechanism of presynaptic blockage, Science 193:1256–1258, 1976.
1018. Coleman ES: Clostridial neurotoxins: tetanus and botulism, Compend Contin Educ Pract Vet 20(10):1089–1097, 1998.
1019. Cherington M: Electrophysiologic methods as an aid in diagnosis of botulism: a review, Muscle Nerve 5(9S):S28–S29, 1982.
1020. van Nes JJ, van der Most van Spijk: Electrophysiological evidence of peripheral nerve dysfunction in six dogs with botulism type C, Res Vet Sci 40(3):372–376, 1986.
1021. Malik R, Farrow BR: Tick paralysis in North America and Australia, Vet Clin North Am Small Anim Pract 21(1):157–171, 1991.
1022. Ilkiw JE, Turner DM: Infestation in the dog by the paralysis tick *Ixodes holocyclus*. 3. Respiratory effects, Aust Vet J 64(5):142–144, 1987.
1023. Ilkiw JE, Turner DM: Infestation in the dog by the paralysis tick *Ixodes holocyclus*. 2. Blood-gas and pH, haematological and biochemical findings, Aust Vet J 64(5):139–142, 1987.
1024. Ilkiw JE, Turner DM, Howlett CR: Infestation in the dog by the paralysis tick *Ixodes holocyclus*. 1. Clinical and histological findings, Aust Vet J 64(5):137–139, 1987.
1025. Holland CT: Asymmetrical focal neurological deficits in dogs and cats with naturally occurring tick paralysis (*Ixodes holocyclus*): 27 cases (1999-2006), Aust Vet J 86(10):377–384, 2008.
1026. Wheeler SJ: Disorders of the neuromuscular junction, Prog Vet Neurol 2(2):129–135, 1991.
1027. Peterson ME: Snake bite: coral snakes, Clin Tech Small Anim Pract 21:183–186, 2006.
1028. Chrisman CL, Hopkins AL, Ford SL, et al: Acute, flaccid quadriplegia in three cats with suspected coral snake envenomation, J Am Anim Hosp Assoc 32(4):343–349, 1996.

1029. Marks SL, Mannella C, Schaer M: Coral snake envenomation in the dog: report of four cases and review of the literature, J Am Anim Hosp Assoc 26:629–634, 1990.
1030. Nafe LA: Selected neurotoxins, Vet Clin North Am Small Anim Pract 18(3):593–604, 1988.
1031. Dorman DC, Fikes JD: Diagnosis and therapy of neurotoxicological syndromes in dogs and cats: selected syndromes induced by pesticides, part 2, Prog Vet Neurol 4(4):111–120, 1993.
1032. Fikes JD, Zachary JF, Parker AJ: Clinical, biochemical, electrophysiologic, and histologic assessment of chlorpyrifos induced delayed neuropathy in the cat, Neurotoxicology 13:663–678, 1992.
1033. Jaggy A, Oliver JE: Chlorpyrifos toxicosis in two cats, J Vet Intern Med 4(3):135–139, 1990.
1034. Levy JK: Chronic chlorpyrifos toxicosis in a cat, J Am Vet Med Assoc 203(12):1682–1684, 1993.
1035. Clemmons RM, Meyer DJ, Sundlof SF, et al: Correction of organophosphate-induced neuromuscular blockade by diphenhydramine, Am J Vet Res 45(10):2167–2169, 1984.
1036. Lindstrom J, Shelton D, Fujii Y: Myasthenia gravis, Adv Immunol 42:233–284, 1988.
1037. Shelton GD, Cardinet GH, Lindstrom JM: Canine and human myasthenia gravis autoantibodies recognize similar regions on the acetylcholine receptor, Neurology 38(9):1417–1423, 1988.
1038. Atwater SW, Powers BE, Park RD, et al: Thymoma in dogs: 23 cases (1980-1991), J Am Vet Med Assoc 205(7):1007–1013, 1994.
1039. O'Dair HA, Holt PE, Pearson GR, et al: Acquired immune-mediated myasthenia gravis in a cat associated with cystic thymus, J Small Anim Pract 32:198–202, 1991.
1040. Rusbridge C, White RN, Elwood CM, et al: Treatment of acquired myasthenia gravis associated with thymoma in two dogs, J Small Anim Pract 37(8):376–380, 1996.
1041. Shelton GD, Schule A, Kass PH: Risk factors for acquired myasthenia gravis in dogs: 1,154 cases (1991-1995), J Am Vet Med Assoc 211(11):1428–1431, 1997.
1042. Kent M, Glass EN, Acierno M, et al: Adult onset acquired myasthenia gravis in three Great Dane littermates, J Small Anim Pract 49(12):647–650, 2008.
1043. Lipsitz D, Berry JL, Shelton GD: Inherited predisposition to myasthenia gravis in Newfoundlands, J Am Vet Med Assoc 215(7):956–958, 1999.
1044. Shelton GD, Ho M, Kass PH: Risk factors for acquired myasthenia gravis in cats: 105 cases (1986-1998), J Am Vet Med Assoc 216(1):55–57, 2000.
1045. Shelton GD, Willard MD, Cardinet GH, et al: Acquired myasthenia gravis. Selective involvement of esophageal, pharyngeal, and facial muscles, J Vet Intern Med 4(6):281–284, 1990.
1046. Dewey CW, Bailey CS, Shelton GD, et al: Clinical forms of acquired myasthenia gravis in dogs: 25 cases (1988-1995), J Vet Intern Med 11(2):50–57, 1997.
1047. King LG, Vite CH: Acute fulminating myasthenia gravis in five dogs, J Am Vet Med Assoc 212(6):830–834, 1998.
1048. Ducoté JM, Dewey CW, Coates JR: Clinical forms of myasthenia gravis in cats, Compend Contin Educ Pract Vet 21(5):440–448, 1999.
1049. Hackett TB, Van Pelt DR, Willard MD, et al: Third degree atrioventricular block and acquired myasthenia gravis in four dogs, J Am Vet Med Assoc 206(8):1173–1176, 1995.
1050. Levine JM, Bergman RL, Coates JR, et al: Myasthenia gravis and hypothyroidism in a dog with meningomyelitis, J Am Anim Hosp Assoc 41(4):247–251, 2005.
1051. Klebanow ER: Thymoma and acquired myasthenia gravis in the dog: a case report and review of 13 additional cases, J Am Anim Hosp Assoc 28(1):63–69, 1992.
1052. Moore AS, Madewell BR, Cardinet GH, et al: Osteogenic sarcoma and myasthenia gravis in a dog, J Am Vet Med Assoc 197(2):226–227, 1990.
1053. Krotje LJ, Fix AS, Potthoff AD: Acquired myasthenia gravis and cholangiocellular carcinoma in a dog, J Am Vet Med Assoc 197(4):488–490, 1990.
1054. Shelton GD: Myasthenia gravis: lessons from the past 10 years, J Small Anim Pract 39(8):368–372, 1998.
1055. Malik R, Ho S, Church DB: The normal response to repetitive motor nerve stimulation in dogs, J Small Anim Pract 30:20–26, 1989.
1056. Sims MH, McLean RA: Use of repetitive nerve stimulation to assess neuromuscular function in dogs. A test protocol for suspected myasthenia gravis, Prog Vet Neurol 1(3):311–319, 1990.
1057. Hopkins AL, Howard JF, Wheeler SJ, et al: Stimulated single fibre electromyography in normal dogs, J Small Anim Pract 34:271–276, 1993.
1058. Shelton GD: How do I treat? Acquired myasthenia gravis in the dog and cat, Prog Vet Neurol 1(3):343–344, 1990.
1059. Abelson AL, Shelton GD, Whelan MF, et al: Use of mycophenolate mofetil as a rescue agent in the treatment of severe generalized myasthenia gravis in three dogs, J Vet Emerg Crit Care 19(4):369–374, 2009.
1060. Dewey CW, Coates JR, Ducote JM, et al: Azathioprine therapy for acquired myasthenia gravis in five dogs, J Am Anim Hosp Assoc 35(5):396–402, 1999.
1061. Bexfield NH, Watson PJ, Herrtage ME: Management of myasthenia gravis using cyclosporine in 2 dogs, J Vet Intern Med 20(6):1487–1490, 2006.
1062. Bartges JW, Klausner JS, Bostwick EF, et al: Clinical remission following plasmapheresis and corticosteroid treatment in a dog with acquired myasthenia gravis, J Am Vet Med Assoc 196(8):1276–1278, 1990.
1063. Lainesse MF, Taylor SM, Myers SL, et al: Focal myasthenia gravis as a paraneoplastic syndrome of canine thymoma: improvement following thymectomy, J Am Anim Hosp Assoc 32(2):111–117, 1996.
1064. Shelton GD, Joseph R, Richter K, Hitt M, et al: Acquired myasthenia gravis in hyperthyroid cats on tapazole therapy, J Vet Intern Med 11(2):120, 1997.
1065. Shelton GD, Lindstrom JM: Spontaneous remission in canine myasthenia gravis: implications for assessing human MG therapies, Neurology 57(11):2139–2141, 2001.
1066. Johnson RP, Watson ADJ, Smith J, et al: Myasthenia in springer spaniel littermates, J Small Anim Pract 16(10):641–647, 1975.
1067. Dickinson PJ, Sturges BK, Shelton GD, LeCouteur RA: Congenital myasthenia gravis in smooth-haired miniature dachshund dogs, J Vet Intern Med 19(6):920–923, 2005.
1068. Wallace ME, Palmer AC: Recessive mode of inheritance in myasthenia gravis in the Jack Russell terrier, Vet Rec 114(14):350, 1984.
1069. Miller LM, Lennon VA, Lambert EH, et al: Congenital myasthenia gravis in 13 smooth fox terriers, J Am Anim Hosp Assoc 182(7):694–697, 1983.
1070. Indrieri RJ, Creighton SR, Lambert EH, et al: Myasthenia gravis in two cats, J Am Vet Med Assoc 182(1):57–60, 1983.

1071. Joseph RJ, Carrillo JM, Lennon VA: Myasthenia gravis in the cat, J Vet Intern Med 2(2):75–79, 1988.
1072. Flagstad A, Trojaborg W, Gammeltoft S: Congenital myasthenic syndrome in the dog breed Gammel Dansk Honsehund: clinical, electrophysiological, pharmacological and immunological comparison with acquired myasthenia gravis, Acta Vet Scand 30(1):89–102, 1989.
1073. Miller LM, Hegreberg GA, Prieur DJ, et al: Inheritance of congenital myasthenia gravis in smooth fox terrier dogs, J Hered 75(3):163–166, 1984.
1074. Thompson PN, Steinlein OK, Harper CK, et al: Congenital myasthenic syndrome of Brahman cattle in South Africa, Vet Rec 153(25):779–781, 2003.

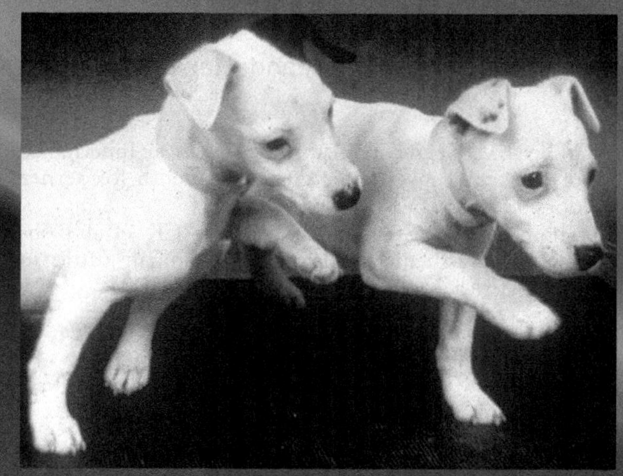

CHAPTER 8

Ataxia of the Head and the Limbs

Ataxia is a lack of coordination that may be present without spasticity, paresis, or involuntary movements. Paresis, when present, is especially useful in localizing lesions. Ataxia is characterized by a broad-based stance and uncoordinated movements of the head, trunk, or limbs. Lesion localization of animals manifesting head and limb ataxia is described in Chapter 2 and is summarized in Figure 8-1. A brief review is presented in this chapter.

LESION LOCALIZATION

For clinical purposes, ataxia can be classified into three major categories: general proprioceptive, vestibular, and cerebellar. Clinical signs result when a disease process interferes with the recognition or coordination of position changes involving the head, trunk, or limbs. Key neurologic signs that are useful for localizing the lesion may be observed. Figure 8-2 is an algorithm for the formulation of a differential diagnosis of ataxia. This algorithm is based largely on a few key differential signs. For example, abnormal movements of the head or the eyes indicate that the lesion is not in the spinal cord but rather in the vestibular system, brainstem, or cerebellum.

General Proprioceptive Ataxia

Loss of proprioceptive impulses from the limbs and, in some cases, the trunk produces general proprioceptive (GP) ataxia. For the purpose of localization, abnormalities of general proprioception in the limbs are interpreted in exactly the same way as motor dysfunction (see Chapters 2, 6, and 7). For example, loss of proprioception in the pelvic limbs with normal proprioception in the thoracic limbs indicates a lesion caudal to T2 involving the large diameter, ascending fibers in the spinal cord or sensory fibers of the peripheral nerve. Further localization is achieved by examining the spinal reflexes and segmental responses to noxious stimuli (e.g., pinching the skin with hemostats). General proprioceptive ataxia is frequently associated with paresis because the pathways (descending upper motor neuron [UMN] pathways and ascending GP pathways) for each are closely related anatomically throughout the nervous system. The primary spinal cord pathways for transmission of GP information are those located in the spinocerebellar tracts of the lateral funiculus and in the dorsal columns (fasciculus gracilis—from the pelvic limbs; fasciculus cuneatus—from the thoracic limbs and neck), which project to the cerebellum and those in the dorsal funiculus that project to the contralateral somesthetic cerebral cortex. Primary neurodegenerative disorders, and compressive and ischemic-related injuries will result in damage and loss of these pathways. Fibers that are longer and larger in diameter are more susceptible to these pathologies.

Vestibular Ataxia

Anatomy

The vestibular system detects linear acceleration and rotational movement of the head. This system does not initiate motor activity; however, its sensory input is used to modify and coordinate movement. The vestibular system primarily controls the muscles involved in maintaining equilibrium, positioning the head, and regulating eye movement.

The peripheral components of the vestibular and cochlear systems are encased by the petrous temporal bone containing a vestibule for the inner ear, hence the name. Receptors for the vestibulocochlear system are located within a membranous labyrinth that is encased within a bony labyrinth (semicircular canals, vestibule, and cochlea). The membranous labyrinth is composed of the cochlear duct, three semicircular ducts, and the otolithic organs (utricle and saccule). The cochlear duct contains the sensory receptors for hearing, the organ of Corti. The semicircular ducts, utricle, and saccule contain sensory receptors for maintaining equilibrium. Perilymph, similar in constituency to cerebrospinal fluid (CSF), separates the bony and membranous labyrinths. The membranous labyrinth is filled with endolymph, which is potassium rich. The endolymph provides a medium by which the receptors of the semicircular ducts and otolithic organs can detect changes in head position.

Two kinds of receptors are present: maculae in the utriculi and sacculi and cristae in the ampullae at the base of the semicircular ducts. The maculae are arranged approximately at right angles to each other. They function to detect head position with respect to gravity and linear acceleration, and help to maintain equilibrium. Any rotation of the head changes the direction of the cristae according to the movement of the endolymph. The cristae are in synaptic contact

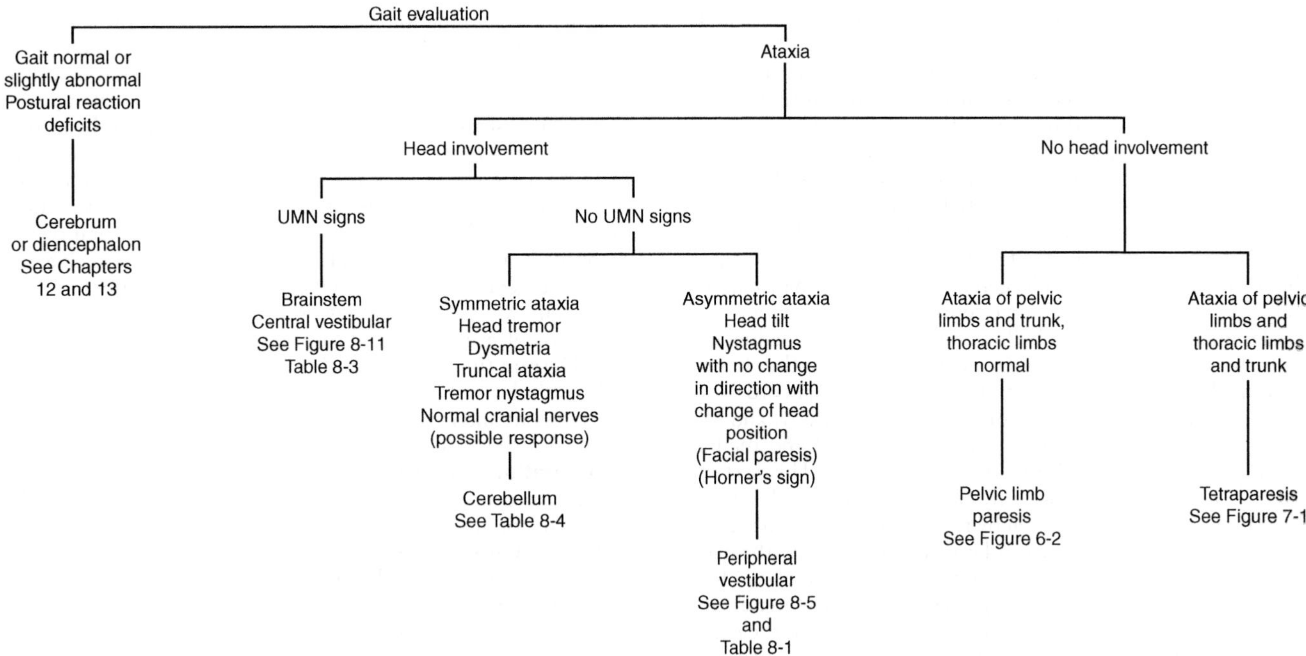

Figure 8-1 Algorithm for the diagnosis of ataxia based on gait, head involvement, and motor function of the limbs.

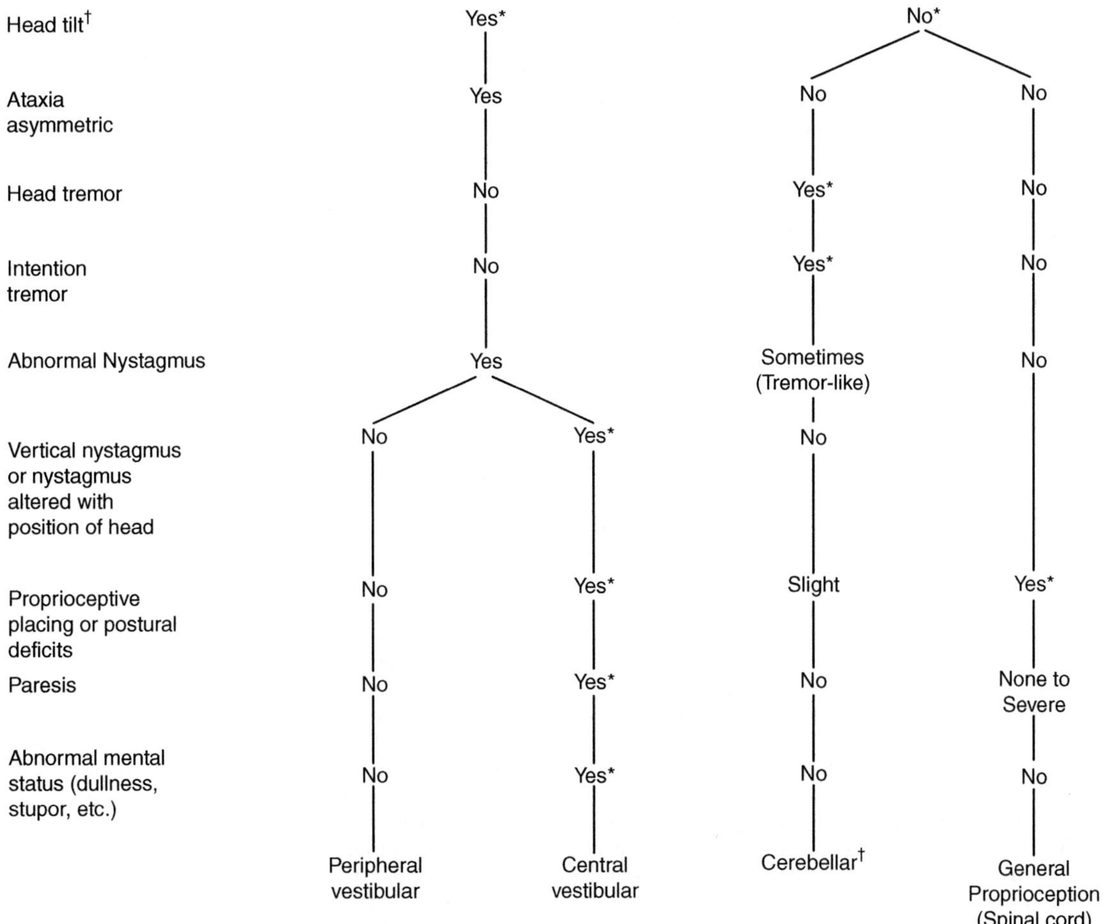

Figure 8-2 Algorithm for the diagnosis of ataxia resulting from vestibular, cerebellar, or spinal cord disease. *Key differential signs. Lesion in the brainstem can cause central vestibular, cerebellar, and upper motor neuron signs. Lesions involving the cerebellar flocculonodular lobe may cause head tilt. When the caudal cerebellar peduncle is involved, head tilt may be opposite (paradoxical) the side of the lesion.

with the afferent nerve fibers of the vestibular nerve, which send impulses to the brainstem. The three semicircular canals are oriented in different planes, which allow the receptors to predict loss of balance and maintain equilibrium during movement regardless of the direction of the movement.

Input to the brain is by way of the vestibular division of cranial nerve (CN) VIII. The vestibular nerve is composed of bipolar neurons, with cell bodies located in the vestibular ganglia contained within the internal acoustic meatus of the petrosal bone. The vestibular nerve enters the brainstem at the level of the rostral medulla and caudal cerebellar peduncle in proximity to CN V and CN VII. The nerve terminates in one of four vestibular nuclei or in the cerebellum via the cerebellar peduncles.

Pathways from the vestibular nuclei project to other brainstem nuclei, cerebellum, cerebral cortex, and spinal cord. Vestibular projections to the motor nuclei of CN III, IV, and VI, which control eye movements travel by way of the medial longitudinal fasciculus (MLF) in the brainstem. This system controls normal (physiologic) nystagmus, which can be demonstrated in the normal animal by moving its head from side to side or up and down. As the head is turned to one side, the eyes move in a slow direction to the opposite side *(slow phase)* followed by a jerk movement *(fast phase)* toward (ipsilateral) the side of the head turn. The slow phase also is known as the *doll's eye response.* The fast phase is akin to the *oculocephalic reflex (or vestibulo-ocular reflex)*, which provides a compensatory adjustment to keep the eyes fixed on one object. The direction of the fast phase is always in the same direction of the head movement. Normal or physiologic nystagmus may be depressed or absent with vestibular dysfunction. This is observed by lagging of the fast phase or dysconjugate eye movements (see Chapter 11). Other ways of eliciting normal nystagmus are caloric testing and assessment of postrotary nystagmus. Both are difficult to perform and interpret and are usually not necessary in the evaluation of vestibular dysfunction. Briefly, with caloric testing, placement of cool water into the external ear canal produces nystagmus to the opposite side and placement of warm water produces nystagmus to the same side (mnemonic—COWS: cool, opposite; warm, same). This test may be useful when assessing vestibular function in the comatose animal.

Projections to the vomiting center of the brainstem are important in the development of motion sickness *(visual-vestibular sensory dissociation)*. The vomiting center is located in the reticular formation of the brainstem and has direct connection with the vestibular nuclei. Vomiting is often a clinical sign of acute vestibular dysfunction.

The vestibular apparatus also works in close association with the cerebellum to maintain balance and coordination. Pathways project directly from CN VIII or from the vestibular nuclei through the caudal cerebellar peduncle to several areas in the cerebellum. Namely the flocculonodular lobe and the fastigial nucleus.

Vestibular impulses reach the cerebral cortex via the medial geniculate nucleus and projection fibers to the cerebral cortex. These pathways inform the animal of its position during movement.

Vestibular information is transmitted to the somatic muscles via the vestibulospinal tracts. These pathways are important for the regulation of antigravity muscles of the limbs and trunk. Basically, the vestibulospinal tracts facilitate the ipsilateral extensor muscles and inhibit the ipsilateral flexors and contralateral extensors.

Signs of Vestibular Dysfunction— Peripheral Versus Central

An animal with vestibular dysfunction manifests abnormalities in eye position/movement, head and body position, muscle tone, and voluntary motor movements. The purpose of the neurologic examination is to determine the neuroanatomic localization as whether the lesion affects the peripheral (sensory receptors or CN VIII) or central (brainstem) vestibular system (see Figure 8-2). In general, common clinical signs of vestibular disease (peripheral or central) are ataxia, head tilt, and abnormal nystagmus. These signs may be present alone or in combination with each other. In general, the determination of central vestibular disease is made through the observation of other signs that implicate a lesion affecting the brainstem. Signs such as abnormal mentation, postural reaction deficits, and other cranial nerve deficits, suggest involvement of the brainstem. Animals not displaying signs suggestive of brainstem involvement are considered to have peripheral vestibular disease. Despite this, some animals with lesions affecting the central vestibular system may not demonstrate signs of brainstem involvement and in doing so appear clinically identical to those with a disorder affecting the peripheral vestibular system.

Mentation. Animals with peripheral vestibular disease should have normal mentation. However, in some animals, severe disorientation and nausea sometimes makes assessment of the mental state difficult. Animals with central vestibular disease may be dull or obtunded because of proximity of the vestibular nuclei and tracts to the reticular activating system in the brainstem. Severely affected animals may be stuporous or comatose.

Gait and Posture. Presence of a head tilt obviously indicates vestibular dysfunction and an asymmetric disease process. Loss of ipsilateral excitatory input to the extensor muscles of the neck causes the head to tilt to the side of the lesion. In subtle cases, blindfolding the animal may accentuate the tilt. In most cases, the head tilt is *toward* the side of the lesion. The head tilt may vary in severity and may be a residual deficit with resolution of a disease process. Similarly, unilateral vestibular lesions cause a loss of ipsilateral extensor tone and animals fall to the side of the lesion. Moreover, because the extensor tone on the contralateral side is no longer inhibited, the increased extensor tone on the contralateral side causes the animal to lean or roll to the side of the lesion.

Vestibular ataxia is generally asymmetric unless bilateral lesions are present. The animal usually falls or drifts toward the side of the lesion. Turning in tight circles is usually a sign of vestibular dysfunction (wide circles accompanied by propulsive walking without an obvious ataxia suggests forebrain dysfunction ipsilateral to the side the animal circles toward), although exceptions may be observed. With circling related to vestibular dysfunction, the movement is usually toward the side of the lesion, but movement in the opposite direction can occur with central vestibular lesions (*paradoxical vestibular disease*; see the following discussion). Signs of paresis or postural reaction deficits in the limbs associated with a head tilt indicate central vestibular disease. Paresis in central vestibular disease is caused by injury of the descending UMN tracts that project through the brainstem. Thus, a *major* way to differentiate between central and peripheral vestibular disease is to evaluate the animal critically for evidence of motor dysfunction or GP ataxia. Careful assessment of postural reactions, especially proprioceptive positioning and the hopping response, is the key factor in localizing vestibular lesions. In some animals with severe vestibular dysfunction, the only postural reaction that can be accurately assessed is proprioceptive positioning. Most important, the side of the postural reaction deficits implicates the side of the lesion in the brainstem. Consequently, postural reactions deficits observed in the right thoracic and pelvic limbs means that the lesion affects the right side of the brainstem, regardless of the side of the head tilt.

Strabismus and Nystagmus. When any component of the vestibular system is disrupted, strabismus or abnormal nystagmus can occur independently (spontaneously) of head movement. When the head is elevated, *ventral strabismus* is often seen ipsilateral to the lesion in either peripheral or central vestibular disease. When the head is returned to its normal position, the strabismus resolves. This type of strabismus is referred to as positional or vestibular strabismus. It is in contradistinction to a fixed strabismus in which the abnormal eye position does not change with changes in the position of the head. Fixed strabismus is observed with lesions affecting CN III, IV, or VI (see Chapter 11). Ventral strabismus can be seen with peripheral and central vestibular disease and is therefore not a localizing sign.

Animals with vestibular dysfunction often display abnormal nystagmus that is constantly present. This is referred to as *spontaneous (or resting) nystagmus*. In some cases, spontaneous nystagmus is absent; however, with changes in head position, abnormal nystagmus may be induced. This may be referred to as *positional or inducible* nystagmus. Because of visual compensation, spontaneous nystagmus often is the first of the clinical signs of vestibular disease to disappear or resolve. Thus a way to induce abnormal nystagmus in an animal suspected to have vestibular disease is to decompensate them. This is accomplished by rapid turning of the head from side to side, tipping the nose in a vertical direction, blindfolding or flipping the animal on its back, size permitting. Hence, positional or induced nystagmus also indicates vestibular dysfunction. Presence of abnormal (spontaneous or positional) nystagmus indicates vestibular dysfunction and may be present in central or peripheral vestibular disease. This can be explained by imbalance of input being relayed from the sensory receptors in the labyrinth or CN VIII (peripheral) to and from the vestibular nuclei (central). For example, asymmetric sensory input, consisting of impulses from the normal side (side opposite of the head tilt) combined with absent or reduced impulses from the affected side into the vestibular nuclei is perceived as head movement; thereby causing the eyes to move in the opposite direction of the perceived rotation (slow phase toward the lesion) followed by a fast reset (fast phase away from the lesion).

Abnormal nystagmus is named according to its orientation (horizontal, rotatory, or vertical). Additionally, the direction of nystagmus is named in accordance with the direction of the fast phase. In peripheral vestibular disease, the nystagmus may be horizontal or rotatory, with the fast phase or jerk directed *away* from the side of the head tilt. The direction of nystagmus should not change in animals with peripheral vestibular disease. With a central vestibular lesion, the nystagmus may be similar to that described for peripheral lesions; however, nystagmus that changes in the direction of the fast phase with alterations in head position, nystagmus in which the fast phase is directed toward the head tilt, or that is *vertical* in direction strongly suggests a central vestibular lesion, although exceptions may occur.

Cranial Nerves. Due to the proximity of CN VIII with CN VII and the postganglionic sympathetic fibers that innervate the eye, which traverse the middle ear, the observation of facial paresis/paralysis and Horner's syndrome (loss of sympathetic innervation to the eye) suggests peripheral vestibular disease. The sympathetic nerve courses through the middle ear in dogs and cats and often is affected in otitis media with associated Horner's syndrome (see Chapter 11).[1,2] In large animals, this is not the case because there is no evidence that the postganglionic sympathetic fibers pass through the tympanic bullae in these species. CN VII and CN VIII dysfunction without Horner's syndrome may occur with either peripheral or central vestibular disease. This is related to the intimate anatomic relationship of CN VII and CN VIII. CN VII exits the brainstem in close association with the vestibular nerve and separates from it within the petrosal bone. CN VII courses through the facial canal, which opens into the middle ear.

Dysfunction of other cranial nerves (V-XII) associated with head tilt suggests a central vestibular lesion that involves other areas of the brainstem. Some syndromes that cause peripheral neuropathy, however, also affect other cranial nerves, including the vestibular nerve. Thus evidence of multiple cranial nerve involvement does not necessarily indicate central vestibular disease.

Deafness, more commonly associated with peripheral vestibular disease, is caused by damage to the tissues for conduction (external or middle ear) or sensorineural transmission (inner ear, organ of Corti, or cochlear nerve) involved in hearing. Brainstem lesions affecting the sympathetic pathways typically affect other structures, and additional signs are seen.

Paradoxical Vestibular Disease. *Paradoxical vestibular disease* is an uncommon presentation of central vestibular disease in which the clinical signs of vestibular dysfunction are directed opposite the side of the anatomic lesion. For example, an animal may display vestibular ataxia directed to the left with a left-sided head tilt with abnormal nystagmus directed to the right, which suggests a left-sided lesion, yet the anatomic lesion is on the right side. In the case of paradoxical vestibular disease, the determination of the side of the anatomic lesion is made based on other localizing signs. The most useful signs to determine the side of the anatomic lesion are postural deficits, which occur ipsilateral to the lesion. Therefore, the side of the lesion in paradoxical vestibular disease is localized according to the side of the postural deficits. Other cranial nerve deficits, such as CN V or CN VII, also help determine the side of the anatomic lesion, which also occur on the side ipsilateral to the lesion. Paradoxical vestibular disease is generally caused by lesions that involve the flocculonodular lobes or the caudal cerebellar peduncles.[3] An explanation is related to loss of the cerebellar inhibitory influence on the ipsilateral vestibular nuclei, resulting in relative excessive discharge (in relationship to the unaffected side in which there is a relative decrease in the frequency of discharges of discharges; the rate of efferent discharges from the normal side appears decreased) from the vestibular nuclei forcing the head tilt and loss of balance to the opposite side.[4] In summary, paradoxical vestibular disease is the observation of clinical signs opposite of the anatomic lesion, which reflects involvement of the central vestibular system.

Bilateral Vestibular Disease. *Bilateral vestibular disease* does not cause a head tilt because of the lesion symmetry. The animal often walks slowly in a crouched position and tends to avoid sudden movements, and often exhibits a characteristic side-to-side swaying of the head. Because of lack of input to the vestibular nuclei on both sides of the brainstem, normal or physiologic nystagmus is absent and abnormal nystagmus is not observed. Bilateral vestibular dysfunction more commonly occurs with peripheral vestibular diseases and less so with central vestibular diseases.

Cerebellar Ataxia

Anatomy

The cerebellum functions as a major coordinator of motor activity. It compares the intent of motor activity with the performance required to complete the activity. The cerebellum receives input through three paired peduncles. The caudal cerebellar peduncles carry sensory and proprioceptive fibers from the vestibular system, basal nuclei, and spinal cord. The middle cerebellar peduncles transmit information from the cerebral cortex by way of the pons. A few fibers relaying proprioceptive information from the head and spinal cord enter through the rostral cerebellar peduncles. The majority of fibers leaving the cerebellum travel through the rostral cerebellar peduncle to project to the cerebral cortex, midbrain, reticular formation, and vestibular nuclei. The

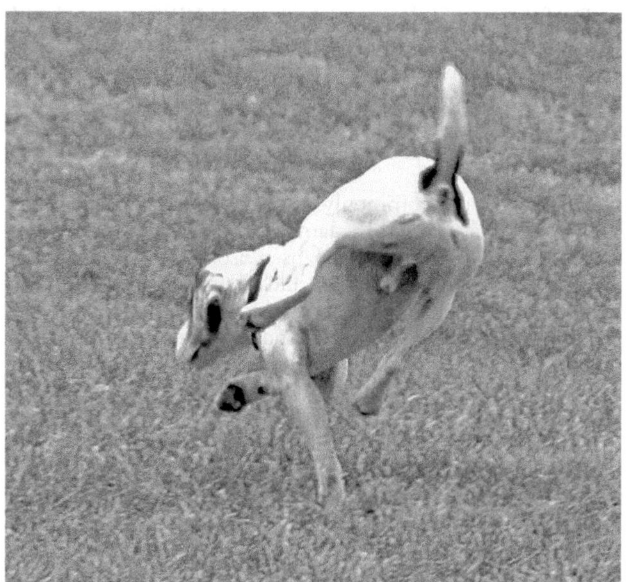

Figure 8-3 A 2-year-old Jack Russell terrier with hereditary spinocerebellar ataxia. Note the severe truncal cerebellar ataxia.

flocculonodular lobes of the cerebellum are important in vestibular system activities. Lesions of the flocculonodular lobe of the cerebellum often can cause paradoxical vestibular dysfunction (see previous discussion of paradoxical vestibular dysfunction).[3]

Signs of Cerebellar Dysfunction

A disease of the cerebellum or its peduncles results in characteristic clinical signs. The cerebellum performs below the level of consciousness to control muscle movements accurately, assist in maintaining equilibrium and proprioception, and control posture. Therefore, behavior and level of consciousness are not affected by pure cerebellar lesions. Because the cerebellum does not initiate motor activity, paresis is not a sign of cerebellar dysfunction unless the brainstem is also affected.

Gait and Posture. The gait is characterized by symmetric truncal ataxia (Figure 8-3) and dysmetria, which is commonly manifested as hypermetria (Figure 8-4). Posture at rest and during movement is basewide for maintaining position and stabilization of the trunk. Cerebellar dysfunction rarely produces head tilt or circling.

Animals with acute onset cerebellar disease can develop a *decerebellate posture*: opisthotonos, tonic extension of the thoracic limbs, and flexion of the pelvis and pelvic limbs. The pelvic limbs may also be extended if the ventral aspect of the rostral lobe of the cerebellum is affected. Spinal reflexes may be exaggerated in the early stages.[3] The spasticity decreases after a few days, and the other signs of chronic lesions, including intention tremor of the head and cerebellar ataxia, develop over a period of several weeks to months.

Intention Tremor. Cerebellar tremor occurs with movement (intention) and at rest (postural). An intention tremor that is most pronounced in the head is very suggestive of cerebellar disease. The intention tremor is most obvious when the animal attempts a purposeful or goal-directed movement, such as eating or drinking. Postural tremor or titubation consists of rocking movements—forward-backward and side-to-side. Cerebellar tremors are absent in relaxed or sleep states and are not considered involuntary movements (see Chapter 10). Ocular movement disorders occur as clinical signs of cerebellar disease.[5] Flutter consisting of eye oscillations and dysmetria occurs

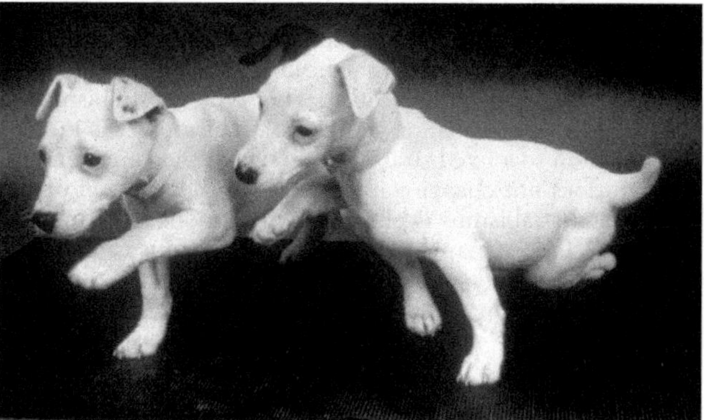

Figure 8-4 Jack Russell terrier puppies with primary cerebellar granule cell degeneration. Note the hypermetric gait.

during movement and gaze fixation. Upbeat and downbeat nystagmus can be induced with a rapid change in head position. Menace response may be impaired in animals with diffuse cerebellar disease, even though vision and facial nerve function are normal. Anisocoria and alterations in the size of the palpebral fissure have been observed with cerebellar lesions.[3]

DISEASES

This chapter discusses diseases that commonly affect the brainstem, cerebellum, and peripheral vestibular system. The disorders that produce GP ataxia because of spinal cord disease are described in Chapters 6 and 7. Diseases with involuntary movements as the primary sign (e.g., tremor, spasticity) are discussed in Chapter 10. As in previous chapters, this section is organized according to the anatomic location of the lesion and the course of the disease (acute versus chronic, progressive versus nonprogressive).

Acute Progressive and Nonprogressive Peripheral Vestibular Diseases

A diagnostic approach to peripheral vestibular disease is outlined in Figure 8-5. A careful history is taken to determine exposure to ototoxic drugs. Using otoscopic examinations and imaging studies (radiographic or cross-sectional imaging computed tomography [CT] or magnetic resonance imaging [MRI]) of the external ear canal and the tympanic bulla, the clinician must decide whether abnormalities exist. CT is more sensitive for evaluation of middle and inner ear diseases than radiography. MRI depicts the inner ear anatomy, especially the hyperintensity of the endolymph on T2-weighted (T2W) images. T1-weighted (T1W) images after intravenous contrast administration can detect inflammatory conditions of the inner ear. If toxic agents have not been administered, the patient's history is used to place the condition in one of two categories: chronic progressive or acute nonprogressive. If the initial otoscopic examination or imaging studies disclose an abnormality, the disorder is classified as inflammatory or noninflammatory based on the results of myringotomy, cytology, and culture and antimicrobial susceptibility testing of material obtained from the tympanic bulla. Certain inflammatory and neoplastic diseases can fall into either broad category, depending on the propensity of the disease to produce detectable lesions that are grossly visible on otoscopic inspection or with imaging studies. The etiologic categories for peripheral vestibular disease include anomalous, neoplastic, inflammatory, idiopathic, and toxic. These disorders according to disease onset and progression are outlined in Table 8-1.

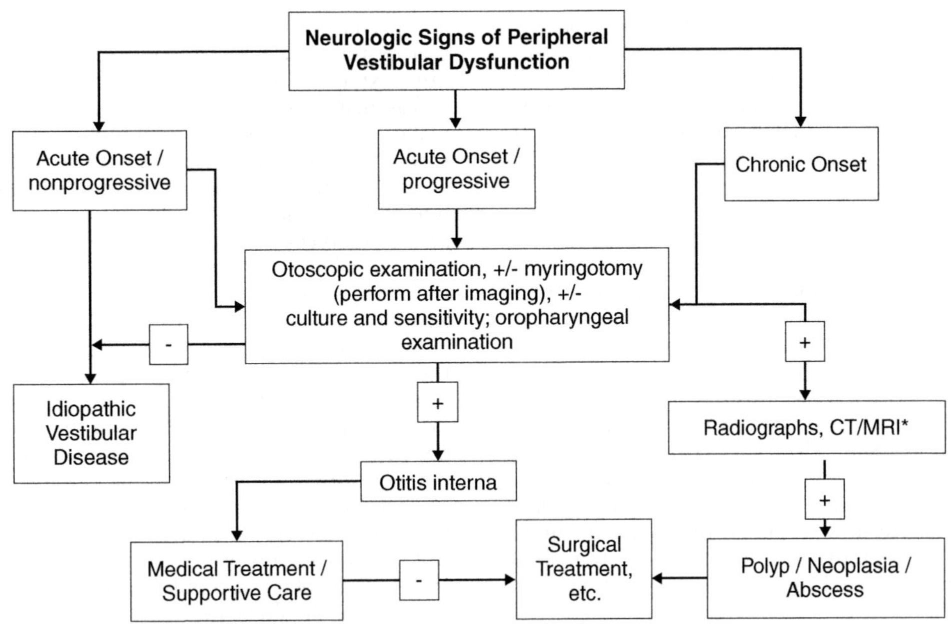

Figure 8-5 Algorithm for the diagnostic approach of peripheral vestibular disease.

TABLE 8-1

*Etiology of Peripheral Vestibular Disease**

Etiologic Category	Acute Nonprogressive	Acute Progressive	Chronic Progressive
Anomalous	Congenital vestibular disease (C, F, B)		
Metabolic			Hypothyroidism (7, 15)
Neoplastic (12)		Metastatic	Primary aural tumors Ceruminous gland adenocarcinoma Sebaceous gland adenocarcinoma Squamous cell carcinoma Bony tumors Neurofibrosarcoma
Inflammatory (15)		Otitis media/interna (all) Inflammatory polyp (C, F)	Otitis media interna (all) Inflammatory polyp (C, F)
Idiopathic	Canine idiopathic Feline idiopathic		
Toxic (15)		Ototoxic drugs (topical and systemic)	
Traumatic (12)	Head injury		Temporohyoid osteoarthropathy (E)
Vascular	*Cuterebra* larval Migration (F)		

C, Canine; F, feline; B, bovine; E, equine.
*Numbers in parentheses refer to chapters in which entities are discussed.

Anomalous

Congenital Vestibular Syndromes. Congenital vestibular syndromes occur sporadically in litters of purebred dogs and cats.[6] They have been reported in beagles, German shepherd dogs, Doberman pinschers, cocker spaniels, smooth fox terriers, Akitas, and several other breeds.[1,7-9] Affected Siamese, Burmese, Persian, and Tonkinese cats also have been identified.[10] Vestibular signs develop from the time of birth until the animal is several weeks of age. Deafness may accompany the vestibular disease and may be unilateral or bilateral. The pathogenesis of the lesion is unknown. Although most of the conditions are assumed to be inherited, a definite pattern of inheritance has not been identified. Lymphocytic labyrinthitis was identified histologically in two litters of affected Doberman pinschers.[11] Some congenitally affected animals gradually improve, whereas others have persistent head tilt and deafness. No effective therapy is known. The pendular nystagmus of Siamese cats is caused by an abnormality of the visual pathways rather than vestibular disease (see Chapter 11). Pendular nystagmus of Holstein and Jersey cattle with no other clinical signs could be a similar syndrome.[12,13]

Metabolic

Hypothyroidism (see Chapter 15). Hypothyroidism can cause signs of peripheral or central vestibular disease.[14,15] Clinical signs may be acute or chronic. Peripheral vestibular dysfunction may be related to the signs of polyneuropathy associated with hypothyroidism or the myxomatous compressive neuropathy and the vestibular nerve exits the skull foramina.[6,14] Diagnosis is based on documenting low T_4, free T_4, and elevated thyroid-stimulating hormone (TSH). Signs of vestibular dysfunction usually resolve within 2 to 4 weeks of thyroid supplementation.

Inflammatory

Otitis Media/Interna

Pathogenesis. The most common cause of peripheral vestibular disease in dogs and cats is an inner ear infection that has originated in the external ear canal and progressed into the middle ear and ultimately affects the inner ear. As such, infections are often referred to as otitis media/interna. Of 83 cases of peripheral vestibular disease in the dog, 49% were attributed to infection.[1] Similarly in cats, otitis media/interna was suspected in 43% of cats with peripheral vestibular disease.[16] Otitis media/interna is also common in food animals but not in horses.[13] The most common risk factor in ruminants for otitis media/interna is respiratory infection, but other factors include infected milk during suckling and ear mite infestation.[17,18]

Otitis media/interna in animals is caused most commonly by bacteria, although yeast and fungal organisms are encountered occasionally. Otitis externa caused by bacteria is the most common cause of otitis media/interna in small animals.[1] The causative bacteria in small animals include *Staphylococcus* spp., *Streptococcus* spp., *Proteus* spp., *Pseudomonas* spp., *Pasteurella* spp., and *Escherichia coli*.[19] In the absence of otitis externa, alternate routes of infection include retrograde spread via the auditory (eustachian) tubes and hematogenous spread. In horses, *Streptococcus* spp., *Actinobacillus* spp., and *Staphylococcus* spp. are most frequent. Lambs and cattle more often have *Pasteurella* spp., *Streptococcus* spp., or *Arcanobacterium* spp.[18,20] Streptococcus organisms are most likely to be found in pigs.[21] In pigs and small ruminants, it is not uncommon for otitis interna to extend through the internal acoustic meatus resulting in meningitis, empyema, and encephalitis.[13]

In dogs, otitis externa can be classified into predisposing, primary, secondary, and perpetuating causes.[22] Predisposing causes include the confirmation of the pinnae and external ear canal. Primary causes include etiologies such as ectoparasites, atopy, food allergies, foreign bodies, and neoplasia. Primary etiologies result in the development of secondary infection. Left untreated, infections become chronic. With chronic infection, pathologic changes develop within the external ear canal, which perpetuate infection. Breeds of dogs that are predisposed to chronic otitis externa (cocker spaniels, poodles, and German shepherd dogs) are at increased risk of developing otitis media/interna. Chronic otitis externa with mite or tick infestation can extend into otitis media with damage to the tympanic membrane from the mites and associated inflammatory response. A primary secretory otitis media (PSOM) has been described in Cavalier King Charles spaniels.[23] These dogs have severe head and neck pain that may be consequence of a the middle ear that contains debris within the tympanic bulla consisting of a mucus plug. Occasionally, otic foreign bodies, such as grass awns, foxtail awns, or spear grass, predispose dogs to otitis externa with progression to otitis media/interna. Recurrent episodes are common. Extension of guttural pouch mycosis in horses is a rare cause of vestibular and facial nerve signs with temporohyoid osteoarthropathy (see Chapter 9) a more likely cause.[24-26]

Clinical Signs. Otitis media/interna may cause the clinical signs of vestibular ataxia as discussed earlier. Head shaking, aural pain, and exudative discharge are often present in cases of otitis externa. Torticollis, circling, positional ventral strabismus (vestibular strabismus), and abnormal nystagmus are specific neurologic signs consistent with peripheral vestibular dysfunction. When present in conjunction with signs of otitis externa, a diagnosis of otitis media/interna is presumed. Occasionally the otitis media/interna can extend into the cranial cavity.[27,28] In most cases of intracranial extension of otitis media/interna, signs consistent with central vestibular disease are present; however, some cases may only display signs consistent with peripheral vestibular disease. Unilateral facial paralysis is common because the inflammatory process often extends to the facial nerve as it passes through the petrosal bone.[29] Otitis media, with no involvement of the inner ear, does not cause vestibular dysfunction. In dogs and cats, Horner's syndrome, either complete or partial (miosis alone or with slight elevation of the nictitating membrane) can be seen on the affected side if the sympathetic nerve in the middle ear is involved.[2] Because the postganglionic fibers of the sympathetic nerve do not enter the middle ear in large animals, Horner's syndrome is not seen with otitis media/interna in these species.

Diagnosis. The diagnosis of otitis media/interna is confirmed by otoscopic examination and imaging studies. If purulent otitis externa is present, cytologic evaluation and culture with antimicrobial susceptibility testing of the material in the external ear should be performed followed by gentle but thorough cleaning. Cattle with otitis media/interna frequently have purulent otorrhea, but this is not the case in sheep.[17] Deep sedation or anesthesia aids in critical otoscopic examination. The tympanic membrane is examined carefully for hyperemia, edema, hemorrhage, and erosion. Fluid in the middle ear makes the tympanic membrane appear opaque and produces bulging of the membrane into the external ear canal. If the tympanic membrane is ruptured or eroded, fluid is aspirated gently from the middle ear for cytology and bacteriologic culture. If the tympanic membrane is intact but abnormal, myringotomy is performed with a 22-gauge spinal needle of appropriate length or with a sterile myringotomy knife. If aspiration of the middle ear fails to yield a small quantity of fluid for evaluation, 0.25 to 0.5 mL of sterile saline is injected and then aspirated. Cytology and microbial culture and antimicrobial susceptibility testing are performed. Brainstem auditory evoked response (BAER) testing can estimate peripheral and central auditory function.

Radiographic examination of the skull is a valuable aid in the diagnosis and prognosis of chronic otitis media/interna. Radiographic projections include lateral, dorsoventral, "open-mouth," and oblique views of each tympanic bulla. Positive findings include fluid opacity in the tympanic bulla and exostosis, sclerosis, or erosion in the tympanic bulla (Figure 8-6). Lysis of the bulla or surrounding structures is more often associated with neoplasia. Despite the presence of otitis media/interna, radiographs may be normal.[30]

Cross-sectional imaging provides for a more sensitive method of imaging the middle and inner ear than radiography. Computed tomography findings in otitis media/interna include thickening of the tympanic bulla and the presence of soft/fluid tissue density within the tympanic bulla.[31,32] Proliferation, sclerosis, or lysis of the tympanic bulla may be observed.[33] Magnetic resonance imaging findings associated with otitis media/interna include observation of material in the tympanic bulla with intermediate signal intensity on T1W and hyperintense signal intensity on T2W images.[16,34-36] T1W images obtained after intravenous contrast administration may reveal peripheral enhancement along the interior of the tympanic bulla.[27] Additionally, absence of signal intensity from the labyrinthine fluid on T2W images may be suggestive of involvement of the inner ear.[37] Meningeal enhancement on T1W postcontrast images has also been described secondary to otitis interna with intracranial extension of the inflammatory process (Figure 8-7).[37] Cerebrospinal fluid (CSF) analysis should be performed in cases in which intracranial extension is

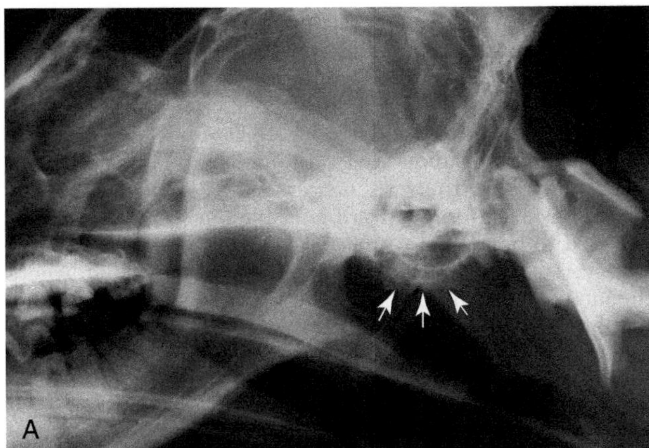

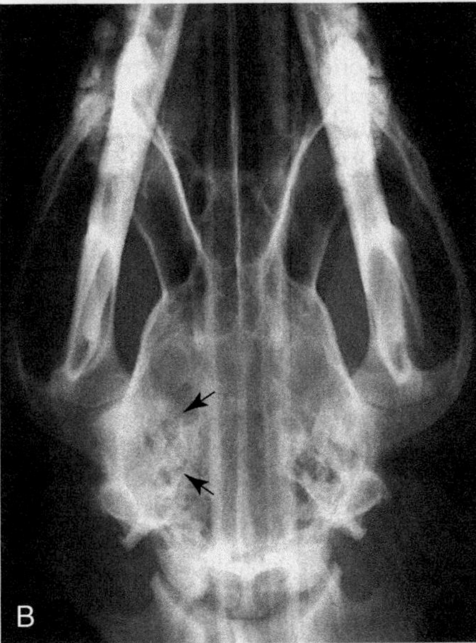

Figure 8-6 **A,** Lateral skull radiograph of a dog with severe otitis media/interna. Note the proliferative bony reaction of the osseous bulla *(arrows)*. **B,** Ventrodorsal skull radiograph of the same dog. Note the opacity of the right tympanic bulla *(arrows)*. A bulla osteotomy was performed to curette the diseased bone and to establish drainage from the middle ear.

suspected to evaluate for bacterial meningitis. Such extension may not be accompanied by clinical signs unless it progresses into brain abscessation.[27]

In horses with temporohyoid osteoarthropathy, radiography may identify stress fractures of the petrosal bone and periosteal proliferative changes around the bulla and hyoid bones.[24,38] However, aural, pharyngeal, and guttural pouch endoscopy is more reliable than radiography, with CT or MRI being the most reliable in confirming a diagnosis.[25] On CT, osseous proliferation of the stylohyoid bone and temporohyoid articulation was the most consistent feature of temporohyoid osteoarthropathy.[39]

Treatment. The medical treatment of otitis media/interna consists of a prolonged course of appropriate parenteral and topical antibiotics chosen on the basis of culture and antimicrobial susceptibility results. Cultures may be insensitive for *Pseudomonas* spp. infection. Initial treatment also should include thorough cleansing and flushing with sterile saline.[40] Penicillinase-resistant penicillins, cephalosporins, chloramphenicol, metronidazole, and high-dose fluoroquinolones are often appropriate choices. We prefer long-term bactericidal antibiotic therapy and in chronic cases, therapy

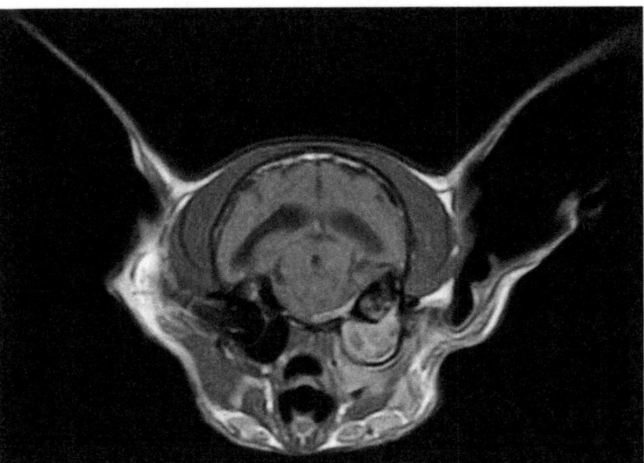

Figure 8-7 A transverse postcontrast T1W MRI from an 11-year-old cat with right-side vestibular disease and chronic otitis externa. Note the hyperintensity in the bulla with meningeal enhancement in the ventral aspect of the right brainstem. A bulla osteotomy confirmed bacterial otitis media/interna.

for 6 to 8 weeks is recommended. Antibiotics and corticosteroids instilled in the external ear canal rarely reach the middle ear and therefore are seldom useful for resolving the inner ear infection. Because ototoxic agents can penetrate into the inner ear from the middle ear, they should be avoided. Unfortunately, this excludes most of the common topical medications (see subsequent discussion of ototoxicity).[41]

In chronic disease or when medical treatment and in animals with worsening of neurologic signs, surgical drainage and débridement of the middle ear and the tympanic bulla often are needed to resolve the infection. Various techniques have been described. In cats, we prefer the ventral bulla osteotomy because it affords the best visibility and exposure for biopsy, débridement, and drainage.[42] In dogs, total ear canal ablation combined with lateral bulla osteotomy may be required with chronic otitis externa and media.[43-45] Nasopharyngeal polyps of the middle ear may result in recurrent infections and must be removed (see subsequent discussion). If there has been intracranial extension of the otitis media/interna, bulla osteotomy should be pursued followed by long-term antibiotic therapy.[27]

Therapy for otitis media/interna must resolve the infection and prevent extension to the brainstem. The prognosis for recovery depends on several factors: (1) the resistance of the organism, (2) the chronicity of disease, (3) the extent of bone involvement, and (4) the reversibility of the neurologic damage. In chronic otitis interna, neurologic deficits, specifically the head tilt may be irreversible; however, most animals soon compensate for their vestibular deficits. Facial paralysis is usually irreversible. Resulting keratoconjunctivitis sicca requires long-term therapy with artificial tears.

Inflammatory Polyp. Inflammatory (aural or nasopharyngeal) polyps of the middle ear are suspected in cats with peripheral vestibular dysfunction in young cats.[46] Cats with inflammatory polyps may present with stridor, nasal discharge, sneezing, and occasionally with dyspnea. Inflammatory polyps are usually unilateral. Polyps can extend into the external ear canal or within the nasopharynx. Diagnosis requires careful examination of the external ear canal and the oropharynx. Otoscopic examination reveals bulging of the tympanic membrane from the fluid or soft tissue mass. Skull radiography may identify a soft tissue opacity in the pharyngeal region or thickening of the osseous bulla secondary to otitis media. CT and MRI are more sensitive than radiography for determining the extent of the mass. Increased fluid and soft tissue mass are observed in the bulla. Polyps that extend into the external ear canal or the nasopharynx usually can be removed by gentle traction and avulsion (Figure 8-8). Exploratory surgery and ventral bulla osteotomy are required with middle ear involvement (Figure 8-9).[47] Appropriate antibiotic therapy is instituted based on culture and antimicrobial susceptibility results. Recurrence rate for traction avulsion alone is 30% and less than 8% for those undergoing a ventral bulla osteotomy.[48] With traction alone, treatment with prednisone for 2 weeks may reduce recurrence, whereas ventral bull osteotomy prevents recurrence in most cats.

Idiopathic

Feline Idiopathic Vestibular Syndrome

Pathogenesis. An acute, idiopathic, nonprogressive peripheral vestibular disease has been commonly recognized in cats.[16,49] Whereas most reports describe this syndrome to have a nonprogressive disease course, a recent study described most cats (69%) affected by presumptive idiopathic vestibular syndrome actually showed progressive clinical signs.[16] There is no breed or sex predilection. The condition occurs sporadically and is not associated with other infectious diseases. The incidence seems to be highest in July and August in the northeastern

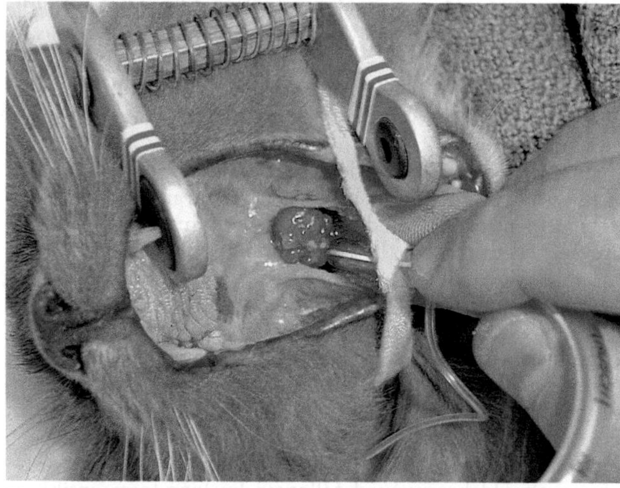

Figure 8-8 A young cat with left-sided peripheral vestibular disease. Oral examination revealed a nasopharyngeal polyp that was subsequently removed by gentle traction. (Copyright 2010 University of Georgia Research Foundation, Inc.)

United States.[49] These observations have not been substantiated in the southern United States, leading some to speculate that the syndrome may be caused by *Cuterebra* fly larvae.[50] In a review of 75 cases, including two necropsies, one cat had hemorrhage in the labyrinth on the affected side, and the other cat had mild nonsuppurative leptomeningitis but no lesions directly involving the vestibular system.[49] An analogous syndrome has been termed lizard poisoning in some areas and is believed to be related to the ingestion of blue-tailed lizards; however, these lizards are not present in the Northeast, where the incidence seems high. There is speculation that idiopathic vestibular disease may represent a self-limiting inflammatory process of the peripheral vestibular apparatus, not identified on MRI.[16]

Clinical Signs. Clinical signs develop acutely and are usually unilateral, although bilateral involvement has been observed. Signs of otitis externa are lacking, and affected cats are usually healthy in all other respects. Cats with unilateral disease develop severe head tilt, disorientation, falling, rolling, and abnormal nystagmus. In bilateral disease, affected cats have little head tilt but have difficulty moving because of severe disorientation. The head may swing in wide excursions from side to side. The cat usually remains in a crouched posture with the limbs widely abducted and may cry out as if extremely frightened. Abnormal nystagmus may not be present; however, normal nystagmus is reduced or absent bilaterally. Some affected cats vomit and are anorextic. Importantly, clinical signs are consistent with peripheral vestibular without any other neurologic deficits. Affected animals should not have facial nerve deficits or Horners syndrome. The finding of neurologic deficits that are not directly attributable to the peripheral vestibular system excludes the diagnosis of feline idiopathic vestibular disease.

Diagnosis. The diagnosis is based on the clinical signs and the absence of evidence supporting a diagnosis of bacterial otitis externa, media, or interna of other causes.

Treatment. Therapy is mainly supportive. Affected cats spontaneously improve within 72 hours and are usually normal in 2 to 3 weeks. Antiemetics are indicated in cats with nausea but do not ease the vestibular signs. Sedation may be necessary during the acute phase of the disease to suppress crying or thrashing. The prognosis for recovery is excellent. Residual vestibular dysfunction is uncommon.

Canine Idiopathic Vestibular Syndrome

Pathogenesis. Acute, idiopathic vestibular syndromes are recognized in older dogs. In a review of 83 cases of peripheral vestibular disease, 39% were considered idiopathic.[1] The disease is not associated with any known infectious agent. Most

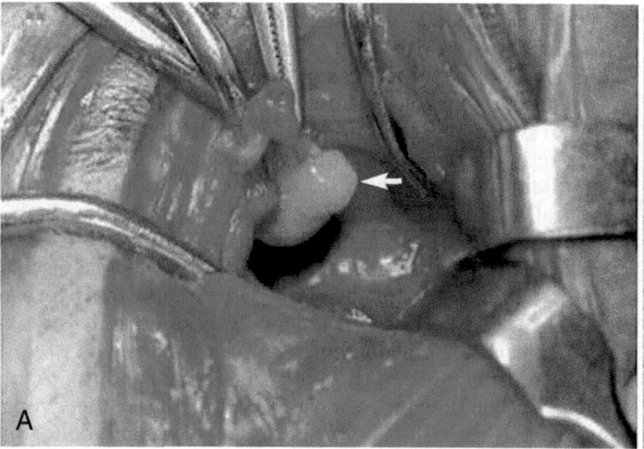

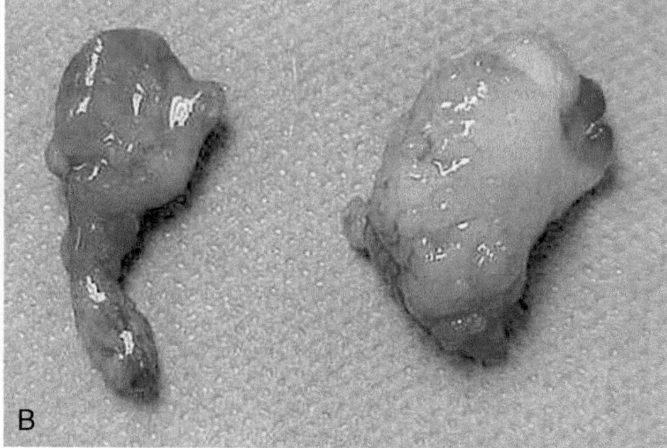

Figure 8-9 **A,** An intraoperative photograph from a young cat with peripheral vestibular disease of an inflammatory polyp *(white arrow)* visualized after a bulla osteotomy. **B,** The polyps displayed after surgical excision.

affected doss are older than 5 years of age with a median age of 12 to 13 years. No breed and sex predilections have been observed.[1,51]

Clinical Signs. Signs develop acutely to peracutely and on occasion may be preceded by vomiting and nausea. As in cats with idiopathic vestibular syndrome, neurologic signs solely reflect peripheral vestibular dysfunction. The observation of other neurologic deficits excludes canine idiopathic vestibular syndrome.

Diagnosis. The diagnosis is based on the clinical signs and the absence of evidence supporting a diagnosis of bacterial otitis media/interna or other disease. We have seen older dogs with peripheral vestibular disease that are hypothyroid and recover with thyroid supplementation. See the discussion of hypothyroidism in Chapters 7 and 15. Because the idiopathic disease is usually self-limiting, cause and effect are difficult to prove.

Treatment. Therapy is symptomatic. Dogs spontaneously improve in 72 hours and are usually normal in 7 to 10 days. Severely affected dogs may take 3 to 4 weeks to return to normal. Head tilt may persist in some cases but it usually does not interfere with function. The condition may recur.

Toxic

Ototoxicity. A large variety of drugs can cause ototoxicity, affecting vestibular function, hearing, or both. Most of these agents initially cause damage to the receptors and eventually cause degeneration of the nerve. Toxicity can occur from either parenteral or topical therapy.[52,53] Topical application is probably safe if the tympanic membrane is intact.[54] Ototoxic agents are listed in Box 8-1.[41] The aminoglycoside antibiotics are most frequently incriminated in ototoxicity. The signs may be unilateral or bilateral. Risk factors for ototoxicity include high drug doses, therapy for longer than 14 days, or their use in treating patients with impaired renal function. Patients receiving these drugs should be monitored closely for signs of renal toxicity and ototoxicity. In patients with decreased renal function, dosages are reduced or ideally, these drugs are replaced by other nontoxic antibiotics. Vestibular signs usually improve once the offending ototoxic agents are discontinued; however, deafness may be permanent.

Flushing of the external ear canal is a relatively common procedure in the treatment of otitis externa. Whereas adverse effects are rarely encountered, ototoxicity can occur.[55] Vestibular dysfunction, facial nerve paresis/paralysis, Horner's syndrome, and hearing loss can occur. Ototoxicity may be the result of mechanical damage from instruments or aggressive irrigation.[55] Additionally, translocation of bacteria or bacterial products through the external acoustic meatus and into the tympanic bulla may occur secondary to flushing the ear. Subsequently, bacterial toxins may penetrate through an intact round or vestibular window to enter the inner ear and lead to ototoxicity.[56] The presence of inflammation may enhance the penetration into the inner ear.[57]

BOX 8-1

Ototoxic Drugs and Chemicals

Antibiotics

Aminoglycosides
Streptomycin
Dihydrostreptomycin
Gentamicin
Neomycin
Kanamycin
Amikacin
Tobramycin

Other
Polymyxin B
Minocycline
Erythromycin
Vancomycin
Chloramphenicol

Antiseptics
Ethanol
Iodine and iodophors
Benzalkonium chloride
Chlorhexidine
Cetrimide
Benzethonium chloride

Antineoplastics
Cisplatin
Nitrogen mustard

Diuretics
Bumetanide
Ethacrynic acid
Furosemide

Heavy Metals
Arsenic
Lead
Mercury

Miscellaneous
Ceruminolytic agents
Detergents
Quinine
Propylene glycol
Salicylates

Data from Mansfield PD: Ototoxicity in dogs and cats, Compend Contin Educ Pract Vet 12:332–337, 1990.

Chronic Progressive Peripheral Vestibular Diseases

Neoplastic

Aural Neoplasms

Pathogenesis. Primary tumors initially can cause peripheral vestibular dysfunction if the tumor originates from or compresses the vestibular nerve. Tumors arising from the vestibular nerve (i.e., neurofibromas, neurofibrosarcomas, malignant nerve sheath tumors) rarely develop in this nerve; when present, a slowly progressive course of vestibular disease evolves over several months. More commonly, tumors can arise from the pinna, externa ear canal, and middle ear and secondarily can cause vestibular dysfunction.[46,58] Tumors of the tympanic bullae or the labyrinth (fibrosarcomas, chondrosarcomas, osteosarcomas) may destroy structures in the inner ear. Ceruminous gland adenocarcinomas, sebaceous gland adenocarcinoma, carcinomas of unknown etiology, and squamous cell carcinoma are the most common tumors of the ear.[59] Squamous cell carcinoma in cats may arise from the epithelial lining of either the middle or inner ear.[60] Tumors arising from the tissues of the ear in cats have a higher likelihood of malignancy than in dogs.[59] Eventually these tumors can grow into the brainstem, and central vestibular signs become apparent.

Diagnosis. Diagnosis is suspected on visual observation and with otoscopic examination. When the mass is exterior, diagnosis is made by fine needle aspiration, impression smears, and tissue biopsy. Bony lysis may be seen on skull radiographs. CT or MRI provides greater anatomic detail and is indicated to

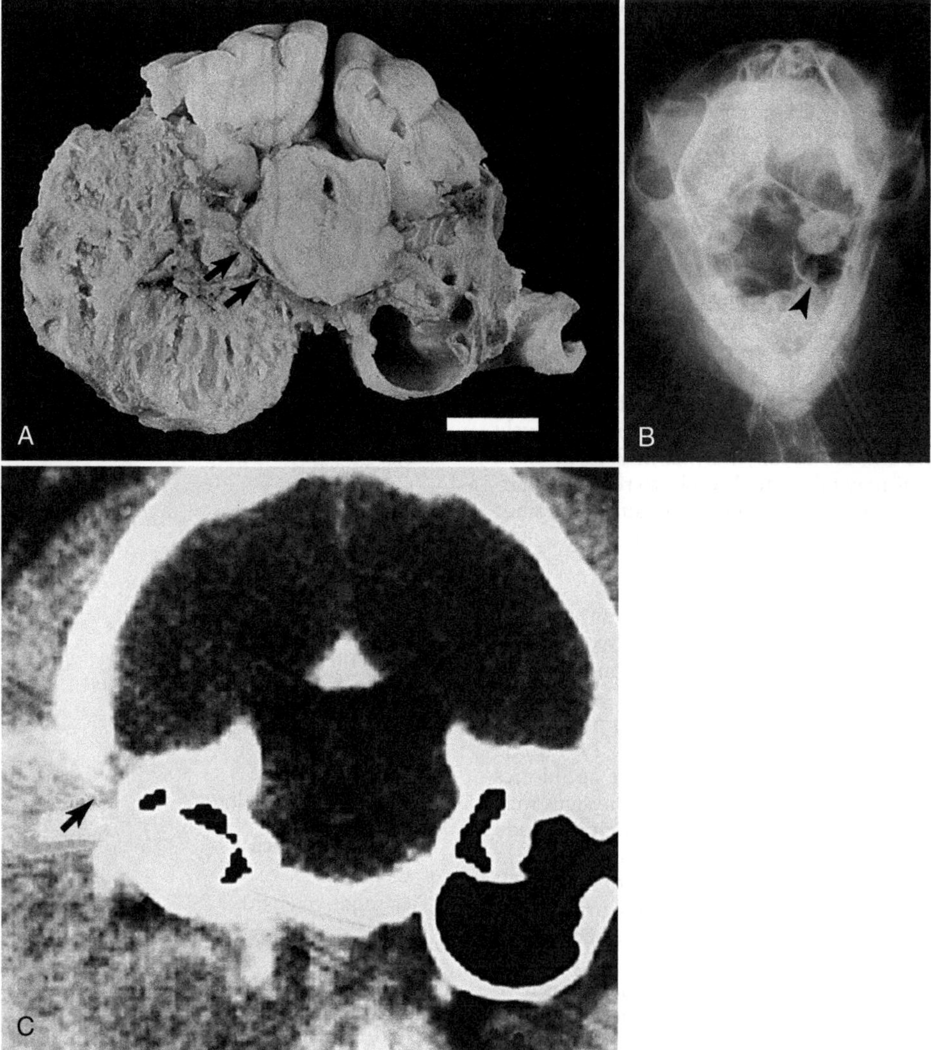

Figure 8-10 Transverse pathologic section of brain and cranium **(A)**, survey skull radiograph **(B)**, and computed tomography image **(C)** from a 5-year-old female domestic cat with initial signs of otitis externa and peripheral vestibular disease and subsequent clinical evidence of brainstem involvement. A mass was palpated at the base of the left ear. A mass has obliterated the left tympanic bulla and invaded the calvaria (*arrows* in **A** and **C**). The left tympanic bulla in **B** is obscured compared with the right tympanic bulla, which can be clearly seen (*arrowhead*). However, the nature of the underlying lesion is poorly defined in the survey radiograph. The cat was euthanized and squamous cell carcinoma was diagnosed on microscopic examination of the lesion. Bar in **A** = 1 cm. (From Kornegay JN: Feline neurology, Philadelphia, 1991, JB Lippincott.)

determine the complete extent of the neoplasm (Figure 8-10). Lysis of the tympanic bulla, petrous temporal bone, and calvaria may be seen along with soft-tissue proliferation. Contrast enhancement may further delineate the extent of the mass. Principles for tumor staging need to be followed for complete assessment of the aural neoplasms.[46,58]

Treatment. Complete and aggressive surgical resection remains the treatment of choice. In dogs, long-term control is possible for completely excised tumors.[59] For more invasive or infiltrative conditions in which a surgical cure is not possible, adjunctive therapies, such as radiation therapy, may extend disease-free intervals and overall survival times. Poor prognostic indicators in cats include neurologic signs at the time of diagnosis, diagnosis of squamous cell carcinoma or carcinoma of unknown cause, and invasion into the lymphatic system.[59] Dogs with extensive tumor involvement tend to have a poor prognosis.[59]

Central Vestibular Diseases

A diagnostic approach to central vestibular (brainstem) disease is outlined in Figure 8-11. MRI is the procedure of choice when evaluating for structural disease in animals with central vestibular dysfunction.[16,37] Unlike CT, in which beam hardening artifact can obscure CT examination of the caudal fossa of the cranium, MRI provides excellent anatomic evaluation of the brainstem (see Chapter 4). Cerebrospinal fluid analysis is useful for confirming inflammatory disease. Molecular-based testing techniques and serology assist with diagnosis of infectious diseases. Of the various categories outlined in Table 8-2, degenerative, metabolic, neoplastic, inflammatory, and vascular conditions are most common. Because of the close functional and anatomic relationship between the vestibular nuclei and cerebellum, the signs of central vestibular disease are often observed either concurrently with signs of cerebellar disease or represent the sole manifestation of a cerebellar

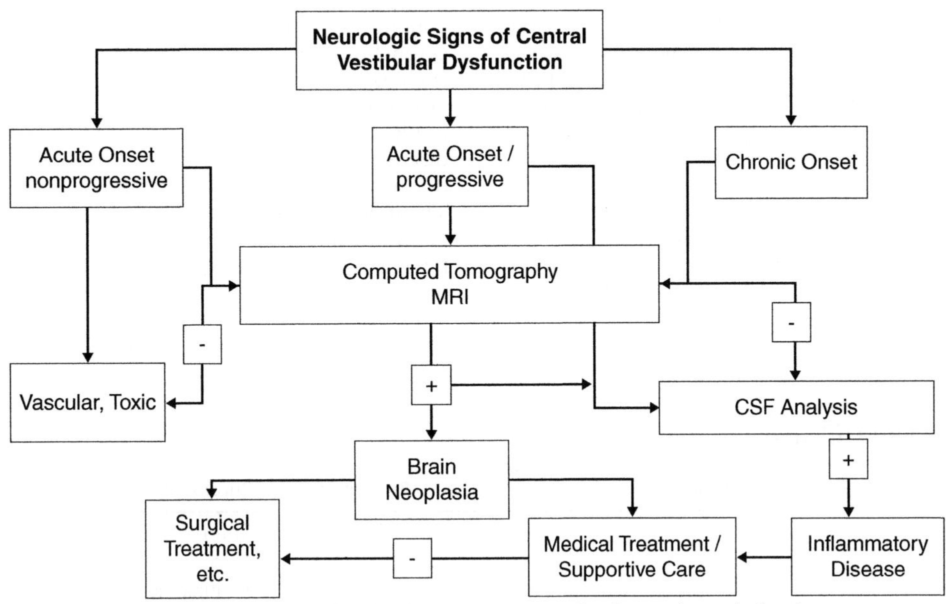

Figure 8-11 Algorithm for the diagnostic approach of central vestibular disease.

TABLE 8-2

Etiology of Central Vestibular (Brainstem) Disease*

Etiologic Category	Acute Nonprogressive	Acute Progressive	Chronic Progressive
Degenerative (all)			Storage diseases Neuronopathies (7) Neuroaxonal dystrophy (7) Demyelinating diseases (7, 10, 15)
Metabolic	Hypothyroidism (C)	Hypoglycemia (15)	Hypothyroidism (C)
Neoplastic (12)		Metastatic	Primary (12) Meningioma Medulloblastoma Glioma Choroid plexus papilloma Epidermoid cyst
Nutritional (15)		Thiamine deficiency (F, C, E)	
Idiopathic			Intracranial arachnoid cyst/diverticulum
Inflammatory (15)		Viral Distemper (C) Equine encephalomyelitis Feline infectious peritonitis Mycotic Bacterial Listeriosis (C, B, O, G, Ca) Various bacteria Pituitary abscess (B, G, O, E) Rickettsial Protozoal Granulomatous meningoencephalitis (C) Necrotizing encephalitis (C)	Viral Distemper (C) Feline infectious peritonitis Bacterial Protozoal Mycotic Granulomatous meningoencephalitis (C)
Toxic (15)		Lead (C, B) Hexachlorophene Metronidazole (C, F) Ivermectin (C)	Lead (C, B) Hexachlorophene
Traumatic (12)	Head injury		
Vascular (12)	Hemorrhage Infarction		

B, Bovine; *C*, canine; *Ca*, camelid; *E*, equine; *F*, feline; *G*, caprine; *P*, porcine.
*Numbers in parentheses refer to chapters in which entities are discussed.

lesion, consequently central vestibular diseases are discussed with the cerebellar diseases. The neoplastic and inflammatory diseases are summarized and discussed in Chapters 12 and 15. Localization of lesions to the caudal brainstem has been discussed previously.

Cerebellar Diseases

The diagnostic approach to cerebellar disease is similar to that of central vestibular disease. Table 8-3 outlines the cerebellar disorders. Of the categories listed, the chronic degenerative conditions, malformations, inflammatory, and vascular conditions are most common. Most diseases that affect the cerebellum are relatively slow in onset, but vascular lesions such as infarction of cerebellar vasculature may cause acute, nonprogressive clinical signs. Vascular and neoplastic diseases are likely to produce other signs of encephalopathy and are discussed in Chapter 12. Steroid-responsive tremor syndrome characterized by tremor is discussed in Chapter 10. The inflammatory disorders are discussed in Chapter 15. Disorders confined to the cerebellum are discussed in the following sections. These conditions are largely congenital or degenerative.

TABLE 8-3

*Etiology of Cerebellar Disease**

Etiologic Category	Acute Nonprogressive	Acute Progressive	Chronic Progressive
Degenerative (all)			Cerebellar cortical degeneration Abiotrophies Multiple system degeneration Neuroaxonal dystrophies (7) Axonopathy (7) Dysmyelinating disease (7, 10, 15) Storage diseases (15) Spongiform encephalopathies (15) Bovine familial convulsions and ataxia (10) Doddler syndrome (1) (B)
Anomalous (all)	Cerebellar malformation Cerebellar hypoplasia inherited Cerebellar hypoplasia viral induced Dandy-Walker syndrome Hypomyelinogenesis (10) Intracranial arachnoid cyst/ diverticulum (C, F) Occipital dysplasia (C, F)		Chiari malformation (7)
Neoplastic (all) (12)		Metastatic	Primary Medulloblastoma Choroid plexus papilloma Epidermoid cyst Glioma Meningioma
Nutritional (15)		See toxic	
Inflammatory (15)	Steroid responsive tremor syndrome (10)	Distemper FIP Other viral Scrapie Louping ill Protozoal GME Rickettsial	Distemper FIP Other viral Protozoal Mycotic GME Rickettsial
Toxic (15)		Ivermectin Metronidazole	Lead Hexachlorophene Organophosphates Grass staggers (B, O, G) Alpha-mannosidosis plant (B, O, G)
Traumatic (12)	Head injury		
Vascular (12)	Infarction Septic emboli Hemorrhage		

C, Canine; *F*, feline; *B*, bovine; *P*, porcine; *Ca*, camelid; *G*, caprine; *E*, equine; *FIP*, feline infectious peritonitis; *GME*, granulomatous encephalomyelitis.

*Numbers in parentheses refer to chapters in which entities are also discussed.

Cerebellar Degenerative Disorders

Primary Cerebellar Cortical Degeneration. In a review of congenital cerebellar diseases, de Lahunta[61,62] grouped these disorders into three categories: (1) in utero or neonatal viral infections; (2) malformations of genetic or unknown cause; and (3) degenerative diseases, referred to as abiotrophies. Clinical signs vary in age of onset, severity, and rate of progression. Specifically, neonatal conditions of cerebellar malformation or degeneration are characterized by signs of cerebellar dysfunction from birth or time of first ambulation.[63] Hereditary ataxias, including the abiotrophies, are a heterogeneous group of cerebellar degenerative diseases that include neonatal, juvenile, and adult onset conditions.[61,62,64] These progressive cerebellar degenerations in animals can vary in clinical presentation and disease distribution. Myelin disorders and spongiform encephalopathies also can affect the cerebellum (see Chapters 7, 10, and 15). Tables 8-4 and 8-5 list the congenital and degenerative disorders occurring in animals. The appendix also has these diseases listed by breed and species.

Pathogenesis. Primary cerebellar cortical degeneration refers to degeneration and loss of Purkinje cells and/or granule cell neurons. Pathologic processes of cerebellar cortical degeneration are classified microscopically as atrophy, abiotrophy, and transsynaptic neuronal degeneration.[64] Atrophy, a term that lacks specificity, refers to loss of cerebellar mass often secondary to a primary degenerative process.[202] Abiotrophy is a process by which cells normally develop but prematurely degenerate due to an intrinsic cellular defect.[61,62,63] The term *abiotrophy* derives its meaning: *a* (absence), *bio* (life), and *trophy* (nourishment). Transsynaptic neuronal degeneration refers to anterograde or retrograde neuronal degeneration subsequent to failure of input to or output from affected cells. In the cerebellar cortical degenerative disorders in dogs, the Purkinje cell neurons often are affected more severely with secondary transsynaptic neuronal degeneration of the granule cell neurons. While many of these disorders are presumably of an autosomal recessive inheritance pattern, the underlying mechanisms of intracellular defect remain undefined. Bernese mountain dogs have a hepatocerebellar degeneration syndrome suggesting an underlying biochemical defect.[98]

These disorders have been most frequently reported in dogs and a few reports exist in cats, horses, cattle, and pigs (see Tables 8-5 and 8-6).[13,62,184,203] Cerebellar cortical atrophy involving Purkinje cell neuronal degeneration has been described in the Wiltshire, Merino, Corriedale, Welsh, Border Leicester, and Charolais breeds of sheep.[204] Cerebellar cortical atrophy occurs in cattle breeds that include the Holstein, Charolais, Limousin, and Angus.[13,170] Age of onset can vary to include neonatal, early, or delayed into adulthood.[61,62,64] Many cerebellar abiotrophies occur with progressive cerebellar ataxia beginning between 2 and 6 months of age.[62] Disease onset later in life in adult dogs has been reported in the Brittany spaniel, American Staffordshire terrier, old English sheepdog, Gordon setter, and a mixed-breed dog.[102-110] There are reports of delayed onset in cats.[124-126] Histopathology in most cerebellar cortical degenerations show Purkinje cell neuron degeneration and loss with secondary granule cell neuron degeneration.[62,69] Primary degeneration of the cerebellar granule cell neurons has been reported in the Bavarian mountain dog, Coton de Tulear, border collie, Italian Spinone, Lagotto Romagnolo, Brittany spaniel, beagle, and Jack Russell terrier.*

Clinical Signs. Clinical signs consist of either an insidious or acute onset. Many animals with cerebellar cortical degeneration become apparent clinically at time of ambulation and are progressive. Dogs with cerebellar cortical degeneration show severe cerebellar ataxia (dysmetria), with intention tremors of the head and trunk as the predominant signs. Gait deficits in canine cerebellar abiotrophy of neonates can vary to the extent that the affected animal is nonambulatory. Beagle dogs,[83,84] Samoyeds,[206] Jack Russell terriers,[111] and Chow chows[72] are able to ambulate at the appropriate age but are ataxic. In contrast, Coton de Tulears,[87] Rhodesian ridgebacks,[93] miniature poodles,[92] and Irish setters[90] are nonambulatory (astasia) and have severe motor deficits. The cerebellar cortical degenerations have been most thoroughly studied in the Gordon setter[108-110] and rough-coated collie[119]; other breeds are listed in Table 8-5. The progression of clinical signs with the primary cerebellar cortical degenerations varies in rate and severity with the different diseases.

Diagnosis. A presumptive diagnosis is based on when a breed at risk or other young, purebred dog develops progressive cerebellar ataxia. Often there are several dogs affected in the litter. Magnetic resonance imaging can provide evidence of cerebellar atrophy based on increased size of the subarachnoid space overlying the cerebellum and between the folia (Figure 8-12).[205,207,208] Cerebrospinal fluid analysis may be helping in ruling out other inflammatory or infectious causes. The final diagnosis is established by histopathologic examination. On examination postmortem, the cerebellum may be smaller in size, which is recognized in the latter disease stage. Variations in types of neuronal cell loss, extension into the brainstem, and distribution within the areas of the cerebellum can be used to establish distinct pathologies for these different breed-related cerebellar cortical distributions.

Treatment. There are no treatments. Eventually the affected animals become severely compromised and euthanasia is recommended when the animal is unable to ambulate. Some dogs maintain the ability to ambulate long term. Modification of the home environment and feeding arrangements may be necessary to allow for accommodation as the disease progresses. The disorders can offer a spontaneous animal model for these neurodegenerative disorders in people. A few dog colonies have been established for further disease study.

Multiple System Degeneration. Canine multiple system degeneration is a fatal movement disorder of dogs characterized by degeneration of the basal nuclei. This disease syndrome was first described in 1968 in Kerry blue terriers.[128-130] This disorder was also recently discovered in the Chinese crested dog.[131] Affected dogs are normal until 3 to 6 months of age, when they develop a cerebellar ataxia. Signs progress over 6 to 12 months to difficulty initiating movement (dyskinesia to akinesia) and postural instability (Figure 8-13). Degeneration of the basal nuclei is visible on MRI as increased signal on T2W images. Histologic characterization includes degeneration of the cerebellar Purkinje neurons early on in the disease course. If the disease is allowed to progress, degeneration also occurs in the olivary nucleus, substantia nigra, putamen, and caudate nuclei. The inheritance pattern is autosomal recessive and the gene has been mapped to a locus on chromosome 1 in the Chinese crested dog and Kerry blue terrier.[131]

Other neurodegenerative disorders including the cerebello-olivary degenerations consist of multiple neuronal degenerations and axonal degeneration involving the long tracts of the spinal cord and cerebellum have been reported in the Cairn terrier, cocker spaniel, golden retriever, Rottweiler, and other breeds (see Chapter 7 and Table 8-4).[132-136]

Neuroaxonal Dystrophy. This disorder of axonal transport affecting multiple systems, including the cerebellum and associated pathways. Signs may be primarily cerebellar in origin in some dogs (rottweilers, collies, Chihuahuas, Jack Russell terrier, papillon) and in domestic cats.* The disease

*References 87, 97, 100, 103, 104, 111, 112, 114, and 205.

*References 140, 142, 143, 146, 148, and 149.

TABLE 8-4

Degenerative Cerebellar Disorders of Dogs and Cats

Diseases	Associated Disease or Breed and (Cell Type)	Onset (Inheritance)	References
Neonatal Syndromes			
Viral-induced cerebellar hypoplasia	Canine herpesvirus	Neonatal (acquired)	65
	Feline panleukopenia	Neonatal (acquired)	66-68
Cerebellar hypoplasia with lissencephaly	Wire fox terrier	Neonatal (possible)	63,69,70
	Irish setter	Neonatal (possible)	63,69,70
	Samoyed	Neonatal (possible)	71
Cerebellar hypoplasia	Chow chows	Neonatal (AR)	72
	Miniature poodle	Neonatal (unknown)	73,74
	St. Bernard	Neonatal (AR?)	75
Cerebellar agenesis	Poodle	Neonatal (unknown)	74
	Siberian husky	Neonatal (unknown)	76
Vermian hypoplasia, agenesis, Dandy-Walker	Various breeds—bull terrier, Boston terrier, Weimaraner, Dachshund, Beagle, silky terrier, Labrador retriever, miniature poodle, mixed breed	Neonatal (single case)	73,77-80
	Cat	Neonatal (single case)	81
Abiotrophies	Australian kelpies (P, G)	Neonatal (unknown)	82
	Beagle (P, G)	Neonatal (possible)	70,83,84
	Bern running dog (P)	Neonatal (unknown)	85
	Bull mastiff (with hydrocephalus) (P, G)	Neonatal (AR?)	86
	Coton de Tulear (G?)	Neonatal (AR)	87
	Dachshund mix (P,G)	Neonatal (unknown)	88
	Irish setter (P, G and MSD)	Neonatal (AR)	89,90
	Labrador retriever	Neonatal (unknown)	91
	Miniature poodle (P, G and MSD)	Neonatal (unknown)	92
	Rhodesian ridgeback (coat dilution) (P, G)	Neonatal (familial)	93
	Samoyeds	Neonatal (unknown)	63
	Cat (P,G)	Neonatal (AR?)	94
Postnatal Syndromes			
Primary cortical cerebellar degeneration	Akita (P,G)	Young (unknown)	62
	Airedale terrier (P,G)	Young (possible)	95
	Bavarian mountain dog (G)	Young (unknown)	96
	Beagle (G)	Unknown onset	97
	Bern running dog	Young (unknown)	85
	Bernese mountain dog (hepatocellular) (P)	Early (AR)	98
	Bernese mountain dog (P,G)	Early (unknown)	99
	Border collie (G or P,G)	Young (AR?)	100,101
	Brittany spaniel (P,G)	Late (possible)	102
	Brittany spaniel (G)	Adult (possible)	103
	Cairn terrier	Early (unknown)	70
	Clumber spaniel	Early (unknown)	70
	Cocker spaniel	Early (unknown)	70
	Coton de Tulear (immune) (G)	Early (unknown)	104
	English bulldog (P,G)	Early (possible)	105
	English pointer (P,G)	Early (X-linked)	106
	Finnish harrier (P)	Early (unknown)	107
	German shepherd dog (P)	Early (unknown)	70
	Golden retriever (P,G)	Early (unknown)	70
	Gordon setter (P,G)	Adult (AR)	108-110
	Great Dane (P,G)	Early (unknown)	70
	Jack Russell terrier (G)	Early (AR?)	111

TABLE 8-4

Degenerative Cerebellar Disorders of Dogs and Cats—cont'd

Diseases	Associated Disease or Breed and (Cell Type)	Onset (Inheritance)	References
	Kerry blue terrier	Early (unknown)	O'Brien, DP personal communication
	Italian hound (G)	Adult (unknown)	112
	Labrador retriever (P,G)	Early (unknown)	70,91,113
	Lagotto Ramagnolo (G or P,G)	Early (unknown)	114
	Miniature schnauzer (P,G)	Early (unknown)	115
	Miniature schnauzer–beagle cross (P,G)	Late (unknown)	116
	Mixed breeds (P,G)	70	70
	Old English sheepdog (P,G)	Adult (AR)	117
	Portuguese Podenco (P,G)	Early (unknown)	118
	Rough-coated collie (P,G)	Early (AR)	119
	Scottish terrier (P,G)	Early (unknown)	120
	Staffordshire terrier (arylsulfatase G deficiency) (P,G)	Adult (AR)	121
	Cats—DSH (P,G)	Early (AR) or Adult (unknown)	70,122-124
	Siamese (P,G)	Adult (unknown)	125
	Persian (P,G)	Adult (unknown)	126
	Havana brown (hepatic microvascular dysplasia) (P)	Early (unknown)	127
Multiple systems degeneration (MSD) (extrapyramidal)	Kerry blue terrier	Early (AR)	128-130
	Chinese crested dog	Early (AR)	131
Multiple neuronal degeneration (with cerebellar signs)	Cairn terrier	Early (unknown)	132,133
	Cocker spaniel	Early (unknown)	134
	Golden retriever	Early (Unknown)	135
	Irish setter	Neonatal (AR)	89,90
	Miniature poodle	Neonatal (unknown)	92
	Rottweiler	Early (unknown)	136
	Swedish Lapland reindeer-herd dog	Early (unknown)	137
	Cats—DSH	Early (unknown)	138
Neuroaxonal dystrophy	Rottweiler	Early-Adult (AR)	139,140
	Chihuahua	Early (unknown)	141
	Working collie sheepdog	Early (AR)	142
	Jack Russell terrier	Early (unknown)	143
	German shepherd dog	Early (unknown)	144
	Papillon	Early (unknown)	145-147
	Cat—DSH	Early (AR)	148,149
	Siamese	Early (unknown)	150

AR, Autosomal recessive; *P*, Purkinje neurons; *G*, granule cell neurons.

has been best characterized in the rottweiler.[139,140] Similar lesions, predominantly in the spinal cord, are seen in many dog breeds, cat, Suffolk sheep, and Morgan horses (see Chapters 7 and 15). Neurons degenerate with prominent axonal swelling called a spheroid. The swelling represents accumulations of the cytoskeleton and can be visualized in the termination of the long proprioceptive tracts of the brainstem nuclei. The age of onset tends to be within a few weeks to months of ase and insidiously progresses over years; rottweilers and German shepherd doss are usually older than 1 year of age. All affected animals have signs of cerebellar ataxia with intention tremor and some also show concurrent signs of neuropathy (LMN paresis). Autosomal recessive or familial inheritance is suspected.

Lysosomal Storage Disorders

Pathogenesis. Lysosomes are intracellular organelles where catabolism takes place for large molecules, including proteins, saccharides, glycogen, nucleic acids, and lipids. Lysosomal storage diseases occur when undigested materials accumulate because of an inherited enzyme deficiency or by ingestion of toxin that inhibits a lysosomal enzyme.[209] In neuronal ceroid lipofuscinoses, the storage products are proteins and enzyme defects, which are thought to occur in the proteolytic pathways or with intracellular transport mechanisms.[210] For most lipofuscinoses, subunit c of the mitochondrial ATP synthase is the major byproduct. The by-products of many lysosomal storage disorders accumulate in neural and visceral tissues. These disorders can be neonatal where the buildup of storage product interferes with

TABLE 8-5

Congenital and Degenerative Cerebellar Diseases in Large Animals

Diseases	Diseases and Breeds	Inheritance	References
Viral-Induced Cerebellar Hypoplasia[13]			
	Akabane virus—calves, lambs		151,152
	Aino virus—calves		153
	Blue tongue virus—calves, lambs		154-156
	Border disease—lambs, kits		157
	Bovine viral diarrhea virus—calves, lambs, kids		158-160
	Cache Valley fever		161
	Hog cholera virus—piglets		162
	Kasba—calves		163
	Rift Valley fever—calves, lambs		164
	Swine fever—piglets		165
	Wesselsbron disease—calves and lambs		166
Cerebellar Malformation			
Dandy-Walker	Calves (Ayrshire, Jersey), lambs, kids, foals		13,78,167-171
Cerebellar hypoplasia	Calves—Ayrshire, Angus, Hereford, shorthorn, Jersey, Charolais, Jersey, unknown	AR (Hereford) or Unknown	172-178
	Piglets—Wessex saddleback x large white pis	Unknown	13,179
	Foals—Paso Fino, thoroughbred		13
Cerebellar Cortical Degeneration (Abiotrophy)			
	Bovine—Holstein, Charolais, Limousin, Angus	Suspect AR	180-186
	Bovine familial convulsions and ataxia—Angus and Angus-crossbred, Charolais, Polled Hereford	AD with incomplete penetrance	172,183,187,188
	Sheep—Merino, Corriedale, Welsh, Border Leicester, Charolais, Wiltshire, daft lamb disease type A	AR or unknown	62,189-192
	Doddler syndrome—(hereditary lethal spasms)—Hereford, Jersey	AR?	193-194
	Pigs—Yorkshire	Unknown	13,70
	Equine—Arabian, Gotland pony, Oldenburg, Eriskay pony	AR or unknown	13,195-197
Neuroaxonal Dystrophy			
	Ovine—Suffolk (1.5-5 mo), Merino (1-4 yr; 4-7 mo)	Uknown	13,198
	Equine—Morgan (4 mo), Hafflinger (4 mo)	Uknown	200,201

AD, Autosomal dominant; *AR*, autosomal recessive.

normal development of brain function. Most lysosomal storage diseases, except for the mucopolysaccharidoses exhibit severe involvement of the neurons, thus manifest as neurologic signs. In many cases, the brain functions normally until the accumulation of storage product becomes toxic. The high metabolic demand in neurons combined with a lack of cell turnover make them susceptible to early degeneration. Because the cerebellum is very dependent on fast conduction for transmission of sensory information and motor output for efficient coordination of movement, cerebellar signs are often the first signs of storage disease. Likewise, the cerebellum is very sensitive to myelin disorders (see Chapter 7). One of the most well-studied myelin disorders, globoid cell leukodystrophy, is the result of the buildup of a by-product, galactocerebroside, which is specifically derived from myelin and accumulates in macrophages. A toxic substrate, psychosine, destroys the myelin, a feature of this disorder.

Microscopic examination of affected tissue reveals vacuolation, which represents lysosomes distended with storage products (Figure 8-14).[202] The ceroid lipofuscinoses are characterized by lysosomal storage of autofluorescent lipopigment with neurons and other cell types. Ultrastructural examination usually reveals membrane-bound vesicles and in some diseases shows distinctive pathologies.[209] The composition of the storage products are detected by biochemical analysis and special staining procedures. Atrophy of the cerebral cortex and the cerebellum is a feature of neuronal ceroid lipofuscinoses but not with the other storage disorders. A large number of murine models and models in dogs and cats have been identified.[211-213,215,216] The lysosomal storage disorders are further reviewed in Table 15-2 and have also been reported in sheep, cattle, goats, and pigs.[209,210,213,214] The inheritance often has been determined as autosomal recessive or is still unknown for many of these disorders.

Clinical Signs. Onset of signs often occurs within a few months of life but can occur later in life as in the case with some of the neuronal ceroid lipofuscinoses. Disease progression is chronic, insidious, and fatal. Clinical signs often

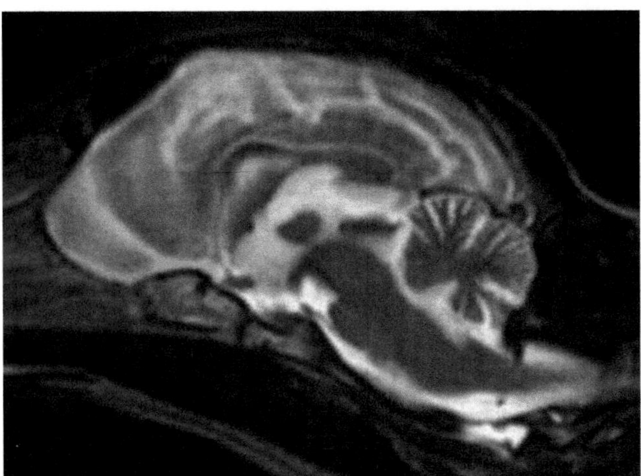

Figure 8-12 A T2W MRI of cerebellar atrophy from a juvenile dachshund with neuronal ceroid lipofuscinosis and cerebellar atrophy demonstrating increased size of the subarachnoid space overlying the cerebellum and between the folia.

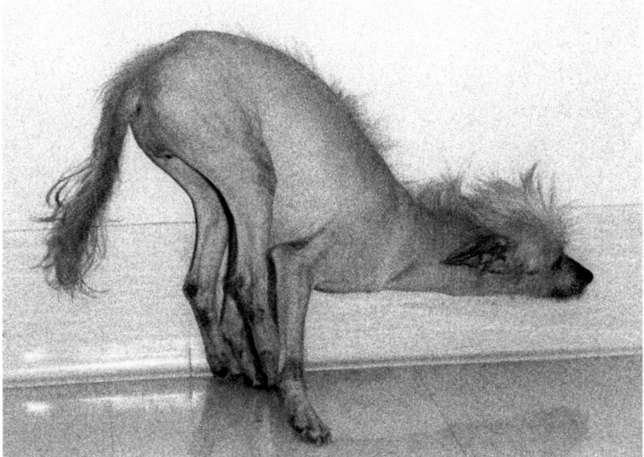

Figure 8-13 A Chinese crested dog with multiple system degeneration, which has progressed from cerebellar ataxia to basal nuclei degeneration and dyskinesia. As these dogs develop difficulty initiating movements, they shift weight forward until they begin to fall and then they are able to move forward. (From O'Brien DP, Coates JR: Brain disease. In Ettinger SJ, Feldman EC, editors: Textbook of veterinary internal medicine: diseases of the dog and cat, ed 7, St Louis, 2010, Elsevier.)

are multifocal and vary from signs of forebrain dysfunction (blindness and seizures) to cerebellar/vestibular signs. Signs often progress to or manifest cognitive abnormalities, ocular abnormalities, and weakness. Cerebellar signs are clinical features for the gangliosidoses, sphingomyelinoses, mannosidoses, glycogenoses, ceroid lipofuscinoses, and globoid cell leukodystrophies.[209,212,215,216] The mucopolysaccharidoses and mucoliposes have clinical features of skeletal and facial malformation.[217] Enlargement of visceral organs is apparent with some glycogen storage disorders, sphingomyelinoses, and mannosidoses.[209,218] The storage disorders sphingomyelinosis type A, mannosidosis, glycogen storage disease type IV, fucosidosis, and globoid cell leukodystrophy may also have peripheral nerve involvement and therefore affected animals may display LMN weakness.[219] The neuronal ceroid lipofuscinoses have a combination of signs that include behavior abnormalities, vision loss, cerebellar ataxia, and seizures or myoclonus.[210] Signs of cerebellar ataxia can predominate in some forms of neuronal ceroid lipofuscinoses.[210,220-222]

Diagnosis. Diagnosis is based on signalment, clinical signs, and ruling out other acquired diseases.[215] Peripheral blood, bone marrow, and CSF may reveal vacuolated leukocytes. Metabolic by-products for some disorders can be measured in the urine. As some storage disorders also affect muscles and nerves, biopsy of these tissues can be useful.[219] Peripheral nerve biopsy is performed in globoid cell leukodystrophy.[223] Some disorders have been evaluated using MRI.[224] Diagnosis can be made by genetic testing for known mutations or confirming the decreased enzyme activity on tissue biopsies or blood leukocytes. Confirmation of diagnosis is based on identifying swollen neurons and that the cells have a vacuolated appearance (see Figure 8-14), and recognizing other histopathologic features for these disorders.[209]

Treatment. There is no treatment for these spontaneous diseases; however, experimental treatment approaches are under study. Therapeutic approaches of the lysosomal storage diseases are based on the knowledge that lysosomal enzymes are secreted and taken up by neighboring cells, thus allowing for cell-to-cell exchange. Three general treatment strategies have been developed: enzyme replacement therapy, cell transplantation, and gene therapy.[211,213]

Anomalous

Cerebellar Malformation. Clinical signs for these neonatal syndromes are present at birth or in the early postnatal period before normal ambulation. Neonatal conditions of the cerebellum have been characterized by malformation or perinatal cellular degeneration of the cerebellum.[61,64] Cerebellar malformations include aplasia and partial agenesis or hypoplasia, which refers to absence or uniform paucity of cerebellar tissue, respectively, without evidence of neuronal degeneration. Clinical signs are usually nonprogressive and may improve with accommodation. These syndromes are usually characterized by symmetric signs and a nonprogressive disease course. Cerebellar hypoplasia is reserved for those diseases in which intrinsic or extrinsic factors alter the normal development of germinal populations of neuroepithelial cells, such as inherited disorders, nutritional deficiencies, and teratogens.[69] The prolonged development of the cerebellum extends into the postnatal period. Thus exposure to viral agents or toxins at a precise stage of fetal or early postnatal life damages the developing cerebellum and results in a cerebellar ataxia from the time of birth.[63]

Viral-Induced Cerebellar Hypoplasia

Parvovirus. The parvovirus responsible for feline infectious enteritis (panleukopenia) can produce a variety of cerebellar malformations, including cerebellar hypoplasia. Although not as common, parvovirus has been isolated from dogs with cerebellar malformations.[225] In utero or perinatal infection of the brain adversely affects development of the cerebellum. Both the cerebellar granule cell and Purkinje neurons are decreased in number or are lacking. The loss of cellularity is due to the cytopathologic effects on the external granule cell layer.[66,226] Destruction of the external germinal cell layer causes hypoplasia of the granule cell layer. Maturing Purkinje neurons also may be destroyed.[227] The destruction may be so severe that the size of the cerebellar cortex is grossly reduced (hence the term cerebellar hypoplasia) (Figure 8-15).[66,228] Cerebellar granule cell and Purkinje neuron layers are reduced microscopically (Figure 8-16). The resulting lesions are irreversible.[67,229] Some affected kittens have concomitant cysts, hydrocephalus, or hydranencephaly (see Chapter 12).[230,231]

The number of kittens affected will vary from one kitten, a portion of the litter, or the entire litter being affected. Symmetric, nonprogressive cerebellar signs typically are present in affected kittens at the time of ambulation. Some kittens appear to improve, apparently because of accommodation through other senses, such as vision and conscious proprioception. No

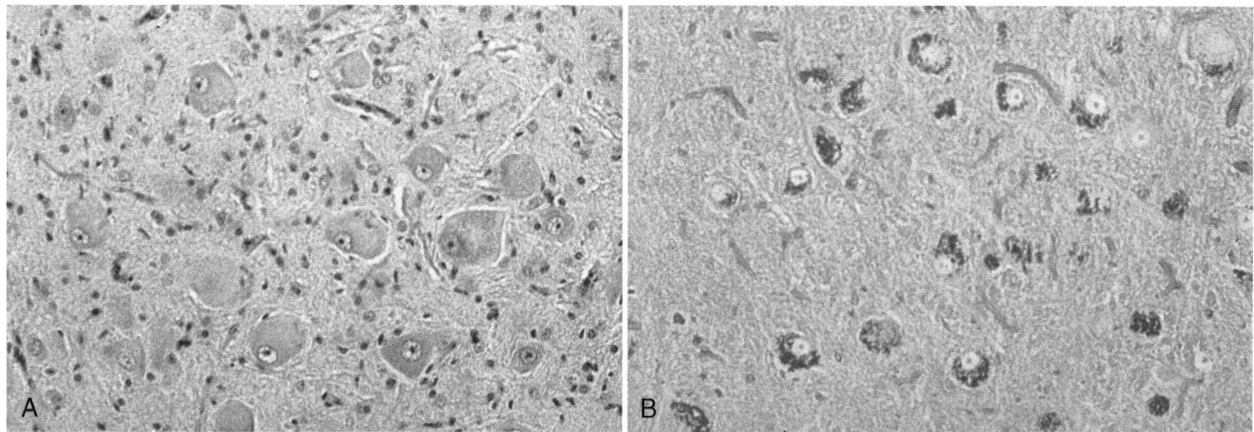

Figure 8-14 Histopathology of brainstem neurons from a Norwegian forest cat with type IV glycogen storage disease. **A,** Photomicrograph showing swollen neurons with eccentric placement of the nuclei (H&E stain; ×20). **B,** Photomicrograph showing presence of PAS (+) storage material within the cytoplasm of neurons (periodic acid–Schiff stain; ×20). (Courtesy Dr. Kyle Braund).

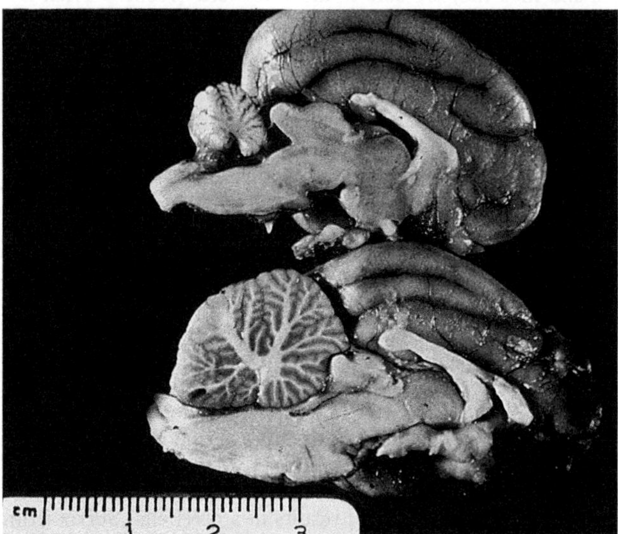

Figure 8-15 Cerebellar hypoplasia in a kitten affected in utero with panleukopenia virus *(top)*. Note the small cerebellum, compared with that of a normal cat *(bottom)*.

systemic signs of feline infectious enteritis are present. Kittens that are infected with the virus after 2 weeks of age rarely develop neurologic signs, even though systemic signs may be severe. In addition to the virulent virus, a modified-live vaccine virus also may produce this syndrome. Pregnant queens and kittens less than 3 weeks of age should be given killed virus vaccines. The presence of nonprogressive signs of strict cerebellar disease in young kittens strongly suggests a diagnosis of cerebellar hypoplasia. No effective therapy for this disease exists. Some kittens can function as pets; however, others have incapacitating disease and should be euthanized.

Bovine Virus Diarrhea. Fetal calves infected with this virus between 100 and 200 days of gestation develop severe cerebellar degeneration and hypoplasia.[159,232] Ocular lesions include retinal atrophy, optic neuritis, cataracts, and microphthalmia with retinal dysplasia. At birth, affected calves have symmetric, nonprogressive cerebellar signs. Some calves improve as they compensate for the cerebellar disease. No treatment is known. The disease can be prevented by vaccinating appropriately.

Canine Herpesvirus. This virus affects puppies less than 2 weeks of age. The disease is characterized by generalized systemic signs, including sudden death. Rarely, puppies survive the systemic effects of the virus and develop residual cerebellar ataxia. The cerebellar ataxia is a residual effect of the inflammatory response.[65] The cerebellar signs are nonprogressive.

Akabane Virus. This virus produces severe destruction of germinal cells in the brains of fetal lambs and calves.[151,152,233] Hydranencephaly also may be seen. The disease has been observed in Australia, Japan, and Israel. Clinical signs are related to the cerebral cortical and cerebellar lesions.

Bluetongue Virus. This virus produces severe destruction of germinal cells in the brains of fetal lambs and calves.[154,234] Hydranencephaly and cerebellar atrophy are the usual lesions. Lambs develop the most severe lesions when infected at 50 to 58 days of gestation.[235]

Border Disease Virus. This virus is a pestivirus, which infects lambs, calves, and kids through transplacental transmission.[170] Infection can lead to developmental disturbances of the brain, including the cerebellum, cause tremors, and affects the wool (see Chapter 10).

Hog Cholera Virus. Hog cholera vaccine virus, when administered to susceptible pregnant sows, produces numerous lesions in fetal pigs, including lesions in the cerebellum.[162] The clinical signs are those of a diffuse whole-body tremor (see Chapter 10).

Inherited Cerebellar Hypoplasia and Dysplasia. Numerous breed-specific syndromes and individual cases of cerebellar dysplasia or aplasia have been described most frequently in dogs but also in cats, horses, cattle, pigs, sheep, and other animals.[61,63,64,170] Cerebellar aplasia has been reported in Siberian huskies[76] and a poodle.[74]

Some congenital cerebellar hypoplasias are inherited. Dysplasia of the cerebral cortex and cerebellar hypoplasia has been reported in wire fox terriers,[63,69,70] Irish setters,[63,69,70] Samoyed, [63,69,70] and St. Bernard.[75] The Irish setters, Samoyeds and wire fox terriers also have lissencephaly. Chow chows and miniature poodles have pure cerebellar hypoplasia.[72-74] The cerebellum is symmetrically small as a result of depletion of Purkinje and cerebellar granule cells. An inherited cerebellar hypoplasia was reported in the cat and was characterized with loss of the Purkinje cells in the cerebellar hemisphere.[122,123] In cattle, cerebellar hypoplasia or aplasia is a presumed autosomal recessive disorder in Hereford, Shorthorn, Angus, Guernsey, Ayrshire, and Holstein.* Pigs with inherited cerebellar hypoplasia had depletion of both granule and Purkinje cells.[179]

*References 13, 71, 170, 173, 236, and 237.

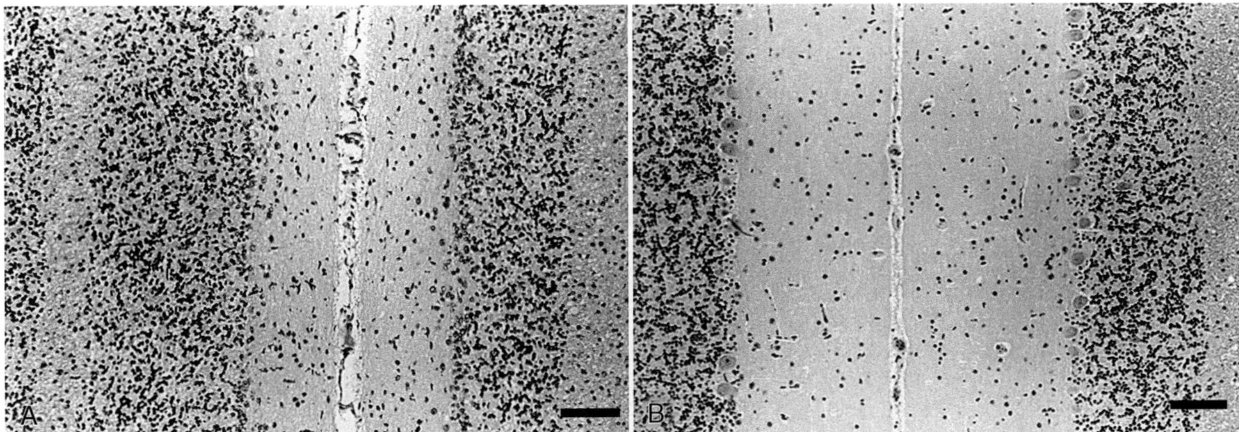

Figure 8-16 Photomicrographs of cerebellum from a 6-week-old female kitten with cerebellar hypoplasia **(A)** and a normal adult cat **(B)**. The cerebellar folia of the affected kitten are hypoplastic. Note particularly the relative thickness of the molecular cell layers at the center of each figure. Granule cell and Purkinje cell numbers are reduced in the affected kitten. Hematoxylin and eosin. Bar = 30 μm in each. (From Kornegay JN: Cerebellar hypoplasia. In August JR, editor: Consultations in feline internal medicine, Philadelphia, 1991, WB Saunders.)

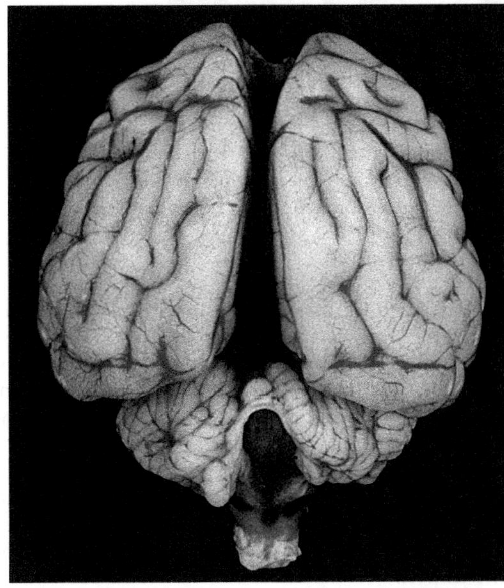

Figure 8-17 Brain from an 8-week-old male dachshund with nonprogressive ataxia and intention tremor. The caudal vermis is hypoplastic. (From Kornegay JN: Congenital cerebellar diseases. In Kirk RW, editor: Current veterinary therapy X, Philadelphia, 1989, WB Saunders.)

Cerebellar vermian agenesis, akin to Dandy-Walker syndrome in humans, has been reported in a number of dog breeds and calves but also in foals, lambs, and kittens (Figure 8-17).[69,73,77-81,167-169] Other congenital brain malformations may be associated with the vermal defects. Mechanisms responsible for preferential caudal cerebellar vermis aplasia have not been defined. The primitive caudal medullary velum may be abnormally impermeable to CSF, thus leading to distention of the embryonic fourth ventricle so that the caudal vermis fails to differentiate properly from the metencephalic alar plates. Some of these animals also have hydrocephalus.[69]

Intracranial Arachnoid Cyst/Diverticulum. Intracranial arachnoid cysts/diverticulum in the quadrigeminal region are subarachnoid fluid accumulations.[238,239] Small and brachycephalic breeds are predisposed to intracranial arachnoid cysts/diverticulum.[240] The cerebellum and occipital lobe of the cerebral cortex are often compressed with occipital lobe compression more likely to be associated with clinical signs.[240] Many are diagnosed as incidental findings in dogs.[240-242] Vestibulocerebellar signs may develop with growth and compression of the surrounding neural tissues. Diagnosis can be made on MRI or CT and by ultrasonography.[238,242,243] Surgical decompression and cystoperitoneal shunt placement are effective treatments for clinically affected animals.[244,245]

Occipital Dysplasia. Enlargement of the foramen magnum and congenital shortening of C1, most often seen in toy breed dogs, has been called occipital dysplasia.[246,247] Concomitant hydrocephalus has been observed. In severe cases, the cerebellum and brainstem are exposed, making these structures vulnerable to compression and causing secondary syringohydromyelia akin to Chiari malformation (see Chapter 7).[248] The clinical signs reported included pain at the craniocervical junction, personality change, and cerebellar ataxia. Often the clinical signs are more related to hydrocephalus. Many dogs remain asymptomatic. The diagnosis is confirmed MRI of the cranium and cervical vertebrae. Other causes of the signs should be pursued because many normal animals have an enlarged foramen magnum.[249] An apparent correlation of the larger opening and brachycephalic skulls has been noted. Marked variation in the shape of the foramen magnum was found in a study of 48 beagle skulls.[250] No impairment of function could be attributed to the change. No brain or spinal cord anomalies were found.

Metabolic

Hypothyroidism. As discussed above, hypothyroidism has been associated with vestibulo-cerebellar dysfunction. Causes for central vestibular dysfunction have been attributed to infarction of the cerebellum.[15,251] However, the pathogenesis in dogs without evidence of infarction remains unknown. Hypercholesterolemia or hyperlipidemia is a consistent clinicopathologic abnormality in dogs that are hypothyroid with signs of central vestibular dysfunction.[15,251] Diagnosis is based on documenting low T_4, free T_4, and elevated TSH. Signs of vestibular dysfunction resolve within 2 to 4 weeks of thyroid supplementation.

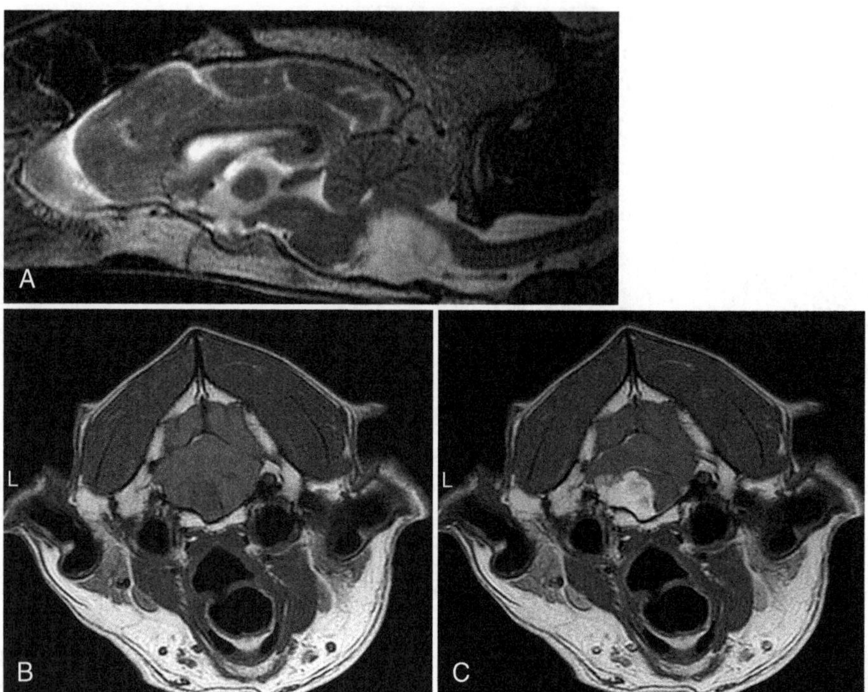

Figure 8-18 An MRI from an 11-year-old German shepherd dog with nonambulatory tetraparesis and central vestibular signs. **A,** T2W sagittal MRI showing a hyperintense mass displacing the brainstem medulla and cerebellum dorsally. **B,** A transverse T1W MRI showing a hypointense to isointense mass in the left brainstem medulla. **C,** The same image after intravenous contrast administration showing homogeneous to heterogeneous enhancement of the mass with irregular margination and compression of the brainstem to the right. The mass was confirmed as a mesothelial meningioma on histopathology.

Neoplasia

Primary and Secondary Cerebellar Neoplasms

Pathogenesis. Primary and metastatic tumors can affect the cerebellum in dogs and cats (see also Chapter 12).[252-254] Medulloblastomas selectively arise in the cerebellum in all species and are most likely to occur in younger dogs and cats.[255,256] Choroid plexus papillomas can occur in any part of the ventricular system but are most common in the fourth ventricle.[257] Gliomas and meningiomas (Figure 8-18) may occur in the caudal fossa of the cranial cavity (caudal tentorium) affecting the cerebellum, but they are more frequent in the rostral fossa (rostral tentorium).[258,259] Lymphoma affecting only the cerebellum has been reported in dogs.[260]

Clinical Signs. Signs of cerebellar neoplasia usually progress slowly, but acute exacerbation may follow hemorrhage, infarction, or obstruction of CSF flow with secondary increased intracranial pressure.

Diagnosis and Treatment. The diagnosis should be made with CT or MRI. Collection of CSF for analysis is contraindicated because of the risk of herniation. Surgical resection of these tumors is difficult because of limited exposure, but debulking and radiation therapy or chemotherapy can provide an alternative to euthanasia.

Nutritional

Thiamine Deficiency. Thiamine deficiency is rare in dogs and cats. Most cases are the result of inappropriate preparation of food, inadequate concentration in the diet, or feeding diets high in thiaminases.[261-264] Other proposed causes of thiamine deficiency include interference with intestinal absorption, abnormal utilization secondary to liver disease, and increased requirements.[265] Clinical signs include abnormal mentation, seizures, dilated unresponsive pupils, opisthotonos, tetraparesis, and vestibular dysfunction.[261,262,264-266] In dogs and cats, pathologic changes include hemorrhage necrosis of specific brainstem nuclei including caudal colliculus, lateral geniculate, and the medial vestibular and oculomotor nuclei.[262-265] The gold standard for diagnosis remains unclear, but MRI may disclose bilaterally and symmetric lesions in affected brainstem nuclei.[265,267] Often a presumptive diagnosis is reached based on dietary history, neurologic examination, cross-sectional imaging studies, and response to therapy.[265,267] Most affected dogs and cats respond rapidly to thiamine supplementation.

Horses can develop thiamine deficiency after ingestion of bracken fern and horsetail, which contain thiaminase.[268,269] Clinical signs include vestibular ataxia, muscle tremors, weight loss, inactivity, bradycardia, and obtunded mentation. Treatment includes thiamine supplementation and removal from abnormal diet and making nutritious forage available. Thiamine deficiency in sheep and cattle results in classical polioencephalomalacia.

Toxic

Plants Toxins. Table 15-4 through 15-8 list common plants and toxins that may cause ataxia, tremors, tetany, and other signs related, at least in part, to cerebellar involvement. For a complete discussion, other references should be consulted (see Chapters 10 and 15).[13]

Ergotism (Grass Staggers). This acute disorder occurs in cattle, sheep, and rarely horses that ingest grasses with toxins or fungi that infest the grasses.[13,270] The fungal alkaloids cause neurologic signs that occur in specific seasons. Many cattle or sheep grazing at one time are affected with signs of ataxia, tremor, tetany, and recumbency. Grasses associated with staggers include rye grass, Dallis grass, Bermuda grass, and canary grass.[271] The sclerotium of the fungus develops in the seed head of Dallis grass and is present in highest concentrations during wet summers.[272] Affected animals are bright and alert and gradually recover when removed from toxic pastures. Severely affected animals may develop extensor rigidity, opisthotonus, and clonic convulsions. Control of the disorder is achieved by removing grazing livestock before the seed heads develop or by mowing affected pastures to remove the seed heads.

Locoweed. These plants represent the *Astragalus* and *Oxytropis* spp. in North America and *Swainsona* spp. in Australia. This is known as blind staggers or locoism in foraging animals that include livestock and horses.[214] Along with weight loss, aggression, and hyperesthesia, cerebellar ataxia is a prominent clinical sign. The alkaloid toxin, swainsonine induces a lysosomal storage disease, alpha-mannosidosis. Removing the animals from the pasture can reverse some of the clinical signs but the behavior changes may be permanent.

Metronidazole Toxicity. Metronidazole is an antimicrobial that can cause acute onset cerebello-vestibular signs in dogs and cats.[273-276] Clinical signs of toxicosis begin with anorexia and progress rapidly to generalized ataxia, tremor, and central vestibular and cerebellar signs. Neurologic signs usually resolve after discontinuation of the drug. Diazepam and its affects on the gamma-aminobutyric acid (GABA) receptor can promote faster recovery times.[277] See Chapter 15 for further discussion.

Vascular

Vascular Infarction. Occlusion of the rostral or caudal cerebellar artery causes infarction of the cerebellum and brainstem, producing signs of paradoxical vestibular or acute cerebellar dysfunctions (see also Chapter 12).[278-280] The disorder is most commonly observed in older dogs. The clinical signs are peracute, severe, lateralizing, and nonprogressive after the first few hours. Neurologic signs include acute cerebelar ataxia, head tilt, menace response deficit, ventral (vestibular) strabismus, mild lateralizing postural deficits, and abnormal nystagmus. Diagnosis is based on MRI of the brain. Diagnostic findings include hyperintense wedge-shaped lesions often in the rostral cerebellum that may extend into the dorsal medulla.[280] Lesions display variable enhancement patterns. A specialized imaging technique called diffusion-weighted imaging can help confirm the diagnosis for an infarct (see Chapters 4 and 12). CSF analysis may be normal or reveal mild increases in mononuclear cells and protein may be present. The lesions correspond to the distribution of the rostral or caudal cerebellar artery. Affected dogs usually improve within 5 to 7 days and may totally recover. There is no definitive treatment. Affected dogs should be carefully evaluated for renal disease, hyperadrenocorticism, pheochromocytoma, hypertension, and hypothyroidism, conditions that predispose to vascular disease and thrombosis.[251,279]

CASE STUDIES

CASE 8-1 TIPSY

▪ Signalment

Canine, Spitz, female, 3 years old.

▪ History

The owner reports a severe lack of coordination and loss of balance since the dog was 6 weeks old. The clinical signs have been nonprogressive.

▪ Physical Examination

Negative except for the neurologic problem.

▪ Neurologic Examination

Mental status

Alert

Gait

Severe symmetric truncal ataxia; hypermetria/dysmetria in all four limbs

Posture

Basewide stance; intention tremor; no head tilt

Postural reactions

Proprioceptive positioning is normal. The dog shows difficulty in coordination of hemistanding and walking.

Spinal reflexes

Patellar reflex is exaggerated in both pelvic limbs.

Cranial nerves

Absent menace response OU; normal PLR and pupil size/symmetry OU; normal palpebral reflex; the dog appears visual OU, Both eyes.

Sensory evaluation

Normal

▪ Lesion Location

The dog has generalized symmetric ataxia characterized by hypermetria in all four limbs. Also there is associated with head tremor and intention tremor implicating the cerebellum. No paresis or cranial nerve dysfunction (specifically, vestibular signs) is present. The signs are consistent with generalized cerebellar disease.

▪ Differential Diagnosis

1. Cerebellar hypoplasia or other congenital/anomalous malformation
2. Cerebellar abiotrophy
3. Degenerative disease (e.g., lysosomal storage disease)
4. Inflammatory (infectious vs. noninfectious) disease

▪ Diagnostic Plan

1. Cross-sectional imaging may provide anatomic evidence of a small cerebellum suggestive of hypoplasia or atrophy.
2. CSF analysis will diagnose inflammatory disease; based on results of culture, serology, and PCR testing for infectious disease
3. Metabolic screening (analysis of intermediate metabolites in urine)
4. Clinical history provides the strongest data for the order of differential diagnosis
5. Histopathology would provide a definitive diagnosis

Continued

CASE 8-1 *TIPSY*—cont'd

▪ Diagnosis

A congenital or early postnatal syndrome is suspected because the signs began at an early age. The signs have been nonprogressive, which tends to rule out abiotrophies, degenerative disease (storage diseases), and inflammatory disease. Based on the early onset of clinical signs and lack of progression, cerebellar hypoplasia or other malformation is most likely. MRI would be necessary for presumptive diagnosis; however, based on treatment options (see later discussion) the value of the information provided by MRI needs to be discussed with the owners. Parvoviral deoxyribonucleic acid (DNA) can be amplified from archival brains (cerebellum) of some dogs with cerebellar hypoplasia. This suggests that in utero parvoviral infection might be associated with cerebellar hypoplasia in dogs.

▪ Treatment

Cerebellar hypoplasia or other malformations are not treatable. One exception is that intracranial arachnoid cysts/diverticula that is occasionally treated surgically. Although improvement is unlikely, the dog can function as a pet. The dog should not be bred because the disease may be hereditary.

CASE 8-2 *TEDDY*

▪ Signalment

Canine, Pekingese, male, 2 years old.

▪ History

Progressive lack of coordination and falling from side to side in past 72 hours. The head swings from side to side and bobs up and down. There is no history of trauma. No other signs are present.

▪ Physical Examination

Normal

▪ Neurologic Examination

Mental status

Alert, panting

Gait

Tetraparesis; unable to stand without support; with support, the dog does display severe hypermetria in all four limbs and truncal ataxia

Posture

Wide excursions of the head with the head swinging to both sides; as well as vertically.

Postural reactions

Abnormal in all four limbs. Proprioceptive placing deficits are in all limbs which may be in the right TL and PLs. The hopping is decreased in all limbs; worse in the right TL and PL; with the right PL most severely affected. Tactile placing is absent in the PLs and decreased in the TLs.

Spinal reflexes

The patellar reflex is exaggerated on both sides and shows clonus on the right side

Cranial nerves

Normal or physiologic nystagmus is absent OU. The eyes are positioned centrally in the palpebral fissures; however, when the head position was altered, a ventrolateral strabismus is present OD. When the head was elevated, abnormal nystagmus was induced, which was horizontal with fast phase directed to the left.

Sensory evaluation

Normal

▪ Lesion Location

This dog displays a relatively common clinical presentation in which both cerebellar (head bob and hypermetria) and vestibular signs (lack of normal or physiologic nystagmus and positional or induced abnormal nystagmus) are present. The absence of normal nystagmus OU while maintaining the ability to move the eyes voluntarily or when abnormal nystagmus is induced means that CN III, IV, and VI remain functional and therefore implicates bilateral involvement of the vestibular system. The presence of ventrolateral strabismus when the head position is altered also suggests vestibular dysfunction. The paresis and postural reaction deficits point toward a central vestibular (brainstem) disease. A lesion or a disease process involving the cerebellomedullary junction could cause both cerebellar and central vestibular signs.

▪ Differential Diagnosis

1. Encephalitis
2. Neoplasia
3. Infarction

▪ Diagnostic Plan

1. CBC, chemistry profile, and UA to rule out polysystemic disease that could lead to the primary differential diagnoses.
2. Magnetic resonance imaging would be ideal for diagnosis of a structural lesion due to neoplasia or inflammation.
3. CSF analysis would assist with diagnosis of inflammatory disease; based on results culture, serology, and polymerase chain reaction (PCR) testing for infectious disease

▪ Diagnostic Results

MRI was normal. CSF analysis revealed white blood cell (WBC) count of 380 cells/uL (88% lymphocytes, 12% neutrophils), protein concentration 120 mg/dL. Culture of CSF was negative. Serology for distemper virus, toxoplasmosis, rickettsial organisms, and *Cryptococcus* was negative.

▪ Diagnosis

Encephalitis of unknown etiology was the diagnosis.

▪ Treatment

While awaiting results of serology, the dog was administered doxycycline and clindamycin antibiotics with no response. The dog was then administered prednisone at immunosuppressive doses for 4 weeks and then the dosage was tapered very slowly for several months until discontinued.

TL, Thoracic limbs; *PL*, pelvic limbs; *OU*, both eyes; *OD*, right eye; *OS*, left eye.

CASE 8-3 PISTOL PETE

▪ Signalment
Feline, domestic shorthair, male, 6 months old.

▪ History
The cat has been ill for 10 days. He is obtunded, disoriented, ataxic, and sleeps most of the time. He has gotten progressively worse.

▪ Physical Examination
The cat is dehydrated, thin, and extremely depressed. His temperature is 102.5° F.

▪ Neurologic Examination
Mental status
Obtunded to stupor; grinds teeth when aroused

Gait
Nonambulatory tetraparesis; when supported in a standing position falls to the left and right; both thoracic limbs are extended.

Posture
Recumbent; slight head tilt to left; the thoracic limbs show spasticity

Postural reactions
Proprioceptive positioning is decreased to absent in all limbs. Postural reactions are decreased in all limbs.

Spinal reflexes
The patellar reflex is increased on both sides. The flexor withdrawal reflexes are brisk in all limbs. A crossed-extensor reflex was present in the left thoracic limb

Cranial nerves
A rotary nystagmus was present in both eyes with the direction of the fast phase changing with change in head position.

Sensory evaluation
Normal

▪ Lesion Location
The predominant signs are those of central vestibular disease (vestibular signs plus postural reaction deficits and abnormal mental status implicate a central vestibular lesion). The severe depression and altered mental attitude also could be related to forebrain disease. Inflammation or degeneration is most probable.

▪ Differential Diagnosis
1. Infectious inflammatory disease
   a. Rabies
   b. Feline infectious peritonitis (FIP)
   c. Toxoplasmosis
   d. Fungal—*Cryptococcus*
   e. Bacterial encephalitis
2. Thiamine deficiency
3. Neurodegeneration

▪ Diagnostic Plan: (activated when rabies possibility has been minimized)
1. A CBC, chemistry profile, and UA to evaluate for polysystemic disease
2. A CSF analysis would diagnose presence of inflammatory disease; based on results of culture, serology, and PCR testing for infectious disease
3. Can observe response to therapy with thiamine administration

▪ Diagnostic Results
The owner was questioned carefully about vaccinating the cat for rabies, which was done when the cat was 12 weeks of age. The CSF analysis revealed 200 WBCs (90% segmented neutrophils, 10% lymphocytes); protein concentration was 200 mg/dL. Culture of CSF was negative. Serology for feline infection peritonitis (FIP) IgG was 1:560.

▪ Diagnosis
Noneffusive FIP was suspected based on CSF analysis results.

▪ Treatment
Viral infection of FIP causes damage to the neural tissues through secondary immune responses. Corticosteroid treatment with an antiinflammatory dosage was attempted but the cat continued to deteriorate. The prognosis is poor and the owner elected euthanasia. Necropsy and histopathology were suggestive for FIP.

CASE 8-4 ELOISE

▪ Signalment
Feline, domestic shorthair, female, 2 years old.

▪ History
The cat developed acute ataxia and lack of coordination. The cat developed a head tilt to the right and circling to the right. Appetite was good. No history of previous ear infection exists.

▪ Physical Examination
No abnormalities noted. Otic examination is normal

▪ Neurologic Examination
Mental status
Alert

Gait
Circles to right; asymmetric ataxia; the cat drifts and falls to the right

Posture
Head tilt to the right

Postural reactions
All within normal limits

Spinal reflexes
All within normal limits

Continued

CASE 8-4 ELOISE—cont'd

Cranial nerves
A ventrolateral strabismus was elicited when the head was elevated. Abnormal nystagmus was present with fast phase to the left.

Sensory evaluation
Normal

▪ Lesion Location
The circling, head tilt, asymmetric ataxia, positional strabismus, and spontaneous nystagmus with the fast phase directed to the left suggest a right-sided vestibular lesion. The absence of abnormal mental state, paresis, or other cranial nerve involvement localizes the lesion to the right peripheral vestibular system.

▪ Differential Diagnosis
1. Acute bacterial otitis media/interna
2. Trauma
3. Idiopathic feline vestibular syndrome by exclusion of differential diagnosis 1 and 2

▪ Diagnostic Plan
1. Otoscopic examination
2. Skull radiography; greater sensitivity for identification of otitis media/interna with cross-sectional imaging (CT or MRI)
3. Hematology

▪ Diagnostic Results
The otoscopic examination was normal. Skull radiography was within normal limits. After imaging a myringotomy was performed with a 22-gauge spinal needle and instilling 0.3 mL sterile saline into the tympanic cavity. The fluid was aspirated and submitted for cytology and culture. Cytology results were unrevealing.

▪ Diagnosis
Feline idiopathic vestibular syndrome is the most likely diagnosis. This is a disease is of unknown cause and no specific therapy is known. Recovery usually takes 3 to 6 weeks.

▪ Treatment
Although otitis media interna is unlikely, one still could choose to empirically treat the cat with the appropriate antibiotics. In this case, the cat was treated with a broad-spectrum antibiotic for 10 days while awaiting culture results (yielded no growth). The cat recovered in 3 weeks. The presumptive diagnosis was feline idiopathic vestibular syndrome.

CASE 8-5 PIPPIN

▪ Signalment
14-year-old female spayed border collie.

▪ History
Three days ago this dog developed acute nonprogressive tetraparesis, severe ataxia, right head tilt, and falling to the right. The dog has a long-standing history of pelvic limb lameness and hormone-responsive urinary incontinence and has been receiving diethylstilbesterone, phenylpropanolamine, and nonsteroidal antiinflammatory agents. Medications were stopped 3 days ago, and the dog has steadily improved.

▪ Physical Examination
No abnormalities were detected.

▪ Neurologic Examination
Mental status
Alert and responsive

Gait
Reluctant to ambulate. The dog prefers to lie in sternal recumbency. During ambulation, the dog was very ataxic in all limbs with hypermetria of the right TL.

Posture
The head is tilted to the left.

Postural reactions
Postural reactions are decreased in all limbs, with deficits worse on the right side.

Spinal reflexes
Spinal reflexes are intact.

Cranial nerves
A ventrolateral strabismus in the right eye was elicited upon elevation of the head. Abnormal nystagmus was evident as rotary to vertical with the fast phase to the left.

Sensory evaluation
Normal

▪ Lesion Location
The clinical signs are those of an acute central vestibular syndrome localized primarily to the right side based on postural reactions. The left-sided head tilt is paradoxical to what one would expect. The presence of paresis detected on examination of postural reactions strongly suggests a right-sided lesion in the brainstem affecting vestibular nuclei. The marked hypermetria noted in the right thoracic limb suggests involvement of the cerebellum or cerebellar peduncles. The signs had an acute onset and were not progressive.

CASE 8-5 PIPPIN—cont'd

▪ Differential Diagnosis

1. Vascular infarction
2. Trauma
3. Inflammatory
4. Neoplasia

▪ Diagnostic Plan

1. Complete blood count (CBC), chemistry profile and urinalysis would rule out polysystemic disease.
2. Thoracic radiography and abdominal ultrasound would rule out metastatic disease.
3. MRI of the brain would be the diagnostic procedure of choice in this case to rule out a cerebellar infarct or neoplasia.
4. CSF analysis would rule out inflammatory disease.
5. Serology would assist with diagnosis of infectious disease.

▪ Diagnostic Results

Chemistry profile revealed hypercholesterolemia. MRI revealed an area of hyperintensity on the T2W images in the right rostral cerebellum and brainstem (rostral medulla). It was not contrast enhancing after intravenous contrast administration. CSF analysis was within normal limits. Serologic testing for toxoplasmosis and rickettsial organisms was negative.

▪ Diagnosis

Categories of neurologic disease with these characteristics include trauma, inflammation (may be progressive), and infarction. Based on the chemistry profile results, thyroid function testing was performed and results were conclusive with hypothyroidism. Hypothyroidism has been associated with secondary infarction. The vascular anatomy of the vessels in the cerebellum makes it more prone to infarction compared with other areas of the brain. Hypertension may also be an underlying cause for infarction. Blood pressure measurements were normal throughout the dog's hospital stay.

▪ Treatment

The dog was administered thyroid supplementation and gradually regained the ability to ambulate without ataxia. Given the history and neurologic findings, infarction of the right dorsal anterior medulla and cerebellum is the leading rule-out in this case.

REFERENCES

1. Schunk KL, Averill DRJ: Peripheral vestibular syndrome in the dog: a review of 83 cases, J Am Vet Med Assoc 182(12):1354–1357, 1983.
2. Kern TJ, Aromando MC, Erb HN: Horner's syndrome in dogs and cats: 100 cases (1975-1985), J Am Vet Med Assoc 195(3):369–373, 1989.
3. Holliday TA: Clinical signs of acute and chronic experimental lesions of the cerebellum, Vet Sci Commun 3:259–278, 1980.
4. Thomas WB: Vestibular dysfunction, Vet Clin North Am Small Anim Pract 30(1):227–249, 2000.
5. Cogan DG, Chu FC, Reingold DB: Ocular signs of cerebellar disease, Arch Ophthalmol 100(5):755–760, 1982.
6. Rossmeisl JH: Vestibular disease in dogs and cats, Vet Clin North Am Small Anim Pract 40:81–100, 2010.
7. Bedford PGC: Congenital vestibular disease in the English cocker spaniel, Vet Rec 105(23):530–531, 1979.
8. Lee M: Congenital vestibular disease in a German shepherd dog, Vet Rec 113(24):571, 1983.
9. Stirling J, Clarke M: Congenital peripheral vestibular disorder in two German shepherd dogs, 57(4):200, 1981.
10. Vernau KM, LeCouteur RA: Feline vestibular disorders. Part II: diagnostic approach and differential diagnosis, J Feline Med Surg 1:81–89, 1999.
11. Forbes S, Cook JRJ: Congenital peripheral vestibular disease attributed to lymphocytic labyrinthitis in two related litters of Doberman pinscher pups, J Am Vet Med Assoc 198(3):447–449, 1991.
12. McConnon JM, White ME, Smith MC, et al: Pendular nystagmus in dairy cattle, J Am Vet Med Assoc 182(8):812–813, 1983.
13. Mayhew IG: Large animal neurology, ed 2, Ames, Iowa, 2009, Wiley-Blackwell.
14. Jaggy A, Oliver JE, Ferguson DC, et al: Neurological manifestations of hypothyroidism: a retrospective study of 29 dogs, J Vet Intern Med 8(5):328–336, 1994.
15. Higgins MA, Rossmeisl JH, Panciera DL: Hypothyroid-associated central vestibular disease in 10 dogs: 1999-2005, J Vet Intern Med 20:1363–1369, 2006.
16. Negrin A, Cherubini GB, Lamb C, et al: Clinical signs, magnetic resonance imaging findings and outcome in 77 cats with vestibular disease: a retrospective study, J Feline Med Surg 12:291–299, 2010.
17. Morin DE: Brainstem and cranial nerve abnormalities: listeriosis, otitis media/interna and pituitary abscess syndrome, Vet Clin North Am Food Anim Pract 20: 243–273, 2004.
18. Jensen R, Maki LR, Lauerman LH, et al: Cause and pathogenesis of middle ear infection in young feedlot cattle, J Am Vet Med Assoc 182(9):967–972, 1983.
19. Colombini S, Merchant SR, Hosgood G: Microbial flora and antimicrobial susceptibility patterns from dogs with otitis media, Vet Dermatol 11(4):235–239, 2000.
20. Jensen R, Pierson RE, Weibel JL, et al: Middle ear infection in feedlot lambs, J Am Vet Med Assoc 181:805–807, 1982.
21. Olson LD: Gross and microscopic lesions of middle and inner ear infections in swine, Am J Vet Res 42(8):1433–1440, 1981.
22. Rosser EJ: Causes of otitis externa, Vet Clin North Am Small Anim Pract 34:459–468, 2004.
23. Stern-Bertholtz W, Sjöström L, Häkanson NW: Primary secretory otitis media in the cavalier King Charles spaniel: a review of 61 cases, J Small Anim Pract 44(6):253–256, 2003.
24. Blythe LL, Watrous BJ, Schmitz JA, et al: Vestibular syndrome associated with temporohyoid joint fusion and temporal bone fracture in three horses, J Am Vet Med Assoc 185(7):775–781, 1984.
25. Walker AM, Sellon DC, Cornelisse CJ, et al: Temporohyoid osteoarthropathy in 33 horses (1993-2000), J Vet Intern Med 16(6):697–703, 2002.
26. Power HT, Watrous BJ, de Lahunta A: Facial and vestibulocochlear nerve disease in six horses, J Am Vet Med Assoc 183(10):1076–1080, 1983.

27. Sturges BK, Dickinson PJ, Kortz GD, et al: Clinical signs, magnetic resonance imaging features, and outcome after surgical and medical treatment of otogenic intracranial infection in 11 cats and 4 dogs, J Vet Intern Med 20(3):648–656, 2006.
28. Spangler EA, Dewey CW: Meningoencephalitis secondary to bacterial otitis media/interna in a dog, J Am Anim Hosp Assoc 36(3):239–243, 2000.
29. Kern TJ, Erb HN: Facial neuropathy in dogs and cats: 95 cases (1975-1985), J Am Vet Med Assoc 191(12):1604–1609, 1987.
30. Remedios AM, Fowler JD, Pharr JW: A comparison of radiographic versus surgical diagnosis of otitis media, J Am Anim Hosp Assoc 27:183–188, 1991.
31. Love NE, Kramer RW, Spodnick GJ, et al: Radiographic and computed tomographic evaluation of otitis media in the dog, Vet Radiol Ultrasound 36(5):375–379, 1995.
32. Detweiler DA, Johnson LR, Kass PH, et al: Computed tomographic evidence of bulla effusion in cats with sinonasal disease: 2001-2004, J Vet Intern Med 20: 1080–1084, 2006.
33. Garosi LS, Dennis R, Schwarz T: Review of diagnostic imaging of ear diseases in the dog and cat, Vet Radiol Ultrasound 44:137–146, 2003.
34. Allgoewer I, Lucas S, Schmitz SA: Magnetic resonance imaging of the normal and diseased feline middle ear, Vet Radiol Ultrasound 41(5):413–418, 2000.
35. Dvir E, Kirberger RM, Terblanche AG: Magnetic resonance imaging of otitis media in a dog, Vet Radiol Ultrasound 41:46–49, 2000.
36. Garosi LS, Lamb CR, Targett MP: MRI findings in a dog with otitis media and suspected otitis interna, Vet Rec 146:501–502, 2000.
37. Garosi LS, Dennis R, Penderis J, et al: Results of magnetic resonance imaging in dogs with vestibular disorders: 85 cases (1996-1999), J Am Vet Med Assoc 218(3):385–391, 2001.
38. Blythe LL: Otitis media and interna and temporohyoid osteoarthropathy, Vet Clin North Am Equine Pract 13(1):21–42, 1997.
39. Hilton H, Puchalski SM, Aleman M: The computed tomographic appearance of equine temporohyoid osteoarthropathy, Vet Radiol Ultrasound 50(2):151–156, 2009.
40. Palmeiro BS, Morris DO, Wiemelt SP, et al: Evaluation of outcome of otitis media after lavage of the tympanic bulla and long-term antimicrobial drug treatment in dogs: 44 cases (1998-2002), J Am Vet Med Assoc 225(4):548–553, 2004.
41. Mansfield PD: Ototoxicity in dogs and cats, Compend Contin Educ Pract Vet 12(3):331–337, 1990.
42. Trevor PB, Martin RA: Tympanic bulla osteotomy for treatment of middle-ear disease in cats: 19 cases (1984-1991), J Am Vet Med Assoc 202(1):123–128, 1993.
43. Mason LK, Harvey CE, Orsher RJ: Total ear canal ablation combined with lateral bulla osteotomy for end-stage otitis in dogs. Results in thirty dogs, Vet Surg 17(5): 263–268, 1988.
44. Matthiesen DT, Scavelli T: Total ear canal ablation and lateral bulla osteotomy in 38 dogs, J Am Anim Hosp Assoc 26:257–268, 1990.
45. Beckman SL, Henry WBJ, Cechner P: Total ear canal ablation combining bulla osteotomy and curettage in dogs with chronic otitis externa and media, J Am Vet Med Assoc 196(1):84–90, 1990.
46. Fan TM, Lorimier LP: Inflammatory polyps and aural neoplasia, Vet Clin North Am Small Anim Pract 34(2):489–509, 2004.
47. Faulkner JE, Budsberg SC: Results of ventral bulla osteotomy for treatment of middle ear polyps in cats, J Am Anim Hosp Assoc 26:496–499, 1990.
48. Anderson DM, Robinson RK, White RAS: Management of inflammatory polyps in 37 cats, Vet Rec 147(24):684–687, 2000.
49. Burke EE, Moise NS, de Lahunta A, et al: Review of idiopathic feline vestibular syndrome in 75 cats, J Am Vet Med Assoc 187(9):941–943, 1985.
50. Glass EN, Cornetta AM, de Lahunta A, et al: Clinical and clinicopathologic features in 11 cats with Cuterebra larvae myiasis of the central nervous system, J Vet Intern Med 12(5):365–368, 1998.
51. Blauch B, Martin CL: A vestibular syndrome in aged dogs, J Am Anim Hosp Assoc 10:37–40, 1974.
52. Merchant SR, Neer TM, Tedford BL, et al: Ototoxicity assessment of a chlorhexidine otic preparation in dogs, Prog Vet Neurol 4(3):72–75, 1993.
53. Merchant SR: Medically managing chronic otitis externa and media, Vet Med 92(6):518–534, 1997.
54. Strain GM, Merchant SR, Neer TM, et al: Ototoxicity assessment of a gentamicin sulfate otic preparation in dogs, Am J Vet Res 56(4):532–538, 1995.
55. Gortel K: Otic flushing, Vet Clin North Am Small Anim Pract 34:557–565, 2004.
56. Schachern PA: The permeability of the round window membrane during otitis media, Arch Otolaryngol Head Neck Surg 113:625–629, 1987.
57. Cureoglu S, Schachern PA, Rinaldo A, et al: Round window membrane and labyrinthine pathological changes: an overview, Acta Otolaryngol 125:9–15, 2005.
58. Wilson HM: Tumors of the ear. In August JR, editor: Consultations in feline internal medicine, ed 6, St Louis, 2010, Elsevier.
59. London CA, Dubilzeig RR, Vail DM, et al: Evaluation of dogs and cats with tumors of the ear canal: 145 cases (1978-1992), J Am Vet Med Assoc 208(9):1413–1418, 1996.
60. Indrieri RJ, Taylor RF: Vestibular dysfunction caused by squamous cell carcinoma involving the middle ear and inner ear in two cats, J Am Vet Med Assoc 184(4):471–473, 1984.
61. de Lahunta A: Diseases of the cerebellum, Vet Clin North Am Small Anim Pract 10(1):91–101, 1980.
62. de Lahunta A: Abiotrophy in domestic animals: a review, Can J Vet Res 54(1):65–76, 1990.
63. de Lahunta A: Comparative cerebellar disease in domestic animals, Compend Contin Educ Pract Vet 2:8–19, 1980.
64. Kornegay JN: Ataxia of the head and limbs: cerebellar diseases in dogs and cats, Prog Vet Neurol 1(3):255–274, 1990.
65. Percy DH, Carmichael LE, Albert DM, et al: Lesions in puppies surviving infection with canine herpes virus, Vet Pathol 8:37–53, 1971.
66. Csiza CK, de Lahunta A, Scott FW, et al: Pathogenesis of feline panleukopenia virus in susceptible newborn kittens. II. Pathology and immunofluorescence, Infect Immun 3(6):838–846, 1971.
67. Herdon R, Margolis G, Kilham L: The synaptic organization of the malformed cerebellum induced by perinatal infection with the feline panleukopenia virus (PLV), J Neuropathol Exp Neurol 30:196–205, 1971.
68. Kilham L, Margolis G, Colby ED: Congenital infections of cats and ferrets by feline panleukopenia virus manifested by cerebellar hypoplasia, Lab Invest 17(5): 465–480, 1967.

69. Summers BA, Cummings JF, de Lahunta A: Malformations of the central nervous system. In Summers BA, Cummings JF, de Lahunta A, editors: Veterinary neuropathology, St Louis, 1995, Mosby.
70. de Lahunta A: Veterinary neuroanatomy and clinical neurology, Philadelphia, 1983, WB Saunders.
71. de Lahunta A, Glass E: Veterinary neuroanatomy and clinical neurology, St Louis, 2009, Saunders Elsevier.
72. Knecht CD, Lamar CH, Schaible R, et al: Cerebellar hypoplasia in chow chows, J Am Anim Hosp Assoc 15(1):51–53, 1979.
73. Oliver JE, Geary JC: Cerebellar anomalies: two cases, Vet Med Small Anim Clin 60:697–702, 1965.
74. Kay WJ, Budzynski AZ: Cerebellar hypoplasia and agenesis in the dog, J Neuropathol Exp Neurol 29:156, 1970.
75. Franklin RJM, Ramsey IK, McKerrel RLE: An inherited neurological disorder of the St. Bernard dog characterised by unusual cerebellar cortical dysplasia, Vet Rec 140:656–657, 1997.
76. Harari J, Miller D, Padgett GA, et al: Cerebellar agenesis in two canine littermates, J Am Vet Med Assoc 182(6):622–623, 1983.
77. Kornegay JN: Cerebellar vermian hypoplasia in dogs, Vet Pathol 23(4):374–379, 1986.
78. Pass DA, Howell JM, Thompson RR: Cerebellar malformation in two dogs and a sheep, Vet Pathol 18(3):405–407, 1981.
79. Dow RS: Partial agenesis of the cerebellum in dogs, J Comp Neurol 72:569–586, 1940.
80. Schmid V, Lang J, Wolf M: Dandy-Walker-like syndrome in four dogs: cisternography as a diagnostic aid, J Am Anim Hosp Assoc 28(4):355–360, 1992.
81. Regnier AM, Ducos de Lahitte MJ, Delisle MB, et al: Dandy-Walker syndrome in a kitten, J Am Anim Hosp Assoc 29(6):514–518, 1993.
82. Thomas JB, Robertson D: Hereditary cerebellar abiotrophy in Australian kelpie dogs, Aust Vet J 66(9):301–302, 1989.
83. Kent M, Glass E, de Lahunta A: Cerebellar cortical abiotrophy in a beagle, J Small Anim Pract 41:321–323, 2000.
84. Yasuba M, Okimoto K, Iida M, et al: Cerebellar cortical degeneration in beagle dogs, Vet Pathol 25(4):315–317, 1988.
85. Good R: Untersuchungen uber eine Kleinhirnrindenatrophie beim hund, Bern, Switzerland, 1962, University of Bern (dissertation).
86. Carmichael S, Griffiths IR, Harvey MJ: Familial cerebellar ataxia with hydrocephalus in bull mastiffs, Vet Rec 112(15):354–358, 1983.
87. Coates JR, O'Brien DP, Kline KL, et al: Neonatal cerebellar ataxia in Coton de Tulear dogs, J Vet Intern Med 16:680–689, 2002.
88. Nesbit JW, Ueckermann JF: Cerebellar cortical atrophy in a puppy, J S Afr Vet Assoc 52(3):247–250, 1981.
89. Sakai T, Harashima T, Yamamura H, et al: Two cases of hereditary quadriplegia and amblyopia in a litter of Irish setters, J Small Anim Pract 35(4):221–223, 1994.
90. Palmer AC, Payne JE, Wallace ME: Hereditary quadriplegia and amblyopia in the Irish setter, J Small Anim Pract 14(6):343–352, 1973.
91. Perille AL, Baer K, Joseph RJ, et al: Postnatal cerebellar cortical degeneration in Labrador retriever puppies, Can Vet J 32:619–621, 1991.
92. Cummings JF, de Lahunta A: A study of cerebellar and cerebral cortical degeneration in miniature poodle pups with emphasis on the ultrastructure of Purkinje cell changes, Acta Neuropathol 75(3):261–271, 1988.
93. Chieffo C, Stalis IH, Van Winkle TJ, et al: Cerebellar Purkinje's cell degeneration and coat color dilution in a family of Rhodesian Ridgeback dogs, J Vet Intern Med 8(2):112–116, 1994.
94. Taniyama H, Takayanagi S, Izumisawa Y, et al: Cerebellar cortical atrophy in a kitten, Vet Pathol 31(6):710–713, 1994.
95. Cordy DR, Snelbaker HA: Cerebellar hypoplasia and degeneration in a family of Airedale dogs, J Neuropathol Exp Neurol 11:324–328, 1996.
96. Flegel T, Matiasek K, Henke D, et al: Cerebellar cortical degeneration with selective granule cell loss in Bavarian mountain dogs, J Small Anim Pract 48(8):462–465, 2007.
97. Tago Y, Katsuta O, Tsuchitani M: Granule cell type cerebellar hypoplasia in a beagle dog, Lab Anim 27(2):151–155, 1993.
98. Carmichael KP, Miller M, Rawlings CA, et al: Clinical, hematologic, and biochemical features of a syndrome in Bernese mountain dogs characterized by hepatocerebellar degeneration, J Am Vet Med Assoc 208(8): 1277–1279, 1996.
99. Fankhauser R, Freudiger U, Vandevelde M, et al: Purkinjezellatrophie nach Masernvirus-Vakzinierung beim Hund, Schweiz Archiv Neurol Neurochir Psychiatr 112:353–363, 1973.
100. Sandy JR, Slocombe RF, Mitten RW, et al: Cerebellar abiotrophy in a family of border collie dogs, Vet Pathol 39:736–739, 2002.
101. Gill JM, Hewland M: Cerebellar degeneration in the border collie, N Z Vet J 28(8):170, 1980.
102. Higgins RJ, LeCouteur RA, Kornegay JN, et al: Late-onset progressive spinocerebellar degeneration in Brittany spaniel dogs, Acta Neuropathol 96(1):97–101, 1998.
103. Tatalick LM, Marks SL, Baszler TV: Cerebellar abiotrophy characterized by granular cell loss in a Brittany, Vet Pathol 30(4):385–388, 1993.
104. Tipold A, Fatzer R, Jaggy A, et al: Presumed immune-mediated cerebellar granuloprival degeneration in the Coton de Tulear breed, J Neuroimmunol 110(1-2): 130–133, 2000.
105. Gandini G, Botteron C, Brini E, et al: Cerebellar cortical degeneration in three English bulldogs: clinical and neuropathological findings, J Small Anim Pract 46(6): 291–294, 2005.
106. O'Brien DP: Hereditary cerebellar ataxia, Proceed of the 11th ACUIM Forum, Washington DC, pp 546–549, 1993.
107. Tontitila P, Lindberg LA: Ett fall av cerebellar ataxi hos finsk stovare, Svomen elainLaakarilehti 77:135–138, 1971.
108. Cork LC, Troncoso JC, Price DL: Canine inherited ataxia, Ann Neurol 9(5):492–498, 1981.
109. de Lahunta A, Fenner WR, Indrieri RJ, et al: Hereditary cerebellar cortical abiotrophy in the Gordon setter, J Am Vet Med Assoc 177(6):538–541, 1980.
110. Steinberg HS, Troncoso JC, Cork LC, et al: Clinical features of inherited cerebellar degeneration in Gordon setters, J Am Vet Med Assoc 179(9):886–890, 1981.
111. Coates JR, Carmichael KP, Shelton D, et al: Preliminary characterization of a cerebellar ataxia in Jack Russell terriers, J Vet Intern Med 10(3):176, 1996.
112. Cantile C, Salvadori C, Modenato M, et al: Cerebellar granuloprival degeneration in an Italian hound, J Vet Med A Physiol Pathol Clin Med 49(10):523–525, 2002.
113. Bildfell RJ, Mitchell SK, Lahunta AD: Cerebellar cortical degeneration in a Labrador retriever, Can Vet J 36(9):570–572, 1995.

114. Jokinen TS, Rusbridge C, Steffen F, et al: Cerebellar cortical abiotrophy in Lagotto Romagnolo dogs, J Small Anim Pract 48(8):470–473, 2007.
115. Berry ML, Blas-Machado U: Cerebellar abiotrophy in a miniature schnauzer, Can Vet J 44(8):657–659, 2003.
116. Chrisman CL, Spencer CP, Crane SW, et al: Late-onset cerebellar degeneration in a dog, J Am Vet Med Assoc 182(7):717–720, 1983.
117. Steinberg HS, Winkle TV, Bell JS, et al: Cerebellar degeneration in Old English sheepdogs, J Am Vet Med Assoc 217(8):1162–1165, 2000.
118. van Tongeren SE, van Vonderen IK, van Nes JJ, et al: Cerebellar cortical abiotrophy in two portuguese podenco littermates, Vet Q 22:172–174, 2001.
119. Hartley WJ, Barker JSF, Wanner RA, et al: Inherited cerebellar degeneration in the rough coated collie, Aust Vet Pract 8(2):79–85, 1978.
120. van der Merwe LL, Lane E: Diagnosis of cerebellar cortical degeneration in a Scottish terrier using magnetic resonance imaging, J Small Anim Pract 42(8):409–412, 2001.
121. Olby N, Blot S, Thibaud JL, et al: Cerebellar cortical degeneration in adult American Staffordshire terriers, J Vet Intern Med 18(2):201–208, 2004.
122. Aye MM, Izumo S, Inada S, et al: Histopathological and ultrastructural features of feline hereditary cerebellar cortical atrophy: a novel animal model of human spinocerebellar degeneration, Acta Neuropathol 96(4):379–387, 1998.
123. Inada S, Mochizuki M, Izumo S, et al: Study of hereditary cerebellar degeneration in cats, Am J Vet Res 57(3): 296–301, 1996.
124. Barone G, Foureman P, deLahunta A: Adult-onset cerebellar cortical abiotrophy and retinal degeneration in a domestic shorthair cat, J Am Anim Hosp Assoc 38:51–54, 2002.
125. Shamir M, Perl S, Sharon L: Late onset of cerebellar abiotrophy in a Siamese cat, J Small Anim Pract 40(7):343–345, 1999.
126. Negrin A, Bernardini M, Baumgärtner W, et al: Late onset cerebellar degeneration in a middle-aged cat, J Feline Med Surg 8(6):424–429, 2006.
127. Carmichael KP, Richey LJ: Cerebellar Purkinje cell degeneration and hepatic microvascular dysplasia in Havana brown kittens, Vet Pathol 42:689, 2005.
128. de Lahunta A, Averill DRJ: Hereditary cerebellar cortical and extrapyramidal nuclear abiotrophy in Kerry blue terriers, J Am Vet Med Assoc 168(12):1119–1124, 1976.
129. Montgomery DL, Storts RW: Hereditary striatonigral and cerebello-olivary degeneration of the Kerry blue terrier. I. Gross and light microscopic central nervous system lesions, Vet Pathol 20(2):143–159, 1983.
130. Montgomery DL, Storts RW: Hereditary striatonigral and cerebello-olivary degeneration of the Kerry blue terrier. II. Ultrastructural lesions in the caudate nucleus and cerebellar cortex, J Neuropathol Exp Neurol 43(3):263–275, 1984.
131. O'Brien DP, Johnson GS, Schnabel RD, et al: Genetic mapping of canine multiple system degeneration and ectodermal dysplasia loci, J Hered 96(7):727–734, 2005.
132. Cummings JF, de Lahunta A, Gasteiger EL: Multisystemic chromatolytic neuronal degeneration in cairn terriers. A case with generalized cataplectic episodes, J Vet Intern Med 5(2):91–94, 1991.
133. Palmer AC, Blakemore WF: A progressive neuronopathy in the young cairn terrier, J Sm Anim Pract 30(2):101–106, 1988.
134. Jaggy A, Vandevelde M: Multisystem neuronal degeneration in cocker spaniels, J Vet Intern Med 2(3):117–120, 1988.
135. da Costa RC, Parent JM, Poma R, et al: Multisystem axonopathy and neuronopathy in Golden retriever dogs, J Vet Intern Med 23:935–939, 2009.
136. Kortz GD, Meier WA, Higgins RJ, et al: Neuronal vacuolation and spinocerebellar degeneration in young Rottweiler dogs, Vet Pathol 34(4):296–302, 1997.
137. Sandefeldt E, Cummings JF, de Lahunta A: Animal model of human disease. Infantile spinal muscular atrophy, Werdnig-Hoffman disease. Animal model: hereditary neuronal abiotrophy in Swedish Lapland dogs, Am J Pathol 82:649–652, 1976.
138. Resibois A, Poncelet L: Olivopontocerebellar atrophy in two adult cats, sporadic cases or new genetic entity, Vet Pathol 41(1):20–29, 2004.
139. Chrisman CL, Cork LC, Gamble DA: Neuroaxonal dystrophy of Rottweiler dogs, J Am Vet Med Assoc 184(4):464–467, 1984.
140. Cork LC, Troncoso JC, Price DL, et al: Canine neuroaxonal dystrophy, J Neuropathol Exp Neurol 42(3): 286–296, 1983.
141. Blakemore WF, Palmer AC: Nervous disease in the Chihuahua characterised by axonal swellings, Vet Rec 117(19):498–499, 1985.
142. Clark RG, Hartley WJ, Burgess GS, et al: Suspected inherited cerebellar neuroaxonal dystrophy in collie sheepdogs, N Z Vet J 30(7):102–103, 1982.
143. Sacre BJ, Cummings JF, de Lahunta A: Neuroaxonal dystrophy in a Jack Russell terrier pup resembling human infantile neuroaxonal dystrophy, Cornell Vet 83(2):133–142, 1993.
144. Duncan ID, Griffiths IR: Canine giant axonal neuropathy, Vet Rec 101:438–441, 1977.
145. Diaz JD, Duque C, Geisel R: Neuroaxonal dystrophy in dogs: case report in 2 litters of papillon puppies, J Vet Intern Med 21:531–534, 2007.
146. Franklin RJM, Jeffery ND, Ramsey IK: Neuroaxonal dystrophy in a litter of papillon pups, J Small Anim Pract 36(10):441–444, 1995.
147. Nibe K, Kita C, Morozumi M, et al: Clinicopathological features of canine neuroaxonal dystrophy and cerebellar cortical abiotrophy in papillon and papillon-related dogs, J Vet Med Sci 69(10):1047–1052, 2007.
148. Carmichael KP, Howerth EW, Oliver JE Jr, et al: Neuroaxonal dystrophy in a group of related cats, J Vet Diagn Invest 5(4):585–590, 1993.
149. Woodard JC, Collins GH, Hessler JR: Feline hereditary neuroaxonal dystrophy, Am J Pathol 74(3):551–566, 1974.
150. Rodriguez F, Espinosa de los Monteros A, Morales M, et al: Neuroaxonal dystrophy in two Siamese kitten littermates, Vet Res 138:548–549, 1996.
151. Konno S, Moriwaki M, Nakagawa M: Akabane disease in cattle: congenital abnormalities caused by viral infection. Spontaneous disease, Vet Pathol 19(3):246–266, 1982.
152. Parsonson IM, Della-Porta AJ, Snowdon WA: Congenital abnormalities in newborn lambs after infection of pregnant sheep with Akabane virus, Infect Immun 15(1):254–262, 1977.
153. Tsuda T, Yoshida K, Ohashi S, et al: Arthrogryposis, hydranencephaly and cerebellar hypoplasia syndrome in neonatal calves resulting from intrauterine infection with Aino virus, Vet Res 35(5):531–538, 2004.
154. Barnard BJH, Pienaar JG: Bluetongue virus as a cause of hydranencephaly in cattle, Onderstepoort J Vet Res 43(3):155–157, 1976.

155. Leipold HW, Dennis SM: Congenital defects of the bovine central nervous system, Vet Clin North Am Food Anim Pract 3(1):159–177, 1987.
156. Osburn BI: Animal model for human disease. Hydranencephaly, porencephaly, cerebral cysts, retinal dysplasia, CNS malformations. Animal model: bluetongue-vaccine-virus infection in fetal lambs, Am J Pathol 67(1):211–214, 1972.
157. Nettleton PF, Gilray JA, Russo P, et al: Border disease of sheep and goats, Vet Res 29(3/4):327–340, 1998.
158. Brown TT, de Lahunta A, Bistner SI, et al: Pathogenetic studies of infection of the bovine fetus with bovine viral diarrhea virus. I. Cerebellar atrophy, Vet Pathol 11(6):486–505, 1974.
159. Kahrs RF, Scott FW, de Lahunta A: Congenital cerebellar hypoplasia and ocular defects in calves following bovine viral diarrhea-mucosal disease infection in pregnant cattle, J Am Vet Med Assoc 156(10):1443–1450, 1970.
160. Ward GM: Experimental infection of pregnant sheep with bovine viral diarrhea-mucosa disease virus, Cornell Vet 61(1):179–191, 1971.
161. Edwards JF, Livingston CW, Chung SI, et al: Ovine arthrogryposis and central nervous system malformations associated with in utero Cache Valley virus infection: spontaneous disease, Vet Pathol 26(1):33–39, 1989.
162. Johnson KP, Ferguson LC, Byington DP, et al: Multiple fetal malformations due to persistent viral infection. I. Abortion, intrauterine death, and gross abnormalities in fetal swine infected with hog cholera vaccine virus, Lab Invest 30(5):608–617, 1974.
163. Miura Y, Kubo M, Goto Y, et al: Hydranencephaly-cerebellar hypoplasia in a newborn calf after infection of its dam with Chuzan virus, Jpn J Vet Sci 52(4):689–694, 1990.
164. Coetzer JAW: Brain teratology as a result of transplacental virus infection in ruminants, J S Afr Vet Assoc 51(3):153–157, 1980.
165. Done JT, Harding JDJ: The relationship of maternal swine fever infection to cerebellar hypoplasia in piglets, Proc R Soc Med 59:1083–1084, 1966.
166. Coetzer JAW, Theodoridis A, Herr S, et al: Wesselsbron disease: a cause of congenital porencephaly and cerebellar hypoplasia in calves, Onderstepoort J Vet Res 46(3):165–169, 1979.
167. Jeffrey M, Preece BE, Holliman A: Dandy-Walker malformation in two calves, Vet Rec 126(20):499–501, 1990.
168. Madarame H, Azuma K, Nozuki H, et al: Dandy-Walker malformation in a Japanese black calf, Vet Pathol 27(4):296–298, 1990.
169. Cudd TA, Mayhew IG, Cottrill CM: Agenesis of the corpus callosum with cerebellar vermian hypoplasia in a foal resembling the Dandy-Walker syndrome: pre-mortem diagnosis by clinical evaluation and CT scanning, Equine Vet J 21(5):378–381, 1989.
170. Washburn KE, Streeter RN: Congenital defects of the ruminant nervous system, Vet Clin North Am Food Anim Pract 20:413–434, 2004.
171. Verhaart WJC: Partial agenesis of the cerebellum and medulla and total agenesis of the corpus callosum in a goat, J Comp Neurol 77:477–478, 1942.
172. Wallace MA, Scarratt WK, Crisman MV, et al: Familial convulsions and ataxia in an Aberdeen Angus calf, Prog Vet Neurol 7(4):145–148, 1996.
173. Innes JRM, Russell DS, Wilsdon AJ: Familial cerebellar hypoplasia and degeneration in Hereford calves, J Pathol Bacteriol 50:455–461, 1940.
174. Saunders LZ, Sweet JD, Martin SM, et al: Hereditary congenital ataxia in Jersey calves, Cornell Vet 42:559–591, 1952.
175. Allen JG: Congenital cerebellar hypoplasia in Jersey calves, Aust Vet J 53(4):173–175, 1977.
176. Edmonds L, Crenshaw D, Selby LA: Micrognathia and cerebellar hypoplasia in an Aberdeen Angus herd, J Hered 64(2):62–64, 1973.
177. Schild AL, Riet-Correa F, Fernandes CG, et al: Cerebellar hypoplasia and porencephaly in Charolais cattle in Southern Brazil, Ciencia Rural 31(1):149–153, 2001.
178. Finnie EP, Leaver DD: Cerebellar hypoplasia in calves, Aust Vet J 41:287–288, 1965.
179. Kidd AR, Done JT, Wrathall AE, et al: A new genetically determined congenital nervous disorder in pigs, Br Vet J 142:275–285, 1986.
180. Johnson KR, Fourt DL, Ross RH, et al: Hereditary congenital ataxia in Holstein-Friesian calves, J Dairy Sci 41:1371–1375, 1958.
181. Kemp J, McOrist S, Jeffrey M: Cerebellar abiotrophy in Holstein Friesian calves, Vet Rec 136(8):198, 1995.
182. Schild AL, Riet-Correa F, Portiansky EL, et al: Congenital cerebellar cortical degeneration in Holstein cattle in southern Brazil, Vet Res Commun 25(3):189–195, 2001.
183. Cho DY, Leipold HW: Cerebellar cortical atrophy in a Charolais calf, Vet Pathol 15(2):264–266, 1978.
184. White ME, Whitlock RH, de Lahunta A: A cerebellar abiotrophy of calves, Cornell Vet 65(4):476–491, 1975.
185. Mitchell PJ, Reilly W, Harper PAW, et al: Cerebellar abiotrophy in Angus cattle, Aust Vet J 70(2):67–68, 1993.
186. Woodman MP, Scott PR, Watt N, et al: Selective cerebellar degeneration in a Limousin cross heifer, Vet Rec 132(23):586–587, 1993.
187. Barlow RM: Further observations on bovine familial convulsions and ataxia, Vet Rec 105:91–94, 1979.
188. Barlow RM: Morphogenesis of cerebellar lesions in bovine familial convulsions and ataxia, Vet Pathol 18:151–162, 1981.
189. Harper RAW, Duncan DW, Plant JW, et al: Cerebellar abiotrophy and segmental axonopathy: two syndromes of progressive ataxia in Merino sheep, Aust Vet J 63:18–21, 1986.
190. Innes JRM, MacNaughton WN: Inherited cortical cerebellar atrophy in Corriedale lambs in Canada identical with daft lamb disease in Britain, Cornell Vet 40:127–135, 1950.
191. Milne EM, Schock A: Cerebellar abiotrophy in a pedigree Charolais sheep flock, Vet Rec 143:224–225, 1998.
192. Johnstone AC, Johnson CB, Malcolm KE, et al: Cerebellar cortical abiotrophy in Wiltshire sheep, N Z Vet J 53(4):242–245, 2005.
193. Gregory DW, Mead SW, Regan WM: Hereditary congenital lethal spasms in Jersey cattle, J Hered 35:195–200, 1944.
194. High JW, Kincaid CM, Smith HJ: Doddler cattle, J Hered 49:250–252, 1958.
195. Baird JD, Mackenzie CD: Cerebellar hypoplasia and degeneration in part-Arab horse, Aust Vet J 50:25–28, 1974.
196. Palmer AC, Blakemore WF, Cook WR, et al: Cerebellar hypoplasia and degeneration in the young Arab horse: clinical and neuropathological features, Vet Rec 93(3):62–66, 1973.
197. Bjorck G, Everz KE, Hansen HJ, et al: Congenital cerebellar ataxia in the Gotland pony breed, Zentralbl Veterinarmed A 20:341–345, 1973.

198. Cordy DR, Richards WP, Bradford GE: Systemic neuroaxonal dystrophy in Suffolk sheep, Acta Neuropathol 8:133–140, 1967.
200. Beech J, Haskins M: Genetic studies of neuraxonal dystrophy in the Morgan, Am J Vet Res 48(1):109–113, 1987.
201. Baumgartner W, Frese K, Elmadfa I: Neuroaxonal dystrophy associated with vitamin E deficiency in two Haflinger horses, J Comp Pathol 103:113–119, 1990.
202. Summers BA, Cummings JF, de Lahunta A: Veterinary neuropathology, St Louis, 1995, Mosby.
203. Shichiro I, Masami M, Shuji I, et al: Study of hereditary cerebellar degeneration in cats, Am J Vet Res 57:296–301, 1996.
204. Jolly RD, Blair HT, Johnstone AC: Genetic disorders of sheep in New Zealand: a review and perspective, N Z Vet J 52(2):52–64, 2004.
205. Flegel T, Matiasek K, Henke D, et al: Cerebellar cortical degeneration with selective granule cell loss in Bavarian mountain dogs, J Small Anim Pract 48(8):462–465, 2007.
206. Cummings JF, Summers BA, de Lahunta A, et al: Tremors in Samoyed pups with oligodendrocyte deficiencies and hypomyelination, Acta Neuropathol 71(3-4):267–277, 1986.
207. Henke D, Bottcher P, Doherr MG, et al: Computer-assisted magnetic resonance imaging brain morphometry in American Staffordshire terriers with cerebellar cortical degeneration, J Vet Intern Med 22(4):969–975, 2008.
208. Thames RA, Robertson ID, Flegel T, et al: Brain morphometry in dogs using magnetic resonance imaging: the effect of breed, age and cerebellar degenerative disease, Vet Radiol Ultrasound , 2010:in press.
209. Jolly RD, Walkley SU: Lysosomal storage diseases of animals: an essay in comparative pathology, Vet Pathol 34(6):527–548, 1997.
210. Jolly RD: Comparative biology of the neuronal ceroid-lipofuscinoses: an overview, Am J Med Genet 57:307–311, 1995.
211. Ellinwood NM, Vite CH, Haskin ME: Gene therapy for lysosomal storage diseases: the lessons and promise of animal models, J Gene Med 6:481–506, 2004.
212. March PA: Neuronal storage disorders. In August JR, editor: Consultations in feline internal medicine, ed 4, Philadelphia, 2001, WB Saunders.
213. Vite CH: Gene therapy for lysomal storage diseases. In August JR, editor: Consultations in feline internal medicine, ed 6, St Louis, 2010, Saunders Elsevier.
214. Jolly RD: Lysosomal storage diseases in livestock, Vet Clin North Am Food Anim Pract 9:41–53, 1993.
215. Skelly BJ, Franklin RJM: Recognition and diagnosis of lysosomal storage diseases in the cat and dog, J Vet Intern Med 16:133–141, 2002.
216. Evans RJ: Lysosomal storage diseases in dogs and cats, J Small Anim Pract 30(3):144–150, 1989.
217. Haskins ME, Bingel SA, Northington JW, et al: Spinal cord compression and hindlimb paresis in cats with mucopolysaccharidosis VI, J Am Vet Med Assoc 182(9):983–985, 1983.
218. Haskins ME, Otis EJ, Hayden JE, et al: Hepatic storage of glycosaminoglycans in feline and canine models of mucopolysaccharidoses I, VI, and VII, Vet Pathol 29(2):112–119, 1992.
219. Coates JR, O'Brien DP: Inherited peripheral neuropathies in dogs and cats, Vet Clin North Am Small Anim Pract 34:1361–1401, 2004.
220. Sisk DB, Levesque DC, Wood PA, et al: Clinical and pathologic features of ceroid lipofuscinosis in two Australian cattle dogs, J Am Vet Med Assoc 197(3):361–364, 1990.
221. Evans J, Katz ML, Levesque D, et al: A variant form of neuronal ceroid lipofuscinosis in American bulldogs, J Vet Intern Med 19(1):44–51, 2005.
222. Wilkie JSN, Hudson EB: Neuronal and generalized ceroid-lipofuscinosis in a Cocker Spaniel, Vet Pathol 19:623–628, 1982.
223. Vicini DS, Wheaton LG, Zachary JF, et al: Peripheral nerve biopsy for diagnosis of globoid cell leukodystrophy in a dog, J Am Vet Med Assoc 192(8):1087–1090, 1988.
224. Cozzi F, Vite CH, Wenger DA, et al: MRI and electrophysiological abnormalities in a case of canine globoid cell leukodystrophy, J Small Anim Pract 39(8):401–405, 1998.
225. Schatzberg SJ, Haley NJ, Barr SC, et al: Polymerase chain reaction (PCR) amplification of parvoviral DNA from the brains of dogs and cats with cerebellar hypoplasia, J Vet Intern Med 17(4):538–544, 2003.
226. Kilham L, Margolis G, Colby ED: Cerebellar ataxia and its congenital transmission in cats by feline panleukopenia virus, J Am Vet Med Assoc 158:888–901, 1971.
227. Csiza CK, Scott FW, de Lahunta A, et al: Feline viruses XIV: transplacental infections in spontaneous panleukopenia of cats, Cornell Vet 61:423–439, 1971.
228. Csiza CK, de Lahunta A, Scott FW, et al: Spontaneous feline ataxia, Cornell Vet 62:300–322, 1972.
229. Carpenter MR, Harter DH: A study of congenital feline cerebellar malformations: an anatomic and physiologic evaluation of agenetic defects, J Comp Neurol 105:51–93, 1956.
230. Greene CE, Gorgasz EJ, Martin CL: Hydranencephaly associated with feline panleukopenia, J Am Vet Med Assoc 180(7):767–768, 1982.
231. Sharp NJH, Davis BJ, Guy JS, et al: Hydranencephaly and cerebellar hypoplasia in two kittens attributed to intrauterine parvovirus infection, J Comp Pathol 121(1):39–53, 1999.
232. Scott FW, Kahrs RF, de Lahunta A: Virus induced congenital anomalies of the bovine fetal. I. Cerebellar degeneration (hypoplasia) ocular lesions and fetal mummification following experimental infection with bovine viral diarrhea-mucosal disease virus, Cornell Vet 63:536–560, 1973.
233. Narita M, Inui S, Hashiguchi Y: The pathogenesis of congenital encephalopathies in sheep experimentally induced by Akabane virus, J Comp Pathol 89(2):229–240, 1979.
234. Osburn BI, Silverstein AM, Prendergast RA, et al: Experimental viral-induced congenital encephalopathies. I. Pathology of hydranencephaly and porencephaly caused by bluetongue vaccine virus, Lab Invest 25(3):197–205, 1971.
235. Osburn BI, Johnson RT, Silverstein AM, et al: Experimental viral-induced congenital encephalopathies. II. The pathogenesis of bluetongue vaccine virus infection in fetal lambs, Lab Invest 25(3):206–210, 1971.
236. Swan RA, Taylor EG: Cerebellar hypoplasia in beef shorthorn calves, Aust Vet J 59(3):95–96, 1982.
237. O'Sullivan BM, McPhee CP: Cerebellar hypoplasia of genetic origin in calves, Aust Vet J 51(10):469–471, 1975.
238. Vernau KM, Kortz GD, Koblik PD, et al: Magnetic resonance imaging and computed tomography characteristics of intracranial intra-arachnoid cysts in 6 dogs, Vet Radiol Ultrasound 38(3):171–176, 1997.
239. Milner RJ, Engela J, Kirberger RM: Arachnoid cyst in cerebellar pontine area of a cat: diagnosis by magnetic resonance imaging, Vet Radiol Ultrasound 37(1):34–36, 1996.

240. Matiasek LA, Platt SR, Shaw S, et al: Clinical and magnetic resonance imaging characteristics of quadrigeminal cysts in dogs, J Vet Intern Med 21(5):1021–1026, 2007.
241. Duque C, Parent J, Brisson B, et al: Intracranial arachnoid cysts: are they clinically significant? J Vet Intern Med 19(5):772–774, 2005.
242. Kitagawa M, Kanayama K, Sakai T: Quadrigeminal cisterna arachnoid cyst diagnosed by MRI in five dogs, Aust Vet J 81(6):340–343, 2003.
243. Saito M, Olby NJ, Spaulding KA: Identification of arachnoid cysts in the quadrigeminal cistern using ultrasonography, Vet Radiol Ultrasound 42:435–439, 2001.
244. Dewey CW, Krotscheck U, Bailey KS, et al: Craniotomy with cystoperitoneal shunting for treatment of intracranial arachnoid cysts in dogs, Vet Surg 36(5):416–422, 2007.
245. Lowrie M, Wessmann A, Gunn-Moore D, et al: Quadrigeminal cyst management by cystoperitoneal shunt in a 4-year-old Persian cat, J Feline Med Surg 11(8):711–713, 2009.
246. Kelly JH: Occipital dysplasia and hydrocephalus in a toy poodle, Vet Med Small Anim Clin 70(8):940–941, 1975.
247. Parker AJ, Park RD: Occipital dysplasia in the dog, J Am Anim Hosp Assoc 10:520–525, 1974.
248. Bagley RS, Harrington ML, Tucker RL, et al: Occipital dysplasia and associated cranial spinal cord abnormalities in two dogs, Vet Radiol Ultrasound 37(5):359–362, 1996.
249. Evans HE: Prenatal development. In Evans HE, editor: Miller's anatomy of the dog, ed 3, Philadelphia, 1993, WB Saunders.
250. Watson AG, de Lahunta A, Evans HE: Dorsal notch of foramen magnum due to incomplete ossification of supraoccipital bone in dogs, J Small Anim Pract 30(12):666–673, 1989.
251. Vitale CL, Olby NJ: Neurologic dysfunction in hypothyroid, hyperlipidemic Labrador retrievers, J Vet Intern Med 21(6):1316–1322, 2007.
252. Troxel MT, Vite CH, Van Winkle TJ, et al: Feline intracranial neoplasia: retrospective review of 160 cases (1985-2001), J Vet Intern Med 17:850–859, 2003.
253. Snyder JM, Shofer FS, Van Winkle TJ, et al: Canine intracranial primary neoplasia: 173 cases (1986-2003), J Vet Intern Med 20:669–675, 2006.
254. Snyder JM, Lipitz L, Skorupski KA, et al: Secondary intracranial neoplasia in the dog: 177 cases (1986-2003), J Vet Intern Med 22:172–177, 2008.
255. Kitagawa M, Koie H, Kanazawa K, et al: Medulloblastoma in a cat: clinical and MRI findings, J Small Anim Pract 44:139–142, 2003.
256. Steinberg H, Galbreath EJ: Cerebellar medulloblastoma with multiple differentiation in a dog, Vet Pathol 35(6):543–546, 1998.
257. Westworth DR, Dickinson PJ, Vernau W, et al: Choroid plexus tumors in 56 dogs (1985-2007), J Vet Intern Med 22(5):1157–1165, 2008.
258. Van Winkle TJ, Steinberg HS, DeCarlo AJ, et al: Myxoid meningiomas of the rostral cervical spinal cord and caudal fossa in four dogs, Vet Pathol 31(4):468–471, 1994.
259. Adamo PF, Clinkscales JA: Cerebellar meningioma with paradoxical vestibular signs, Prog Vet Neurol 2(2):137–142, 1991.
260. Lefbom BK, Parker GA: Ataxia associated with lymphosarcoma in a dog, J Am Vet Med Assoc 207(7):922–923, 1995.
261. Read DH, Harrington DD: Experimentally induced thiamine deficiency in beagle dogs: clinical observations, Am J Vet Res 42(6):984–991, 1981.
262. Read DH, Harrington DD: Experimentally induced thiamine deficiency in beagle dogs: pathologic changes of the central nervous system, Am J Vet Res 47(10):2281–2289, 1986.
263. Studdert VP, Labuc RH: Thiamin deficiency in cats and dogs associated with feeding meat preserved with sulphur dioxide, Aust Vet J 68:54–57, 1991.
264. Loew FM: Thiamine deficiency in dogs, Vet Pathol 14:650–653, 1977.
265. Garosi LS, Dennis R, Platt SR, et al: Thiamine deficiency in a dog: clinical, clinicopathologic and magnetic resonance imaging findings, J Vet Intern Med 17:719–723, 2003.
266. Steenbeck S, Fischer A: Clinically suspected thiamine deficiency encephalopathy in two cats fed with a commercial cat foot, Tierarztl Prax 35:55–58, 2007.
267. Penderis J, McConnell JF, Calvin J: Magnetic resonance imaging features of thiamine deficiency in a cat, Vet Rec 160:270–272, 2007.
268. Evans TR, Evans WC, Roberts HE: Studies on bracken poisoning in the horse, Br Vet J 107:364–371, 1951.
269. Henderson JA, Evans MA: The antithiamine action of, Equisetum, J Am Vet Med Assoc 120:375–378, 1952.
270. Plumlee KH, Galey FD: Neurotoxic mycotoxins: a review of fungal toxins that cause neurological disease in large animals, J Vet Intern Med 8(1):49–54, 1994.
271. Scarratt WK: Cerebellar disease and disease characterized by dysmetria or tremors, Vet Clin North Am Food Anim Pract 20:275–289, 2004.
272. Tyler JW: Naturally occurring neurologic disease in calves fed *Claviceps* sp. infected Dallis grass hay and pasture, Prog Vet Neurol 3:101–106, 1990.
273. Caylor KB, Cassimatis MK: Metronidazole neurotoxicosis in two cats, J Am Anim Hosp Assoc 37:258–262, 2001.
274. Dow SW, LeCouteur RA, Poss ML, et al: Central nervous system toxicosis associated with metronidazole treatment of dogs: five cases (1984-1987), J Am Vet Med Assoc 195(3):365–368, 1989.
275. Olson EJ, Morales SC, McVey AS, et al: Putative metronidazole neurotoxicosis in a cat, Vet Pathol 42:665–669, 2005.
276. Saxon B, Magne ML: Reversible central nervous system toxicosis associated with metronidazole therapy in three cats, Prog Vet Neurol 4(1):25–27, 1993.
277. Evans J, Levesque D, Knowles K, et al: Diazepam as a treatment for metronidazole toxicosis in dogs: a retrospective study of 21 cases, J Vet Intern Med 17(3):304–310, 2003.
278. Garosi L, McConnell JF, Platt SR, et al: Clinical and topographic magnetic resonance characteristics of suspected brain infarction in 40 dogs, J Vet Intern Med 20(2):311–321, 2006.
279. Garosi L, McConnell JE, Platt SR, et al: Results of diagnostic investigations and long-term outcome of 33 dogs with brain infarction (2000-2004), J Vet Intern Med 19(5):725–731, 2005.
280. McConnell JF, Garosi L, Platt SR: Magnetic resonance imaging findings of presumed cerebellar cerebrovascular accident in twelve dogs, Vet Radiol Ultrasound 46(1): 1–10, 2005.

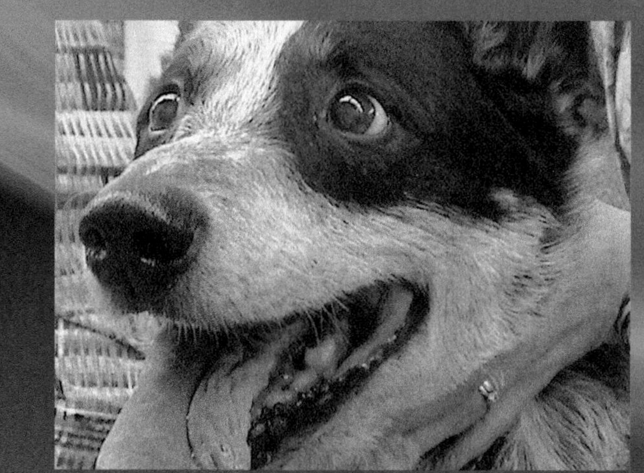

CHAPTER 9

Disorders of the Face, Tongue, Esophagus, Larynx, and Ear

LESION LOCALIZATION

The problems described in this chapter result from dysfunction of cranial nerves (CNs) V, VII, VIII (cochlear), IX, X, XI, and XII. Disorders of CN VIII (vestibular) are discussed in Chapter 8, and disorders of the cranial nerves associated with vision and the eyes are discussed in Chapter 11. The localization of cranial nerve lesions is presented in Chapters 1 and 2 and is reviewed briefly in this chapter (see Table 2-4 and Figure 1-5).

Lesions affecting cranial nerves may be peripheral (nerve fibers) or central (neurons in the brainstem). Differentiation is based on the results of a careful neurologic examination and diagnostics tests such as cross-sectional imaging. Clinically, peripheral cranial nerve disorders are characterized by specific nerve deficits with no evidence of involvement of the brainstem.

Cranial nerve dysfunction resulting from brainstem lesions is characterized by isolated or multiple cranial nerve involvement and, more importantly, by specific signs referable to the brainstem, such as ipsilateral postural reaction deficits, paresis of the ipsilateral limbs, central vestibular disease, and changes in mentation. Occasionally, the generalized lower motor neuron (LMN) diseases may predominantly affect specific cranial nerves (e.g., laryngeal paralysis). These diseases usually are recognized because of other LMN signs in the limbs. In some cases, electromyography (EMG) is needed to establish the generalized nature of the LMN disease.

Cranial Nerve V (Trigeminal Nerve)

Anatomy

The trigeminal nerve (CN V) contains both sensory and motor fibers. The trigeminal nerve is divided into three main branches: ophthalmic, maxillary, and mandibular nerves. All three branches contain sensory fibers, whereas only the mandibular nerve contains motor fibers. The general somatic efferent (GSE), neurons (motor) are located in the pons. Axons emerge from the lateral aspect of the pons and together with sensory fibers form the trigeminal nerve. After exiting the pons, the trigeminal nerve courses in the trigeminal canal within the petrous portion of the temporal bone. Upon leaving the trigeminal canal, the trigeminal nerve divides into its three main branches. The mandibular nerve leaves the cranial cavity via the oval foramen to innervate the muscles of mastication (temporalis, masseter, pterygoids, rostral digastricus, and mylohyoideus muscles). Sensation to the surface of the head is supplied by CN V through all branches. The ophthalmic nerve innervates the eyelid, nasal mucosa, globe of the eye, and the cornea. The ophthalmic nerve enters the cranial cavity via the orbital fissure. The maxillary nerve provides sensation to the lateral side of the face overlying the maxilla from the nasal plane to the level of the rostral aspect of the zygomatic arch. The maxillary nerve receives sensory input from the calvaria via the round foramen. The mandibular nerve provides sensation to the skin of the lower jaw, teeth of the lower jaw, tongue, and buccal cavity. The ophthalmic nerve is the sensory arc of the corneal reflex and, together with the maxillary nerve, the palpebral reflex. The cell bodies for the general somatic afferent (GSA) (sensory) neurons are located in the trigeminal ganglion within the trigeminal canal. Axons enter the pons to form the spinal tract of the trigeminal nerve, which courses caudally through the medulla to the level of the first cervical spinal cord segment. GSA axons in the spinal tract of the trigeminal nerve synapse on neurons immediately adjacent to the tract in the nucleus of the spinal tract of the trigeminal nerve. At its rostral end, this nucleus is contiguous with the pontine sensory nucleus of the trigeminal nerve. From these nuclei, axons decussate and extend to the contralateral thalamus. From the thalamus, GSA information is distributed via the internal capsule and corona radiata to the contralateral somatosensory cerebral cortex for conscious perception.

The anatomic distribution of GSA fibers in CN V is of considerable importance in the identification of lesions involving the trigeminal nerve and brainstem. Lesions in the medulla involving the spinal tract of CN V result in ipsilateral loss of facial sensation but no impairment of the masticatory muscles. Loss of both sensory and motor function of the trigeminal nerve usually results from pontine lesions affecting cranial nerve nuclei or extramedullary disorders that affect both motor and sensory nerve fibers. Loss of motor function with no sensory impairment is associated with discrete lesions in the trigeminal motor nucleus in the pons or preferential involvement of the motor nerve fibers or the muscle of mastication.

Clinical Signs

For the reasons just described, facial sensation may be absent (analgesia) ipsilateral to lesions involving the trigeminal nerve and brainstem. In addition, corneal and palpebral reflexes may be diminished because of interference with the sensory arcs of these reflexes. The pinna of the dog (and probably other species) is innervated by the facial nerve (CN VII) on the concave surface and by branches of C2 on the convex surface, not by the trigeminal nerve (Figure 9-1).[1,2] Diminished conscious response to facial stimulation can also be caused by lesions of the forebrain. In this case, response to a noxious stimulus is decreased (hypalgesia) but usually not totally absent on the side of the face contralateral to the lesion. This is best appreciated by noxious stimulation of the nasal mucosa such as with stimulation of the nasal mucosa with a hemostat. Importantly, palpebral and corneal reflexes are normal with lesions involving the forebrain (Figure 9-2). In addition to facial hypalgesia, affected animals also demonstrate other signs compatible with forebrain lesions (see Chapter 12). Bilateral involvement of motor nerves results in a "dropped jaw" (mouth open) that cannot be closed voluntarily (mandibular paralysis). The jaw muscles are atonic and become atrophic if the paralysis persists for longer than 7 days. Unilateral motor lesions are difficult to detect until specific muscle atrophy develops ipsilaterally (Figure 9-3).

Cranial Nerve VII (Facial Nerve)

Anatomy

The facial nerve innervates the muscles of facial expression. Its neurons are located in the facial nuclei of the rostral medulla (Figure 9-4). Within the medulla, fibers leave the facial nuclei and course dorsomedially and around the abducent nucleus. The fibers leave the ventrolateral surface of the medulla ventral to CN VIII. The facial nerve enters the petrosal bone through the internal acoustic meatus on the dorsal side of CN VIII. The nerve emerges from the calvaria through the stylomastoid foramen to innervate the muscles of facial expression. Inflammatory or neoplastic disease involving the inner ear may extend to the facial nerve, resulting in ipsilateral facial paralysis. The facial nerve is the main motor pathway for the corneal and palpebral reflexes. Lesions of the upper motor neurons (UMNs) to the facial nucleus may cause abnormal facial expression without loss of facial reflexes.[3]

Clinical Signs

Lesions of CN VII result in ipsilateral facial paresis or paralysis. The lip may droop on the affected side, and food or saliva may fall from that side of the mouth. In horses, the nasal philtrum may deviate to the normal side due to the unopposed muscle tone of the facial muscles on the unaffected side. Drooping of the ear may be observed in animals with erect ears (Figure 9-5). Closure of the palpebral fissure when performing the palpebral and corneal reflexes will be diminished to absent. In small animals, the palpebral fissure may be wider, whereas in large animals ptosis may occur. Exposure keratitis is a common sequela of facial nerve injury in dogs, especially in breeds that tend to have ectropion or exophthalmic globes. In small animals with chronic facial paralysis, the palpebral fissure may become narrowed, the nose deviates toward the affected side, and the ear on the affected side is drawn dorsally as a result of atrophy of the muscles of facial expression. However, given the normally small-sized muscles of facial expression, the atrophy may not be evident on visual inspection.

Vestibular signs are commonly associated with facial paresis or paralysis because of the close anatomic relationship of the facial and vestibular nerves at the brainstem and in their course through the petrosal bone. These two locations must be differentiated because of the difference in prognosis and therapy. Lesions at the brainstem result in central vestibular disease, whereas lesions in the petrosal bone cause peripheral vestibular disease. See Chapter 8 for a discussion of these disorders.

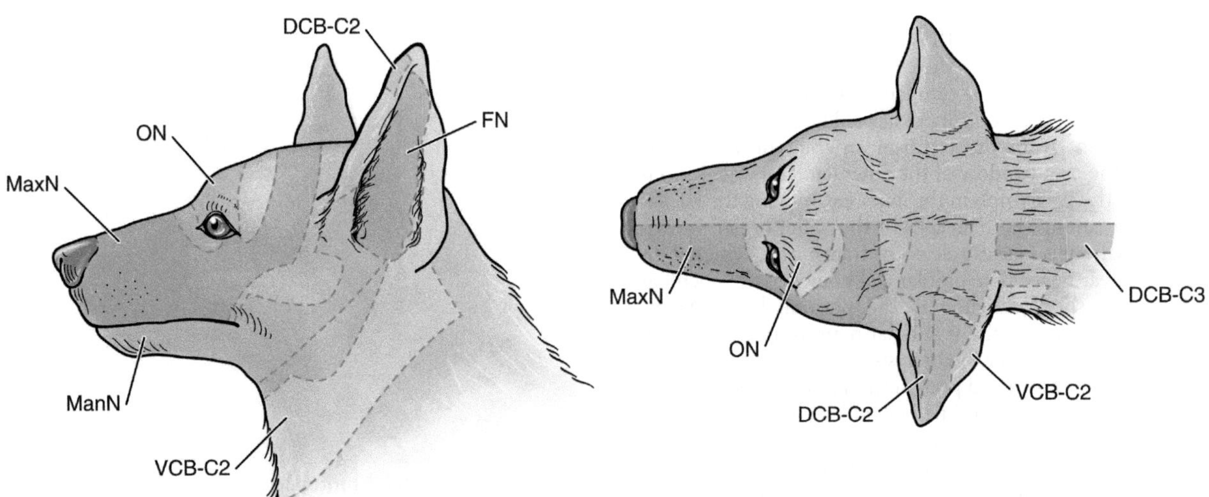

Figure 9-1 Areas of cutaneous innervation of the head that are supplied by one nerve (autonomous zones). **A,** Lateral view. **B,** Dorsal view. *DCB-C2,* Dorsal cutaneous branch of the second cervical nerve; *VCB-C2,* ventral cutaneous branch of the second cervical nerve; *DCB-C3,* dorsal cutaneous branch of the third cervical nerve; *FN,* facial nerve; *MaxN,* maxillary nerve, *CN V; ManN,* mandibular nerve, CN V; *ON,* ophthalmic nerve. (From Whalen LR, Kitchell RL: Electrophysiologic studies of the cutaneous nerves of the head of the dog, Am J Vet Res 44:615, 1983.)

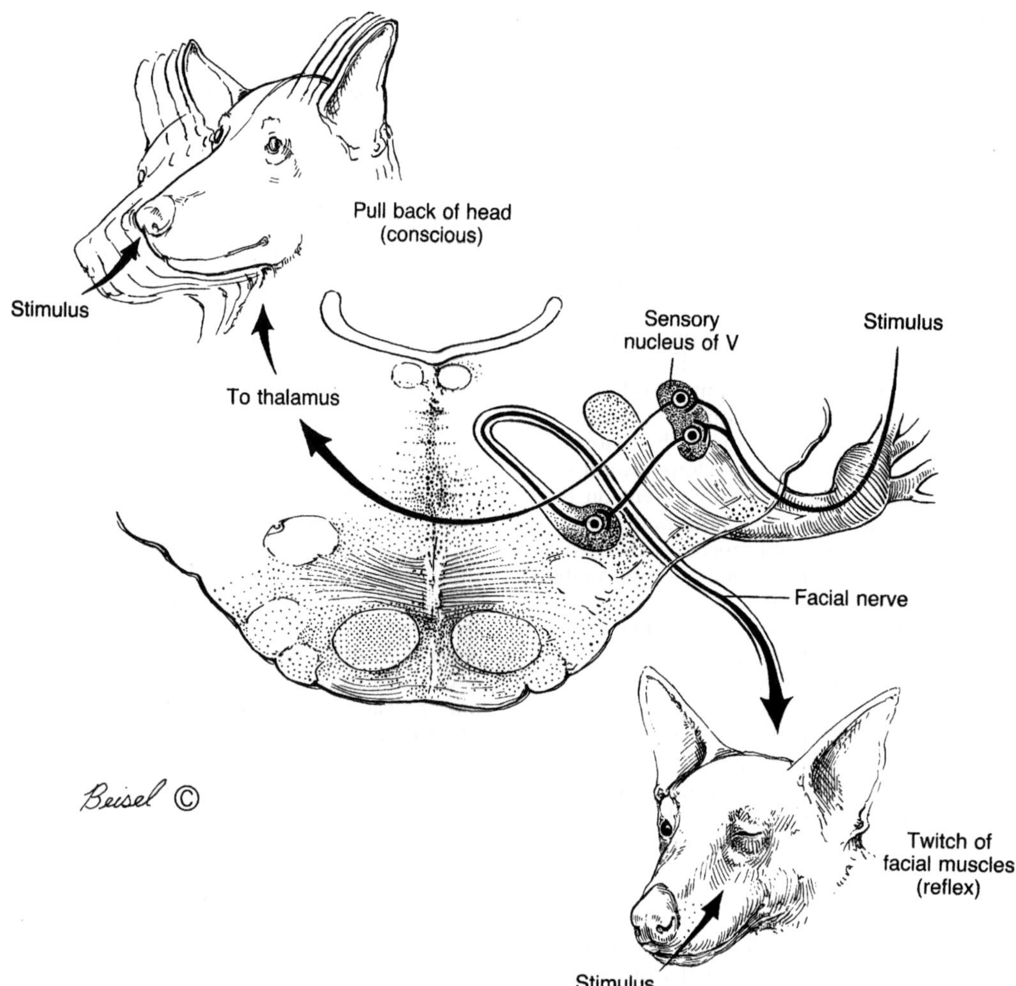

Figure 9-2 Reflex and conscious pain perception pathways of the trigeminal nerve (CN V). (From Greene CE, Oliver JE: Neurologic examination. In Ettinger SJ, editor: Textbook of veterinary internal medicine, ed 2, Philadelphia, 1983, WB Saunders.)

Cranial Nerve VIII (Cochlear Nerve)

Anatomy

The vestibular branch of CN VIII is discussed in Chapter 8. The tympanic membrane separates the external ear from the middle ear. Sound waves striking the tympanic membrane vibrate the membrane and attached auditory ossicles. The auditory ossicles transmit vibrations from the tympanic membrane across the middle ear to the oval window of the inner ear. The waveform is transmitted to the perilymph in the inner ear, moving the basilar membrane containing the hair cells of the spiral organ. Movement of the hair cells causes release of transmitter, which activates the cochlear nerve. The bipolar cell bodies of the cochlear nerve form the spiral ganglion in the petrosal bone. Axons extend proximally to join the vestibular neurons in the internal acoustic meatus. They enter the brainstem at the junction of the rostral medulla oblongata and pons, terminating on the cochlear nuclei. The central pathway is bilateral and multisynaptic. From the cochlear nuclei, axons project to several brainstem nuclei, in particular, the caudal colliculi. Axons from the caudal colliculi project to LMN nuclei in the brainstem and cervical spinal cord completing reflex arcs involved in auditory function. Additionally, axons from the caudal colliculi project to the medial geniculate nuclei of the thalamus. Conscious perception of sound is served by the projection from the medial geniculate nuclei to the temporal lobes of the cerebral cortex (auditory cortex). Although the pathway has significant bilateral components, the cortical projection is largely from the contralateral ear.[4]

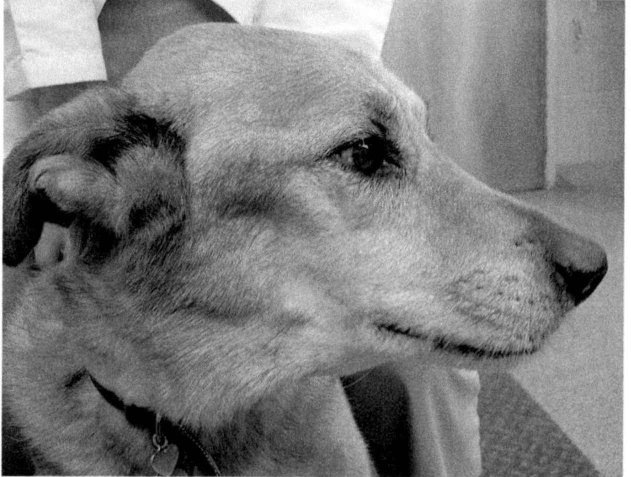

Figure 9-3 Unilateral motor lesions are difficult to detect until specific muscle atrophy develops ipsilaterally. (Copyright 2010 University of Georgia Research Foundation, Inc.)

Clinical Signs

Deafness can be classified as either conductive or sensorineural. Conductive deafness occurs due to lesions of the external or middle ear cavities, whereas inner ear lesions

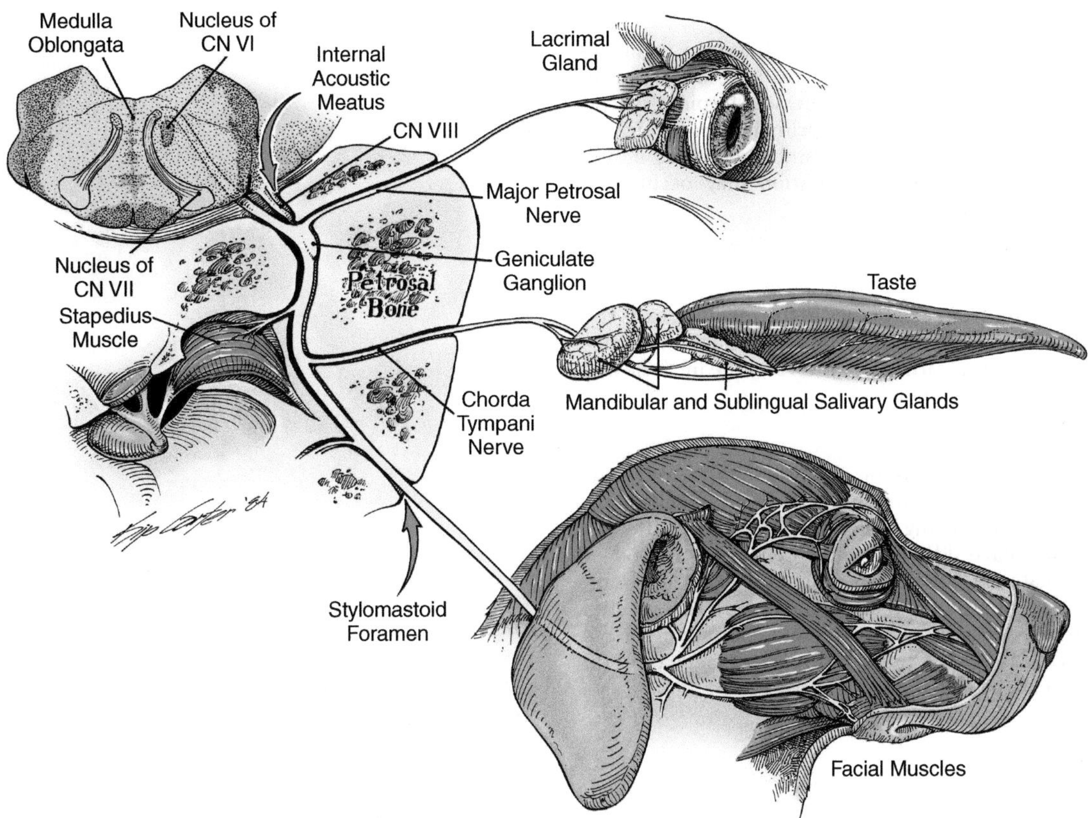

Figure 9-4 The facial nerve originates in the medulla oblongata and enters the internal acoustic meatus of the petrosal bone with vestibulocochlear nerve (CN VIII). Branches include nerves to the lacrimal glands, stapedius muscle, mandibular and sublingual salivary glands, and sensory fibers for taste. The major component exits the stylomastoid foramen and innervates the muscles of facial expression. Testing for function of the various branches can localize the site of the lesion in facial paralysis.

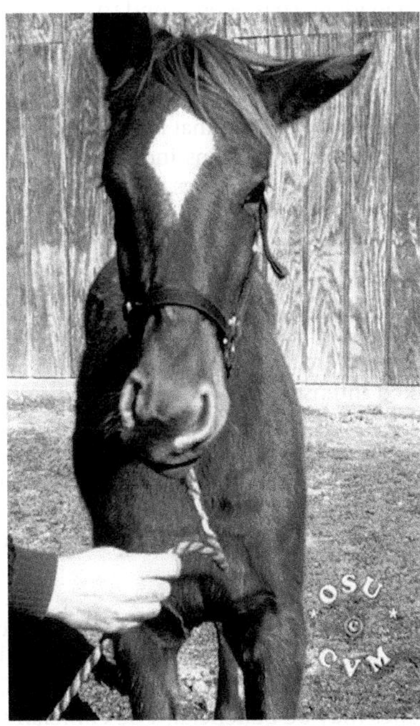

Figure 9-5 A horse with left facial nerve paralysis. Note the drooped ear and deviation of the nose to the right.

lead to sensorineural deafness. Chronic otitis externa or otitis media is the most common cause of conductive deafness. In sensorineural deafness, receptor cells generally fail to develop, develop and then subsequently degenerate, or are damaged. Conductive deafness typically causes partial hearing loss and only rarely total loss. Lesions of the cochlear nerve or the receptors cause complete deafness. Unilateral deafness is difficult to recognize clinically without electrophysiologic tests. Central lesions rarely cause clinically detectable hearing loss. Tests for hearing are discussed in Chapter 4.

Cranial Nerve IX (Glossopharyngeal Nerve), Cranial Nerve X (Vagus Nerve), and Cranial Nerve XI (Accessory Nerve)

Anatomy

These cranial nerves are discussed as a group because their nerve fibers originate from the same medullary nuclei and because they interact to control pharyngeal and laryngeal motor activity. They originate in the nucleus ambiguus in the medulla. The rostral two thirds of this nucleus are involved in swallowing by means of motor impulses through the glossopharyngeal and vagus nerves. The caudal nucleus ambiguus controls the laryngeal and esophageal muscles through the accessory and vagus nerves and branches of the vagus nerves (recurrent laryngeal nerves). These nerves enter the jugular foramen from within the cranial cavity and emerge from the calvaria through the tympano-occipital fissure.

Clinical Signs

Dysphagia is the primary clinical sign of lesions involving the rostral nucleus ambiguus or its nerves (glossopharyngeal, vagus). The gag reflex is absent or depressed. Inspiratory dyspnea from laryngeal paralysis is the primary clinical sign of lesions involving the caudal nucleus ambiguus or its nerves (vagus, recurrent laryngeal). Regurgitation may occur as a result of megaesophagus.

Cranial Nerve XII (Hypoglossal Nerve)

Anatomy

This nerve originates from cell bodies in the medulla, exits the medulla just caudal to the accessory nerve through the hypoglossal foramen of the calvaria, and innervates the intrinsic and extrinsic muscles of the tongue.

Clinical Signs

With bilateral lesions, paresis or paralysis of the tongue is the main clinical sign. Affected animals have difficulty with the oral phase of swallowing (see later discussion). Affected animals may also have difficulty with prehension of food or water. With unilateral lesions, clinical signs may be inapparent. When protruded, the tongue will deviate toward the affected side as a result of denervation atrophy and contracture of the tongue muscles. Often the affected side of the tongue takes on a wrinkled appearance (Figure 9-6).

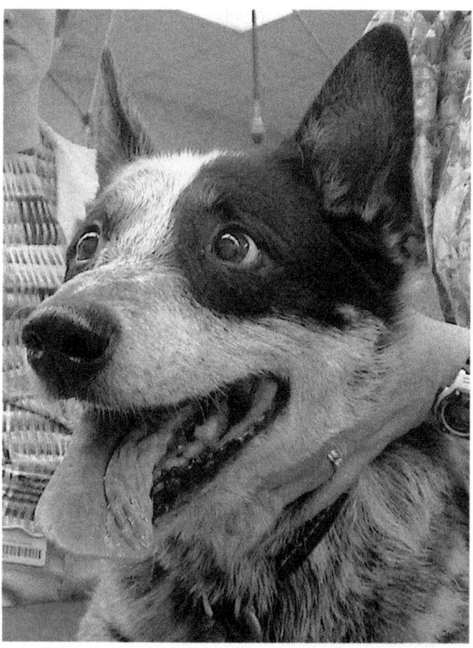

Figure 9-6 Dog with unilateral lesions. When protruded, the tongue will deviate toward the affected side as a result of denervation atrophy and contracture of the tongue muscles. Note the wrinkled appearance. (Copyright 2010 University of Georgia Research Foundation, Inc.)

DISEASES

Bilateral Trigeminal Nerve Lesions

Idiopathic trigeminal neuropathy that results in acute bilateral paralysis of the masticatory muscles has been observed in dogs and cats.[5,6] Although clinical signs often reflect mandibular nerve dysfunction, concurrent sensory deficits have been noted in approximately 35% of affected dogs.[6] Extensive bilateral, nonsuppurative inflammation, demyelination, and some axonal degeneration of all portions of the trigeminal nerve and the ganglion, with no brainstem lesions, have been observed at necropsy.[4] Rarely, sensory deficits isolated to the areas of cutaneous innervation of all the branches of the trigeminal nerve without motor deficits have been observed.[7] Axonal loss in all branches of the trigeminal nerve, in the brainstem in the spinal tract of the trigeminal nerve, and trigeminal ganglion was seen at necropsy. Panciera et al[8] reported a case of polyradiculoganglioneuritis in a 9-year-old Airedale terrier with left-sided Horner's syndrome and left-sided atrophy of the masticatory muscles. Extensive nonsuppurative inflammation was identified in the preganglionic and postganglionic segments of the trigeminal nerve along with scattered degenerative neurons in the motor nucleus of the trigeminal nerve. The lesions were more severe on the left side. Horner's syndrome likely occurred due to the close anatomic relationship of the ocular sympathetics with the inflamed left trigeminal nerve. In addition, less intense inflammatory lesions were identified in spinal nerve roots and in sciatic and radial nerves, consistent with polyradiculoneuritis and ganglionitis. The nature of the inflammatory response supports the notion that the lesions were immune-mediated.

Importantly, idiopathic trigeminal neuropathy must be differentiated from other causes of bilateral trigeminal dysfunction. Occasionally, hematopoietic neoplasms such as lymphoma and myelomonocytic leukemia can involve the trigeminal nerves bilaterally.[9,10] Signs may be limited to involvement of the trigeminal nerves or may involve other cranial nerves. Occasionally, head trauma can result in bilateral trigeminal paralysis without signs indicative of brainstem injury, suggesting trauma to the mandibular nerves.

Clinical Signs

The onset of clinical signs is acute or subacute. The jaw hangs open (drop jaw), and the mouth cannot be closed voluntarily. The dog cannot grasp food and has difficulty drinking water. Mild dysphagia may be present. Dehydration and drooling are associated signs. Facial hypalgesia or analgesia may be noted.[6] Corneal ulcerations also can occur. Horner's syndrome is seen in some dogs.[6] Affected dogs are alert and responsive and have no other detectable neurologic deficits. The clinical signs are suggestive of brainstem paralysis, which is observed with rabies. Until sufficient evidence has been found to exclude rabies, clinicians should be extremely careful when examining these dogs.

Diagnosis

A diagnosis of idiopathic trigeminal neuropathy is based on the clinical signs, the absence of signs indicative of brainstem disease, and exclusion of other causes. Cerebrospinal fluid (CSF) analysis may reveal a mild to moderate elevation in protein with a mild lymphocytic and monocytic pleocytosis.[6] EMG abnormalities may be observed in the muscles of mastication. Bilateral enlargement of the trigeminal nerves has been observed on magnetic resonance imaging (MRI). The affected trigeminal nerves were hypointense on T-1 weighted (T1W) and had a mixed intensity on T-2 weighted (T2W) images and demonstrated variable contrast enhancement.[11] The disease should not be confused with masticatory myositis. In the latter disease, the mouth is closed, and the animal resents having its jaw moved or manipulated. Pain may be associated with muscle palpation in animals in the acute phase of masticatory myositis.

Treatment

No definitive treatment is available. Corticosteroids do not seem to hasten recovery. Affected animals should be given fluid therapy and enteral caloric support. Esophagotomy or gastrotomy tubes may be beneficial. The clinician should exercise caution to prevent aspiration pneumonia, especially in dysphagic animals. Performing frequent physical therapy by opening and closing the mouth helps to delay muscle atrophy. Recovery is usually complete in 2 to 3 weeks. Multiple episodes may occur in the same dog. The prognosis is good.

Unilateral Trigeminal Nerve Lesions

Neoplasia affecting the trigeminal nerve produces progressive ipsilateral atrophy of the masticatory muscles.[12] Ipsilateral alterations in facial sensation may also be present. Affected dogs tend to be older and are usually presented for examination because of profound unilateral atrophy of the temporalis and masseter muscles. MRI is the best imaging modality to identify lesions involving the trigeminal nerve or brainstem[11,12] (Figure 9-7). However, caution should be exercised when interpreting trigeminal nerve lesions on MRI because the normal trigeminal nerves and ganglia enhance with contrast administration, whereas elsewhere contrast enhancement often suggests pathology.[13] Computed tomography (CT) can also be used but is less sensitive. Most commonly, lesions are found in the proximal trigeminal nerve extending into the adjacent brainstem or in the trigeminal ganglion (Figure 9-8). Nerve sheath tumors and meningiomas are the most common tumors causing this syndrome. Surgical resection of the neoplastic process has been reported.[12] Most affected animals are treated palliatively with corticosteroids to reduce tumoral edema. Alternatively, radiation therapy may be considered in affected animals.

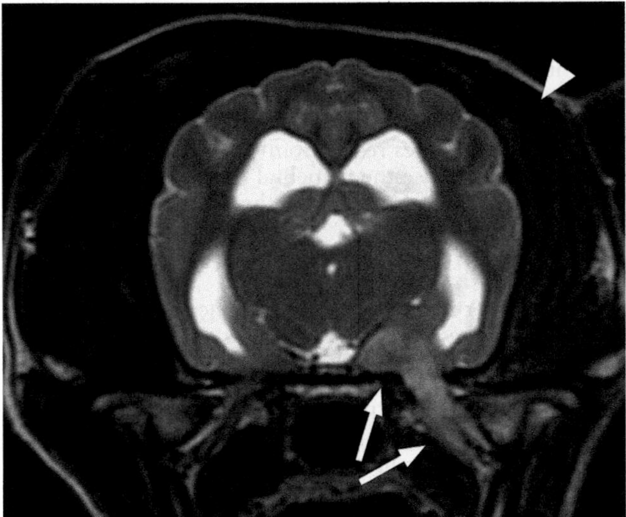

Figure 9-7 A transverse plane T2W MRI of the brain of a dog with a suspected nerve sheath tumor of cranial nerve V. The affected nerve is enlarged and hyperintense *(arrows)*. Note the atrophy of the left temporalis muscle *(arrow head)*. (Copyright 2010 University of Georgia Research Foundation, Inc.)

Recently, Palmer reported a dog with ischemic infarction affecting the motor nucleus of the trigeminal nerve and corticospinal tracts.[14] The affected dog developed unilateral atrophy of the masticatory muscles and hemiparesis secondary to damage of the motor nucleus of the trigeminal nerve and corticospinal tracts, respectively.

Abnormal Facial Sensation

Hyperesthesia of the face is a common problem in humans but is rarely observed in animals. Orofacial pain has been reported in cats, particular the Burmese cat.[15] Apparently self-inflicted excoriations were observed on the face. Nonsuppurative meningoencephalitis that involved the trigeminal nerve and ganglion was found on necropsy. Hypesthesia (reduced sensation) is seen with many causes of trigeminal nerve disorders.

Facial Paralysis

The most common disease that produces facial nerve injury is otitis media/otitis interna (see Chapter 8). Polyneuropathies also can affect the facial nerve (see Chapter 7).

Idiopathic Facial Paralysis

This idiopathic disease occurs in the absence of otitis media/interna. The clinical signs are similar to those of human facial neuritis (Bell's palsy), the cause of which often is not known.[16] In people, many cases are caused by viral inflammation, with herpes zoster and herpes simplex viruses suspected. Swelling of the nerve in the petrosal bone causes compression and ischemia, presumably leading to degenerative change.

In a study of 95 cases of facial paralysis in dogs and cats, the condition was judged idiopathic because of lack of any other findings in 75% of dogs and 25% of cats.[17] Otitis media/interna was the most frequently associated disease in dogs. Hypothyroidism was found in some.[18] In dogs, the cocker spaniel has an increased incidence of facial paralysis.[17,19] Cocker spaniels are also at greater risk of otitis media or interna than is the

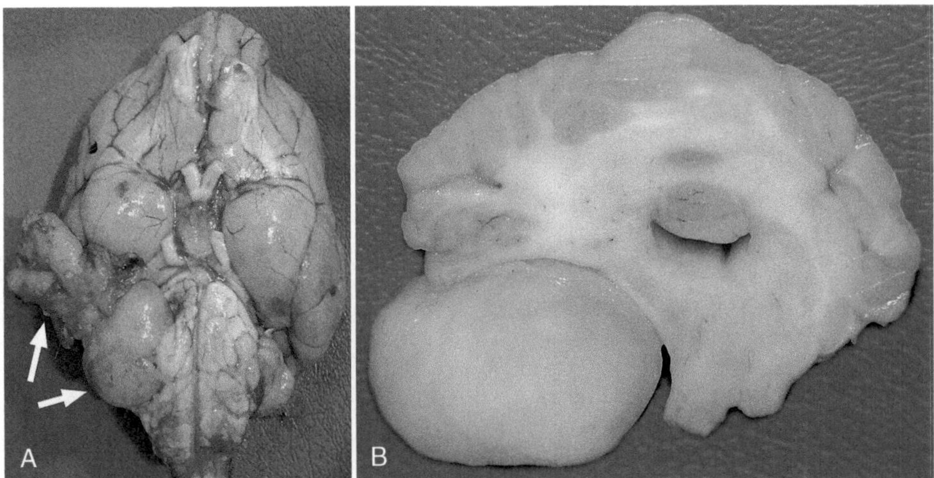

Figure 9-8 **A,** Ventral gross image of a West highland white terrier with a nerve sheath tumor involving cranial nerve V. The lesion extends into and compresses the pons and medulla oblongata **B,** Transverse section of the brain from **A.** The mass is compressing the medulla oblongata. (Copyright 2010 University of Georgia Research Foundation, Inc.)

general canine population. Biopsy of facial nerves in two cases showed nerve fiber degeneration and loss of large-diameter myelinated fibers.[19]

Clinical Signs. Paralysis of the muscles of facial expression usually occurs acutely, is unilateral, and is not associated with vestibular disease or otitis media/interna (Figure 9-9). Affected animals are afebrile and have no systemic signs of illness. The course is variable; however, the clinical signs are maximal in 7 days. Recovery takes 3 to 6 weeks. Exposure keratitis occurs commonly because of improper lubrication of the cornea. The contralateral nerve may become involved subsequently.[19]

Diagnosis. The diagnosis is made by exclusion of other diseases that can affect the facial nerve. As otitis media or interna are the most common problems, a thorough otoscopic examination and imaging of the bulla should be performed. MRI is the imaging modality of choice. Enhancement of the facial nerve through its course in the temporal bone has been observed in idiopathic facial paralysis.[20] In addition to exclusion of other diseases, the benefit of MRI is that the extent of enhancement of the facial nerve within the temporal bone may be prognostic. Dogs with no enhancement recover more quickly than those with enhancement of a single segment of the facial nerve. Dogs with extensive enhancement may not recover. Additionally, hypothyroidism may be associated with facial paralysis; thyroid function should be critically evaluated.[21] Electromyography of the face and other muscles helps to exclude polyneuropathy.

Treatment. No specific treatment is known. The prognosis for recovery, with or without therapy, is good. If tear production is decreased, artificial tears should be prescribed.

Hemifacial Spasm (Constant Contraction of the Muscles of Facial Expression)

Hemifacial spasm is rarely observed in dogs or cats (Figure 9-10). The condition represents tetany of the facial musculature. Signs include blepharospasm, elevation of the ear, deviation of the nose to the affected side, and wrinkling or displacement of the upper lip. In humans, hemifacial spasm occurs most commonly as a result of compression of the facial nerve at its exit from the medulla by an ectopic or aberrant vessel in the caudal cranial fossa (posterior inferior cerebellar artery). [22] Neurovascular compression may lead to demyelination ultimately resulting in ectopic discharges within the facial nerve.[23] Concurrent hypertension may also play a role.[24] Hemifacial spasms have been reported in dogs with otitis media/interna and presumed facial neuritis and a degenerative lesion of the medulla.[25,26] Ipsilateral Horner's syndrome has been reported concurrently.[25] This condition may precede signs of facial paralysis. Hemifacial spasm has been reported as a consequence of intracranial disease in two dogs.[27] Presumptive neoplastic lesions were observed in the caudal cranial fossa in one dog and middle cranial fossa in the other dog. Although speculative, the lesion in the caudal cranial fossa was proposed to be exciting the facial motor nucleus directly. The lesion in the middle cranial fossa was thought to have resulted in an increased excitement from a lack of UMN inhibition. Hemifacial spasm in this instance occurred as a sign of UMN dysfunction. Lesions that isolate the facial nuclear motor neurons from UMN control can result in hemifacial spasm as a result of the loss of inhibitory interneuronal activity. The palpebral reflex may be hyperactive in that spasm of the eyelids may be observed when the reflex is elicited. This form of hemifacial spasm is associated with other signs of brainstem dysfunction. In humans, CT and MRI play a role in the diagnosis.[28] Treatment in humans consists of medical therapy and surgical microvascular decompression.[29] Hemifacial spasm must be differentiated from contractures secondary to denervation. Muscular contractures result from denervation atrophy and fibrosis, in which case the palpebral reflex should be absent. The diagnosis and treatment are the same as described for facial nerve paralysis.

Facial Nerve Trauma

Injury to one or more branches of the facial nerve can occur in all species. The most common causes are recumbency during anesthesia and tight halters in large animals.[3,30] Closed injury to the facial nerve causes varying degrees of neurapraxia and axonotmesis (Figure 9-11). Clinical signs caused by neurapraxia usually improve in 2 weeks or less. Axonotmesis requires regrowth of the axon from the site of injury at an approximate rate of 1 mm per day.

Temporohyoid Osteoarthropathy

Temporohyoid osteoarthropathy is a condition in middle-aged horses in which there is a proliferative osteoarthropathy and ankylosis of the temporohyoid joint. Although both sides are typically affected, clinical signs typically relate to unilateral neurologic signs.[31-33] The pathogenesis of the condition

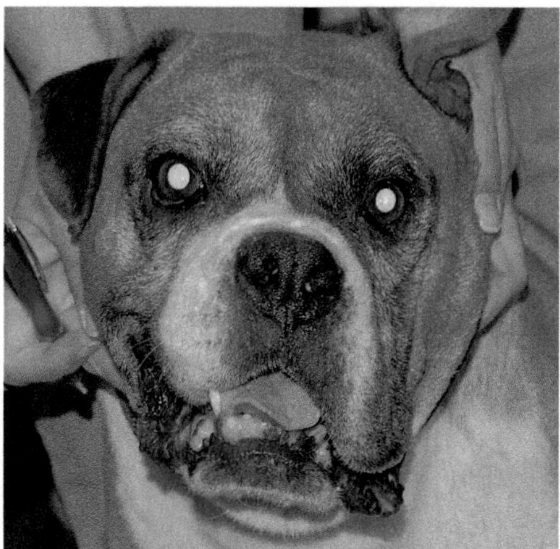

Figure 9-9 Facial paralysis in a boxer dog. Note the drooping left upper and lower lip. The left eye has slight ectropion of the ventral eyelid. (Copyright 2010 University of Georgia Research Foundation, Inc.)

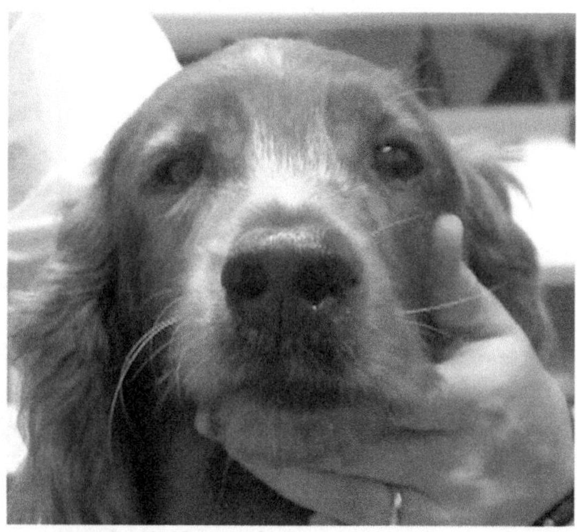

Figure 9-10 Hemifacial spasm in a dog. Note the deviation of the nose to the affected side, and displacement of the upper lip. (Copyright 2010 University of Georgia Research Foundation, Inc.)

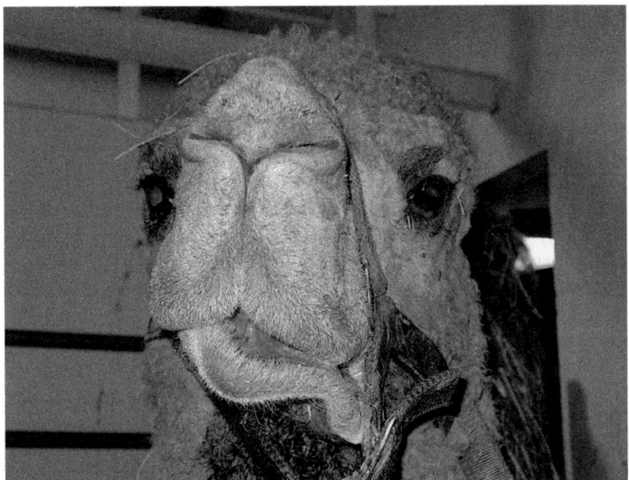

Figure 9-11 Injury to one or more branches of the facial nerve can occur in all species. A traumatic facial paralysis on the left side occurred during restraint. Neuropraxia was suspected because recovery occurred 10 days later.

remains unknown; however, both traumatic and infectious etiologies have been proposed.[34,35] With behaviors such as forced head jerking, falling, teeth floating, nasogastric intubation, and vocalization, acute fractures of the petrous temporal bone can occur, resulting in acute onset of vestibular and facial nerve dysfunction.[32,35] Presumptive diagnosis is made through a combination of typical signalment, history, and signs of CN VII and VIII dysfunction. Hearing may also be affected based on brainstem auditory evoked response (BAER) testing.[36] Rarely CN IX and X also may be involved. The diagnosis is established with endoscopic evaluation of the guttural pouch during which visualization of an enlarged proximal stylohyoid bone is detected.[32,35] Radiography may also be used in the diagnosis. Cross-sectional imaging using CT has also been used to establish a diagnosis.[37] Both medical and surgical therapies exist for the treatment of temporohyoid osteoarthropathy. Medical therapy involves supportive care and antiinflammatories. Partial stylohyoid ostectomy can be performed in an attempt to prevent recurrence. In one study of 33 affected horses, 70% returned to prior usage, which in some cases required up to 2 years before maximal improvement was achieved.[32] Despite this, many horses continued to have neurologic deficits.

Deafness

Most of the information on deafness in animals relates to cats and dogs. Deafness can be acquired or congenital.

Acquired Deafness

Older animals often have some degree of hearing loss. Loss of cells in the spiral ganglion appears to be the primary cause.[38] Attempts have been made to fit dogs with hearing aids, but training dogs to wear them is difficult.

Some polyneuropathies, especially that of hypothyroidism, affect the cochlear nerve.[18] Severe hypoxia may also cause damage to the cochlear nerve or receptors. Neoplasms and trauma may cause deafness in rare cases. Toxic agents and drugs cause progressive cochlear damage (see Table 8-2). Common agents include aminoglycoside antibiotics, salicylates, loop diuretics such as furosemide, and topically applied antiseptics such as chlorhexidine and cetrimide.[39] Severe middle ear infections may cause conduction problems, but toxins that reach the inner ear may produce receptor or nerve degeneration.

TABLE 9-1

Hereditary Deafness in Animals and Associated References

Breed	Reference
Canine	
Akita	54
American Staffordshire terrier	54
Australian heeler	47
Australian shepherd	47, 49
Beagle	78
Border collie	49
Boston terrier	47
Boxer	47
Bull terrier	49
Catahoula	54
Cocker spaniel	47
Collie	46, 51
Dalmatian	48-52, 54, 68, 71-77, 83, 84
Dappled dachshund	54
Doberman pinscher	56, 57
Dogo Argentino	44, 54
English bulldog	47
English setter	47, 53
Fox terrier	45
Great Dane	46
Great Pyrenees	43, 54
Jack Russell terrier	58
Maltese	54
Miniature poodle	54
Mongrel	54
Norwegian dunkerhound	54, 78
Old English sheepdog	47
Papillon	54
Pointer	41
Rhodesian ridgeback	54
Rottweiler	42
Scottish terrier	45
Sealyham terrier	45
Shetland sheepdog	49
Shropshire terrier	49
Walker foxhound	40
West Highland white terrier	54
Numerous other breeds	78
Feline	
White, blue eyes	59-65,69, 85-88
Horse	67
Llama, alpaca	66

Modified from Oliver JE: Deafness. In Lorenz MD, Cornelius LM, editors: Small animal medical diagnosis, ed 2, Philadelphia, 1993, JB Lippincott.

Congenital Sensorineural Deafness

Congenital sensorineural deafness occurs in the dog,[40-58] cat,[59-65] llama,[66] alpaca,[66] and horse[67] (Table 9-1). Congenital sensorineural deafness typically is the result of a defect in the end organ (hair cells of the organ of Corti). Pathology solely affecting the hair cells has been observed in the Doberman.[57] Affected pups display concurrent signs of vestibular dysfunction. An autosomal recessive pattern of inheritance is suggested. Likewise, lesions restricted to the organ of Corti and spiral ganglion have been observed in a deaf rottweiler pup.[42] More commonly, congenital sensorineural deafness occurs as a consequence of degeneration of the stria vascularis and secondary loss of neuroepithelial structures known as cochlea-saccular degeneration (Scheibe type). The stria vascularis is the main vascular supply to the cochlea and is responsible for endolymph production needed for maintenance of the health and function of the hair cells. Degeneration of the stria vascularis results in collapse of Reissner's membrane, and ultimately degeneration of hair cells of the organ of Corti.[50,68] Loss of neurons in the spiral ganglion also occurs.[50,68] An association with pigmentation, coat color, and iris color has been made in affected small and large animals. This has been most extensively studied in the Dalmatian dog and white cat.[61,69] Normally, melanocytes are found in the stria vascularis. Although their exact role is unknown, melanocytes are necessary to maintain a normal electrical potential through K^+ ions in the endolymph, which is essential for the health of the stria vascularis.[70] An absence of melanocytes has been observed in deaf Dalmatian dogs.[50,68] Interestingly, albinism is not associated with deafness. In albinism, melanocytes are present but unable to produce melanin yet otherwise are functional in the stria vascularis. In deaf Dalmatian pups, the inner ear structures are normal from birth up to 1 to 4 weeks of age at which time the degeneration of the stria vascularis occurs.[50,68] In general, the earliest development of deafness occurs at 4 weeks of age. However, in some dogs, deafness may not develop until 16 weeks of age.[48,51,68,71] Deafness may be unilateral or bilateral. The prevalence of deafness in Dalmatians ranges from 16% to 29%, with 21% unilaterally and 7% bilaterally affected.[72-77]

In Dalmatian dogs, two genes play a role in coat color: the S gene (S), which determines the distribution of pigmented and nonpigmented areas, and the merle gene (M). Both genes have been associated with deafness.[78] Homozygosity for the merle gene (MM) results in an almost white animal with an association for deafness, blindness, and microophthalmia.[79] The S gene has 4 alleles, S (nonspotted), s^i (Irish spotting), s^p(piebald), and s^w(extreme piebald). While several specific genes have been investigated, the exact genetic locus or loci involved in deafness has not been identified.[80-82] Congenital sensorineural deafness in Dalmatians has been associated with both the mm and S genes.[76] The coat color of Dalmatians is determined by the expression of the extreme recessive allele of the piebald gene (s^w, s^w) creating the white coat combined with the a dominant flecking and ticking gene with alleles for either black (B) or brown (b) spot or rarely lemon (ee) or tricolor (a^ta^t) spots.[73] Weak expression of the piebald gene results in patches. Dogs with patches are more likely to have normal hearing.[74] True patches must be differentiated from coalescence of spots. Normally, Dalmatian pups are born all white and later develop spots. True patches are present at birth. In Dalmatians, blue irises are a strong indication of expression of the extreme piebald allele (s^w, s^w) of the S gene. Consequently, Dalmatians with blue irises have a greater prevalence of deafness than those with brown irises.[83,84] In contrast, blue irises are not associated with deafness in dogs with merle coat color.[79] Although the exact mode of inheritance of congenital sensorineural deafness in Dalmatian dogs is unknown, deafness is thought to be a polygenic trait in which a single locus provides a major contribution to hearing.[76,83]

Other dog breeds associated with the piebald allele include bull terriers, English setters, and Dogo Argentinos. Dogs with the merle pattern coat color include the collie, Australian shepherd, Shetland sheepdog, border collie, catahoula leopard dog, Cardigan Welsh corgi, dachshund, and Great Dane breeds, and less commonly the Old English sheepdog and American cocker spaniel.

In cats, a high prevalence of deafness is observed in white cats with blue irises.[85,86] In cats, the white gene (W) is autosomal dominant over color. Often, blue irises are present in white cats. Seventeen registered cat breeds carry the W gene.[65] Like deaf Dalmatian dogs, deaf white cats are born with normal cochlear anatomy with degeneration beginning on postnatal day 5 and rapidly progressing to complete degeneration of the organ of Corti by postnatal day 21. Whereas the typical pathologic changes in deaf cats are similar to those observed in deaf Dalmatian dogs, a second type of pathology also has been observed.[87] In this form, there was hypertrophy of the Reissner's membrane, the supporting cells of the organ of Corti, and the epithelial cells of the basilar membrane, which filled the scala media obscuring the stria vascularis and affecting the differentiation of the hair cells. The overall prevalence of deafness in client-owned pure-bred cats is approximately 20%.[65] The prevalence in experimental colonies of cats is much greater.[65,85,86] The exact mode of inheritance is unknown. It is unlikely that a pleiotropic effect (one gene with several phenotypes) of one major gene is responsible for deafness in white cats with blue irises.[88]

Clinically, bilaterally deaf animals demonstrate a decreased behavioral response to noise such as turning, looking, or moving their ears in relation to sounds. Affected animals are also more difficult to rouse from sleep. However, they are normal in all other regards. Unilaterally deaf animals are difficult to detect. Consequently, determination of hearing should not be made based on a behavioral response to noise. BAER testing is a reliable and effective method of evaluation of hearing. Importantly, the BAER can be used to determine unilateral deafness. The presence of a normal BAER does not exclude deafness because a lesion may affect neuroanatomic structures involved in hearing (i.e., medial geniculate nuclei and temporal lobes of the cerebrum) that are not evaluated with the BAER. However, given the site of pathology involved in congenital sensorineural deafness, an absent BAER is diagnostic for deafness in most dogs with congenital deafness. Thorough screening of breeding animals from breeds associated with congenital sensorineural deafness should be performed to eliminate affected animals from breeding stocks. Dogs can be tested with BAER at about 5 to 6 weeks of age. The BAER is normally not present until 3 weeks of age. No treatment is available for congenital sensorineural deafness.

Laryngeal Paralysis

Unilateral and bilateral paresis or paralysis of the laryngeal muscles has been reported in dogs, cats, and horses. Unilateral paralysis results in moderate inspiratory dyspnea and inspiratory noise. Bilateral paralysis leads to episodes of gagging, cyanosis, severe inspiratory dyspnea, and collapse. The intrinsic muscles of the larynx are innervated by the recurrent laryngeal nerve, which consists of branches of the vagus nerve. The neurons that give rise to the vagus are located in the caudal portion of the nucleus ambiguus. These neurons are topographically oriented with those involved in adductors of the larynx residing dorsally and those involved in abduction of the larynx residing ventrally in the nucleus ambiguus.[89] Injury to these nerve fibers or their cell bodies in the caudal nucleus ambiguus results in the clinical signs.

The diagnosis of laryngeal paralysis is relatively straightforward and is based on the observation of the larynx during all phases of respiration. Normally, the vocal cords and arytenoid cartilage abducts during inspiration. The observation of the vocal cords and arytenoids displaying inadequate abduction during inspiration or remaining in a paramedian position is consistent with a diagnosis of laryngeal paresis or paralysis, respectively. Paradoxical movement of the vocal cords can occur in animals with pronounced inspiratory effort giving the false impression of motion. Consequently, an assistant should aid in evaluation by telling the examiner when the animal inhales and exhales. Observation of laryngeal function in dogs and cats is performed by direct visualization per os. Alternatively, transnasal laryngoscopy has been performed in dogs.[90] Transnasal laryngoscopy is commonly performed in horses.[91,92] Ultrasonographic evaluation of laryngeal function has also been performed in dogs and cats.[93,94] In dogs and cats, laryngeal examination is performed under sedation or a light plane of anesthesia. The depth of anesthesia and choice of anesthetics are critical for proper evaluation. For dogs and cats, acceptable sedatives include acepromazine and butorphanol.[95] Acceptable anesthetics include ketamine alone or in combination with diazepam, thiopental, or propofol.[95] Doxapram, a centrally acting respiratory stimulant, may aid in the diagnosis of laryngeal paralysis in dogs by increasing the respiratory effect and possibly increasing arytenoid cartilage movements.[96,97]

Dogs

Congenital and acquired forms of laryngeal paralysis have been described in dogs. The acquired form of laryngeal paralysis occurs as part of a generalized polyneuropathy or myopathy.[98] Alternatively, laryngeal paralysis may occur in the absence of other neurologic clinical signs in which it is often referred to as idiopathic laryngeal paralysis. Congenital causes accounted for 21% and 30% of the cases reported in two studies.[99,100]

Congenital Laryngeal Paralysis. Congenital laryngeal paralysis most often occurs in conjunction with more diffuse signs of neuromuscular disease (see Chapter 7). Rarely, congenital laryngeal paralysis occurs in isolation.

Bouvier des Flanders. Congential laryngeal paralysis in Bouvier des Flandres dogs is inherited as an autosomal dominant trait and results in unilateral or bilaterally laryngeal paralysis.[101,102] In a study of 105 affected Bouvier dogs, the dogs ranged in age from 4 months to 7 years of age with most affected dogs being 4 to 8 months of age. The onset of clinical signs occurs between 4 months and 6 months of age. Laryngeal examination revealed bilateral laryngeal paralysis in 28 dogs and unilaterally laryngeal paralysis in 71 dogs with the affected side always being the left. Three dogs displayed slight motion of both arytenoids, whereas three dogs displayed normal abduction. In the three dogs with normal abduction, abnormal adduction was identified. Three dogs also had pelvic limb weakness consistent with neuromuscular disease. Electromyography of the larynx was consistent with denervation of at least one muscle group of the larynx. In many dogs, both normal motor unit potentials and abnormal denervation potentials were identified. Electrophysiologic abnormalities were present as early as 8 weeks of age. Histologic evaluation of the many of the intrinsic laryngeal muscles including the cricoarytenoideus muscle was consistent with denervation atrophy. Evaluation of the recurrent laryngeal nerves revealed wallerian degeneration. Degeneration of the neurons of the nucleus ambiguous also was observed.[103]

Siberian Husky and Siberian Husky–Alaskan Malamute Crosses. Laryngeal paralysis has been observed in Siberian husky dogs and husky crosses.[104,105] Affected pups were under 6 months of age with some pups demonstrating clinical signs at 4 to 8 weeks of age. Bilateral and left-sided unilateral laryngeal paralysis was observed. Like the Bouvier, degeneration and loss of neurons in the nucleus ambiguus were observed. Peripheral nerves, including the recurrent laryngeal nerves were normal.

White German Shepherds. Four all-white German shepherds with a presumed congenital form of laryngeal paralysis have been reported.[106] Affected dogs ranged in age from 9 months to 2 years. The earliest age of onset of inspiratory stridor was 5 months of age, whereas exercise intolerance was noted at 3 months of age in one dog. Concurrent megaesophagus was present in one dog. None of the dogs had other signs of neuromuscular disease.

Rottweilers. Three neurologic diseases—laryngeal paralysis-polyneuropathy complex (LPPC), neuronal vacuolation, and neuroaxonal dystrophy have been associated with laryngeal paralysis in young rottweilers.[107-109] Affected dogs with LPPC were presented between 11 and 16 weeks of age.[109] The dogs were evaluated primarily for inspiratory stridor; however, mild to moderate tetraparesis, delayed postural reactions, and reduced spinal reflexes also were observed. The onset of clinical signs occurred between 9 and 13 weeks of age. Megaesophagus was observed in one dog with regurgitation. Most of the affected pups also had lenticular cataracts. One pup had sensorineural deafness based on an absent potentials with BAER testing. Electrophysiology consistent with denervation potentials was identified in the appendicular musculature and intrinsic laryngeal musculature along with decreased compound muscle action potentials (CMAPs) with direct nerve stimulation studies. Histologic lesions were consistent with neurogenic atrophy of appendicular and intrinsic laryngeal muscles secondary to axonal degeneration of peripheral nerves, including the recurrent laryngeal nerves. Abnormalities were more severe distally consistent with a distal peripheral neuropathy.

Laryngeal paralysis has also been observed in conjunction with neuronal vacuolation and spinocerebellar tract degeneration in rottweiler dogs.[108] Affected dogs displayed subtle tetraparesis and general proprioceptive ataxia. Over several weeks, progressive weakness and inspiratory stridor were observed. Histologically, vacuolation was observed in neurons of the cerebral cortex and in nuclei of the thalamus, midbrain, cerebellum, medulla oblongata, and spinal cord gray matter. Additionally, axonal necrosis of the dorsolateral and ventromedial white matter of the spinal cord was observed. In the peripheral nervous system, neuronal vacuolation occurred in the spinal ganglia. Denervation atrophy was observed in the intrinsic laryngeal muscles and axonal degeneration predominantly affecting the distal aspect of the large caliber, myelinated axons of the recurrent laryngeal nerves were observed.[110,111] Muscles innervated by the cranial laryngeal nerves (cricothyroideus and thyrohyoideus) were normal. Findings were consistent with a dying-back neuropathy. Similar clinicopathologic findings were observed in a mixed-breed dog.[112] An analogous clinicopathologic syndrome has been observed in two, 6-month old boxer puppies.[113] The dogs displayed progressive pelvic limb paresis and ataxia, upper airway stridor, and visual deficits. Neurologic findings were consistent with a combined myelopathy and neuropathy. Interestingly, the dogs also had ocular abnormalities including microphthalmia, cataracts, and retinal dysplasia.

Dalmatian Dogs. Laryngeal paralysis polyneuropathy complex has been reported in Dalmatian dogs.[114] The condition was presumed to be an autosomal recessive trait. The age of onset of clinical signs ranged from 2 months to 6 months of age. One dog was 12 months old at the time of onset of clinical signs. Along with typical signs of laryngeal paralysis, some dogs had laryngeal spasms necessitating emergency treatment. Almost all affected dogs had concurrent neurologic deficits consisting of megaesophagus and generalized neuromuscular signs. The onset of other neurologic signs preceded, occurred simultaneously, or after the development of laryngeal paralysis. Histologic evaluation revealed denervation atrophy of the laryngeal and appendicular muscles along with axonal degeneration of recurrent laryngeal nerve and nerves of the and appendicular musculature. The distal appendicular muscles and nerves, specifically large, myelinated axons, were preferentially affected. Prognosis was grave. Most affected dogs die from or are euthanized for aspiration pneumonia.

Pyrenean Dogs. Laryngeal paralysis has been observed in Pyrenean mountain dogs.[115] Affected dogs were between 2½ and 6 months of age. Affected dogs also displayed generalized weakness and regurgitation. Bilateral and left unilateral laryngeal paralysis were observed. Electrophysiology disclosed reduced CMAP with mild reduction in nerve conduction velocity consistent with an axonopathy. An autosomal pattern of inheritance was suspected.

Acquired Laryngeal Paralysis. Laryngeal paralysis has been associated with chronic polyneuropathy (see Chapter 7), injury to the vagus nerve during neck surgery, lead and organophosphate toxicity, and retropharyngeal infection.[99,116,117]

Middle-aged to older large and giant-breed dogs, specifically the Labrador retriever, are most commonly affected. Males may be predisposed. In one study, 25% of all dogs undergoing general anesthesia had some degree of laryngeal paresis based on examination via laryngoscopy.[118] However, only 5% of dogs had clinical signs of respiratory obstruction related to laryngeal paralysis.[118] In addition to respiratory signs related to laryngeal paralysis, affected dogs often cough or gag when eating. Exercise intolerance is common. Importantly, affected dogs should be carefully evaluated for other neurologic deficits. Acquired laryngeal paralysis may be the most prominent or sole clinical manifestation of an underlying generalized neuromuscular disorder.[98,117] Based on neurologic deficits and electrophysiology, concurrent neuromuscular signs are likely related to a distal axonopathy, which may be progressive.[98] Hypothyroidism may cause polyneuropathy with concurrent laryngeal paralysis.[18] Dogs without an identifiable underlying neuromuscular disease are classified as idiopathic laryngeal paralysis.

Severely affected dogs are treated by surgical correction aimed at enlarging the rim glottis without altering the ability to close the glottis during swallowing. There are a variety of surgical techniques.[100,119-125] In general, unilateral arytenoid cartilage lateralization is preferred over bilateral arytenoid lateralization or partial laryngotomy. Postoperatively, most dogs experience improvement or resolution of clinical signs.[119,120,122,126] Aspiration pneumonia is the most common complication associated with surgical correction of laryngeal paralysis.[119,120,122,126,127] In one study, dogs with underlying neurologic disease were significantly more likely to experience complications with surgical correction and suffer a higher mortality rate.[120] Likewise, dogs having had bilateral arytenoid lateralization had a greater incidence of complications and mortality than dogs having undergone unilateral arytenoid lateralization or partial laryngectomy.[120] Dogs weighing less than 10 kg may be less likely to improve postoperatively.[126] Dogs may have a lifelong risk for respiratory complications.

Cats

Laryngeal paralysis is uncommon in cats as compared with dogs and horses. Laryngeal paralysis in cats does not have a sex or breed predilection. Reported causes of laryngeal paralysis include iatrogenic trauma to the vagus or recurrent laryngeal nerves related to thyroidectomy, surgical correction of patent ductus arteriosus and perineural injection of irritating chemicals, along with neuromuscular disease, neoplasia, and idiopathic Laryngeal paralysis.[128-132] Tumors may invade or compress the vagus or recurrent laryngeal nerve anywhere along its course. Laryngeal paralysis has been associated with tumors involving the osseous bulla, which may compress the vagus nerve exiting the tympano-occipital fissure.[133] In one cat, lymphoma was found infiltrating the cervical portion of the vagus nerve.[134] In another cat, pulmonary squamous cell carcinoma had affected the vagus resulting in laryngeal paralysis.[135] Unlike dogs, idiopathic laryngeal paralysis affects cats of all ages.[93,128-131] Idiopathic laryngeal paralysis in young cats (<2 years of age) is speculated to be congenital, although definitive documentation is lacking.[93,128-130,136] Cats with unilateral laryngeal paralysis in which respiratory signs are not life threatening may be treated conservatively by restricted activity and remaining indoors.[129] Surgery should be considered in bilaterally affected cats or those with severe respiratory compromise. Surgical options are similar to those in dogs.[129-131] Complications include aspiration pneumonia, laryngeal swelling, and implant failure. In a study of 16 cats, 12 with bilateral disease were treated. Of these 12 cats, 5 were treated medically because of concurrent dysphagia, megaesophagus, or laryngeal cancer. Of the 7 cats treated surgically, 2 died within 3 days after surgery, 4 had long-term successful outcomes, and 1 was lost to follow-up.[129]

Horses

There are a variety of causes of laryngeal paralysis in the horse. An underlying cause of laryngeal paralysis is found in only a small proportion of affected horses.[137,138] Isolated lesions involving structures associated along the course of the vagus and recurrent laryngeal nerve include guttural pouch disorders, pharyngeal and laryngeal disease, perineural injections of irritant drugs and trauma to the neck. As in dogs, laryngeal paralysis in horses may be a manifestation of an underlying polyneuropathy or myopathy. In such instances, laryngeal paralysis is often observed in conjunction with other signs of generalized neuromuscular dysfunction. For example, laryngeal paralysis can occur secondary to hyperkalemic periodic paresis.[139,140] Laryngeal paralysis also may occur as the result of lead or delayed organophosphate intoxication.[137,141] Bilateral laryngeal paralysis may occur with hepatic encephalopathy (HE) in the horse.[142] In such cases, laryngeal paralysis may improve with resolution of HE.[142] Postanesthetic laryngeal paralysis also has been observed.[143,144]

In most affected horses, an underlying cause is not identified, which is referred to as recurrent laryngeal neuropathy (RLN). Young, mature thoroughbred, hunter types, and draft horses are most commonly affected.[137,145] The disease tends to affect horses with a tall and long neck phenotype. Although a pattern of inheritance has not be proven, pathologic changes observed in foals suggest a hereditary basis.[146]

Pathologic changes are found primarily in the distal portion of left recurrent laryngeal nerve but also can be observed in the right recurrent laryngeal nerve.[147] Axonal degeneration with demyelination and regeneration are noted pathologically in the left and, to a lesser degree, in the right recurrent laryngeal nerves. The recurrent laryngeal nerves appear to be the only nerves affected.[147] However, nerves of the limbs and axons of the long fiber tracts of the central nervous system (CNS) may be involved in some animals.[148,149] The disease has been characterized as a distal axonopathy that preferentially affects the longest and largest fibers. Alternatively, RLN may be a dying-back neuropathy beginning distally and progressing to involve the proximal aspect of the nerve.[147] The cause of RLN remains unknown. However, a neuronal metabolic dysfunction would presumably place distal axons of longer nerves at greater risk and also explain the fact that larger horses are predisposed.

Clinical signs relate to upper airway dysfunction. Because of paralysis of the muscles innervated by the left recurrent laryngeal nerve, the vocal fold cannot be abducted during inspiration and an audible sound ("roaring") is produced. In addition to abnormal respiratory noise, affected horses demonstrate poor performance and exercise intolerance.

The diagnosis is made by observing abnormal laryngeal function with transnasal endoscopy. Affected horses are graded based on the severity of laryngeal dysfunction observed endoscopically. There are several different grading schemes used in the evaluation of RLN.[91,92,150] In horses with suspected RLN in which resting laryngeal endoscopy is normal, high-speed treadmill laryngeal endoscopy may be a more sensitive method of establishing a diagnosis.[151] Additionally, unilateral atrophy of the muscles of the larynx may be palpable.[152] Although technically challenging, electrophysiologic testing, including EMG and measurement of recurrent laryngeal nerve latency, have been used to assess laryngeal function. The thoraco-laryngeal reflex (TLR), or "slap test," has been used in the diagnosis of RLN. Slapping the horse just caudal to the withers should elicit adduction of the contralateral arytenoid cartilage. It has been used in conjunction with laryngeal endoscopy and electrophysiology but given a lack of sensitivity, this test is not considered reliable for diagnosis.[153] Surgical treatment usually is effective.[3,154,155] In Thoroughbred racing horses, performance following surgery improves but not necessarily to predisease status in older animals.[156]

Dysphagia

The process of swallowing is a complex function that requires normal anatomy and neurologic function. Abnormalities involving anatomy or neurologic function result in swallowing disorders referred to as dysphagia. Knowledge of the anatomy involved in swallowing is important to understanding the clinical signs associated with dysphagia and interpretation of diagnostic tests. Relevant anatomy includes the mouth or oral cavity, tongue, pharynx, and esophagus. The oral cavity and pharynx serve respiratory and digestive functions. The pharynx is composed of three areas, the oropharynx (area between the soft palate and base of the tongue), the nasopharynx (area between the soft palate and the ventral aspect of the calvaria extending from the choanae [rostral] to the end of the soft palate [caudal]), and the laryngopharynx (area of the pharynx dorsal to the larynx, which leads to the esophagus). The intrapharyngeal opening exists between the oropharynx and nasopharynx rostrally and the laryngopharynx caudally. At the caudal end of the laryngopharynx is the cricopharyngeus muscle, which serves as the upper esophageal sphincter (UES).

Normal swallowing has been divided into three different phases: oropharyngeal, esophageal, and gastroesophageal.[157] The oropharyngeal phase can be further subdivided into oral (prehension and formation of a food bolus), pharyngeal (movement of the food bolus to the laryngopharynx), and pharyngoesophageal (movement of the food bolus into the proximal esophagus) phases. During the oral phase, food is masticated, formed into a bolus by the tongue compressing food against the palate, and moved to the base of the tongue. During the pharyngeal phase, peristaltic waves move the food to the laryngopharynx, where during the final phase, pharyngoesophageal, the UES relaxes and the food bolus is moved into the cranial esophagus. These last two phases proceed with rapid and well-coordinated timing. Within the esophagus, primary and secondary peristaltic waves move the bolus of food to the lower esophageal sphincter (LES), which relaxes allowing the bolus to enter the stomach. Neurologically, swallowing requires normal function of CNs V, VII, IX, X, XI, and XII. The oral phase of swallowing requires the normal function of CNs V, VII, and XII for prehension, mastication, and formation of a food bolus. The pharyngeal and pharyngoesophageal phases require normal function of CNs IX, X, and XI. Normal function of the esophagus requires CN X function. Coordinated function of these motor nuclei is under control of the swallowing center located in the medulla between the facial and olivary nuclei.[158] Abnormalities in any one phase of swallowing can result in dysphagia. Consequently, swallowing disorders are classified as problems of (1) bolus formation and passage from the mouth to the cranial esophagus (oropharyngeal dysphagia), (2) passage of the bolus from the cranial esophagus to the gastroesophageal junction, (3) disturbances in passage of the bolus from the esophagus into the stomach, and (4) mixed swallowing problems.[159]

Although some clinical signs are indicative of disorders involving a specific phase of swallowing, most clinical signs are nonspecific. Dogs with oral-stage deficits commonly have a reduced ability to hold food in the mouth or transport food to the base of the tongue, whereas dogs with pharyngeal and cricopharyngeal dysfunction more commonly have a cough, have aspiration pneumonia, and make repeated unsuccessful attempts to swallow. Other clinical signs include gagging, difficulty in drinking water or forming a solid bolus, excessive mandibular or head motion, persistent forceful ineffective swallowing efforts, foaming from the mouth, salivation, nasal regurgitation, dropping food from the mouth, coughing, failure to thrive, aspiration pneumonia, and reluctance to eat.[159]

Dysphagia is a common problem in large animals and frequently results from nonneurologic disorders, such as pharyngitis, objects obstructing the esophagus ("choke"), and abscesses.[3,160,161] Likewise, structural abnormalities can result in dysphagia in dogs and cats. Importantly, the structural cause of dysphagia should be eliminated before evaluation of neurologic (functional) disorders. In general, definitive identification of the affected phase of swallowing in animals with dysphagia requires positive contrast videofluoroscopy.[159,162] Quantification of the timing and duration of the various phases of swallowing have been described in the dog.[162]

Neurologic causes of dysphagia include polyneuropathies (see Chapter 7), botulism (see Chapter 7), rabies (see Chapter 15), and other infectious diseases such as listeriosis and protozoal encephalitis (see Chapter 15). The following disorders are categorized according to which phase of swallowing they affect.

Oropharyngeal Phases

Disorders involving the oral and pharyngeal phases of swallowing are often the result of disorders involving one or more cranial nerves. Myasthenia gravis also may selectively affect the pharyngeal muscles and the esophagus.[163]

Guttural Pouch Disease. Infections of the guttural pouch, usually by *Aspergillus* spp. or *Streptococcus equi*, may cause dysphagia, epistaxis, nasal discharge, and pain. Horner's syndrome and laryngeal and facial paresis may be present. The infection tends to localize in the dorsal wall of the guttural pouch close to the course of the glossopharyngeal nerve, the pharyngeal branch of the vagus nerve, and the internal carotid artery and closely associated sympathetic nerves.[3,4]

Diagnosis is made by endoscopy, radiography, and culture of material from the pouch. Treatment with topical antifungal agents has not been successful. Surgical removal or cauterization of lesions may be effective. Occlusion of the internal carotid artery may lessen or prevent epistaxis. Mycotic infections have a poorer prognosis than do bacterial infections.[3,4]

Nigropallidal Encephalomalacia. Nigropallidal encephalomalacia is characterized by acute dysfunction of muscles innervated by the motor fibers of CNs V, VII, and XII. It was first described in horses from northern California and southern Oregon that grazed on pastures containing large quantities of yellow star thistle *(Centaurea solstitialis)*.[164] Because of the typical clinical signs and the association with yellow star thistle, the disease also is called chewing disease and yellow star thistle poisoning. This condition also has been reported in horses from Colorado and Utah that grazed on pastures containing abundant Russian knapweed *(Centaurea repens)*, a plant related to yellow star thistle.[165,166] The disease occurs in the western United States and in Australia, where the offending plants are endemic.

Bilateral symmetric necrosis develops in the brainstem in the region of the globus pallidus and the substantia nigra, both components of the extrapyramidal system. Interestingly, the disease affects dopaminergic neurons. The toxic principle has not been definitively identified. However, several substances have been isolated from these plants. Glutathione deficiency and subsequent oxidative stress; toxicity secondary to excessive excitatory neurotransmitters, such as aspartate and glutamate; and high levels of tyramine, a biologically active amine, may play a role in toxicity.[167-169]

Clinical Signs. Although affected horses range in age from 4 months to 10 years, younger horses are most commonly affected.[166] Foals that are nursed by clinically normal mares have been affected and conversely, foals of affected mares have remained normal.[166]Affected horses are acutely unable to grasp food or drink water. The mouth is held partially open, the lips are retracted, and rhythmic tongue movements and purposeless chewing motions are apparent.[166] Lip and tongue movements are similar to "pill-rolling" movements of humans with Parkinson disease. Affected horses are drowsy and have a fixed facial expression. The facial muscles are hypertonic. Facial muscle flaccidity and gait impairment do not develop. Food or water placed in the caudal pharynx can be swallowed. The clinical signs suggest specific UMN dysfunction of CNs V, VII, and XII. Some horses may improve, but complete recovery has not been reported. Most horses die of starvation or aspiration pneumonia.

Diagnosis. The diagnosis is based on history and clinical signs. The facial hypertonicity and the lack of ataxia or paresis differentiate nigropallidal encephalomalacia from other diseases. MRI of the brain has been performed in an affected horse.[170] Lesions in the area of the globus pallidus and substantia nigra were observed. On T1W images, a hyperintense ring circumscribed the lesions. On T2W images, the lesions were hyperintense. Contrast enhancement was not observed.

Treatment. No specific treatment is known and the prognosis for recovery is poor. Feeding affected horses by tube prolongs life, allowing time for clinical improvement. Horses should not be allowed to graze on pastures where the offending plants are abundant.

Glossopharyngeal Neuralgia. In humans, glossopharyngeal neuralgia is a rare condition of paroxysms of pain in the distribution of the glossopharyngeal nerve.[171] On occasion, it is associated with cardiac syncope.[172] When associated with autonomic dysfunction such as bradycardia and syncope, the syndrome is referred to as vagoglossopharyngeal neuralgia.[171] A brainstem tumor causing a sensory and autonomic syndrome associated with the glossopharyngeal nerve has been reported.[173] A 7-year-old male miniature poodle initially evaluated for cervical spinal pain later progressed to episodes of syncope and seizures associated with pharyngeal stimulation via palpation and eating. Dysphagia was observed with eating, but not with drinking. Severe bradycardia, cyanosis, weak pulse pressure, and miotic pupils were observed during episodes. No EMG or CSF abnormalities were present. Serum catecholamine metabolites were low, suggestive of decreased sympathetic tone. CT demonstrated a mass in the caudal brainstem. Necropsy was not performed. The syndrome was apparently caused by stimulation of the afferents in the glossopharyngeal nerves. The afferent stimulation results in activation the carotid sinus reflex via vagal efferents leading to bradycardia, inhibition of vasomotor centers leading to peripheral vasodilation and hypotension, and inhibition of sympathetic output.

Cricopharyngeal Dysfunction. An uncommon cause of dysphagia involves the cricopharyngeus muscle, which together with the thyropharyngeus muscles forms the UES. Coordinated relaxation of this sphincter occurs during the pharyngoesophageal phase. Disorders involving the cricopharyngeal muscles, such as cricopharyngeal dysfunction (CD), include the inability to relax the sphincter (achalasia), delayed relaxation of the cricopharyngeus muscle as the bolus of food moves caudally (asynchrony), and failure to close the sphincter (chalasia).[174] Often a combination of abnormalities is present in CD. Clinical signs consist of repeated attempts to swallow, gagging, coughing, and nasopharyngeal reflux, excessive salivation, and regurgitation, and weight loss.[175] Positive contrast-enhanced videofluoroscopic evaluation of swallowing liquids and solid food is used to confirm the diagnosis.[159,162] Using liquid barium, a mean time ±SD between closure of the epiglottis and opening of the UES is 0.09 ± 0.02 second in normal dogs.[162] The observation of a delay and/or a complete or partial obstruction in the UES is consistent with CD.

Cricopharyngeal dysfunction can be acquired or congenital. Acquired CD often occurs in conjunction with other neuromuscular disorders including myasthenia gravis, laryngeal paralysis, masticatory myositis, and endocrine-associated neuromuscular disorders such as hypothyroidism.[176,177] Congenital CD has been observed in the cocker spaniel, springer spaniel, miniature poodles, and golden retriever dogs.[175,176,178] In the golden retriever, CD appears to be a genetic trait although the exact mode of inheritance is unknown.[178]

Treatment involves cricopharyngeal myotomy or myectomy, alone or in combination with thyropharyngeal myotomy or myectomy.[176,179] It is imperative to confirm CD before performing surgery because myotomy/myectomy may exacerbate other disorders, especially those involving the pharyngeal phase of swallowing. Successful outcome occurs in younger dogs with congenital CD. Surgery is less successful in older dogs and dogs with associated disease processes due to recurrence of clinical signs and/or aspiration pneumonia.[176]

Esophageal Phase. Megaesophagus Esophageal dysfunction, with or without megaesophagus (ME), results in an inability to transport food from the pharynx to the stomach. ME involves the loss of esophageal motor function and is characterized by ineffective esophageal peristalsis and esophageal dilation.[180] ME is common in dogs, infrequent in cats, and rare in large animals. Regurgitation is the primary sign of megaesophagus. The diagnosis is made radiographically (Figure 9-12). Unless a specific underlying cause is documented, treatment of esophageal dysfunction entails feeding the animal with the head elevated. Aspiration pneumonia is a common complication. The prognosis for functional recovery is poor in many cases.

The causes of esophageal dysfunction may be primary (congenital, idiopathic) or secondary (acquired). Secondary (acquired) esophageal dysfunction is common in generalized neuropathies and myopathies, including myasthenia gravis, hypothyroidism, hypoadrenocorticism, and intoxications such as lead toxicity (see Chapter 7). ME also can occur in dogs treated with potassium bromide. Withdrawal of the drug results in resolution of ME. ME may occur alone, without generalized weakness, in dogs with myasthenia gravis.[163] An increased prevalence of acquired ME is reported in German shepherd dogs, golden retrievers, Great Danes, and Irish setters.[181-183] The diagnosis of acquired ME necessitates identification of an underlying disorder. In myasthenia gravis, the diagnosis is made by identifying serum antibodies to acetylcholine receptors. Other causes require documenting an underlying endocrine disorder or toxicity. EMG of the esophageal muscles can be done by passing a stomach tube to define the cervical esophageal wall. The examination should include representative muscles of the limbs and face to rule out generalized neuropathies and myopathies. The prognosis

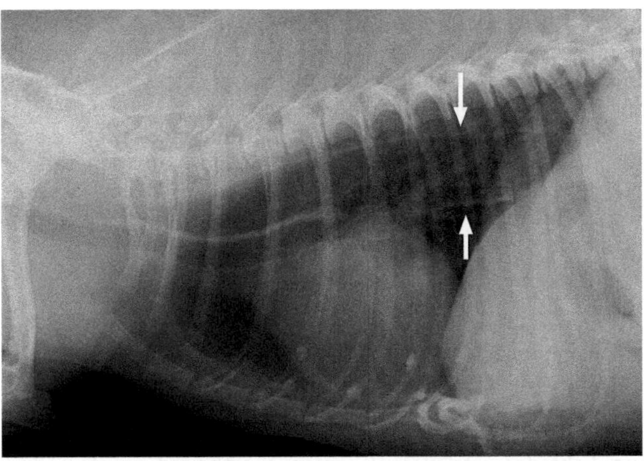

Figure 9-12 Radiographic diagnosis of esophageal dysfunction. *Arrow* highlights dorsal and ventral walls of the esophagus. (Copyright 2010 University of Georgia Research Foundation, Inc.)

for acquired ME is guarded and depends on the ability to treat the underlying disease.

Primary (idiopathic) ME occurs frequently in young dogs and consequently has been referred to as congenital idiopathic ME. In cats, idiopathic ME accounts for approximately 20% of cases.[184] The diagnosis is made by excluding other causes. Esophageal dysfunction without ME appears to affect young dogs, especially terriers.[185] Congenital ME has been reported in litters of Newfoundlands, Shar-Peis, and Siamese cats.[186-188] ME is reported as an inherited disease in miniature schnauzers and wire fox terriers.[189,190] In congenital idiopathic ME, vagal motor nerve function and esophageal motor performance appear to be normal.[191] Instead, the disease appears to be a consequence of abnormal afferent innervation of the esophagus.[192,193] Whereas most affected animals remain affected lifelong, in some young terriers, improved esophageal motility occurs with age.[185] Likewise, spontaneous resolution of ME can occurs suggesting a delay in the development of afferent innervation of the esophagus.

Gastroesophageal Phase

Esophageal achalasia has been documented in a 5-year-old, male golden retriever presented for regurgitation.[194] Although initial thoracic radiographs were normal, over time esophageal dilation occurred. On fluoroscopic examination of swallowing, the lower esophageal sphincter failed to open. The dog underwent a distal esophagomyotomy, which resolved the clinical signs.

Hypoglossal Paralysis

Paralysis of the tongue usually results from neoplastic and inflammatory diseases affecting the medulla. Hypoglossal paralysis is a common sign in rabies. The tongue may be affected in generalized neuropathies (see Chapter 7). Specific inflammatory disease of the hypoglossal nerve has not been reported. Bilateral sectioning of the hypoglossal nerves causes oral dysphagia (see preceding discussion).[159]

Dysautonomia

Dysfunction of the autonomic nervous system has been termed dysautonomia. The syndrome has been primarily reported in the horse, cat, and dog, and rarely in llamas. Clinical and pathologic similarities exist in all affected species; however, there are several clinical signs that differ between species. Pathologically, the disease is characterized by neuronal degeneration (chromatolysis) of neurons in postsynaptic sympathetic and parasympathetic ganglia, spinal ganglia, and the ventral and intermediate gray matter of the spinal cord, and numerous brainstem nuclei (CNs III, V, VI, VII, X, XII).[195]

Regardless of species, the presumptive diagnosis is based on history, signalment, and clinical signs. Additionally, pharmacologic testing of the autonomic nervous system may aid in establishing a presumptive diagnosis. Ocular pharmacology typically employs direct-acting and indirect-acting parasympathomimetic drugs. Topical ocular application of a dilute concentration (0.1%) pilocarpine results in miosis in affected animals while it causes no changes in pupil size in normal animals supporting denervation hypersensitivity in dysautonomia. Similarly, topical ocular administration of physostigmine (an indirect-acting parasympathomimetic) results in no change in pupil size in affected animals and miosis in normal animals suggesting a lack of postganglionic parasympathetic innervations in dysautonomia. Similarly, failure of the heart rate to increase after intravenous injection of atropine (0.02 mg/kg in dogs and cats) supports a lack of parasympathetic nervous innervations to the heart. The heart rate may not increase in affected animals due to a lack of sympathetic innervations to the heart. Cardiovascular testing employing direct-acting sympathomimetics is contraindicated given the potential for development of severe or life-threatening arrhythmias. Schirmer tear testing may disclose a lack of tear production implicating loss of parasympathetic innervation to the lacrimal glands. Intradermal (ID) injection of histamine in normal animals results in a skin wheal. Development of a wheal requires sympathetic innervations to the skin. A lack of wheal formation after ID histamine injection supports a loss of sympathetic tone. Other less commonly employed tests include identification of orthostatic hypotension and measurement of serum or urinary catecholamines or their metabolites. Ultimately, definitive diagnosis requires histopathologic identification of neuronal chromatolysis involving postganglionic autonomic neurons and specific cranial nerve nuclei and spinal cord gray matter.

Horses (Grass Sickness)

Grass sickness is a severe debilitating and almost always fatal condition in horses. The disease primarily is reported in Scotland, although cases have also been reported in England, Wales, and the European mainland.[196] A clinical and pathologically identical disease has been reported in South America and is referred to as *mal seco*.[197,198] Clinical signs largely reflect dysfunction of the gastrointestinal tract. Bladder paralysis may also occur. Grass sickness is characterized by three clinical forms: acute, subacute, and chronic. The acute form is characterized by an acute onset (<48 hours) of lethargy, colic due to severely decreased gut motility resulting in small intestinal distention and gastric reflux. Affected horses also have difficulty swallowing, ptosis, muscle tremors, patchy sweating, and tachycardia. The subacute form (<7 days) presents as a milder condition in addition to colonic impactions and a "tucked up" stance. The chronic form presents as chronic weight loss, weakness, mild dysphagia and ileus, and rhinitis sicca.[199]

Although numerous causes have been speculated including insects, fungi, viruses, toxic plants, and bacterial toxins, the definitive cause remains unknown.[196] The current most plausible explanation is a toxico-infectious etiology resulting from *Clostridium botulinum type* C, in which intestinal infection with *C. botulinum* leads to production of the neurotoxin, (BoNT/C) in affected horses. Supportive evidence is provided by the fact that *C. botulinum* neurotoxin can be isolated from 75% of acute and 67% of subacute and chronic cases whereas isolation of the neurotoxin is found in only 10% of normal horses.[200] Moreover, affected horses tend to have low serum IgG antibodies levels to BoNT/C and the surface antigens of *C. novyi* type A (phenotypically similar to *C. botulinum* type C) suggesting a lack of a protective effect.[201] These findings are in conjunction with certain epidemiologic data. Horses at risk tend to be young and/or have had a recent move to a new location.[196] Similarly, there is an increased risk if previous cases, in particular recent cases, have occurred on the farm. Conversely, there is a decreased risk for horses having been exposed to an affected horse, which suggests that low-grade chronic exposure to the potential cause of the disease may be protective. Additionally, cases tend to occur during spring and summer months. Density of horses, cutting of grasses, soil type, and concurrent grazing animals such as cattle may also play a role.[202]

Presumptive diagnosis is made through a combination of signalment, history, and physical examination findings. Definitive diagnosis requires histopathologic identification of neuronal chromatolysis of submucosal and myenteric nerve plexus (antemortem) or peripheral autonomic ganglia and brainstem nuclei (postmortem). Antemortem diagnosis can be obtained through biopsy of the ileum; however, given the necessity for general anesthesia and laparotomy, this procedure is associated with significant risks.[203] Treatment is largely supportive. With intensive supportive and nursing care, some chronically affected horses can recover.[204]

Cats

Dysautonomia in cats, referred to as Key-Gaskell syndrome, was first reported in 1982 in England, where the disease in large part has been confined.[205] With the exception of Norway and Sweden, individual reports or small numbers of cases have been reported in other European countries, New Zealand, and the United States.[206,207] Many of the cases in the United States occurred in cats that had been recently imported from the United Kingdom.[208] Since the late 1980s, subsequent reports have declined. Younger cats tend to be affected. In multicat households, both single and multiple cats may be affected. The underlying etiology remains unknown. However, increased levels of fecal IgA antibodies directed against *C. botulinum* C/D neurotoxin, BoNT/C toxoid and IgA directed against surface antigens of *C. botulinum* C/D were noted in affected cats compared with control cats, suggesting a similar toxico-infectious etiology involving *C. botulinum* as thought to occur in grass sickness.[209] Like equine dysautonomia, affected cats display signs related to gastrointestinal dysfunction.[206,210] Most cats develop clinical signs acutely over a 48-hour period, but other cats become progressively affected over 7 days. The disease affects indoor and outdoor cats. Signs include anorexia, constipation, ME, and consequent regurgitation and weight loss. Affected cats appear dull and lethargic. Other common clinical signs include dry external nares and oral cavity, reduced tear production, dilated pupils with reduced pupillary reflex, and elevated nictitating membranes. Urinary and fecal incontinence associated with reduced to absent perineal reflex may be observed. Unlike horses, affected cats are often bradycardic (<120 beats/min) and in a few cases syncope may occur.[210] In a few cases, mild postural reaction deficits were noted in the pelvic limbs. To aid in assessing affected cats, a grading system based on clinical signs has been proposed in which signs are divided into those uncommon or seen only with dysautonomia and those that occur with other conditions.[211] Scoring provides for inconclusive, probably, and positive presumptive diagnosis. Complete blood count, biochemical profile, and urinalysis largely reflect secondary dehydration and hypovolemia. Radiographs may disclose ME, a distended gastrointestinal tract, and enlarged urinary bladder. Presumptive diagnosis is made through a combination of history, clinical signs, and pharmacologic testing of the autonomic system. Treatment is supportive. Affected cats require intensive care including nutritional support and drug therapy to improve gastrointestinal and urinary function. The prognosis is guarded for severely affected cats. Prognosis may be better in cats with higher heart rates.[212] Approximately 25% to 50% of cats may survive with intensive care. Recovery takes weeks but may require up to a year for complete resolution of signs.

Dogs

As occurs in the horse and cat, dysautonomia in the dog affects animals in a specific geographic region. Most affected dogs in the United states are primarily from eastern Kansas and western and southern Missouri.[213,214] Affected dogs tend to be younger than 2 years old. Large-breed dogs, including Labrador retrievers, German shorthaired pointers, and German shepherds, are among the most common breeds affected.[213-215] Several risk factors have been identified.[213] Affected dogs tend to live in more rural environments, spend a greater time outdoors, and have a greater opportunity to roam unattended than unaffected dogs. Although cases are identified year-round, most cases occur between February and April with fewer cases occurring in the summer and early fall. Clinical signs tend to occur acutely. Vomiting, diarrhea, and anorexia are the most common clinical signs. Decreased anal tone appears to be a common nonautonomic sign in dogs. Additional clinical signs reflected autonomic dysfunction affecting the urinary, gastrointestinal, and ocular systems. Affected dogs may have altered systolic cardiac function based on echocardiography.[216] Similar to dysautonomia in cats, signs in dogs include oculonasal discharge, xanthostoma, decreased tear production, regurgitation, anorexia, weight loss, constipation, tenesmus, dysphagia, dysphonia, dysuria, urinary retention, and mydriasis (Figure 9-13). Radiographic studies often reveal aspiration pneumonia, ME, or a distended stomach, small bowel, or urinary bladder.[217] Presumptive diagnosis is based on history, signalment, clinical signs, and pharmacologic testing of the autonomic nervous system. Definitive diagnosis requires histopathologic evaluation. Treatment involves intensive supportive care. Pharmacologic therapy is aimed

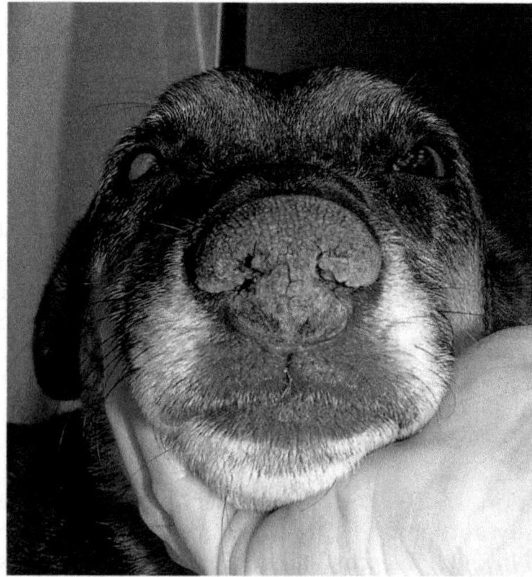

Figure 9-13 Dysautonomia in a dog. There is dry crusting of the nose as a consequence of xanthostoma and decreased tear production. There is also anisocoria. The left nictitating membrane is elevated compared with the right.

at improving urinary and gastrointestinal tract function. The prognosis for affected dogs is poor. Most dogs are euthanized based on the severity of clinical signs

Unilateral Cranial Polyneuropathy

Unilateral tumors extending along the floor of the cranial cavity may produce chronic compressive polyneuropathy that affects primarily CNs III, V, VII, and VIII. Animals are usually presented because of unilateral facial nerve paralysis, unilateral masticatory muscle atrophy, vestibular signs, alone or in combination. Sometimes animals are presented for unilateral pupillary dilation or ventrolateral strabismus. Examination of cranial nerve reflexes reveals multiple cranial nerve involvement and decreased facial sensation ipsilateral to the lesion. MRI or CT reveals a mass lesion that extends along the floor of the cranial cavity. In our experience, meningioma and lymphoma are the most common tumors producing this syndrome. In some cases, compression of the brainstem may result in paresis and ataxia. Because of the extensive nature of the tumor and the inaccessibility to surgery, the prognosis is poor for most dogs. Chemotherapy and/or radiation treatment may be beneficial.

CASE STUDIES

Key: *0*, Absent; *+1*, decreased; *+2*, normal; *+3*, exaggerated; *+4*, very exaggerated or clonus; *PL*, pelvic limb; *TL*, thoracic limb; *NE*, not evaluated.

CASE STUDY 9-1 *EVA*

▪ Signalment

11 year old Australian shepherd female spayed dog

▪ History

Approximately 9-month progressive history of inspiratory stridor. Initially, inspiratory noise was audible only when the dog was panting. Over time, the stridor became more audible. The owners have noticed a change in the sound of the dog's bark. In the last 2 to 3 months, the dog has become exercise intolerant. After a few minutes of walking, the dog will begin to pant heavily during which time harsh noise is audible during both inspiration and expiration. Twenty-four hours before presentation, the dog was taken to an emergency service after exercise for dyspnea and cyanosis. With time and supplemental oxygen, the dog's condition improved.

▪ Neurologic Examination

Mental status

Normal

Gait

Normal

Posture

Slightly flexed at the hocks bilaterally

Postural reactions

Normal in all four limbs

Spinal reflexes

Thoracic limbs; normal flexor reflex, tone, and muscle mass—bilaterally; pelvic limbs; +2 patellar, slightly reduced flexor reflexes—bilaterally (not flexing at the hock with normal strength), mild atrophy of the gastrocnemius and cranial tibialis muscles with normal muscular tone, bilaterally. All other spinal reflexes are normal.

Cranial nerves

All normal

Sensory examination

Normal

Palpation

Normal

▪ Lesion Location

The history is suspicious for upper airway dysfunction such as laryngeal paresis/paralysis. Given the history of an acute exacerbation leading to dyspnea and cyanosis, bilaterally laryngeal paresis/paralysis is suspected. Physical obstruction from structural disease (i.e., neoplasia affecting the airway) cannot be excluded. Abnormalities appreciated in the pelvic limbs are consistent with LMN dysfunction, which together with laryngeal paralysis may indicate a diffuse LMN disorder.

▪ Differential Diagnosis

1. Polyneuropathy—degenerative
2. Polyneuropathy—secondary to endocrine or neoplasia
3. Polymyopathy—degenerative or inflammatory/infectious
4. Myasthenia gravis

▪ Diagnostic Plan

1. MDB including creatine kinase (CK) level—may detect underlying endocrine disorder, inflammatory, or infectious etiologies
2. Three view thoracic radiographs—to evaluate for concurrent megaesophagus, exclude structural disease from consideration (e.g., identify abnormality in the upper airway), and evaluate for the presence of a primary or metastatic neoplasia
3. Direct laryngeal examination under sedation or light anesthesia to detect the presence of laryngeal paresis/paralysis or a structural cause of the respiratory noise
4. Electrophysiologic testing (EMG, direct nerve stimulation and conduction studies, F-wave evaluation)
5. Based on result of electrophysiologic tests may consider nerve or muscle biopsy
6. Based on results of steps 1 through 5, may consider measurement of antibodies directed at the acetylcholine receptor (MG titer)
7. Based on results of steps 1 through 6, may consider pursuing specific endocrine testing (i.e., hypothyroidism)

▪ Diagnostic Results

1. MDB—normal
2. Thoracic radiographs—normal
3. Direct laryngeal examination—bilaterally laryngeal paralysis; no evidence of structural disease
4. EMG disclosed fibrillation potentials and positive sharp waves in the muscle distal to the stifle and elbow. Markedly reduced CMAP with motor nerve conduction velocity (NCV) of the sciatic-tibial and ulnar nerves.

Continued

CASE STUDY 9-1 *EVA—cont'd*

Mild prolongation of the minimal latency of the F wave of the sciatic-tibial and ulnar nerves.

▪ Diagnosis

The electrophysiologic data were consistent with a diffuse axonal disorder primarily affecting the distal portion of the axon. The owners declined nerve and muscle biopsies; however, a degenerative process was suspected. A poor prognosis was given. After counseling the owners about the likelihood of further decline, which may result in appendicular weakness, the owner opted to pursue surgical correction of the laryngeal paralysis.

▪ Treatment

Unilateral arytenoids lateralization was performed. The dog recovered from surgery uneventfully. Despite continued respiratory noise, no further episodes of dyspnea occurred. However, the dog continued to progress with LMN weakness over the following 6 months.

CASE STUDY 9-2 *OSCAR*

▪ Signalment

9-year-old cat DSH, male castrated

▪ History

1-month history of ptosis and miosis OS. Two weeks before presentation, the owner noticed that food would fall out of the cat's mouth on the left side. Additionally, when the owner made a noise, the left ear would not move in response to noise.

▪ Neurologic Examination

Mental status
Normal

Gait
Normal

Posture
Normal

Postural reactions
Normal in all four limbs

Spinal reflexes
All normal

Cranial nerves
Menace response—0 OS (however, the cat would retract the eye in response to the menacing gesture), +2 OD; palpebral reflex—0 OS, +2 OD, response to noxious stimulation of the nasal mucosa—normal bilaterally. There was miosis, ptosis of the dorsal eyelid, elevation of the nictitating membrane OS. The left ear did not move in response to noise or touch.

Sensory Examination
Normal

Palpation
The cat was painful with pressure applied to the left tympanic bulla and with opening of the mouth.

▪ Lesion Location

CN VII (peripheral), and loss of sympathetic innervations to the eye OS (Horner's syndrome)

▪ Differential Diagnosis

1. Otitis media/interna
2. Neoplasia
3. Inflammatory polyp

▪ Diagnostic Plan

1. Otoscopic examination—to evaluate for evidence of otitis externa or neoplasia affecting the external ear canal.
2. MDB—assess the general health of the cat in preparation for CT or MR imaging
3. Three view thoracic radiographs—evaluate for the presence of metastatic disease
4. MRI or CT of the head

▪ Diagnostic Results

1. Brown waxy debris in the external ear canals bilaterally
2. MDB—normal
3. Thoracic radiographs—normal
4. MRI disclosed a contrast enhancing soft tissue mass causing lysis of the left osseous bulla

▪ Diagnosis

MRI findings were consistent with a neoplasm affecting the tympanic bulla

▪ Treatment

A left-sided ventral bulla osteotomy was performed. Biopsy was consistent with adenocarcinoma. Postoperatively, the cat underwent radiation therapy.

CASE STUDY 9-3 *BEACON*

▪ Signalment

10-year-old Weimaraner, male neutered

▪ History

An acute onset of multiple episodes of "vomiting"; episodes occurred shortly after eating. The dog would lower its head and undigested food and liquid would passively come out. Twenty-four hours before presentation, the dog became lethargic and reluctant to get up and walk. The owner also noticed an increase in the dog's respiratory rate and effort.

▪ Neurologic Examination

Mental status
Quiet but appropriately responding to stimuli

CASE STUDY 9-3 *BEACON*—cont'd

Gait
Severe exercise intolerance. The dog required assistance to stand. The gait was short strided and choppy. The dog could only walk 3 to 4 feet and then would lie down.

Posture
When standing, places the thoracic limbs more adducted under and caudally placed under the thorax. Pelvic limbs were slightly flexed at the hock, stifle, and hips, bilaterally.

Postural reactions
When dog's weight was supported, postural reactions are mildly reduced in all four limbs.

Spinal reflexes
Thoracic limbs— +1 flexor reflex, normal muscular tone and muscle mass; pelvic limbs— +2 patellar, +1 flexor reflex, normal muscular tone and muscle mass, bilaterally

Cranial nerves
Normal

Sensory examination
Normal

Palpation
Normal

▪ Lesion location
Signs consistent with diffuse LMN disease: Although the owner stated that the dog was vomiting, the description is more consistent with regurgitation. The episodes are passive and not associated with an abdominal effort as is seen with vomiting. Regurgitation is indicative of dysphagia associated with the esophageal phase of swallowing consistent with decreased esophageal motility or ME. Given the history of frequent episodes of regurgitation, the increased respiratory rate and effort may reflect aspiration pneumonia. Appendicular weakness was consistent with diffuse LMN weakness.

▪ Differential Diagnosis
1. Myasthenia gravis
2. Polyneuropathy
3. Polymyopathy
4. Intoxication (lead, organophosphates)

▪ Diagnostic Plan
1. MDB including CK level—to identify a systemic disorder that may result in a polyneuropathy or polymyopathy and to detect evidence of systemic inflammation (i.e., pneumonia)
2. Thoracic radiographs—to document ME and possible aspiration pneumonia
3. An edrophonium hydrochloride test (Tensilon test) to observe for improvement in muscle strength
4. Measurement of antibodies directed at the acetylcholine receptor (MG titer)
5. Based on results of steps 1 through 4, consider endoscopic evaluation of the esophagus to exclude structural causes of esophageal dysfunction (i.e., esophageal stricture or neoplasia)
6. Based on results of steps 1 through 4, consider electrophysiologic testing (EMG, direct nerve stimulation, and conduction studies, F-wave evaluation)

▪ Diagnostic Results
Mild neutrophilic leukocytosis was observed. CK was normal. Thoracic radiographs disclosed an enlarged, air-filled esophagus from the caudal cervical region through to the stomach consistent with ME. There was single round soft tissue opacity in the cranial mediastinum. An air bronchogram pattern was observed in the right middle lung lobe. There was minimal improvement in strength after administration of edrophonium hydrochloride. The MG titer was 3.41 nmol/L (reference range <0.06 nmol/L), which is consistent with acquired myasthenia gravis. Based on the thoracic radiographic findings, acquired myasthenia gravis was likely secondary to thymoma.

▪ Diagnosis
Myasthenia gravis secondary to a presumptive thymoma

▪ Treatment
Despite initiation of parenteral cholinergic drugs and immunosuppression, the dog's condition declined. The owner elected euthanasia. At necropsy, a thymoma was identified in the mediastinum.

CASE STUDY 9-4 *DARLA*

▪ Signalment
9-year-old Labrador retriever, female spayed

▪ History
3-month history of atrophy of the temporalis muscle on the right

▪ Neurologic Examination
Mental status
Quiet to dull

Gait
Mild general proprioceptive ataxia of the right thoracic and pelvic limbs

Posture
Normal; occasionally would stand on the dorsum of the foot of the right pelvic limb. Mild right head tilt

Postural reactions
Markedly delayed in the right thoracic and pelvic limbs; normal in the left thoracic and pelvic limbs

Continued

CASE STUDY 9-4 *DARLA—cont'd*

Spinal reflexes
All normal

Cranial nerves
Menace response—0 OD, +2 OS; with the left eye covered, the dog would track objects with the right eye; palpebral reflex—0 OD, +2 OS; response to noxious stimulation of the nasal mucosa—0 right, +2 left; mild right head tilt, no abnormal nystagmus, normal physiologic nystagmus, positional ventral strabismus OD when the head was elevated. The commissure of the lips on the right was drooping. Ptyalism was evident from the right commissure of the lips. There was less tone in the lips on the right. The right ear did not move in response to noise or touch. No other abnormalities were noted.

Sensory examination
Analgesia of the right nasal mucosa and skin over the maxilla

Palpation
Severe atrophy of the temporalis and masseter muscles on the right

▪ Lesion Location
Signs consistent with deficits in CN V (atrophy of the muscles of mastication and facial analgesia), VII (facial paralysis), VIII on the right (right head tilt and positional strabismus) nuclei or nerves. However, the change in mental state and ipsilateral postural reaction deficits suggests a lesion affected the right pons and rostral medulla oblongata.

▪ Differential Diagnosis
1. Neoplasia
2. Granuloma
3. Hemorrhage
4. Infarction (ischemic)

▪ Diagnostic Plan
1. MBD—evaluation of the general health and to identify evidence of systemic involvement of the underlying disorder
2. Three view thoracic radiographs—assess for underlying primary or metastatic neoplasm
3. MRI of the head

▪ Diagnostic Results
1. MDB—stress leukogram
2. Thoracic radiographs—within normal limits
3. MRI disclosed a solitary, strongly contrast-enhancing mass at the level of the right cerebellopontine medullary angle. Rostrally, the mass was contiguous with an enlarged trigeminal nerve. The mass severely compressed the adjacent pons and rostral medulla oblongata.

▪ Diagnosis
Neoplasia—presumptive trigeminal nerve sheath tumor

▪ Treatment
Given the guarded prognosis associated with this neoplasm, the owner declined further therapy.

CASE STUDY 9-5 *ABBY*

▪ Signalment
5-year-old cocker spaniel, female spayed

▪ History
An acute onset of a right-head tilt, falling, stumbling, and circling to the right. One month before presentation, the dog had started drooling and dropping food from the right side of the mouth. The owner also noted that the dog was not blinking the right eye.

▪ Neurologic Examination
Mental status
Normal

Gait
Moderate vestibular ataxia on the right side

Posture
Right head tilt

Postural reactions
Normal in all four limbs

Spinal reflexes
All normal

Cranial nerves
Menace response—0 OD, +2 OS; with the left eye covered, the dog would track objects with the right eye; palpebral reflex—0 OD, +2 OS; response to noxious stimulation of the nasal mucosa—normal bilaterally. Mild right head tilt, spontaneous horizontal nystagmus with the fast phase directed to the left. The commissure of the lips on the right was drooping and the mucosa was slightly everted. There was less tone in the lips on the right. The right ear did not move in response to noise or touch.

Sensory examination
Normal

Palpation
Normal

▪ Lesion Location
Peripheral CN VII and VIII

▪ Differential Diagnosis
1. Otitis media/interna
2. Neoplasia
3. Hypothyroidism

CASE STUDY 9-5 *ABBY*—cont'd

▪ Diagnostic Plan
1. Otoscopic examination
2. Schirmer tear test
3. MDB
4. MRI or CT

▪ Diagnostic Results
1. Evidence of chronic proliferative changes to the epithelium of the external ear canal. There was purulent discharge in the right external ear canal obscuring visualization of the tympanic membrane. Cytologic evaluation disclosed degenerative neutrophils with intracellular and extracellular mixed population of bacteria.
2. Schirmer tear test—0 mm OD, 7 mm OS
3. MDB—normal
4. MRI disclosed a fluid/soft tissue mass of mixed intensity within the right tympanic bulla. There was peripheral enhancement of the inner surface of the tympanic bulla.

▪ Diagnosis
Otitis interna/otitis media

▪ Treatment
Given the chronic proliferative changes of the external ear canal, a total ear canal ablation and lateral bulla osteotomy was performed. Postoperatively, the dog was placed on antibiotics based on culture and sensitivity testing of the material of the tympanic bulla. The vestibular dysfunction gradually improved. Facial nerve paralysis remained. The owners also were instructed to administer artificial tears in the right eye.

CK, Creatine kinase; *CMAP,* compound muscle action potential; *CN,* cranial nerve; *CT,* computed tomography; *EMG,* electromyography; *LMN,* lower motor neuron; *MDB,* minimum database; *ME,* megaesophagus; *MG,* myasthenia gravis; *MRI,* magnetic resonance imaging; *NCV,* nerve conduction velocity; *OD,* right eye; *OS,* left eye.

REFERENCES

1. Whalen LR, Kitchell RL: Electrophysiologic studies of the cutaneous nerves of the head of the dog, Am J Vet Res 44:615–627, 1983.
2. Whalen LR, Kitchell RL: Electrophysiologic and behavioral studies of the cutaneous nerves of the concave surface of the pinna and the external ear canal of the dog, Am J Vet Res 44:628–634, 1983.
3. Mayhew IG: Large animal neurology, ed 2, Oxford, 2008, Blackwell.
4. De Lahunta A, Glass EN: Veterinary neuroanatomy and clinical neurology, ed 3, St Louis, 2008, Saunders Elsevier.
5. Hoelzle RJ: Idiopathic trigeminal neuropathy in a dog, Vet Med Small Anim Clin 78:345, 1983.
6. Mayhew PD, Bush WW, Glass EN: Trigeminal neuropathy in dogs: a retrospective study of 29 cases (1991-2000), J Am Anim Hosp Assoc 38:262–270, 2002.
7. Carmichael S, Griffiths IR: Case of isolated sensory trigeminal neuropathy in a dog, Vet Rec 109:280–282, 1981.
8. Panciera RJ, Ritchey JW, Baker JE, et al: Trigeminal and polyradiculoneuritis in a dog presenting with masticatory muscle atrophy and Horner's syndrome, Vet Pathol 39:146–149, 2002.
9. Carpenter JL, King NW Jr, Abrams KL: Bilateral trigeminal nerve paralysis and Horner's syndrome associated with myelomonocytic neoplasia in a dog, J Am Vet Med Assoc 191:1594–1596, 1987.
10. Pfaff AMD, March PA, Fishman C: Acute bilateral trigeminal neuropathy associated with nervous system lymphosarcoma in a dog, J Am Anim Hosp Assoc 36:57–61, 2000.
11. Schultz RM, Tucker RL, Gavin PR, et al: Magnetic resonance imaging of acquired trigeminal nerve disorders in six dogs, Vet Radiol Ultrasound 48:101–104, 2007.
12. Bagley RS, Wheeler SJ, Klopp L, et al: Clinical features of trigeminal nerve-sheath tumor in 10 dogs, J Am Anim Hosp Assoc 34:19–25, 1998.
13. Pettigrew R, Rylander H, Schwarz T: Magnetic resonance imaging contrast enhancement of the trigeminal nerve in dogs without evidence of trigeminal neuropathy, Vet Radiol Ultrasound 50:276–278, 2009.
14. Palmer AC: Pontine infarction in a dog with unilateral involvement of the trigeminal motor nucleus and pyramidal tract, J Small Anim Pract 48:49–52, 2007.
15. Heath S, Rusbridge C, Johnson N, et al: Orofacial pain syndrome in cats, Vet Rec 149:660, 2001.
16. Asbury AK, McKhann GM, McDonald WI: Diseases of the nervous system: clinical neurobiology, Philadelphia, 1986, Ardmore Medical Books.
17. Kern TJ, Erb HN: Facial neuropathy in dogs and cats: 95 cases (1975-1985), J Am Vet Med Assoc 191:1604–1609, 1987.
18. Jaggy A, Oliver JE, Ferguson DC, et al: Neurological manifestations of hypothyroidism: a retrospective study of 29 dogs, J Vet Intern Med 8:328–336, 1994.
19. Braund KG, Luttgen PJ, Sorjonen DC, et al: Idiopathic facial paralysis in the dog, Vet Rec 105:297–299, 1979.
20. Couturier L, Degueurce C, Ruel Y, et al: Anatomical study of cranial nerve emergence and skull foramina in the dog using magnetic resonance imaging and computed tomography, Vet Radiol Ultrasound 46:375–383, 2005.
21. Jaggy A, Oliver JE: Neurologic manifestations of thyroid disease, Vet Clin North Am Small Anim Pract 24:487–494, 1994.
22. Tan NC, Chan LL, Tan EK: Hemifacial spasm and involuntary facial movements, QJM 95:493–500, 2002.
23. Nielsen VK: Pathophysiology of hemifacial spasm: I. Ephaptic transmission and ectopic excitation, Neurology 34:418–426, 1984.
24. Oliveira LD, Cardoso F, Vargas AP: Hemifacial spasm and arterial hypertension, Mov Disord 14:832–835, 1999.
25. Roberts SR, Vainisi SJ: Hemifacial spasm in dogs, J Am Vet Med Assoc 150:381–385, 1967.
26. Parker AJ, Cusick PK, Park RD, et al: Hemifacial spasms in a dog, Vet Rec 93:514–516, 1973.
27. Van Meervenne SA, Bhatti SF, Martle V, et al: Hemifacial spasm associated with an intracranial mass in two dogs, J Small Anim Pract 49:472–475, 2008.
28. Jager L, Reiser M: CT and MR imaging of the normal and pathologic conditions of the facial nerve, Eur J Radiol 40:133–146, 2001.
29. Kenney C, Jankovic J: Botulinum toxin in the treatment of blepharospasm and hemifacial spasm, J Neural Transm 115:585–591, 2008.

30. Renegar WR: Auriculopalpebral nerve paralysis following prolonged anesthesia in a dog, J Am Vet Med Assoc 174:1007–1009, 1979.
31. Power HT, Watrous BJ, de Lahunta A: Facial and vestibulocochlear nerve disease in six horses, J Am Vet Med Assoc 183:1076–1080, 1983.
32. Walker AM, Sellon DC, Cornelisse CJ, et al: Temporohyoid osteoarthropathy in 33 horses (1993-2000), J Vet Intern Med 16:697–703, 2002.
33. Blythe LL, Watrous BJ, Schmitz JA, et al: Vestibular syndrome associated with temporohyoid joint fusion and temporal bone fracture in three horses, J Am Vet Med Assoc 185:775–781, 1984.
34. Blythe LL: Otitis media and interna and temporohyoid osteoarthropathy, Vet Clin North Am Equine Pract 13:21–42, 1997.
35. Divers TJ, Ducharme NG, de Lahunta A, et al: Temporohyoid osteoarthropathy, Clin Tech Equine Pract 5:17–23, 2006.
36. Aleman M, Puchalski SM, Williams DC, et al: Brainstem auditory-evoked responses in horses with temporohyoid osteoarthropathy, J Vet Intern Med 22:1196–1202, 2008.
37. Pease AP, van Biervliet J, Dykes NL, et al: Complication of partial stylohyoidectomy for treatment of temporohyoid osteoarthropathy and an alternative surgical technique in three cases, Equine Vet J 36:546–550, 2004.
38. Knowles K, Blauch B, Leipold H, et al: Reduction of spiral ganglion neurons in the aging canine with hearing loss, Zentralbl Veterinarmed A 36:188–199, 1989.
39. Mansfield PD: Ototoxicity in dogs and cats, Compend Contin Educ Pract Vet 12:331–337, 1990.
40. Adams EW: Hereditary deafness in a family of foxhounds, J Am Vet Med Assoc 128:302–303, 1956.
41. Coppens AG, Gilbert-Gregory S, Steinberg SA, et al: Inner ear histopathology in "nervous Pointer dogs" with severe hearing loss, Hear Res 200:51–62, 2005.
42. Coppens AG, Kiss R, Heizmann CW, et al: An original inner ear neuroepithelial degeneration in a deaf Rottweiler puppy, Hear Res 161:65–71, 2001.
43. Coppens AG, Resibois A, Poncelet L: Bilateral deafness in a Maltese terrier and a great Pyrenean puppy: inner ear morphology, J Comp Pathol 122:223–228, 2000.
44. Coppens AG, Steinberg SA, Poncelet L: Inner ear morphology in a bilaterally deaf Dogo Argentino pup, J Comp Pathol 128:67–70, 2003.
45. Erickson F, Saperstein G, Leipold HW, et al: Congenital defects of dogs—Part 3, Canine Pract 4:40–53, 1977.
46. Gwin RM, Wyman M, Lim DJ, et al: Multiple ocular defects associated with partial albinism and deafness in the dog, J Am Anim Hosp Assoc 17:401–408, 1981.
47. Hayes HM Jr, Wilson GP, Fenner WR, et al: Canine congenital deafness: epidemiologic study of 272 cases, J Am Anim Hosp Assoc 17:473–476, 1981.
48. Hudson WR, Ruben RJ: Hereditary deafness in the Dalmatian dog, Arch Otolaryngol 75:213–219, 1962.
49. Igarashi M, Alford BR, Cohn AM, et al: Inner ear anomalies in dogs, Ann Otol Rhinol Laryngol 81:249–255, 1972.
50. Johnsson LG, Hawkins JE Jr, Muraski AA, et al: Vascular anatomy and pathology of the cochlea in Dalmatian dogs. In Vascular disorders and hearing defects, University Park, MA, 1973, University Park Press.
51. Lurie MH: The membranous labyrinth in the congenitally deaf collie and Dalmatian dog, Laryngoscope 58:279–287, 1948.
52. Marshall AE: Use of brain stem auditory-evoked response to evaluate deafness in a group of Dalmatian dogs, J Am Vet Med Assoc 188:718–722, 1986.
53. Sims MH, Shull-Selcer E: Electrodiagnostic evaluation of deafness in two English setter littermates, J Am Vet Med Assoc 187:398–404, 1985.
54. Strain GM: Congenital deafness in dogs and cats, Compend Contin Educ Pract Vet 13:245–250, 1991:252–253.
55. Suga F, Hattler KW: Physiological and histopathological correlates of hereditary deafness in animals, Laryngoscope 80:81–104, 1970.
56. Wilkes MK, Palmer AC: Congenital deafness in Dobermans, Vet Rec 118:218, 1986.
57. Wilkes MK, Palmer AC: Congenital deafness and vestibular deficit in the Doberman, J Small Anim Pract 33:218–224, 1992.
58. Famula TR, Cargill EJ, Strain GM: Heritability and complex segregation analysis of deafness in Jack Russell terriers, BMC Vet Res 3:31, 2007.
59. Bosher SK, Hallpike CS: Observations on the histogenesis of the inner ear degeneration of the deaf white cat and its possible relationship to the aetiology of certain unexplained varieties of human congenital deafness, J Laryngol Otol 80:222–235, 1966.
60. Creel D, Conlee JW, Parks TN: Auditory brainstem anomalies in albino cats. I. Evoked potential studies, Brain Res 260:1–9, 1983.
61. Delack JB: Hereditary deafness in the white cat, Compend Contin Educ Pract Vet 6:609–617, 1984.
62. Elverland HH, Mair IW: Hereditary deafness in the cat. An electron microscopic study of the spiral ganglion, Acta Otolaryngol 90:360–369, 1980.
63. Rebillard G, Rebillard M, Carlier E, et al: Histophysiological relationships in the deaf white cat auditory system, Acta Otolaryngol 82:48–56, 1976.
64. Wolff D: Three generations of deaf white cats, J Hered 33:39–43, 1942.
65. Cvejic D, Steinberg TA, Kent MS, et al: Unilateral and bilateral congenital sensorineural deafness in client-owned pure-breed white cats, J Vet Intern Med 23:392–395, 2009.
66. Gauly M, Vaughan J, Hogreve SK, et al: Brainstem auditory-evoked potential assessment of auditory function and congenital deafness in llamas *(Lama glama)* and alpacas (*L. pacos*), J Vet Intern Med 19:756–760, 2005.
67. Harland MM, Stewart AJ, Marshall AE, et al: Diagnosis of deafness in a horse by brainstem auditory evoked potential, Can Vet J 47:151–154, 2006.
68. Anderson H, Henricson B, Lundquist PG, et al: Genetic hearing impairment in the Dalmatian dog. An audiometric, genetic and morphologic study in 53 dogs, Acta Otolaryngol 232(suppl):231–234, 1968.
69. Bosher SK, Hallpike CS: Observations on the histological features, development and pathogenesis of the inner ear degeneration of the deaf white cat, Proc R Soc Lond B Biol Sci 162:147–170, 1965.
70. Steel KP: Inherited hearing defects in mice, Annu Rev Genet 29:675–701, 1995.
71. Mair IW: Hereditary deafness in the Dalmatian dog, Arch Otorhinolaryngol 212:1–14, 1976.
72. Holliday TA, Nelson HJ, Williams DC, et al: Unilateral and bilateral brainstem auditory-evoked response abnormalities in 900 Dalmatian dogs, J Vet Intern Med 6:166–174, 1992.
73. Strain GM, Kearney MT, Gignac IJ, et al: Brainstem auditory-evoked potential assessment of congenital deafness in Dalmatians: associations with phenotypic markers, J Vet Intern Med 6:175–182, 1992.
74. Famula TR, Oberbauer AM, Sousa CA: A threshold model analysis of deafness in Dalmatians, Mamm Genome 7:650–653, 1996.

75. Juraschko K, Meyer-Lindenberg A, Nolte I, et al: Analysis of systematic effects on congenital sensorineural deafness in German Dalmatian dogs, Vet J 166:164–169, 2003.
76. Muhle AC, Jaggy A, Stricker C, et al: Further contributions to the genetic aspect of congenital sensorineural deafness in Dalmatians, Vet J 163:311–318, 2002.
77. Wood JLN, Lakhani KH: Prevalence and prevention of deafness in the Dalmatian: assessing the effect of parental hearing status and gender using ordinary logistic and generalized random litter effect models, Vet J 154:121–133, 1997.
78. Strain GM: Deafness prevalence and pigmentation and gender associations in dog breeds at risk, Vet J 167:23–32, 2004.
79. Strain GM, Clark LA, Wahl JM, et al: Prevalence of deafness in dogs heterozygous or homozygous for the merle allele, J Vet Intern Med 23:282–286, 2009.
80. Brenig B, Pfeiffer I, Jaggy A, et al: Analysis of the 5′ region of the canine PAX3 gene and exclusion as a candidate for Dalmatian deafness, Anim Genet 34:47–50, 2003.
81. Mieskes K, Distl O: Evaluation of ESPN, MYO3A, SLC26A5 and USH1C as candidates for hereditary nonsyndromic deafness (congenital sensorineural deafness) in Dalmatian dogs, Anim Genet 38:533–534, 2007.
82. Stritzel S, Wohlke A, Distl O: Elimination of SILV as a candidate for congenital sensorineural deafness in Dalmatian dogs, Anim Genet 38:662–663, 2007.
83. Famula TR, Oberbauer AM, Sousa CA: Complex segregation analysis of deafness in Dalmatians, Am J Vet Res 61:550–553, 2000.
84. Greibrokk T: Hereditary deafness in the Dalmatian: relationship to eye and coat color, J Am Anim Hosp Assoc 30:170–176, 1994.
85. Bergsma DR, Brown KS: White fur, blue eyes, and deafness in the domestic cat, J Hered 62:171–185, 1971.
86. Mair IW: Hereditary deafness in the white cat, Acta Otolaryngol Suppl 314:1–48, 1973.
87. Ryugo DK, Cahill HB, Rose LS, et al: Separate forms of pathology in the cochlea of congenitally deaf white cats, Hear Res 181:73–84, 2003.
88. Geigy CA, Heid S, Steffen F, et al: Does a pleiotropic gene explain deafness and blue irises in white cats? Vet J 173:548–553, 2007.
89. Gacek RR: Localization of laryngeal motor neurons in the kitten, Laryngoscope 85:1841–1859, 1975.
90. Radlinsky MG, Mason DE, Hodgson D: Transnasal laryngoscopy for the diagnosis of laryngeal paralysis in dogs, J Am Anim Hosp Assoc 40:211–215, 2004.
91. Hackett RP, Ducharme NG, Fubini SL, et al: The reliability of endoscopic examination in assessment of arytenoid cartilage movement in horses. Part I: subjective and objective laryngeal evaluation, Vet Surg 20:174–179, 1991.
92. Rakestraw PC, Hackett RP, Ducharme NG, et al: Arytenoid cartilage movement in resting and exercising horses, Vet Surg 20:122–127, 1991.
93. Rudorf H, Barr F: Echolaryngography in cats, Vet Radiol Ultrasound 43:353–357, 2002.
94. Bray JP, Lipscombe VJ, White RA, et al: Ultrasonographic examination of the pharynx and larynx of the normal dog, Vet Radiol Ultrasound 39:566–571, 1998.
95. Jackson AM, Tobias K, Long CD, et al: Effects of various anesthetic agents on laryngeal motion during laryngoscopy in normal dogs, Vet Surg 33:102–106, 2004.
96. Miller CJ, McKiernan BC, Pace J, et al: The effects of doxapram hydrochloride (Dopram-V) on laryngeal function in healthy dogs, J Vet Intern Med 16:524–528, 2002.
97. Tobias KM, Jackson AM, Harvey RC: Effects of doxapram HCl on laryngeal function of normal dogs and dogs with naturally occurring laryngeal paralysis, Vet Anaesth Analg 31:258–263, 2004.
98. Jeffery ND, Talbot CE, Smith PM, et al: Acquired idiopathic laryngeal paralysis as a prominent feature of generalized neuromuscular disease in 39 dogs, Vet Rec 158:17–21, 2006.
99. Greenfield CL: Canine laryngeal paralysis, Compend Contin Educ Pract Vet 9:1011–1017, 1987.
100. Harvey CE, O'Brien JA: Upper airway obstruction surgery. 5. Treatment of laryngeal paralysis in dogs by partial laryngectomy, J Am Anim Hosp Assoc 18:551–556, 1982.
101. Venker-van Haagen AJ, Bouw J, Hartman W: Hereditary transmission of laryngeal paralysis in Bouviers, J Am Anim Hosp Assoc 17:75–76, 1981.
102. Venker-van Haagen AJ, Hartman W, Goedegebuure A, et al: The source of normal motor unit potentials in supposedly denervated laryngeal muscles of dogs, Zentralbl Veterinarmed A 25A:751–761, 1978.
103. Venkar-van-Heagen AJ: Investigation of pathogenesis of hereditary laryngeal paralysis in the Bouvier, The Netherlands, 1980, University of Utrecht.
104. O'Brien JA, Hendriks J: Inherited laryngeal paralysis. Analysis in the husky cross, Vet Q 8:301–302, 1986.
105. Polizopoulou ZS, Koutinas AF, Papadopoulos GC, et al: Juvenile laryngeal paralysis in three Siberian husky x Alaskan malamute puppies, Vet Rec 153:624–627, 2003.
106. Ridyard AE, Corcoran BM, Tasker S, et al: Spontaneous laryngeal paralysis in four white-coated German shepherd dogs, J Small Anim Pract 41:558–561, 2000.
107. Bennett PF, Clarke RE: Laryngeal paralysis in a Rottweiler with neuroaxonal dystrophy, Aust Vet J 75:784–786, 1997.
108. Kortz GD, Meier WA, Higgins RJ, et al: Neuronal vacuolation and spinocerebellar degeneration in young Rottweiler dogs, Vet Pathol 34:296–302, 1997.
109. Mahony OM, Knowles KE, Braund KG, et al: Laryngeal paralysis-polyneuropathy complex in young Rottweilers, J Vet Intern Med 12:330–337, 1998.
110. de Lahunta A, Summers BA: The laryngeal lesion in young dogs with neuronal vacuolation and spinocerebellar degeneration, Vet Pathol 35:316–317, 1998.
111. Salvadori C, Tartarelli CL, Baroni M, et al: Peripheral nerve pathology in two Rottweilers with neuronal vacuolation and spinocerebellar degeneration, Vet Pathol 42:852–855, 2005.
112. Salvadori C, Tartarelli CL, Baroni M, et al: Neuronal vacuolation, myelopathy and laryngeal neuropathy in a mixed-breed dog, J Vet Med A Physiol Pathol Clin Med 54:445–448, 2007.
113. Geiger DA, Miller AD, Cutter-Schatzberg K, et al: Encephalomyelopathy and polyneuropathy associated with neuronal vacuolation in two boxer littermates, Vet Pathol 46:1160–1165, 2009.
114. Braund KG, Shores A, Cochrane S, et al: Laryngeal paralysis-polyneuropathy complex in young Dalmatians, Am J Vet Res 55:534–542, 1994.
115. Gabriel A, Poncelet L, Ham Lv, et al: Laryngeal paralysis-polyneuropathy complex in young related Pyrenean mountain dogs, J Small Anim Pract 47:144–149, 2006.
116. Gaber CE, Amis TC, LeCouteur RA: Laryngeal paralysis in dogs: a review of 23 cases, J Am Vet Med Assoc 186:377–380, 1985.
117. Braund KG, Steinberg HS, Shores A, et al: Laryngeal paralysis in immature and mature dogs as one sign of a more diffuse polyneuropathy, J Am Vet Med Assoc 194:1735–1740, 1989.

118. Broome C, Burbidge HM, Pfeiffer DU: Prevalence of laryngeal paresis in dogs undergoing general anaesthesia, Aust Vet J 78:769–772, 2000.
119. Hammel SP, Hottinger HA, Novo RE: Postoperative results of unilateral arytenoid lateralization for treatment of idiopathic laryngeal paralysis in dogs: 39 cases (1996-2002), J Am Vet Med Assoc 228:1215–1220, 2006.
120. MacPhail CM, Monnet E: Outcome of and postoperative complications in dogs undergoing surgical treatment of laryngeal paralysis: 140 cases (1985-1998), J Am Vet Med Assoc 218:1949–1956, 2001.
121. Payne JT, Martin RA, Rigg DL: Abductor muscle prosthesis for correction of laryngeal paralysis in 10 dogs and one cat, J Am Anim Hosp Assoc 26:599–604, 1990.
122. Schofield DM, Norris J, Sadanaga KK: Bilateral thyroarytenoid cartilage lateralization and vocal fold excision with mucosoplasty for treatment of idiopathic laryngeal paralysis: 67 dogs (1998-2005), Vet Surg 36:519–525, 2007.
123. Smith MM, Gourley IM, Kurpershoek CJ, et al: Evaluation of a modified castellated laryngofissure for alleviation of upper airway obstruction in dogs with laryngeal paralysis, J Am Vet Med Assoc 188:1279–1283, 1986.
124. Gourley IM, Paul H, Gregory C: Castellated laryngofissure and vocal fold resection for the treatment of laryngeal paralysis in the dog, J Am Vet Med Assoc 182:1084–1086, 1983.
125. Rosin E, Greenwood K: Bilateral arytenoid cartilage lateralization for laryngeal paralysis in the dog, J Am Vet Med Assoc 180:515–518, 1982.
126. Snelling SR, Edwards GA: A retrospective study of unilateral arytenoid lateralisation in the treatment of laryngeal paralysis in 100 dogs (1992-2000), Aust Vet J 81:464–468, 2003.
127. Burbidge HM, Goulden BE, Jones BR: Laryngeal paralysis in dogs: an evaluation of the bilateral arytenoid lateralisation procedure, J Small Anim Pract 34:515–519, 1993.
128. Hardie EM, Kolata RJ, Stone EA, et al: Laryngeal paralysis in three cats, J Am Vet Med Assoc 179:879–882, 1981.
129. Schachter S, Norris CR: Laryngeal paralysis in cats: 16 cases (1990-1999), J Am Vet Med Assoc 216:1100–1103, 2000.
130. White RA, Littlewood JD, Herrtage ME, et al: Outcome of surgery for laryngeal paralysis in four cats, Vet Rec 118:103–104, 1986.
131. White RN: Unilateral arytenoid lateralisation for the treatment of laryngeal paralysis in four cats, J Small Anim Pract 35:455–458, 1994.
132. Wells AL, Long CD, Hornof WJ, et al: Use of percutaneous ethanol injection for treatment of bilateral hyperplastic thyroid nodules in cats, J Am Vet Med Assoc 218:1293–1297, 2001.
133. Busch DS, Noxon JO, Miller LD: Laryngeal paralysis and peripheral vestibular disease in a cat, J Am Anim Hosp Assoc 28:82–86, 1992.
134. Schaer M, Zaki FA, Harvey HJ, et al: Laryngeal hemiplegia due to neoplasia of the vagus nerve in a cat, J Am Vet Med Assoc 174:513–515, 1979.
135. Nestor DD, Rosenstein DS: Radiographic diagnosis: laryngeal paralysis secondary to pulmonary squamous cell carcinoma in a cat, Vet Radiol Ultrasound 45:325–326, 2004.
136. Campbell D, Holmberg DL: Surgical treatment of laryngeal paralysis in a cat, Can Vet J 25:414–416, 1984.
137. Dixon PM, McGorum BC, Railton DI, et al: Laryngeal paralysis: a study of 375 cases in a mixed-breed population of horses, Equine Vet J 33:452–458, 2001.
138. Goulden BE, Anderson LJ: Equine laryngeal hemiplegia part II: some clinical observations, N Z Vet J 29:194–198, 1981.
139. Traub-Dargatz JL, Ingram JT, Stashak TS, et al: Respiratory stridor associated with polymyopathy suspected to be hyperkalemic periodic paralysis in four quarter horse foals, J Am Vet Med Assoc 201:85–89, 1992.
140. Carr EA, Spier SJ, Kortz GD, et al: Laryngeal and pharyngeal dysfunction in horses homozygous for hyperkalemic periodic paralysis, J Am Vet Med Assoc 209:798–803, 1996.
141. Rose RJ, Hartley WJ, Baker W: Laryngeal paralysis in Arabian foals associated with oral haloxon administration, Equine Vet J 13:171–176, 1981.
142. Hughes KJ, McGorum BC, Love S, et al: Bilateral laryngeal paralysis associated with hepatic dysfunction and hepatic encephalopathy in six ponies and four horses, Vet Rec 164:142–147, 2009.
143. Abrahamsen EJ, Bohanon TC, Bednarski RM, et al: Bilateral arytenoid cartilage paralysis after inhalation anesthesia in a horse, J Am Vet Med Assoc 197:1363–1365, 1990.
144. Dixon PM, Railton DI, McGorum BC: Temporary bilateral laryngeal paralysis in a horse associated with general anaesthesia and post anaesthetic myositis, Vet Rec 132:29–32, 1993.
145. Bohanon TC, Beard WL, Robertson JT: Laryngeal hemiplegia in draft horses. A review of 27 cases, Vet Surg 19:456–459, 1990.
146. Duncan ID: Determination of the early age of onset of equine recurrent laryngeal neuropathy. 2. Nerve pathology, Acta Neuropathol 84:316–321, 1992.
147. Hahn CN, Matiasek K, Dixon PM, et al: Histological and ultrastructural evidence that recurrent laryngeal neuropathy is a bilateral mononeuropathy limited to recurrent laryngeal nerves, Equine Vet J 40:666–672, 2008.
148. Cahill JI, Goulden BE: Equine laryngeal hemiplegia. Part I. A light microscopic study of peripheral nerves, N Z Vet J 34:161–169, 1986.
149. Cahill JI, Goulden BE: The pathogenesis of equine laryngeal hemiplegia: a review, N Z Vet J 35:82–90, 1987.
150. Ducharme NG, Hackett RP, Fubini SL, et al: The reliability of endoscopic examination in assessment of arytenoid cartilage movement in horses. Part II. Influence of side of examination, reexamination, and sedation, Vet Surg 20:180–184, 1991.
151. Morris EA, Seeherman HJ: Evaluation of upper respiratory tract function during strenuous exercise in racehorses, J Am Vet Med Assoc 196:431–438, 1990.
152. Cook WR: Diagnosis and grading of hereditary recurrent laryngeal neuropathy in the horse, J Equine Vet Sci 8:432–455, 1988.
153. Hawe C, Dixon PM, Mayhew IG: A study of an electrodiagnostic technique for the evaluation of equine recurrent laryngeal neuropathy, Equine Vet J 33:459–465, 2001.
154. Fulton IC, Derksen FJ, Stick JA, et al: Treatment of left laryngeal hemiplegia in standardbreds, using a nerve muscle pedicle graft, Am J Vet Res 52:1461–1467, 1991.
155. Tulleners EP, Harrison IW, Raker CW: Management of arytenoid chondropathy and failed laryngoplasty in horses: 75 cases (1979-1985), J Am Vet Med Assoc 192:670–675, 1988.
156. Strand E, Martin GS, Haynes PF, et al: Career racing performance in thoroughbreds treated with prosthetic laryngoplasty for laryngeal neuropathy: 52 cases (1981-1989), J Am Vet Med Assoc 217:1689–1696, 2000.
157. Shelton GD: Swallowing disorders in the dog, Compend Contin Educ Pract Vet 4:607–614, 1982.
158. Weisbrodt NW: Neuromuscular organization of esophageal and pharyngeal motility, Arch Intern Med 136:524–531, 1976.

159. Suter PF, Watrous BJ: Oropharyngeal dysphagias in the dog: a cinefluorographic analysis of experimentally induced and spontaneously occurring swallowing disorders. I. Oral stage and pharyngeal stage dysphagias, Vet Radiol 21:24–39, 1980.
160. Baum KH, Halpern NE, Banish LD, et al: Dysphagia in horses: the differential diagnosis-Part II, Compend Contin Educ Pract Vet 10:1405–1410, 1988.
161. Greet T: Dysphagia in the horse, In Pract 11:256–262, 1989.
162. Pollard RE, Marks SL, Davidson A, et al: Quantitative videofluoroscopic evaluation of pharyngeal function in the dog, Vet Radiol Ultrasound 41:409–412, 2000.
163. Shelton GD, Willard MD, Cardinet GH III, et al: Acquired myasthenia gravis. Selective involvement of esophageal, pharyngeal, and facial muscles, J Vet Intern Med 4:281–284, 1990.
164. Fowler ME: Nigropallidal encephalomalacia in the horse, J Am Vet Med Assoc 147:607–616, 1965.
165. Larson KA, Young S: Nigropallidal encephalomalacia in horses in Colorado, J Am Vet Med Assoc 156:626–628, 1970.
166. Young S, Brown WW, Klinger B: Nigropallidal encephalomalacia in horses caused by ingestion of weeds of the genus, *Centaurea*. J Am Vet Med Assoc 157:1602–1605, 1970.
167. Tukov FF, Anand S, Gadepalli RSVS, et al: Inactivation of the cytotoxic activity of repin, a sesquiterpene lactone from *Centaurea repens*, Chem Res Toxicol 17:1170–1176, 2004.
168. Moret S, Populin T, Conte LS, et al: HPLC determination of free nitrogenous compounds of *Centaurea solstitialis* (Asteraceae), the cause of equine nigropallidal encephalomalacia, Toxicon 46:651–657, 2005.
169. Roy DN, Peyton DH, Spencer PS: Isolation and identification of two potent neurotoxins, aspartic acid and glutamic acid, from yellow star thistle *(Centaurea solstitialis)*, Nat Toxins 3:174–180, 1995.
170. Sanders SG, Tucker RL, Bagley RS, et al: Magnetic resonance imaging features of equine nigropallidal encephalomalacia, Vet Radiol Ultrasound 42:291–296, 2001.
171. Teixeira MJ, de Siqueira SR, Bor-Seng-Shu E: Glossopharyngeal neuralgia: neurosurgical treatment and differential diagnosis, Acta Neurochir (Wien) 150:471–475, 2008:discussion 475.
172. Rushton JG, Stevens JC, Miller RH: Glossopharyngeal (vagoglossopharyngeal) neuralgia. A study of 217 cases, Arch Neurol 38:201–205, 1981.
173. Shores A, Vaughn DM, Holland M, et al: Glossopharyngeal neuralgia syndrome in a dog, J Am Anim Hosp Assoc 27:101–104, 1991.
174. Watrous BJ: Clinical presentation and diagnosis of dysphagia, Vet Clin North Am Small Anim Pract 13:437–459, 1983.
175. Ladlow J, Hardie RJ: Cricopharyngeal achalasia in dogs, Compend Contin Educ Pract Vet 22:750–755, 2000.
176. Warnock JJ, Marks SL, Pollard R, et al: Surgical management of cricopharyngeal dysphagia in dogs: 14 cases (1989-2001), J Am Vet Med Assoc 223:1462–1468, 2003.
177. Bruchim Y, Kushnir A, Shamir MH: L-thyroxine responsive cricopharyngeal achalasia associated with hypothyroidism in a dog, J Small Anim Pract 46:553–554, 2005.
178. Davidson AP, Pollard RE, Bannasch DL, et al: Inheritance of cricopharyngeal dysfunction in golden retrievers, Am J Vet Res 65:344–349, 2004.
179. Niles JD, Williams JM, Sullivan M, et al: Resolution of dysphagia following cricopharyngeal myectomy in six young dogs, J Small Anim Pract 42:32–35, 2001.
180. Washabau RJ, Hall JA: Diagnosis and management of gastrointestinal motility disorders in dogs and cats, Compend Contin Educ Pract Vet 19:721–737, 1997.
181. Gaynor AR, Shofer FS, Washabau RJ: Risk factors for acquired megaesophagus in dogs, J Am Vet Med Assoc 211:1406–1412, 1997.
182. Harvey CE, O'Brien JA, Durie VR, et al: Megaesophagus in the dog: a clinical survey of 79 cases, J Am Vet Med Assoc 165:443–446, 1974.
183. Strombeck DR: Pathophysiology of esophageal motility disorders in the dog and cat. Application to management and prognosis, Vet Clin North Am 8:229–244, 1978.
184. Moses L, Harpster NK, Beck KA, et al: Esophageal motility dysfunction in cats: a study of 44 cases, J Am Anim Hosp Assoc 36:309–312, 2000.
185. Bexfield NH, Watson P, Herrtage ME: Esophageal dysmotility in young dogs, J Vet Intern Med 20:1314–1318, 2006.
186. Knowles KE, O'Brien DP, Amann JF: Congenital idiopathic megaesophagus in a litter of Chinese Shar-Peis: clinical, electrodiagnostic, and pathological findings, J Am Anim Hosp Assoc 26:313–318, 1990.
187. Schwartz A, Ravin CE, Greenspan RH, et al: Congenital neuromuscular esophageal disease in a litter of Newfoundland puppies, J Am Vet Radiol Soc 17:101–105, 1976.
188. Guilford WG: Megaesophagus in the dog and cat, Semin Vet Med Surg (Small Anim) 5:37–45, 1990.
189. Cox VS, Wallace LJ, Anderson VE, et al: Hereditary esophageal dysfunction in the miniature schnauzer dog, Am J Vet Res 41:326–330, 1980.
190. Osborne CA, Clifford DH, Jessen C: Hereditary esophageal achalasia in dogs, J Am Vet Med Assoc 151:572–581, 1967.
191. Holland CT, Satchell PM, Farrow BR: Vagal esophagomotor nerve function and esophageal motor performance in dogs with congenital idiopathic megaesophagus, Am J Vet Res 57:906–913, 1996.
192. Holland CT, Satchell PM, Farrow BR: Vagal afferent dysfunction in naturally occurring canine esophageal motility disorder, Dig Dis Sci 39:2090–2098, 1994.
193. Holland CT, Satchell PM, Farrow BR: Selective vagal afferent dysfunction in dogs with congenital idiopathic megaoesophagus, Auton Neurosci 99:18–23, 2002.
194. Boria PA, Webster CR, Berg J: Esophageal achalasia and secondary megaesophagus in a dog, Can Vet J 44:232–234, 2003.
195. Pollin MM, Griffiths IR: A review of the primary dysautonomias of domestic animals, J Comp Pathol 106:99–119, 1992.
196. McCarthy HE, Proudman CJ, French NP: Epidemiology of equine grass sickness: a literature review (1909-1999), Vet Rec 149:293–300, 2001.
197. Araya O, Vits L, Paredes E, et al: Grass sickness in horses in southern Chile, Vet Rec 150:695–697, 2002.
198. Uzal FA, Robles CA, Olaechea FV: Histopathological changes in the coeliaco-mesenteric ganglia of horses with "mal seco," a grass sickness-like syndrome, in Argentina, Vet Rec 130:244–246, 1992.
199. Doxey DL, Milne EM, Gilmour JS, et al: Clinical and biochemical features of grass sickness (equine dysautonomia), Equine Vet J 23:360–364, 1991.
200. Hunter LC, Miller JK, Poxton IR: The association of *Clostridium botulinum* type C with equine grass sickness: a toxicoinfection? Equine Vet J 31:492–499, 1999.
201. Hunter LC, Poxton IR: Systemic antibodies to *Clostridium botulinum* type C: do they protect horses from grass sickness (dysautonomia)? Equine Vet J 33:547–553, 2001.

202. Newton JR, Hedderson EJ, Adams VJ, et al: An epidemiological study of risk factors associated with the recurrence of equine grass sickness (dysautonomia) on previously affected premises, Equine Vet J 36:105–112, 2004.
203. Scholes SF, Vaillant C, Peacock P, et al: Diagnosis of grass sickness by ileal biopsy, Vet Rec 133:7–10, 1993.
204. Doxey DL, Milne EM, Ellison J, et al: Long-term prospects for horses with grass sickness (dysautonomia), Vet Rec 142:207–209, 1998.
205. Key TJ, Gaskell CJ: Puzzling syndrome in cats associated with pupillary dilatation, Vet Rec 110:160, 1982.
206. Sharp NJ: Feline dysautonomia, Semin Vet Med Surg (Small Anim) 5:67–71, 1990.
207. Kidder AC, Johannes C, O'Brien DP, et al: Feline dysautonomia in the Midwestern United States: a retrospective study of nine cases, J Feline Med Surg 10:130–136, 2008.
208. Sharp NJH: Feline dysautonomia, Semin Vet Med Surg (Small Anim) 5:67–71, 1990.
209. Nunn F, Cave TA, Knottenbelt C, et al: Association between Key-Gaskell syndrome and infection by *Clostridium botulinum* type C/D, Vet Rec 155:111–115, 2004.
210. Sharp NJH, Nash AS, Griffiths IR: Feline dysautonomia (the Key-Gaskell syndrome): a clinical and pathological study of forty cases, J Small Anim Pract 25:599–615, 1984.
211. Sharp NJH: Visceral dysfunction. In Wheeler SJ, editor: Manual of small animal neurology, Cheltenham, 1989, British Small Animal Veterinary Association.
212. Cave TA, Knottenbelt C, Mellor DJ, et al: Outbreak of dysautonomia (Key-Gaskell syndrome) in a closed colony of pet cats, Vet Rec 153:387–392, 2003.
213. Berghaus RD, O'Brien DP, Johnson GC, et al: Risk factors for development of dysautonomia in dogs, J Am Vet Med Assoc 218:1285–1290, 2001.
214. Harkin KR, Andrews GA, Nietfeld JC: Dysautonomia in dogs: 65 cases (1993-2000), J Am Vet Med Assoc 220:633–639, 2002.
215. Longshore RC, O'Brien DP, Johnson GC, et al: Dysautonomia in dogs: a retrospective study, J Vet Intern Med 10:103–109, 1996.
216. Harkin KR, Bulmer BJ, Biller DS: Echocardiographic evaluation of dogs with dysautonomia, J Am Vet Med Assoc 235:1431–1436, 2009.
217. Detweiler DA, Biller DS, Hoskinson JJ, et al: Radiographic findings of canine dysautonomia in twenty-four dogs, Vet Radiol Ultrasound 42:108–112, 2001.

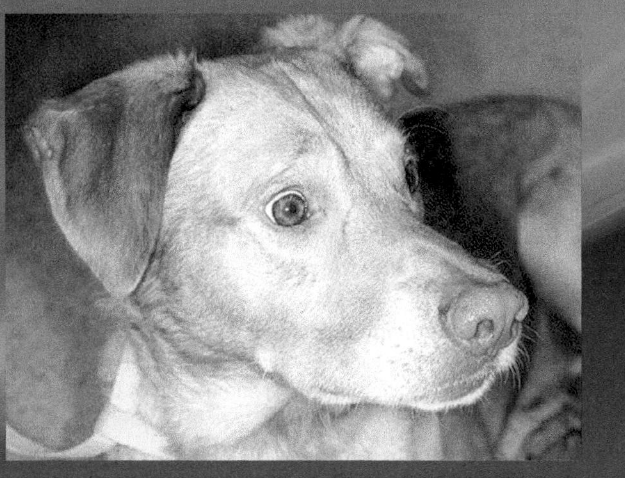

CHAPTER 10

Disorders of Involuntary Movement

Involuntary movement disorders encompass a wide range of diseases that result from *involuntary* muscle contractions. Many occur in specific breeds and often an underlying genetic pattern of inheritance is suspected. In this chapter, disorders of involuntary movements are classified employing categories based on acceptable medical terminology used in describing the clinical manifestations of abnormal movements.[1]

The term *involuntary movement* not only implies muscle contractions without volition, but importantly, the muscle contractions and therefore movements occur in *conscious* animals. Abnormal movements are also observed in unconscious animals or during sleep as occur with seizures or movements during rapid eye movement (REM) sleep. Abnormal movements associated with seizures are discussed in Chapter 13. Likewise, abnormal movements may be associated with voluntary movements as occurs with ataxia, abnormal posture, and intention tremor related to cerebellar disease. Abnormal movements associated with voluntary movement are discussed in Chapter 8.

TERMINOLOGY AND CLASSIFICATION

Overall, involuntary movement disorders are a result of alterations in either the muscle or nerve membrane potential leading to hyperexcitability and therefore represent disorders of muscle or disorders involving the lower motor neuron (LMN) (cell body, axon, or neuromuscular junction).[1] Several clinical syndromes are associated with disorders of muscle (myotonia) and with disorders involving the lower motor neuron, including tetanus, tetany, myoclonus, and a group of disorders referred to as movement disorders. An overview is presented in Box 10-1.

Myotonia

Myotonia is a clinical sign of sustained muscle contraction after a physiologic, mechanical, or chemical stimulation.

Tetanus

Tetanus is a state of sustained muscular contraction without periods of relaxation caused by repetitive stimulation of the motor nerve trunk at frequencies so high that individual muscle twitches are fused and cannot be distinguished from one another.[2] In clinical medicine, the term *tetanus* is generally used to describe the disease caused by *Clostridium tetani* toxin.

Tetany

Tetany is a condition that is similar to tetanus but characterized by intermittent tonic muscular contractions.

Rigidity

Rigidity is a descriptive term that is used to convey an increased resistance to changes in the position or angle of a single joint or multiple joints (i.e., difficulty in flexing or extending a joint). This may occur as a consequence of either increased muscular tone, or a mechanical defect involving the muscles, tendons, or ligaments such that joint movement is restricted (i.e., ankylosis).

Spasm

A spasm is an involuntary contraction of a muscle or group of muscles.

Spasticity

Spasticity is a descriptive term often used for disorders that have increased muscular tone. Spasticity is characterized by an increase in tonic stretch reflexes ("muscle tone") with exaggerated myotatic reflexes resulting from hyperexcitability of the stretch reflex.[2] It is often associated with disturbances involving the upper motor neurons (UMNs), resulting in reduced inhibition of the extensor motor neurons. With UMN disease, paresis or paralysis and increased myotatic and other segmental spinal reflexes occur. Lesion localization for UMN disease is described in Chapter 2.

Decerebrate and Decerebellate Postures

Lesions of the rostral brainstem (midbrain, rostral pons) produce a posture called *decerebrate rigidity* in which all limbs are extended with increased extensor tone. Forced flexion of the limb is met with increased resistance to a point, then an abrupt loss of resistance and flexion occurs, called the clasp-knife reflex. If the cerebellum, particularly the rostral lobe, is also damaged the head and neck are extended and the back

BOX 10-1

Classification Scheme for Involuntary Movement Disorders

Disorders involving muscle
- Myotonia—the clinical sign of prolonged contraction or delayed relaxation following stimulation of the muscle
  - Congential
  - Acquired

Disorders involving the neuron
- Tetanus—the clinical syndrome of sustained muscular contraction without relaxation. Used synonymously with the disease caused by the toxin produced by *Clostridium tetani.*
- Tetany—similar to tetanus, tetany is the clinical syndrome of intermittent muscular contractions
- Myoclonus—the clinical manifestation of sudden contraction of a group of muscles followed by its relaxation
  - Spontaneous
  - Repetitive—sometimes referred to as a tremor
    - Constant
    - Action-related
    - Postural
    - Episodic
    - Resting
- Movement disorders—a variety of abnormal movement; syndromes often involve complex movements, which may be stereotypic or varied and involve specific body parts or are generalized.

is arched (lordosis) in a posture called *opisthotonos*.[3] The posture is generally accompanied by increased extensor tone in the limbs. Acute lesions of the cerebellum without damage to the brainstem cause a posture termed *decerebellate rigidity* that is similar to decerebrate posture, but the pelvic limbs are flexed and uncoordinated movements may occur (Figure 10-1).

Myoclonus

Myoclonus is the rhythmic movement of the portion of a body that is the result of a sudden involuntary contraction of a group of muscles followed by its relaxation. When occurring in a limb, it is appreciated as a rhythmic flexion or extension of the affected limb(s). The movement can be further qualified based on its frequency (i.e., rapid or slow) and excursion (i.e., gross or fine movement). When occurring in a muscle of the axial skeleton such as the temporalis muscles, it appears as rhythmic muscle contractions.

Tremor

Tremor is a term that is often used to describe the resultant involuntary movements of rapid, repetitive myoclonus. The term *tremor* is applied to the observation of rapid, repetitive rhythmic flexion of joints, which appears as a vibration or shivering that may be diffuse or limited to specific anatomy such as a limb. Tremor can be qualified based on rate and degree of excursion of the joint giving rise to such terms as "fine" or "coarse" tremors with minute or large joint movements, respectively. As such, tremors may be a normal physiologic response. Referred to as *physiologic tremors,* rapid and repetitive fine oscillations may be observed during periods of stress (e.g., a frightened animal) or during periods of hypothermia. Conversely, *pathologic tremors* occur as a consequence

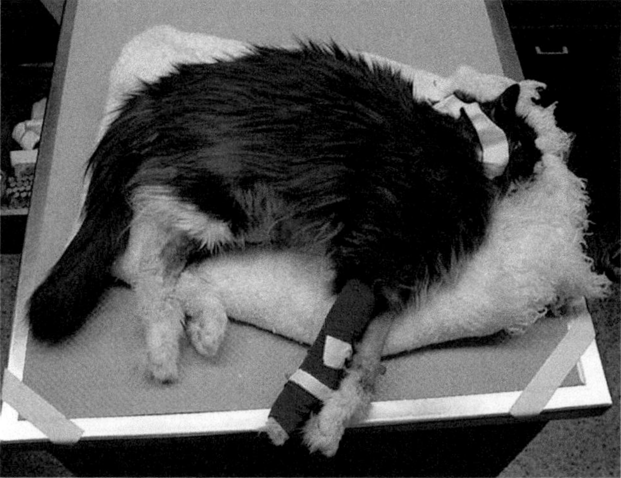

Figure 10-1 A 3-year-old FS domestic long hair presented after a traumatic fall. Note the decerebellate posture. There is opisthotonus. The thoracic limbs are extended and the pelvic limbs are flexed.

of a disease process. Pathology of any part of the motor unit may manifest tremors as part of the clinical disease spectrum. Pathologic tremors may be the result of hyperexcitability of the LMN in which tremors are the manifestation of an involuntary movement. Due to their involuntary nature, these conditions are discussed in this chapter. Alternatively, pathologic tremors may occur during voluntary movements. Tremors may be associated with diseases of the cerebellum, basal ganglia, and related pathways. For example, intention tremors occur with voluntary (purposeful) movements such as movement of the head when an animal attempts to eat or drink. Intention tremors are further described in Chapter 8. Similarly, tremors are often observed as a consequence of weakness from neuromuscular disease. In this instance, fine tremors are observed when the animal is attempting to support its weight against gravity when standing

Fasciculation

Fasciculation is visible as irregular movements over the surface of the affected muscle caused by spontaneous contractions of individual motor units suggestive of lower motor neuron lesion.[1] Muscle fasciculations do not produce rhythmic limb or body movements as seen with tremor. Fasciculation is common in motor neuron disease.

Myokymia

Movements associated with myokymia have been described as rippling and vermicular (wormlike) and may also appear as tremors. Myokymia is not affected by motion and can persist during sleep. Myokymia can be generalized or focal. Neuromyotonia is characterized by muscle stiffness and persistent contraction.[1]

Dyskinesia

Numerous syndromes resulting in involuntary movement, referred to simply as movement disorders, are described in humans and nonhuman primates. Most of these disorders have not been reproduced in quadrupeds, even with experimental lesions in areas thought to or known to cause the disorder in humans or primates. The term *dyskinesia* denotes abnormal movement and several movement disorders are included in this category.

Chorea is the contraction of random muscles throughout the body, occurring at random times and for random durations.[4]

Dystonia is contraction of muscles, either focal or generalized, often including antagonist muscles that contract simultaneously. In humans, dystonia is frequently described as twisting on the long axis of the body part.

Athetosis is a slow, writhing movement of the fingers, sometimes described as pill-rolling movements in humans. The movements of the lips in horses with nigropallidal encephalomalacia caused by a plant toxin have been compared with athetosis. A related movement disorder has been produced in cats with lesions in the caudate nucleus in which affected cats displayed slow kneading movements of the paws and abrupt, exaggerated movements of the thoracic limbs.[5]

Ballismus denotes wild, large-amplitude, irregular limb movements. It frequently occurs on one side of the body and is then referred to as hemiballismus. Ballismus is apparently related to chorea because humans often have ballismus after a stroke, which then gradually changes to chorea over days.[4]

EXAMINATION, LESION LOCALIZATION, AND DIFFERENTIAL DIAGNOSIS

Although signs may be constant in affected animals, some of the disorders of involuntary movement are episodic in nature. As a result, some affected animals may appear normal at the time of examination making lesion localization difficult. Hence, a thorough anamnesis is paramount to defining disorders of involuntary movements. Helpful information includes whether the movement was isolated to a single anatomic location or occurred diffusely, whether the movement was triggered by specific stimuli, and whether the movement was associated with increased muscular tone. Moreover, knowing whether the movement persisted during relaxation or sleep may help to better define the event. If possible, analyzing video recordings of the episodic movements may be helpful when evaluating affected animals that are normal during examination. Occasionally, the diagnosis of an involuntary movement disorder is supported by excluding from consideration other conditions in which similar movements occur. Most important, a seizure disorder should be eliminated as the underlying disease process when evaluating episodic involuntary movement disorders. Characterization and diagnostic work up for seizure disorders are described in Chapter 13.

Disorders of involuntary movement involve hyperexcitability of the LMN unit and therefore provide the foundation for lesion localization. Lower motor neuron hyperexcitability may be caused by an imbalance of facilitation and inhibition on the LMN related to imbalances in excitatory neurotransmitters such as glutamate, and inhibitory neurotransmitters such as gamma-aminobutyric acid (GABA) and glycine, respectively. The firing pattern of an individual LMN is determined by synaptic connections from the primary peripheral afferents, descending UMN pathways from the brain, and local interneuron connections. Loss of adequate facilitation causes decreased muscle tone and reflexes typical of LMN disease, (see Chapter 7). Loss of inhibitory control causes increased firing of the LMN and intermittent or continuous contraction of the muscles it innervates.

DISORDERS INVOLVING THE MUSCLE MEMBRANE

Disorders involving the muscles:

Congenital Myotonia—General

Myotonia is defined as the clinical sign related to prolonged contraction or delayed relaxation following voluntary stimulation of the muscle or stimulation evoked mechanically,

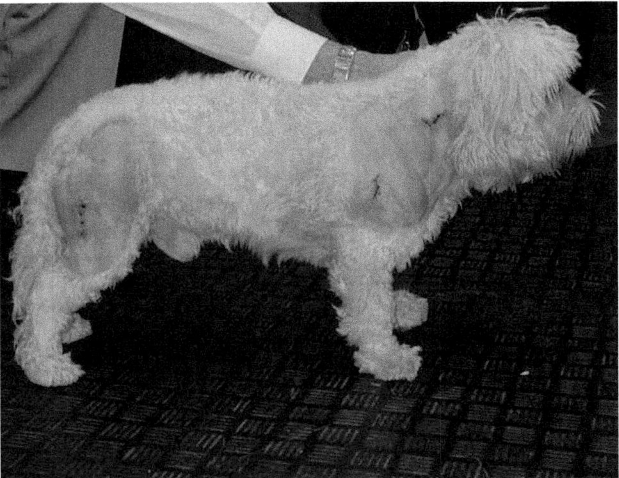

Figure 10-2 A 2-year-old mixed-breed dog that was evaluated for difficulty standing up from a lying position, frequently falling, and a "stiff gait." Myotonic discharges were observed with EMG. Findings were consistent with myotonia congenita. Note the prominent muscular hypertrophy of the proximal limbs and cervical muscles. (Copyright 2010 University of Georgia Research Foundation, Inc.)

electrically, or chemically.[6] Myotonia displays as muscle stiffness. Muscle stiffness can occur with activity (action myotonia) or occur after percussion of the muscle with a reflex hammer, which results in dimpling of the muscle (percussive myotonia).[6] In long-haired animals, the dimple is easily seen on the tongue. With time, the muscles may become hypertrophied, especially in the proximal parts of the limbs and in the neck (Figure 10-2). Electrophysiologically, electromyography (EMG) reveals complex multiphasic discharges that wax and wane in amplitude over a range of 10 μV to 1 mV, with a frequency range of 50 to 100 Hz discharges.[7] Acoustically, the sound produced by myotonic discharges that waxe and wane, which are often likened to an airplane "dive bomber," or revving of a motorcycle engine. Myotonic discharges observed with EMG may occur in the presence or absence of clinical signs of myotonia.

Based on light microscopic changes observed in muscle, clinical syndromes that result in myotonia can occur in disorders (1) without obvious muscle pathology (nondystrophic myopathies associated with myotonia) or (2) in conjunction with pathologic changes in muscle (dystrophic myopathies associated with myotonia).

The latter may be referred to as muscular dystrophies. Historically, the term muscular dystrophy has defined the disease process involving an abnormality of the dystrophin protein (in humans, Duchenne muscular dystrophy and in dogs, golden retriever muscular dystrophy). With the development and the increased use of molecular techniques, several disorders have been identified that may result not only from abnormalities in the dystrophin protein but also from other protein associated dystrophin-glycoprotein complexes.[8] These disorders are collectively known as congenital muscular dystrophies.[8] The term *muscular dystrophy* can be applied to any condition that results in light microscopic changes in myofibers consisting of a pattern of small group muscle necrosis and regeneration associated with a predominance of type 1 fibers and fiber type grouping. Myofiber size variation occurs due to myofiber hypertrophy and regenerating fibers. Muscular dystrophies span a wide spectrum of microscopic changes in muscle ranging from minimal to quite severe. Congenital muscular dystrophies are discussed in Chapter 7. Often these disorders result in clinical signs consistent with LMN disease such as weakness, reduced to absent reflexes, and muscular atrophy. However, some cases of muscular dystrophy can share clinical similarities including muscle hypertrophy, myotonia, and electrophysiologic changes with nondystrophic myopathies associated with myotonia disorders.

Nondystrophic myopathies associated with myotonia largely reflect diseases associated with abnormal ion channels (ion channelopathy) that function in muscle. The most well-recognized channelopathy involves chloride channels, but sodium channel disorders can also result in myotonia. In these disorders, myofibers appear normal (nondystrophic) microscopically, albeit hypertrophied.

Nondystrophic Myopathies Associated With Myotonia

Myotonia Congenita. Myotonia congenita is caused by abnormal chloride ion transfer across the muscle sarcolemma. Decreased chloride conductance leads to myofiber hyperexcitability and spontaneous myofiber action potentials.[9] Normally, muscle contraction begins with an action potential spreading across the muscle sarcolemma. This action potential is the result of the influx of sodium through open sodium channels (depolarization). Ultimately, depolarization of the sarcolemma results in an intracytosolic influx of calcium, which drives the contractile elements. For the myofiber to relax, repolarization must occur. In general, repolarization of excitable tissue occurs as a result of potassium (K^+) efflux. Over a cell membrane as large as that of a myofiber, repolarization due to K^+ efflux would result in an extracellular buildup of K^+ over time. Such buildup would lead to subsequent depolarization after the termination of the initial action potential, "afterdepolarizations."[9] As a consequence, the muscle becomes unable to relax due to continued contractions generated by afterdepolarizations. To effectively repolarize, chloride ion exchange helps buffer the need for K^+ efflux. Myofibers are rich in chloride channel 1 (CLC-1) protein, which is composed of two identical protein channels, produced from the CLCN-1 gene.[10] Both channels function together and allow the influx of chloride ions through the sarcolemma. Abnormalities in the CLC-1 protein result in impaired chloride ion conductance leading to an inability to relax the muscle.

In humans, myotonia congenita is inherited as an autosomal dominant (Thomsen disease) or recessive (Becker myotonia) condition. Myotonia congenita has been studied extensively in the goat.[9,11-13] Affected goats have been erroneously referred to as "fainting goats." Initial studies showed that affected goats had decreased chloride conductance in myofibers.[13] Later, a defect in the *CLC-1* gene in which a substitution of a highly conserved alanine residue with proline leading to decreased chloride conductance was documented.[9] In addition to the goat, myotonia congenita has been observed in the dog,[14-21] horse,[22] and cat[23,24](see Table 10-1).

Canine Myotonia Congenita. Myotonia congenita has been reported most frequently in the chow chow[19,25,26] and miniature schnauzer.[20,27,28] Individual dogs of various other breeds also have been described.[14-18,21] Clinical signs are similar in all reports. Although clinical signs are present at birth, muscle stiffness is more evident at the time pups begin to walk. In addition to generalized muscle stiffness, signs consist of difficulty rising, abnormal postures (sawhorse stance with the limbs abducted), bunny hopping, muscle hypertrophy, particularly of the proximal limb musculature, stridorous breathing, dysphagia, and regurgitation. With excitement or stimulation, affected dogs can develop profound extensor rigidity causing the dog to fall over and be unable to right itself. Some affected dogs appear to improve with mild to moderate exercise ("warm-up" phenomenon). Dental and craniofacial abnormalities have been observed in affected miniature schnauzers.[27] Abnormalities include delayed eruptions of deciduous and permanent dentition, increased interdental spaces, malocclusions, difficulty opening and closing the mouth, mandibular brachygnathism, protrusion of the tongue, and flattening of the zygomatic arch. These malformations have not been observed in other affected breeds. The diagnosis is made through recognition of clinical signs in young animals and exclusion of other conditions resulting in similar clinical signs. Electrophysiologic testing may provide supportive data. EMG is useful to detect the characteristic "myotonic" discharges. However, these potentials can be confused with a more common abnormality referred to as complex repetitive discharges, which are observed in other neuromuscular diseases (see Chapter 4). In dogs, polymerase chain reaction (PCR) testing for the *CLC-1* gene mutation observed in the miniature schnauzer can be performed. However, not all cases of myotonia congenita relate to this mutation; therefore, a negative result does not exclude the diagnosis. Procainamide or mexiletine may provide some reduction in clinical signs.

Feline Myotonia Congenita. Affected cats show signs at an early age.[23,24] Signs are similar to those in dogs. Distortion of the face, elevated nictitating membranes, and ear position occurred when startled or when hissing. Affected cats show some improvement with exercise (warm-up phenomenon).

Hyperkalemic Periodic Paralysis. Similar to myotonia congenita, hyperkalemic periodic paralysis (HPP) is an ion channel disorder of muscles.[29] However, HPP is the consequence of a sodium channel defect that results in increased sodium permeability and a subsequent increase in the resting membrane potential of muscle cells. This allows K^+ to diffuse extracellularly, accounting for the observed hyperkalemia causing further depolarization of the muscle cell. As the resting membrane potential nears threshold, myofibers become hyperexcitable (myotonia). With further depolarization, the resting membrane potential becomes so abnormal that excitability and muscle contractions decline. Clinically, this results in paralysis.

Hyperkalemic periodic paralysis has been observed in the quarter horse and a dog (see Chapter 7).[30,31] At the onset of signs, affected horses display brief episodes of myotonia, muscle fasciculation, and elevation of the nictitating membranes. During episodes, affected horses excessively sweat, have normal to increased muscle tone, and elevated heart and respiratory rates. Once the episodes are over, the affected animals appear normal.

Acquired Myotonia

Acquired Myopathy With Characteristics of Myotonia

Several forms of acquired myopathy may have myotonic features. Inflammatory myopathy, whether immune mediated or caused by an infectious agent such as toxoplasmosis, may have complex repetitive discharges on the EMG and some increased contraction of the muscles. On occasion, endocrine-related myopathy develops that is caused by increased circulating corticosteroids with affected dogs displaying clinical signs consistent with myotonia. This has been referred to as pseudomyotonia and has been associated degenerative changes in muscle.[32] The pathophysiology is unknown. Given the degenerative changes present in muscle and the lack of myotonic discharges, the condition should be referred to as pseudomyotonia. Hyperadrenocorticism (Cushing syndrome) may be caused by adrenal tumors, pituitary tumors, or exogenous administration of corticosteroids. Microscopically, the pathologic changes in muscle occur late in the course of the syndrome. Often, affected dogs demonstrate mild clinical signs typically associated with hyperadrenocorticism. A stiff gait or weakness with exercise may be recognized. The pelvic limbs are frequently more obviously affected than the thoracic limbs. The pelvic limbs are extended and directed slightly caudally. Pelvic limb movement is characterized by decreased flexion of the coxofemoral and stifle joints with most of the advancement of the pelvic limbs occurring by flexion of the hock, giving the impression of paddling movements while walking. Proximal appendicular muscle hypertrophy is often pronounced. Microscopic evaluation of muscle reveals variability in fiber size, increased numbers of nuclei, myofiber necrosis and atrophy (primarily of type II fibers), and increased amounts of perimysial connective tissue. The diagnosis of pseudomyotonia related to hyperadrenocorticism is made through a combination of clinical signs in the presence of hyperadrenocorticism, and electrophysiology and microscopic evaluation of muscle. In general, signs may persist despite resolution of hyperadrenocorticism. Procainamide or mexiletine may improve clinical signs.[33]

Drugs and Toxins

Certain chemicals and drugs have been associated with myotonia related to the effects of chloride conductance. The commonly used postemergent herbicide 2,4 dichlorophenoxyacetic acid (2,4 D) may result in myotonia. Experimentally, dogs administered 2,4 D orally developed gastrointestinal signs and electrophysiologic evidence of myotonia.[34] Percussive myotonia was appreciated in the tongue but the gait was unaffected. In humans, cholesterol-lowering drugs (statins) such as clofibrate, simvastatin, and pravastatin may result in myotonia.[35]

Dystrophic Myopathies Associated With Myotonia

Myotonia has been associated with dystrophic myopathies in the dog, cat, and horse.[36-39] Unlike myotonia congenita, dystrophic pathologic changes are observed histologically. In the dog and cat, the clinical sign of myotonia can be associated with dystrophin-deficient muscular dystrophy and other congential disorders involving the dystrophin-glycoprotein complex.[39-41] Despite this, clinical signs typical of LMN disease predominate. However, electrophysiologic evidence of muscle membrane excitability (complex repetitive discharges) along with the clinical observation of myotonia and muscular hypertrophy (especially in the cat) can be observed. In a few instances, microscopic evidence of dystrophic change in muscle is minimal. In the veterinary literature, these disorders have been termed *myotonic dystrophies* based on similarities to the condition in humans. Although the exact pathogenesis in these cases remains unknown, based on the observed pathology they are presumed to be related to other muscular dystrophies. Their inclusion here is based on a similar clinical presentation as occurs with the nondystrophic myotonias and the lack of severe dystrophic microscopic changes typical of most disorders involving the dystrophin-glycoprotein complex.

Humans

In humans, myotonic dystrophy is a genetic condition. Two forms are known: DM1 and DM2. Affected individuals suffer from progressive weakness and display clinical signs and electrophysiologic evidence of myotonia.[42] DM1 is the result of an expanded repeat of an unstable trinucleotide (CTG) in the *DMPK* (myotonic dystrophy protein kinase) gene in chromosome 19q.[43] DM2, also known as proximal myotonic myopathy (PROMM), is a CCTG expansion in the *ZNF9* gene in chromosome 3q.[44] Although not fully understood, it appears that the RNA produced by transcription of the expanded repeat results in the pathophysiology.[45] Affected individuals may have concurrent cataracts, cardiac, gastrointestinal, and endocrine disorders.[42]

Myotonic dystrophy similar to that in humans has been observed in the horse and dog.[36-38] Table 7-11 lists the hereditary and muscular changes in these animals. Myotonic dystrophies are associated with moderate to severe, progressive weakness (see chapter 7).

TABLE 10-1

Myotonia Congenita

Species/Breed	Heredity	References
Caprine	Autosomal dominant or recessive	9, 11-13
Canine		
Miniature schnauzer	Autosomal recessive	20, 27, 28
Chow chow	Autosomal recessive (?)	19, 25, 26
Staffordshire terrier	Autosomal recessive (?)	18
Australian cattle dog	Autosomal recessive	14
Cocker spaniel	Unknown	15
West Highland white terrier	Unknown	20
Great Dane	Unknown	16
Jack Russell terrier	Unknown	17
Cat		
Siamese	Unknown	23, 24
Equine	Unknown	22

Equine

This condition is typically evident within a few months of birth.[36] Affected foals suffer progressive weakness, difficulty rising, and a stiff gait. There is increased tone in the limbs with proximal limb muscle hypertrophy especially in the superficial gluteal, semimembranosus, semitendinosus, and longissimus muscles. Percussive myotonia is evident. Electrophysiologically, myotonic discharges are observed, which persist with neuromuscular blockade suggesting a primary muscle defect. Pathologic changes observed in muscle include internalized nuclei, sarcoplasmic masses, and occasional ring fibers. Additionally, gonadal hypoplasia and reduced testosterone levels were identified in one affected foal.[36] The condition shares obvious similarities to that observed in humans.

Canine

There are two reported cases of myotonic dystrophy in the dog.[37,38] Signs developed at 3 to 6 months of age in one dog and 28 months of age in the other. Both affected dogs were young and showed clinical and electrophysiologic abnormalities similar to affected horses. In one dog, dysphagia resulted in weight loss due to inadequate caloric intake and progressive muscular atrophy, which leads to euthanasia.[37] Muscular atrophy rather than hypertrophy was observed in the affected dogs.

DISORDERS INVOLVING THE LMN

Pathology of any part of the motor neuron may result in an involuntary muscle contraction or movement. These conditions are divided into four categories: tetanus, tetany, myoclonus, and conditions referred to as movement disorders. Tetanus, the sustained contraction of muscle, is a single disease process related to exposure to the toxin produced by *Clostridium tetani*. Like tetanus, tetany involves contractions of muscle; however, between contractions there are periods of relaxation. Clinically, contractions may be described as spasms or the observation of episodes of muscle spasticity. Myoclonus is a broad category of diseases that involve a sudden muscle contraction followed by relaxation. Disorders involving myoclonus are grouped according to whether they occur sporadically or repetitively; repetitive myoclonus is further grouped based on whether myoclonus occurs constantly or in association with actions, or posture, or occur episodically or at rest. Lastly, movement disorders are conditions in which there are complex movements involving numerous muscle groups of multiple limbs.

Tetanus

Pathophysiology

Tetanus is caused by the toxin (tetanospasmin) produced by *C. tetani*, a spore-bearing anaerobic bacillus.[46] The spores are resistant to most sporicidal agents and can remain viable for years.[47] The organisms may be found in soil and are common in the feces of many species. Bacteria gain access to the animal's tissues through open wounds, proliferate, and produce the toxin. Deep wounds with poor oxygenation are most susceptible. The toxin is composed of a heavy (H) and light (L) chain.[48] The H chain is responsible for binding to gangliosides on nerves and subsequent internalization. The toxin ascends via retrograde transport within the axons of nerves to the spinal cord where it transsynaptically invades the inhibitory interneurons and then disseminates throughout the central nervous system (CNS). The L chain is a metalloprotease, which cleaves synaptobrevin, a membrane protein in synaptic vesicles necessary for the release of neurotransmitters.[48] Ultimately, tetanus toxin blocks the release of the inhibitory neurotransmitters glycine and GABA. Glycine is the neurotransmitter for primary inhibitory interneurons such as the Renshaw cell; GABA is the inhibitory transmitter for descending pathways. The result is an uninhibited firing of the LMN. Tetanus toxin can also block sympathetic preganglionic neurons resulting in autonomic dysfunction. Finally, tetanus toxin may bind directly at neuromuscular junctions and cause neuromuscular facilitation. Although all domestic animals are susceptible to tetanus, horses are most sensitive whereas dogs and ruminants are more resistant. Cats appear to be very resistant.

Clinical Signs

Clinical signs relate not only to the amount of toxin but also to species susceptibility. In dogs, younger dogs appear to be at greater risk for developing more severe clinical signs.[49] The clinical signs of tetanus occur 3 to 10 days after infection but may be delayed for up to 3 weeks in dogs and cats. If the toxin ascends in a nerve of a limb, that limb shows tetanus first, followed by the opposite limb and eventually the entire body. If the toxin circulates in the blood, signs of tetanus start in the head and then become generalized. Elevation of the nictitating membrane and contraction of the facial and mastication muscles are seen before development of tetanus in the rest of the body[49] (Figure 10-3). Generalized signs include increased muscle tone and stiffness, usually in all the limbs and in the muscles of the head. The lips are drawn in an exaggerated "grin" often referred to as *ris sardonicus*; in erect-eared breeds, the ears are drawn toward each other and the jaws are tightly closed. Other early signs are a stiff gait and tail elevation. In the later stages, the animal is recumbent with extension of all four limbs and opisthotonus. Signs are enhanced by stimulation (auditory or tactile). Death may occur from respiratory complications related to inability to breathe due to rigidity of the respiratory muscles, aspiration pneumonia, or from cardiac arrhythmias.

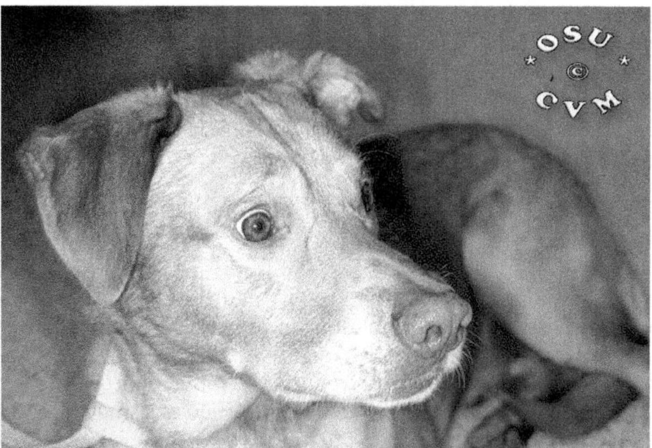

Figure 10-3 Elevation of the nictitating membrane and contraction of the facial and mastication muscles are seen before development of tetanus in the rest of the body. Note the muscle tone and stiffness in the head and that the ears are drawn toward each other.

In some rare cases, signs may stay localized to one limb, which may confuse the diagnosis. Localized tetanus is seen more commonly in cats.[50] Invariably, clinical signs of localized tetanus demonstrate as extensor rigidity in a limb. In general, when localized to the thoracic limb, the limb is directed caudally, the elbow is extended, and the carpus flexed.[51]

Autonomic effects may include cardiac arrhythmias such as the bradyarrhythmias including atrioventricular blocks, and atrial standstill.[49,52,53] Conversely, tachyarrhythmias, including supraventricular tachycardia and accelerated idioventricular arrhythmias, may occur.[52] Tachypnea and increased inspiratory stridor may occur as a result of laryngeal paralysis.[52] Respiratory failure due to respiratory muscle paralysis may necessitate mechanical ventilation. Hiatal hernia and megaesophagus may be present and result in regurgitation. Secondary aspiration pneumonia may result from laryngeal paralysis or dysphagia related to paralysis of muscles involving eating and swallowing. Some dogs experience urinary retention. Affected animals often are hyperthermic likely due to continuous muscle activity. Clinicopathologic data reflect nonspecific abnormalities. Affected animals often have elevated creatinine kinase activity as a consequence of sustained muscle activity or recumbency.

Diagnosis

The diagnosis is based on the characteristic clinical signs and evidence of infection. EMG has been used to support the diagnosis.[51,54,55] EMG has been particularly helpful in diagnosis of focal tetanus. EMG abnormalities include prolonged insertional activity, and spontaneous continuous motor unit discharges that occur in both the agonist-antagonistic muscle groups.[54] Serum antibody titers to tetanus toxin can be used to confirm the diagnosis, but they are rarely used in clinical practice. Identifying clostridial organisms cytologically or with culture from infected wounds is supportive of the diagnosis. However, in many cases, the source of infection is not always evident. Intraabdominal infections, such as metritis, enteritis, and abscesses, may be a cause. Infection of the reproductive tract may cause tetanus localized to the pelvic limbs. Tetanus has been observed after spaying or neutering. It is possible that spores from the environment may penetrate into the healing surgical wound. Alternatively, infection at the surgical site such as with uterine stump infections can result in tetanus.[52] In young dogs, the loss of deciduous teeth may also provide a source of infection.[49]

Treatment

Treatment includes wound débridement, systemic administration of antibiotics, and potentially administration of antitoxin to neutralize unbound, circulating toxin. Historically, penicillin was considered the antibiotic of choice in the treatment of tetanus. However, the structure of penicillin is similar to GABA and therefore it may act as a competitive inhibitor. At high concentrations, penicillins can cause CNS hyperexcitability and seizures. Although hypothetical, penicillins may potentiate inhibition of GABA in tetanus. Consequently, metronidazole has become the drug of choice for treatment of tetanus because it is bactericidal against C. *tetani*, it is able to penetrate into necrotic tissue, and is effective in anaerobic environments. Antibiotics used in the treatment of tetanus include metronidazole (10 mg/kg of body weight, administered orally every 8 hours), penicillin G (20,000 to 100,000 IU/kg of body weight, administered intramuscularly [IM] or subcutaneously [SQ] [penicillin K can be administered intravenously; IV] every 6 to 8 hours), tetracycline (22 mg/kg, administered *per os* (PO) or IV every 8 hours), and clindamycin (3 to 10 mg/kg of body weight, administered (PO, IV, or IM every 8 to 12 hours). Antibiotics should be administered for a minimum of 10 to 14 days.

Tetanus antitoxin (TAT) is available as antitetanus equine serum and may be beneficial in treatment. Tetanus antitoxin neutralizes only circulating, unbound toxin. Since clinical signs are related to toxin already bound and internalized within CNS neurons, TAT does not speed recovery. Tetanus antitoxin can be given IM, SQ, or IV. Intravenous administration of TAT gives a rapid increase in circulating antitoxin and is the preferred route of administration. However, use of TAT intravenously should be done cautiously. A dose of 100 to 1000 IU/kg is recommended for dogs and 10,000 IU for horses. Intravenous TAT is associated with a high incidence of anaphylaxis. An intradermal (ID) test injection of (0.1 to 0.2 mL) of antitoxin should be performed before IV administration. However, animals not demonstrating a skin reaction with ID testing still may have an adverse systemic reaction when treated intravenously.[49,56] Likewise, some animals with skin reactions with ID testing may not develop adverse reactions when administered antitoxin intravenously. Pretreatment with antihistamines and cortico steroids is recommended. Intravenous fluid therapy and epinephrine (0.1 mL/kg of 1:10,000 dilution) are used in the treatment of anaphylactic reactions. In horse, intrathecal administration of TAT has been used. In adult horses, a dose between 5000 and 10,000 units has been recommended.[57] The benefit to intrathecal administration is unknown. In one study, the recovery rate of horses treated intrathecally was 77% as opposed to 50% in those treated IV or IM.[58] However, another study failed to demonstrate a similar benefit.[56] Intrathecal administration in small animals is not recommended. Instead, the goal of TAT therapy is to prevent further binding of any circulating unbound toxin.

Sedation may be required to control severe muscle spasms, hyperexcitable states, and seizures. Phenothiazine tranquilizers such as acepromazine or chlorpromazine depress descending excitatory neurons in the brainstem. Phenothiazines are not contraindicated in animals with tetanus-induced seizures. Phenobarbital is used to control seizures. It can be combined with the phenothiazines, but its dose should be reduced. Glycopyrrolate can be used to treat bradycardia. The benzodiazepines, such as diazepam or clonazepam, may be helpful because they work though GABA transmission and block polysynaptic reflexes in the medulla and spinal cord.

Nursing care must include a quiet environment, frequent turning if the animal is recumbent, and skin cleanliness. Oral intake may be impossible; hence, parenteral fluids and nutrients may be necessary. Nasogastric, esophagotomy, or gastric tubes may be used. Radiographic evaluation of the thoracic cavity before feeding should be performed to identify the presence of hiatal hernia, megaesophagus, or aspiration pneumonia. Abdominal distention should be monitored in ruminants not able to maintain sternal recumbency and eructate, and breeds of dogs susceptible to bloat. In young animals surviving the disease, before epiphysial closure is complete, tetanus may cause a variety of growth abnormalities in long bones.

Prognosis

The prognosis is usually good for dogs and cats. The prognosis is best for dogs with less severe clinical signs. In dogs, reported survival rates include 50%, 77%, and 92%.[49,52,59] Horses or cows that become recumbent have poor prognoses. In a retrospective study of 20 horses, the mortality rate was 75%.[56] Prognosis was best for horses that had been vaccinated with toxoid within a year of developing tetanus, that remained ambulatory, able to eat and drink, responded to phenothiazine tranquilizers, and had clinical signs that stabilized in 2 to 3 days.[56] Horses that received intravenous tetanus antitoxin did better than those that received antitoxin subcutaneously. Immunization with toxoid is recommended in horses. It is given to newborn foals and boosters are given every few years. Toxoid is given at the time of injury or surgery or before parturition.[57]

Tetany

Tetany shares clinical similarities to tetanus. However, tetany is the clinical sign of intermittent increased extensor tone. Tetany may be congenital or acquired as a result of metabolic disturbances, presumed immune mediated disease, or intoxication.

Congenital Tetany

Congenital tetany has been observed in cattle, dogs, and horses. Regardless of the species, clinical signs are similar. At birth, affected animals display variable degrees of extensor rigidity in all limbs and opisthotonus. Affected animals may not be able to stand or walk without assistance. If capable, affected animals adopt a sawhorse stance and walk with a stiff gait. With external stimuli, increased extensor rigidity occurs. Although these congenital syndromes have been referred to as congenital myoclonus, the clinical picture is dominated by tetany; therefore, these congenital syndromes are hereto referred to as congenital tetany.

Cattle-Inherited Congenital Myoclonus. This syndrome has also been erroneously described as neuraxial edema.[60] Healy and colleagues differentiated two syndromes found in Hereford and Polled Hereford cattle.[61] Congenital tetany occurs primarily in Polled Herefords and their crossbreeds. It is inherited as an autosomal recessive trait with onset before birth. Clinical signs consist of increased extensor tone in all limbs, opisthotonus, hyperesthesia, and seizures. Affected animals appear mentally normal. They are unable to stand without assistance. Various external stimuli result in increased extensor tone. Many of the calves have traumatic lesions of the hip joints, suggesting the presence of clinical signs in affected calves in utero. No histologic lesions are present in the CNS in these animals. A deficiency in functional glycine receptors in the spinal cord has been identified.[62] A nonsense mutation in the α_1 subunit of the glycine receptor resulting in loss of function and its expression on the cell has been demonstrated.[63] The second disease, neuraxonal edema, was found in polled Herefords and Herefords. Clinical signs developed after birth and consisted of dullness, opisthotonus, and recumbency. The animals had a characteristic histologic evidence of status spongiosus of the nervous system. Ketone concentrations were high in the urine, with a distinct aroma of burnt sugar. Healy and colleagues compared this syndrome with maple syrup urine disease in humans, one of several disorders of amino acid metabolism. The disease appears to be inherited as an autosomal recessive trait. The exact nature of the amino acid abnormality is not known. Neuraxonal edema has also been reported in conjunction with hypomyelinogenesis in Hereford calves, but subsequent studies demonstrated that this was only hypomyelinogenesis.[64,65]

Labrador Retrievers—Familial Reflex Myoclonus. Congenital tetany has been observed in Labrador retriever pups and has many characteristics of the congenital myoclonus of Hereford cattle.[66] The abnormality was recognized in pups at 3 weeks of age. Affected pups were unable to rise without assistance. Extensor muscle tone was increased in all limbs making evaluation of reflexes difficult, but the neurologic examination was otherwise normal. Resistance to manipulation of the limbs or neck was present. Muscles were of normal size, and no dimpling occurred with percussion. The characteristic finding was increased muscle contraction with any tactile or auditory stimulus or with voluntary activity. The muscle activity included all four limbs, opisthotonus, and contractures of the muscles of facial expression and the muscles of mastication. Episodes of cyanosis occurred during severe and prolonged tetany of the diaphragm and intercostal muscles.[67] Laboratory values were normal. Resting EMG was normal. However, with auditory, tactile, and electrical stimuli, EMG showed intermittent bursts of large motor-unit potentials (0.5 to 15 mV).[67] Electrical stimulation resulted in EMG activity in other limbs.[67] Normal dogs had no response to the same stimulus. Necropsy revealed mild esophageal dilation, but no other gross or histologic lesions. A similarity was suggested to the spastic mutant mouse that has a deficiency in glycine receptors.[66] Clonazepam, diazepam, and phenobarbital therapy resulted in minimal relaxation.[66,67] Interestingly, upon recovery from pentobarbital and inhalant anesthesia, affected dogs remained refractory to stimulus-induced tetany for 12 to 14 hours.[67]

Horses. Two Peruvian Pasos foals have been reported with clinical signs identical to polled Herefords and Labrador retrievers.[68] Foals displayed tetany in response to external stimuli from birth. No histologic abnormalities were observed in muscle specimens. The affected foals had approximately 40% less functional glycine receptors in the spinal cord than controls. In comparison, affected Herefords have 80% loss of glycine receptors, which may account for the greater severity of clinical signs in affected cattle.[68] A similar clinical syndrome occurs in Egyptian Arabian foals born with a color coat dilution.[69] Foals are unable to stand. Histologic lesions are lacking. Pedigree analysis suggests an autosomal recessive inheritance.

Spasticity Syndromes

As mentioned previously, spasticity is most commonly associated with lesions involving the upper motor neuron system. Increased extensor tone is the result of a lack of extensor inhibition of the LMN. The term *spasticity* has also been applied to involuntary movement disorders in which the main clinical sign is tetany. Hence, these syndromes are described here.

Spastic Paresis of Calves. Spastic paresis, also called Elso heel and spastic paralysis, occurs in young cattle of many breeds. Affected calves are typically recognized before 3 to 4 months of age but signs can occur anytime between the ages of 1 week and 12 months. The disease is suspected to have a genetic basis modified by environmental factors. Clinically, there is increased muscle tone in the gastrocnemius and superficial digital flexors causing hyperextension of the hock. In severe cases, increased tone is also present in the biceps femoris, semimembranosus, semitendinosus, and quadriceps muscles. The signs are usually bilateral, but one side is often worse. The pelvic limbs are held caudally in extension, especially at the hock. The limb is advanced like a pendulum. Some improvement occurs with walking, but movement never becomes normal. Forceful attempts to flex the limb cause increased tone and clonic contractions of the extensors.[70] Secondary osteoarthritis of the hock may develop. The pathogenesis appears to be an increase in the activity of the gamma efferent system. Sectioning of the dorsal roots or blocking of the small gamma motor neurons reduces the clinical signs.[71] Lowered levels of homovanillic acid, the main metabolite of dopamine, were found in the cerebrospinal fluid (CSF), suggesting a primary defect in dopamine metabolism.[72] Various treatments have been proposed. In one study, medical therapy using lithium and copper supplementation was associated with a high success rate if used soon after onset of signs.[73] Partial neurectomy of the tibial nerve at the level of the stifle alleviates clinical signs with few complications in a majority of affected animals.[74]

Spastic Syndrome of Adult Cattle. Periodic spasticity, crampiness, stretches, or standing disease are names given a syndrome that affects the extensor muscles of the lumbar region and pelvic limbs. The condition is similar to spastic paresis except that it occurs in older animals and is more episodic. Clinical signs are recognized in animals older than 6 years.[75] The Holstein-Friesian and Guernsey cattle are among the most commonly reported breeds.[75] Affected animals develop episodic increased extensor tone of the pelvic limbs and thoracolumbar muscles. The affected limb is raised and extended caudally or forcefully flexed. With time, the episodes increase in severity. Episodes occur when the animal stands up or with movement but are not seen at rest. One or both limbs may be affected; in the latter case the movements alternate from side to side. Evidence for an autosomal dominant inheritance with incomplete penetrance is reported.[76]

A similar syndrome has been reported in a 2-year-old blue-faced Leicester ram.[77] Progressive increased extensor tone and tremors were observed in the pelvic limbs. Extensor tone increased with auditory stimuli. Signs remained unchanged for 6 months.

Metabolic Causes of Tetany

The resting membrane and threshold potential of a neuron is maintained by balances between sodium, potassium, calcium, and chloride.[78] Excess or depletion of these electrolytes can alter membrane conductance leading to hyperexcitability.

Hypocalcemia. In the dog, hypocalcemia is a common cause of tetany. In plasma, calcium exists as ionized (~50%), protein bound (~40%), or chelated (~10%). Only ionized calcium concentration is biologically active. The distribution of calcium between these three forms is affected by such things as serum protein content, acid-base status, and the presence of anions that act as chelators (e.g., Mg^{++} or phosphate). Hypocalcemia results in tetany when serum total calcium concentrations drop below 6 mg/dL or an ionized concentration of approximately 0.6 to 0.7 mmol/L. Although several formulas exist for correction of total calcium concentration in hypoproteinemic dogs, these formulas are inaccurate, especially in animals with renal disease.[79] At best, corrective formulas may guide a crude estimation of ionized calcium levels. Physiologically, calcium ion concentrations control neuronal membrane permeability to sodium ions. With low calcium concentrations, there is increased permeability to sodium. Consequently the nerve becomes hyperexcitable and neuronal discharges are capable of developing with little to no stimulus. Regardless of the cause, clinical signs reflect peripheral nervous system hyperexcitability resulting in spontaneous discharges of nerve fibers resulting in spontaneous muscle contractions. However, CNS hyperexcitability may also play a role. Affected animals display varying degrees of muscle stiffness, fasciculations, and cramping in different muscle groups. In addition, affected animals may display shifting limb lameness, stiff gait, and decreased activity. Other clinical signs include hyperthermia, abnormalities in behavior (aggression, lethargy, vocalization), facial rubbing, and painful appearance. Over time, increased muscle contractions lead to tetany and seizures. In some animals, clinical signs are not present at rest, requiring external stimuli or exercise to develop. Hyperventilation secondary to panting can precipitate tetany.

The common causes of hypocalcemia in dogs and cats include postparturient hypocalcemia, hypoparathyroidism, renal failure, and protein-losing enteropathies.

Postparturient Hypocalcemia. Postparturient eclampsia (puerperal tetany) in the bitch usually occurs within 14 days after whelping.[80] The exact mechanism of postparturient hypocalcemia in the bitch is not known; however, calcium losses from fetal ossification and lactation combined with deficient osteoclastic activity or calcium absorption are probably responsible for altered calcium homeostasis. Although some dogs become hypoglycemic, low blood glucose probably is not important in the production of tetany. Small-breed dogs with nervous temperaments appear more susceptible to this disorder. Nervous dogs may be predisposed because they hyperventilate during parturition, inducing respiratory alkalosis, which favors protein binding of calcium, thus lowering ionized calcium concentrations.

Diagnosis of postparturient hypocalcemia is based on clinical signs and low ionized calcium concentrations. Treatment includes 10% calcium gluconate administered slowly IV at a dose of 0.5 to 1.5 mL/kg or 5 to 15 mg/kg (over 10 to 30 minutes) and *to effect* as individual requirements vary; simultaneously heart rate and rhythm are monitored for bradyarrhythmias.[81] In mildly affected animals or those requiring repeated intravenous administration to correct clinical signs, 10% calcium gluconate (not calcium chloride) can be given subcutaneously. The dose is 60 to 90 mg/kg/day or alternatively the intravenous dose needed to stop clinical signs can be used.[81] Dosages are diluted with 1 to 4 parts 0.9% NaCl and then divided and given every 6 to 8 hours subcutaneously. Animals that continue to have seizures or that remain excessively irritable or restless can be mildly sedated with benzodiazepines. For maintenance therapy, puppies are separated from the bitch for 24 hours and supplemented with the bitch's milk or puppy formula. Full nursing is restricted for an additional 48 hours. If possible the puppies should be weaned. Oral calcium lactate or gluconate is given in dosages of 0.5 to 2.0 g/day in divided doses.

Eclampsia of Mares. Eclampsia of mares is rarely encountered except in draft horses. Most cases occur in lactating mares near the 10th day after parturition or 1 to 2 days after weaning. Factors that may predispose the animal to eclampsia in mares include grazing on a lush pasture, strenuous work, and prolonged transport. Affected mares tend to sweat profusely and develop muscle spasticity. Rapid respiration, muscular fasciculations, and trismus are evident. The rectal temperature is normal or mildly elevated, and the pulse may be rapid and irregular. Swallowing may be affected. The diagnosis is based on clinical signs and the presence of reduced serum ionized calcium concentrations. Treatment with IV calcium solutions produces rapid, complete recovery.

Hypoparathyroidism. Hypoparathyroidism results in decreased secretion of parathormone (PTH) with subsequent hypocalcemia and hyperphosphatemia. This condition has been recognized most frequently in dogs. Hypoparathyroidism can be divided into primary and secondary causes. Although the exact cause is unknown, primary hypoparathyroidism in dogs is likely a primary autoimmune disease. Acute primary hypoparathyroidism is characterized by a sudden onset of tetany or seizures or both. A chronic form of the disease is associated with recurrent depression, lethargy, anorexia, vomiting, intermittent facial and thoracic limb spasm, and latent tetany. Primary hypoparathyroidism is suspected in a dog with persistent hypocalcemia and hyperphosphatemia in the presence of normal renal function. Less commonly, secondary hypoparathyroidism occurs as a result of destruction of the parathyroid glands related to treatment of thyroid disease or hyperparathyroidism. Decreased concentrations of intact PTH in the presence of hypocalcemia substantiate the diagnosis. Treatment involves administration of vitamin D analogs, such as dihydrotachysterol, ergocalciferol (vitamin D_2), or calcitriol (1,25 dihydroxycholecalciferol). Approximate dosages of these drugs are dihydrotachysterol, 0.01 mg/kg of body weight daily initially followed by 0.02 to 0.03 mg/kg/day as a maintenance dose; ergocalciferol (vitamin D_2), 1000 to 2000 U/kg daily to once weekly depending on effect; and calcitriol, 0.03 to 0.06 mcg/kg/day. Dosing varies between individual animals. Therefore, clinicians must individualize the dosage by monitoring the serum calcium levels twice a week to prevent hypocalcemia or hypercalcemia until the correct dosage is established. Calcium supplementation must be administered with caution because its use with vitamin D increases the probability of hypercalcemic toxicity.

Chronic Renal Failure. Chronic renal failure may cause hypocalcemia based on ionized calcium concentrations.[82,83] Despite this, clinical signs related to hypocalcemia are rarely observed. Caution should be exercised when correcting hypocalcemia in animals with CRF due to the presence of concurrent hyperphosphatemia.

Protein-losing enteropathy. Protein-losing enteropathies (PLE) can lead to hypoalbuminemia which affects calcium concentrations leading to clinical signs of hypocalcemia.[84] Hypocalcemia in dogs with PLE may be related to hypoparathyroidism secondary to poor vitamin D absorption in the intestine or hypomagnesium.[85,86]

Hypomagnesemic Tetany. These syndromes occur primarily in pregnant and lactating cattle pastured on highly fertilized, lush spring pastures. This tetany also occurs in pregnant and lactating ewes and occasionally in feeder cattle.[87] Several hypomagnesemic conditions have been described, including grass tetany, wheat pasture poisoning, milk tetany of calves, and transport tetany. The basic pathophysiology of each is similar and probably is related to decreased dietary intake and mobilization or increased excretion of magnesium. In addition to low dietary magnesium, dietary potassium and sodium concentration also play a role in the development of grass tetany.[88]

Early signs include restlessness, extreme alertness, and muscular twitching. Animals may become excitable, belligerent, and even aggressive. Stimulation may induce severe signs of tetany, ataxia, and bellowing. Animals may become recumbent with opisthotonus and paddling movements. The diagnosis of grass tetany is supported by laboratory findings of hypomagnesemia (<1 mg/dL), hypocalcemia (<7 mg/dL), and high normal levels of potassium. Therapy should correct the immediate ionic imbalance and should supplement the dietary intake of magnesium. Magnesium lactate in a 3.3% solution (2.2 mL/kg), magnesium gluconate in a 15% solution (0.44 mL/kg), and magnesium sulfate in a 20% solution (0.44 mL/kg) can be given slowly via intravenous or subcutaneous routes. Commercial combination solutions may also be used effectively. Magnesium oxide, 1 g/45 kg daily, should be force fed or supplied in blocks containing protein supplements and molasses. Animals on high-risk pastures should be given magnesium oxide or chloride supplements.

Wheat pasture poisoning is similar to grass tetany, except it occurs in cattle and sheep that graze on a cereal grain pasture during its early growth. Diagnosis and treatment are the same as those for grass tetany.

Milk tetany occurs in 2- to 4-month-old calves that are fed only milk. Signs may occur after episodes of diarrhea. Digestive disorders may decrease magnesium absorption, thus complicating the magnesium deficiency. Clinical signs include hyperesthesia, nervousness, recumbency, and seizures. Repeated attacks may occur. Diagnosis is based on the history, clinical signs, and serum magnesium concentrations below 0.7 mg/dL. Calves respond to parenteral magnesium ionic therapy. Susceptible calves should be given magnesium oxide supplements, 1 g/day.

Transport tetany occurs after stressful events such as transportation, vaccination, deworming, adverse weather, and marked dietary changes. Transport tetany occurs in both cattle and sheep. Dietary reduction in calcium, magnesium, and potassium coupled with stress produces ionic imbalances that result in a wide range of clinical signs, from spastic to flaccid paralysis. The signs usually begin within 24 hours of the stress but may be delayed for 72 hours. Early manifestations include restlessness, anorexia, and excitement. These signs progress to muscular trembling, teeth grinding, ataxia, and recumbency. Opisthotonus, paddling, and coma may develop. Treatment consists of parenteral administration of polyionic glucose solutions and attentive nursing care.

Muscle Cramping With Hypoadrenocorticism. Two standard poodles were reported with muscle cramping of the limbs.[89] The clinical presentation most closely resembled tetany and therefore is included here. Both dogs episodically exhibited acute onset of rigid extension of a single limb lasting several seconds. Episodes were observed with all limbs. During the episodes, the appendicular muscles were rigid with palpable fasciculations. Percussive myotonia was not detectable. EMG was normal in one dog. Both dogs were diagnosed with hypoadrenocorticism. At the time of diagnosis, both dogs were dehydrated, hypovolemic, hyponatremic, hypochloremic, hyperkalemic, and azotemic. Ionized calcium was normal. With adequate supplementation of mineralocorticoids, episodes resolved. The exact cause of the syndrome was undetermined but given resolution with treatment, the episodes were likely the result of electrolyte and fluid imbalances.

Immune-Mediated Causes of Tetany: Stiff Horse Syndrome

A syndrome characterized by increased extensor tone in the pelvic limbs, paraspinal muscle contracture, and pain on palpation of the affected muscles has been observed in an 11-year-old horse.[90] Similar signs had occurred 1 year prior. Clinical signs improved with corticosteroid therapy. Serum autoantibodies directed against glutamic acid decarboxylase, a cytosolic enzyme, which converts glutamate to GABA in the nerve terminal, were detected. It was postulated that autoantibodies interfered with the production of GABA, resulting in a loss of function of spinal inhibitory interneurons. The disorder was thought similar to stiff man syndrome in humans.

Toxic Cause of Tetany: Strychnine

Strychnine is a rodenticide that is sometimes implicated in malicious or accidental poisonings of small animals. It produces tetanic spasms that are exacerbated by auditory or tactile stimuli. In dogs, intoxication is seen more commonly in young, less than 2 years of age, male large-breed dogs in rural areas.[91] This may simply reflect a greater likelihood of exposure in such dogs. The signs may appear within 10 minutes to 2 hours after ingestion.[92] In one report, signs did not manifest for 10 hours.[93] The toxic dose in most animals ranges from 0.3 to 1.0 mg/kg with the lethal dose being 2.0 mg/kg in cats.[94] Clinical signs typically begin with nervousness, restlessness, and apprehension rapidly progressing to increased muscle rigidity causing a stiff gait. Increased muscle rigidity quickly progresses to lateral recumbency with the limbs held in extension and opisthotonus. Facial muscle rigidity also occurs. At this stage, tetanic seizures occur. Between seizures, there is partial relaxation. The pupils may be fixed and mydriatic. Seizures can be stimulated by touch or noise. Eventually, respiratory failure and death occurs. Presumptive diagnosis is based on clinical signs. Although there are many toxins that can cause similar clinical signs, strychnine intoxication seems to be most severe and occurs most rapidly. Definitive diagnosis is based on toxicologic analysis of stomach contents, urine, blood, or liver tissue. Antemortem, stomach contents and urine are most likely to provide a diagnosis. However, over time stomach contents decline in concentration as the toxin moves out into the intestinal tract. Blood levels may be low as strychnine is readily metabolized or excreted unchanged in the urine.

Treatment is directed at limiting absorption and controlling the tetany. Induction of vomiting or gastric lavage followed by activated charcoal administration reduces the absorption. Caution should be exercised before inducing vomiting as stimulation may induce seizures. Tetany is controlled with pentobarbital sodium given intravenously to effect. Six to 12 hours may be necessary to allow for the toxin to be metabolized in dogs.[95] Caution must be used to prevent overdosing. Endotracheal intubation and maintenance of respiration are mandatory. Inhalation anesthesia, benzodiazepines, and methocarbamol can be used to reduce the need for large doses of barbiturates. Fluid diuresis promotes renal excretion of the toxin. Acidification of the urine is recommended to enhance elimination, which should be completed in 24 to 48 hours.

Myoclonus

Myoclonus is the clinical manifestation of a sudden contraction of a group of muscles followed by its relaxation. Historically, myoclonus has been used to describe contractions of muscle groups that result in a relatively low frequency (slow) rhythmic jerking movements of the limb or gross contractions of muscle groups of the axial skeleton. The observation of similar movements in association with other conditions had led to the use of myoclonus as a descriptive term to qualify events such as seizures, as in myoclonic seizures (see Chapter 13). Here, myoclonus is used more broadly to describe a condition in which contraction followed by relaxation of muscle groups occurs. As such, myoclonus can be qualified as to the nature of its occurrence (sporadic or repetitive), when occurring repetitively, whether or not cycles of contraction and relaxation occur constantly or episodically, when associated with action/movement or rest or posture. Additionally, myoclonus may manifest as fine or gross movements.

In general, myoclonus can occur sporadically or repetitively. Sporadic forms are likely benign conditions in which myoclonus may be observed and then not recur for prolonged periods of time giving the impression of an isolated event. Sporadic forms have received little attention in the veterinary literature. Given the infrequency of each event, the diagnosis of sporadic myoclonus is problematic. Often the diagnosis is one of exclusion. Importantly, it may be difficult to differentiate sporadic myoclonus from simple focal seizures (see Chapter 13). Therefore the diagnosis of sporadic myoclonus frequently entails exclusion of simple partial seizures.

As the name implies, repetitive myoclonus is the recurring cycles of contraction followed by relaxation. Repetitive myoclonus may be constant, episodic, action-related, postural, and resting.

When appearing as a recurring fine movement, it may be described clinically as a tremor. Consequently, the two terms are used synonymously in the context of rapid, repetitive myoclonus in which rhythmic flexion of joints occur with a frequency such that they appear as a vibration or shivering (fine tremor) or may involve slower more gross movements (coarse tremor). These movements may be diffuse or limited to specific anatomy such as a limb.

Constant Repetitive Myoclonus

Canine Distemper. The most widely known disease process associated with constant myoclonus is secondary to canine distemper infection. However, constant repetitive myoclonus can occur with other causes of CNS inflammation.[96] Constant repetitive myoclonus secondary to canine distemper virus was recognized and described as early as 1862.[97] Any group of muscles may be affected. Frequently myoclonus is confined to a flexor group in one limb, but myoclonus involving a combination of muscle groups in more than one limb, the facial muscles, or the muscles of mastication also can occur. Clinically, the affected dog displays constant, rhythmic contractions of the affected limb or muscle group. Although difficult to appreciate with movement, myoclonus often continues with activity, rest, sleep, or with light anesthesia. During rest and sleep, the frequency and severity of the myoclonus lessens. The syndrome may occur before, during, or after the overt encephalitis typical of canine distemper. Most often myoclonus develops after all other clinical sign of infection have resolved.[97] Occasionally, myoclonus is the only clinical signs implicating prior canine distemper infection. Experimental studies have demonstrated that the abnormality lies in the spinal cord or brainstem within intrinsic neural circuits.[98] In some dogs, IV bolus administration of lidocaine may stop or reduce the frequency of myoclonus. In those demonstrating a response, oral procainamide may provide continued suppression of myoclonus. Anticonvulsants have no benefit. Some dogs seem to improve with time. If the myoclonus does not interfere with eating or locomotion, the dog can live with it.

Drug Induced. Constant repetitive myoclonus is occasionally observed in other conditions. Drugs including morphine, etomidate, and propofol can induce constant repetitive myclonus.[99-101] In such cases, myoclonus resolves as the drugs are metabolized. Rarely, lead toxicity can induce myoclonus in dogs.[102] Myoclonus resolves with chelation therapy.

Tic in a Horse. A myoclonic twitch in the thoracic limb of an 18-month-old quarter horse occurred after a traumatic accident.[103] The affected limb was paretic. The horse stood with the affected limb abducted, slightly flexed at the carpus, and with the toe on the ground and the elbow dropped. A week after the injury, constant repetitive myoclonus developed in the triceps and latissimus dorsi muscles. Myoclonus was present when standing or lying, and when asleep but was absent under anesthesia. Various drugs were tried; however, only xylazine resulted in temporary resolution. The myoclonus progressively decreased in intensity and resolved by 11 weeks.

Episodic Repetitive Myoclonus

Shivers. This disorder is seen most often in draft horses; however, it has also been reported in a quarter horse and Thoroughbred.[104,105] The syndrome is characterized by exaggerated flexion and abduction of one or both pelvic limbs successively.[105,106] The affected limb is held in flexion and abduction for several seconds. In addition, tremors may be present in the gluteal and tail muscles. The tail may be raised. The abnormal movements can occur while standing but are more pronounced when the animal is made to back up. Consequently, they also may be considered an episodic, postural repetitive tremor. The gait may appear stiff or choppy or may be normal. Affected animals may appear uncomfortable or painful during an episode. Signs are often present for years and progress slowly to the point of incapacitation. No lesions have been identified in nerves or the CNS.[106] Affected horses may have muscle pathology characteristic of equine polysaccharide storage myopathy; however, its role in shivers is uncertain.[106,107] No treatment has been defined.

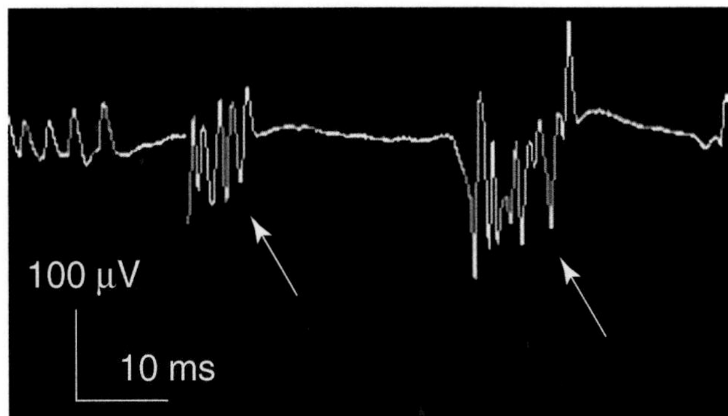

Figure 10-4 EMG tracing from the limb of a 2-year-old Jack Russell terrier with myokymia, which is visualized as rippling skin movements across the muscle. The EMG reveals rhythmic bursts of single motor unit potentials appearing as doublets or triplets myokymic discharges *(arrows)*. Myokymia sounds like soldiers marching during the EMG recording.

Myokymia. This syndrome is also known as continuous muscle fiber activity or myokymia.[108,109] Myokymia denotes a specific clinical phenomenon of rhythmic, undulating, vermiform (wormlike) or wavelike movements of the skin overlying contracting muscle fibers. Movements are continuous and importantly persist during sleep and general anesthesia. Movements can be generalized or affect isolated muscle groups, particularly facial muscles.[110] Signs begin acutely and can have a progressive course. Affected animals with generalized disease may develop hyperthermia, progressive stiffness, limb contractures, and collapse.[108] Myokymia likely represents the clinical manifestation of motor axon or motor nerve terminal hyperexcitability (known as neuromyotonia). In humans, a variety of etiologies can result in myokymia including Guillain-Barré syndrome, multiple sclerosis, radiation plexopathy, brainstem tumors, timber rattle snake envenomation, and a variety of autoimmune diseases, in particular one directed against voltage-gated potassium channels.[111] The etiology has not been defined in dogs and cats.[109-111] The condition has been reported in the Jack Russell terrier and other dog breeds and in cats.[108-111]

Diagnosis is based on characteristic appearance of the movement of the overlying skin. Affected animals may have an elevated serum creatinine kinase (CK) activity. Definitive diagnosis entails EMG identification of myokymic and neuromyotonic discharges. Myokymic discharges are short, rhythmic, or semirhythmic bursts of doublet, triplet, or multiplets of motor unit potentials (MUP) occurring at a rate of 5 to 62 Hz (Figure 10-4). Neuromyotonic discharges are long bursts of MUPs occurring at rates of 150 to 300 Hz that wax and wane in amplitude. Treatment involves drugs that stabilize the muscle membrane potential. Drugs include phenytoin, carbamazepine, procainamide, mexiletine hydrochloride, and corticosteroids. The prognosis is good for focal syndromes as muscle activity may not affect the quality of life. Prognosis in generalized syndromes is guarded because response to therapy is variable.

Action-Related Repetitive Myoclonus

Action-related repetitive myoclonus tremors occur with muscular activity but abate at rest. In most cases, clinical signs relate to diffuse muscle tremors that occur rapidly. Most disorders are either congenital or acquired.

Congenital Action-Related Repetitive Myoclonus

CNS Myelin Disorders. Abnormalities involving CNS myelin can be broadly categorized into reduced or absent myelin production (hypomyelinogenesis, hypomyelination), abnormal myelination (dysmyelination—leukodystrophy, myelinolysis), and demyelination. Developmental disorders of normal myelin cause thinly myelinated and some nonmyelinated axons (hypomyelinogenesis) or abnormal myelin (dysmyelination).[112] Hypomyelinogenesis and dysmyelination can be inherited in some species and breeds and also occurs secondary to in utero infection with several viral agents.[112] These disorders are distinct from primary demyelinating diseases in which myelin develops normally and is later destroyed by external agents (e.g., canine distemper). Primary demyelinating diseases frequently cause cerebellar signs. Demyelination can be secondary to axonal degeneration. These diseases are discussed in Chapter 7, which lists the primary disorders of myelin development.

The clinical signs of syndromes (hypomyelination and dysmyelination) are usually noticed in the first few weeks of life or as the affected animals begin to walk. The signs are similar in all species. Signs consist of action-related repetitive myoclonus. When standing or walking, affected animals display what appears as a diffuse coarse (large-amplitude) tremor causing the animal to "bounce up and down" in a rhythmic manner. In dogs, the pelvic limbs are generally more affected than the thoracic limbs. Some affected dogs fall frequently, giving the impression of ataxia. Severely affected animals may be unable to walk. With sleep or relaxation, the tremor is not present. These congenital disorders of myelination have been extensively studied in the pig, sheep, mouse, and dog.

The presumptive diagnosis is based on the history, presenting signs, and lack of positive findings on any diagnostic test. Generally more than one animal in the litter is affected. Distinguishing developmental disorder of myelination from cerebellar disease or demyelination is difficult. Although often confused with the intention tremor observed with cerebellar disease, animals with these developmental disorders do not display the dysmetria seen with cerebellar disease. Likewise, most of the demyelinating diseases are not apparent at such an early age.

Six different myelin disorders have been defined in pigs.[113-118] Only two of these—type A-III, which is sex-linked in Landrace, and type A-IV, which is an autosomal recessive trait in Saddlebacks—are inherited. Affected pigs develop signs at 2 to 3 days of age. Myelin is abnormal in the Saddlebacks, and oligodendrocytes are reduced in the Landrace. No treatment for the inherited forms is known.

In sheep the disorder is called *Border disease*. Affected lambs have a characteristic hairy fleece and are called hairy shaker lambs.[119,120] Border disease is caused by a pestivirus antigenetically similar to bovine viral diarrhea virus.[121] Infection occurs in utero. Infected lambs remain persistently viremic, and antibody negative, and continually excrete virus.[121] In addition to hypomyelination, affected lambs are often stunted and may have skeletal deformities. Similar to Border disease in sheep, calves born from cows infected with bovine viral diarrhea virus at 100 days' gestation may be born with cerebellar dysplasia and hypomyelination.[122] In addition, Hereford calves have a rare degenerative disorder characterized by neurofilament accumulation in neurons. Tremor is a prominent sign seen hours after birth.[123]

Hypomyelination has been observed in several different breeds of dog, including the springer spaniel, Weimaraner, chow chow, Samoyed, lurcher hound, and Bernese mountain dog.[124-129] The best studied is the springer spaniel ("shaking pup") in which the disease is X-linked. In the springer spaniel, a point mutation in the *PLP1* gene, which encodes for myelin proteolipid protein, a major protein necessary for myelination results in diffuse CNS hypomyelination.[130] In addition to abnormal myelin, there are decreased numbers of oligodendrocytes.[131] Remaining oligodendrocytes are immature.[131]

Hypomyelination has been reported in two Siamese cat littermates.[132] Normal at birth, affected cats developed signs within weeks. Action-related myoclonus predominated in the clinical syndrome. Diffuse hypomyelination of the spinal cord was evident at necropsy. Subjectively oligodendrocyte numbers were normal.

Many animals that are not severely affected improve with age, but assistance with feeding is usually necessary because they cannot nurse properly. In Springer spaniels, males do not show much improvement, but the carrier females are less severely affected and improve considerably with maturation. Chow chow and Weimaraner dogs improve to near normal with maturity. Sheep and pigs may recover if assisted with nutrition. Cattle may also improve, but the degenerative disease in Herefords is progressive and fatal. No treatment exists.

Central Axonopathy. Enlargement of axons in the CNS without dystrophic changes such as spheroids has been associated with diffuse tremors. Secondary to enlarged axons, decreased myelin content, spongy changes, and gliosis are also present. A generalized axonopathy occurred in three Scottish terriers with generalized tremor and ataxia.[133] The dogs had a common sire. Age at presentation was 4 to 5 months, and all were euthanized within 2 months due to progression. Axonopathies also have been reported in the quarter horse and Holstein-Friesian cattle.[134,135]

Acquired Action-Related Repetitive Myoclonus

Inflammatory. Steroid-responsive tremor syndrome (SRTS, idiopathic tremors, little white shakers, idiopathic cerebellitis is an acute, generalized tremor syndrome responsive to glucocorticoids occurs in young small-breed adult dogs. Initially the syndrome was observed in small white breeds, such as Maltese, poodles, and West Highland white terriers, hence the term little white shakers. However, the condition also affects other small breeds that are not white.[136-138] In a study, 22 of 24 dogs with generalized tremors diagnosed with SRTS based on excellent and rapid response to treatment with prednisone, most dogs were 1 to 5 years of age, and all weighed less than 15 kg, and more than 50% of the dogs were nonwhite mixed breeds.[138] The tremor worsens with movement, decreases at rest, and is absent during sleep. The disease is nonprogressive after the first 2 to 3 days. Spontaneous remission may occur. With the exception of tremors, neurologic examination is normal in most instances. Less commonly, paraparesis and tetraparesis have been observed.[137] Other concurrent clinical signs include opsoclonus (rapid multidirectional involuntary eye movements), head tilt, hypermetria, and decreased menace response. Although cerebellovestibular signs are uncommon, observation of such signs has implicated the cerebellum as a neuroanatomic site of origin of the tremors. However, the tremor is more rapid than usually expected with cerebellar disease and ataxia absent. More likely, diffuse inflammation of the CNS accounts for the tremors. In the few cases in which dogs were necropsied, mild nonsuppurative inflammation of the nervous system, not confined to the cerebellum, was found.[139] Speculated causes include viral or immune-mediated inflammatory disease. The relation to white coat color has led to hypotheses involving a relation to tyrosine metabolism; however, these are not albino animals.[140]

The diagnosis is made through exclusion of other diseases combined with CSF fluid analysis. About 50% of affected dogs have mild to moderate mixed or mononuclear inflammatory changes in the CSF.[138] Treatment is with immunosuppressive doses of corticosteroids, diazepam, or both.[137,138] In dogs not responding to immunosuppression, propranolol, a beta-adrenergic blocker may be effective. The corticosteroids should be given in decreasing doses for 8 to 12 weeks. Stopping therapy early may lead to relapse, which may be more difficult to control. Clinical improvement is expected in 2 to 3 days but may take up to 10 days to occur. Relapses after recovery have been seen.

Toxins. Tremors are often associated with toxicosis involving numerous compounds. Therefore the presence of tremors is not pathognomonic for a particular intoxication. In addition to tremors, clinical signs involving other organ systems are usually present.

Toxins may exert effects at the neuromuscular junction through increased release of acetylcholine and increased receptor stimulation and subsequent muscular fatigue. Other toxins can cause imbalances of neurotransmitters in the CNS to cause tremors. In particular neurotoxic agents that stimulate the CNS will manifest signs of hyperactivity, hyperesthesia, muscle tremors and fasciculation, and behavior changes. Toxicants affecting the autonomic nervous system induce clinical signs by interference with cholinergic neurotransmission. Stimulation of the cholinergic neurotransmission will result in bronchoconstriction, muscle tremors, exocrine gland stimulation, bradycardia, and other CNS effects. Signs of blockade of cholinergic neurotransmission depend upon the type of cholinergic receptor involved. Nicotinic blockage results in skeletal muscle paralysis and often tremors. Toxins like bromethalin and hexachlorophene affect myelin causing intramyelinic edema and alter conduction of the action potential. Discussed here are a select group of compounds in which tremors are the main feature of intoxication.

Mycotoxicoses. A mycotoxin, penitrem A is produced by several *Penicillium* spp., *Aspergillus*, and *Claviceps*. Ingestion results in severe generalized tremors, opsoclonus, and seizures in dogs.[138,141] Numerous sources associated with the production of mycotoxin include mold contamination of cream cheese, macaroni and cheese, walnuts, bread, rice, and compost.[142] Tremors occur approximately 2 to 3 hours following the ingestion.[141] The severity of the tremors may be related to the amount of mycotoxin ingested. Vomiting often precedes tremors. Affected dogs may be hyperthermic due to muscular activity. Rarely, ventilatory failure may occur.[143] The presumptive diagnosis is based on observing the ingestion of spoiled foods or compost, elimination of other causes of tremors, and response to therapy. Definitive diagnosis is made by measuring penitrem A concentrations in stomach contents. Treatment is directed at reducing absorption, reducing tremors, and supportive care. Induction of emesis or gastric lavage should be considered. The tremors lessen in severity with IV bolus of benzodiazepines. In severely affected dogs, bolus administration of a benzodiazepine drug followed by a constant rate infusion may be necessary for several hours. In dogs not responding to benzodiazepines, pentobarbital sodium may be required.[144] Methocarbamol (55 to 200 mg/kg IV) to effect and at a rate of 2 mL/min) may also be helpful in controlling tremors.[145] Animals requiring pentobarbital require close monitoring due to the respiratory depression associated with pentobarbital. Sedated animals that continue to vomit are at risk of aspiration pneumonia. Supportive care involves intravenous fluid therapy and temperature monitoring. Most dogs recover quickly but severely affected animals may take up to several weeks.[141] Mycotoxins associated with plants in large animals are discussed in the next section and are listed in Chapter 15.

Poisonous Plants. Plant toxicoses causing tremors usually affect multiple animals in a group, are seasonal, and often occur late in the growth period of the plants.[146] Food animals are affected more frequently than horses. Tremors are often associated with ataxia, dysmetria, and in some cases seizures. The diagnosis is based on clinical signs and identification of the toxic plant in pastures where affected animals graze. Dallis grass and some other similar grasses are infested with *Claviceps paspali*, which produces a neurotoxin. Phalaris neurotoxicity is caused by alkaloids that interfere with serotonin release. Perennial ryegrass is infested with mycotoxins, and annual ryegrass has a toxin produced by a *Corynebacterium*.[136] See Table 15-17 for details.

Heavy-Metal Poisoning. Lead is the most common heavy metal causing toxicosis in animals. Gastrointestinal and CNS signs dominate the clinical picture in most cases. Horses seem to be more resistant and generally have peripheral neuropathy and respiratory problems.[147] In cats and dogs, vomiting and diarrhea may occur, especially with acute poisoning. Cattle may bloat and have diarrhea. CNS signs include seizures, blindness, abnormal behavior, and tremors.[148,149] Tremors are usually associated with chronic low-grade poisoning and probably are caused by the demyelinating effects of lead. The acute cases often have laminar cerebrocortical necrosis accounting for the predominance of cerebral signs. Lead poisoning and other heavy-metal toxicities, including diagnosis and management, are discussed in Chapter 15.

Hexachlorophene. Hexachlorophene, an ingredient in antiseptic soaps (pHisoHex), may cause generalized tremors, especially in young animals. Oral administration of hexachlorophene in an attempt to reproduce the clinical syndrome cause vomiting and diarrhea, salivation, tachypnea, and depression.[150] Clinical cases of hexachlorophene toxicity have resulted from both topical contact and ingestion.[150-152] Lesions are primarily vacuolation of the white matter. Treatment is eliminating exposure and supportive care. Acute intoxication may be helped by osmotic diuresis.[151] Dogs often recover with time.

Organophosphates and Chlorinated Hydrocarbons. Organophosphate compounds may cause tremors in some cases of chronic intoxication. Tremors usually precede the more common findings of seizures and neuromuscular weakness. Organophosphates potentiate effects of acetylcholine at the neuromuscular junction by binding acetylcholinesterase. Tremors and fasciculations associated with muscle weakness occur as depolarizing neuromuscular junction blockade effects take place.[153] Chlorinated hydrocarbons often produce tremors as a major component of toxicity. Fine tremors or fasciculations of the muscles may be accompanied by seizures, tonic spasms, and autonomic manifestations. These toxicities are discussed in Chapter 15.

Other Tremorogenic Agents. Carbamates, pyrethrins, pyrethroids, ivermectin, bromethalin, and theobromine may cause tremors.[138] Pyrethrins and pyrethroid insecticides alter both sodium and chloride conductance causing tremors. Class I and II pyrethrins and pyrethroid compounds act on gated sodium channels in nerve and muscle causing persistent depolarization and failure of membrane repolarization.[154,155] Class II pyrethroids inhibit binding of GABA to the $GABA_A$ receptor, which prevents influx of chloride. This causes further membrane depolarization and blockade of action potential and failure of membrane repolarization. Young cats are more frequently affected. Clinical signs include hyperexcitability, seizures, and muscle weakness manifesting as tremors and fasciculation.[156,157]

Postural-Related Repetitive Myoclonus (Tremor)

As suggested by the name, postural repetitive myoclonus affects specific muscles involved in weight support. Clinical signs are present only with weight bearing and are absent during activity or at rest while lying down (i.e., non–weight bearing).

Postural Repetitive Myoclonus in Geriatric Dogs. A very rapid, fine tremor occurs in the pelvic limbs of some older dogs. Occasionally, it also involves the thoracic limbs. The severity may progress slowly over months to years or remain static. The tremor is present only when the dog is standing. When not weight bearing or during activity, tremors are not observed. There is preservation of strength and gait. The dogs do not appear to be in pain or bothered by the tremor. The diagnosis is based on signalment, typical characteristics, and elimination of other causes of tremors. Treatment is unnecessary.

Orthostatic Postural Myoclonus in Great Danes and Scottish Deerhounds. Orthostatic postural myoclonus has been observed in young otherwise healthy Great Danes and Scottish deerhounds.[158,159] Affected dogs are usually under 2 years of age. Fine, rapidly progressive tremors occur in all limbs only when the dogs are weight supporting. In one dog, the thoracic limbs were more affected when eating while in another dog, the pelvic limbs were more affected when attempting to sit. Moreover, the severity of the tremor increased dramatically when posturing to sit. Tremors are absent with movement such as walking, when not supporting weight, when leaning against their owners for support, or when lifted off the ground. Neurologic examination was normal. Under anesthesia, EMG and motor nerve studies were normal. However, surface EMG performed in awake, standing animals demonstrated the presence of repetitive motor unit potentials occurring regularly at a frequency of 13 to 16 Hz. Such potentials are absent when affected dogs are in a non–weight supporting position (lying down). Using a stethoscope over the muscles, low-pitched noise can be heard coinciding with the tremor. Histologic lesions were absent in the muscle and nerve specimens. The diagnosis is based on signalment, characteristic tremors, and electrophysiologic demonstration of motor unit potential occurring at a frequency of 13 to 16 Hz when weight bearing. Treatment consists of benzodiazepines or phenobarbital. Given the potential to develop tolerance to benzodiazepines, phenobarbital therapy may be preferred.[158]

A similar condition has been reported in the Pietrain pig.[160] Affected piglets displayed a tremor while standing and walking but not when lying down. EMG burst activity in the semitendinosus muscles occurred at 14 Hz. Other electrophysiologic data were normal. Piglets were sired by a phenotypically normal boar known to produce offspring with an autosomal recessive myopathy. Despite this, histologic lesions were not identified in the nervous system or muscle of affected piglets.

Head Tremor. A coarse tremor, often called a "head bob," has been described in the Doberman pinscher, boxer, and English bulldog.[161] Similar movements were reported in a Shetland sheepdog.[162] The tremor usually develops in young dogs. Affected dogs display a rapid, coarse tremor of the neck and head that may oscillate vertically or horizontally. Tremor episodes appear randomly. Some owners feel that affected dogs have tremor episodes after prolonged strenuous exercise, but the tremors tend to occur during periods of relaxation. During episodes, dogs are responsive and can stand and walk, and in all other regards the dogs appear normal. The tremor can be stopped by getting the dog to change the tone and posture of the neck and head. Neurologic examination and diagnostic tests, including hematology, biochemistry, thyroid function testing, cross-sectional imaging, and CSF analysis are normal. The tremor may persist for many years and in rare occasions, the tremor resolves spontaneously. Treatments with corticosteroids, anticonvulsants, or benzodiazepines are ineffective and unnecessary.

Movement Disorders (Dyskinesia/Dystonia)

Movement disorders are sudden, involuntary contractions of specific muscle groups that may persist over a period of time either at rest or during activity in an awake, conscious animal. These conditions also can be referred to as dyskinesia. The most common clinical presentation is dystonia, a sustained contraction of a group of muscles involving the pelvic limb, which appears as increased extensor tone. Even when all limbs are involved, signs often predominate in the pelvic limbs. Abnormal movements can be triggered by excitement or exercise. The pathogenesis may involve a functional or absolute deficiency in neurotransmitters or their receptors as structural lesions are usually absent.

Focal Dyskinesia/Dystonia

Scotty Cramp. Scottish terriers are affected by an inherited disorder characterized primarily by episodic dystonia primarily involving the pelvic limbs but also involving the thoracic limbs in severely affected dogs. The syndrome is inherited as a recessive trait with variable expression.[163,164] Signs occur between 1 and 3 years of age. Episodes are precipitated by exercise, fear, and excitement. With excitement, the pelvic limbs assume a hypertonic, extended position or may occasionally display exaggerated flexion of one or both limbs. Thoracic limbs may become abducted and develop extensor tone. Signs progress over several minutes. Severely affected dogs assume lordosis and may fall into lateral recumbency. The severity varies from mildly affected to incapacitated. Structural nervous system lesions are lacking. A functional deficiency in serotonin modulation of motor neuron function has been postulated.[165,166] Disease severity varies inversely with CNS serotonin levels. Drugs such as methysergide or methionine that decrease CNS serotonin result in more severe signs.[167] Diagnosis is based on signalment and characteristic clinical signs. Treatment is aimed at muscle relaxation or increasing serotonin levels, which reduce severity and duration of episodes. Oral diazepam at a dose of 0.5 to 1.5 mg/kg every 8 hours (or other benzodiazepine derivatives) or acepromazine is most frequently used. Recently, fluoxetine, a serotonin reuptake inhibitor was used to treat an affected dog.[168] The disease is not life threatening unless it severely incapacitates the dog.

Hypertonicity in Cavalier King Charles Spaniels. This condition is also known as episodic falling, deer stalking, and tetany in Cavalier King Charles spaniels.[169] Affected dogs display clinical signs between 1 and 4 years of age. Affected dogs progressively develop pelvic limb dystonia, appearing as increased extensor tone over several minutes. Thoracic limbs may also be involved. Excitement and exercise are associated with development of clinical signs. Although the pathogenesis is unknown, the disease is thought to be similar to a human condition called hyperexplexia, which is a glycine receptor abnormality.[170] As the major inhibitory neurotransmitter in the spinal cord, glycine affects α-motor neurons. As occurs in polled Hereford cattle, abnormalities in glycine or its receptor lead to excitation of α-motor neurons. Diagnosis is based on signalment and characteristic clinical signs. Treatment with oral diazepam or other benzodiazepine derivatives may help control the severity of episodes. The disease is not life threatening. Syndromes similar to that observed in the Scottish terrier and Cavalier King Charles spaniel have been reported in the Dalmatian and Norwich terrier in which clinical signs of pelvic limb dystonia have been observed.[171,172]

Dyskinesia/Dystonia

Bread-Related

Bichon Frise. A movement disorder has been reported in young bichon frise dogs.[173] The episodes occur randomly. They can be precipitated by excitement or occur at rest. The severity, duration, and frequency vary within an individual dog and between dogs. Movements may involve the facial musculature and the trunk and limbs. Affected dogs may display unilateral facial dystonia resulting in a grimacing expression. Dystonia of a single limb may appear as sustained hyperflexion or extension of the affected limb. Chorea-like movement of a limb consisting of rapid flexion and extension of a limb may occur. Affected dogs may assume a kyphotic posture due to dystonia of the muscles of the thoracic vertebral column.

Boxer Dog. A condition similar to that in the bichon frise dog has been observed in young boxer puppies.[174] Multiple pups of both genders were affected. Episodes could be provoked by excitement or by stimuli. Movements were not stereotypic, varying between episodes in a single pup and between different pups. Episodes consisted of combinations of facial, truncal, and limb movements. Facial muscle dystonia resulted in a grimacing expression. Athetosis of the neck musculature resulted in torticollis. Chorea-like movements of the limbs consisting of holding up a limb in extension, slapping a limb toward the ground in rapid succession, or sustained hyperflexion of a limb were observed.

Dancing Doberman. This disease is characterized by intermittent flexion of one or both pelvic limbs while standing. Signs begin in a single limb.[175] The contralateral pelvic limb may become affected. Affected dogs develop weakness and atrophy of the distal pelvic limb musculature. Signs are limited to the pelvic limbs and consist of exaggerated reflexes. Chronically affected dogs may develop postural reaction deficits. EMG may reveal positive sharp waves, fibrillation potentials, and complex repetitive discharges involving the gastrocnemius muscles. In some dogs, histologic study was consistent with a primary myopathy with features consistent with myotonic myopathy. In others, abnormalities were noted in the spinal cord suggesting underlying or concurrent spinal cord pathology.

Stringhalt. Affected horses display a gait characterized by hyperflexion of one or both pelvic limbs with the affected limb being held in flexion for up to several minutes. Signs occur especially during the start of walking but also occur during movement. Severity ranges from mild, occurring occasionally, to severe incapacitation in which both pelvic limbs flex simultaneously resulting in bunny hopping or an inability to stand without assistance. Rarely, exaggerated flexion of the thoracic limbs may occur. Two forms of stringhalt are described. The classic form occurs spontaneously in single individuals worldwide without a known cause.[176-178] Affected horses do not recover. The second form is referred to as Australian stringhalt and occurs in epidemics affecting multiple horses in a single area or farm. Cases occur in late summer to early fall after a dry or drought season. Affected horses have grazed on poor quality pastures. Outbreaks have been reported in Australia, New Zealand, and South and North America.[176-182] Many horses improve slowly over weeks to a year. Australian stringhalt is a distal axonopathy that is presumed to be related to toxicity or a metabolic deficiency.[183] An association with ingestion of the weed, *Hypochoeris radicata* has been proposed.[176,179,182,184] Affected animals should be removed from access to toxic plants and rested. Tenectomy of the lateral digital extensor tendon may help in severe cases.[184] Phenytoin improves clinical signs.[185] Recently, Botox injections into the motor end plate region of the digital extensor muscles has been proposed as a treatment.[186]

Acquired Dyskinesia/Dystonia

Several drugs have been reported to cause dyskinesia. The mechanism by which they cause abnormal movement is known. Phenobarbital administration has been associated with dyskinesia in a dog.[187] The clinical signs consist of severe, whole body jerking movements that cause the affected dog to fall. Intermittent fine tremors of the facial, neck, and shoulder musculature were also observed. The affected dog was agitated and restless. Signs gradually diminished and resolved as phenobarbital was tapered and discontinued. Propofol administration has been associated with a variety of abnormal movements including opsoclonus (rapid abnormal eye movements) and myoclonus.[99,188] Clinical signs resolve with discontinuation of the drug.

CASE STUDIES

Key: *0*, Absent; *+1*, decreased; *+2*, normal; *+3*, exaggerated; *+4*, very exaggerated or clonus; *PL*, pelvic limb; *TL*, thoracic limb; *NE*, not evaluated.

CASE STUDY 10-1 *JACK*

▪ Signalment

12-year-old Dachshund, female spayed

▪ History

Several month progressive history of a stiff gait. Signs initially were noticed in the pelvic limbs and have progressed to affect the thoracic limbs. The dog has a history of polydipsia and polyuria (PD/PU). The dog's hair coat has been poor for approximately 1 to 2 years.

▪ Neurologic Examination

Mental status

Normal

Gait

Stiff gait in the pelvic and thoracic limbs. When advancing the thoracic limbs, the dog does not flex normally at the shoulder and elbow. Likewise, the coxofemoral and stifle joints do not flex adequately when the pelvic limbs are advanced. To advance the thoracic limbs, the dog tends to circumduct the limbs. The pelvic limbs are mainly advanced through flexion of the hocks.

Posture

Normal

Postural reactions

Although performed stiffly, postural reactions are normal.

Spinal reflexes

Reduced flexor reflexes due to extensor rigidity, increased tone, proximal musculature hypertrophy in all four limbs; +2 patellar reflexes bilaterally

Cranial nerves

Normal

Sensory examination

Normal

Palpation

Proximal muscle hypertrophy, slight paraspinal muscle atrophy

Continued

CASE STUDY 10-1 *JACK—cont'd*

■ Lesion Location
LMN disorder

■ Differential Diagnosis
1. Myotonia (acquired)—endocrine related, intoxication
2. Polymyositis

■ Diagnostic Plan
1. MDB including CK measurement—assess for endocrine disorder
2. Electrophysiologic testing
3. Muscle biopsy

■ Diagnostic Results
1. Chemistry profile disclosed a mild SAP elevation; UA disclosed isosthenuria
2. Electrophysiology: EMG disclosed positive sharp waves, fibrillation potentials, and complex repetitive discharges in the musculature of the thoracic and pelvic limbs. Direct motor nerve stimulation tests and conduction studies were normal.

■ Diagnosis
Given the history of PU/PD and abnormalities identified on the MDB, a low dose dexamethasone suppression test was performed. Results were consistent with pituitary dependent hyperadrenocorticism. Based on the finding of hyperadrenocorticism combined with the examination findings and electrophysiologic data, a diagnosis of acquired myopathy with characteristics of myotonia (pseudomyotonia) secondary to hyperadrenocorticism was made.

■ Treatment
The dog received medical treatment for hyperadrenocorticism (mitotane) and mexiletine for the secondary pseudomyotonia. Despite control of the endocrinopathy, clinical signs of pseudomyotonia persisted.

CK, Creatine kinase; *CSF*, cerebrospinal fluid; *EMG*, electromyography; *LMN*, lower motor neuron; *MDB*, minimum database; *MRI*, magnetic resonance imaging; *NPO*, nothing per os; *PU/PD*, polyuria/polydipsia; *SAP*, serum allkaline phosphatase; *UA*, urinalysis; *WBC*, white blood cell count

CASE STUDY 10-2 *BELLA*

■ Signalment
8-month-old Labrador retriever, female spayed

■ History
Acute onset of vomiting. Within hours of vomiting, the dog developed a change in gait consisting of difficulty rising and generalized stiffness when walking. Fourteen days before presentation, the dog had undergone a routine ovariohysterectomy (OHE) by the referring veterinarian. No complications were observed from the surgery.

■ Neurologic Examination

Mental status
Normal

Gait
Mild to moderate generalized stiff gait

Posture
Normal, except that the dog's tail was held elevated and slightly curled up compared with normal. The dog's facial muscles were "drawn" caudally, resulting in a grimacing expression and the dog's ears were positioned more dorsal and medial (adducted) on the head. The nictitating membranes were mildly elevated in both eyes.

Postural reactions
Normal

Spinal reflexes
Increased musculature tone in all four limbs

Cranial nerves
All normal

Sensory examination
Normal

Palpation
Normal

■ Lesion Location
Diffuse LMN disorder

■ Differential Diagnosis
1. Tetanus
2. Tetany—secondary to intoxication (strychnine or 2,4 D herbicide)
3. Tetany—electrolyte disorder (hypocalcemia)

■ Diagnostic Plan
1. MDB including CK measurement—assess for underlying systemic disorder
2. Abdominal and thoracic radiographs—identify underlying reason for vomiting

■ Diagnostic Results
1. MDB—Normal
2. Abdominal radiographs were normal
3. Thoracic radiographs—evidence of a hiatal hernia

■ Diagnosis
Based on the history of recent OHE surgery and classical clinical signs, a presumptive diagnosis of tetanus was made. Abdominal ultrasonography of the abdomen did not disclose any abnormalities consistent with intraabdominal infection. With the exception of the healed incision from OHE, no other wounds or sources of infection were found. The dog's condition rapidly deteriorated to the point of

CASE STUDY 10-2 BELLA—cont'd

recumbency, rigid extension of the limbs, and opisthotonus. With any stimuli, signs would worsen.

▪ Treatment

The dog was treated with diazepam, acepromazine, and phenobarbital for muscle relaxation and sedation. Cotton balls were placed in the external ear canals to lessen auditory stimuli. Metronidazole was administered in case of an unidentified clostridial infection. After intradermal skin testing, the dog was administered intravenous equine tetanus antitoxin. Clinical signs reached maximum intensity over 24 hours, remained static for 3 to 4 days, and then gradually improved. Approximately 10 days after onset, the dog was discharged with minimal clinical signs.

CK, Creatine kinase; *LMN*, lower motor neuron; *MDB*, minimum database; *OHE*, ovariohysterectomy.

CASE STUDY 10-3 LULU

▪ Signalment

4-year-old cairn terrier, female spayed

▪ History

Acute onset of generalized constant, repetitive action-related myoclonus (tremors). The owners reported that the tremors would lessen when the dog was resting and was absent when the dog was sleeping.

▪ Neurologic Examination

Mental status

Normal

Gait

Difficult to discern due to generalized coarse tremor involving the body, limbs, and head; no obvious ataxia or weakness appreciated. However, when dog was excited, tremors worsened to the point where the dog would occasionally stumble and fall.

Posture

Difficult to determine if abnormal. The dog could not remain still when standing.

Postural reactions

Normal

Spinal reflexes

All Normal

Cranial nerves

Rapid, irregular, random direction, jerking movements of the eyes (opsoclonus)

Sensory examination

Normal

Palpation

Normal

▪ Lesion Location

Diffuse CNS disorder

▪ Differential Diagnosis

1. Steroid-responsive tremor syndrome ("little white shaker syndrome")
2. Intoxication (penitrem A, lead, hexachlorophene, organophosphates, pyrethrins, carbamates)
3. Electrolyte disorder (i.e., hypocalcemia)
4. Degenerative (i.e., globoid cell leukodystrophy, myelin disorder, axonopathy)

▪ Diagnostic Plan

1. MDB
2. MRI
3. CSF analysis
4. Measurement of serum lead level

▪ Diagnostic Results

1. MDB—Normal
2. MRI—Normal
3. CSF—Mild pleocytosis (11 WBC; normal < 5 cells/mcL; primarily mononuclear; normal protein content)

▪ Diagnosis

Based on signalment (small-breed dog), typical clinical signs, exclusion of other disease processes, and mild mononuclear pleocytosis in CSF, a presumptive diagnosis of steroid-responsive tremor syndrome was made.

▪ Treatment

The dog was started on prednisone (2 mg/kg orally twice daily). Clinical signs gradually improved over 3 days. The dosage of prednisone was tapered gradually over 3 months and then discontinued. No recurrences were noted.

CSF, Cerebrospinal fluid; *MDB*, minimum database; *MRI*, magnetic resonance imaging; *WBC*, white blood cell count.

CASE STUDY 10-4 *KATE*

▪ Signalment
2-year-old English bulldog, female spayed

▪ History
Acute onset of episodic tremors of the head and neck. The owners reported that during each episode the dog would shake its head as one would do when saying "no." The movement was rapid. Episodes would randomly occur multiple times daily. During the episodes, the dog was responsive and acted otherwise normal. When offered a treat, the tremor would stop temporarily as the dog accepted the treat from the owner but then would resume. The tremor would also stop if the dog rested with its head on the ground.

▪ Neurologic Examination
Mental status
Normal

Gait
Normal

Posture
Normal

Postural reactions
Normal

Spinal reflexes
Normal

Cranial nerves
Normal

Sensory examination
Normal

Palpation
Normal

▪ Lesion Location
Unknown (CNS or PNS)

▪ Differential Diagnosis
1. Postural repetitive myoclonus—head tremors
2. Cerebellar disease (although other signs of cerebellar disturbance not present)

▪ Diagnostic Plan
MDB to exclude underlying systemic disorder

▪ Diagnostic Results
MDB—Normal

▪ Diagnosis
Postural repetitive myoclonus—head tremors based on the signalment, history, classical characteristic appearance of the movement, and normal neurologic examination.

▪ Treatment
None

CNS, Central nervous system; *MDB*, minimum database; *PNS*, peripheral nervous system.

CASE STUDY 10-5 *LOGAN*

▪ Signalment
5-year-old golden retriever, male castrated

▪ History
Acute history of vomiting and diarrhea, which rapidly progressed to generalized action-related repetitive myoclonus (tremors). The owners have reported that the dog had been roaming loose unattended hours before developing vomiting and diarrhea.

▪ Neurologic Examination
Mental status
Normal

Gait
Normal; obvious coarse tremor involving the entire body, limbs, and head.

Posture
Normal

Postural reactions
Normal

Spinal reflexes
Normal

Cranial nerves
Normal

Sensory examination
Normal

Palpation
Normal

▪ Lesion Location
Diffuse CNS

▪ Differential Diagnosis
1. Intoxication (penitrem A, lead, hexachlorophene, organophosphates, pyrethrins, carbamates)
2. Steroid-responsive tremor syndrome ("little white shaker syndrome")
3. Electrolyte disorder (i.e., hypocalcemia)

Continued

CASE STUDY 10-5 *LOGAN*—cont'd

▪ Diagnostic Plan

1. MDB including CK level—assess electrolytes
2. Abdominal radiograph
3. Based on potential for exposure:
   a. Measurement of penitrem A in stomach contents
   b. Measurement of serum lead levels
   c. Measurement of acetylcholinesterase activity in serum
4. Based on results of diagnostic tests 1 and 2 and potential for exposure to intoxicants:
   a. MRI
   b. CSF analysis

▪ Diagnostic Results

1. MDB was normal
2. Abdominal radiographs—normal

▪ Diagnosis

Upon further discussions with the owners, the dog had had a history of dietary indiscretion (eating garbage). Presumptive diagnosis of intoxication of the mycotoxin penitrem A based on the potential given the history of being loose and unattended, vomiting and diarrhea shortly preceding the onset of tremors, and exclusion of other disease processes. Measurement of penitrem A levels was not pursued.

▪ Treatment

The dog was treated with activated charcoal orally and parenteral diazepam and methocarbamol for 24 hours. Additionally, the dog was treated with supportive care (NPO and intravenous fluids). Gastric lavage was not performed given the dog's mild clinical signs and the risk of aspiration pneumonia associated with orogastric intubation and lavage. The dog gradually improved over 48 hours and was discharged from the hospital.

CK, Creatine kinase; *CNS*, central nervous system; *CSF*, cerebrospinal fluid; *MDB*, minimum database; *MRI*, magnetic resonance imaging; *NPO*, nothing per os; *PU/PD*, polyuria/polydipsia; *WBC*, white blood cell count.

REFERENCES

1. Lahunta Ad, Glass EN, Kent M: Classifying involuntary muscle contractions, Compend Contin Educ Pract Vet 28:516–518, 520-522, 524-525, 528–529, 2006.
2. Dorland WAN: Dorland's illustrated medical dictionary, Philadelphia, 2007, WB Saunders.
3. Roberts T: Neurophysiology of postural mechanisms, New York, 1967, Plenum Press.
4. Hallet M, Ravits J: Involuntary movements. In Asbury AK, McKhann GM, McDonald WI, editors: Diseases of the nervous system: clinical neurobiology, Philadelphia, 1986, Ardmore Medical Books.
5. Liles SL, Davis GD: Athetoid and choreiform hyperkinesias produced by caudate lesions in the cat, Science 164:195–197, 1969.
6. Vite CH: Myotonia and disorders of altered muscle cell membrane excitability, Vet Clin North Am Small Anim Pract 32:169–187, 2002.
7. Kimura J: Electrodiagnosis in diseases of nerve and muscle—principles and practice, New York, 2001, Oxford University Press.
8. Schatzberg SJ, Shelton GD: Newly identified neuromuscular disorders, Vet Clin North Am Small Anim Pract 34:1497–1524, 2004.
9. Beck CL, Fahlke C, George AL Jr: Molecular basis for decreased muscle chloride conductance in the myotonic goat, Proc Natl Acad Sci U S A 93:11248–11252, 1996.
10. Jentsch TJ: CLC chloride channels and transporters: from genes to protein structure, pathology and physiology, Crit Rev Biochem Mol Biol 43:3–36, 2008.
11. Bryant SH: Myotonia in the goat, Ann N Y Acad Sci 317:314–325, 1979.
12. Bryant SH, Lipicky RJ, Herzog WH: Variability of myotonic signs in myotonic goats, Am J Vet Res 29:2371–2381, 1968.
13. Lipicky RJ, Bryant SH: Sodium, potassium, and chloride fluxes in intercostal muscle from normal goats and goats with hereditary myotonia, J Gen Physiol 50:89–111, 1966.
14. Finnigan DF, Hanna WJ, Poma R, et al: A novel mutation of the CLCN1 gene associated with myotonia hereditaria in an Australian cattle dog, J Vet Intern Med 21:458–463, 2007.
15. Hill SL, Shelton GD, Lenehan TM: Myotonia in a cocker spaniel, J Am Anim Hosp Assoc 31:506–509, 1995.
16. Honhold N, Smith DA: Myotonia in the Great Dane, Vet Rec 119:162, 1986.
17. Lobetti RG: Myotonia congenita in a Jack Russell terrier, J S Afr Vet Assoc 80:106–107, 2009.
18. Shires PK, Nafe LA, Hulse DA: Myotonia in a Staffordshire terrier, J Am Vet Med Assoc 183:229–232, 1983.
19. Jones BR, Anderson LJ, Barnes GR, et al: Myotonia in related chow chow dogs, N Z Vet J 25:217–220, 1977.
20. Vite CH, Melniczek J, Patterson D, et al: Congenital myotonic myopathy in the miniature schnauzer: an autosomal recessive trait, J Hered 90:578–580, 1999.
21. Griffiths IR, Duncan ID: Myotonia in the dog: a report of four cases, Vet Rec 93:184–188, 1973.
22. Steinberg S, Botelho S: Myotonia in a horse, Science 137:979–980, 1962.
23. Hickford FH, Jones BR, Gething MA, et al: Congenital myotonia in related kittens, J Small Anim Pract 39:281–285, 1998.
24. Toll J, Cooper B, Altschul M: Congenital myotonia in 2 domestic cats, J Vet Intern Med 12:116–119, 1998.
25. Farrow BR, Malik R: Hereditary myotonia in the chow chow, J Small Anim Pract 22:451–465, 1981.
26. Shores A, Redding RW, Braund KG, et al: Myotonia congenita in a chow chow pup, J Am Vet Med Assoc 188:532–533, 1986.
27. Gracis M, Keith D, Vite CH: Dental and craniofacial findings in eight miniature schnauzer dogs affected by myotonia congenita: preliminary results, J Vet Dent 17:119–127, 2000.
28. Rhodes TH, Vite CH, Giger U, et al: A missense mutation in canine C1C-1 causes recessive myotonia congenita in the dog, FEBS Lett 456:54–58, 1999.
29. Meyer TS, Fedde MR, Cox JH, et al: Hyperkalaemic periodic paralysis in horses: a review, Equine Vet J 31: 362–367, 1999.

30. Jezyk PF: Hyperkalemic periodic paralysis in a dog, J Am Anim Hosp Assoc 18:977–980, 1982.
31. Spier SJ, Carlson GP, Holliday TA, et al: Hyperkalemic periodic paralysis in horses, J Am Vet Med Assoc 197:1009–1017, 1990.
32. Greene CE, Lorenz MD, Munnell JF, et al: Myopathy associated with hyperadrenocorticism in the dog, J Am Vet Med Assoc 174:1310–1315, 1979.
33. Swinney GR, Foster SF, Church DB, et al: Myotonia associated with hyper-adrenocorticism in two dogs, Aust Vet J 76:722–724, 1998.
34. Dickow LM, Podell M, Gerken DF: Clinical effects and plasma concentration determination after 2,4-dichlorophenoxyacetic acid 200 mg/kg administration in the dog, J Toxicol Clin Toxicol 38:747–753, 2000.
35. Lossin C, George AL Jr: Myotonia congenita, Adv Genet 63:25–55, 2008.
36. Reed SM, Hegreberg GA, Bayly WM, et al: Progressive myotonia in foals resembling human dystrophia myotonica, Muscle Nerve 11:291–296, 1988.
37. Simpson ST, Braund KG: Myotonic dystrophy-like disease in a dog, J Am Vet Med Assoc 186:495–498, 1985.
38. Smith BF, Braund KG, Steiss JE, et al: Possible adult onset myotonic dystrophy in a boxer, J Vet Intern Med 12:120, 1998.
39. Howard J, Jaggy A, Busato A, et al: Electrodiagnostic evaluation in feline hypertrophic muscular dystrophy, Vet J 168:87–92, 2004.
40. Gaschen FP, Hoffman EP, Gorospe JR, et al: Dystrophin deficiency causes lethal muscle hypertrophy in cats, J Neurol Sci 110:149–159, 1992.
41. Valentine BA, Cooper BJ, Cummings JF, et al: Progressive muscular dystrophy in a golden retriever dog: light microscope and ultrastructural features at 4 and 8 months, Acta Neuropathol 71:301–310, 1986.
42. Machuca-Tzili L, Brook D, Hilton-Jones D: Clinical and molecular aspects of the myotonic dystrophies: a review, Muscle Nerve 32:1–18, 2005.
43. Mahadevan M, Tsilfidis C, Sabourin L, et al: Myotonic dystrophy mutation: an unstable CTG repeat in the 3' untranslated region of the gene, Science 255:1253–1255, 1992.
44. Ranum LP, Rasmussen PF, Benzow KA, et al: Genetic mapping of a second myotonic dystrophy locus, Nat Genet 19:196–198, 1998.
45. Day JW, Ranum LP: RNA pathogenesis of the myotonic dystrophies, Neuromuscul Disord 15:5–16, 2005.
46. Bleck TP: Pharmacology of tetanus, Clin Neuropharmacol 9:103–120, 1986.
47. Hagan WA, Bruner DW, Timoney JF: Hagan and Bruner's microbiology and infectious diseases of domestic animals: with reference to etiology, epizootiology, pathogenesis, immunity, diagnosis, and antimicrobial susceptibility, Ithaca, NY, 1988, Comstock.
48. Coleman ES: Clostridial neurotoxins: tetanus and botulism, Compend Contin Educ Pract Vet 20:1089–1097, 1998.
49. Burkitt JM, Sturges BK, Jandrey KE, et al: Risk factors associated with outcome in dogs with tetanus: 38 cases (1987-2005), J Am Vet Med Assoc 230:76–83, 2007.
50. Baker JL, Waters DJ, DeLahunta A: Tetanus in two cats, J Am Anim Hosp Assoc 24:159–164, 1988.
51. Malik R, Church DB, Maddison JE, et al: Three cases of local tetanus, J Small Anim Pract 30:469–473, 1989.
52. Bandt C, Rozanski EA, Steinberg T, et al: Retrospective study of tetanus in 20 dogs: 1988-2004, J Am Anim Hosp Assoc 43:143–148, 2007.
53. Panciera DL, Baldwin CJ, Keene BW: Electrocardiographic abnormalities associated with tetanus in two dogs, J Am Vet Med Assoc 192:225–227, 1988.
54. De Risio L, Zavattiero S, Venzi C, et al: Focal canine tetanus: diagnostic value of electromyography, J Small Anim Pract 47:278–280, 2006.
55. Polizopoulou ZS, Kazakos G, Georgiadis G, et al: Presumed localized tetanus in two cats, J Feline Med Surg 4:209–212, 2002.
56. Green SL, Little CB, Baird JD, et al: Tetanus in the horse: a review of 20 cases (1970 to 1990), J Vet Intern Med 8:128–132, 1994.
57. Mayhew IG: Toxic disease. Large animal neurology, Oxford, 2009, Wiley-Blackwell.
58. Muylle E, Oyaert W, Ooms L, et al: Treatment of tetanus in the horse by injections of tetanus antitoxin into the subarachnoid space, J Am Vet Med Assoc 167:47–48, 1975.
59. Adamantos S, Boag A: Thirteen cases of tetanus in dogs, Vet Rec 161:298–302, 2007.
60. Harper PA, Healy PJ, Dennis JA: Inherited congenital myoclonus of polled Hereford calves (so-called neuraxial oedema): a clinical, pathological and biochemical study, Vet Rec 119:59–62, 1986.
61. Healy PJ, Harper PA, Dennis JA: Diagnosis of neuraxial oedema in calves, Aust Vet J 63:95–96, 1986.
62. Gundlach AL, Dodd PR, Grabara CS, et al: Deficit of spinal cord glycine/strychnine receptors in inherited myoclonus of poll Hereford calves, Science 241:1807–1810, 1988.
63. Pierce KD, Handford CA, Morris R, et al: A nonsense mutation in the alpha1 subunit of the inhibitory glycine receptor associated with bovine myoclonus, Mol Cell Neurosci 17:354–363, 2001.
64. Duffell SJ: Neuraxial oedema of Hereford calves with and without hypomyelinogenesis, Vet Rec 118:95–98, 1986.
65. Duffell SJ, Harper PA, Healy PJ, et al: Congenital hypomyelinogenesis of Hereford calves, Vet Rec 123:423–424, 1988.
66. Fox JG, Averill DR, Hallett M, et al: Familial reflex myoclonus in Labrador retrievers, Am J Vet Res 45:2367–2370, 1984.
67. March PA, Knowles K, Thalhammer JG: Reflex myoclonus in two Labrador retriever littermates: a clinical, electrophysiological, and pathological study, Prog Vet Neurol 4:19–24, 1993.
68. Gundlach AL, Kortz G, Burazin TCD, et al: Deficit of inhibitory glycine receptors in spinal cord from Peruvian Pasos: evidence for an equine form of inherited myoclonus, Brain Res 628:263–270, 1993.
69. Fanelli HH: Coat colour dilution lethal ("lavender foal syndrome"): a tetany syndrome of Arabian foals, Equine Vet Educ 17:260–263, 2005.
70. Denniston JC, Shive RJ, Friedli U, et al: Spastic paresis syndrome in calves, J Am Vet Med Assoc 152:1138–1149, 1968.
71. De Ley G, De Moor A: Bovine spastic paralysis: results of surgical deafferentation of the gastrocnemius muscle by means of spinal dorsal root resection, Am J Vet Res 38:1899–1900, 1977.
72. De Ley G, De Moor A: Bovine spastic paralysis: cerebrospinal fluid concentrations of homovanillic acid and 5-hydroxyindoleacetic acid in normal and spastic calves, Am J Vet Res 36:227–228, 1975.
73. Arnault GA: Bovine spastic paresis. An epidemiologic, clinical and therapeutic study in a Charolais practice in France. Efficacy of lithium therapy, Bovine Pract 18: 236–240, 1983.

74. Vlaminck L, De Moor A, Martens A, et al: Partial tibial neurectomy in 113 Belgian blue calves with spastic paresis, Vet Rec 147:16–19, 2000.
75. Roberts SJ: Hereditary spastic diseases affecting cattle in New York state, Cornell Vet 55:637–644, 1965.
76. Sponenberg DP, Vleck LDV, McEntee K: The genetics of the spastic syndrome in dairy bulls, Vet Med 80: 92–94, 1985.
77. Kyles KWJ, Sargison ND: Spastic syndrome in a blue-faced Leicester ram, Vet Rec 150:380–381, 2002.
78. Shelton GD: Disorders of neuromuscular transmission, Semin Vet Med Surg (Small Anim) 4:126–132, 1989.
79. Schenck PA, Chew DJ: Prediction of serum ionized calcium concentration by use of serum total calcium concentration in dogs, Am J Vet Res 66:1330–1336, 2005.
80. Drobatz KJ, Casey KK: Eclampsia in dogs: 31 cases (1995-1998), J Am Vet Med Assoc 217:216–219, 2000.
81. Feldman EC, Nelson RW: Hypocalcemia and primary hypoparathyroidism. Canine and feline endocrinology and reproduction, St Louis, 2004, Saunders.
82. Barber PJ, Elliott J: Feline chronic renal failure: calcium homeostasis in 80 cases diagnosed between 1992 and 1995, J Small Anim Pract 39:108–116, 1998.
83. Kogika MM, Lustoza MD, Notomi MK, et al: Serum ionized calcium in dogs with chronic renal failure and metabolic acidosis, Vet Clin Pathol 35:441–445, 2006.
84. Kimmel SE, Waddell LS, Michel KE: Hypomagnesemia and hypocalcemia associated with protein-losing enteropathy in Yorkshire terriers: five cases (1992-1998), J Am Vet Med Assoc 217:703–706, 2000.
85. Bush WW, Kimmel SE, Wosar MA, et al: Secondary hypoparathyroidism attributed to hypomagnesemia in a dog with protein-losing enteropathy, J Am Vet Med Assoc 219:1732–1734, 2001.
86. Mellanby RJ, Mellor PJ, Roulois A, et al: Hypocalcaemia associated with low serum vitamin D metabolite concentrations in two dogs with protein-losing enteropathies, J Small Anim Pract 46:345–351, 2005.
87. Sargison ND, Macrae AI, Scott PR: Hypomagnesaemic tetany in lactating Cheviot gimmers associated with pasture sodium deficiency, Vet Rec 155:674–676, 2004.
88. Dua K, Care AD: Impaired absorption of magnesium in the aetiology of grass tetany, Br Vet J 151:413–426, 1995.
89. Saito M, Olby NJ, Obledo L, et al: Muscle cramps in two standard poodles with hypoadrenocorticism, J Am Anim Hosp Assoc 38:437–443, 2002.
90. Nollet H, Sustronck B, Deprez P, et al: Suspected case of stiff-horse syndrome, Vet Rec 146:282–284, 2000.
91. Olsen TF, Allen AL: Causes of sudden and unexpected death in dogs: a 10-year retrospective study, Can Vet J 41:873–875, 2000.
92. Grauer GF, Hjelle JJ: Toxicology. In Morgan RV, editor: Handbook of small animal practice, New York, 1988, Churchill Livingstone.
93. Meiser H, Hagedorn HW: Atypical time course of clinical signs in a dog poisoned by strychnine, Vet Rec 151:21–24, 2002.
94. Atkins CE, Johnson RK: Clinical toxicities of cats, Vet Clin North Am 5:623–652, 1975.
95. Harris WF: Clinical toxicities of dogs, Vet Clin North Am 5:605–622, 1975.
96. Tipold A: Diagnosis of inflammatory and infectious diseases of the central nervous system in dogs: a retrospective study, J Vet Intern Med 9:304–314, 1995.
97. Whittier JR: Flexor spasm syndrome in the carnivore. I. Review of its occurrence in the literature as "canine chorea," Am J Vet Res 17:720–723, 1956.
98. Breazile JF, Blaugh BS, Nail N: Experimental study of canine distemper myoclonus, Am J Vet Res 27: 1375–1379, 1966.
99. Brooks DE: Propofol-Induced movement disorders, Ann Emerg Med 51:111–112, 2008.
100. Kona-Boun JJ, Pibarot P, Quesnel A: Myoclonus and urinary retention following subarachnoid morphine injection in a dog, Vet Anaesth Analg 30:257–264, 2003.
101. Muir WW III, Mason DE: Side effects of etomidate in dogs, J Am Vet Med Assoc 194:1430–1434, 1989.
102. O'Brien DP: Lead toxicity in a dog, J Am Anim Hosp Assoc 17:845–850, 1981.
103. Beech J: Forelimb tic in a horse, J Am Vet Med Assoc 180:258–260, 1982.
104. Davies PC: Shivering in a thoroughbred mare, Can Vet J 41:128–129, 2000.
105. Deen T: Shivering, a rare equine lameness, Equine Pract 6:19–21, 1984.
106. Valentine BA, de Lahunta A, Divers TJ, et al: Clinical and pathologic findings in two draft horses with progressive muscle atrophy, neuromuscular weakness, and abnormal gait characteristic of shivers syndrome, J Am Vet Med Assoc 215: 1621, 1661–1665, 1999.
107. Andrews FM, Spurgeon TL, Reed SM: Histochemical changes in skeletal muscles of four male horses with neuromuscular disease, Am J Vet Res 47:2078–2083, 1986.
108. Van Ham L, Bhatti S, Polis I, et al: "Continuous muscle fibre activity" in six dogs with episodic myokymia, stiffness and collapse, Vet Rec 155:769–774, 2004.
109. Galano HR, Olby NJ, Howard JF Jr, et al: Myokymia and neuromyotonia in a cat, J Am Vet Med Assoc 227:1608–1612, 2005.
110. Walmsley GL, Smith PM, Herrtage ME, et al: Facial myokymia in a puppy, Vet Rec 158:411–412, 2006.
111. Oh SJ, Alapati A, Claussen GC, et al: Myokymia, neuromyotonia, dermatomyositis, and voltage-gated K^+ channel antibodies, Muscle Nerve 27:757–760, 2003.
112. Duncan ID: Abnormalities of myelination of the central nervous system associated with congenital tremor, J Vet Intern Med 1:10–23, 1987.
113. Done JT: Congenital nervous diseases in pigs: a review, Lab Anim 2:207–217, 1968.
114. Done JT: The congenital tremor syndrome in pigs, Vet Annu 16:98–102, 1976.
115. Done JT, Woolley J, Upcott DH, et al: Porcine congenital tremor type AII: spinal cord morphometry, Br Vet J 142:145–150, 1986.
116. Emerson JL, Delez AL: Cerebellar hypoplasia, hypomyelinogenesis, and congenital tremors of pigs, associated with prenatal hog cholera vaccination of sows, J Am Vet Med Assoc 147:47–54, 1965.
117. Harding JD, Done JT, Harbourne JF, et al: Congenital tremor type A 3 in pigs: an hereditary sex-linked cerebrospinal hypomyelinogenesis, Vet Rec 92:527–529, 1973.
118. Patterson DS, Sweasey D, Brush PJ, et al: Neurochemistry of the spinal cord in British Saddleback piglets affected with congenital tremor, type A-IV, a second form of hereditary cerebrospinal hypomyelinogenesis, J Neurochem 21:397–406, 1973.
119. Clarke GL, Osburn BI: Transmissible congenital demyelinating encephalopathy of lambs, Vet Pathol 15:68–82, 1978.
120. Saperstein G, Leipold HW, Dennis SM: Congenital defects of sheep, J Am Vet Med Assoc 167:314–322, 1975.
121. Nettleton PF, Gilray JA, Russo P, et al: Border disease of sheep and goats, Vet Res 29:327–340, 1998.

122. Otter A, Welchman D de B, Sandvik T, et al: Congenital tremor and hypomyelination associated with bovine viral diarrhoea virus in 23 British cattle herds, Vet Rec 164:771–778, 2009.
123. Rousseaux CG, Klavano GG, Johnson ES, et al: "Shaker" calf syndrome: a newly recognized inherited neurodegenerative disorder of horned Hereford calves, Vet Pathol 22:104–111, 1985.
124. Cummings JF, Summers BA, de Lahunta A, et al: Tremors in Samoyed pups with oligodendrocyte deficiencies and hypomyelination, Acta Neuropathol 71:267–277, 1986.
125. Griffiths IR, Duncan ID, McCulloch M, et al: Shaking pups: a disorder of central myelination in the spaniel dog. Part 1. Clinical, genetic and light-microscopical observations, J Neurol Sci 50:423–433, 1981.
126. Kornegay JN, Goodwin MA, Spyridakis LK: Hypomyelination in Weimaraner dogs, Acta Neuropathol 72:394–401, 1987.
127. Mayhew IG, Blakemore WF, Palmer AC, et al: Tremor syndrome hypomyelination in lurcher pups, J Small Anim Pract 25:551–559, 1984.
128. Palmer AC, Blakemore WF, Wallace ME, et al: Recognition of "trembler," a hypomyelinating condition in the Bernese mountain dog, Vet Rec 120:609–612, 1987.
129. Vandevelde M, Braund KG, Walker TL, et al: Dysmyelination of the central nervous system in the chow chow dog, Acta Neuropathol 42:211–215, 1978.
130. Nadon NL, Duncan ID, Hudson LD: A point mutation in the proteolipid protein gene of the "shaking pup" interrupts oligodendrocyte development, Development 110:529–537, 1990.
131. Griffiths IR, Duncan ID, McCulloch M: Shaking pups: a disorder of central myelination in the spaniel dog. II. Ultrastructural observations on the white matter of the cervical spinal cord, J Neurocytol 10:847–858, 1981.
132. Stoffregen DA, Huxtable CR, Cummings JF, et al: Hypomyelination of the central nervous system of two Siamese kitten littermates, Vet Pathol 30:388–391, 1993.
133. Van Ham L, Vandevelde M, Desmidt M, et al: A tremor syndrome with a central axonopathy in Scottish terriers, J Vet Intern Med 8:290–292, 1994.
134. Harper PA, Healy PJ: Neurological disease associated with degenerative axonopathy of neonatal Holstein-Friesian calves, Aust Vet J 66:143–144, 145–146, 1989.
135. Seahorn TL, Fuentealba IC, Illanes OG, et al: Congenital encephalomyelopathy in a quarter horse, Equine Vet J 23:394–396, 1991.
136. Cuddon PA: Tremor syndromes, Prog Vet Neurol 1: 285–299, 1990.
137. Bagley RS, Kornegay JN, Wheeler SJ, et al: Generalized tremors in Maltese: clinical findings in seven cases, J Am Anim Hosp Assoc 29:141–145, 1993.
138. Wagner SO, Podell M, Fenner WR: Generalized tremors in dogs: 24 cases (1984-1995), J Am Vet Med Assoc 211:731–735, 1997.
139. DeLahunta A, Glass E: Veterinary neuroanatomy and clinical neurology, St Louis, 2009, Saunders Elsevier.
140. Parker AJ: How do I treat? "Little white shakers," Prog Vet Neurol 2:151, 1991.
141. Hocking AD, Holds K, Tobin NF: Intoxication by tremorgenic mycotoxin (penitrem A) in a dog, Aust Vet J 65:82–85, 1988.
142. Tiwary AK, Puschner B, Poppenga RH: Using roquefortine C as a biomarker for penitrem A intoxication, J Vet Diagn Invest 21:237–239, 2009.
143. Boysen SR, Rozanski EA, Chan DL, et al: Tremorgenic mycotoxicosis in four dogs from a single household, J Am Vet Med Assoc 221:1420, 1441–1444, 2002.
144. Lowes NR, Smith RA, Beck BE: Roquefortine in the stomach contents of dogs suspected of strychnine poisoning in Alberta, Can Vet J 33:535–538, 1992.
145. Young KL, Villar D, Carson TL, et al: Tremorgenic mycotoxin intoxication with penitrem A and roquefortine in two dogs, J Am Vet Med Assoc 222:35, 52–53, 2003.
146. Mayhew IG: Large animal neurology, Oxford, UK; Ames, Iowa, 2008, Blackwell.
147. Dollahite JW, Younger RL, Crookshank HR, et al: Chronic lead poisoning in horses, Am J Vet Res 39: 961–964, 1978.
148. Knecht CD, Crabtree J, Katherman A: Clinical, clinicopathologic, and electroencephalographic features of lead poisoning in dogs, J Am Vet Med Assoc 175:196–201, 1979.
149. Zook BC, Carpenter JL, Leeds EB: Lead poisoning in dogs, J Am Vet Med Assoc 155:1329–1342, 1967.
150. Scott DW, Bolton GR, Lorenz MD: Hexachlorophene toxicosis in dogs, J Am Vet Med Assoc 162:947–949, 1973.
151. Thompson JP, Senior DF, Pinson DM, et al: Neurotoxicosis associated with the use of hexachlorophene in a cat, J Am Vet Med Assoc 190:1311–1312, 1987.
152. Bath ML: Hexachlorophene toxicity in dogs, J Small Anim Pract 19:241–244, 1978.
153. Jaggy A, Oliver JE: Chlorpyrifos toxicosis in two cats, J Vet Intern Med 4:135–139, 1990.
154. Vijverberg HP, van den Bercken J: Annotation. Action of pyrethroid insecticides on the vertebrate nervous system, Neuropathol Appl Neurobiol 8:421–440, 1982.
155. de Weille JR, Brown LD, Narahashi T: Pyrethroid modifications of the activation and inactivation kinetics of the sodium channels in squid giant axons, Brain Res 512: 26–32, 1990.
156. Whittem T: Pyrethrin and pyrethroid insecticide intoxication in cats, Compend Contin Educ Pract Vet 17: 489–495, 1995.
157. Hansen SR, Stemme KA, Villar D, et al: Pyrethrins and pyrethroids in dogs and cats, Compend Contin Educ Pract Vet 16:707–710, 1994:712.
158. Garosi LS, Rossmeisl JH, de Lahunta A, et al: Primary orthostatic tremor in Great Danes, J Vet Intern Med 19:606–609, 2005.
159. Platt SR, De Stefani A, Wieczorek L: Primary orthostatic tremor in a Scottish deerhound, Vet Rec 159:495–496, 2006.
160. Wissel J, Harlizuis B, Richter A, et al: A new tremor mutant in the Pietrain pig: an animal model of orthostatic tremor? Clinical and neurophysiological observations, Mov Disord 12:743–746, 1997.
161. Bagley RS: Tremor syndromes in dogs: diagnosis and treatment, J Small Anim Pract 33:485–490, 1992.
162. Nakahata K, Uzuka Y, Matsumoto H, et al: Hyperkinetic involuntary movements in a young Shetland sheepdog, J Am Anim Hosp Assoc 28:347–348, 1992.
163. Meyers KM, Padgett GA, Dickson WM: The genetic basis of a kinetic disorder of Scottish terrier dogs, J Hered 61:189–192, 1970.
164. Clemmons RM, Peters RI, Meyers KM: Scotty cramp: a review of cause, characteristics, diagnosis, and treatment, Compend Contin Educ Pract Vet 2:385–388, 1980.
165. Andersson B, Andersson M: On the etiology of "Scotty Cramp" and "Splay": two motoring disorders common in the Scottish terrier breed, Acta Vet Scand 23:550–558, 1982.

166. Schaub RG, Meyers KM: Evidence for a small functional pool of serotonin in neurohumoral transmission, Res Commun Chem Pathol Pharmacol 10:29–36, 1975.
167. Roberts DD, Hitt ME: Methionine as a possible inducer of Scotty cramp, Canine Pract 13:29–31, 1986.
168. Geiger KM, Klopp LS: Use of a selective serotonin reuptake inhibitor for treatment of episodes of hypertonia and kyphosis in a young adult Scottish terrier, J Am Vet Med Assoc 235:168–171, 2009.
169. Herrtage ME, Palmer AC: Episodic falling in the cavalier King Charles spaniel, Vet Rec 112:458–459, 1983.
170. Rusbridge C: Neurological diseases of the cavalier King Charles spaniel, J Small Anim Pract 46:265–272, 2005.
171. Woods CB: Hyperkinetic episodes in two Dalmatian dogs, J Am Anim Hosp Assoc 13:255–257, 1977.
172. Furber RM: Cramp in Norwich terriers, Vet Rec 115:46, 1984(letter).
173. Penderis J, Franklin RJ: Dyskinesia in an adult bichon frisé, J Small Anim Pract 42:24–25, 2001.
174. Ramsey IK, Chandler KE, Franklin RJ: A movement disorder in boxer pups, Vet Rec 144:179–180, 1999.
175. Chrisman CL: Dancing Doberman disease: clinical findings and prognosis, Prog Vet Neurol 1:83–90, 1990.
176. Cahill JI, Goulden BE: Stringhalt: current thoughts on aetiology and pathogenesis, Equine Vet J 24:161–162, 1992.
177. Cahill JI, Goulden BE, Pearce HG: A review and some observations on stringhalt, N Z Vet J 33:101–104, 1985.
178. Huntington PJ, Jeffcott LB, Friend SC, et al: Australian stringhalt: epidemiological, clinical and neurological investigations, Equine Vet J 21:266–273, 1989.
179. Araujo JA, Curcio B, Alda J, et al: Stringhalt in Brazilian horses caused by *Hypochaeris radicata*, Toxicon 52:190–193, 2008.
180. Araya O, Krause A, Solis de Ovando M: Outbreaks of stringhalt in southern Chile, Vet Rec 142:462–463, 1998.
181. Galey FD, Hullinger PJ, McCaskill J: Outbreaks of stringhalt in northern California, Vet Hum Toxicol 33:176–177, 1991.
182. Gay CC, Fransen S, Richards J, et al: *Hypochaeris*-associated stringhalt in North America, Equine Vet J 25:456–457, 1993.
183. Slocombe RF, Huntington PJ, Friend SC, et al: Pathological aspects of Australian stringhalt, Equine Vet J 24:174–183, 1992.
184. Torre F: Clinical diagnosis and results of surgical treatment of 13 cases of acquired bilateral stringhalt (1991-2003), Equine Vet J 37:181–183, 2005.
185. Huntington PJ, Seneque S, Slocombe RF, et al: Use of phenytoin to treat horses with Australian stringhalt, Aust Vet J 68:221–224, 1991.
186. Wijnberg ID, Schrama SE, Elgersma AE, et al: Quantification of surface EMG signals to monitor the effect of a Botox treatment in six healthy ponies and two horses with stringhalt: preliminary study, Equine Vet J 41: 313–318, 2009.
187. Kube SA, Vernau KM, LeCouteur RA: Dyskinesia associated with oral phenobarbital administration in a dog, J Vet Intern Med 20:1238–1240, 2006.
188. Smedile LE, Duke T, Taylor SM: Excitatory movements in a dog following propofol anesthesia, J Am Anim Hosp Assoc 32:365–368, 1996.

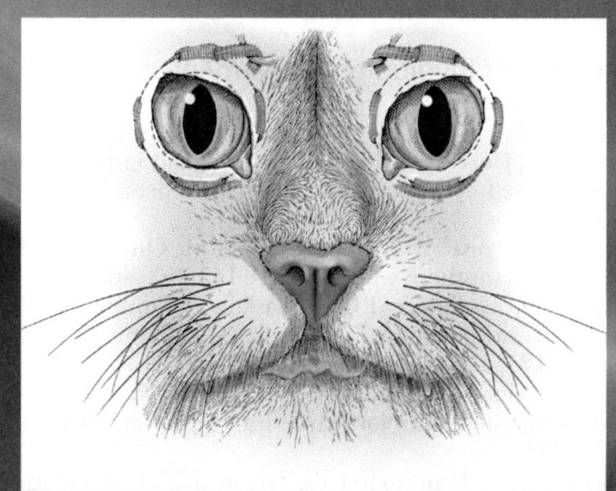

CHAPTER 11

Blindness, Anisocoria, and Abnormal Eye Movements

Disorders involving the eye are common in veterinary practice. Although conscious perception of light (vision) is often discussed in isolation, given the intimate relationship between vision, autonomic control of the pupil, and voluntary ocular movements, this chapter discusses disorders related to these functions together. These complex functions require integration of multiple areas of the brain and spinal cord and consequently numerous diseases may cause visual deficits, abnormal pupil function, or abnormal ocular movements. Imperative to establishing a correct anatomic diagnosis is the integration of findings related to vision, pupil size, and function and ability to move the globe voluntarily.

LESION LOCALIZATION

Vision

The visual pathway is presented in Figures 11-1 and 11-2 and Table 11-1. Methods of testing vision are discussed in Chapter 1. The visual pathway begins with the retina. The outermost layer of the retina is composed of the photoreceptors, dendritic processes of the rod and cone neurons. Photoreceptors are distributed throughout the retina, but a greater density of receptors is located in the area centralis, which is important for acute vision. Excited by light, photoreceptors are in synaptic relationship with the second neurons of the visual pathway, bipolar neurons. In turn, bipolar neurons interact with the third neuron in the visual pathway, ganglion neurons. Axons of the retinal ganglion cell neurons coalesce to form the optic disc and course in the optic nerve. At the optic chiasm, axons originating from the medial (nasal) retina decussate and continue as the contralateral optic tract. Axons from the lateral (temporal) retina remain ipsilateral (do not cross at the chiasm) and course in the ipsilateral optic tract.

The degree of decussation of optic nerve fibers at the optic chiasm varies in different species. As a general rule, the more lateral the eyes are placed on the head, the greater the degree of decussation and the less vision is binocular. In primates, essentially all the fibers from the medial half of the retina cross, while all the fibers from the lateral half of the retina remain ipsilateral enabling binocular vision. In carnivores, all of the fibers from the medial retina decussate in addition to approximately half the fibers of the lateral retina. In most herbivores, 80% or more of the fibers cross. In horses, only about 17% of fibers cross.[1] Almost all the fibers cross in rabbits.

Approximately 80% of the axons of each optic tract synapse in the lateral geniculate nucleus (LGN) of the thalamus. From the LGN, axons project via the optic radiation to the occipital cortex of the cerebrum. Throughout the visual pathway, there is a retinotopic organization whereby axons from specific regions of the retina project to a specific area of the LGN and also the occipital cortex. The importance of this retinotopic organization of the LGN and occipital cortex is exemplified in the Siamese cat (see later discussion).

Pupillary Light Reflexes

The pathway for pupillary light reflexes (PLRs) is outlined and illustrated in Figures 11-1 and 11-2 and in Table 11-1. The methods of testing pupillary reflexes are described in Chapter 1. The afferent limb of the pupillary light reflex is largely the same as for vision. However, axons in the optic tract not involved in vision diverge from the visual pathway at the LGN. Rather than synapsing, axons project over the LGN to the pretectal nuclei at the level of the midbrain. The majority of axons of the pretectal nuclei cross to synapse on the contralateral general visceral efferent (GVE, parasympathetic division) neurons of the oculomotor nerve (cranial nerve [CN] III) nuclei, which provide parasympathetic innervation to the pupil. Some axons of the pretectal nuclei remain ipsilateral. Additionally, axons originating from the lateral retina and therefore remaining ipsilateral at the chiasm also project to the pretectal nuclei. In doing so, stimulation of the retina projects to the oculomotor nerve nuclei bilaterally. Axons from GVE neurons course in CN III, exit the cranial cavity via the orbital fissure, and synapse in the ciliary ganglion. Postganglionic neurons from the

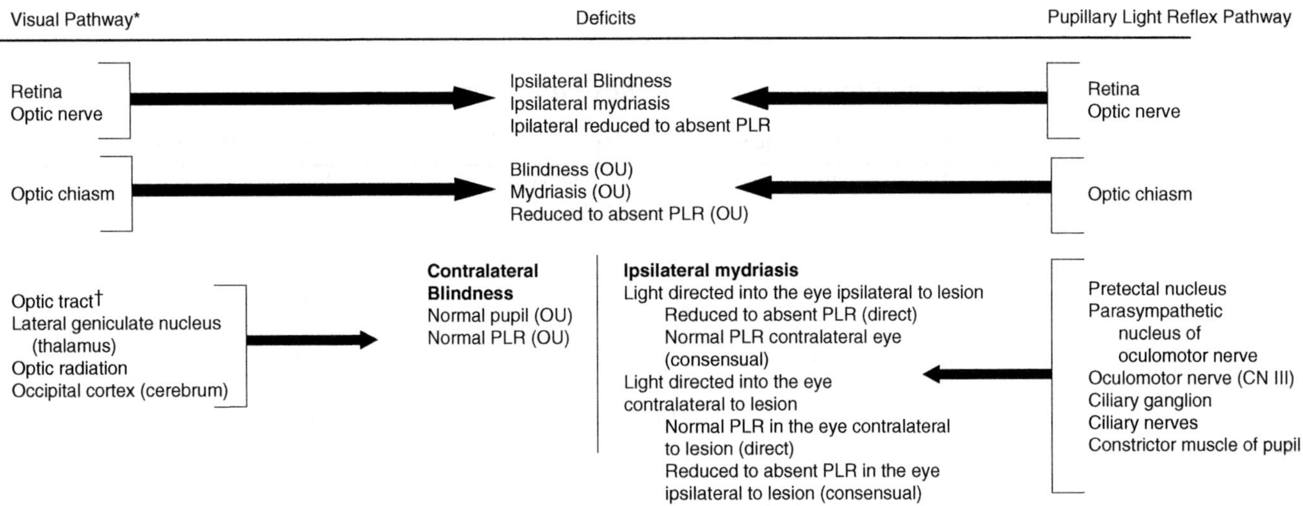

Figure 11-1 Deficits from a unilateral lesion of the visual and pupillary light reflex (PLR) pathways.

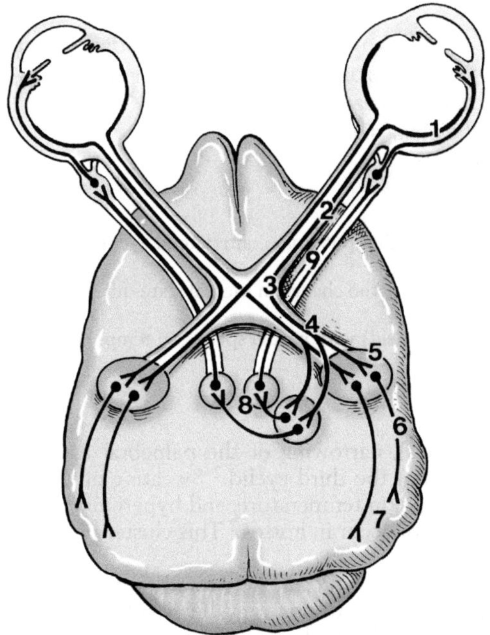

Figure 11-2 Pathways for vision and the pupillary light reflex pathway. *1*, Retina/optic nerve; *2*, orbit (cranial nerve [CN] II, III); *3*, optic chiasma; *4*, optic tract; *5*, lateral geniculate nucleus (thalamus); *6*, optic radiation; *7*, occipital cortex; *8*, parasympathetic nucleus of CN III (midbrain); *9*, CN III (oculomotor).

ciliary ganglion innervate the constrictor muscle of the pupil via the short ciliary nerve. Stimulation results in constriction of the pupil. Ultimately, there is bilateral input to the pretectal nuclei and therefore bilateral projections to the autonomic division of CN III nuclei. As a result, light directed into one eye results in constriction of both pupils. Constriction of the pupil in response to light directed in that eye is referred to as the direct response. Constriction of the contralateral pupil is referred to as the consensual or indirect response. The anatomic organization of the afferent limb of the PLR provides multiple means for input of afferent information allowing minimal stimulation for normal function and preservation of function in many disease processes.

As can be deduced from the discussion above, evaluation of the menace response and pupillary light reflex is critical in determining an anatomic diagnosis in an animal with visual dysfunction. Unilateral lesions involving the retina or optic nerve result in an ipsilateral absent menace response, mydriasis, and decreased or absent PLR. Unilateral lesions involving the optic chiasm typically produce bilateral absence of the menace response, mydriasis, and decreased or absent PLR. Unilateral lesions caudal to the optic chiasm, affecting the optic tract, LGN, optic radiation, or occipital lobe of the cerebrum result in a contralateral absent menace response with normal pupil size and PLR. As a general rule with unilateral lesions in the optic tract, stimulation of the contralateral retina with a bright light provides enough stimulus to activate the lateral retina (whose axons remain ipsilateral at the chiasm). The ispilateral projections from the lateral retina of the affected eye combined with the projections from the unaffected eye provide ample activation of both pretectal nuclei and therefore both oculomotor nerve nuclei to maintain a normal PLR with unilateral lesions caudal to the optic chiasm. Lesions involving the optic tract, LGN, optic radiation, or occipital lobe of the cerebrum cause loss of one half of the visual field, referred to as hemianopsia. The visual field can be defined as the image of the environment that is projected on to the retina when fixed in one position. Therefore, objects or light from the right side of the animal will stimulate the medial aspect of the retina of the right eye and the lateral aspect of the retina of the left eye. Despite this, lesions caudal to the chiasm typically result in visual deficits only in the contralateral eye. This may be a reflection of the greater percentage of axons from the retina that cross at the chiasm.

Additionally, axons from the retina also project to a wide array of brainstem nuclei, in particular the rostral colliculus. The rostral colliculi are involved in the coordination of head movements and movement of the extraocular eye muscles with visual input. From the rostral colliculi, axons project directly or indirectly to the cerebrum, cerebellum, and spinal cord. This allows for visual tracking of objects and moving the eye to ensure light focuses on the area centralis for acute vision.

Caution must be exercised in the interpretation of visual deficits. Because the examiner must rely on motor or behavioral reactions, several tests should be used to confirm an impression that an animal has visual dysfunction. See Chapter 1 for details.

TABLE 11-1

Signs of Lesions in the Visual and Pupillary Light Reflex Pathways

Lesion Location	Vision/Menace Response	Pupil Size	Pupillary Light Reflexes
Retina/optic nerve (unilateral lesion)	Absent on affected side	Usually mydriasis of the affected side*	*When testing affected eye* Direct PLR—reduced to absent Consensual—reduced to absent *When testing the unaffected eye* Direct PLR—normal Consensual—reduced to absent
Bilateral retina/optic nerve/optic chiasm	Absent in both eyes	Bilateral mydriasis	Absent in both eyes
Unilateral optic tract, lateral geniculate nucleus, optic radiation, occipital cortex	Absent in contralateral eye‡ Normal in ipsilateral eye	Normal in both eyes	Normal in both eyes
Midbrain (bilateral) parasympathetic nucleus of CN III†	Normal in both eyes	Bilateral mydriasis	Absent in both eyes
Unilateral CN III	Normal in both eyes	Mydriasis of the affected side Normal in contralateral eye	*When testing affected eye* Direct PLR—reduced to absent Consensual—normal *When testing the unaffected eye* Direct PLR—normal Consensual—reduced to absent
Sympathetic innervation to the eye	Normal in both eyes	Constricted on affected side and does not dilate in dark Normal on contralateral side and dilates in dark	Normal in both eyes

CN, Cranial nerve.

*Depending on the degree of room light, may appear normal; in bright light, may receive enough input from contralateral eye to maintain normal pupil size.

†Lesions affecting the midbrain would result in severe changes in mental state (see Chapter 12); the change in mental state differentiates midbrain lesion from CN III lesion.

‡Depending on how menace response is tested, loss of vision occurs in nasal retina (temporal field) with partial sparing in temporal retina (nasal field). See Figure 11-2.

Lesions of CN III (including the ciliary ganglion and the short ciliary nerves) or of the constrictor muscle of the pupil cause ipsilateral loss of PLR and mydriasis without affecting vision. Bilateral lesions are unusual except in lesions of the brainstem. Lesions of the pretectal nucleus or the parasympathetic nucleus of CN III cause loss of pupillary constriction.

Sympathetic control of the dilator muscle of the pupil is illustrated in Figure 11-3 and Tables 11-1 and 11-2. Note that these pathways originate in the hypothalamus, and axons course ipsilaterally down the brainstem and cervical spinal cord via the lateral tectotegmental tracts (midbrain) to synapse on lower motor neurons (LMNs) located in the intermediate gray matter of the spinal cord segments T1 through T3. This is considered the UMN pathway. It provides facilitatory input. Preganglionic (first order neuron) fibers leave the spinal cord with roots of the brachial plexus. In the thorax, fibers compose the cranial sympathetic trunk, which courses cranially in the neck with the vagus nerve (vagosympathetic trunk) synapsing in the cranial cervical ganglion located near the tympanic bulla. Postganglionic (second-order neuron) sympathetic axons then follow other cranial nerves to innervate structures in the head. Sympathetic activation is produced by emotional reactions such as fear and rage. Sympathetic nerves also innervate smooth muscle in the periorbital fascia and the eyelids, including the third eyelid in some species. Lesions of this pathway result in a constricted pupil (miosis), slight retraction of the globe because of loss of tone in the periorbita (enophthalmos), narrowing of the palpebral fissure (ptosis), and elevation of the third eyelid.[2] Sweating of the ipsilateral face, increased skin temperature, and hyperemia of the nostril and conjunctiva occur in horses.[3] This cluster of signs is called Horner's syndrome.

Differentiation of preganglionic and postganglionic lesions using pharmacologic testing may be possible in the first few weeks of Horner's syndrome. Denervation hypersensitivity causes exaggerated responses with stimulation using direct-acting agents when the postganglionic neuron is involved. Indirect-acting agents require an intact postganglionic neuron for an effect. Instillation of 1% hydroxyamphetamine, an indirect-acting agent, causes good dilation of a normal eye, an eye with a preganglionic lesion, or one with an UMN neuron lesion, but it causes minimal dilation of an eye with a postganglionic lesion. Instillation of 1% phenylephrine, a direct-acting agent, causes minimal dilation of a normal eye or one with a preganglionic lesion but good dilation of an eye with a postganglionic lesion.[4,5] Unfortunately, pharmacologic testing is often unreliable.[6]

Dazzle Reflex

When a bright light is shined in the eye, the animal squints or completely closes the palpebral fissure. This is referred to as the dazzle reflex. Although not well defined, the anatomic pathways involve the retina, optic nerve, and tract to the level of the LGN. From the LGN, axons project to the rostral colliculi from which tectonuclear pathways stimulate CN VII for eyelid

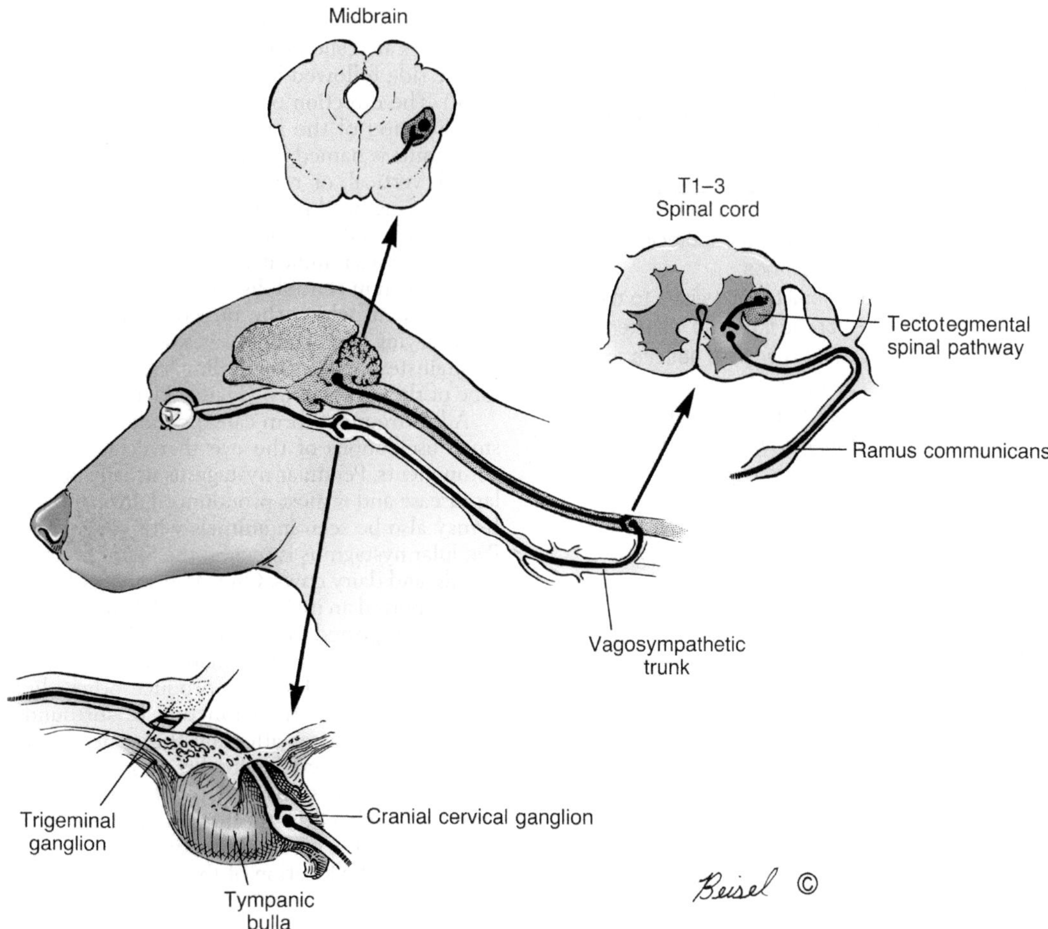

Figure 11-3 Pathway of sympathetic innervation of the eye. (From Greene CE, Oliver JF Jr: Neurologic examination, In Ettinger SJ, editor: Textbook of veterinary medicine, ed 2, 1982, Philadelphia, WB Saunders.)

closure. Because the pathway does not involve the cerebrum, animals that are blind from cerebral disease maintain this reflex, while animals with lesions involving the afferent pathway (retina, optic nerve, and tract to the level of the LGN, and rostral colliculi) or the efferent pathway (CN VII) lack this reflex.

Anisocoria

Anisocoria or unequal pupils may be caused by ocular or neurologic disorders. Ocular diseases include abnormalities of the iris, cornea, lens, or retina. Ocular pain, especially if uveitis is present, causes miosis. Atrophy of the iris results in mydriasis. Increased intraocular pressure also causes mydriasis. Unilateral blindness from a retinal disorder may cause only a mild dilation of the affected eye in dogs and cats because of weaker consensual stimulation. Moving a light source from eye to eye (the swinging "flashlight" test), the pupil of the affected eye will constrict when light is directed into the unaffected eye. When the light is swung to the affected eye, the pupil of the affected eye will dilate.

Eye Movements

The extraocular eye muscles are innervated by CN III (oculomotor), CN IV (trochlear), and CN VI (abducent) (Figure 11-4). Eye movements are controlled by UMNs from the cerebral cortex and through brainstem vestibular reflexes. The eye muscles normally act in a synergistic or an antagonistic manner to provide coordinated conjugate movements. Testing of eye movements is discussed in Chapter 1. Abnormalities of eye position include paralysis of gaze in a direction related to a muscle or a group of muscles, strabismus, or globe deviation. Abnormalities of eye movement include loss of normal nystagmus (conjugate eye movements with movement of the head) and abnormal nystagmus.

When the globe is fixed in a deviated position (strabismus), regardless of head position, a lesion of CN III, IV, or VI is suspected. Lesions of the trochlear nerve (CN IV) may cause slight rotation of the globe, which is difficult to evaluate in animals that have a round pupil. Lesions of CN III and VI cause ventrolateral and medial strabismus, respectively. Several weeks after an injury, the globe may return to its normal midposition, but loss of movement occurs dorsally, medially, and ventrally with a lesion of CN III and laterally with a lesion of CN VI (see Figures 11-4 and 11-5). Positional strabismus (disconjugate deviation of the eye in certain head positions) is characteristic of lesions of the vestibular system. Typically, the eye ipsilateral to the vestibular abnormality is ventrally deviated in the palpebral fissure when the nose is elevated. In this case, eye movements can be elicited in all directions by appropriate movements of the head (normal nystagmus), demonstrating that all extraocular muscles are functional (see Chapter 8). In food animals, both eyes tend to maintain a horizontal position; therefore, they are ventrally placed when the head is elevated, although the affected side may be more deviated relative to the normal side. If CNs III, IV, *and* VI are affected, the eye remains in a normal position within the orbit. However, normal nystagmus will be absent.

TABLE 11-2

Clinical Signs Expected With a Unilateral Lesion Involving the Sympathetic Innervations to the Eye

Site of the Lesion	Clinical Signs
Lateral tectotegmental tract	Ipsilateral GP ataxia/UMN deficits to the thoracic and pelvic limbs
T1-3 spinal cord segment	Ipsilateral LMN deficits to the thoracic limb and ipsilateral GP ataxia/UMN deficits to the pelvic limb
Brachial plexus lesion	Ipsilateral LMN deficits to the thoracic limb and normal pelvic limb
Vagosympathetic trunk	Ipsilateral laryngeal paralysis*
Postganglionic extension (tympanic bulla)	Ipsilateral CN VII and VIII deficits (facial paralysis and vestibular dysfunction)
Orbital fissure/retrobulbar extension	Ipsilateral CN III, IV, V (ophthalmic branch), VI deficits (ptosis of the upper eyelid, paralysis of the extraocular eye muscles, analgesia to the medial canthus of the eye)

CN, Cranial nerve.
*Laryngeal paralysis may occur if the lesion affects the GVE fibers of the CN V (vagus).

Conjugate and Disconjugate Eye Movements

Conjugate eye movements require coordination of the three cranial nerves and their muscles. The pathway responsible for this coordination is the medial longitudinal fasciculus (MLF), which runs in the center of the brainstem and conveys afferent information from the vestibular nuclei to the nuclei of CN III, CN IV, and CN VI for ocular movements. Lesions in several anatomic areas can result in an absence of normal nystagmus with the globe remaining in a central position without strabismus (ophthalmoplegia). Lesions of the MLF may cause disconjugate movements or, more commonly, a lack of eye movements in response to moving the head (external ophthalmoplegia; paralysis of the extraocular musculature). Lesions of the MLF are seen most commonly after an acute head injury that produces hemorrhage in the center of the brainstem (see Chapter 12). Similarly, a lesion affecting CN III, CN IV, and CN VI nuclei, their respective nerves, or extraocular muscles will result in external ophthalmoplegia. Referred to as cavernous sinus syndrome, lesions involving the cavernous sinus (connected, paired venous sinuses located ventrally in the middle cranial fossa) may affect CN III, CN IV, and CN VI and sensory and autonomic functions of the ocular structures given the close anatomic relationship between these CNs and the cavernous venous sinus.[7,8] Diagnosis involves magnetic resonance imaging (MRI) or computed tomography (CT) of the head.[9,10] External ophthalmoplegia also has been reported from thyroid adenocarcinoma invading the cavernous sinus intracranially and affecting the three cranial nerves.[11]

Nystagmus

Nystagmus is involuntary rhythmic movement of the eyes. Normal nystagmus (also known as physiologic nystagmus or doll's eye reflex) may be visual in origin (i.e., watching telephone poles go by from a moving car), or it may be vestibular in origin (e.g., turning the head rapidly). The visual and vestibular types are called jerk nystagmus because of the slow phase to one side followed by the fast or rapid recovery movement (jerk). The direction of the nystagmus is named according to the direction of the fast component. Abnormal (pathologic) nystagmus is named by the direction of the movement (horizontal, vertical, or rotatory) and by any change in direction with varying head positions. Jerk nystagmus that is horizontal or rotatory and that does not change direction with varying head positions is indicative of peripheral vestibular disease but may be seen in central disease. Vertical jerk nystagmus or with nystagmus in which the direction of the fast phase changes with varying head positions is associated with central vestibular brainstem lesions (including lesions of the flocculonodular lobe of the cerebellum) (Figure 11-6; see also Chapter 8).

A less frequent form called pendular nystagmus consists of small oscillations of the eye that do not have fast and slow components. Pendular nystagmus usually occurs with cerebellar disease and is most pronounced during fixation of the gaze. It may also be seen in animals with congenital visual deficits. Pendular nystagmus is seen in the Siamese cat, other Asian cat breeds, and dairy cows. One large survey of cows in New York State reported an incidence of 0.51% in several breeds.[12] It has also been reported as a familial problem in Ayrshire bulls.[13]

Except for lesions of the globe and the orbit, most diseases affecting the visual system produce other clinical signs that are related to abnormal function of surrounding structures. For example, masses affecting the optic chiasm or the optic tracts usually affect the forebrain, specifically related to the hypothalamus. Lesions of CN III, CN IV, or CN VI cause other signs related to the brainstem. Lesions of the occipital lobe affects other cerebral functions. The combination of signs helps define the location of the lesion (see Chapter 2).

DISEASES

Diseases causing blindness, pupillary abnormalities, and ocular movement disorders are listed in Tables 11-3 through 11-5. The history and the physical and neurologic examinations should provide the clinician with a list of the most probable diseases to be considered. Most of the diseases presented in the figures are also discussed in other chapters. Only those that are related primarily to the visual system are discussed here. Many disorders affect multiple anatomic locations in the visual system. However, this may be difficult to appreciate clinically. For the purposes of discussion, diseases are grouped based on their primary clinical effect. Therefore, disorders are divided into those involving (1) the eye, optic nerve, or optic chiasm and (2) those involving the LGN, optic radiations, or occipital lobe of the cerebrum despite an often multifocal pathologic distribution.

Disorders of the Eye (Retina), Optic Nerve, and Chiasm

Degenerative Diseases

Retinal Dystrophy. Retinal dystrophies are degenerative disorders that result in a loss of photoreceptors. The most well studied are a group of inherited canine retinal dystrophies known as progressive retinal atrophy (PRA).[14] In general, affected animals develop progressive blindness. Initially, the rod cell photoreceptors deteriorate causing night blindness but with time, cone cell function declines resulting in daytime blindness. Most dogs are affected at an early age; however, late onset forms also exist. Clinically, there is an absent menace response, mydriasis, and decreased to absent PLR, bilaterally. Funduscopic examination reveals a hyperreflective tapetum secondary to retinal atrophy, attenuation of the retinal vasculature, and atrophy of the optic disc. In some dogs, secondary cataracts develop. Most forms of PRA display autosomal recessive pattern of inheritance; however, there are also X-link and dominantly inherited forms. Autosomal recessive PRA has been observed in the Abyssinian cat.[15] Affected kittens display the same clinical signs and examination findings as affected dogs. PRA is uncommon in horses, but the thoroughbred horse may be predisposed.[16] The diagnosis is based on clinical examination. Electroretinogram (ERG) may provide supportive data. Importantly, whereas ERG may not provide a definitive diagnosis, it does help eliminate other disease processes from consideration. Definitive diagnosis may be obtained in some breeds using available DNA tests.[14] In dogs, there are 12 known causative mutant genes involved in PRA (*PDE6, RPE65, PDE6, RPGR, RHO, CNGB3, PRCD, RPGRIP1, VMD2, RD3, STK38L, and NPHP4*).[17]

Retinal degeneration and an adult onset cerebellar abiotrophy has been observed in a 4-year-old cat.[18] The affected cat displayed progressive signs of cerebellar disease over several years in addition to bilateral blindness, mydriatic pupils, and absent PLR. Funduscopic examination revealed diffuse hyperreflectivity of the tapetum lucidum and attentuation of the retinal vasculature. Histologically, there was a loss of rod and cone photoreceptors. In the cerebellum there was a loss of Purkinje neurons and granular cell neurons. The cause was unknown.

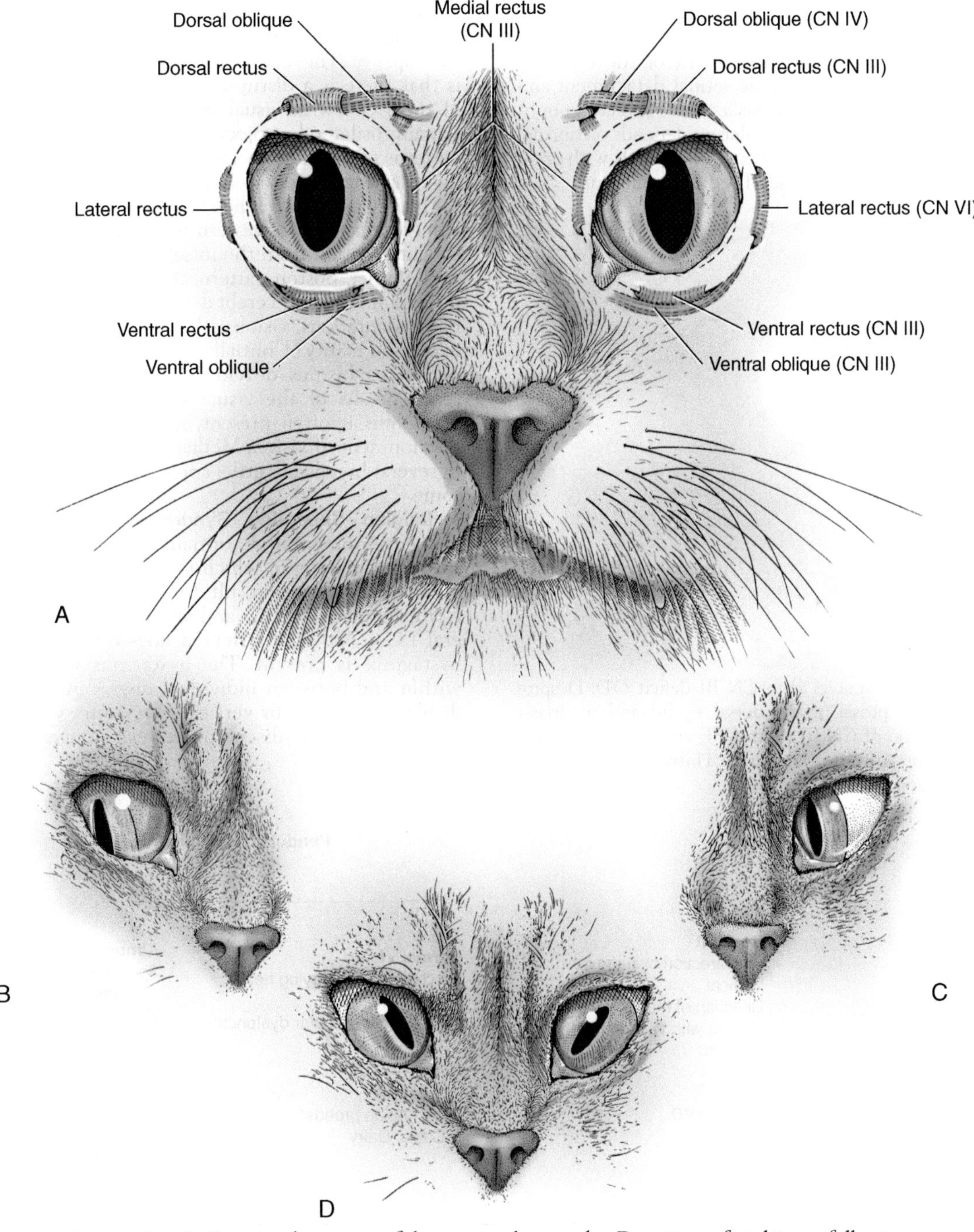

Figure 11-4 **A,** Functional anatomy of the extraocular muscles. Directions of strabismus following **B,** paralysis of the oculomotor neurons; **C,** paralysis of the abducent neurons; and **D,** paralysis of the trochlear neurons. *CN III,* Oculomotor nerve; *CN IV,* trochlear nerve; *CNVI,* abducent.

Anomalies

Retinal and Optic Nerve Aromalies. Primary retinal anomalies are relatively common in dogs but are less common in other species. Anomalies include coloboma, optic nerve hypoplasia, collie eye anomaly/syndrome, and various forms of retinal dysplasia. The types of anomaly and the breeds affected are listed in several reviews and other textbooks.[16,19-21] While many anomalies do not affect vision, some cause blindness and in some cases nystagmus and pupillary abnormalities.

Optic nerve hypoplasia and aplasia has been observed in a number of species.[22-25] In the dog, the shih tzu and miniature poodle are commonly affected breeds.[23,26] Optic nerve hypoplasia may affect one or both eyes. Clinical signs relate to blindness, mydriasis, and absent PLR in the affected eye. Some dogs may retain vision. Funduscopic examination reveals decreased size or absence of the optic disc. A variety of malformations affecting the posterior segment of the eye may coexist.[23] Secondary changes include retinal detachment and vitreal hemorrhage. Optic nerve aplasia occurs less commonly. Development of normal retinal vasculature depends on normal development of the retina. Consequently in animals with optic nerve aplasia, the fundus is devoid of retinal vasculature.[23]

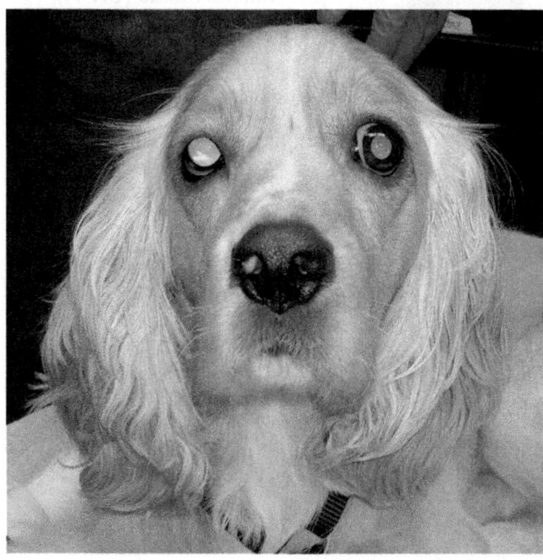

Figure 11-5 A cocker spaniel with CN III deficit OD. Despite minimal strabismus, ptosis of the dorsal eyelid and mydriasis implicate dysfunction of CN III (both GSE and GVE (parasympathetic) innervations. (Copyright 2010 University of Georgia Research Foundation, Inc.)

Two congenital abnormalities are worth mention despite having limited clinical effects on vision. Both conditions are discussed here given their effect on eye position and nystagmus.

Siamese Cat Syndrome. Siamese, Birman, and Himalayan cats have a congenital defect entailing the routing of axons involved in the visual system. The defect is related to a mutation at the albino locus for coat color that leads to an imperfect tyrosinase-negative albinism.[27] In Siamese cats, some axons originating from the lateral (temporal) retina incorrectly decussate at the chiasm rather than remaining ipsilateral.[28,29] In fact, in most normal cats the medial (nasal) retina with axons that project to the contralateral LGN is sharply demarcated with limited overlap from the lateral retina with axons that project to the ipsilateral LGN. In Siamese cats, this line of demarcation is less distinct with greater overlap.[28,29] The consequence of this misrouting of axons is that there is a disruption of the retinotopic organization of the LGN with visual information that should normally remain ipsilateral, projecting to the contralateral LGN. Two patterns of adaptations (named based on the location of the investigating laboratory where they were initially described) in the occipital cortex have developed to accommodate this defect.[30] In the Midwestern pattern, there is suppression of the information from the misdirected lateral retina, whereas in the other, Boston pattern, there is a reorganization of the projections to the cerebral cortex.[30] As a consequence of both adaptations, vision is less binocular and therefore has decreased acuity.[31] Initially born with normal eye position, medial strabismus develops to compensate for the misdirected axons of the visual system.[32] Similarly, pendulous nystagmus is often present, likely related to the abnormal development of vision. Medial strabismus has been reported in several breeds of cattle, apparently as an inherited trait in some.[33]

Belgian Sheepdog Syndrome. An autosomal recessive developmental abnormality has been observed in the Belgian sheepdog in which there is a congenital lack of an optic chiasm.[34] As a result, there is no decussation of axons from the medial retina and all axons project to the ipsilateral LGN. Although affected dogs retain vision, abnormal nystagmus is present. The nystagmus varies considerably within and between individual dogs.[35] Affected dogs may display horizontal or vertical nystagmus, which may occur as conjugate or disconjugate eye movements. Vertical

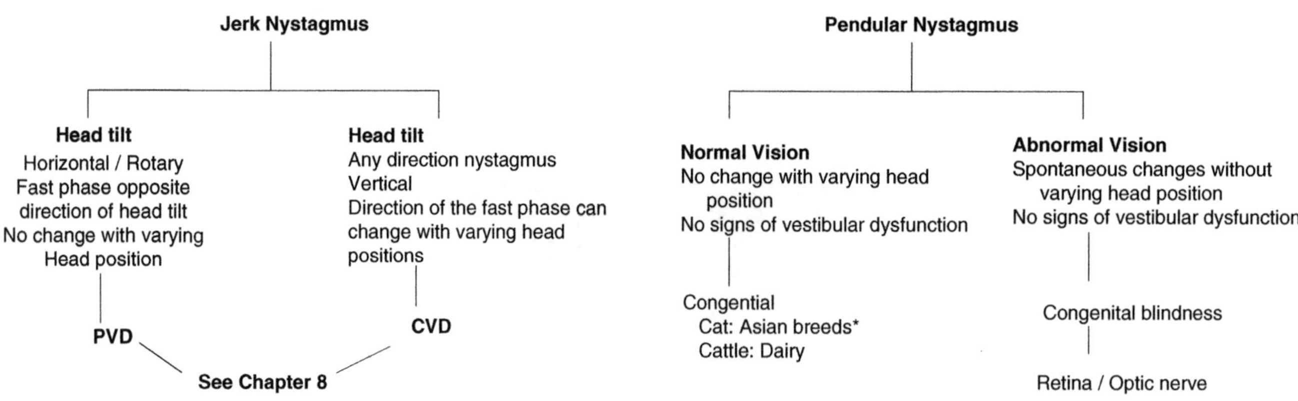

Figure 11-6 Nystagmus. *Vision appears normal clinically, however, nystagmus may develop from abnormal visual acuity related to congenital disturbance in the retinotopic organization of the visual pathway.[27] *PVD*, peripheral vestibular dysfunction; *CVD*, central vestibular dysfunction.

TABLE 11-3

*Etiology of Blindness**

Disease Category	Nonprogressive	Acute Progressive	Chronic Progressive
Degenerative			Storage diseases (R, C) (8, 15) Retinal dystrophy/degeneration (R) Demyelinating diseases (O, X, C) (7, 8, 15)
Anomalous	Hydrocephalus (C) (12) Optic nerve hypoplasia (O) Retinal dysplasia (R) Cerebral malformations (C) (12) Coloboma‡ (O) Collie eye syndrome† (R)		Hydrocephalus (C) (12)
Metabolic	Hyperthermia (C) (15) Hypoxia (C) (12)	Hypoglycemia (C) (12) Hepatic encephalopathy (C) (12)	Hypoglycemia (C) (12) Hepatic encephalopathy (C) (12)
Neoplastic (12)		Lymphoma/Hematopoietic neoplasia (R) Melanoma (R)	Primary (12) Meningioma (O, X, C) Gliomas (O, X, C) Ependymoma (C) Choroid plexus papilloma (C) Secondary (12) Metastatic (R, O, X, C) Pituitary adenoma (O, X, C) Lymphoma/hematopoietic neoplasia (R, O, X, C) Calvaria (O, X, C)
Nutritional		Thiamine deficiency— ruminants (O) (12)	Hypovitaminosis A (R, O) Taurine deficiency—cats (R)
Inflammatory/ infectious (15)		Canine distemper (R, O, X, C) Feline infectious peritonitis (R, O, X, C) Toxoplasmosis (R, C) Thromboembolic meningoencephalitis— bovine (R, C) Bovine virus diarrhea (R, O) Systemic mycoses (O, X, C) Bacterial infections (O, X, C)	Canine distemper (R, O, X, C) Feline infectious peritonitis (R, O, X, C) Toxoplasmosis (R, C) Systemic mycoses (O, X, C) Bacterial infections (O, X, C) GME/Necrotizing encephalitides— dogs (O, X, C) Protothecosis (C) Immune mediated (O)
Toxic (15)		Lead and other heavy metals (C) Hexachlorophene (C)	Lead and other heavy metals (C) Hexachlorophene (C)
Traumatic	Retinal detachment Retinal hemorrhage Edema (O, X, C) Hemorrhage (O, X, C)	Edema (O, X, C) Hemorrhage (O, X, C)	
Vascular	Infarcts (R, C) Hemorrhage (R, O, X, C)		

R, Retina; O, optic nerve; X, optic chiasm; C, optic tract and cerebral cortex.
*Numbers in parentheses refer to chapters in which entities are discussed.
†Collie eye syndrome and coloboma typically do not affect vision.

disconjugate nystagmus is sometimes referred to as see-saw nystagmus.[36]

Metabolic Syndromes

The retina is highly dependent on oxygen to support its high metabolic rate.[37] Consequently, diseases that result in hypoxia, ischemia, or other metabolic dysfunction may also affect vision. However, adverse affects to other body systems predominate given the wide spectrum of effects caused by these metabolic derangements. Depending on the degree and duration of the disturbance, blindness may be temporary or permanent.

Nutritional

Vitamin A Deficiency. A derivative of vitamin A, 11-*cis*-retinal combines with opsin to form rhodopsin, the pigment in rod cells that is necessary for vision. Deficiency of vitamin A is rare, affecting calves and captive raised exotic cats more than companion animals.[38] Hypovitaminosis A has been reported in feedlot cattle fed grain that was deficient in vitamin A and

TABLE 11-4

Etiology of Pupillary Abnormalities*

Disease Category	Nonprogressive	Acute Progressive	Chronic Progressive
Degenerative	Hypoplasia of optic nerve (O) Retinal dysplasia (R) Coloboma (O)‡ Collie eye syndrome (R)‡		Retinal dystrophy (R) Hydrocephalus† (12)
Metabolic		Diffuse metabolic abnormalities	
Neoplastic			Rostrotentorial tumor† (12)
Nutritional		Thiamine deficiency—dogs and cats (15)	
Idiopathic	Pupillotonia/Pourfour du Petit syndrome Anisocoria/Dyscoria— cats (FeLV associated)	Dysautonomia (9, 15)	
Inflammatory/ Infectious (15)		Retrobulbar abscess Several infectious diseases (15) Middle ear infections (8)	
Toxic	Organophosphates	Lead† (15)	
Traumatic	Brainstem hemorrhage (12) Brachial plexus lesions (5)	Hematoma† (12)	Cerebral edema† (12)

R, Retina; O, optic nerve; *FeLV*, feline leukemia virus.
*Numbers in parentheses refer to chapters in which entities are discussed.
†Signs referable to the oculomotor nerve are secondary to tentorial herniation. More commonly associated with acquired hydrocephalus.
‡Collie eye syndrome and coloboma typically do not affect vision unless extensive involvement of the optic nerve.

TABLE 11-5

Etiology of Ocular Movement Disorders*

Disease Category	Nonprogressive	Acute Progressive	Chronic Progressive
Degenerative			Storage diseases (R, C) (8, 15) Demyelinating diseases (O, C) (7, 8, 15)
Anomalous	Hydrocephalus (C) (12) Strabismus with optic pathway anomalies—cats		Hydrocephalus (C) (12)
Neoplastic			Any tumor affecting the brainstem, cerebellum, vestibular system, or CN III, IV, VI (8, 12,)
Nutritional		Thiamine deficiency—dogs and cats (15)	
Inflammatory/ infectious		Any disease affecting the brainstem, cerebellum, vestibular system, or CN III, IV, VI (8, 15)	
Toxic		Hexachlorophene (15)	
Traumatic (12)	Lesions of the brainstem, cerebellum, vestibular system, or CN III, IV, VI		
Vascular (12)	Lesions of the brainstem, cerebellum, vestibular system, or CN III, IV, VI		

CN, Cranial nerve.
*Numbers in parentheses refer to chapters in which entities are discussed.

calves born from cattle grazed on foliage deficient in vitamin A.[39-41] In addition to blindness from abnormal rod cell function, compression of the optic nerve occurs secondary to abnormal skeletal growth of the calvaria. Affected calves also have increased intracranial pressure and communicating hydrocephalus from abnormal development of the arachnoid villi.[41]

Vitamin E Deficiency. Vitamin E deficiency results in retinal degeneration and lipopigment accumulation beginning in the central area of the tapetum lucidum and progressing peripherally and is related to the role of vitamin E as an antioxidant. Regardless of the species, funduscopic examination reveals central retinal degeneration and patchy brown pigmentation of the retina (lipofuscin accumulation). Experimentally, vitamin E deficiency consistently results in visual defects in dogs.[42] Naturally occurring hypovitaminosis E has been reported in a group of hunting dogs fed a deficient diet.[43] Retinal pigment epithelial dystrophy (RPED) has been reported in a number of breeds of dog including the English cocker and Briard.[44,45] Funduscopic examination is identical to dogs with vitamin E deficiency. Although not fully understood, dogs with RPED have abnormally low serum vitamin E levels unrelated to diet or malabsorption.[46] Similarly, approximately 40% of horses with equine motor neuron disease, a disorder likely related to abnormal antioxidant properties possibly due to abnormal vitamin E metabolism, have observable lipofuscin accumulation in the retina despite rare visual deficits (see Chapter 7).[47]

Taurine Deficiency. Cats have an obligate need for taurine in their diet due to an inability to synthesize it. Feline central retinal degeneration (FCRD) can be produced by diets that are deficient in the amino acid taurine.[48] Classically, funduscopic examination reveals a horizontal, linear area of hyperreflectivity.[49] Cats that are exclusively fed commercial dog food develop FCRD.[38]

Neoplasia

Neoplasia affecting the eye, optic nerve, or chiasm is commonly encountered in dogs and cats.[50] Lymphoma can involve all portions of the globe or optic nerves. Neoplasms also can arise in adjacent anatomic areas and extend into the orbit. This is observed with tumors involving the nasal cavity and paranasal sinuses. A variety of primary neoplasms also occur in the retrobulbar area. In dogs, orbital meningioma has been reported.[51] The average age of affected dogs is 9 years, with no breed or sex predilection. Clinical signs relate to a retrobulbar mass, including exophthalmos, orbital swelling, and prolapsed globe. Visual deficits are common. Long-term success can be achieved with surgical resection. Postoperatively, average follow-up time is 1.5 years, with some dogs surviving much longer. Local recurrence can occur and may cause visual deficits in the contralateral eye. In cats, squamous cell carcinoma, lymphoma, and melanoma are most commonly reported.[52] Ocular fibrosarcoma can develop after trauma, leading to blindness.[53] Extension along the optic nerve to the chiasm can affect vision in the contralateral eye.

Tumors of the pituitary gland can cause visual-field deficits from compression of the optic chiasm; however, most pituitary tumors grow dorsally into the hypothalamus instead of spreading out rostrally and caudally. Therefore, signs of visual dysfunction occur when masses are quite large.[54]

Idiopathic

Sudden acquired retinal degeneration syndrome (SARDS) causes acute blindness, mydriasis, and decreased PLR.[55] Affected dogs typically have acute bilateral blindness. Early in the disease course on the fundus, pupil size, and PLR may appear normal. With time, retinal atrophy results in hyperreflectivity of the tapetum lucidum, mydriasis, and decreased to absent PLR. Dogs with SARDS also may display signs consistent with Cushing disease.[55] The ERG reveals absence of a response of the retina, which helps differentiate SARDS from other disorders. There is no effective treatment.

Inflammatory

Optic neuritis is inflammation of the optic nerve. Sudden blindness may be noticed if both eyes are affected. Papilledema and vascular congestion are seen on funduscopic examination if that portion of the nerve is affected. Atrophy of the disc is noted as the process resolves. Chorioretinitis may also be present. ERG can help to differentiate primary retinal disease from optic nerve disease. The diagnostic workup should include MRI and cerebrospinal fluid (CSF) analysis. Serologic testing for infectious disease should be pursued based on the presence of systemic involvement, MRI, and CSF analysis. Canine distemper, toxoplasmosis, and cryptococcosis are among the infectious diseases that cause optic neuritis. Granulomatous meningoencephalomyelitis (GME) can affect the optic nerves.[56] The prognosis for optic neuritis depends on the underlying condition; however, in many cases an underlying etiology is not identified. Edema and inflammation may lead to permanent loss of function of the nerve. In cases without an infectious etiology, early treatment should include corticosteroids at an immunosuppressive dosage. Adjunctive therapy using cytosine arabinoside or cyclosporine may provide long-term control. Other supportive therapies or antibiotic therapy are given as indicated by the animal's condition. Prognosis for return of vision is guarded to poor. In one report of 12 dogs with optic neuritis, 7 remained alive, 5 were permanently blind, and 2 had partial vision.[57]

Sinusitis of the sphenopalatine sinuses in the horse can compress the optic nerve, resulting in optic nerve atrophy.[58] A similar disease process has been reported in the dog and cat.[59] Affected animals displayed abnormalities involving both vision and PLR. In addition, exophthalmos was observed in some animals. The presumptive diagnosis was based on MRI findings, CSF analysis, and response to antibiotics. Typical MRI findings consisted of loss of the normal hyperintense signal on T1-weighted images of the bone marrow and enlargement of the sphenoid bones. In addition, there was marked enhancement of the sphenoid bones and meninges of the ventral portion of the brain. Cerebrospinal fluid analysis varied among animals; however, a marked neutrophilic pleocytosis with intracellular bacteria was observed in one case. Long-term treatment with antibiotics resulted in resolution of clinical signs.

Toxic

Enrofloxacin has been associated with retinal degeneration in cats.[60] Signs develop acutely, often within a few days of initiating antibiotic therapy but may take up to 12 weeks to develop. Signs consist of bilateral blindness, mydriasis, and decreased PLR. Funduscopic examination reveals tapetal hyperreflectivity and attenuation of retinal vasculature. Dosages known to cause the retinal degeneration range from 4.6 mg/kg per os (PO) administered once daily to 27 mg/kg PO administered twice daily. Recovery of vision is guarded but may occur if the drug is discontinued promptly. The mechanism of toxicity is unknown. Factors such as increasing dosage and age of the cat may play a role.[61] Other quinolones may also cause toxicity, consequently caution should be exercised when using fluoroquinolones in cats, especially older cats.

Several cows developed retinal degeneration secondary to a chemical sealant containing acrylamide. Exposure to the chemical occurred after an accidental environmental contamination of the water supply. Retinal and optic nerve axonal degeneration was observed.[62]

Trauma

Any portion of the visual system can be affected by trauma. Most injuries affect the CNS caudal to the chiasm. In horses, trauma can result in injury to one or both optic nerves.[63] With head trauma, the brain may shift caudally in the cranial cavity. This places traction on the optic nerves, which are fixed in place within the optic canals resulting in stretching (tethering) of the nerves.

Disorders Involving the Optic Tract, LGN, Optic Radiations, or Occipital Lobe

Degenerative

An abnormality of the intracellular enzyme systems causes an accumulation of the products of metabolism in the neurons (neuronal storage diseases). Affected neurons function abnormally and eventually die. This group of diseases is listed in Tables 11-2 through 11-4 as storage diseases (see Chapters 8 and 15). Because neurons of higher metabolic demand are more susceptible, the retina, the lateral geniculate nucleus, and the occipital cortex are the most common targets in the visual system. Cranial nerve nuclei usually are not affected until late in the disease. The diseases are hereditary, progressive, and invariably fatal. Presumptive diagnosis is made by assessment of the history, knowledge of the breed selectivity, and exclusion of other diagnoses. Antemortem diagnosis may be established by identification of abnormal organic acids in the urine or blood. Definitive diagnosis can be made through DNA testing, which is available for a number of storage diseases. Frequently, definitive diagnosis is made at necropsy via histologic evaluation of the CNS. Antemortem brain biopsy can be performed in some cases. Likewise, biopsy of tissues other than brain may provide a diagnosis in some of the systemic storage diseases.

Demyelinating diseases as an example, globoid cell leukodystrophy, is caused by an enzymatic deficiency of galactocerebrosidase activity resulting in an intracellular accumulation of psychosine, a toxic metabolite to myelin forming oligodendrocytes and Schwann cells. Signs of cerebellar and spinal cord dysfunction (UMN signs, proprioceptive deficits) are characteristic of the clinical syndrome. However, the visual pathways (optic nerve, optic tract, optic radiation) may be affected. Demyelination occurs secondary to many inflammatory diseases (e.g., canine distemper virus), which can also affect the visual pathways (see Chapters 7 and 8).

Anomalies

Hydrocephalus may be the result of a congenital anomaly often in small and toy breed dogs or may be secondary to mass lesions or inflammation leading to obstruction of the ventricular system and secondary ventricular dilation. Enlargement of the lateral ventricles may compress the optic radiation and the occipital cortex resulting in visual deficits. Hydrocephalus should always be considered in young, small, or toy breed dogs with blindness, normal PLR, and normal pupil size. A diagnosis of hydrocephalus requires MRI or CT. In young dogs with a persistent fontanelle, ultrasonography may be performed through the fontanelle to visualize ventriculomegaly (see Chapter 12).

Metabolic Syndromes

Metabolic-related diseases that affect cerebral cortical function may produce blindness with intact pupillary light reflexes. Examples include hypoglycemia, hepatic encephalopathy, and uremia. Acute metabolic problems such as hypoxia and hyperthermia usually affect the cerebral cortex most severely. Cortical blindness frequently follows severe hypoxic episodes such as cardiac arrest (see Chapters 12 and 15). It is not uncommon for animals that are postictal to have blindness with normal pupil size and pupillary light reflexes (Chapter 13).

Neoplasia

Visual deficits commonly occur with intracranial tumors.[64] Consequently, visual pathway abnormalities are often helpful for localizing intracranial tumors. Neoplasia of the CNS is discussed in Chapter 12.

Nutritional Deficiencies

Polioencephalomalacia (PEM) of ruminants is characterized by cerebral necrosis and edema. Signs of cerebral dysfunction, including blindness, are noted. The pupillary light reflexes are usually normal, unless edema has caused tentorial herniation with compression of the oculomotor nerves. Extorsion of the globe, supposedly from damage to the trochlear nucleus (CN IV), is seen in this syndrome, but the pathogenesis is not clear. An excess of thiaminase in the rumen, producing an acute thiamine deficiency, commonly underlies this condition. However, other causes of PEM include lead toxicity, water deprivation/hypernatremia, and sulfur associated PEM.[65] Thiamine deficiency in small animals, primarily in cats, causes hemorrhages and malacia in the brainstem. Eye movements and pupillary light reflexes may be affected (see Chapter 15).

Inflammatory

Systemic infectious diseases with CNS involvement frequently affect the visual system. Lesions often affect the retina and visual pathways in the CNS. Common infectious diseases include canine distemper, feline infectious peritonitis, toxoplasmosis, rickettsial diseases, systemic mycoses, and thromboembolic meningoencephalitis.[38,66-68] Presumptive diagnosis is based on clinicopathologic data including MRI, CSF analysis, and where available, serology and measurement of antibody titers in CSF, or PCR testing of infectious diseases. Evidence of fundic inflammatory lesions (chorioretinitis) can support the diagnosis.

Granulomatous meningoencephalomyelitis, necrotizing leukoencephalitis, and necrotizing meningoencephalitis are suspected immune-mediated inflammatory diseases. Visual deficits are commonly observed in affected dogs. In addition, an ocular form of GME may predominantly affect the optic nerves.[69]

Toxic

Heavy-metal poisoning, especially lead poisoning, may produce cortical blindness. Toxins that affect the brainstem or cerebellum, such as hexachlorophene, may cause nystagmus (see Chapter 15).

Trauma

Any portion of the visual system can be affected by trauma. Assessing mental state along with oculomotor nerve function is of primary importance in evaluating an animal with head injury. Initially, miosis may be observed as a result of damage to inhibitory UMN function to the oculomotor nerve. These UMNs are located in the cerebrum. With increased brain swelling, tentorial herniation of the occipital lobes compresses the oculomotor nerve nucleus in the midbrain. As a result, a fixed, dilated pupil usually ipsilateral to the herniation (if it is unilateral) occurs. A paralysis of the extraocular muscles that produces a ventrolateral strabismus follows the mydriasis. Hemorrhage in the brainstem also produces abnormal pupils. Midbrain hemorrhage may cause fixed, dilated pupils if the oculomotor nucleus is destroyed with the sympathetic pathway intact, but in most cases the pupils are fixed and midposition because both sympathetic and parasympathetic pathways are affected. Serial assessment of pupillary function, together with mental status, motor function, and other cranial nerve function is important for evaluation of animals with head trauma. Bilateral, fixed, dilated, or midposition pupils along with severe obtundation from the time of injury strongly suggest brainstem injury or hemorrhage that is often irreversible. Progressive dilation of the pupils suggests a developing tentorial herniation that may be treatable (see Chapter 12).

Vascular

Feline ischemic encephalopathy related to *Cuterebra* larval infection may cause contralateral vision loss[70] (see Chapter 12). Similarly, cerebral infarction in dogs may affect the visual system.

Disorders Involving Pupil Function

Dysautonomia

Dysautonomia is a diffuse degeneration of the autonomic nervous system; its cause is unknown[71-76] (see Chapters 9 and 15). The clinical signs include dysuria, bladder distention, decreased anal tone, mydriasis with absent pupillary light reflexes, elevated membrane nictitans, intestinal ileus, vomiting or regurgitation, xerostomia, decreased tear production, and dry nose. Animals are visual, and the menace response is normal. Definitive diagnosis necessitates histologic identification of chromatolytic degeneration of autonomic ganglia, brainstem nuclei, and lateral and ventral horns of the spinal cord. Presumptive diagnosis involves identification of autonomic dysfunction. Denervation hypersensitivity of the iris muscle can be detected in many dogs by instilling 0.1% pilocarpine in one eye and observing for miosis. The test is positive in 85% to 100% of affected dogs.[73,74] Intradermal histamine (0.05 mL of 1:10,000 histamine) produces a wheal, but the expected flare response is often blunted in affected dogs.[73] Administration of atropine (0.02 mg/kg administered intravenously) is not predictable for increasing heart rate.[73] Schirmer tear testing may detect decreased tear production in many affected dogs. The prognosis for recovery is poor. Although the cause is unknown, toxico-infectious etiology may underlie the disease (see Chapters 3, 9, and 15).

Pupillotonia

Pupillotonia is a pupil that is slow to react to light, both on direct and consensual responses. It is thought to be immune mediated. Primary abnormalities of the visual and oculomotor pathways must be excluded. Only one case has been reported.[77]

Horner's Syndrome

Horner's syndrome can result from a lesion affecting any aspect of the pathway supplying sympathetic innervation to the eye (Figure 11-3 and Table 11-2). Horner's syndrome is not associated with visual deficits. Localization is dependent on associated clinical signs. For example, lesions involving the UMN pathway result in ipsilateral general proprioceptive (GP) ataxia/UMN signs to the thoracic and pelvic limbs. A lesion involving the T1-T3 spinal cord segments cause ipsilateral GP ataxia/UMN signs in the pelvic limb and LMN signs in the thoracic limb. Horner's, as a result of disruption of the descending UMN axons (lateral tectotegmental spinal tracts) in the cervical spinal cord or the intermediate gray matter of the T1-T3 spinal cord segments, is commonly observed in animals secondary to fibrocartilaginous embolic myelopathy.[78,79] Injury or neoplasia of the brachial plexus may cause monoparesis and Horner's syndrome on the same side. Middle ear disease is frequently associated with Horner's syndrome in dogs because the sympathetic fibers pass through the tympanic bulla. Guttural pouch infections may cause Horner's syndrome in horses. In dogs and cats, the most common causes of Horner's syndrome include head, neck, or chest trauma; chronic otitis media or otitis interna; brachial plexus avulsion; intracranial and intrathoracic neoplasia; and vigorous ear cleaning.[6,80] The condition is thought to be idiopathic in 42% to 55% of cases.[6,80] Horner's syndrome spontaneously resolves in a large percentage of cases.[80] Depending on the specific cause, time to resolution varies but on average resolution occurs in approximately 8 weeks.[80]

Horner's syndrome with no detectable cause was found in 62 golden retrievers in a 6-year period.[81] The lesion was of the preganglionic neuron based on pharmacologic testing. The investigators reported only 25 cases of Horner's syndrome in other breeds in the same period. Of those, 20 had specific diseases causing the signs. In horses, Horner's syndrome can secondarily result from intravenous injections in the neck, cervical trauma, neoplasia, and ligation of the carotid artery for treatment of guttural pouch mycosis.[82-85] Most of the cases result from surgical or external trauma.

Other Pupil Abnormalities

Diffuse forebrain disease of acute onset such as that with traumatic brain injury can cause bilateral miotic pupils. The most likely mechanism relates to loss of UMN inhibition on the parasympathetic oculomotor neurons. Brain herniation also affects pupil size and is discussed in Chapter 12.

Pourfour du Petit Syndrome

Pupil dilation, widened palpebral fissure, exophthalmos, and retraction of the nictitating membrane were observed in three cats immediately after the tympanic bulla was flushed with saline for the treatment of otitis media.[86] Visual, facial nerve, and vestibular deficits were not noted. The signs were consistent with hyperactivity of the sympathetic innervation of the eye. Signs resolved within hours in one cat and days in another. Horner's syndrome developed 4 days later and eventually resolved in the third cat. The syndrome resembled a similar condition in humans called Pourfour du Petit syndrome.

Dyscoria

Dyscoria is an abnormally shaped pupil. Oftentimes, dyscoria is associated with structural abnormalities of the pupil. The development of dyscoria involves either the medial or lateral branch of the short ciliary nerves of one eye. In cats, the pupil will take on "D" or "reverse D" shape. Feline leukemia virus and lymphoma have been associated with dyscoria in cats.[87,88] Reduced PLR has been associated with feline immunodeficiency virus.[89] The exact pathogenesis is unknown but may be related to a CNS lesion rather than peripherally affecting the parasympathetic branches of CN III or the iris.[89]

Toxins

Organophosphates and carbamates are acetylcholinesterase inhibitors that produce severe miosis along with other signs that include salivation, gastrointestinal signs, urination, and muscle fasciculation and weakness.

CASE STUDIES

CASE STUDY 11-1 *ARES*

 veterinaryneurologycases.com

Neurologic Examination

Menace response

Normal OU

Pupil size

Mydriatic pupil OD; Normal pupil size OS

Pupillary light reflexes (PLR)

	Reaction	
Shine light	OS	OD
OS	+	–
OD	+	–

Eye Position and Movement

Fixed ventrolateral strabismus OD; normal eye position OS; normal nystagmus OS

Assessment

Right oculomotor nerve (CN III) lesion. The unilateral clinical signs suggest a lesion after the nerve leaves the brainstem. The nuclei are only millimeters apart, and lesions at this level usually affect both sides. Both the GVE (parasympathetic innervation) and GSE (voluntary motor function) are affected as evidenced by mydriasis/lack of PLR and fixed strabismus, respectively.

CASE STUDY 11-2 *GOLIATH*

 veterinaryneurologycases.com

Neurologic Examination

Menace response

Normal OS; absent OD

Pupil size

The right pupil is mydriatic compared to the left pupil.

PLR

	Reaction	
Shine light	OS	OD
OS	+	+
OD	–	–

Eye Position and Movement

Normal eye position OU; normal nystagmus OU

Assessment

Right optic nerve or retinal lesion. A funduscopic examination may help differentiate a lesion between these two anatomic localizations. An electroretinogram may be necessary if no retinal lesions are visible. MRI may be necessary to identify a lesion affecting the optic nerve.

CASE STUDY 11-3 *LINCOLN*

 veterinaryneurologycases.com

Neurologic Examination

Menace response

Absent OU

Pupil size

Normal OU

PLR

Normal OU

	Reaction	
Shine light	OS	OD
OS	+	+
OD	+	+

Eye Position and Movement

Normal eye position OU; normal nystagmus OU; the animal does not follow moving objects

Assessment

The findings are consistent with a lesion affecting either the white matter of the optic radiations or occipital cortex of the cerebrum bilaterally. Consideration should be given to a bilateral optic tract lesion or bilateral lateral geniculate nuclei; however, lesions at these anatomic locations may affect PLR pathways. Etiologies may include degenerative disease, anomalous (hydrocephalus, congenital lesions of the cerebrum), metabolic, or toxic disorders; neoplastic or inflammatory (infectious or noninfectious) diseases do not typically have symmetric deficits. Signalment, history, and other aspects of the neurologic examination may help further refine the differential diagnosis.

CASE STUDY 11-4 *MARVEL*

veterinaryneurologycases.com

▪ Neurologic Examination

Menace response
Normal in both eyes

Pupil size
Normal OU

PLR
Normal OU

Shine light	Reaction OS	Reaction OD
OS	+	+
OD	+	+

Eye Position and Movement
Medial strabismus OS; normal eye positions OD; dorsal and ventral movements can be elicited OS by moving the head; normal nystagmus OD

▪ Assessment

Left abducent nerve (CN VI) lesion. Isolated lesions of CN VI are rare. In a clinical case, other signs of brainstem disease may be present.

CASE STUDY 11-5 *SPIKE*

 veterinaryneurologycases.com

▪ Neurologic Examination

Menace response
Absent OU

Pupil size
Mydriatic OU

PLR

Shine light	Reaction OS	Reaction OD
OS	−	−
OD	−	−

Eye Position and Movement
Normal eye position OU; normal nystagmus OU; the animal does not follow moving objects

▪ Assessment

Bilateral retina or bilateral optic nerve lesions, or a lesion affecting the optic chiasm. This situation is one in which lesions affecting both retinas or optic nerves are more common than a single lesion affecting the chiasm. Retinopathies and optic neuropathies are seen more often than are primary lesions of the optic chiasm.

CASE STUDY 11-6 *TUNA*

veterinaryneurologycases.com

▪ Neurologic Examination

Menace response
Normal OU

Pupil size
Normal OU

PLR

Shine light	Reaction OS	Reaction OD
OS	+	+
OD	+	+

Eye Position and Movement
The eyes are in the normal midposition, but no vestibular eye movements can be elicited.

▪ Assessment

There are two possible anatomic explanations to account for the observed deficits. (1) A lesion affecting the MLF or vestibular system bilaterally. The MLF is the tract connecting the vestibular nuclei to the nuclei of CN III, IV, and VI. (2) Alternatively, a lesion could exist that affects the CN III, IV, and VI bilaterally. In this case, one would expect there to be an abnormality in the PLR, bilaterally. Other neurologic deficits may help differentiate between these two anatomic sites. With a lesion affecting the MLF, one would expect a severe change in mental state (i.e., stupor or coma; see Chapter 12). Typical lesions that affect the MLF include severe brainstem lesions, such as a hemorrhage or tumor. Multiple cranial neuropathies include inflammatory (infectious or noninfectious) disease, neoplastic disease (lymphoma or other infiltrative tumor), or idiopathic conditions.

CN, cranial nerve; *GSE*, general somatic efferent; *GVE*, general visceral efferent; *MLF*, medial longitudinal fasciculus; *MRI*, magnetic resonance imaging; *OD*, right eye; *OS*, left eye; *OU*, both eyes.

REFERENCES

1. Timney B, Macuda T: Vision and hearing in horses, J Am Vet Med Assoc 218:1567–1574, 2001.
2. van den Broek AHM: Horner's syndrome in cats and dogs: a review, J Small Anim Pract 28:929–940, 1987.
3. Sweeney RW, Sweeney CR: Transient Horner's syndrome following routine intravenous injections in two horses, J Am Vet Med Assoc 185:802–803, 1984.
4. Neer TM: Horner's syndrome: anatomy, diagnosis, and causes, Compend Contin Educ Pract Vet 6:740–746, 1984.
5. De Resio L: Second order Horner's syndrome in a cat, J Fel Med Surg 11:714–716, 2009.
6. Kern TJ, Aromando MC, Erb HN: Horner's syndrome in dogs and cats: 100 cases (1975-1985), J Am Vet Med Assoc 195:369–373, 1989.
7. Rossmeisl JH Jr, Higgins MA, Inzana KD, et al: Bilateral cavernous sinus syndrome in dogs: 6 cases (1999-2004), J Am Vet Med Assoc 226:1105–1111, 2005.
8. Theisen SK, Podell M, Schneider T, et al: A retrospective study of cavernous sinus syndrome in 4 dogs and 8 cats, J Vet Intern Med 10:65–71, 1996.
9. Fransson B, Kippenes H, Silver GE, et al: Magnetic resonance diagnosis: cavernous sinus syndrome in a dog, Vet Radiol Ultrasound 41:536–538, 2000.
10. Hernandez-Guerra AM, Del Mar Lopez-Murcia M, Planells A, et al: Computed tomographic diagnosis of unilateral cavernous sinus syndrome caused by a chondrosarcoma in a dog: a case report, Vet J 174:206–208, 2007.
11. Lewis GT, Blanchard GL, Trapp AL, et al: Ophthalmoplegia caused by thyroid adenocarcinoma invasion of the cavernous sinuses in the dog, J Am Anim Hosp Assoc 20:805–812, 1984.
12. McConnon JM, White ME, Smith MC, et al: Pendular nystagmus in dairy cattle, J Am Vet Med Assoc 182:812–813, 1983.
13. Nurmio P, Remes E, Talanti S, et al: Familial undulatory nystagmus in Ayrshire bulls in Finland, Nord Vet Med 34:130–132, 1982.
14. Lin CT, Gould DJ, Petersen-Jonest SM, et al: Canine inherited retinal degenerations: update on molecular genetic research and its clinical application, J Small Anim Pract 43:426–432, 2002.
15. Narfström K: Hereditary and congenital ocular disease in the cat, J Feline Med Surg 1:135–141, 1999.
16. Cutler TJ, Brooks DE, Andrew SE, et al: Disease of the equine posterior segment, Vet Ophthalmol 3:73–82, 2000.
17. Beltran WA: The use of canine models of inherited retinal degeneration to test novel therapeutic approaches, Vet Ophthalmol 12:192–204, 2009.
18. Barone G, Foureman P, deLahunta A: Adult-Onset cerebellar cortical abiotrophy and retinal degeneration in a domestic shorthair cat, J Am Anim Hosp Assoc 38:51–54, 2002.
19. Barnett KC: Inherited eye disease in the dog and cat, J Small Anim Pract 29:462–475, 1988.
20. Whitley RD: Focusing on eye disorders among purebred dogs, Vet Med 83:50–63, 1988.
21. Maggs DJ, Miller PE, Ofri R, et al: Slatter's fundamentals of veterinary ophthalmology, ed 4, St Louis, 2008, Saunders Elsevier.
22. Barnett KC, Grimes TD: Bilateral aplasia of the optic nerve in a cat, Br J Ophthalmol 58:663–667, 1974.
23. da Silva EG, Dubielzig R, Zarfoss MK, et al: Distinctive histopathologic features of canine optic nerve hypoplasia and aplasia: a retrospective review of 13 cases, Vet Ophthalmol 11:23–29, 2008.
24. Gelatt KN: Congenital ophthalmic anomalies in cattle, Mod Vet Pract 57:105–109, 1976.
25. Cutler TJ, Brooks DE, Andrew SE, et al: Disease of the equine posterior segment, Vet Ophthalmol 3:73–82, 2000.
26. Kern TJ, Riis RC: Optic nerve hypoplasia in three miniature poodles, J Am Vet Med Assoc 178:49–54, 1981.
27. Johnson BW: Congenitally abnormal visual pathways of Siamese cats, Compend Contin Educ Pract Vet 13:374–378, 1991.
28. Cooper ML, Pettigrew JD: The retinothalamic pathways in Siamese cats, J Comp Neurol 187:313–348, 1979.
29. Stone J, Campion JE, Leicester J: The nasotemporal division of retina in the Siamese cat, J Comp Neurol 180:783–798, 1978.
30. Shatz CJ, LeVay S: Siamese cat: altered connections of visual cortex, Science 204:328–330, 1979.
31. Kalil RE, Jhaveri SR, Richards W: Anomalous retinal pathways in the Siamese cat: an inadequate substrate for normal binocular vision, Science 174:302–305, 1971.
32. Blake R, Crawford ML: Development of strabismus in Siamese cats, Brain Res 77:492–496, 1974.
33. Power EP: Bilateral convergent strabismus in two Friesian cows, Ir Vet J 41:357–358, 1987.
34. Williams RW, Garraghty PE, Goldowitz D: A new visual system mutation: achiasmatic dogs with congenital nystagmus, Abstr Soc Neurosci 17:187, 1991.
35. Dell'Osso LF, Williams RW: Ocular motor abnormalities in achiasmatic mutant Belgian sheepdogs: unyoked eye movements in a mammal, Vision Res 35:109–116, 1995.
36. Dell'Osso LF, Williams RW, Jacobs JB, et al: The congenital and see-saw nystagmus in the prototypical achiasma of canines: comparison to the human achiasmatic prototype, Vision Res 38:1629–1641, 1998.
37. Yu DY, Cringle SJ: Oxygen distribution and consumption within the retina in vascularised and avascular retinas and in animal models of retinal disease, Prog Retin Eye Res 20:175–208, 2001.
38. Aguirre GD, Gross SL: Ocular manifestations of selected systemic diseases, Compend Contin Educ Vet 2:144–153, 1980.
39. Booth A, Reid M, Clark T: Hypovitaminosis A in feedlot cattle, J Am Vet Med Assoc 190:1305–1308, 1987.
40. Divers TJ, Blackmon DM, Martin CL, et al: Blindness and convulsions associated with vitamin A deficiency in feedlot steers, J Am Vet Med Assoc 189:1579–1582, 1986.
41. Hill B, Holroyd R, Sullivan M: Clinical and pathological findings associated with congenital hypovitaminosis A in extensively grazed beef cattle, Aust Vet J 87:94–98, 2009.
42. Riis RC, Sheffy BE, Loew E, et al: Vitamin E deficiency retinopathy in dogs, Am J Vet Res 42:74–86, 1981.
43. Davidson MG, Geoly FJ, Gilger BC, et al: Retinal degeneration associated with vitamin E deficiency in hunting dogs, J Am Vet Med Assoc 213:645–651, 1998.
44. Bedford PGC: Retinal pigment epithelial dystrophy (CPRA): a study of the disease in the briard, J Small Anim Pract 25:129–138, 1984.
45. McLellan GJ, Cappello R, Elks R, et al: Clinical and pathological observations in English cocker spaniels with primary metabolic vitamin E deficiency and retinal pigment epithelial dystrophy, Vet Rec 153:287–292, 2003.
46. McLellan GJ, Elks R, Lybaert P, et al: Vitamin E deficiency in dogs with retinal pigment epithelial dystrophy, Vet Rec 151:663–667, 2002.
47. Riis RC, Jackson C, Rebhun W, et al: Ocular manifestations of equine motor neuron disease, Equine Vet J 31:99–110, 1999.

48. Hayes KC, Carey RE, Schmidt SY: Retinal degeneration associated with taurine deficiency in the cat, Science 188:949–951, 1975.
49. Leon A, Levick WR, Sarossy MG: Lesion topography and new histological features in feline taurine deficiency retinopathy, Exp Eye Res 61:731–741, 1995.
50. Attali-Soussay K, Jegou JP, Clerc B: Retrobulbar tumors in dogs and cats: 25 cases, Vet Ophthalmol 4:19–27, 2001.
51. Mauldin EA, Deehr AJ, Hertzke D, et al: Canine orbital meningiomas: a review of 22 cases, Vet Ophthalmol 3:11–16, 2000.
52. Willis MA, Wilkie DA: Ocular oncology, Clin Tech Small Anim Pract 16:77–85, 2001.
53. Barrett P, Merideth R, Alarcon F: Central amaurosis induced by an intraocular, posttraumatic fibrosarcoma in a cat, J Am Anim Hosp Assoc 31:242–245, 1995.
54. Davidson MG, Nasisse MP, Breitschwerdt EB, et al: Acute blindness associated with intracranial tumors in dogs and cats: eight cases (1984-1989), J Am Vet Med Assoc 199:755–758, 1991.
55. Montgomery KW, van der Woerdt A, Cottrill NB: Acute blindness in dogs: sudden acquired retinal degeneration syndrome versus neurological disease (140 cases, 2000-2006), Vet Ophthalmol 11:314–320, 2008.
56. Nafe LA: Canine optic neuritis, Compend Contin Educ Pract Vet 3:978–981, 1981.
57. Fischer CA, Jones GT: Optic neuritis in dogs, J Am Vet Med Assoc 160:68–79, 1972.
58. Barnett KC, Blunden AS, Dyson SJ, et al: Blindness, optic atrophy and sinusitis in the horse, Vet Ophthalmol 11(suppl 1):20–26, 2008.
59. Busse C, Dennis R, Platt SR: Suspected sphenoid bone osteomyelitis causing visual impairment in two dogs and one cat, Vet Ophthalmol 12:71–77, 2009.
60. Gelatt KN, van der Woerdt A, Ketring KL, et al: Enrofloxacin-associated retinal degeneration in cats, Vet Ophthalmol 4:99–106, 2001.
61. Wiebe V, Hamilton P: Fluoroquinolone-induced retinal degeneration in cats, J Am Vet Med Assoc 221:1568–1571, 2002.
62. Godin AC, Dubielzig RR, Giuliano E, et al: Retinal and optic nerve degeneration in cattle after accidental acrylamide intoxication, Vet Ophthalmol 3:235–239, 2000.
63. Martin L, Kaswan R, Chapman W: Four cases of traumatic optic nerve blindness in the horse, Equine Vet J 18:133–137, 1986.
64. Bagley RS, Gavin PR, Moore MP, et al: Clinical signs associated with brain tumors in dogs: 97 cases (1992-1997), J Am Vet Med Assoc 215:818–819, 1999.
65. Gould DH: Polioencephalomalacia. J Anim Sci 76:309–314, 1998.
66. Ellett EW, Playter RF, Pierce KR: Retinal lesions associated with induced canine ehrlichiosis: a preliminary report, J Am Anim Hosp Assoc 9:214–218, 1973.
67. Gelatt KN, Whitley RD, Samuelson DA, et al: Ocular manifestations of viral diseases in small animals, Compend Contin Educ Pract Vet 7:968–977, 1985.
68. Martin CL: Retinopathies of food animals. In Howard JL, editor: Current veterinary therapy: food animal practice, Philadelphia, 1981, WB Saunders.
69. Adamo PF, Adams WM, Steinberg H: Granulomatous meningoencephalomyelitis in dogs, Compend Contin Educ Pract Vet 29:678–690, 2007.
70. Williams KJ, Summers BA, de Lahunta A: Cerebrospinal cuterebriasis in cats and its association with feline ischemic encephalopathy, Vet Pathol 35:330–343, 1998.
71. Edney ATB, Gaskell CJ, Sharp NJH: Waltham symposium no. 6: feline dysautonomia-an emerging disease, J Small Anim Pract 28:333–416, 1987.
72. Guilford WG, O'Brien DP, Allert A, et al: Diagnosis of dysautonomia in a cat by autonomic nervous system function testing, J Am Vet Med Assoc 193:823–828, 1988.
73. Harkin KR, Andrews GA, Nietfeld JC: Dysautonomia in dogs: 65 cases (1993-2000), J Am Vet Med Assoc 220:633–639, 2002.
74. Longshore RC, O'Brien DP, Johnson GC, et al: Dysautonomia in dogs: a retrospective study, J Vet Intern Med 10:103–109, 1996.
75. Pollin M, Sullivan M: A canine dysautonomia resembling the Key-Gaskell syndrome, Vet Rec 118:402–403, 1986.
76. Presthus J, Bjerkas I: Canine dysautonomia in Norway, Vet Rec 120:463–464, 1987.
77. Gerding PA, Brightman AH, Brogdon JD: Pupillotonia in a dog, J Am Vet Med Assoc 189:1477, 1986.
78. MacKay AD, Rusbridge C, Sparkes AH, et al: MRI characteristics of suspected acute spinal cord infarction in two cats, and a review of the literature, J Feline Med Surg 7:101–107, 2005.
79. Cauzinille L: Fibrocartilaginous embolism in dogs, Vet Clin North Am Small Anim Pract 30:155–167, 2000:vii.
80. Morgan RV, Zanotti SW: Horner's syndrome in dogs and cats: 49 cases (1980-1986), J Am Vet Med Assoc 194:1096–1099, 1989.
81. Boydell P: Idiopathic Horner's syndrome in the golden retriever, J Small Anim Pract 36:382–384, 1995.
82. Green SL, Cochrane SM, Smith-Maxie L: Horner's syndrome in ten horses, Can Vet J 33:330–333, 1992.
83. Bacon CL, Davidson HJ, Yvorchuk K, et al: Bilateral Horner's syndrome secondary to metastatic squamous cell carcinoma in a horse, Equine Vet J 28:500–503, 1996.
84. Milne JC: Malignant melanomas causing Horner's syndrome in a horse, Equine Vet J 18:74–75, 1986.
85. Murray MJ, Cavey DM, Feldman BF, et al: Signs of sympathetic denervation associated with a thoracic melanoma in a horse, J Vet Intern Med 11:199–203, 1997.
86. Boydell P: Iatrogenic pupillary dilation resembling Pourfour du Petit syndrome in three cats, J Small Anim Pract 41:202–203, 2000.
87. Brightman AH III, Ogilvie GK, Tompkins M: Ocular disease in FeLV-positive cats: 11 cases (1981-1986), J Am Vet Med Assoc 198:1049–1051, 1991.
88. Nell B, Suchy A: "D-shaped" and "reverse-D-shaped" pupil in a cat with lymphosarcoma, Vet Ophthalmol 1:53–56, 1998.
89. Phillips TR, Prospero-Garcia O, Puaoi DL, et al: Neurological abnormalities associated with feline immunodeficiency virus infection, J Gen Virol 75:979–987, 1994.

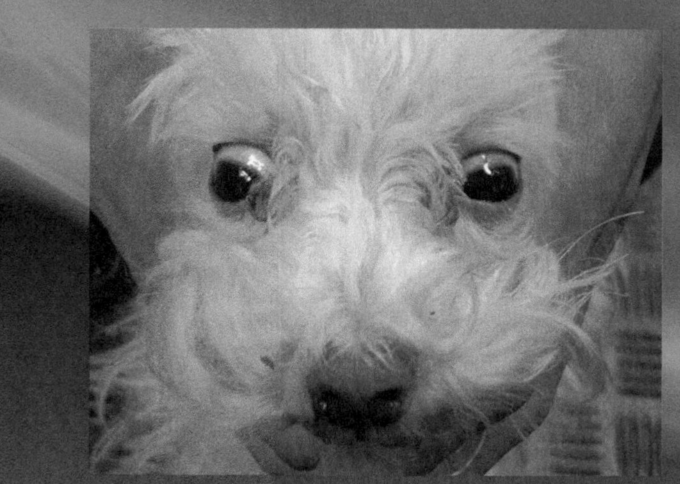

CHAPTER 12

Stupor or Coma

Altered states of consciousness are always related to abnormal brain function. Assessment of an animal's level of consciousness, often referred to as mentation, mental state, or sensorium, is a crucial yet frequently underappreciated aspect of a thorough neurologic examination. While animals in stupor or coma are readily identified, subtle changes in mental state may not be easily recognized. However, in some instances, identification of a subtle change in the mental state may be the only clue that helps to establish an intracranial neuroanatomic localization. This has an enormous impact on the differential diagnosis and diagnostic workup of an affected animal. Consequently, clinicians should devote adequate time to critically assess the mental state of every neurologic animal.

Nomenclature involving abnormal mental states is often confusing because the terminology is not based on objective criteria. Instead, terms extend beyond simple medical analysis and encompass the clinician's subjective interpretation of an animal's behavioral response. Confounding this assessment is the effect caused by the animal being in an unfamiliar environment such as a veterinary hospital. Even normal animals may behave differently in the hospital environment. This is especially true for cats. In some cases, the pet owner may play a critical role in an accurate assessment of the mental state. In the end, the determination of an abnormal mental state requires careful integration of behavior, owner assessment, and the impact of an unfamiliar environment and stimuli.

For clinical purposes, the following definitions are adequate:

Normal: The animal is alert, responds to external stimuli, is aware of its surroundings, and responds to commands as expected.

Dull: The animal is lethargic and less responsive to its environment but still has the capability to become responsive in a normal manner. Most sick animals are depressed.

Disoriented, confused: Although the animal can respond to its environment, it may do so in an inappropriate manner.

Obtunded: The animal is mild to moderately less wakeful or less responsive to the environment or external stimuli.

Stuporous: The animal appears to be asleep when undisturbed but can be aroused by strong stimulation, especially noxious stimuli. No clear boundary separates dullness, obtundation, and stupor.

Comatose: The animal is unconscious and does not respond to any stimulus except for reflex activity. For example, a strong toe pinch may elicit a flexion reflex or may increase extensor posturing but does not cause a behavioral reaction such as crying, biting, or turning the head.

Vegetative: The animal lacks awareness of the environment but shows arousal. Brainstem function is present, but forebrain responses are absent.[1]

Brain dead: The animal is in a coma, is apneic, lacks all brainstem reflexes, and has electrocerebral silence.

LESION LOCALIZATION

Consciousness or mental state is maintained by sensory stimuli that act through the ascending reticular activating system (ARAS) on the cerebral cortex (Figure 12-1). The ARAS is a group of neurons that extend to the caudal diencephalon from the medulla oblongata.[2] Sensory information originating from the spinal cord or cranial nerve afferents projects to the ARAS, which in turn projects to the thalamus and ultimately to the cerebral cortex. In fact, all sensory pathways have collateral input to the ARAS of the pons and the midbrain. The ARAS projects diffusely to the cerebral cortex, maintaining a background of activity through cholinergic synapses on cortical neurons.[3] A balance is maintained between the ARAS and an adrenergic system that projects from nuclei in the midbrain and the diencephalon, which may be considered the sleep system.[4-6] Alterations in the balance of these two systems can produce signs ranging from hyperexcitability to coma. Narcolepsy, a syndrome of sleep attacks, is discussed in Chapter 13.

Decreasing levels of consciousness indicate abnormal function of the cerebrum or brainstem, causing interference with the cerebrocortical activation by the ARAS. Stupor and coma are caused by (1) diffuse, bilateral forebrain (cerebrum and diencephalon) lesions; (2) metabolic or toxic encephalopathies;

and (3) disorders affecting the brainstem, in particular, the midbrain and pons.

An anatomic diagnosis can be made on the basis of mental status, motor function, and brainstem reflexes. Of particular importance are neuro-ophthalmologic signs (vision, pupils, and eye movements) (see Chapter 11 and Table 12-1). Alterations in the respiratory pattern may be correlated with levels of brainstem abnormalities, but they are less reliable than the other signs.

Diffuse bilateral forebrain disease usually does not produce localizing signs, although some inflammatory processes may be somewhat asymmetric. With diffuse cerebral disease, voluntary motor activity and postural reactions may be absent or severely depressed. Rhythmic walking movements, reflecting brainstem and spinal cord activity, may be elicited if the animal is suspended in a normal standing posture. Vision and the menace responses may be absent, although the pupillary light reflexes (PLR) are normal. Normal or Physiologic nystagmus is normal, but the animal does not follow moving objects. Normal pupil size and vestibular eye movements indicate an intact brainstem, whereas the loss of vision and voluntary motor activity indicates abnormal forebrain function. Lesions

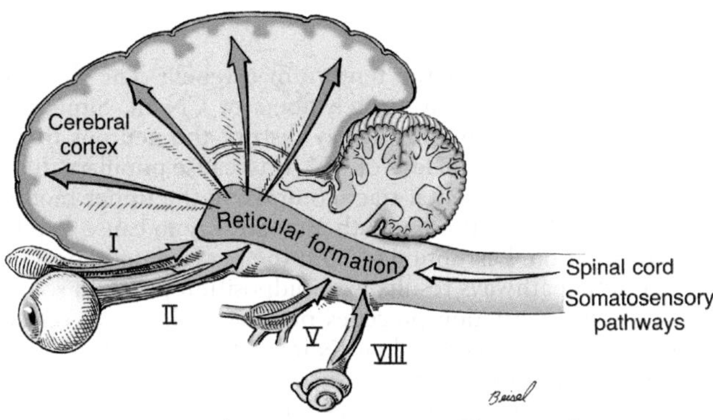

Figure 12-1 Reticular activating system. The reticular activating system of the brainstem receives input from most sensory systems. Diffuse projections from the reticular activating system to the cerebral cortex maintain consciousness.

in the diencephalon also cause in a similar signs. The pupillary light reflex may be abnormal if the lesion involves the optic chiasm. The animal may also have other signs of endocrine disease.

In its most severe form, diffuse forebrain involvement produces the chronic vegetative state, wherein the animal has brainstem reflexes but no behavioral reactions. Signs of inflammation involving the meninges (meningitis) may also be present and include pain on palpation of the head and the neck, rigidity of the neck muscles, and resistance to flexion of the neck. Infection, immune-mediated inflammation, or blood in the subarachnoid space can cause meningeal inflammation.

Metabolic or toxic encephalopathies usually depress cerebral functions early, whereas brainstem functions are affected later. Importantly, metabolic or toxic encephalopathies do not produce focal or lateralizing signs. Signs are generally the same as those of diffuse cerebral lesions but may have other components, depending on the cause. For example, barbiturates also can cause depression of the spinal reflexes; organophosphate insecticides can cause muscle fasciculation, peripheral neuropathy, and autonomic signs; and a number of toxins can cause seizures. Specific entities for toxins are discussed in Chapter 15.

Disorders affecting the brainstem cause alteration in mental state in conjunction with dysfunction of brainstem reflexes. Lesions may be focal resulting in asymmetric signs. In general, bilateral or diffuse lesions involving the brainstem result in severe obtundation, stupor, or coma. There are a variety of disease processes that can affect the brainstem. In most instances, the disease process (tumor, infection, inflammation, infarction) directly impacts the brainstem. However, in certain instances, brainstem dysfunction is the result of compression related to herniation (displacement) of the cerebrum or cerebellum.

The calvaria form an inelastic case around the brain. Within the cranial cavity exists only brain parenchyma, cerebrospinal fluid (CSF), and blood. The volume of these components determines the intracranial pressure (ICP). With an increase in volume of one or more of these intracranial constituents, there must be a corresponding decrease in volume of the others. For example, with brain swelling, there may be compression of the ventricles lessening the volume of CSF within the cranial cavity. Moreover, certain pathologies, such as a tumor, abscess, hematoma, or

TABLE 12-1

Signs of Lesions Causing Stupor and Coma

Lesion	Motor Function	Vision	Pupils	Eye Movements
Diffuse bilateral forebrain disease	Tetraparesis; postural deficits, reflexes are normal	Absent	Normal	Normal; however, animal does not track objects
Metabolic or toxic encephalopathy	Tetraparesis; postural deficits, reflexes may be depressed	Absent	Normal or pinpoint in size Responsive PLRs	Normal; however, animal does not track objects, particularly if in coma
Bilateral lesions of rostral brainstem*	Tetraparesis; postural deficits, reflexes are exaggerated,increased extensor tone (decerebrate rigidity)	Absent with caudal tentorial herniation; present in primary brainstem lesions	Dilated or midposition, absent PLRs	Ventrolateral strabismus; decreased vestibular eye movements
Unilateral compression of rostral brainstem*	Hemiparesis or tetraparesis; postural deficits, reflexes are exaggerated, increased extensor tone on affected side	Present; may be contralateral loss with caudal tentorial herniation	Dilated, ipsilateral	Ipsilateral ventrolateral strabismus, decreased vestibular eye movements

PLRs, Pupillary light reflexes.
*More severe signs are expected with intra-axial lesions compared to extra-axial lesions that result in compression

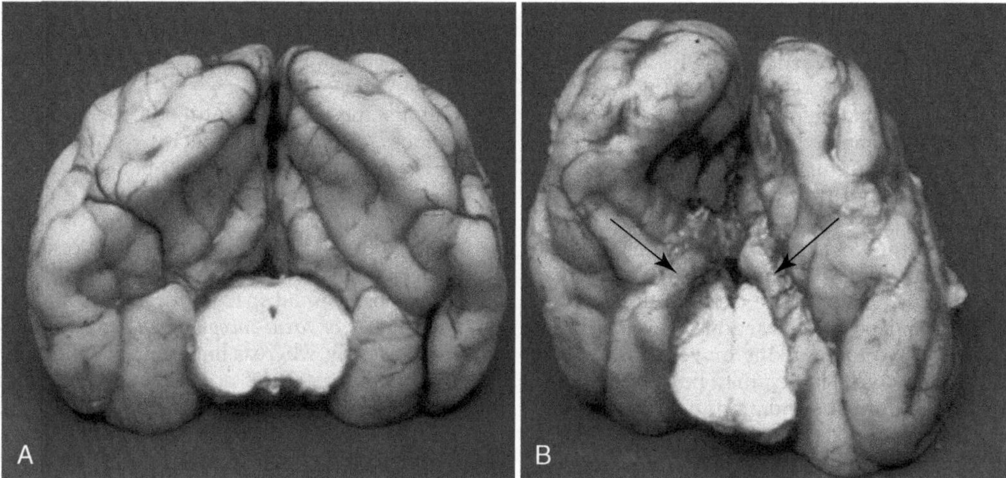

Figure 12-2 Caudal view of the brains of two dogs sectioned at the midbrain. **A,** Normal brain. Note the patent mesencephalic aqueduct. **B,** Caudal tentorial herniation has occurred in which the cerebrum has herniated caudally through the tentorial notch *(arrows)* causing compression of the rostral colliculi and obstruction of the mesencephalic aqueduct. (Copyright 2010 University of Georgia Research Foundation, Inc.)

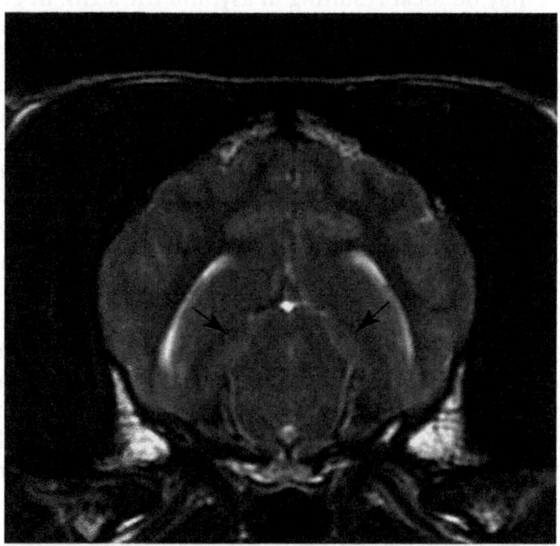

Figure 12-3 Axial T2W image of the brain of a mixed-breed dog. As in Figure 12-2, *B,* there is caudal tentorial herniation of the cerebrum *(arrows)* resulting in compression of the rostral colliculi (Copyright 2010 University of Georgia Research Foundation, Inc.)

edema, also must be accommodated. Since the cranial cavity is rigid, increased volume of the intracranial constituents can be tolerated to a certain degree but beyond this there is a rapid increase in ICP.[7] Increased ICP can cause displacement of the cerebral hemisphere(s) caudally under the tentorium cerebelli, resulting in compression of the brainstem[8] (Figures 12-2 and 12-3). Other types of herniations also can occur. Unilateral masses cause a herniation on the same side, whereas diffuse cerebral edema usually causes a bilateral herniation. If the ICP continues to rise, or if the mass starts in the caudotentorial compartment (caudal cranial fossa), the cerebellum may herniate through the foramen magnum, compressing the medulla oblongata. The respiratory pathways are blocked, resulting in death.

The signs of brainstem compression from tentorial herniation are outlined in Table 12-2. Masses that compress the brainstem usually cause similar signs. Abnormal pupil size and symmetry implicating involvement of cranial nerve (CN) III or disruption of the tectum and tegmentum of the midbrain are particularly important to the clinician because pupillary changes are one of the earliest detectable signs of herniation of the cerebrum under the tentorium cerebelli. The shift in intracranial contents may stretch fibers of CN III. Similarly, compression on the midbrain may disrupt the neurons from the parasympathetic nucleus of CN III to cause pupillary dilation or the tectotegmental tract comprising the upper motor neurons (UMNs) of the sympathetic pathway to cause pupillary constriction. Disruption of both the parasympathetic and sympathetic pathways results in a midposition pupil. In some cases, pupil constriction precedes pupillary dilation as result of disruption of the cerebral UMN input that normally inhibits CN III.[9] Mydriasis or miosis in conjunction with abnormal mental status indicates impending deterioration of the animal. In both cases, rapid assessment and treatment are imperative.

DISEASES

The causes of stupor and coma are classified according to the presence or absence of focal or lateralizing signs and the onset and progression. Accordingly, diseases are categorized as diseases with focal or lateralizing signs: acute onset with progressive history, acute onset with nonprogressive history, and chronic onset; or disease with no focal or lateralizing signs: acute or chronic onset (Table 12-3).

Focal or Lateralizing Signs

Acute Progressive

Traumatic brain injury (TBI).

Pathophysiology. Head injuries in dogs and cats are most often the result of motor vehicle crashes.[10,11] In horses, direct blows to the frontal region, collision with a solid object, or impact to the poll when a horse flips over backward are the most common causes of TBI.[12] Pathophysiologically, TBI can be divided into primary and secondary injury. Primary TBI occurs at the time of injury. The terms that are commonly used in describing TBI are defined in Box 12-1. The clinical differentiation of concussion from contusion is not clear and has no significance for clinical management. Concussions represent physiologic disruptions of cells and are completely reversible. Contusions cause structural disruption of cells and tracts and may not be reversible. Fractures of the calvaria may result in laceration of brain parenchyma or disruption of the vasculature of the brain or meninges leading to hematoma formation. Often intracranial hemorrhage and edema develop as part of the primary insult.

TABLE 12-2

Signs of Progressive Bilateral Caudal Tentorial Herniation*

Level	Mental State	Pupils	Eye Movements	Motor Function	Respiratory
Initial onset	Dull/Obtunded	Small, responsive	Normal	Tetraparesis; postural deficits	Normal
Increased severity	Severe obtundation or stupor	Midposition, responsive	Normal	Tetraparesis; postural deficits, Reflexes are normal or exaggerated	Cheyne-Stokes respiration
Severe midbrain† compression	Stupor or Coma	Dilated or midposition, decreased responsive	Decreased, possible ventrolateral strabismus	Decerebrate rigidity, tetraplegia Reflexes are normal or exaggerated	Hyperventilation
Pontine compression†	Coma	Pinpoint or midposition unresponsive	Absent, ventrolateral strabismus	Same as with midbrain compression	Rapid shallow respirations
Medullary compression†	Coma	Dilated, unresponsive	Absent, ventrolateral strabismus	Same as with midbrain compression	Irregular to apnea, slow pulse

Modified from Oliver JE Jr: Neurologic emergencies in small animals. Vet Clin North Am 2:341–357, 1972.
*With unilateral lesions, ipilateral deficits in pupil size, pupillary light reflex, and motor function would be expected.
†Difficult to distinguish clinically.

Anatomically, hemorrhage may occur in an epidural, subdural, subarachnoid, or intraaxial (parenchymal) location. The most common locations for intracranial hemorrhage are subarachnoid and intraaxial. In humans, diffuse axonal injury (DAI) is the result of specific forces applied to the head during the injury.[13] Although DAI is a histologic diagnosis, it is suspected in cases in which the mechanism of injury is consistent with the development of DAI, severe neurologic deficits are present, and there is no focal lesion observed on computed tomography (CT) or magnetic resonance imaging (MRI) despite evidence of brain swelling.[14] At the present time, DAI is poorly described in veterinary medicine but is likely to exist. In addition to these primary injuries, brain edema often develops.

Three types of brain edema may occur, cytotoxic, vasogenic, or interstitial. Cytotoxic edema results from fluid accumulation in neurons and astrocytes secondary to cellular hypoxia that disrupts cell membrane function. Vasogenic edema results from damage to the blood-brain barrier (BBB), and the fluid accumulation is extracellular. Resolution of vasogenic edema is the focus of most antiedema therapies. The third type of edema, interstitial, occurs in hydrocephalus. Cerebral edema can be assumed to exist in any patient with neurologic signs after head injury.

These primary injuries may result in increased ICP. As a result of increased ICP, alterations in cerebral blood flow (CBF) and brain metabolism develop, which may exacerbate brain edema. Abnormalities in CBF and metabolism lead to secondary brain injury. Other possible biochemical events central to the development and progression of secondary injury include increases in intracellular calcium concentrations, free radical production, and excitotoxicity related to glutamate.[13] Hyperglycemia, a sympathoadrenal response, may occur in dogs and cats following TBI.[15] The degree of hyperglycemia may be associated with increased mortality rates or decreased prognosis, but the exact relationship is not known. Hyperglycemia may potentiate neurologic injury by increasing free radical production, cerebral edema, excitatory amino acid (glutamate) release, and cerebral acidosis.[15] Likewise, hypoglycemia can have deleterious effects on neuronal function. Consequently, care should be taken to avoid creating hyperglycemia or hypoglycemia. Secondary brain injury develops quickly following the initial injury and may cause irreversible central nervous system (CNS) pathology. Medical treatment for TBI is directed at preventing or decreasing the severity of the secondary injury.

Assessment. A thorough physical examination is imperative to establish the existence of concurrent or contributing factors that may impact the nervous system. Animals involved in traumatic events often have multiple organ injuries. Careful attention and treatment of concurrent injuries are necessary for a successful outcome. A complete and thorough neurologic examination should be performed in all animals experiencing trauma, regardless of whether or not overt neurologic deficits are observed. Differentiation of the signs of diffuse and focal CNS lesions from the signs of tentorial herniation is discussed earlier. Differentiation between acute brainstem hemorrhage and tentorial herniation is summarized in Table 12-4.

Treatment. The treatment of traumatic brain injury cannot be separated from the management of the animal as a whole because multiple organ injuries are common. Moreover, many of the treatments used to stabilize systemic disturbances have effects that are beneficial in limiting the secondary effects of TBI. Consequently, treatment can be divided into therapies aimed at correction of extracranial derangements and therapies directed at correction of intracranial alterations.

The priorities for assessment of an animal presented to the veterinary clinic are (1) assessment of oxygenation and ventilation, (2) assessment of hemodynamic status, (3) assessment for multisystemic injuries, (4) neurologic examination and lesion localization, (5) medical or surgical treatment for neurologic injury, and (6) monitor patient for worsening signs.

In general, treatment is focused on maintaining CBF, which is tightly regulated in normal animals. In a process of pressure autoregulation, CBF remains constant through a wide range of mean arterial pressures (MAPs). During times when MAP is outside the range of pressure autoregulation, CBF becomes solely related to MAP.[16] Consequently, arterial pressures below 50 mm Hg result in hypoperfusion and ischemia of the brain while pressures above 150 mm Hg may exacerbate

TABLE 12-3

Etiology of Stupor and Coma

Condition	Acute Nonprogressive	Acute Progressive	Chronic Progressive
Focal or Lateralizing Signs			
Neoplastic (12)		Secondary Metastatic Lymphoma	Primary brain tumors Meningiomas Gliomas Pituitary Calvarial tumors (MLO)
Inflammatory/infectious (15)	Meningoencephalomyelitis	Meningoencephalomyelitis	Meningoencephalomyelitis
Traumatic (12)	Intraaxial hemorrhage	Epidural, subdural hematoma	Subdural hematoma
Vascular (12)	Infarction		
No Focal or Lateralizing Signs			
Degenerative (15)			Storage diseases (8, 15)
Anomalous	Brain malformations	Acquired hydrocephalus	Congenital hydrocephalus
Metabolic (15)	Hydroencephaly Intracranial Intraarachnoid cyst/diverticulum	Hypoglycemia (15) Electrolyte imbalances Liver failure; hepatic encephalopathy (15) Renal failure (15) Diabetic coma Adrenal disorders Thyroid disorders Acid-base disorders Hypothyroid coma (15) Heat stroke Hypoxia Equine hypoxic/ischemic encephalopathy Inborn errors of metabolism	Brain malformations
Neoplasia		Pituitary, hypothalamic tumors	
Nutritional (15)		Thiamine deficiency	
Idiopathic (13)		Postictal seizure Narcolepsy	
Inflammatory / infectious (15)	Meningoencephalomyelitis	Meningoencephalomyelitis	Meningoencephalomyelitis
Toxic (15)		Heavy metals Barbiturates Carbon monoxide Hypertensive encephalopathy Enterotoxemia	Water intoxication Plants Salt poisoning
Traumatic		Cerebral edema	

Numbers in parentheses refer to chapters in which conditions are discussed.

hemorrhage and edema.[17] Although CBF cannot be easily assessed in clinical practice, CBF depends heavily on cerebral perfusion pressure (CPP), which can be indirectly assessed. Cerebral perfusion pressure is determined by the formula: CPP = MAP – ICP. From this equation, it is clear that MAP plays a substantial role in CPP. Consequently, measures that support MAP positively affect CPP. A second aspect in the regulation of CBF is chemical autoregulation related to partial pressure of carbon dioxide ($Paco_2$). Cerebral vasculature is responsive to CO_2 concentration. Vasodilation occurs with increased CO_2 concentration, whereas vasoconstriction occurs with decreased CO_2 concentration. In states of severe hypocapnia, ischemia can develop secondary to vasoconstriction, which exacerbates secondary brain injury. Conversely, hypercapnia also can negatively impact secondary brain injury by increasing ICP. As $Paco_2$ increases, vasodilation results in increased blood volume within the cranial cavity, which increases ICP. From this understanding of the cerebral vascular physiology, it becomes evident that the most important aspects of assessment and treatment of TBI involve assessment and normalization of oxygenation, ventilation, and hemodynamic parameters such as blood pressure.

Specific treatments should initially be directed at correction of extracranial derangements. Standard protocols for treating hypovolemic shock or hypotension are recommended. Fluid therapy should be vigorous if shock is present, but excessive fluid therapy should be avoided because it can contribute to cerebral edema. Supplemental oxygenation should be provided in animals experiencing hypoxemia. Supplemental oxygenation may be provided in the form of nasal cannulas or oxygen cages. In severely anemic animals, red blood cell transfusion may be necessary to provide adequate O_2 carrying capacity. Careful and judicious use of analgesics should be

BOX 12-1

Terminology of Head Injury

Concussion: Transient loss of consciousness without structural lesions

Contusion: Pathologic alterations in the brain including edema, petechial hemorrhage, disruption of nerve fibers, and so forth

Coup and Contrecoup: Injuries at the point of impact (coup) and at the opposite pole of the brain (contrecoup)

Cerebral Edema: An increase in intracellular/cytotoxic (gray matter) and extracellular/vasogenic (white matter) fluid, present in most head injuries

Hemorrhage:

- *Epidural:* Bleeding between the dura and the calvaria, usually caused by a fracture with laceration of a meningeal artery
- *Subdural:* Bleeding between the dura and the arachnoid layers of the meninges, usually caused by disruption of the bridging veins, so it develops slowly
- *Subarachnoid:* Bleeding into the subarachnoid space, usually caused by disruption of the veins or the arteries of the arachnoid; relatively common in animals
- *Intraaxial* (parenchymal): Bleeding into the tissue of the brain, usually caused by disruption of the parenchymal vessels; relatively common in animals

Diffuse axonal injury: disruption of axons secondary to specific forces applied to the head during trauma; in humans, identified based on type of trauma involved, presence of diffuse edema without a primary lesion (i.e., hemorrhage)

Calvarial fractures:

- *Linear:* Fractures of the calvaria that are not displaced
- *Depressed:* Fractures of the calvaria that encroach on the brain
- *Compound (open):* Fractures of the calvaria that have a laceration of the skin

used in severely painful animals to help avoid hypocapnia related to panting.[16] Importantly, analgesics may confound the clinician's ability to adequately assess the mental state of affected animals. Therefore, a careful balance between providing adequate pain relief without obscuring objective monitoring of the level of consciousness must be reconciled.

The patient should be appropriately evaluated for thoracic and abdominal injuries. Radiography and ultrasonography (US) are useful aids in the diagnosis of a variety of thoracic and abdominal injuries. The extent of the injuries must be determined and addressed.

The nervous system should then be evaluated as described previously (see Chapters 1 and 2). Evaluations of the level of consciousness, pupillary function and eye movements, dysfunction of other CNs, and motor function are adequate for the assessment of the level and the extent of damage to the CNS. Serial neurologic examinations are imperative because worsening of the neurologic status should prompt further diagnostic and therapeutic interventions.

In severely affected animals failing to improve or those declining in the face of correction of systemic disturbances, treatment directed at lowering ICP should be instituted.

TABLE 12-4

Comparison of Acute Brainstem Hemorrhage with Tentorial Herniation After Head Injury

Feature Compared	Brainstem Hemorrhage	Tentorial Herniation
Onset	Immediate or early	Delayed
Course	Usually static	Progressive
Mental status	Coma, stupor if small lesion	Obtundation, progressing to coma
Pupils	Poor to unresponsive midposition, may be dilated if a small lesion	Miosis, progressing to midposition and unresponsive
Eye movements	Absent	Normal progressing to unresponsive
Motor function	Tetraplegia Decerebrate posture	Normal or tetraparesis or hemiparesis, progressing to plegia with decerebrate posture

Mannitol, a nonmetabolizable 6-carbon polyalcohol, is an osmotic diuretic that can lower ICP likely through two mechanisms. Mannitol increases plasma volume, which produces the rheologic effect of decreasing the hematocrit and blood viscosity, which improves CBF—ultimately causing vasoconstriction related to autoregulation, which decreases ICP.[18] The second mechanism is a reduction in intracellular water related to an osmotic effect, which ultimately reduces brain volume.[19] Mannitol may also act as a free radical scavenger.[20] Its use is contraindicated in dehydration, hypovolemia, anuria, and hyperosmolality.[21] It is used with caution in animals with concurrent heart failure. A 20% mannitol solution is administered at a dosage of 0.5 to 1.0 g/kg of body weight, administered intravenously (IV) over 15 to 20 minutes. It can be repeated every 4 to 6 hours. Mannitol will precipitate in solution at cool temperatures. Consequently, mannitol should be warmed and administered through a filter to remove potential precipitates. Given the diuretic and osmotic effects of mannitol, careful monitoring of the hydration status and serum sodium concentration should be done to prevent dehydration. This is especially important with repeated use. Administration of furosemide (0.7 mg/kg IV 15 minutes after mannitol administration) may prolong the beneficial effects of mannitol.[22,23]

Hypertonic saline (HTS, 7.5% NaCl) can also be used to reduce ICP. The effects of HTS are similar to those of mannitol. Hypertonic saline has a rheological effect similar to mannitol that increases CBF. By reducing intracellular water, HTS decreases endothelial cell volume, which increases capillary diameter and it reduces red blood cell size, which ultimately increases CBF.[14] Intracranial pressure also is decreased by a reduction of cerebral edema by an osmotic effect. Although there is no clear beneficial effect of HTS over mannitol, HTS may be preferred over mannitol given its ability to expand the intravascular volume to greater extent than mannitol, which helps better support MAP.[14] Another advantage of HTS is that it has less of a diuretic effect than mannitol. Hypertonic saline may be used in animal refractory to the effects of mannitol. Hypertonic saline is administered intravenously at a dosage of 4 mL/kg of body weight.

In animals requiring mechanical ventilation, hyperventilation to maintain a normal to slightly low Pa_{CO_2} (30 to 35 mm Hg)

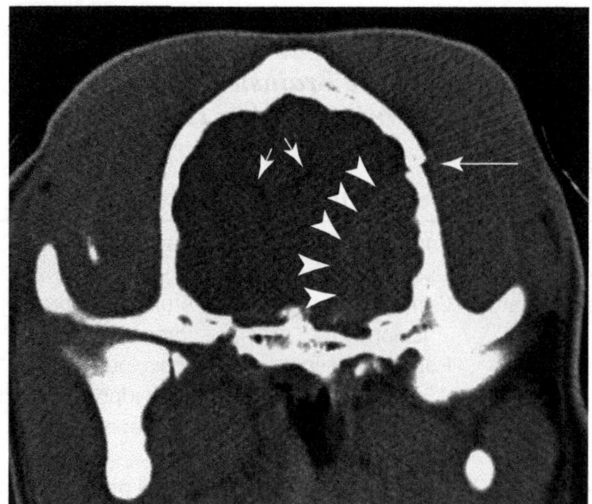

Figure 12-4 Axial CT image of the brain of a Labrador retriever that sustained head trauma. There is a fracture of the left parietal bone *(large arrow)*. Within the cranial cavity, there is a large, hyperattenuating mass consistent with an epidural hematoma (outlined by *arrowheads*), which is displacing the brain as evidenced by deviation of the lateral ventricles *(small arrows)*. (Copyright 2010 University of Georgia Research Foundation, Inc.)

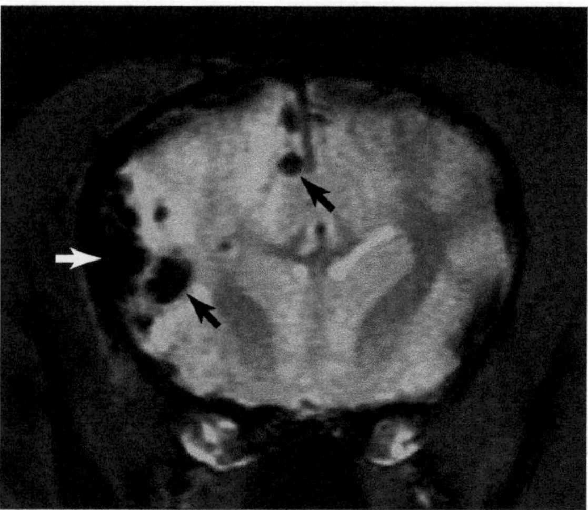

Figure 12-5 Axial T2*W (GRE) image of the brain of a Boston terrier that sustained head trauma. There are multiple signal voids *(black areas)* that are consistent with hemorrhages. Some of the hemorrhages are likely subdural *(white arrow)* and others are intraparenchymal *(small black arrows)*. (Copyright 2010 University of Georgia Research Foundation, Inc.)

may be used to reduce ICP through vasoconstriction of the intracranial vasculature.[17,24]

In recumbent animals, maintaining the head elevated approximately 30 degrees above the rest of the body may help reduce ICP by promoting venous drainage.[17] Care must be taken to not compress the jugular veins.

Seizures may occur anytime following TBI. Seizures should be controlled with intravenous diazepam at a dose of 0.5 to 1.0 mg/kg of body weight. It can be repeated at 5- to 10-minute intervals for three or four doses. Injectable phenobarbital may be required in some cases, but it may increase CNS depression. See Chapter 13 for additional information on seizure management.

After the patient is stabilized, frequent monitoring of the severity of signs is imperative. The use of a standardized coma scale is useful for comparison between examinations. The animal should be observed closely for 24 to 48 hours for progressive signs. In stable animals, imaging studies may be performed to establish the existence of fractures of the calvaria and pathology affecting the brain. Due to the complexity of the calvaria, plain radiography is difficult to interpret, which may lead to underdiagnosis or overdiagnosis of calvarial fractures. Cross-sectional imaging studies (CT or MRI) provide a more detailed evaluation of the brain and calvaria. However, cross-sectional imaging does require general anesthesia. Consequently, cross-sectional imaging should only be pursued in stable animals. The clinician must balance the value of the information gained with imaging against the risk of general anesthesia to the animal. (See Chapter 4 for information regarding cross-sectional imaging.) CT is commonly performed in humans with TBI. Although CT provides excellent delineation of calvarial defects, soft tissue injury to the brain may not be appreciated in animals. The major advantage of CT is that imaging is performed rapidly often taking seconds to minutes (Figure 12-4). MRI provides detailed imaging of the brain. Edema, hemorrhage, presence of brain herniation, and calvarial deficits can be observed with MRI (Figure 12-5). Although MRI is preferred over CT for imaging of the brain, the major disadvantage of MRI is that imaging does require substantial time to perform. In the end, surgical intervention is rarely necessary so imaging is not commonly pursued. Fractures are infrequently treated surgically. However, open skull fractures should be débrided and closed as early as possible. Surgical evacuation of intracranial hemorrhage has been performed. The main indication to consider surgical evacuation of intracranial hemorrhage is lack of response or rapid decline in the face of appropriate medical therapy to improve CBF and reduce ICP.

Stuporous or comatose animals require more critical assessment and care, and have a worse prognosis. Animals with severe alterations in consciousness (stupor or coma) are more likely to have lesions affecting the brainstem than cerebrum. Brainstem hemorrhage usually can be differentiated from tentorial herniation from the time course of the neurologic signs (see Table 12-4). Intraaxial brainstem hemorrhage, which usually occurs in the midbrain or the pons, often produces coma immediately after the trauma. Little or no improvement usually occurs in this case. Tentorial herniation may develop from cerebral edema (usually bilateral) or from rostrotentorial hemorrhage. The progression of signs is usually characteristic (see Table 12-2). Animals with brainstem hemorrhage rarely recover, and those that do usually have severe neurologic deficits. Tentorial herniation must be managed early with aggressive measures to decrease ICP to be successful. Severe tentorial herniation with compression and distortion of the brainstem produces multiple small brainstem hemorrhages (Duret hemorrhages) that may be irreversible. In addition, increased intracranial pressure transmitted to the caudal fossa may produce cerebellar herniation through the foramen magnum, causing death by interference with the medullary respiratory centers.

Management of the comatose patient must include maintaining hydration and nutrition; regulating body temperature; providing adequate ventilation (including hyperventilation in the early stages); preventing decubital ulcers by frequent changes in recumbency, meticulous cleaning of the skin, and cushioning; and maintaining urinary and fecal elimination. Management of the comatose patient can be time-consuming and expensive but is rewarding when successful.

Equine Head Trauma. Two types of cranial fractures in horses result in serious brain injury.[25] Frontal bone fractures result from direct impact and are often open, depressed fractures with direct cerebral laceration and hemorrhage from the fracture fragments. Neurologic signs include contralateral blindness, facial hypalgesia, depression, compulsive wandering toward the side of the lesion, and generalized seizures.

TABLE 12-5

MRI Findings in Brain Tumors

Ischemic Infarction

Signal Intensity

T1W	T2W	T2W FLAIR	Contrast Enhancement	DWI	ADC Map
Hypo	Hyper	Hyper	Noncontrast enhancing Mild to moderate (rare) Marked enhancement (rare)	Hyper	Hypo (acute) Hyper (chronic)

Anatomic Location	Vascular Supply	Clinical Signs
Cerebellum		
Rostral	Rostral cerebellar artery (branch off caudal communicating artery)	Ipsilateral cerebellovestibular signs, decerebellate posture Occasionally episodic vestibular signs
Caudal	Caudal cerebellar artery (branch off basilar artery)	Ipsilateral hemiparesis, postural deficits
Forebrain		
Cerebrum Cerebral cortex	Rostral, middle, or caudal artery (depending on location)	Abnormal mental state; contralateral postural deficits, hemiparesis,† and menace response deficits
Caudate nucleus/internal capsule	Striate arteries	Same as with cerebral cortex
Diencephalon (Thalamus)	Perforating artery (proximal, distal, caudal) (branch of basilar or caudal communicating artery	Abnormal mental state Ipsilateral or contralateral hemiparesis or tetraparesis; Ipsilateral or contralateral postural deficits Occasionally head tilt/turn, nystagmus

Hemorrhagic Infarction

Time	State of Hb	Cellular Location	Signal Intensity		
			T1W	T2W	T2*W (presence of signal void)
<24 hr	OxyHb	Intra	Iso	Slightly hyper	None
1-3 days	DeoxyHb	Intra	Iso to Hypo	Hypo	Present
>3 days	MetHb	Intra	Hyper	Hypo	Present
>7 days	MetHb	Extra	Hyper	Hyper	None
>2 wk	Hemosiderin	Intra	Hypo	Hypo	Present

Modified from Garosi L, McConnell JF, Platt SR, et al: Clinical and topographic magnetic resonance characteristics of suspected brain infarction in 40 dogs. J Vet Intern Med 20:311–321, 2006 and Bradley WG Jr: MR appearance of hemorrhage in the brain, Radiology 189:15–26, 1993.
Iso, Isointense; *hypo,* hypointense; *hyper,* hyperintense; *OxyHb,* oxyhemoglobin; *Deoxy Hb,* deoxyhemoglobin; *MetHb,* methemoglobin; *Intra,* intracellular; *Extra,* extracellular.
†Hemiparesis and postural deficits are transient. Typically resolve within 1-2 days of onset.
Intensity is compared with normal brain parenchyma.

Development of anisocoria or mydriasis with decreased PLR may indicate increasing ICP and risk of caudal tentorial herniation. Loss of consciousness and development of mydriatic, unresponsive pupils indicate herniation of the occipital lobes of the cerebrum under the tentorium cerebelli.

Basilar fractures occur when horses flip over backward and strike the poll. These fractures result in compression and hemorrhage of the brainstem. Occipital bone fractures may lacerate the basilar artery and venous sinuses and produce massive hemorrhage into the cranial cavity, guttural pouch, or inner ear. Neurologic signs include coma that lasts from minutes to days. Horses that regain consciousness demonstrate depression, vestibular dysfunction, facial nerve paralysis, tetraparesis, and hemorrhage from the nostrils and ear. Leakage of CSF or blood from the external ear canal is evidence of petrous temporal bone fracture. Epistaxis may result from fracture of the cribriform plate, basisphenoid/basioccipital bones, or hemorrhage into the guttural pouch.

In some cases, trauma to the poll or frontal area may cause bilateral blindness with mydriatic, unresponsive pupils. This injury results from damage to the optic nerves or optic chiasm. The prognosis for recovery of vision is poor.

Radiographs of the head or cross-sectional imaging are required to determine the type, location, and displacement of fractures and fracture fragments. Depressed, comminuted fractures of the frontal and parietal bones are readily identified radiographically. Petrous temporal bone fractures are difficult to identify, and multiple oblique views are necessary to identify the fracture line. Absence of an obvious fracture line radiographically does not preclude a diagnosis of basilar skull fracture. Hemorrhage from the guttural pouch, nose, or external ear canal following a traumatic poll injury is presumptive evidence of a basilar fracture.

Medical treatment is similar to that in dogs and cats; hyperosmolar fluids (mannitol or HTS), furosemide, corticosteroids, and dimethyl sulfoxide (DMSO) may be used. Broad-spectrum antibiotics that cross the blood-brain and blood-CSF barriers are indicated for basilar skull fractures, petrosal bone fractures, and open frontal bone fractures. Cefotaxime is bactericidal, has broad-spectrum antibacterial activity, and penetrates into the CSF in good concentrations (see Chapter 15). Surgical therapy may be indicated for horses with depressed frontal fractures that penetrate nervous tissue and open fractures that communicate with nervous tissue. Animals that deteriorate in the face of appropriate medical therapy also may be surgical candidates. However, without imaging, appropriate surgical intervention may be difficult to ascertain. Even with correct surgical intervention, the prognosis for horses requiring surgery remains poor.[26]

Prognosis. Based on the coma scale used in assessing humans (Glasgow Coma Scale), a modified Glasgow Coma Scale (MGCS) has been developed for use in small animals (Box 12-2).[27] The animal's status in each of three categories—motor activity, brainstem reflexes, and level of consciousness—is assessed. Proposed prognosis has been ascribed to three categories based on the total score; category I (score of 3 to 8) indicates a grave prognosis, category II (scores of 9 to 14) indicates a poor to guarded prognosis, and category III (scores of 15 to 18) indicates a good prognosis. In a retrospective application of the MGCS, score predicted probability of survival in the first 48 hours in a linear fashion with a 50% survival rate being observed in dogs with a score of 8.[28] Unfortunately, the MGCS does not take into account concurrent systemic injuries, changes in neurologic status over time, or effects of treatment. Consequently, the prognosis for animals with TBI likely depends on multiple factors.

As with small animals, the prognosis for horses with TBI likely is dependent on the severity of the clinical signs. In one study of 34 horses, 62% survived to discharge; risk factors for nonsurvivors included elevated packed cell volume (PCV) (40% [nonsurvivors] vs. 33% [survivors]), recumbency lasting more than 4 hours, and basilar fractures.[12] Horses that survive may return to normal function. Some horses are able to return to their intended use despite persistent neurologic deficitis.[12]

BOX 12-2

Small Animal Coma Scale*

Neurologic Function Assessed	Score
Motor Activity	
Normal gait, normal spinal reflexes	6
Hemiparesis, tetraparesis, or decerebrate activity	5
Recumbent, intermittent extensor rigidity	4
Recumbent, constant extensor rigidity	3
Recumbent, constant extensor rigidity with opisthotonos	2
Recumbent, hypotonia of muscles, depressed or absent spinal reflexes	1
Brainstem Reflexes	
Normal PLR and physiologic nystagmus	6
Slow pupillary light reflexes and normal to reduced physiologic nystagmus	5
Bilateral unresponsive miosis with normal to reduced physiologic nystagmus	4
Pinpoint pupils with reduced to absent physiologic nystagmus	3
Unilateral unresponsive mydriasis with reduced to absent physiologic nystagmus	2
Bilateral, unresponsive mydriasis with reduced to absent physiologic nystagmus	1
Level of Consciousness	
Occasional periods of alertness, responsive to environment	6
Depression or delirium, capable of responding to environment but response may be inappropriate	5
Stupor, responsive to visual stimuli	4
Stupor, responsive to auditory stimuli	3
Stupor, responsive only to repeated noxious stimuli	2
Coma, unresponsive to repeated noxious stimuli	1
Assessment	
Good prognosis	15-18
Guarded prognosis	9-14
Grave prognosis	3-8

Modified from Shores A: Craniocerebral trauma. In Kirk RW, editor: Current veterinary therapy X, Philadelphia, 1989, WB Saunders.
*Neurologic function is assessed for each of the three categories and a grade of 1 to 6 is assigned according to the descriptions for each grade. The total score is the sum of the three category scores.

Acute Nonprogressive

Infarction

Pathophysiology The brain has a high metabolic demand, which necessitates an adequate blood supply. A reduction in blood supply results in insufficient delivery of oxygen and glucose that creates an anoxic state and leads to neuronal ischemia and death. Infarctions also are known as strokes or cerebrovascular accidents. Brain infarctions can be produced by disruption of the vasculature leading to a *hemorrhagic infarction* or by occlusion of the vasculature leading to *ischemic infarction*. Occlusion of an intracranial blood vessel may occur due to a *thrombus* or an *embolus*. *Cerebral vasospasm* is a temporary constriction of an intracranial artery, producing transient ischemia. Vasospasm is difficult to document clinically. Transient loss of consciousness due to inadequate cerebral perfusion (syncope) is usually caused by a cardiac arrhythmia, not by vasospasm (see Chapter 13). Typically, brain infarctions result in an acute to peracute onset of neurologic signs. In most instances, signs are nonprogressive. However, in some animals, deterioration may represent the development of edema or an enlarging hematoma.

Hemorrhage in the brain is usually due to trauma. All other causes of hemorrhage combined have a much lower incidence. Hemorrhage-producing stroke syndromes are seen most often with neoplasms that have compromised an artery. Various primary and metastatic tumors have been associated with hemorrhage.[29] Among metastatic tumors, hemangiosarcoma is common[30,31] (Figure 12-6). Small hemorrhages (petechiae) are seen on examination of the brain with inflammation as the primary problem, but other changes predominate.[32] The exceptions to this occurs with infections such as Rocky Mountain spotted fever that cause thrombocytopenia and vasculitis.[33] *Angiostrongylus vasorum* infection also may cause intracranial hemorrhage in dogs.[34-36] Systemic coagulation disorders such as disseminated intravascular coagulopathy (DIC) and idiopathic thrombocytopenic purpura (ITP) usually are recognized by systemic signs.[37] Intraventricular hemorrhage has been observed with von Willebrand disease.[38] Hemorrhage may occur secondary to vascular malformations.[39,40] Occasionally, intracranial hemorrhage occurs without an underlying cause.[39,41]

In comparison to hemorrhagic infarction, ischemic infarction is relatively more common in dogs. For humans, multiple classifications schemes have been proposed, which are based on etiology, anatomic location within the brain, affected vasculature, and diameter of the affected vasculature. Occlusion of a small-diameter vessel affects a small amount of brain

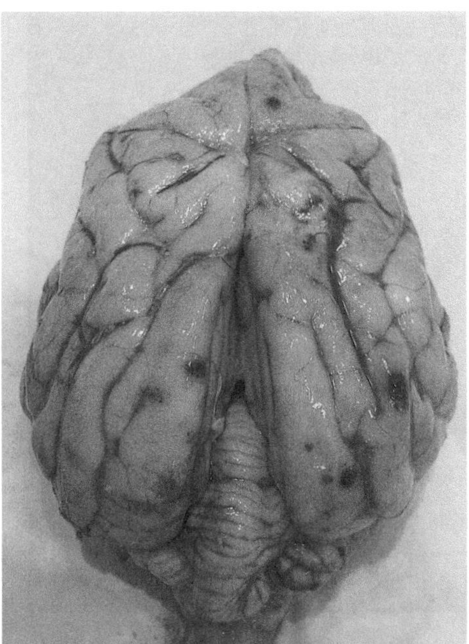

Figure 12-6 Dorsal view of a gross specimen of brain of a rottweiler. There are multiple dark lesions in the cerebral cortex bilaterally and in the caudal right cerebellar hemisphere. Microscopic evaluation was consistent with metastatic hemangiosarcoma. (Copyright 2010 University of Georgia Research Foundation, Inc.)

parenchyma resulting in a lacunar infarct and typically occurs in the thalamus, whereas occlusion of a large diameter vessel affects a greater amount of brain parenchyma resulting in a territorial infarct and typically occurs in the cerebrum or cerebellum.[42] In dogs, both lacunar and territorial infarcts occur. Anatomically, the cerebellum is most commonly affected followed by the cerebrum and thalamus.[43]

Concurrent illness is often present in affected dogs. Chronic renal disease, pheochromocytoma and hyperadrenocorticism are common concurrent illnesses although their exact relationship with the development of infarction is unknown.[44] The cause of most vascular lesions is unknown.[44] Primary vascular changes, such as arteriosclerosis, are rare in animals.[29,45] Atherosclerosis can be produced with atherogenic diets and may be more common in animals with hypothyroidism.[46] Hypothyroidism and hyperlipidemia has been associated with ischemic brain lesions in Labrador retrievers.[47] Fibrocartilaginous emboli from degenerating intervertebral disks cause infarction in the spinal cord; however, involvement of the medulla oblongata has been observed.[48] Infarcts can also occur from septic emboli secondary to bacterial valvular endocarditis.[49] Cardiac disease should be considered in small animals with suspected cerebral infarctions. Metastatic neoplasia or parasites, including the microfilaria of *Dirofilaria immitis*, are less common causes of vascular occlusion in dogs.[50,51] Air, fat, or blood clots may be introduced into the circulation during surgical procedures. Air emboli are of particular concern during vascular surgery of the head and the neck. The causes of infarction are listed in Box 12-3.

Thromboembolic meningoencephalitis (TEME) is an acute disease of cattle that is characterized by infarcts produced by septic emboli. Disseminated coagulopathy may develop subsequently. The disease is caused by *Histophilus somni* and usually is seen in feedlot cattle. Cerebral signs predominate, but brainstem infarcts may produce focal signs (see Chapter 15).

Assessment. Presumptive diagnosis is based on the history and clinical signs in affected animals combined with imaging findings. The imaging modality of choice in animals with suspected brain infarction is MRI. Differentiation between hemorrhagic and ischemic infarction can be made based on MRI characteristics (Table 12-5). Although MRI may accurately identify both ischemic and hemorrhagic infarcts, MRI may not help ascertain an underlying etiology. For example, a hemorrhage infarct secondary to metastatic lesions may appear similar to hemorrhagic infarcts secondary to another cause.

With MRI, ischemic infarcts are hyperintense on T2-weighted (T2W) and T2W fluid attenuated inversion recovery images and are hypointense on T1-weighted (T1W) images in comparison to normal brain tissue.[43] Although most lesions do not enhance after intravenous contrast administration, some lesions display mild to marked enhancement.[43] In addition to imaging characteristics, topography plays an important role in the presumptive diagnosis. Lesions occur in the distribution of certain arterial blood vessels such as those involving the cerebellum (rostral or caudal cerebellar arteries), caudate nucleus (perforating arteries), and the median and paramedian aspect of the thalamus (caudal perforating arteries).[43] As with infarction in other organs, lesions are typically well-circumscribed and occasionally wedge shaped. Diffusion weighted MRI (DWI) has been designed to identify ischemic infarctions soon after onset when conventional imaging sequences may not appear abnormal. DWI is an imaging modality that detects the restriction of molecular movement of water that occurs with cytotoxic edema secondary to infarction. Combining information from DWI with another

BOX 12-3

Etiology of Vascular Disease in the Brain*

- Hemorrhage infarction
  - Trauma
  - Infectious disease (15)
    - Rickettsial, viral, parasitic *(Angiostrongylus vasorum)*
  - Toxins (warfarin) (15)
  - Neoplasia (12)
  - Disseminated intravascular coagulopathy
  - Idiopathic thrombocytopenic purpura
  - Intracarotid injections (equine)
  - Equine hypoxic/ischemic encephalopathy
  - Vascular anomalies
- Ischemic infarction
  - Septic emboli (endocarditis, septicemia, thromboembolic meningoencephalitis) (15)
  - Neoplasia (metastases) (12)
  - Parasites *(Cuterebra* larval migration, *Dirofilaria immitis)* (15)
  - Arteriosclerosis, vasospasm, vascular insufficiency, heart failure
  - Emboli secondary to surgery (air, fat, clot)
- Commonly encountered secondary diseases†
  - Chronic kidney disease
  - Untreated hyperadrenocorticism
  - Diabetes mellitus
  - Hypothyroidism
  - Pheochromocytoma

*Numbers in parentheses refer to chapters in which the conditions are discussed.

†From Garosi L, McConnell JE, Platt SR, et al: Results of diagnostic investigations and long-term outcome of 33 dogs with brain infarction (2000-2004), J Vet Intern Med 19:725–731, 2005 and Vitale CL, Olby NJ: Neurologic dysfunction in hypothyroid, hyperlipidemic Labrador retrievers, J Vet Intern Med 21:1316–1322, 2007.

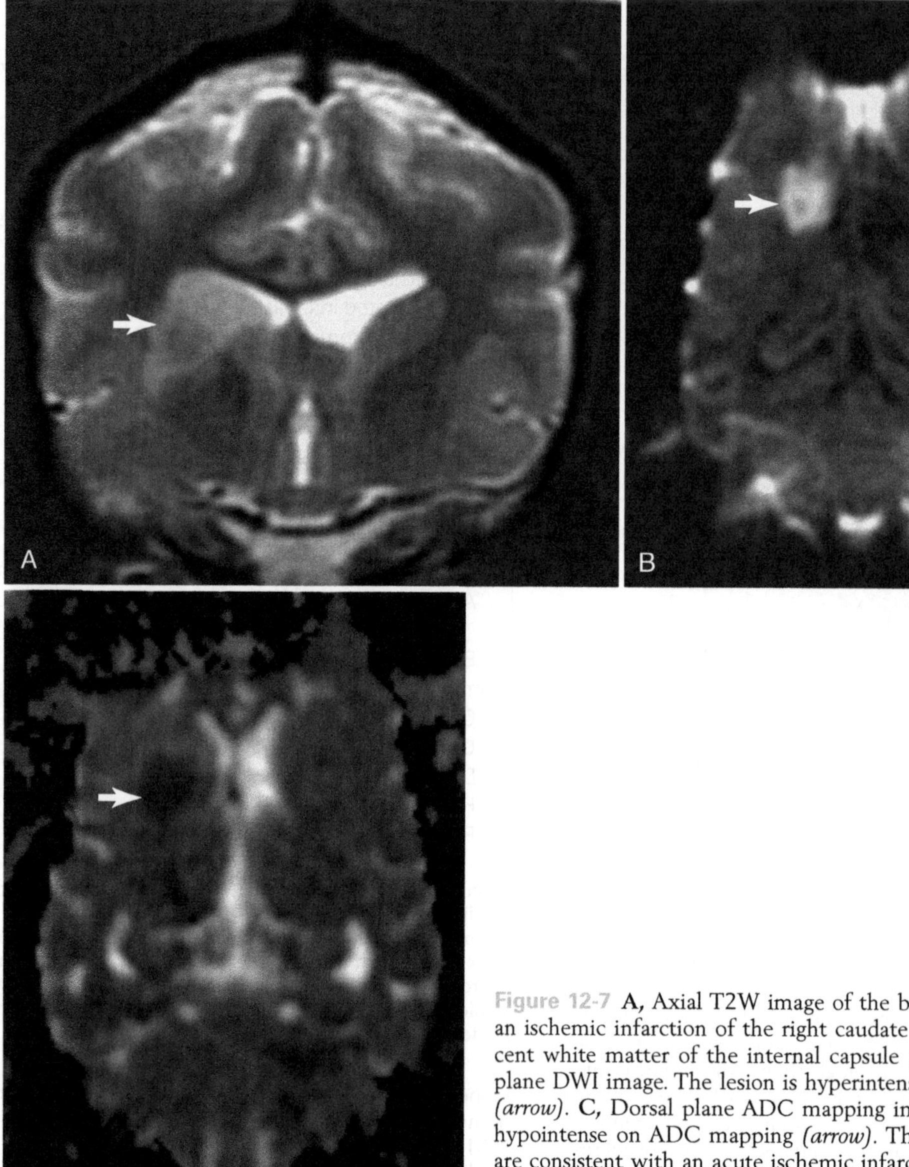

Figure 12-7 **A,** Axial T2W image of the brain of a dog with an ischemic infarction of the right caudate nucleus and adjacent white matter of the internal capsule *(arrow)*. **B,** Dorsal plane DWI image. The lesion is hyperintense on DWI images *(arrow)*. **C,** Dorsal plane ADC mapping image. The lesion is hypointense on ADC mapping *(arrow)*. These characteristics are consistent with an acute ischemic infarction. The affected area is supplied by a perforating artery. (Copyright 2010 University of Georgia Research Foundation, Inc.)

sequenced derived from the DWI sequence, the apparent diffusion coefficient map (ADC map), ischemic infarction can be accurately identified. With DWI and ADC mapping, ischemic infarctions appear hyperintense and hypointense, respectively (Figure 12-7).

Hemorrhagic infarction can also be accurately identified with MRI (Figure 12-8). Imaging characteristics are related to the reduction-oxidation state of iron and the oxygen content of hemoglobin. As extravasated blood progresses from oxyhemoglobin to deoxyhemoglobin to methemoglobin and finally to hemosiderin, the T1W and T2W imaging characteristics observed change due to the magnetic properties of iron, which affects the magnetic field of the tissue around it creating an artifact on MR images.[52] Gradient images (referred to as GRE or T2*W images) take advantage of this effect, allowing identification of lesions not conspicuous on conventional imaging sequences. Hemorrhagic infarction also can be identified with CT. Extravasated blood present in hemorrhage appears as a hyperattenuation or hyperdensity in comparison to normal brain tissue.[41]

Treatment. Management of the unconscious animal is discussed in the section on trauma in this chapter. Less severe lesions are usually not life threatening; however, the amount of residual damage likely depends on the size and location of the lesion. Lesions involving the cerebellum and brainstem are likely to result in more severe clinical signs than those involving the cerebrum or thalamus. Anticoagulants generally are not given unless a hypercoagulable state can be identified. Ultimately, the prognosis varies depending on the extent of neurologic damage and the underlying etiology. Most animals with ischemic infarction recover with supportive care.[44] In some cases, affected dogs die or are euthanized due to lack of improvement or as a result of concurrent illnesses.[44]

Feline Ischemic Encephalopathy

Pathophysiology. Feline ischemic encephalopathy is a distinct syndrome of cerebral myiasis related to *Cuterebra* larval migration through the cerebrum.[53,54] It is believed that the instar (first stage larva) gains entrance to the brain via migration through the nasal cavity and cribriform plate.[54] There is no breed or sex predilection. Young to middle-aged

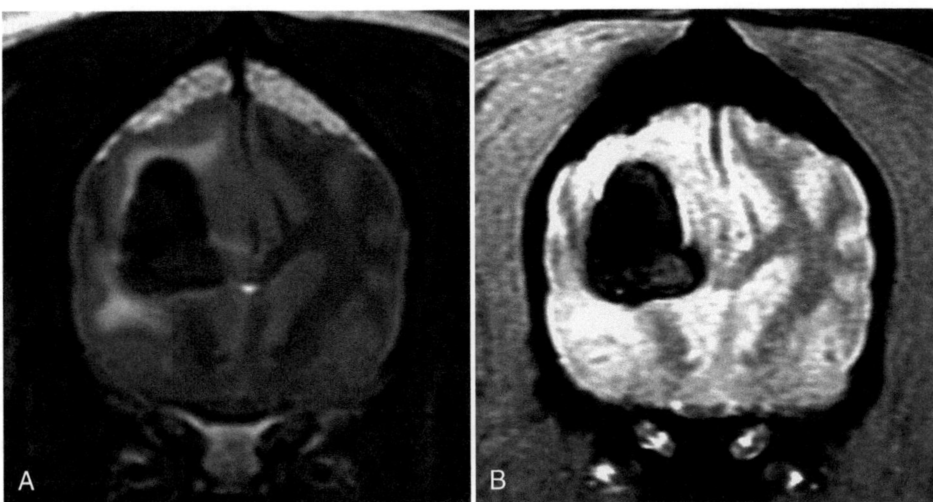

Figure 12-8 **A,** Axial T2W image of the brain of a mixed-breed dog at the level of the caudate nuclei. There is a well-circumscribed, ovoid hypointense mass in the right cerebrum at the level of the centrum semiovale. The lesion is surrounded by edema. **B,** Axial T2*W (GRE) images of the lesion is hypointense. In addition, the lesion was hypointense on T1W images. The MRI characteristics were consistent with an intraaxial hemorrhage. (Copyright 2010 University of Georgia Research Foundation, Inc.)

indoor-outdoor cats develop acute or peracute neurologic deficits during the months from July to September.[53,54]

Clinical Signs. Typically, affected cats display signs consistent with a unilateral (focal) lesion involving the forebrain. Neurologic signs consist of seizures, unilateral blindness, circling, abnormal mental state and behavior, with contralateral postural reactions deficits, menace response deficits, and facial hypalgesia.[53,54] Often affected cats display signs of acute upper respiratory disease such as sneezing or nasal discharge shortly prior (= 48 hours).[53] Abnormal body temperature (hyper- or hypothermia) is observed in most affected cats.[53]

Assessment. Presumptive antemortem diagnosis is based on clinical suspicion and MRI findings. Hyperintensities on T2W images consistent with edema may be observed in the frontal/parietal lobes. Lesions occur in the topography of the vasculature supplied by the middle cerebral artery (Figures 12-9 and 12-10). Also, parasitic tracks may be observed extending from the cribriform plate through the olfactory bulbs and tracks. Cerebrospinal fluid analysis may reveal a mixed pleocytosis including eosinophils.[53] Definitive diagnosis necessitates gross or microscopic identification of the parasite at postmortem. Five characteristic histologic features define the disease process: (1) parasitic tracks, (2) superficial laminar necrosis of the cerebrum, (3) cerebral infarction, (4) subependymal and subpial changes such as astrogliosis, and (5) identification of the parasite.[54]

Treatment. Cats surviving the first 48 hours after the onset of neurologic signs generally improve over time. Blindness and abnormal behavior may persist. Treatment consists of supportive care. Corticosteroids may help reduce the inflammatory response. Additional proposed empirical therapies include ivermectin, broad-spectrum antibiotics, and antihistamines.[53] The benefit of these therapies is unproven. *Cuterebra* larval migration has occasionally been reported in the dog.[55] Similar clinicopathologic findings have been observed.

Chronic Progressive

Primary Brain Tumors. Neoplasia that affects the nervous system is classified into two groups: primary and secondary tumors. Primary tumors arise from structures that normally are found in the cranial cavity, vertebral canal, or peripheral nerves. Secondary tumors metastasize to the CNS from a primary tumor located distant from the CNS. Alternatively, secondary tumors may arise from surrounding structures, such as the nose, ear, calvaria, pituitary gland, or vertebrae and may affect the nervous system by invasion or compression of neural tissue. In this chapter, tumors affecting the brain are discussed. Peripheral nerve and spinal cord tumors were discussed in Chapters 5 and 6, respectively.

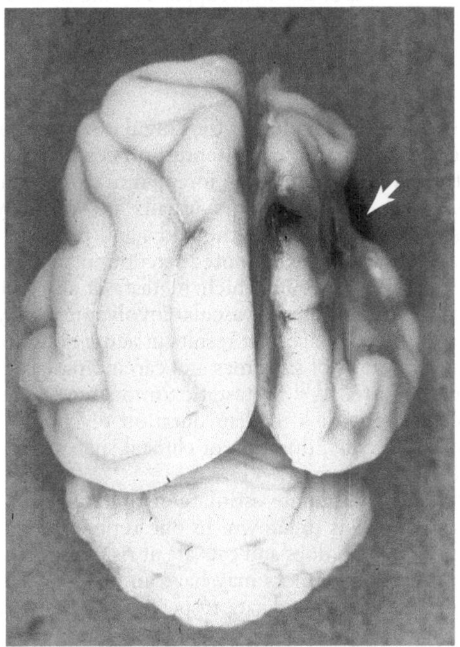

Figure 12-9 Chronic infarction of the left cerebral hemisphere of a cat *(arrow)*. (Copyright 2010 University of Georgia Research Foundation, Inc.)

Pathogenesis. In general, tumors affect the function of the nervous system by (1) the compression of nervous tissue, (2) invasion of the nervous tissue, (3) interference with circulation and subsequent development of vasogenic edema, and (4) disturbance of CSF circulation. Increased intracranial pressure resulting from the combination of the mass effect of the tumor, vasogenic edema, and CSF accumulation may cause

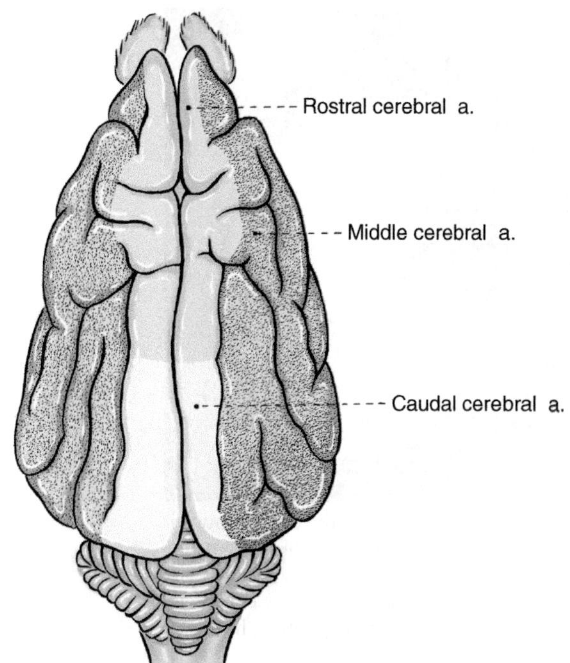

Figure 12-10 Areas of the brain supplied by the cerebral arteries. *a*, Artery. (From Evans HE, Christensen GC: Miller's anatomy of the dog, ed 2, Philadelphia, 1979, WB Saunders.)

brain herniation. Herniation of the cingulate gyrus, herniation of the cerebrum ventral to the tentorium cerebelli, or herniation of the cerebellum into the foramen magnum may occur. In most cases, primary tumors usually grow slowly, rarely metastasize to other areas of the body, and produce chronic, progressive clinical signs. A noted exception to this is with choroid plexus tumors in which metastasis along the CNS can occur.[56-60] Occasionally, vascular involvement may lead to infarction or hemorrhage that results in acute neurologic deficits. CNS metastasis of sarcomas and carcinomas are the most commonly reported.[31,61] Metastatic tumors tend to be aggressive biologically with a median duration of clinical signs to diagnosis and median duration of clinical signs to death both being 21 days[31] (Figure 12-11).

Incidence. An accurate estimate of the incidence of brain tumors in animals is unknown. In one report, a rate of 14.5 and 3.5 per 100,000 dogs and cats are at risk, respectively.[62] In other reports, brain tumors may have an incidence as high as 2.8% and 2.2% in dogs and cats, respectively.[63,64] Brain tumors are infrequently reported in food animals and horses. Consequently, the following discussion pertains to dogs and cats.

The most common primary brain tumor that affects dogs and cats is meningioma.[65,66] Meningioma arises from meninges, specifically the arachnoid cap cells and arachnoid granulations.[67] The second most common primary brain tumors are the glial tumors: astrocytoma and oligodendroglioma.[65,66] Primary brain tumors typically occur as a single mass. In cats, meningioma may be found as an incidental finding, occur as multiple meningiomas, or occur concurrent with another tumor type.[65] In dogs, multiple meningiomas occur uncommonly.[68] Likewise, multiple tumor types occurring simultaneously in dogs are uncommon.[69,70]

The golden retriever and boxer appear predisposed to the development of brain tumors as a whole and meningoma as a specific tumor type.[66,71-73] Additional breeds overrepresented include Labrador retriever, Scottish terrier, Old English sheepdog, Doberman pinscher, and dolichocephalic breeds such as the German shepherd dog and collie.[71-76] The boxer, Boston terrier, and other brachycephalic breeds appear predisposed to the development of glial tumors.[66,76-78] Moreover, the golden retriever, Labrador retriever, German shepherd, and boxer dogs are breeds most commonly affected by secondary tumors.[31] The most common secondary tumor in dogs is hemangiosarcoma, while in cats the most common secondary tumor is lymphoma.[31,65] Pituitary tumors are the second most common secondary tumor[31,65] (see later discussion).

Most dogs with primary brain tumors are 5 years of age, with the mean age of 9.5 years.[66,74,79] Similarly, the mean age of cats with primary brain tumors is 11.3 years.[65] Dogs and cats with meningioma are significantly older than those with other primary brain tumors; meningioma occurs in dogs with a mean age of 11.1 years versus a mean age of 8.0 years for other tumors while meningioma occurs in cats with a mean age of 12.2 years versus 8.2 years with other primary brain tumors.[65,66] The mean age of dogs with secondary brain tumors is 9.6 years.[31] The mean age of cats with secondary tumors is the same as for primary brain tumors.[65]

Clinical Signs. The clinical signs depend on the location of the tumor (Table 12-6). In addition to signs related to the location of the lesion (see Table 12-6), signs due to increased intracranial pressure (depression, papilledema) are frequently present.[80] Sites of predilection for tumors are given in Table 12-7.

The majority of primary brain tumors are located rostral to the tentorium cerebelli.[65,66] Consequently, primary brain tumors often cause clinical signs consistent with a focal lesion involving the forebrain. The most common clinical signs include seizures and a change in mental state or behavior.[65,66,74,81] Blindness from compression of the optic nerves does not occur frequently, but it can occur.[82] Other signs include propulsive circling with preservation of gait, contralateral deficits in postural reactions, menace response, and facial hypalgia. Tumors involving the brainstem caudal to the tentorium cerebelli result in an abnormal mental state, gait deficits such as vestibular, cerebellar, or general proprioceptive ataxia, ipsilateral postural reaction deficits, and ipsilateral deficits in cranial nerve function. On occasion, dogs with intracranial neoplasia may display neck pain.[83] Clinical signs may be present from 1 to 3 months before presenting for evaluation; however, affected animals may display clinical signs for much longer periods of time.[65,66,81] Secondary brain tumors such as metastatic disease or lymphoma may cause multifocal signs. Alternatively, secondary brain tumors arising from structures neighboring the brain may invade the cranial cavity and cause clinical signs related to their effect on the adjacent nervous tissue. Pituitary tumors in animals tend to expand dorsally into the hypothalamus, producing changes in mental state, seizures, and changes in metabolic and endocrine function in the early stages. Nasal tumors that invade may be associated with seizures and abnormal mentation.[84] Affected animals may display clinical signs of nasal disease, epistaxis and discharge, which may be continuous or transient. Occasionally, respiratory signs may be lacking.

Diagnosis. The diagnosis begins by exclusion of other disease processes that may result in similar clinical signs. This is particularly important in animals without evidence of asymmetric neurologic deficits or those solely displaying vague signs, mentation changes, or seizures. A complete blood count, chemistry profile, and urinalysis should be performed to exclude extracranial disease as a primary or concurrent disease process. Three view thoracic radiographs should be performed to evaluate for metastatic disease. Thoracic radiograph abnormalities such as metastatic lesions from a concurrent or unassociated neoplastic processes may be observed in approximately 20% of dogs with primary brain tumors.[66] Thoracic

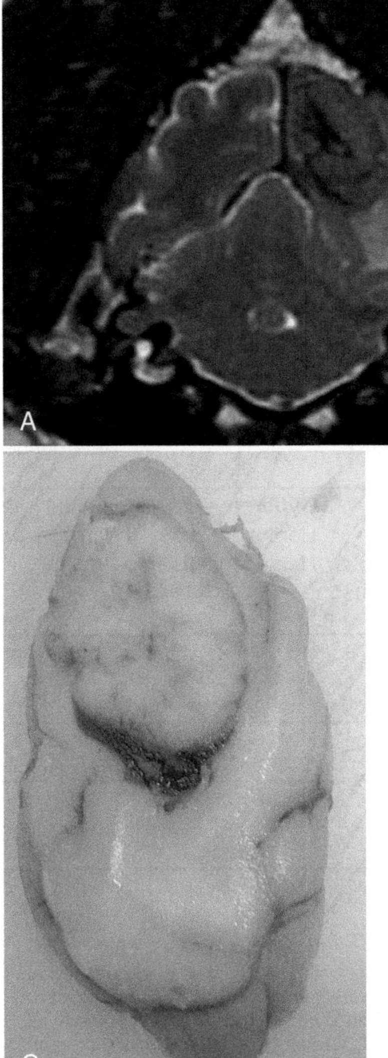

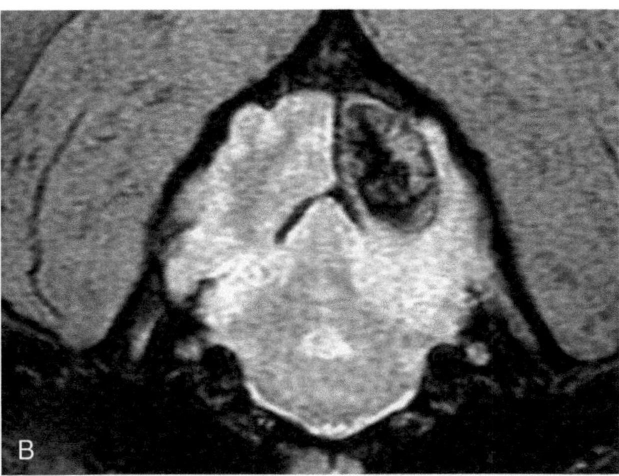

Figure 12-11 **A,** Axial T2W image of the brain of a Labrador retriever at the level of the medulla oblongata. In the left occipital lobe of the cerebrum there is an single, well-circumscribed mass that displays heterogeneous signal intensity (areas of hypointensity and isointensity) surrounded by hyperintensity in the white matter (perilesional edema). **B,** T2*W (GRE) images in which the mass has areas that are hypointense consistent with areas of hemorrhage. **C,** Gross cross section of the left occipital lobe of the cerebrum. The mass is primarily composed of tissue with areas of hemorrhage. Microscopic evaluation of the mass disclosed adenocarcinoma. The dog had a history of prostatic carcinoma for over a year before developing the single metastasis in the brain. (Copyright 2010 University of Georgia Research Foundation, Inc.)

radiographic abnormalities may be present in 54% of dogs with secondary tumors in which 72% of the abnormalities represent a metastatic pattern.[31]

The most important diagnostic step in the evaluation of animals in which a brain tumor is suspected is cross-sectional imaging. Imaging may provide a relatively accurate presumptive diagnosis. MRI is the imaging modality of choice. Imaging characteristics of a lesion such as the location, the size and shape, the border definition (well defined vs. poorly defined borders), intensity of the lesion, and the degree of enhancement (strong enhancement versus no enhancement) and pattern of contrast enhancement (homogeneous, heterogeneous, peripherally enhancing [ring enhancing]) may suggest tumor type (Table 12-7; Figures 12-12 through 12-14). However, nonneoplastic lesions share similarities with a variety of neoplasms, therefore a definitive diagnosis cannot be based entirely on imaging characteristics. Definitive diagnosis requires histologic or cytologic evaluation. Specimens for microscopic evaluation may be obtained surgically via craniectomy or through CT-guided biopsy procedures.[85,86]

CSF analysis may provide limited information in the diagnosis of primary brain tumors. Tumors may cause an increased ICP, which is a contraindication for CSF collection. As with any disease process, the risks of CSF collection should be

TABLE 12-6

Common Sites and Signs of Brain Tumors

Site	Signs
Cerebrum	Seizures, abnormal behavior, normal gait, propulsive circling, contralateral postural reaction deficits, contralateral menace response, and facial sensory deficits
Pituitary-hypothalamus	Behavioral, autonomic, and endocrine signs: polyuria, polydipsia, anorexia Changes in sleeping and behavior patterns; later visual deficits
Brainstem	Abnormal gait and ipsilateral postural reaction and cranial nerve (CN) deficits
Cerebellopontine angle	Ipsilateral CN V, CN VII, and CN VIII deficits, ipsilateral hemiparesis

TABLE 12-7

Magnetic Resonance Features in Canine Brain Tumors

Tumor	Intraaxial/ Extramedullary	Anatomic Location(s)	Shape	T1W Intensity	T2W Intensity	Postcontrast Intensity
Mening	E	Olfactory Cerebral convexities CP angle Basilar/Tentorial Cerebellar convexity	Distinct margin Dural tail Cystic (occasionally)	**Iso-** Hyper- Hypo-	**Hyper-** Iso- Mixed	Intense Homogeneous
Oligo	I	Rostrotentorial Piriform lobe Internal capsule	Distinct margin Round to ovoid	Hypo-	Hyper-	Mild enhancing Ring enhancing
Astro	I	Rostrotentorial Internal capsule Thalamus	Irregular margins Irregular shape	Iso-	Hyper-	None to mild Heterogeneous
CPT	I	Rostrotentorial Intraventricular Lateral/3rd ventricle (75%) 4th ventricle (25%) Metastasis-Carcinoma	Globular Papilliform Hyper- Ventriculomegaly	**Hypo-** Iso- Heterogeneous Homogeneous	**Hyper-** Homogeneous Homogeneous	Intense Homogeneous
GBM	I	Rostrotentorial Cerebrum	Distinct margins Round to ovoid Irregular/ill-distinct	Iso- to hypo-	Hyper-	Ring enhancing
Epend	I	Rostrotentorial	Distinct margins	Hypo-	Hyper-	Intense Homogeneous
Pit	E	Middle cranial fossa Sella turcica	Distinct margins Round to ovoid Extend dorsally	Iso- to hypo-	Hyper-	Intense Homogeneous
LSA	I	Multifocal	Indistinct margins	Iso-	Hyper-	Moderate Heterogeneous

Based on: Kraft SL, Gavin PR, DeHaan C, et al: Retrospective review of 50 canine intracranial tumors evaluated by magnetic resonance imaging, J Vet Intern Med 11:218–225, 1997; Sturges BK, Dickinson PJ, Bollen AW, et al: Magnetic resonance imaging and histologic classification of intracranial meningiomas in 112 dogs, J Vet Intern Med 22:586–595, 2008; Snyder JM, Shofer FS, Van Winkle TJ, et al: Canine intracranial primary neoplasia: 173 cases (1986-2003), J Vet Intern Med 20:669–675, 2006; Troxel MT, Vite CH, Massicotte C, et al: Magnetic resonance imaging features of feline intracranial neoplasia: retrospective analysis of 46 cats, J Vet Intern Med 18:176–189, 2004; Westworth DR, Dickinson PJ, Vernau W, et al: Choroid plexus tumors in 56 dogs (1985-2007), J Vet Intern Med 22:1157–1165, 2008; Lipsitz D, Higgins RJ, Kortz GD, et al: Glioblastoma multiforme: clinical findings, magnetic resonance imaging, and pathology in five dogs, Vet Pathol 40:659–669, 2003; Vural SA, Besalti O, Ilhan F, et al: Ventricular ependymoma in a German shepherd dog, Vet J 172:185–187, 2006.
Mening, Meningioma; *oligo,* oligodendroglioma; *astro,* astrocytoma; *CPT,* choroid plexus tumor; *GBM,* glioblastoma multiforme; *Epend,* ependymoma; *Pit,* pituitary; *LSA,* lymphoma; intensity is compared with normal brain parenchyma. *Iso,* isointense; *hypo,* hypointense; *hyper,* hyperintense.
Bold text denotes most commonly encountered signal intensity.

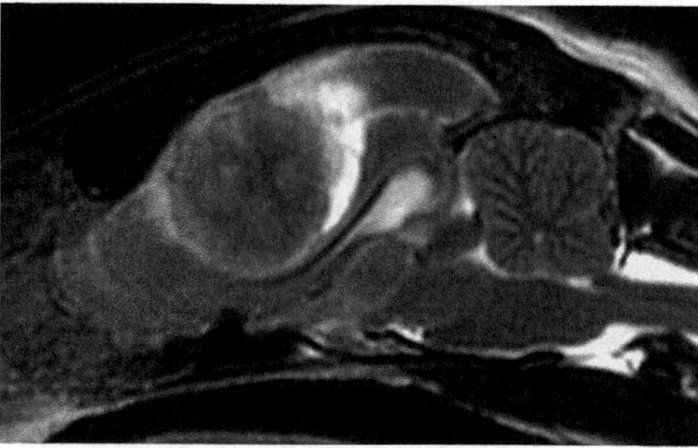

Figure 12-12 A sagittal T2W image of the brain of a cat. There is a large dorsal extradural mass with a broad based attachment to the calvaria that is compressing the cerebrum. The lesion is consistent with a meningioma. (Copyright 2010 University of Georgia Research Foundation, Inc.)

weighed against the potential diagnostic value of CSF analysis. In most dogs with primary brain tumors, CSF analysis is normal or contains increased protein content with a normal WBC count, which is referred to as albuminocytologic dissocation.[87] However, inflammation may be seen with meningiomas.[87] Neutrophilic pleocytosis may occur in 19% to 25% of dogs with intracranial meningiomas.[87,88] Neutrophilic pleocytosis is more frequently associated with meningiomas located in the caudal cranial fossa. Pleocytosis may portend a worse prognosis.[75]

Treatment and Prognosis. Treatment can be divided into palliative and definitive therapy. *Palliative therapy* is directed at controlling the secondary consequences of the tumor in an effort to alleviate clinical signs. Palliative therapy is not aimed at controlling or eliminating the tumor. For animals with brain tumors, palliative therapy is often focused on controlling vasogenic edema and seizures. Prednisone (0.5 to 1.0 mg/kg/day) may be effective at reducing vasogenic edema. If improvement is observed, the dosage may be gradually reduced to the lowest effective dosage to control signs. In acutely affected animals, intravenous formulations of corticosteroids, such as methylprednisolone or prednisolone sodium succinate or dexamethasone sodium phosphate, may be used until the animal is able to receive oral medication. Mannitol or HTS administration is also effective in rapidly reducing vasogenic edema. In animals experiencing seizures, anticonvulsants also should be administered. Phenobarbital or potassium bromide is effective at controlling seizures; however, animals with intracranial neoplasia may experience excessive sedation with these drugs. Levetiracetam may also be used to control seizures without sedative effects. (See Chapter 13 for details regarding anticonvulsant therapy.)

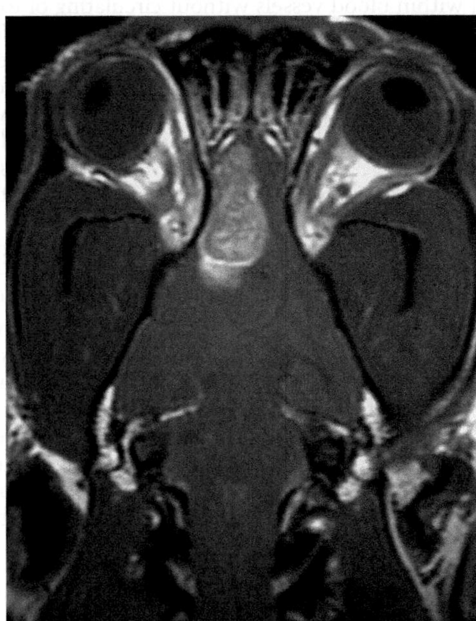

Figure 12-13 A dorsal T1W image of the brain of a golden retriever after intravenous contrast administration. There is a well circumscribed, strongly and uniformly enhancing mass in the right frontal/olfactory lobe of the cerebrum. Microscopic evaluation disclosed a meningioma. (Copyright 2010 University of Georgia Research Foundation, Inc.)

In animals with suspected or confirmed increased ICP, intravenous hypertonic fluids may be used to reduce ICP (see section on traumatic brain injury). Corticosteroids may also alleviate increased ICP by reducing CSF production and stabilizing the endothelial membrane. In animals with ventriculomegaly involving the lateral ventricles related to obstruction of CSF, ventriculoperitoneal shunting may help control intracranial pressure and improve clinical signs (see Hydrocephalus section). Median survival for dogs receiving palliative treatment for brain tumors is approximately 1 to 2 months.[75,89] Longer survival times may occur depending on tumor size and location, severity of clinical signs, response to palliative therapy, and the owner's willingness to continue therapy.

Definitive therapy consists of surgery, radiation therapy, and chemotherapy, alone or in combination. Combination therapy may provide longer control of clinical signs. Surgical resection entails craniectomy. Surgical approaches to the canine brain have been defined and can be applied to the cat.[90-92] The criteria for successful surgery include (1) a solitary, noninvasive tumor; (2) tumors located on or near the surface rostral to the tentorium cerebelli (cerebral hemisphere); (3) minimal neurologic impairment; (4) tumors that appear noninvasive on MRI; (5) a careful and complete surgical resection or debulking; and (6) an intensive anesthetic monitoring and postoperative care regimen. Meningiomas are most likely to meet these requirements. Consequently, most data regarding surgical intervention and prognosis involve meningiomas. In dogs with meningioma affecting the cerebrum, the median survival time with surgery alone is 7 months.[93] Shorter survival times for dogs with meningioma treated by surgical resection alone also have been reported; however, this may reflect the influence of lesion location.[75,94,95] It is probable that dogs with small tumors located rostral and those dogs with minimal clinical signs are likely to experience longer survival times. Similarly, the completeness of gross resection has a positive impact on survival. Several techniques can be used to improve the extent of resection and visualization during surgery, which leads to longer survival times. Intraoperative use of an ultrasound surgical aspirator, an instrument that can ablate tumor tissue while sparing vasculature and minimizing damage to normal brain parenchyma, enables a more complete gross

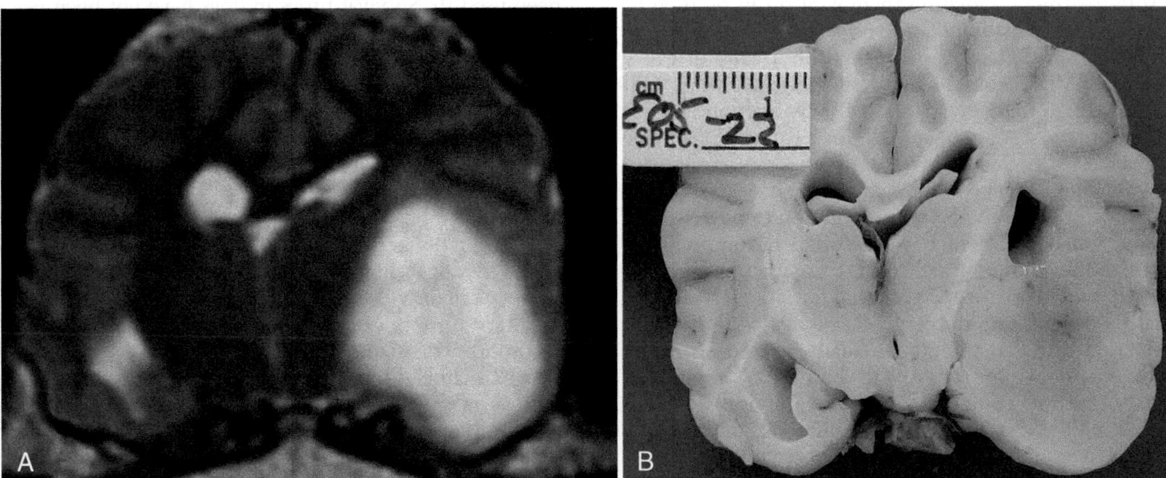

Figure 12-14 **A,** Axial TW image of the brain of an American bulldog at the level of the thalamus. There is a well-circumscribed, uniformly hyperintense intraaxial mass in left piriform lobe of the cerebrum. Secondary compression of the thalamus and lateral ventricle on the left is evident. **B,** Gross section of the brain of the same dog. The mass is affecting the piriform lobe of the cerebrum and displacing the left hemisphere to the right. Microscopic evaluation disclosed an oligodendroglioma. (**A,** Copyright 2010 University of Georgia Research Foundation, Inc. **B,** Courtesy Alexander deLahunta, DVM, PhD.)

resection.[96] Intraoperative ultrasound may provide better delineation of a lesion not grossly apparent on visual inspection.[97] Using a surgical aspirator, the median survival time in dogs with meningioma is 1254 days.[96] Similarly, endoscopic-assisted tumor resection may provide improved visualization and therefore aid in achieving a more complete resection.[98,99] Using intraoperative endoscopy to help visualize margins and areas of incompletely resected tumor, the median survival for dogs with meningioma is 2104 days (median survival for dogs with tumors located rostral to the tentorium cerebelli is 2104 days, whereas median survival for dogs with tumors located caudal to the tentorium cerebelli is 702 days).[98] If accessible by craniectomy, surgery is the treatment of choice for cats with meningioma. Long-term survival is commonly obtained with surgery alone. The median survival time for cats with cerebral meningioma is 21 months.[100] However, many cats live longer than 2 years postoperatively.[100,101]

Radiation therapy may be used adjunctively with surgery or as sole treatment. As adjunctive therapy, dogs receiving postoperative radiation for meningioma have longer survival times than with surgery alone.[75,93] In dogs with meningioma treated with surgery followed by radiation therapy, the median survival time is 16.5 months.[93] Several factors may influence survival with surgery and radiation for meningioma. Proliferating cell nuclear antigen (PCNA) staining can be used to calculate the proliferating fraction (PF_{PCNA}) of tumors, which may reflect the radiosensitivity of the tumor.[102] In dogs treated with surgery and radiation for cerebral meningioma, low PF_{PCNA} was associated with a 9 times greater control of tumors. In one study, the median duration of progression free survival (time to recurrence of signs or death) was 30 months, with dogs with low PF_{PCNA} having both a 1- and 2-year survival rate of 93% versus a 1- and 2-year survival rate of 62% and 42%, respectively, in dogs with high PF_{PCNA}. The extent and intensity of vascular endothelial growth factor (VEGF) expression also has been associated with prolonged survival in dogs treated with surgery and radiation for cerebral meningioma.[103] In one study, the overall median survival was 14.6 months. However, in those dogs with tumors with a low percent expression of VEGF, a median survival time was 25 months versus a median survival time of 14.7 months for those dogs with high VEGF expression.[103]

As a sole treatment, radiation therapy also can be used to treat brain tumors that might not be accessible by surgery. Typically, radiation therapy is performed on a daily or every other day basis. Most protocols are designed to deliver a total radiation dose of 46 to 48 Gy in 2.0 to 4.0 Gy fractions. Hypofractionated or course-fractionated dosing protocols also have been utilized in the treatment of primary brain tumors.[104] Alternatively, radiosurgery using a stereotactic system allows for a single fraction (10 to 15 Gy) of radiation to be delivered through multiple portals, which allows sufficient tumor dosing yet minimizes the amount of radiation to the surrounding normal tissue thereby reducing the potential for radiation damage to normal tissues.[105] Radiosurgery necessitates computerized planning based off of a stereotactic headframe construct.[105] The median survival for dogs with brain tumors treated with radiation therapy alone range from 4.7 months to 23.3 months.[75,89,102-109] The difference in survival times likely reflects differences in radiation therapy protocols, tumor types, size and location of tumors, and clinical signs.

There are few reports detailing the use of chemotherapy for primary brain tumors in animals. Hydroxyurea (30 to 50 mg/kg 3 days a week) has been used in the treatment of meningioma in dogs.[96,110] Preliminary data suggest that hydroxyurea may be effective in dogs with meningioma.[96,110] Similarly, lomustine (50 to 80 mg/m^2 of body surface area at intervals of 6 to 8 weeks) also has been used for dogs with brain tumors.[111,112] Secondary brain tumors such as lymphoma may be treated with multidrug protocols.

Secondary Tumors

CNS Lymphoma

Pathophysiology. Lymphoma may involve the CNS, peripheral nervous system, or both. In dogs, primary CNS lymphoma (lymphoma confined to the CNS) does not appear to be common.[66] More commonly involvement of the CNS occurs as part of multicentric disease. The presentation of CNS lymphoma is similar in cats.[65,113] One specific presentation, intravascular lymphoma in which neoplastic lymphocytes are confined within blood vessels without circulating or extravascular cellular infiltration, has a predilection for the CNS.[114]

In one study, the rottweiler dog appears overrepresented in cases of CNS lymphoma.[31] Most cats with LSA are domestic short-haired cats. The median age of affected dogs was 7.4 years in two studies; however, in another study the median age was 4 years old.[31,66,115] The median age of affected cats ranges from 7 to 10.5 years of age.[65,113] Few cats test positive for feline leukemia virus.[65,113]

Clinical Signs. In most affected animals, clinical signs suggest multifocal nervous system involvement. Signs are usually present for fewer than 30 days before presentation.[31,65,66,115] Common clinical signs include seizures, vestibular dysfunction, and changes in mental state.[31,66,115] Neck pain as a consequence of lymphoma solely affecting the meninges also has been reported.[116] Dogs with intravascular lymphoma may display clinical signs and MRI findings consistent with ischemic infarction.[117] In some affected dogs, no neurologic signs may be present despite CNS involvement.[31] Affected dogs frequently have lymphadenopathy.[115] Similar signs are observed in cats; however, affected cats also may have signs of cranial nerve involvement.[65,115] In the majority of dogs, CSF analysis discloses malignant lymphocytes, whereas fewer cats have malignant lymphocytes in the CSF.[66,113,115] Anatomically, approximately 50% of dogs with lymphoma have multifocal CNS involvement typically affecting the cerebrum or thalamus as common sites.[31,66]

Teatment. Treatment includes multidrug chemotherapy protocols. Often drugs that cross the BBB such as lomustine or cytosine arabinoside are included in protocols. Cranial or craniospinal radiation therapy and intrathecal cytosine arabinoside have also been used.[115] Survival times in dogs have not been well established. In two studies of cats treated with corticosteroids alone, the median survival was 21 and 35 days.[65] In cats treated with chemotherapy and radiation, median survival was 125 days.[113] Too few studies exist detailing long-term survival with treatment to define optimal therapy in affected animals. Despite this, chemotherapy and radiation therapy likely play a role in treatment.

Pituitary Tumors

Pathophysiology. Tumors arising from the pituitary gland may result in neurologic deficits, endocrine dysfunction, or both. In dogs, pituitary tumors are the second most common secondary brain tumor observed.[31] Based on size, pituitary tumors can be divided into microtumors and macrotumors. The size of the normal pituitary gland of dogs is approximately 4 to 6 mm in height, 6 to10 mm in length, and 5 to 9 mm in width.[118,119] The size of the normal pituitary gland of cats is approximately 3.2 mm in height, 5.4 mm in length, and 5 mm in width. Arbitrarily, tumors larger than 10 mm in height or those extending dorsally above the sella turcica are considered macrotumors.[120] Histologically, pituitary tumors are usually adenomas or adenocarcinomas, which occur in equal frequency.[31] Subclassification is based on the cell of origin. Likewise, in cats pituitary tumors are the second most commonly encountered secondary brain tumor. In dogs, breed and sex predilection are not observed.[121] In cats, a male predilection is observed.[122-124]

Clinical Signs. Neurologic signs develop out of a consequence of compression or invasion of the tumor dorsally into the hypothalamus and diencephalon resulting in abnormal behavior and changes in mental state.[120,125-127] Depending on the lesion extent, additional neurologic signs include circling, ataxia, cranial nerve deficits involving vestibular, facial, trigeminal, and oculomotor nerves.[120,125-127] Although in humans blindness occurs commonly with pituitary tumors, in dogs and cats visual deficits rarely occur due to anatomic differences, including an incomplete diaphragma sella and frequent involvement of the par distalis.[124,128,129] Despite this, blindness can occur.[82] Nonspecific signs such as lethargy and anorexia also may be present.

Pituitary tumors often cause endocrine disorders as many tumors remain functionally active. In dogs, hyperadrenocorticism is the most commonly encountered endocrine disorder. Central diabetes insipidus and diabetes mellitus (DM) also have been reported in dogs with pituitary tumors.[130-134] Approximately 80% to 85% of dogs with hyperadrenocorticism have pituitary dependent hyperadrenocorticism (PDH).[135] By definition, dogs with PDH have pituitary tumors. The prevalence of an identifiable pituitary tumor in dogs with PDH is approximately 30%.[136] Moreover, approximately 50% of dogs with PDH develop neurologic signs suggestive of a macrotumor at a mean of 7 months (range 0.5 to 24 months) from a diagnosis of PDH.[136] Interestingly, the presence or absent of neurologic signs in dogs with PDH does not predict the presence of a pituitary tumor.[126] Furthermore, the size of the tumor does not consistently correlate with the presence of neurologic signs.[136] In cats, acromegaly (hypersomatotropism) in which excessive growth hormone (GH) secretion leads to DM is the most commonly encountered concurrent endocrine disorder.[122,124] Hyperadrenocorticism can also occur in cats.[122]

Animals with signs suggestive of an endocrine disorder and neurologic signs should undergo appropriate testings because therapy often entails treatment of the endocrine dysfunction along with definitive therapy directed toward control of the pituitary tumor. In dogs, testing of the pituitary adrenal axis should include low-dose dexamethasone suppression test or ACTH stimulation.[137] Additional tests may include a urinary cortisol to creatinine ratio, high dose dexamethasone suppression test, serum ACTH concentration, and abdominal US.[137] In cats, DM occurs in all cats with acromegaly. In addition, mandibular prognathism, broadening of the frontal bones of the calvaria, cardiomyopathy, and glomerulopathies also may be observed.[124] Unfortunately, assays for feline GH are not widely available.[123] The anabolic consequences of excessive GH are mediated through insulin-like growth factor I (IGF-I; also known as somatomedin C), which is produced by the liver.[123] Consequently, IGF-I serves as a biologic surrogate for GH concentrations and measurement of serum IGF-I concentrations are used to establish the existence of acromegaly. Unfortunately, elevated IGF-I levels have been documented in cats receiving long-term insulin for diabetes mellitus without acromegaly.[138] Additionally, normal IGF-I has been reported in a cat with acromegaly.[139] Ultimately, the definitive diagnosis of acromegaly requires cross-sectional imaging in conjunction with endocrine testing.

Assessment. The diagnosis of a pituitary tumor is established with cross-sectional imaging. Dogs with PDH that develop neurologic signs should undergo cross-sectional imaging.[136] Likewise, cats with DM that are resistant to insulin therapy in which another cause is not identified, those that display physical characteristics along with elevated IGF-I levels, or those that develop neurologic signs should undergo cross-sectional imaging.[123,140] As with other brain tumors, MRI is the imaging modality of choice.[141,142] With MRI, the pituitary gland is easily identifiable. In the normal pituitary gland, a central area of hyperintensity may be observed on MRI in 64% of dogs.[119] Although unknown, the increased signal intensity may represent vasopressin (antidiuretic hormone) since a decrease in the signal intensity occurs with release/depletion vasopressin.[143] Typically, tumors are well circumscribed and demonstrate strong, uniform contrast enhancement (Figure 12-15). CT can also be used in the diagnosis of pituitary tumors.[118] With CT, pituitary tumors typically demonstrate similar characteristics and patterns of contrast enhancement as observed with MRI. In addition to standard imaging procedures, dynamic imaging (MRI or CT) in which rapid imaging of the pituitary is performed during IV contrast administration can be used in the diagnosis of pituitary tumors and may increase the sensitivity of identifying microadenomas.[144,145]

Treatment—Radiation Therapy. Dogs. Radiation therapy is the optimal treatment for dogs with pituitary tumors. Radiation therapy can result in a decrease in the size of a pituitary tumor.[146,147] In one study of dogs with pituitary tumors treated with RT, the median survival time was not reached because dogs lived longer than the study period.[121] The mean

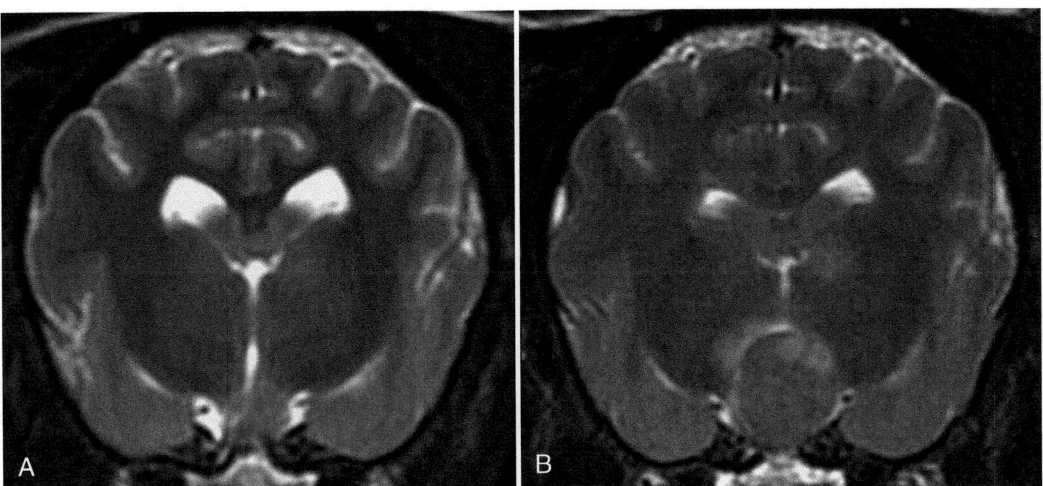

Figure 12-15 **A,** Axial T2W images of the brain of a Boston terrier at the level of the pituitary gland. There is enlargement of the pituitary gland consistent with a macrotumor. **B,** Nine months after initial imaging, repeated images show growth of the pituitary macrotumor. Microscopic evaluation was consistent with a pituitary adenoma. (Copyright 2010 University of Georgia Research Foundation, Inc.)

survival time was 1045 days compared with a median and mean survival of 359 days and 551 days, respectively, in dogs with pituitary tumors not treated with RT.[121] The 1-, 2-, and 3-year survival estimates for dogs treated with RT were 93%, 87%, and 55%, respectively.[121] In another study of dogs with pituitary tumors having undergone RT, median survival time was 1308 days with deaths related to tumor or radiation complications.[106] Despite these prolonged survival times, shorter times also have been reported, which may reflect variation in tumor biology or the presence and severity of neurologic signs.[104,147,148] The impact of neurologic signs on survival is unclear. The presence or absence of neurologic signs did not affect survival in some studies.[106,121] In other studies, shorter survival times have been observed in dogs with neurologic signs in which the median and mean survival times were 355 days and 477 day, respectively.[120] Less severe neurologic impairment was associated with longer survival times.[120] In addition, endocrine active tumors (i.e., those with hyperadrenocorticism) had longer survival times than those with endocrine inactive tumors.[120] Radiation therapy does not appear to predictably control endocrine function in dogs because many dogs continue to require medical therapy for hyperadrenocorticism.[120,121,147] In dogs experiencing initial control or resolution of endocrine dysfunction, recurrence of hyperadrenocorticism may occur months after RT.[120,147] Complications associated with RT for pituitary tumors include hearing loss, vestibular dysfunction, facial paralysis, and seizures.[120,147,148] In eight untreated dogs with pituitary tumors that developed neurologic signs, mean survival time was 141 days with five dogs surviving less than 2 months.[125]

Cats. As in dogs, RT appears to be the treatment of choice for cats with pituitary tumors. In most cats with pituitary tumors treated with RT, clinical signs have consisted of DM secondary to acromegaly without concurrent neurologic signs. In the two largest studies containing 14 and 12 cats each, the median survival was 28 and 18 months, respectively.[149,150] All cats had significant reduction in insulin requirements with approximately 50% of cats having experienced resolution of DM allowing discontinuation of insulin therapy. Although only a few reports exist detailing RT for the treatment of cats solely demonstrating neurologic signs, response to treatment and overall survival times have been similar to cats without neurologic signs.[149,151] Medical therapy for cats with acromegaly treated with exogenous administration of synthetic somatostatin or L-deprenyl does not appear to be effective.[124,152,153]

Tratment—Surgery. Several techniques for transsphenoidal hypophy-sectomy have been described in dogs.[154-156] Similar techniques have been used in cats.[157] Postoperatively, dogs must be supplemented with corticosteroids, thyroxine, and vasopressin to prevent crises related to hypoadrenocorticism, hypothyroidism, and diabetes insipidus, respectively.[158] Diabetes insipidus is usually transient but may require lifelong therapy.[158] Keratoconjunctivitis sicca may also occur.[158] Dehiscence of the incision in the soft palate occurs more commonly in cats.[157] Currently, availability of the procedure is extremely limited. Evaluation of the procedure in a large number of dogs has been limited to a single institution. In the largest case series of 180 dogs with PDH treated by transsphenoidal hypophysectomy, 155 dogs (85%) went into endocrine remission, with 119 dogs (77%) maintaining long-term remission.[159] The 1-, 2-, 3-, and 4-year estimated survival rates were 86%, 83%, 80%, and 79%, respectively. An enlarged pituitary gland was documented by imaging in 63 dogs (53%) that achieved remission suggesting a utility for surgery even in dogs with macrotumors. Fourteen dogs died within 4 weeks postoperatively. In dogs achieving remission, 36 dogs (23%) experienced recurrence after a median of 16 months likely as a result of the presence of residual pituitary tissue postoperatively. Factors that influenced survival and risk of recurrence included age, pituitary size, endocrine factors, and thickness of the sphenoid bone. Fewer cats have been treated with transsphenoidal hypophysectomy.[157,160,161] In one report of seven cats, two died of concurrent disease, five were alive 6 months postoperatively; all experienced remission of PDH with two cats also experiencing a resolution in DM.[157]

Tumors of the Calvaria. The two most common tumors that affect the calvaria are osteosarcoma (OSA) and multilobulated tumor of bone (multilobulated osteochondrosarcoma [MLO]) (Figure 12-16). Typically, tumors occur as a soft tissue or bony mass easily palpable on the head. Severe facial or ocular deformity may occur with tumors affecting the frontal bone or orbit. Definitive diagnosis requires histologic evaluation. Cross-sectional imaging is warranted when considering definitive treatment such as surgery or radiation therapy. Information regarding treatment and survival of dogs with OSA affecting the calvaria is derived from studies detailing tumors involving multiple anatomic areas of the

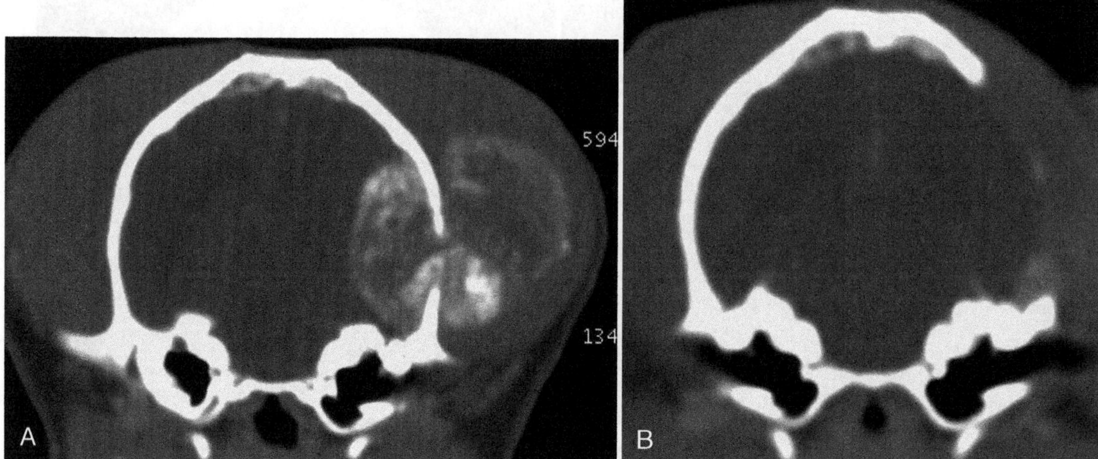

Figure 12-16 **A,** Axial CT image of the brain of a terrier mix. There is a large mass on the left parietal bone that has resulted in bone lysis of the calvaria. The mass extends into the cranial cavity. **B,** Axial CT image obtained after craniectomy for mass removal. Microscopic evaluation was consistent with a multilobulated tumor of bone. (Copyright 2010 University of Georgia Research Foundation, Inc.)

axial skeleton. Similar to appendicular OSA, affected dogs tend to be large breed dogs such as the German shepherd, Labrador retriever, and golden retriever, with a median age of 9 years.[162-164] At the time of presentation, the prevalence of metastatic disease ranges from 11% to 18%.[163-165] When combined with those dogs developing metastasis after diagnosis, the overall metastatic rate for OSA involving the skull is 40%.[164] Treatment involves surgery along with chemotherapy or radiation therapy. Despite multimodal therapy, most dogs die or are euthanized due to local recurrence.[163,164] Median survival ranges from 120 days to 154 days.[162-164] Prognostic factors include weight (longer survival in smaller dogs) and completeness of resection.[163]

Multilobulated tumor of bone occurs in large-breed dogs with a median weight of 29 kg and a median age of 8 years.[166] Often MLO results in a large mass.[167] Multilobulated tumor of bone demonstrates characteristic imaging features. With CT, MLO is characterized as a round to ovoid mass consisting of a nonhomogeneous bone density with well-defined margins and a granular appearance along with bony lysis of the calvaria.[168] With MRI, MLO appear hypointense on T1W images, mixed intensity consisting of areas of hypointensity and hyperintensity on T2W images, and demonstrates nonhomogeneous contrast enhancement (peripheral enhancement with central areas of strong uniform enhancement and areas without enhancement).[169] Unlike OSA, metastasis at the time of presentation is uncommon with MLO.[166] Surgery is the treatment of choice in tumors deemed resectable. In dogs with massive tumors, resection results in large calvarial defects necessitating cranioplasty. Multiple techniques have been employed using methylmethacrylate or titanium mesh to accomplish cranioplasty.[170-172] Only two studies have reported the clinical findings and survival times in a large number of dogs with MLO.[166,173] All dogs were treated with surgery. Given the difficulty in obtaining complete margins, local recurrence was 47% and 58% of affected dogs. Median time to local recurrence was 14 months and 26 months. Metastatic disease developed in 56% and 58% of dogs. In two studies, dogs treated with surgery alone or in combination with chemotherapy or radiation therapy, had an overall median survival time of 21 months and 26 months.[166,173] Histologic grade and degree of resection were prognostic factors for survival.[166]

No Focal or Lateralizing Signs

Acute Progressive

Inflammation (see Chapter 15). Inflammatory disease of the CNS may be the result of infection or immune-mediated inflammation (i.e., granulomatous meningoencephalomyelitis). Inflammatory disease of the CNS often results in an abnormal mental state. Stupor or coma results from a direct effect on neurons, cerebral edema, increased ICP, hypoxia from vasculitis, or systemic metabolic abnormalities.

Viral agents tend to have a greater effect on the nervous tissue. Vasculitis is common with rickettsial and some viral infections. Bacterial and fungal agents produce a greater meningeal reaction. Formulation of a diagnosis requires analysis of CSF analysis for cell counts, protein content, microbiologic testing, antibody or antigen titers, and PCR testing (see Chapter 4).

The management of animals with stupor or coma secondary to inflammatory disease includes treatment of the primary disease, if possible, management of increased ICP, and suppression of the inflammatory response. Increased ICP from cerebral edema and CNS inflammation should be treated with corticosteroids. Whereas suppression of the immune system by corticosteroids in an animal with an infectious disease may seem counterintuitive, the consequences of not treating the increased ICP and CNS inflammation are worse, namely, death. After an initial response to corticosteroids, rapid tapering of the dosage should be attempted. Ultimately, the least amount of corticosteroids should be used to control clinical signs in conjunction with antimicrobial drugs. See Chapter 15 for a complete discussion of inflammatory diseases.

Metabolic Diseases. The brain is the most energy demanding organ in the body and depends on a continuous supply of glucose and oxygen for normal function. It is protected from toxic substances by the BBB and requires a balance of electrolytes and neurotransmitters for appropriate excitability of the neurons. Alterations in brain metabolism can cause severe clinical signs ranging from depression to coma and from tremors to seizures. The most common metabolic problems causing stupor or coma are listed in Table 12-3. Hypoglycemia is discussed in Chapter 15. Hepatic encephalopathy, uremic encephalopathy, and diabetic coma are discussed in Chapter 15.

Heat Stroke. Heat stroke is an acute failure of the heat-regulating mechanisms of the body that results in a body temperature exceeding 40° C (105° F).[174,175] High ambient temperature, high humidity, and poor ventilation are the inciting factors. Brachycephalic breeds of dogs are especially susceptible. A long-haired coat, obesity, and high fever may also predispose the animal to heat stroke.

The primary mechanism for dissipation of heat in dogs and cats is panting. The airflow is unidirectional—in through the nose and out through the mouth.[176] The large surface area of the nasal turbinates promotes heat exchange. Prolonged panting causes respiratory alkalosis that later is modified by metabolic acidosis, presumably from increased muscular activity or dehydration. If hyperthermia continues, cerebral edema and DIC occur frequently, either of which can cause death. Although all of the CNS is involved, the neurons of the cerebral cortex and the cerebellum seem most susceptible to permanent damage.[177,178] The diagnosis of heat stroke is based on the clinical signs and elevation of the body temperature.

The three major objectives of treatment are to reduce body temperature, prevent cerebral edema, and manage DIC if it develops. The body temperature is decreased by administration of cool intravenous fluids or bathing the animal in cold or iced water. The rectal temperature should be monitored continuously or at 10-minute intervals. To prevent hypothermia, cooling is stopped when the rectal temperature reaches 39.5° C (103° F). Iced-water enemas may be used in refractory cases, but they prevent accurate monitoring of body temperature.

If the animal shows evidence of cerebral edema, especially if signs of tentorial herniation are present (see Table 12-2), mannitol or HTS should be administered intravenously. Coagulation function should be monitored and addressed if abnormal. Hemorrhagic diarrhea, petechiae, or excessive bleeding from venipuncture sites may signify thrombocytopenia or the onset of DIC. Fluids should be given intravenously to maintain cardiac output and renal function. Overhydration must be avoided.

The animals should be monitored carefully for at least 24 hours after normothermia is achieved so that recurrences can be prevented. The prognosis with heat stroke is relatively good if treated early (i.e., before signs of cerebral edema or DIC develop).

Hypoxia. Hypoxia is an inadequate supply of oxygen for normal brain function. Arterial oxygen tension levels below 50 mm Hg are detrimental to brain function. Increased levels of carbon dioxide have a profound effect on cerebral blood flow (see Traumatic Brain Injury section). Because no oxygen reserves are present in the brain, merely a few minutes of hypoxia can cause irreversible damage. More than 10 minutes of hypoxia will produce neuronal death. The cerebral cortex and cerebellum are most susceptible to hypoxic damage, and the lower brainstem is most resistant.

The most frequent causes of hypoxia in animals are anesthesia accidents, cardiopulmonary failure, suffocation, smoke inhalation, paralysis of respiration, carbon monoxide poisoning, cyanide poisoning, and near drowning. Despite the almost universal use of inhalation anesthesia with controlled ventilation, complications of anesthesia are common. Cardiac arrhythmias, overdoses of the anesthetic agent, improper intubations, and faulty apparatuses are but a few of the problems encountered. Meticulous attention to detail in the administration and the monitoring of anesthesia is essential.

Heart, lung, and peripheral circulatory failure rival anesthesia and are also frequent causes of hypoxia. Heart and lung disease may cause a mild to severe hypoxemia. If the condition does not cause unconsciousness, the danger of cerebral damage is low. Hypotensive shock may cause profound decreases in cerebral blood flow and cerebral hypoxia, which may lead to irreversible neuronal loss. A primary concern in the management of hypotensive shock is the restoration of blood pressure, ventilation, and oxygenation. Management of the various forms of cardiopulmonary failure, however, is beyond the scope of this text.

Suffocation is a less frequent problem in animals. Examples of causes are aspiration of vomitus, especially in injured or anesthetized animals; aspiration of foreign bodies; and near drowning. Although many animals experiencing near drowning have loss of consciousness, and an abnormal mental state including stupor or coma, neurologic dysfunction may not impact survival.[179]

Paralysis of respiration may occur with lesions of the CNS between the medullary respiratory centers and the origin of the phrenic nerve at C5-7 spinal cord segments (sometimes C4). Occasionally, ventilatory failure is severe enough to require mechanical ventilation.[180] The lesion may affect the respiratory center directly, or it may interrupt the descending pathway in the cervical spinal cord and produce the same effect: apnea. Lesions in the lower cervical spinal cord (C7) or the cranial thoracic region may block these UMN pathways to the intercostal lower motor neurons, but the intact phrenic pathway allows diaphragmatic ("abdominal") breathing to occur. The most common cause of this lesion is trauma. Occasionally, cervical intervertebral disk herniation may also impair respiration.[181] Generalized lower motor neuron (LMN) disease also may cause respiratory paralysis through its effect on both the intercostal and phrenic nerves (see Chapter 7).

Carbon Monoxide. Carbon monoxide (CO) poisoning occurs occasionally in animals exposed in house fires.[182,183] CO preferentially and competitively binds to hemoglobin, forming carboxyhemoglobin. CO has 200 to 230 times greater affinity for hemoglobin (Hb) than oxygen.[184] With CO binding, the O_2 carrying capacity of Hb is reduced, which leads to hypoxemia and hypoxia. In addition to displacing O_2, the Hb molecule undergoes a conformational change, which causes a greater affinity for oxygen at heme sites not binding CO, which shifts the O_2-dissociation curve to the left.[185] The shift in the O_2-dissociation curve to the left further impairs O_2 delivery.[185] Affected animals typically have bright red mucous membranes and rapid, shallow respiration. In dogs, CO toxicity results in ataxia, menace response deficits, loss of consciousness, alterations in mental state, head tremors, twitching, and seizures.[182,183,186-189] Neurologic consequences of CO toxicity are divided into acute and delayed toxicity. Delayed toxicity involves a myelinopathy affecting the cerebral deep white matter such as the centrum semiovale, periventricular white matter, and the corpus callosum symmetrically.[189-191] Recovery from delayed toxicity is possible.[189] Acute toxicity involves neuronal necrosis of the pallidum, substantia nigra, cerebellum, and the hippocampus and demyelination and necrosis of the deep white matter of the cerebral hemispheres.[190] Recovery from acute toxicity likely depends on the severity. In most animals, the respiratory tract also is involved. Treatment is mainly supportive and is aimed at correction of respiratory pathology, hypotension, and hypoxemia. Fluid therapy and supplemental oxygen should be provided. Although not widely available, hyperbaric oxygen chambers may aid in recovery of affected animals by increasing the elimination rate of CO.

Equine Hypoxic and Ischemic Encephalopathy. Equine hypoxic and ischemic encephalopathy (neonatal maladjustment syndrome, peripartum asphyxia syndrome, dummy foal) has been recognized for many years in newborn foals. Ischemic or hypoxic damage of many organs is the suspected cause.[192] Neurologic abnormalities usually develop within 24 hours after birth but may occur up to a week postpartum. The severity of neurologic signs depends on the degree and duration of hypoxia. Mild signs include loss of attentiveness toward the mare, jitteriness, and hyperalertness. More severe signs include irregular respirations, apnea, random intermittent tongue protrusions and sucking behavior, drooling, strabismus, and nystagmus. Some foals may show stiff, rhythmic marching behavior; others may wander aimlessly, may be depressed or stuporous, and may circle in one direction.[192]

Generalized seizures are a common finding. Vocalizations of severely affected foals may sound like a dog's bark (barker foals), and this sign is often accompanied by generalized seizures. The most severely affected foals may be comatose and completely hypotonic, showing seizures and apnea.[192] Pathologically, ischemic necrosis of the cerebral cortical neurons, multifocal areas of brain and meningeal hemorrhages, and edema are observed in affected foals.[193,194]

In addition to the CNS signs, other signs of systemic organ failure may be present. Renal hypoxia produces elevated serum creatinine levels, oliguria, hypocalcemia, hyponatremia, and hypochloridemia. Gastrointestinal signs include colic, ileus, bloody diarrhea, and gastric reflux. Cardiac signs include arrhythmia, tachycardia, murmur, hypotension, and generalized edema. Icterus may develop in foals with hypoxic liver injury.

The diagnosis is based on the characteristic clinical signs of multiple organ dysfunction occurring within 24 to 48 hours of birth. Septic meningitis (see Chapter 15) may cause similar neurologic signs. CSF is normal in foals with hypoxic and ischemic encephalopathy, and neutrophilic pleocytosis and elevated protein concentrations are typical CSF findings in foals with septic meningitis.

Treatment is supportive. Phenobarbital and diazepam may be used to control seizures. The prognosis is poor for severely affected foals with multiple organ involvement. Less severely affected foals that survive the first few days may regain vision and suckling ability, and some make complete recoveries.[192]

Hypertensive Encephalopathy

Pathophysiology. The prevalence of hypertension (HT) has become increasingly recognized in dogs and cats. Normal systolic blood pressure ranges between 118 to 162 mm Hg in healthy cats.[195-197] In dogs, normal systolic blood pressure values range from 131 to 154 mm Hg.[197-199] Many factors can alter the measurement of blood pressure including technical reasons such as the type of recording device, cuff size, and operator skill, and patient factors such as size and demeanor of the animal. Although the prevalence of hypertension in healthy animals has not been definitively established, estimates in dogs range from 0.5% to 10% while in cats an estimate of 2% has been reported.[197] In cats evaluated for signs related to HT or for evaluation of disease associated with HT, a 30% prevalence of HT was found.[200] In dogs, the prevalence of HT may be as high as 93% and 87% with such diseases as renal disease and hyperadrenocorticism, respectively.[197]

There are three main etiologic classifications for HT: white coat, secondary, and idiopathic hypertension. White coat hypertension is an artifactual increase in blood pressure secondary to activation of the sympathetic nervous system associated with fear, excitement, or anxiety.[201] While white coat hypertension does not cause a clinical problem, it does complicate definitive documentation of HT. Secondary hypertension develops as a consequence of systemic disease. In cats, secondary HT is commonly associated with renal disease and hyperthyroidism.[202-208] In dogs, secondary HT is commonly associated with renal disease and hyperadrenocorticism.[197,209] Idiopathic HT is defined as the presence of HT in the absence of other disease conditions associated with HT. It has also been called primary or essential hypertension. Although the prevalence of idiopathic HT is unknown in dogs, approximately 20% of cats with HT are consider idiopathic.[203,210]

Chronic systemic hypertension has a variety of pathologic consequences, referred to as end organ or target organ damage (TOD). Importantly TOD involves the kidneys, eyes, heart, and nervous system.[211] In the kidney, TOD leads to an accelerated decline in renal function and proteinuria. Hypertension can exist at any stage of renal disease including non-azotemic animals.[197] In the eye, HT leads to hypertensive retinopathy and choroidopathy, which commonly causes blindness.[203,205,210,212-215] In the heart, HT may result in cardiomegaly and left ventricular hypertrophy.[205,210,214,216] In the nervous system, HT may result in a hypertensive encephalopathy.[205,207,208,210,217] Neurologic signs have been reported in 29% and 46% of cats with hypertension.[205,210] In one study in hypertensive dogs, 3 of 14 dogs had developed neurologic signs.[218]

Neurologic signs reflect forebrain and vestibular dysfunction. Signs of forebrain involvement include seizures and changes in mentation, whereas vestibular dysfunction includes head tilt, vestibular ataxia, and abnormal nystagmus.[205,207,208,210,217] Other neurologic signs include blindness, weakness, ataxia, tremors, episodes of the paraparesis, and decerebrate postures.[205,207,208,210,217]

The pathophysiology of hypertensive encephalopathy likely involves vasogenic edema affecting the white matter.[219,220] Edema develops when the autoregulatory capacity of the brain vasculature is exceeded leading to hyperperfusion and breakdown of the BBB, which leads to edema.[219,221] In experimentally induced acute HT in cats, coning of the vermis of the cerebellum, cerebellar herniation into the foramen magnum, rostral displacement of the colliculi, and widening and flattening of the cerebral gyri develop as a consequence to increased intracranial pressure.[217] With chronic HT, there is hypertrophy and hyperplasia of the smooth muscle of the brain vasculature from chronic vasoconstriction.[210] These degenerative changes predispose to microhemorrhages.[210] Multifocal cerebral arteriosclerosis with hemorrhages has been observed in naturally occurring HT in cats.[205]

Assessment. A diagnosis of HT encephalopathy is suggested in hypertensive animals (systolic blood pressure of 160 to 170 mm Hg) demonstrating signs of forebrain dysfunction alone or in combination with vestibular dysfunction. As most cases are considered secondary hypertension, affected animals should also be screened for an underlying condition. Cross-sectional imaging should be considered in animals not demonstrating neurologic improvement concurrent with a reduction in systolic blood pressure. Moreover, cross-sectional imaging helps rule out other disease processes that may result in similar neurologic signs. Although not documented in animals, abnormalities associated with HT in humans consist of hyperintensities on T2W images in the white matter of the cerebrum.[219] Similar lesions may be present in the brainstem.[222]

Treatment. Immediate treatment is reserved for animals with severe hypertension that have neurologic abnormalities. In dogs, angiotensin-converting enzyme inhibitors are the drug of choice for the treatment of HT.[223] In cats, amlodipine besylate, a calcium channel blocker, is the drug of choice for HT.[223]

In acute HT, subcutaneous hydralazine has been effective at reducing blood pressure without significant risk of hypotension.[206,223] While parenteral hypotensive medications such as nitroprusside may be preferable in the setting of severe hypertensive encephalopathy, the use of parenteral hypotensive medications is associated with significant risk of hypotension and therefore requires continuous, direct arterial blood pressure measurement.

Inborn Errors of Metabolism. These are diseases that interfere with function at the biochemical level or lead to death of neurons. Some are caused by a deficiency in a key enzyme causing buildup of byproducts (e.g., lysosomal storage diseases) and neuronal dysfunction (see Chapter 15). Diagnosis of these diseases is based on suspicion in cases of young, purebred animals and exclusion of other diseases that may have similar clinical signs. Chemistry profiles with abnormalities in lactic acid, anion gap, bicarbonate, and glucose may raise the index of suspicion for these disorders. Elevated ketone concentrations may be identified in urinalysis. The urine can be screened for organic acid abnormalities. Typically, brain MRI demonstrates diffuse and symmetric changes that predominate in the gray or white matter. Some of these diseases can be managed with dietary adjustments.

Organic acidurias are characterized by presence of abnormal organic acids as a result of an error in a metabolic pathway. Maltese dogs from a family with malonic aciduria developed seizures and stupor.[224] Hypoglycemia, acidosis, and ketonuria were identified. The clinical signs resolved after the diet was altered to feed one that was high in carbohydrate and low in fat.[224] Cobalamin (vitamin B_{12}) is a necessary cofactor for the Krebs cycle. Cobalamin deficiency has been associated with methylmalonic aciduria and encephalopathic signs in cats with a deficiency of intrinsic factor necessary for cobalamin absorption.[225,226] Similar signs were reported in cats with gastrointestinal disease, which also interfered with cobalamin absorption.[227] D-lactic acidosis also has been reported in cats with gastrointestinal disease. Bacterial overgrowth led to the overproduction of the D-isoform of lactic acid.[228]

L-2-hydroxyglutaric aciduria is an inborn error of metabolism that affects humans and Staffordshire bull terriers.[229] In Staffordshire bull terriers, neurologic signs developed between 4 months and 7 years of age. Four of six dogs had chronic progressive disease, and two dogs experienced an acute onset of seizures between 4 and 6 months of age.[29] Neurologic signs include seizures, ataxia, dementia, and head tremor. Levels of L-2-hydroxyglutaric acid and lysine were elevated in urine, CSF, and plasma. MRI disclosed symmetrical and extensive polioencephalopathy suggestive of a metabolic or toxic disorder. CSF analysis was normal. A mutation in the dehydrogenase that metabolizes L-2-hydroxyglutaric acid has been described.[230] No definitive treatment is available.

Nutritional Diseases. Thiamine deficiency may cause stupor or coma, especially in ruminants. Polioencephalomalacia, a symmetric laminar necrosis of the cerebral cortex, occurs in cattle, sheep, and goats. Increased ICP is common. Thiamine deficiency is discussed in Chapter 15.

Chronic Progressive

Degenerative Diseases. Storage diseases, which are inherited degenerative diseases with accumulation of metabolic products in neurons, can cause depression or stupor. The animal may be in a coma terminally. Other signs, such as cerebellar ataxia or seizures, are more common in the early stages of the disease (see Chapters 8 and 15).

Anomalous Conditions. The nervous system has been reported as the most frequently affected organ system by congenital defects.[231] Malformations of the CNS are often caused by abnormalities of morphogenesis that include defects in neural tube closure and abnormalities in neuronal migration. Other malformations result from an altered inductive influence controlled by specific genes of a regionally specified mesoderm.[232] Programmed cell death refers to a process by which cells die during normal development, is an expression of terminal differentiation, and involves new gene expression. This process is critical for achieving correct population size and proper morphogenesis of brain structures. Table 12-8 summarizes common malformations of the forebrain. Cerebellar malformations are described in Chapter 8.

Early in development, the embryo consists of three germ cell layers: ectoderm, mesoderm, and endoderm. The outermost layer, ectoderm, becomes the epidermal, neural and skeletal, and connective tissues of the head. The mesoderm becomes muscle and skeletal tissues and is divided into somites. Each somite separates into dermatomal, myotomal, and sclerotomal regions. The endoderm forms into structures and lining of the respiratory and alimentary tracts.

The neural tube is the progenitor of the CNS and is surrounded by the axial skeleton. Precise timing of embryogenesis must occur for successful neural tube development.[233] The cephalic portion of the neural tube is delineated into three primary vesicles: forebrain (prosencephalon), midbrain (mesencephalon), and hindbrain (rhombencephalon).[234] The forebrain expands to form the prosencephalon that develops into paired telencephalic and optic structures, the diencephalon and third ventricle. The telencephalon subsequently becomes the cerebrum and lateral ventricles. The midbrain remains a small undifferentiated structure, which encompasses the mesencephalic aqueduct. The hindbrain subdivides rostrally into the metencephalon and caudally into the myelencephalon. The metencephalon develops further to become the pons and cerebellum. The myelencephalon forms into the medulla oblongata. After primary neurulation, the neuroblasts proliferate, differentiate into neurons, and migrate. Most of the reported developmental anomalies usually occur during this stage of development.

Neural tube defects result in brain or spinal cord malformations and occur early in gestation as a direct result of defective closure or reopening of the neural tube. Nomenclature of neural tube closure defects provides a description of the type and location of the defect. Neural tube defects are classified as open if neural tissue is exposed or covered only by membrane, or as closed if the defect is covered by normal skin. Neural tube defects also are divided into cranial (brain) and caudal (terminal spinal cord) types. Caudal defects represent anomalies associated with the secondary neurulation process, which produce the neural tube in the sacral and coccygeal regions (see Chapter 6). Embryologic abnormalities of the neural tube often are accompanied by secondary bony defects.

Neural crest cells are condensations of neuroepithelium that form dorsal to the neural tube and give rise to peripheral and autonomic nervous systems, the adrenal medulla, and pigmentary cells. In the cranial region, the population of neural crest cells is quite large. Cranial neural crest cells are a prerequisite for folding of the neural tube and migrate from the neural folds early in embryogenesis.[233] These neural crest cells become the mesenchyme of the face and base of the calvaria. The cells also contribute to the spiral septum in the outflow tract of the heart; therefore agents affecting this tissue migration process are likely to cause defects of the face and heart.

Major differentials for congenital cranial and brain malformations include prenatal or perinatal exposure to infectious diseases and toxins. Some conditions are inherited. Teratogens are external factors that adversely affect embryonic development during the critical period for an organ system.[235] Commonly recognized teratogens include toxins, drugs, viral infections, oversupplementation and undersupplementation of nutrients and environmental factors (e.g., radiation exposure and maternal hyperthermia). The CNS is sensitive to teratogenic insult throughout prenatal and early postnatal development.[235] For many congenital nervous system defects, the cause is difficult to determine, thus is unknown. Other diseases that can mimic congenital defects include lysosomal storage diseases, inborn errors of metabolism, and other inherited degenerative disorders (see Chapters 8 and 15).

TABLE 12-8

Classification of Forebrain Malformations in Domestic Animals

Congenital Defect	Description
Hydrocephalus	Communicating/noncommunicating (obstructive) Internal/external Hydrocephalus ex-vacuo (compensatory) Congenital
Hydranencephaly/Porencephaly	
Primary neural tube defects	Exencephaly/anencephaly Craniorachischisis (cranium bifidum)
Primary axial mesodermal defects	Encephalocele Meningocele Craniofacial mesodermal defects Cleft palate
Disorders of forebrain induction	Holoprosencephaly Arrhinencephaly Cyclopia Agenesis of corpus callosum Microencephaly
Disorders of neuronal migration	Lissencephaly/pachygyria Polymicrogyria Heterotopia

Hydrocephalus

Pathophysiology. Hydrocephalus is the presence of excessive CSF within the brain or cranial cavity. CSF flows from the lateral ventricles through the interventricular foramina to the third ventricle. It continues caudally through the mesencephalic aqueduct to the fourth ventricle and into the subarachnoid space through the lateral apertures of the fourth ventricle. In the subarachnoid space, most of the fluid moves around the brainstem into the rostrotentorial compartment. Most of the absorption occurs through the arachnoid villi in the dorsal sagittal sinus. Absorption also can occur via venous and lymphatic drainage around spinal and cranial nerves. Most of the CSF is produced by the choroid plexus in the lateral, third, and fourth ventricles, but a substantial portion is also produced by the ependyma lining the ventricles, vasculature of the leptomeninges, and pia overlying the brain and spinal cord. Production of CSF is independent of hydrostatic pressure within the ventricles. However, production of CSF is dependent on osmotic pressure, an aspect used in the treatment of

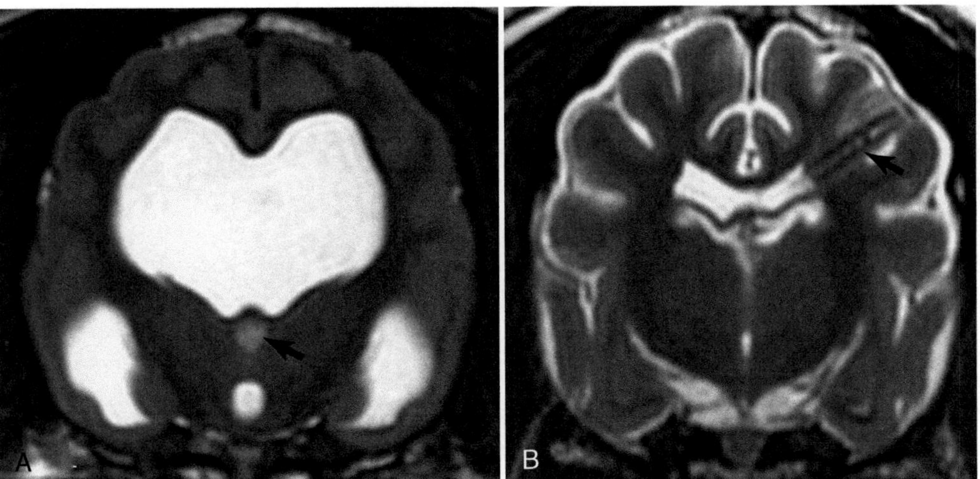

Figure 12-17 **A,** Axial T2W images of the brain of a bulldog with severely dilated lateral ventricles. The third ventricle was also dilated and contained a lesion that extended into the mesencephalic aqueduct *(arrow)*. **B,** Two months after placement of a ventriculoperitoneal (VP) shunt, the ventricular dilation has resolved. The VP shunt can be observed penetrating the left parietal lobe of the cerebrum as it courses toward the lateral ventricle *(arrow)*. (Copyright 2010 University of Georgia Research Foundation, Inc.)

hydrocephalus. Overproduction of CSF by choroid plexus tumors is rare.

Hydrocephalus can be categorized based on the location of excessive CSF and pathogenesis. When CSF accumulates within the ventricular system, it is known as *internal hydrocephalus*. When CSF accumulates within an enlarged area of the subarachnoid space, it is referred to as *external hydrocephalus*. Additionally, excessive CSF may be the result of obstruction to flow (noncommunicating or obstructive hydrocephalus), decreased absorption, or increased production (communicating hydrocephalus). Hydrocephalus also may occur secondary to loss or destruction of CNS parenchyma. Secondary ventricular dilation or expansion of the subarachnoid space occurs in order to occupy the void created by the absence of CNS parenchyma. The term hydrocephalus *ex vacuo* or secondary hydrocephalus describes this process. Based on etiology, hydrocephalus may be acquired or congenital. Hydrocephalus may be seen in any species and is more often congenital than acquired.

Communicating hydrocephalus from decreased absorption of CSF is usually the result of inflammation of the meninges. Inflammation is usually caused by infectious diseases such as occurs with viral infections like canine distemper or feline infectious peritonitis viruses but may be secondary to subarachnoid hemorrhage or to the presence of foreign materials such as radiographic contrast materials that are injected in the subarachnoid space.[236] Congenital absence of the lateral apertures also has been documented.[237] Communicating hydrocephalus has been observed in dogs with ciliary dyskinesia.[238] A lack of CSF flow due to dysfunction of the cilia of the ependyma is thought to explain the development of hydrocephalus. Noncommunicating hydrocephalus secondary to obstruction of CSF flow occurs frequently. Although obstruction can be present at any site, most commonly it is located at the mesencephalic aqueduct. Malformations of the aqueduct range from complete absence to stenosis. Obstruction of the aqueduct also can be secondary to inflammation, infection, or compression by a mass. For example, brainstem tumors that cause obstruction of the aqueduct produce hydrocephalus[239] (Figure 12-17).

Hydrocephalus is a common malformation in domestic animals and most cases of hydrocephalus that are seen in veterinary practice are congenital. The disorder may be caused by environmental (toxic, infectious, deficiencies) or genetic factors. In calves, vitamin A deficiency can result in decreased absorption of CSF via the arachnoid villi and consequent hydrocephalus.[240] Deformities of the temporal bone can obstruct CSF flow, producing hydrocephalus. In foals, a variety of neurologic signs may be seen.[241] Some foals may be normal behaviorally and neurologically. Other foals may display signs such as depression, dementia, and seizures. Inherited conditions have been reported in a number of dairy and beef cattle breeds.[242] Ingestion of plants like *Veratrum californicum* and *Astragalus* spp. by ewes and cows has been shown to cause hydrocephalus in lambs and calves.[243,244]

Congenital hydrocephalus in dogs and cats is usually recognized in the very young animal. The increase in intracranial volume occurs before the sutures of the calvaria have closed, allowing for enlargement of the cranial cavity. In most animal species, the enlargement of the head, the open sutures and persistent fontanelles, and the poor development of the animal may be recognized shortly after birth.

Clinical Signs. Affected dogs are usually taken to the veterinarian when they are between 2 and 3 months of age, sometimes when they are older. Palpation of the skull may reveal the persistent sutures and fontanelles. The prominent frontal areas encroach on the orbits, causing ventrolateral deviation of the eyes (Figure 12-18). Oculomotor nerve function (pupils and eye movements) (see Chapter 11) is usually normal, indicating that the eye deviation is mechanical, not neurologic, in origin. The widening of the skull is detected by palpation of the parietal area, where the space between the skull and the zygomatic arch is narrowed. Additionally, the width of the cranium may extend beyond the zygomatic arches. Head pain may be evident in some animals when the head is palpated.

Puppies and kittens with hydrocephalus usually are smaller and less developed than their littermates. They are often dull, have episodic behavioral changes such as aggression or confusion, and frequently have seizures (see Chapter 13). Because their mental development is poor, they do not learn as readily as their littermates. Visual deficits with normal PLRs are common because of damage to the optic radiation and the occipital cortex (see Chapter 11). Motor function may range from an almost normal gait to severe tetraparesis. Occasionally, asymmetric signs may occur. Despite the fact that ventricular enlargement is limited to the lateral ventricles, episodes

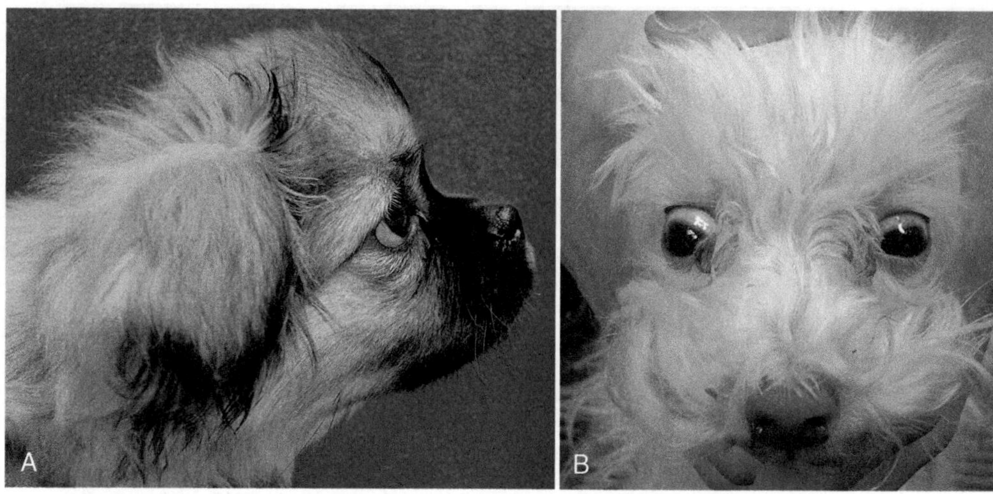

Figure 12-18 **A,** A young Pekingese dog with congenital hydrocephalus. Note the large, domed head, which is characteristic. **B,** A young Maltese terrier with congenital hydrocephalus. Ventrolateral strabismus is the result of encroachment of the orbits by the frontal bones. (Copyright 2010 University of Georgia Research Foundation, Inc.)

of vestibular dysfunction can occur. Papilledema may be seen on fundic examination in a small percentage of cases. Hydrocephalus can lead to abnormal hypothalamic function. Hypodipsic hypernatremia, possibly as a result of pressure atrophy of hypothalamic osmoreceptors, has been observed.[245,246]

In dogs, too few studies of congenital hydrocephalus have been performed to determine the primary defect.[247] A statistically significant correlation between breed, size, and body weight of the dam and hydrocephalus has been demonstrated in dogs (Table 12-9).[248] Some patients have stenosis or atresia of the mesencephalic aqueduct, but others do not.[237,249] In addition to hydrocephalus, other prevalent abnormalities include the formation of diverticula and clefts in periventricular white matter.[237] Concurrent periventricular encephalitis has accompanied such lesions.[237,247] Inflammation may represent a response to necrotic tissue.[237] Alternatively, the presence of periventricular inflammation has led to the suggestion of an underlying etiologic agent.[250]

Ventricular enlargement without clinical signs is a common finding in some toy breeds, especially Chihuahuas, Yorkshire terriers, and Maltese dogs. A kennel of Chihuahuas was studied by Redding.[251] Subclinical hydrocephalus was common. Behavioral changes could be correlated with abnormal electrical encephalography (EEG) in many instances. A selective breeding program in which the EEG was used to screen breeding animals reduced the incidence of hydrocephalus. Redding concluded that the dogs had a compensated hydrocephalus (a balance between production and absorption of CSF) that could be decompensated by relatively mild changes such as trauma or infection. Redding also observed a high incidence of enlargement of the foramen magnum (occipital dysplasia) in these dogs. Whether this abnormality is related to the cause of hydrocephalus or whether it is secondary to increased ICP is unknown. The clinical signs were related to the (1) age at onset, (2) degree of imbalance between production and absorption of CSF, and (3) location of the defect (communicating or noncommunicating).

Simpson[252] studied a series of hydrocephalic Maltese dogs. Fewer than 20% had seizures, with most seizures occurring during the first year of life. Behavioral problems were the most frequent findings. Learned responses such as house training were difficult or impossible to achieve in 75% of the dogs.

Bull terriers affected with complex focal seizures also have a high incidence of moderate to severe hydrocephalus.[253] It is unlikely that the behavioral signs in these dogs are directly related to the concurrent hydrocephalus.

TABLE 12-9

Breeds of Dogs at Increased Risk of Hydrocephalus

Maltese
Yorkshire terrier
English bulldog
Chihuahua
Lhasa apso
Pomeranian
Toy poodle
Cairn terrier
Boston terrier
Pug
Pekingese

Data from Selby LA, Hayes HM, Becker SV: Epizootiologic features of canine hydrocephalus, Am J Vet Res 40:411–414, 1979.

External hydrocephalus is the accumulation of CSF in the subarachnoid space. Often present as a consequence of CNS parenchymal loss, external hydrocephalus as a primary entity has been reported in a dog and two cats.[254,255] Cerebrospinal fluid analysis disclosed pleocytosis and elevated protein content in all affected animals. Bacterial meningoencephalitis was suspected in the dog and may have played a role in one cat. Successful outcome occurred following surgical placement of a CSF shunting device (see later discussion).

Based on clinical signs alone, hydrocephalus in the adult animal is more difficult to recognize. In animals having reached skeletal maturity, the size of the cranial cavity remains normal because the sutures have fused before the increase in ICP. The clinical signs develop more rapidly and are more severe, but they are dependent on the relative balance of production and absorption of CSF. Seizures are a frequent sign in the early stages. Dullness, which may progress to stupor or coma, is common. Because hydrocephalus in the adult is usually secondary to inflammation or a mass, signs of the primary problem may predominate early in the course of the disease. Complete obstruction of the CSF causes a rapidly progressive hydrocephalus, which may cause tentorial herniation, cerebellar herniation, or both.

Assessment. The presumptive diagnosis of hydrocephalus in the young animal is relatively straightforward if the characteristic signs are present. Although the clinical signs of severe hydrocephalus are typical, less severe involvement may produce a more subtle picture. Behavioral changes or seizures may be the only complaint. In most cases, ancillary studies are necessary to confirm the diagnosis.

The definitive diagnosis can be confirmed with imaging procedures. Magnetic resonance imaging is the imaging modality of choice because it not only allows identification of ventricular or subarachnoid dilation but also because it allows identification of an underlying etiology (e.g., mass obstructing CSF flow) or existence of concurrent disease (e.g., meningoencephalitis). This is particularly important in the evaluation of animals in which ventriculomegaly is a common finding, such as in toy breed dogs. In congenital hydrocephalus, MRI discloses enlarged ventricles containing fluid with MRI characteristics consistent with CSF (Figure 12-19). Ventriculomegaly is often confined to the lateral ventricles and may be asymmetric. Secondary parenchymal changes may be observed. Frequently, the periventricular white matter is hyperintense compared with normal white matter on T2W images. Changes in periventricular white matter are more conspicuous on T2W fluid attenuated inversion recovery sequences and likely represent interstitial edema. Although less sensitive in discrimination of soft tissues, CT may also be used in the diagnosis of hydrocephalus. In young animals or those with persistent fontanelles, US using a persistent fontanelle as an acoustic window can be used in the diagnosis of hydrocephalus.[256,257] The main benefit of US is that it can be performed without the need for sedation or general anesthesia, thereby allowing examination of very young animals with little to no morbidity. However, US lacks the sensitivity in discriminating a primary or concurrent disease process. Following US examination, MRI or CT should be performed in affected animals before pursuing therapeutic interventions, especially surgical treatments. Radiography of the head can confirm persistent suture lines and fontanelles. In congenital hydrocephalus, thinning of the calvaria with loss of the normal digitate impressions of the cerebral gyri on the inner surface of the calvaria is absent. The cranial cavity may have a ground–glasslike appearance.

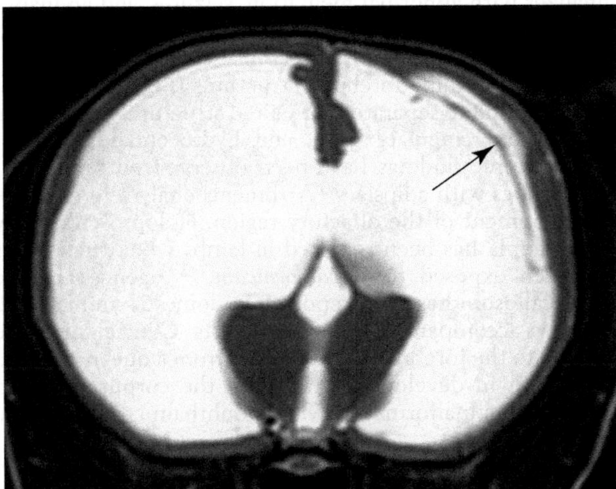

Figure 12-19 Axial T2W image of the brain of a Maltese terrier at the level of the thalamus. The lateral ventricles are extremely dilated as is the third ventricle. There is severe loss of the overlying cerebral cortex. The gyrations of the cerebral cortex are not evident. A cleft is evident in the periventricular white matter *(arrow)*. (Copyright 2010 University of Georgia Research Foundation, Inc.)

Given the wide variation and size and morphology of the canine head, ventricular dimensions likely vary among breeds. Ventricular size, symmetry, and volume have been reported in a few breeds using MRI and US.[258-263] Ventricular size has been defined in kittens up to 5.5 months of age using ultrasonographic evaluation via the bregmatic fontanelle.[264]

Analysis of the CSF may be useful for identifying an etiologic diagnosis. Caution should be exercised before performing a CSF collection in animals with suspected increased ICP (see Chapter 4). Therapeutic measures directed at lowering intracranial pressure should be performed before pursuing a spinal tap. In rare instances, CSF can be obtained by a ventricular tap under general anesthesia.

Treatment. The treatment of hydrocephalus depends on the cause of the disorder and the status of the animal. Acquired hydrocephalus in the adult animal requires resolution of the inciting factor. An inflammatory disease may cause permanent reduction of absorptive capacity, and the hydrocephalus must be managed separately. Treatment involves medical, surgical, or combined therapies. Affected animals usually are in one of the following three categories: (1) mild to severe static signs, (2) acute with rapidly progressive signs (in an animal that was previously normal or previously static tearing of parenchyma may be associated with sudden decline in neurologic status or may exhibit a chronicity of several days[237]), and (3) chronic progressive deterioration.

Animals with mild signs that are static may not require treatment. Animals with severe static or acute progressive signs indicate a poor prognosis and the need for intensive treatment aimed at reducing CSF production and vasogenic or interstitial edema. Unfortunately, animals with severe static signs are unlikely to improve. Initial therapy is directed at medical treatment. Hyperosmolar fluids (mannitol or HTS) can be given to reduce CSF production and vasogenic edema in severely affected animals. Furosemide (0.7 mg/kg intravenously given 15 minutes after completion of the mannitol infusion) may be administered to prolong the effect of mannitol. Hyperosmolar fluids can be repeated as needed every 4 to 6 hours based on clinical signs. Before administration of hyperosmolar fluids or furosemide, assessment of hydration is necessary. If possible, these drugs should not be used in dehydrated animals. Corticosteroids also may be administered at an antiinflammatory dosage (prednisone 0.5 to 1.0 mg/kg) to reduce CSF production and interstitial edema. Anticonvulsant drugs (i.e., phenobarbital) should be used if needed. Animals displaying improvement should be considered for the same long-term treatment as provided for chronic progressive cases.

Animals with chronic progressive deterioration of hydrocephalus, as indicated by the history and serial neurologic examinations, may be treated medically or surgically. Although therapy may stop progression and result in improvement in clinical signs, owners must be made aware that the animal will not likely be totally normal. Following initial therapy, if the neurologic status prevent the animal from functioning as a pet, continued treatment should not be considered. Medical treatment as defined above usually is tried first. Clinical improvement is expected within 3 days. If improvement is seen, the dosage of corticosteroids should be reduced by half after 1 week. After another week, corticosteroids are given once every other day. If signs are stable, medication may be discontinued and repeated only as signs develop. Many animals stabilize in remission and only occasionally require medication. Others require continuous medication. Low-dose, alternate-day therapy can be used for extended periods without problems.

Acetazolamide, a carbonic anhydrase inhibitor, can be used to reduce CSF production. The dosage is 10 mg/kg orally every 6 to 8 hours. Acetazolamide should be used short term. Electrolyte and acid-base status should be monitored. Acetazolamide alone or in combination with corticosteroids or other diuretics can cause metabolic acidosis and hypokalemia.[265] Alternatively, omeprazole (0.7 mg/kg/day or 10 mg/day for dogs <20 kg or 20 mg/day for dogs >20 kg), H^+/K^+ pump inhibitor can be used alone or in combination with other medications to reduce CSF production.[266] The objective of medical treatment is to provide remission of signs with the least possible amount of medication.

Surgical treatment is reserved for animals that require medical therapy to maintain clinical remission yet experience side effects that achieve only partial remission with medical therapy, or that cannot be stabilized medically. Surgical treatment entails placement of a CSF drainage device (shunt) that diverts CSF from the lateral ventricle through a one-way pressure valve and reservoir to the peritoneal cavity. Such shunts are used in humans and can be used in animals. Ultralow pressure valves should be used in dogs and cats (Figure 12-20). The major disadvantages of surgery are the expense and the postoperative complications. The complications include the need to replace the tubing as the animal grows, and occlusion of the tubes by fibrous tissue, choroid epithelium, or ependyma, and infection.[267] The shunts can be very effective for long-term control of clinical signs.[268]

Hydranencephaly/Porencephaly. Hydranencephaly and porencephaly are congenital cavitary anomalies of the brain resulting from failure of cell growth or necrosis. In hydranencephaly, loss of the neuroepithelial cells reduces the thickness of the cerebrum to a thin layer of glial and meningeal cells.[234] As a result, CSF fills the defect because the defect is contiguous with the lateral ventricles but not completely lined by ependyma. In some animals, the defect is limited to a portion of the cerebrum. In severe cases, the cerebral hemispheres are reduced to fluid-filled sacs. An anatomic distinction from hydrocephalus is that the head is of normal size with hydranencephaly. Porencephaly is characterized by multiple discrete cystic defects in the cerebrum, which may or may not communicate with the ventricles or subarachnoid space.

Hydranencephaly and porencephaly often are associated with secondary destructive processes that represent hypoplasia and secondary atrophy in early and later stages of brain development, respectively.[269] In utero viral infections have been implicated as a cause of hydranencephaly in many domestic animal species.[269] A focal or multifocal lesion distribution depends upon the stage of embryogenesis during viral infection. Hydranencephaly in kittens has been reported as a distinct disease entity secondary to in utero feline parvovirus infection (feline panleukopenia virus).[270] However, cerebellar hypoplasia more commonly occurs with this infection. Bluetongue virus, bovine viral diarrhea virus, Cache Valley virus, Akabane virus, and others have been reported to cause hydranencephaly in ruminants.[242,271-274]

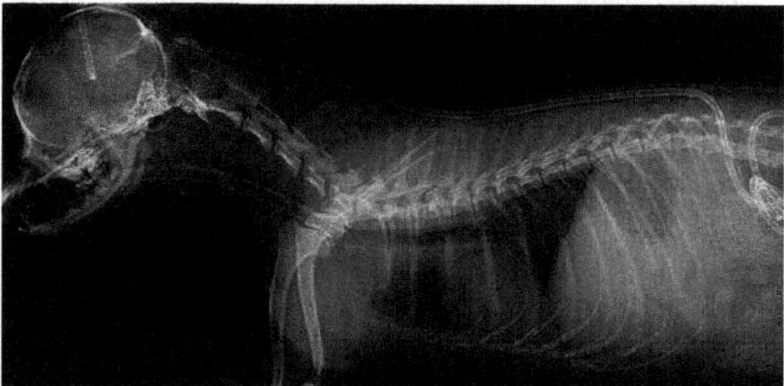

Figure 12-20 Lateral radiograph of a Chihuahua with congenital hydrocephalus obtained postoperatively after ventriculoperitoneal (VP) shunt placement is visualized entering the cranial cavity and coursing subcutaneously to the abdominal cavity. (Copyright 2010 University of Georgia Research Foundation, Inc.)

Cranial Mesodermal Defects. Development of head and facial structures is induced by brain growth.[234] Development of the axial skeleton begins when sclerotomal components of the mesodermal somites migrate around the neural tube soon after closure has been completed. In the cranial region, only the calvaria are formed by axial mesoderm. Primary axial mesodermal defects are a result of abnormal bony mesodermal development without a persistently open neural tube.[235] Encephaloceles and cranial meningoceles consist of a protrusion of brain or meninges through the calvarial defect. Pregnant queens treated with griseofulvin in early pregnancy will produce kittens with cranium bifidum and meningoencephalocele of varying severity.[275] Cranial malformations in Burmese cats is linked to continuous selection since the 1970s for a rounded, brachycephalic facial appearance. These selection processes have produced kittens with lethal neonatal facial deformities.[276] The inheritance pattern is autosomal dominant with incomplete expression.[277] The genetic defect causes abnormal migration of neural crest cells. Affected kittens have varying severities of telencephalic meningoencephalocele and hydrocephalus. Heterozygotes also express a range of facial dimensions.

Cleft palate is one of the most common gross anatomic defects in neonatal kittens and can be associated with other cranial anomalies.[278] Cleft palate alone has been reported as a fetal anomaly when queens were dosed with diphenylhydantoin or griseofulvin.

Disorders of Forebrain Induction. The cerebral cortical neurons undergo maximal development late in the third trimester and during the first two weeks of postnatal growth.[235] Disorders associated with abnormal development of the prosencephalon are termed holoprosencephaly, arrhinencephaly, and cyclopia.[269] Holoprosencephaly refers to a single, nondivided cerebrum over the diencephalon. Holoprosencephaly has been reported in a young miniature schnauzer with abnormal mentation, seizures, and an inability to house train.[279] The affected dog also had adipsia and developed hypernatremia. At necropsy, there was absence or reduction in midline forebrain structures (i.e., corpus callosum), incomplete separation of paired structures (i.e., lateral ventricle and cingulate gyri), and hydrocephalus. Similar gross anatomic findings have been observed on brain MRI in other dogs with adipsia.[280] Arrhinencephaly refers to lack of development of the olfactory region. Holoprosencephaly with cyclopia has been reported in lambs when their dams have been exposed to *V. californicum*.[243] Agenesis of the corpus callosum has been reported in domestic animals and usually is accompanied by other defects. Clinical signs are referable to the forebrain. Kittens born from a queen exposed to griseofulvin developed agenesis of the corpus callosum and cyclopean malformation with anophthalmia and absence of optic nerves.[275]

Disorders of Neuronal Migration. Brain malformations can be caused by abnormalities in neuronal migration. Neuronal migration begins near the periventricular zone. One hypothesis is that during migration, neuroblasts establish synaptic contacts and organize into layers from the ventricle to the pial surface of the cortex. Simultaneously, apoptosis and glial cell proliferation and differentiation occur. Cerebral cortical migrational abnormalities can be grouped into three categories: lissencephaly/pachygyria (lack or partial lack of gyri and sulci), polymicrogyria (extensive folds of cerebral cortex), and heterotopia (disorganized gray matter in inappropriate places).[281]

Lissencephaly (agyria and pachygyria) are reflected by gross abnormalities of the cerebral cortical surface and by microscopic thickening of the cortical laminae/layers. Agyria implies absence of gyri whereas pachygyria implies reduced numbers of broadened gyri. The lesions are caused by arrest neuroblast migration. Lissencephaly with microencephaly has been reported in ruminants, cats, and several dog breeds (Lhasa apso, Irish setter, wire fox terrier, Samoyed).[269] Affected animals manifest abnormal behavior and seizures. Lissencephaly can be identified with MRI.[282]

Polymicrogyria is a disorder of cerebrocortical development resulting in increased numbers of small, disorganized gyri and often accompanied by hydrocephalus. This disorder has been reported in standard poodles and cattle.[283,284] Clinical signs reflect the area of cerebrocortical involvement but often manifest with blindness with normal PLRs and pupil size and seizures.

Other anomalies of the brain may cause alterations in mental status. Some are so grossly abnormal that they are not usually compatible with life. Others are more typically characterized by seizures and are discussed in Chapter 13.

Toxic Disorders. A large number of toxic agents may produce stupor and coma, especially in the terminal stages (see Chapter 15). An overdose of certain drugs, including barbiturates, tranquilizers, narcotics, or avermectins may produce stupor or coma as a primary effect.[285] The drugs may have been given deliberately or may have been ingested accidentally. Occasionally, barbiturate intoxication has occurred after ingestion of a carcass of an animal euthanized by barbiturate overdose. A comparison of the signs of coma caused by drugs with those of coma caused by structural changes in the brain is provided in Table 12-1. Spinal reflexes and respirations are depressed more severely by sedative drugs than by most structural lesions, whereas pupillary responses are less affected.

Most animals that are toxic from CNS depressants can be saved with proper management. If the animal is not in a coma, attentive nursing is usually all that is necessary. Gastric lavage and activated charcoal are useful if the drug was recently ingested. Maintenance of adequate respiration is the most important consideration for an animal in a coma. Mechanical ventilation may be necessary for animals hypoventilating in a coma.

Diuresis is promoted by the intravenous administration of glucose or mannitol. Urine output must be monitored through an indwelling urethral catheter. The excretion of many agents (e.g., barbiturates) is dependent on the rate of urine formation. Hydration and acid-base balance must be maintained. Periodic evaluation of serum electrolytes and blood gases is of great benefit in the management of persistent coma.

CASE STUDIES

CASE STUDY 12-1 *HEATH*

 veterinaryneurologycases.com

▪ Signalment
2 year old male castrated Labrador retriever

▪ History
The owner witnessed the dog being hit by a car. Immediately after the accident, the dog was recumbent and nonresponsive. After 10 minutes, the dog became somewhat responsive but remained obtunded. The dog was taken directly to an emergency clinic.

▪ Physical Examination
The dog's heart rate and respiratory rate were high. Mucous membrane color was pale and the CRT was less than 2 seconds. Auscultation of the chest cavity was normal. The abdomen was nonpainful. There were no obvious fractures or luxations involving the appendicular skeleton. There were mild skin abrasions on the left side of the dog's face.

▪ Neurologic Examination
Mentation
The dog was responsive but obtunded.

Gait
With support the dog was ambulatory with a relatively normal gait.

Postural reactions
Abnormal in the right TL and PLs

Reflex
Normal in all four limbs

Cranial nerve examination
Decreased palpebral OS when stimulated at the medial canthus of the eye; normal palpebral reflex when stimulated at the lateral canthus of the eye; mydriasis OS; absent normal nystagmus OS; present OD

Normal menace response OU
Light directed OS, PLR absent OS; consensual present OD
Light directed OD, PLR present OD; consensual absent OS

Sensory evaluation
Normal

▪ Laboratory Examination
PCV = 48%, TS = 7.2 g/dL; electrolytes were normal.
Chest and abdominal radiographs were normal.

▪ Assessment
The dog's abnormal mentation suggests an intracranial lesion. The dog's gait and postural reaction deficits suggest a lesion at or caudal to the midbrain; postural reaction deficits would suggest a right-sided lesion. However, such abnormalities also may occur with acute lesion involving the forebrain; if related to a forebrain lesion, deficits would be contralateral to the lesion and therefore suggest a left-sided lesion. The decreased palpebral reflex and a

Continued

CASE STUDY 12-1 *HEATH*—cont'd

normal menace response were consistent with CN V dysfunction; specifically the ophthalmic branch. Mydriasis and abnormal PLR OS with a normal menace response is consistent with CN III dysfunction. Finally, the findings of an abnormal palpebral reflex OS, an absence of normal nystagmus OS with normal nystagmus present OD, and no other signs of vestibular dysfunction are consistent with a lesion affecting CN III, IV, VI, and the ophthalmic branch of CN V.

Ultimately there are several possible neuroanatomic localizations that can be made in this case.

(1) A single lesion ventral to the forebrain at the level of the orbital fissure

(2) Multifocal disease, affecting several areas of the brainstem to account for the multiple cranial nerves affected

Given the dog's history, the only disorder to consider in this case is traumatic brain injury.

▪ Treatment

Treatment should initially be directed at stabilizing the dog's systemic condition. Assessment of ventilation, oxygenation, and the cardiovascular system should be performed. The dog should be treated for systemic shock if indicated. Repeated neurologic examination should be conducted once the dog has become systemically stable. If the dog's neurologic condition does not improve once cardiovascular support has been provided or declines in the face of such support, intravenous mannitol or hypertonic saline should be administered for the treatment of increased intracranial pressure.

In the present case, the dog received 90 mL/kg of crystalloid fluids intravenously over the first 30 minutes. The dog's mentation improved. Once stabilized, CT was performed, which revealed a large extradural hematoma at the level of the thalamus on the left (see Figure 12-4). Additionally, a left-sided fracture of the calvaria was evident that extended from the parietal bone at the level of the zygomatic arch rostrally to the orbital fissure. The mentation, gait, and postural reaction deficits were thought to relate to the hematoma directly or through secondary compression of the midbrain. The CN deficits were thought to be related to the fracture through the orbital fissure. The following day a left-sided rostrotentorial craniectomy was performed to remove the hematoma. Recovery from surgery was uneventful. The dog made steady improvement postoperatively. Four weeks after the trauma, the dog was normal except for persistent cranial deficits involving CNs III, IV, VI, and the ophthalmic branch of CN V OS.

CASE STUDY 12-2 *SCOTTY*

 veterinaryneurologycases.com

▪ Signalment

A 3-year-old male castrated DSH cat

▪ History

The owner reported an acute onset of abnormal mentation. The cat experienced generalized seizures. Since the onset of abnormal mentation, the cat has been circling to the right. Two days before the onset of neurologic signs, the owner reported that the cat had been excessively sneezing. The cat has access to the outdoors. No other medical problems were reported. The cat is current on vaccinations.

▪ Physical Examination

Normal except for a rectal temperature of 99° F

▪ Neurologic Examination

Mentation

Obtunded

Gait

Normal; circling to the right

Postural reactions

Abnormal in the left TL and PLs

Reflexes

All normal

Cranial nerve examination

Absent menace response OS; normal pupil size and PLR OU, decreased response to stimulation (hypalgesia) of the left nares

Sensory evaluation

Normal except for the nasal hypalgesia

▪ Laboratory Examination

The complete blood cell count (CBC) revealed a mild neutrophilic leukocytosis. Chemistry profile and urinalysis (UA) were normal.

▪ Assessment

Neuroanatomic localization is consistent with a right-sided forebrain lesion. Acute disorders that result in asymmetric neurologic deficits should be considered in this case. The primary differential diagnoses include vascular, trauma, inflammatory, and neoplastic diseases. For vascular disorders, the acute onset of forebrain signs in conjunction with a history of sneezing and hypothermia is consistent with feline ischemic encephalopathy secondary to cuterebra larval migration. Although there is no history of trauma, the cat does have access to the outdoors and could have sustained a traumatic brain injury. Despite the lack of systemic signs of illness or inflammation, inflammatory (primarily infectious etiologies in cats) disease should be considered. Although the cat is young and has an acute history, neoplasia is a remote possibility. Lymphoma occurs in young cats and is often associated with acute onset of signs. The asymmetric deficits exclude degenerative, metabolic, and toxic disorders from consideration. The acute onset of signs excludes anomalous disorders.

MRI disclosed a lesion affecting the right caudate nucleus and adjacent white matter, right olfactory/frontal and parietal cerebral cortex. The MRI characteristics were consistent with ischemic infarction. CSF analysis revealed a neutrophilic pleocytosis.

The cat was treated with corticosteroids with the intention of reducing vasogenic edema secondary to the infarction and the inflammatory response noted in the CSF analysis. Approximately 3 weeks after the onset of neurologic signs, the cat was normal.

CASE STUDY 12-3 *MAX*

veterinaryneurologycases.com

▪ Signalment
9-year-old male castrated golden retriever

▪ History
The owner reports a chronic progressive change in behavior over the course of 6 weeks. Initially the dog seemed lethargic. Over time, the dog began to wander aimlessly in the house. He seemed to be sleeping more than normal. In the last week, the dog had stopped responding to its name being called. Additionally, the dog has experienced two generalized seizures in the last 2 weeks.

▪ Physical Examination
Normal

▪ Neurologic Examination
Mentation
Obtunded

Gait
Normal

Postural reactions
Normal in all four limbs

Reflexes
Normal in all four limbs

Cranial nerves
Absent menace OS; normal pupil size and PLR, OS

Sensory
Normal

▪ Laboratory Examination
The CBC, chemistry profile, urinalysis (UA) were normal. Chest radiographs were normal.

▪ Assessment
The abnormal mentation suggests an intracranial lesion. The normal gait with presence of normal postural reactions suggest that the lesion is affecting the forebrain. The absent menace response is consistent with a lesion involving the right forebrain. Consequently, the neuroanatomic diagnosis is consistent with a right-sided forebrain lesion.

The dog's history is consistent with a chronic progressive disorder. Given the dog's age, breed, neuroanatomic localization, neoplasia (primary or secondary [metastatic]) is the most likely differential diagnosis. The lack of systemic signs of illness and the lack of laboratory examination abnormalities reduces the likelihood of secondary (metastatic) disease. Inflammatory disease (infectious and noninfectious) should also be considered. The lack of systemic signs of illness and the focal nature of the neurologic deficits make these etiologies of lesser priority. The asymmetry in the neurologic examination excludes degenerative, metabolic, and toxic disorders. Although trauma and vascular disorders are associated with asymmetric neurologic deficits, the lack of history and chronicity exclude these etiologies, respectively.

MRI was performed. A large, extraaxial lesion was observed in the right olfactory/frontal lobe of the cerebrum with vasogenic edema affecting the white matter of the internal capsule. The lesion has MRI characteristics consistent with a meningioma. A transfrontal craniotomy was performed and the mass removed. Microscopic evaluation of the mass was consistent with meningioma. The dog's neurologic signs resolved; however, he continued to have intermittent seizures, which were controlled with anticonvulsant medication.

CASE STUDY 12-4 *LEAH*

veterinaryneurologycases.com

▪ Signalment
8-year-old Female spayed English bulldog

▪ History
Six weeks before presentation, the owner noted an acute onset of lethargy. The dog was evaluated by the referring veterinarian. No physical or neurologic abnormalities were noted. Laboratory examinations, CBC, and chemistry profile were normal. The following day a CT of the head was performed. No lesions were identified. CSF analysis revealed a mild increase in protein content with normal WBC. The dog was started on prednisone therapy (0.5mg/kg orally per day). The dog remained lethargic for approximately 4 weeks, after which time the owner noted a 2-week progressive worsening of the lethargy, intermittent circling to the right, and a recent onset of aggressive behavior (i.e., the dog would growl when petted).

▪ Physical Examination
Normal with the exception of mild muscle wasting of the epaxial, temporal, and appendicular musculature.

▪ Neurologic Examination
Mentation
Dull/obtunded

Gait
Normal: Tendency to circle to the right but not consistently

Postural reactions
Normal in all four limbs

Reflexes
TL, normal; PL, normal

Continued

CASE STUDY 12-4 *LEAH*—cont'd

Cranial nerve examination
All normal

Sensory
Normal

▪ Laboratory Examination

CBC revealed a mild neutrophilic leukocytosis and mild lymphopenia.
Chemistry profile was normal except for increased SAP (548 U/L; normal = 10-119 U/L)
Urine specific gravity was 1.016; urinalysis was otherwise normal.
Chest radiographs were normal

▪ Assessment

As in case 12C, the abnormal mentation suggests an intracranial lesion. The normal gait and postural reactions suggest a neuroanatomic diagnosis of a forebrain lesion. Without evidence of asymmetry, a diffuse forebrain disease should be suspected. However, a focal structural disease also needs to be considered. Therefore a list of differentials should include diseases that affect the forebrain diffusely and focal lesions. Although the initial onset of clinical signs was acute, chronic progressive disorders should be the primary consideration at this time. Diffuse disorders that affect the forebrain include degenerative, metabolic diseases, and some intoxications (i.e., lead toxicity, ethylene glycol). Degenerative disorders (i.e., storage diseases) typically occur in younger animals. The laboratory data are consistent with exogenous corticosteroid administration (i.e., stress leukogram, Serum alkaline phosphatase enzyme induction, and reduced urine specific gravity); however, hepatic encephalopathy related to a primary liver disorder should be considered. Specialized liver function tests such as preprandial and postprandial bile acid concentrations and a fasting serum ammonia level would be needed to document liver dysfunction. Chronic progressive focal forebrain lesions that should be considered are neoplasia and inflammatory disorders. Anomalous, traumatic, and vascular causes are excluded based on age, lack of history, and the chronic progressive nature, respectively.

MRI of the brain was performed and disclosed hydrocephalus involving both lateral ventricles and the third ventricle. A contrast enhancing mass lesion consistent with neoplasia was identified within the third ventricle. The mass lesion extended into and obstructed the mesencephalic aqueduct, which resulted in an obstructive hydrocephalus. Clinical signs were thought to reflect increased intracranial pressure secondary to obstructive hydrocephalus. Consequently, a ventriculoperitoneal (VP) shunt was placed into the left lateral ventricle of the cerebrum in an effort to relieve intracranial pressure (see Figure 12-17). The dog experienced an acute and dramatic improvement in her neurologic deficits after surgery. As is relatively common, the dog had several recurrences of clinical signs related to malfunction of the VP shunt (obstruction of the shunt), which necessitated repeated surgeries to repair the device. Additionally, the dog underwent radiation therapy for the mass lesion in the third ventricle. Despite the initial complications with the VP shunt, the dog did well following radiation therapy. The long-term prognosis remains unknown.

REFERENCES

1. Cartlidge NEF: States of altered consciousness. In Swash M, Kennard C, editors: Scientific basis of clinical neurology, Edinburgh, 1985, Churchill Livingstone.
2. deLahunta A, Glass E: Diencephalon. Veterinary neuroanatomy and clinical neurology, ed 3, St Louis, 2009, Saunders Elsevier.
3. Shute CC, Lewis PR: The ascending cholinergic reticular system: neocortical, olfactory and subcortical projections, Brain 90:497–520, 1967.
4. Hendricks JC, Morrison AR: Normal and abnormal sleep in mammals, J Am Vet Med Assoc 178:121–126, 1981.
5. Siegel JM, Tomaszewski KS, Nienhuis R: Behavioral states in the chronic medullary and midpontine cat, Electroencephalogr Clin Neurophysiol 63:274–288, 1986.
6. Kaitin KI, Kilduff TS, Dement WC: Evidence for excessive sleepiness in canine narcoleptics, Electroencephalogr Clin Neurophysiol 64:447–454, 1986.
7. Milhorat TH: Cerebrospinal fluid and the brain edemas, ed New York, 1987, Neuroscience Society of New York.
8. Kornegay JN, Oliver JE Jr, Gorgacz EJ: Clinicopathologic features of brain herniation in animals, J Am Vet Med Assoc 182:1111–1116, 1983.
9. deLahunta A, Glass E: Lower motor neuron: general visceral efferent system. Veterinary neuroanatomy and clinical neurology, St Louis, 2009, Saunders Elsevier.
10. Kolata RJ, Kraut NH, Johnston DE: Patterns of trauma in urban dogs and cats: a study of 1,000 cases, J Am Vet Med Assoc 164:499–502, 1974.
11. Streeter EM, Rozanski EA, Laforcade-Buress AD, et al: Evaluation of vehicular trauma in dogs: 239 cases (January-December 2001), J Am Vet Med Assoc 235:405–408, 2009.
12. Feary DJ, Magdesian KG, Aleman MA, et al: Traumatic brain injury in horses: 34 cases (1994-2004), J Am Vet Med Assoc 231:259–266, 2007.
13 Greve MW, Zink BJ: Pathophysiology of traumatic brain injury, Mount Sinai J Med 76:97–104, 2009.
14. Helmy A, Vizcaychipi M, Gupta AK: Traumatic brain injury: intensive care management, Br J Anaesth 99:32–42, 2007.
15. Syring RS, Otto CM, Drobatz KJ: Hyperglycemia in dogs and cats with head trauma: 122 cases (1997-1999), J Am Vet Med Assoc 218:1124–1129, 2001.
16. Shapiro HM: Intracranial hypertension: therapeutic and anesthetic considerations, Anesthesiology 43:445–471, 1975.
17. Hopkins AL: Head trauma, Vet Clin North Am Small Anim Pract 26:875–891, 1996.
18. Knapp JM: Hyperosmolar therapy in the treatment of severe head injury in children: mannitol and hypertonic saline, AACN Clin Issues: Advanced Pract Acute Crit Care 16:199–211, 2005.
19. Rangel-Castilla L, Gopinath S, Robertson CS: Management of intracranial hypertension, Neurol Clin 26:521–541, 2008.
20. Bullock R: Mannitol and other diuretics in severe neurotrauma, New Horiz 3:448–452, 1995.
21. Jandrey KE: Using mannitol to treat traumatic brain injuries, Vet Med 94:717–721, 724–725, 1999.

22. Roberts PA, Pollay M, Engles C, et al: Effect on intracranial pressure of furosemide combined with varying doses and administration rates of mannitol, J Neurosurg 66:440–446, 1987.
23. Wilkinson HA, Rosenfeld SR: Furosemide and mannitol in the treatment of acute experimental intracranial hypertension, Neurosurgery 12:405–410, 1983.
24. Proulx J, Dhupa N: Severe brain injury. Part II. Therapy, Compend Contin Educ Pract Vet 20:993–1006, 1998.
25. MacKay RJ: Brain injury after head trauma: pathophysiology, diagnosis, and treatment, Vet Clin North Am Equine Pract 20:199–216, 2004.
26. Rayner SG: Traumatic cerebral partial lobotomy in a thoroughbred stallion, Aust Vet J 83:674–677, 2005.
27. Shores A: Craniocerebral trauma. In Kirk RW, editor: Current veterinary therapy X, Philadelphia, 1989, WB Saunders.
28. Platt SR, Radaelli ST, McDonnell JJ: The prognostic value of the modified Glasgow coma scale in head trauma in dogs, J Vet Intern Med 15:581–584, 2001.
29. Fankhauser R, Luginbuhl H, McGrath JT: Cerebrovascular disease in various animal species, Ann N Y Acad Sci 127:817–860, 1965.
30. Waters DJ, Hayden DW, Walter PA: Intracranial lesions in dogs with hemangiosarcoma, J Vet Intern Med 3:222–230, 1989.
31. Snyder JM, Lipitz L, Skorupski KA, et al: Secondary intracranial neoplasia in the dog: 177 cases (1986-2003), J Vet Intern Med 22:172–177, 2008.
32. Braund KG, Brewer BD, Mayhew IG: Inflammatory, infectious, immune, parasitic, and vascular diseases. In Oliver JE, Hoerlein BF, Mayhew IG, editors: Veterinary neurology, Philadelphia, 1987, Saunders.
33. Rutgers C, Kowalski J, Cole CR, et al: Severe Rocky Mountain spotted fever in five dogs, J Am Anim Hosp Assoc 21:361–369, 1985.
34. Denk D, Matiasek K, Just FT, et al: Disseminated angiostrongylosis with fatal cerebral haemorrhages in two dogs in Germany: a clinical case study, Vet Parasitol 160:100–108, 2009.
35. Garosi LS, Platt SR, McConnell JF, et al: Intracranial haemorrhage associated with *Angiostrongylus vasorum* infection in three dogs, J Small Anim Pract 46:93–99, 2005.
36. Wessmann A, Lu D, Lamb CR, et al: Brain and spinal cord haemorrhages associated with *Angiostrongylus vasorum* infection in four dogs, Vet Rec 158:858–863, 2006.
37. Putsche JC, Kohn B: Primary immune-mediated thrombocytopenia in 30 dogs (1997-2003), J Am Anim Hosp Assoc 44:250–257, 2008.
38. Dunn KJ, Nicholls PK, Dunn JK, et al: Intracranial haemorrhage in a Doberman puppy with von Willebrand's disease, Vet Rec 136:635–636, 1995.
39. Joseph RJ, Greenlee PG, Carrillo JM, et al: Canine cerebrovascular disease: clinical and pathological findings in 17 cases, J Am Anim Hosp Assoc 24:569–576, 1988.
40. Thomas WB, Adams WH, McGavin MD, et al: Magnetic resonance imaging appearance of intracranial hemorrhage secondary to cerebral vascular malformation in a dog, Vet Radiol Ultrasound 38:371–375, 1997.
41. Tidwell AS, Mahony OM, Moore RP, et al: Computed tomography of an acute hemorrhagic cerebral infarct in a dog, Vet Radiol Ultrasound 35:290–296, 1994.
42. Rovira A, Grive E, Alvarez-Sabin J: Distribution territories and causative mechanisms of ischemic stroke, Eur Radiol 15:416–426, 2005.
43. Garosi L, McConnell JF, Platt SR, et al: Clinical and topographic magnetic resonance characteristics of suspected brain infarction in 40 dogs, J Vet Intern Med 20:311–321, 2006.
44. Garosi L, McConnell JE, Platt SR, et al: Results of diagnostic investigations and long-term outcome of 33 dogs with brain infarction (2000-2004), J Vet Intern Med 19:725–731, 2005.
45. Detweiler DK, Ratcliffe HL, Luginbühl H: The significance of naturally occurring coronary and cerebral arterial disease in animals, Ann N Y Acad Sci 149:868–881, 1968.
46. Patterson JS, Rusley MS, Zachary JF: Neurologic manifestations of cerebrovascular atherosclerosis associated with primary hypothyroidism in a dog, J Am Vet Med Assoc 186:499–503, 1985.
47. Vitale CL, Olby NJ: Neurologic dysfunction in hypothyroid, hyperlipidemic Labrador retrievers, J Vet Intern Med 21:1316–1322, 2007.
48. Axlund TW, Isaacs AM, Holland M, et al: Fibrocartilaginous embolic encephalomyelopathy of the brainstem and midcervical spinal cord in a dog, J Vet Intern Med 18:765–767, 2004.
49. Cook LB, Coates JR, Dewey CW, et al: Vascular encephalopathy associated with bacterial endocarditis in four dogs, J Am Anim Hosp Assoc 41:252–258, 2005.
50. Patton CS, Garner FM: Cerebral infarction caused by heartworms *(Dirofilaria immitis)* in a dog, J Am Vet Med Assoc 156:600–605, 1970.
51. Segedy AK, Hayden DW: Cerebral vascular accident caused by *Dirofilaria immitis* in a dog, J Am Anim Hosp Assoc 14:752–756, 1978.
52. Bradley WG Jr: MR appearance of hemorrhage in the brain, Radiology 189:15–26, 1993.
53. Glass EN, Cornetta AM, deLahunta A, et al: Clinical and clinicopathologic features in 11 cats with *Cuterebra* larvae myiasis of the central nervous system, J Vet Intern Med 12:365–368, 1998.
54. Williams KJ, Summers BA, deLahunta A: Cerebrospinal cuterebriasis in cats and its association with feline ischemic encephalopathy, Vet Pathol 35:330–343, 1998.
55. Tieber LM, Axlund TW, Simpson ST, et al: Survival of a suspected case of central nervous system cuterebrosis in a dog: clinical and magnetic resonance imaging findings, J Am Anim Hosp Assoc 42:238–242, 2006.
56. Cantile C, Campani D, Menicagli M, et al: Pathological and immunohistochemical studies of choroid plexus carcinoma of the dog, J Comp Pathol 126:183–193, 2002.
57. Lipsitz D, Levitski RE, Chauvet AE: Magnetic resonance imaging of a choroid plexus carcinoma and meningeal carcinomatosis in a dog, Vet Radiol Ultrasound 40:246–250, 1999.
58. Patnaik AK, Erlandson RA, Lieberman PH, et al: Choroid plexus carcinoma with meningeal carcinomatosis in a dog, Vet Pathol 17:381–385, 1980.
59. Westworth DR, Dickinson PJ, Vernau W, et al: Choroid plexus tumors in 56 dogs (1985-2007), J Vet Intern Med 22:1157–1165, 2008.
60. Zaki FA, Nafe LA: Choroid plexus tumors in the dog, J Am Vet Med Assoc 176:328–330, 1980.
61. Fenner WR: Metastatic neoplasms of the central nervous system, Semin Vet Med Surg (Small Anim) 5:253–261, 1990.
62. Vandevelde M: Brain tumors in domestic animals. In Proceedings of a conference on brain tumors in man and animals: an overview, Research Triangle Park, NC, 1984.
63. Zaki FA: Spontaneous central nervous system tumors in the dog, Vet Clin North Am 7:153–163, 1977.
64. Zaki FA, Hurvitz AI: Spontaneous neoplasms of the central nervous system of the cat, J Small Anim Pract 17:773–782, 1976.
65. Troxel MT, Vite CH, Winkle TJ, et al: Feline intracranial neoplasia: retrospective review of 160 cases (1985-2001), J Vet Intern Med 17:850–859, 2003.

66. Snyder JM, Shofer FS, Van Winkle TJ, et al: Canine intracranial primary neoplasia: 173 cases (1986-2003), J Vet Intern Med 20:669–675, 2006.
67. Summers BA, Cummings JF, DeLahunta A: Tumors of the central nervous system. Veterinary neuropathology, St Louis, 1995, Mosby.
68. McDonnell JJ, Kalbko K, Keating JH, et al: Multiple meningiomas in three dogs, J Am Anim Hosp Assoc 43:201–208, 2007.
69. Alves A, Prada J, Almeida JM, et al: Primary and secondary tumours occurring simultaneously in the brain of a dog, J Small Anim Pract 47:607–610, 2006.
70. Stacy BA, Stevenson TL, Lipsitz D, et al: Simultaneously occurring oligodendroglioma and meningioma in a dog, J Vet Intern Med 17:357–359, 2003.
71. Sturges BK, Dickinson PJ, Bollen AW, et al: Magnetic resonance imaging and histological classification of intracranial meningiomas in 112 dogs, J Vet Intern Med 22:586–595, 2008.
72. Sessums K, Mariani C: Intracranial meningioma in dogs and cats: a comparative review, Compend Contin Educ Vet Pract 31:330–339, 2009.
73. Adamo PF, Forrest L, Dubielzig R: Canine and feline meningiomas: diagnosis, treatment, and prognosis, Compend Contin Educ Pract Vet 26:951–965, 2004.
74. Bagley RS, Gavin PR, Moore MP, et al: Clinical signs associated with brain tumors in dogs: 97 cases (1992-1997), J Am Vet Med Assoc 215:818–819, 1999.
75. Heidner GL, Kornegay JN, Page RL, et al: Analysis of survival in a retrospective study of 86 dogs with brain tumors, J Vet Intern Med 5:219–226, 1991.
76. LeCouteur RA: Current concepts in the diagnosis and treatment of brain tumours in dogs and cats, J Small Anim Pract 40:411–416, 1999.
77. Gavin PR, Fike JR, Hoopes PJ: Central nervous system tumors, Semin Vet Med Surg (Small Anim) 10:180–189, 1995.
78. Braund KG: Neoplasia of the nervous system, Compend Contin Educ Pract Vet 6:717–722, 1984.
79. Higgins RJ, LeCouteur RA, Vernau KM, et al: Granular cell tumor of the canine central nervous system: two cases, Vet Pathol 38:620–627, 2001.
80. Palmer AC, Malinowski W, Barnett KC: Clinical signs including papilloedema associated with brain tumours in twenty-one dogs, J Small Anim Pract 15:359–386, 1974.
81. Foster ES, Carrillo JM, Patnaik AK: Clinical signs of tumors affecting the rostral cerebrum in 43 dogs, J Vet Intern Med 2:71–74, 1988.
82. Davidson MG, Nasisse MP, Breitschwerdt EB, et al: Acute blindness associated with intracranial tumors in dogs and cats: eight cases (1984-1989), J Am Vet Med Assoc 199:755–758, 1991.
83. Coates JR, Dewey CW: Cervical spinal hyperesthesia as a clinical sign of intracranial disease, Compend Contin Educ Pract Vet 20:1025–1037, 1998.
84. Smith MO, Turrel JM, Bailey CS, et al: Neurologic abnormalities as the predominant signs of neoplasia of the nasal cavity in dogs and cats: seven cases (1973-1986), J Am Vet Med Assoc 195:242–245, 1989.
85. Koblik PD, LeCouteur RA, Higgins RJ, et al: CT-guided brain biopsy using a modified Pelorus Mark III stereotactic system: experience with 50 dogs, Vet Radiol Ultrasound 40:434–440, 1999.
86. Koblik PD, LeCouteur RA, Higgins RJ, et al: Modification and application of a Pelorus Mark III stereotactic system for CT-guided brain biopsy in 50 dogs, Vet Radiol Ultrasound 40:424–433, 1999.
87. Bailey CS, Higgins RJ: Characteristics of cisternal cerebrospinal fluid associated with primary brain tumors in the dog: a retrospective study, J Am Vet Med Assoc 188:414–417, 1986.
88. Dickinson PJ, Sturges BK, Kass PH, et al: Characteristics of cisternal cerebrospinal fluid associated with intracranial meningiomas in dogs: 56 cases (1985-2004), J Am Vet Med Assoc 228:564–567, 2006.
89. Turrel JM, Fike JR, LeCouteur RA, et al: Radiotherapy of brain tumors in dogs, J Am Vet Med Assoc 184:82–86, 1984.
90. Klopp LS, Simpson ST, Sorjonen DA, et al: Ventral surgical approach to the caudal brain stem in dogs, Vet Surg 29:533–542, 2000.
91. Glass EN, Kapatkin A, Vite C, et al: A modified bilateral transfrontal sinus approach to the canine frontal lobe and olfactory bulb: surgical technique and five cases, J Am Anim Hosp Assoc 36:43–50, 2000.
92. Oliver JE: Jr: Surgical approach to the canine brain, Am J Vet Res 29:353–378, 1968.
93. Axlund TW, McGlasson ML, Smith AN: Surgery alone or in combination with radiation therapy for treatment of intracranial meningiomas in dogs: 31 cases (1989-2002), J Am Vet Med Assoc 221:1597–1600, 2002.
94. Kostolich M, Dulisch ML: A surgical approach to the canine olfactory bulb for meningioma removal, Vet Surg 16:273–277, 1987.
95. Niebauer GW, Dayrell-Hart BL, Speciale J: Evaluation of craniotomy in dogs and cats, J Am Vet Med Assoc 198:89–95, 1991.
96. Greco JJ, Aiken SA, Berg JM, et al: Evaluation of intracranial meningioma resection with a surgical aspirator in dogs: 17 cases (1996-2004), J Am Vet Med Assoc 229:394–400, 2006.
97. Gallagher JG, Penninck D, Boudrieau RJ, et al: Ultrasonography of the brain and vertebral canal in dogs and cats: 15 cases (1988-1993), J Am Vet Med Assoc 207:1320–1324, 1995.
98. Klopp LS, Rao S: Endoscopic-assisted intracranial tumor removal in dogs and cats: long-term outcome of 39 cases, J Vet Intern Med 23:108–115, 2009.
99. Klopp LS, Ridgway M: Use of an endoscope in minimally invasive lesion biopsy and removal within the skull and cranial vault in two dogs and one cat, J Am Vet Med Assoc 234:1573–1577, 2009.
100. Gordon LE, Thacher C, Matthiesen DT, et al: Results of craniotomy for the treatment of cerebral meningioma in 42 cats, Vet Surg 23:94–100, 1994.
101. Gallagher JG, Berg J, Knowles KE, et al: Prognosis after surgical excision of cerebral meningiomas in cats: 17 cases (1986-1992), J Am Vet Med Assoc 203:1437–1440, 1993.
102. Theon AP, Lecouteur RA, Carr EA, et al: Influence of tumor cell proliferation and sex-hormone receptors on effectiveness of radiation therapy for dogs with incompletely resected meningiomas, J Am Vet Med Assoc 216:701–707, 2000.
103. Platt SR, Scase TJ, Adams V, et al: Vascular endothelial growth factor expression in canine intracranial meningiomas and association with patient survival, J Vet Intern Med 20:663–668, 2006.
104. Brearley MJ, Jeffery ND, Phillips SM, et al: Hypofractionated radiation therapy of brain masses in dogs: a retrospective analysis of survival of 83 cases (1991-1996), J Vet Intern Med 13:408–412, 1999.
105. Lester NV, Hopkins AL, Bova FJ, et al: Radiosurgery using a stereotactic headframe system for irradiation of brain tumors in dogs, J Am Vet Med Assoc 219(1550):1562–1567, 2001.

106. Bley CR, Sumova A, Roos M, et al: Irradiation of brain tumors in dogs with neurologic disease, J Vet Intern Med 19:849–854, 2005.
107. Evans SM, Dayrell-Hart B, Powlis W, et al: Radiation therapy of canine brain masses, J Vet Intern Med 7:216–219, 1993.
108. Spugnini EP, Thrall DE, Price GS, et al: Primary irradiation of canine intracranial masses, Vet Radiol Ultrasound 41:377–380, 2000.
109. Thrall DE, Larue SM, Powers BE, et al: Use of whole body hyperthermia as a method to heat inaccessible tumours uniformly: a phase III trial in canine brain masses, Int J Hyperthermia 15:383–398, 1999.
110. Tamura S, Tamura Y, Ohoka A, et al: A canine case of skull base meningioma treated with hydroxyurea, J Vet Med Sci 69:1313–1315, 2007.
111. Fulton LM, Steinberg HS: Preliminary study of lomustine in the treatment of intracranial masses in dogs following localization by imaging techniques, Semin Vet Med Surg (Small Anim) 5:241–245, 1990.
112. Jung DI, Kim HJ, Park C, et al: Long-term chemotherapy with lomustine of intracranial meningioma occurring in a miniature schnauzer, J Vet Med Sci 68:383–386, 2006.
113. Noonan M, Kline KL, Meleo K: Lymphoma of the central nervous system: a retrospective study of 18 cats, Compend Contin Educ Pract Vet 19:497–504, 1997.
114. McDonough SP, Van Winkle TJ, Valentine BA, et al: Clinicopathological and immunophenotypical features of canine intravascular lymphoma (malignant angioendotheliomatosis), J Comp Pathol 126:277–288, 2002.
115. Rosin A: Neurologic diseases associated with lymphosarcoma in ten dogs, J Am Vet Med Assoc 181:50–53, 1982.
116. Britt JO Jr, Simpson JG, Howard EB: Malignant lymphoma of the meninges in two dogs, J Comp Pathol 94:45–53, 1984.
117. Kent M, Delahunta A, Tidwell AS: MR imaging findings in a dog with intravascular lymphoma in the brain, Vet Radiol Ultrasound 42:504–510, 2001.
118. van der Vlugt-Meijer RH, Voorhout G, Meij BP: Imaging of the pituitary gland in dogs with pituitary-dependent hyperadrenocorticism, Mol Cell Endocrinol 197:81–87, 2002.
119. Kippenes H, Gavin PR, Kraft SL, et al: Mensuration of the normal pituitary gland from magnetic resonance images in 96 dogs, Vet Radiol Ultrasound 42:130–133, 2001.
120. Theon AP, Feldman EC: Megavoltage irradiation of pituitary macrotumors in dogs with neurologic signs, J Am Vet Med Assoc 213:225–231, 1998.
121. Kent MS, Bommarito D, Feldman E, et al: Survival, neurologic response, and prognostic factors in dogs with pituitary masses treated with radiation therapy and untreated dogs, J Vet Intern Med 21:1027–1033, 2007.
122. Elliott DA, Feldman EC, Koblik PD, et al: Prevalence of pituitary tumors among diabetic cats with insulin resistance, J Am Vet Med Assoc 216:1765–1768, 2000.
123. Hurty CA, Flatland B: Feline acromegaly: a review of the syndrome, J Am Anim Hosp Assoc 41:292–297, 2005.
124. Peterson ME, Taylor RS, Greco DS, et al: Acromegaly in 14 cats, J Vet Intern Med 4:192–201, 1990.
125. Sarfaty D, Carrillo JM, Peterson ME: Neurologic, endocrinologic, and pathologic findings associated with large pituitary tumors in dogs: eight cases (1976-1984), J Am Vet Med Assoc 193:854–856, 1988.
126. Wood FD, Pollard RE, Uerling MR, et al: Diagnostic imaging findings and endocrine test results in dogs with pituitary-dependent hyperadrenocorticism that did or did not have neurologic abnormalities: 157 cases (1989-2005), J Am Vet Med Assoc 231:1081–1085, 2007.
127. Kipperman BS, Feldman EC, Dybdal NO, et al: Pituitary tumor size, neurologic signs, and relation to endocrine test results in dogs with pituitary-dependent hyperadrenocorticism: 43 cases (1980-1990), J Am Vet Med Assoc 201:762–767, 1992.
128. Moore SA, O'Brien DP: Canine pituitary macrotumors, Compend Contin Educ Vet Pract 30:33–37, 2008:40.
129. Capen CC, Martin SL, Koestner A: Neoplasms in the adenohypophysis of dogs. A clinical and pathologic study, J Am Vet Med Assoc 4:301–325, 1967.
130. Ferguson DC, Biery DN: Diabetes insipidus and hyperadrenocorticism associated with high plasma adrenocorticotropin concentration and a hypothalamic/pituitary mass in a dog, J Am Vet Med Assoc 193:835–839, 1988.
131. Goossens MM, Rijnberk A, Mol JA, et al: Central diabetes insipidus in a dog with a pro-opiomelanocortin-producing pituitary tumor not causing hyperadrenocorticism, J Vet Intern Med 9:361–365, 1995.
132. Goossens MM: Diabetes insipidus in a dog with an alpha MSH-producing pituitary tumor, Vet Q 16 suppl 1, 61s, 1994.
133. van Keulen LJ, Wesdorp JL, Kooistra HS: Diabetes mellitus in a dog with a growth hormone-producing acidophilic adenoma of the adenohypophysis, Vet Pathol 33:451–453, 1996.
134. Harb MF, Nelson RW, Feldman EC, et al: Central diabetes insipidus in dogs: 20 cases (1986-1995), J Am Vet Med Assoc 209:1884–1888, 1996.
135. Feldman EC, Nelson RW: Canine hyperadrenocorticism. Canine and feline endocrinology and reproduction, ed 3, St Louis, 2004, Saunders.
136. Nelson RW, Ihle SL, Feldman EC: Pituitary macroadenomas and macroadenocarcinomas in dogs treated with mitotane for pituitary-dependent hyperadrenocorticism: 13 cases (1981-1986), J Am Vet Med Assoc 194:1612–1617, 1989.
137. Peterson ME: Diagnosis of hyperadrenocorticism in dogs, Clin Tech Small Anim Pract 22:2–11, 2007.
138. Starkey SR, Tan K, Church DB: Investigation of serum IGF-I levels amongst diabetic and non-diabetic cats, J Feline Med Surg 6:149–155, 2004.
139. Norman EJ, Mooney CT: Diagnosis and management of diabetes mellitus in five cats with somatotrophic abnormalities, J Feline Med Surg 2:183–190, 2000.
140. Peterson ME: Acromegaly in cats: are we only diagnosing the tip of the iceberg?, J Vet Intern Med 21:889–891, 2007.
141. Bertoy EH, Feldman EC, Nelson RW, et al: Magnetic resonance imaging of the brain in dogs with recently diagnosed but untreated pituitary-dependent hyperadrenocorticism, J Am Vet Med Assoc 206:651–656, 1995.
142. Duesberg CA, Feldman EC, Nelson RW, et al: Magnetic resonance imaging for diagnosis of pituitary macrotumors in dogs, J Am Vet Med Assoc 206:657–662, 1995.
143. Teshima T, Hara Y, Masuda H, et al: Relationship between arginine vasopressin and high signal intensity in the pituitary posterior lobe on T1-weighted MR images in dogs, J Vet Med Sci 70:693–699, 2008.
144. Tyson R, Graham JP, Bermingham E, et al: Dynamic computed tomography of the normal feline hypophysis cerebri *(Glandula pituitaria)*, Vet Radiol Ultrasound 46:33–38, 2005.
145. Van der Vlugt-Meijer RH, Meij BP, Voorhout G: Dynamic helical computed tomography of the pituitary gland in healthy dogs, Vet Radiol Ultrasound 48:118–124, 2007.

146. Goossens MM, Feldman EC, Theon AP, et al: Efficacy of cobalt 60 radiotherapy in dogs with pituitary-dependent hyperadrenocorticism, J Am Vet Med Assoc 212:374–376, 1998.
147. Dow SW, LeCouteur RA, Rosychuk RAW, et al: Response of dogs with functional pituitary macroadenomas and macrocarcinomas to radiation, J Small Anim Pract 31:287–294, 1990.
148. Mauldin GN, Burk RL: The use of diagnostic computerized tomography and radiation therapy in canine and feline hyperadrenocorticism, Probl Vet Med 2:557–564, 1990.
149. Brearley MJ, Polton GA, Littler RM, et al: Coarse fractionated radiation therapy for pituitary tumours in cats: a retrospective study of 12 cases, Vet Comp Oncol 4:209–217, 2006.
150. Dunning MD, Lowrie CS, Bexfield NH, et al: Exogenous insulin treatment after hypofractionated radiotherapy in cats with diabetes mellitus and acromegaly, J Vet Intern Med 23:243–249, 2009.
151. Kaser-Hotz B, Rohrer CR, Stankeova S, et al: Radiotherapy of pituitary tumours in five cats, J Small Anim Pract 43:303–307, 2002.
152. Morrison SA, Randolph J, Lothrop CD Jr: Hypersomatotropism and insulin-resistant diabetes mellitus in a cat, J Am Vet Med Assoc 194:91–94, 1989.
153. Abraham LA, Helmond SE, Mitten RW, et al: Treatment of an acromegalic cat with the dopamine agonist L-deprenyl, Aust Vet J 80:479–483, 2002.
154. Axlund TW, Behrend EN, Sorjonen DC, et al: Canine hypophysectomy using a ventral paramedian approach, Vet Surg 34:179–189, 2005.
155. Meij BP, Voorhout G, van den Ingh TS, et al: Transsphenoidal hypophysectomy in beagle dogs: evaluation of a microsurgical technique, Vet Surg 26:295–309, 1997.
156. Niebauer GW, Eigenmann JE, Van Winkle TJ: Study of long-term survival after transsphenoidal hypophysectomy in clinically normal dogs, Am J Vet Res 51:677–681, 1990.
157. Meij BP, Voorhout G, Van Den Ingh TS, et al: Transsphenoidal hypophysectomy for treatment of pituitary-dependent hyperadrenocorticism in 7 cats, Vet Surg 30:72–86, 2001.
158. Hanson JM, van't HM, Voorhout G, et al: Efficacy of transsphenoidal hypophysectomy in treatment of dogs with pituitary-dependent hyperadrenocorticism, J Vet Intern Med 19:687–694, 2005.
159. Hanson JM, Teske E, Voorhout G, et al: Prognostic factors for outcome after transsphenoidal hypophysectomy in dogs with pituitary-dependent hyperadrenocorticism, J Neurosurg 107:830–840, 2007.
160. Abrams-Ogg AC, Holmberg DL, Stewart WA, et al: Acromegaly in a cat: diagnosis by magnetic resonance imaging and treatment by cryohypophysectomy, Can Vet J 34:682–685, 1993.
161. Blois SL, Holmberg DL: Cryohypophysectomy used in the treatment of a case of feline acromegaly, J Small Anim Pract 49:596–600, 2008.
162. Dickerson ME, Page RL, LaDue TA, et al: Retrospective analysis of axial skeleton osteosarcoma in 22 large-breed dogs, J Vet Intern Med 15:120–124, 2001.
163. Hammer AS: Prognostic factors in dogs with osteosarcomas of the flat or irregular bones, J Am Anim Hosp Assoc 31:321–326, 1995.
164. Heyman SJ, Diefenderfer DL, Goldschmidt MH, et al: Canine axial skeletal osteosarcoma. A retrospective study of 116 cases (1986 to 1989), Vet Surg 21:304–310, 1992.
165. Hardy WDJ, Brodey RS, Riser WH: Osteosarcomas of the canine skull, J Am Vet Radiol Soc 8:5–16, 1967.
166. Dernell WS, Straw RC, Cooper MF, et al: Multilobular osteochondrosarcoma in 39 dogs: 1979-1993, J Am Anim Hosp Assoc 34:11–18, 1998.
167. Gallegos J, Schwarz T, McAnulty JF: Massive midline occipitotemporal resection of the skull for treatment of multilobular osteochondrosarcoma in two dogs, J Am Vet Med Assoc 233:752–757, 2008.
168. Hathcock JT, Newton JC: Computed tomographic characteristics of multilobular tumor of bone involving the cranium in 7 dogs and zygomatic arch in 2 dogs, Vet Radiol Ultrasound 41:214–217, 2000.
169. Lipsitz D, Levitski RE, Berry WL: Magnetic resonance imaging features of multilobular osteochondrosarcoma in 3 dogs, Vet Radiol Ultrasound 42:14–19, 2001.
170. Bordelon JT, Rochat MC: Use of a titanium mesh for cranioplasty following radical rostrotentorial craniectomy to remove an ossifying fibroma in a dog, J Am Vet Med Assoc 231:1692–1695, 2007.
171. Bryant KJ, Steinberg H, McAnulty JF: Cranioplasty by means of molded polymethylmethacrylate prosthetic reconstruction after radical excision of neoplasms of the skull in two dogs, J Am Vet Med Assoc 223(59):67–72, 2003.
172. Moissonnier P, Devauchelle P, Delisle F: Cranioplasty after en bloc resection of calvarial chondroma rodens in two dogs, J Small Anim Pract 38:358–363, 1997.
173. Straw RC, LeCouteur RA, Powers BE, et al: Multilobular osteochondrosarcoma of the canine skull: 16 cases (1978-1988), J Am Vet Med Assoc 195:1764–1769, 1989.
174. Kornegay JN, Mayhew IG: Metabolic, toxic, and nutritional diseases of the nervous system. In Oliver JE, Hoerlein BF, Mayhew IG, editors: Veterinary neurology, Philadelphia, 1987, Saunders.
175. Schall WD: Heat stroke. In Kirk RW, ed: Current veterinary therapy VII, Philadelphia, 1980, Saunders, pp. 202–205.
176. Schmidt-Nielsen K, Bretz WL, Taylor CR: Panting in dogs: unidirectional air flow over evaporative surfaces, Science 169:1102–1104, 1970.
177. Mehta AC, Baker RN: Persistent neurological deficits in heat stroke, Neurology 20:336–340, 1970.
178. Krum SH, Osborne CA: Heatstroke in the dog: a polysystemic disorder, J Am Vet Med Assoc 170:531–535, 1977.
179. Heffner GG, Rozanski EA, Beal MW, et al: Evaluation of freshwater submersion in small animals: 28 cases (1996-2006), J Am Vet Med Assoc 232:244–248, 2008.
180. Beal MW, Paglia DT, Griffin GM, et al: Ventilatory failure, ventilator management, and outcome in dogs with cervical spinal disorders: 14 cases (1991-1999), J Am Vet Med Assoc 218:1598–1602, 2001.
181. Kube S, Owen T, Hanson S: Severe respiratory compromise secondary to cervical disk herniation in two dogs, J Am Anim Hosp Assoc 39:513–517, 2003.
182. Drobatz KJ, Walker LM, Hendricks JC: Smoke exposure in dogs: 27 cases (1988-1997), J Am Vet Med Assoc 215:1306–1311, 1999.
183. Drobatz KJ, Walker LM, Hendricks JC: Smoke exposure in cats: 22 cases (1986-1997), J Am Vet Med Assoc 215:1312–1316, 1999.
184. Rodkey FL, O'Neal JD, Collison HA, et al: Relative affinity of hemoglobin S and hemoglobin A for carbon monoxide and oxygen, Clin Chem 20:83–84, 1974.
185. Roughton F, Darling F: The effect of carbon monoxide on oxy-hemoglobin dissociation curve, Am J Physiol 141:17–31, 1944.

186. Fitzgerald KT, Flood AA: Smoke inhalation, Clin Tech Small Anim Pract 21(4): 205–214, 2006.
187. Farrow CS: Smoke inhalation in the dog: current concepts of pathophysiology and management, Vet Med Small Anim Clin 70(4): 404–414, 1975.
188. Jackson CB, Drobatz K: Neurologic dysfunction associated with smoke exposure in dogs, J Vet Emerg Crit Care 12:193, 2004.
189. Mariani CL: Full recovery following delayed neurologic signs after smoke inhalation in a dog, J Vet Emerg Crit Care 13:235–239, 2003.
190. Lapresle J, Fardeau M: The central nervous system and carbon monoxide poisoning. II. Anatomical study of brain lesions following intoxication with carbon monoxide (22 cases), Prog Brain Res 24:31–74, 1967.
191. Ginsberg MD, Myers RE, McDonagh BF: Experimental carbon monoxide encephalopathy in the primate. II. Clinical aspects, neuropathology, and physiologic correlation, Arch Neurol 30:209–216, 1974.
192. Vaala WE: Peripartum asphyxia, Vet Clin North Am Equine Pract 10:187–218, 1994.
193. Palmer AC, Leadon DP, Rossdale PD, et al: Intracranial haemorrhage in pre-viable, premature and full term foals, Equine Vet J 16:383–389, 1984.
194. Palmer AC, Rossdale PD: Neuropathological changes associated with the neonatal maladjustment syndrome in the thoroughbred foal, Res Vet Sci 20:267–275, 1976.
195. Brown SA, Langford K, Tarver S: Effects of certain vasoactive agents on the long-term pattern of blood pressure, heart rate, and motor activity in cats, Am J Vet Res 58:647–652, 1997.
196. Mishina M, Watanabe T, Fujii K, et al: Non-invasive blood pressure measurements in cats: clinical significance of hypertension associated with chronic renal failure, J Vet Med Sci 60:805–808, 1998.
197. Brown S, Adkins R, Bagley A, et al: Guidelines for the identification, evaluation, and management of systemic hypertension in dogs and cats, J Vet Intern Med 21:542–558, 2007.
198. Bodey AR, Michell AR: Epidemiological study of blood pressure in domestic dogs, J Small Anim Pract 37:116–125, 1996.
199. Chalifoux A, Dallaire A, Blais D, et al: Evaluation of the arterial blood pressure of dogs by two noninvasive methods, Can J Comp Med 49:419–423, 1985.
200. Sparkes AH, Caney SM, King MC, et al: Inter- and intra-individual variation in Doppler ultrasonic indirect blood pressure measurements in healthy cats, J Vet Intern Med 13:314–318, 1999.
201. Belew AM, Bartlett T, Brown SA. : Evaluation of the white-coat effect in cats, J Vet Intern Med 13:134–142, 1999.
202. Bodey AR, Sansom J: Epidemiological study of blood pressure in domestic cats, J Small Anim Pract 39:567–573, 1998.
203. Elliott J, Syme HM, Rawlings JM, et al: Feline hypertension: clinical findings and response to antihypertensive treatment in 30 cases, J Small Anim Pract 42:122–129, 2001.
204. Kobayashi DL, Peterson ME, Graves TK, et al: Hypertension in cats with chronic renal failure or hyperthyroidism, J Vet Intern Med 4:58–62, 1990.
205. Littman MP: Spontaneous systemic hypertension in 24 cats, J Vet Intern Med 8:79–86, 1994.
206. Andrew E, Kyles CRG, John D, et al: Management of hypertension controls postoperative neurologic disorders after renal transplantation in cats, Vet Surg 28:436–441, 1999.
207. Gregory CR, Matthews KG, Aronson LR, et al: Central nervous system disorders after renal transplantation in cats, Vet Surg 26:386–392, 1997.
208. Mathews KG, Gregory CR: Renal transplants in cats: 66 cases (1987-1996), J Am Vet Med Assoc 211:1432–1436, 1997.
209. Ortega TM, Feldman EC, Nelson RW, et al: Systemic arterial blood pressure and urine protein/creatinine ratio in dogs with hyperadrenocorticism, J Am Vet Med Assoc 209:1724–1729, 1996.
210. Uchino M, Haga D, Nomoto J, et al: Ocular lesions associated with systemic hypertension in cats: 69 cases (1985–1998), J Am Vet Med Assoc 217:695–702, 2000.
211. Bartges JW, Willis AM, Polzin DJ: Hypertension and renal disease, Vet Clin North Am Small Anim Pract 26:1331–1345, 1996.
212. Turner JL, Brogdon JD, Lees GE, et al: Idiopathic hypertension in a cat with secondary hypertensive retinopathy associated with a high-salt diet, J Am Anim Hosp Assoc 26:647–651, 1990.
213. Stiles J, Polzin DJ, Bistner SI: The prevalence of retinopathy in cats with systemic hypertension and chronic renal failure or hyperthyroidism, J Am Anim Hosp Assoc 30:564–572, 1994.
214. Morgan RV: Systemic hypertension in four cats: ocular and medical findings, J Am Anim Hosp Assoc 22:615–621, 1986.
215. Sansom J, Dunn KA, Smith KC, et al: Ocular disease associated with hypertension in 16 cats, J Small Anim Pract 35:604–611, 1994.
216. Henik RA, Stepien RL, Bortnowski HB: Spectrum of M-mode echocardiographic abnormalities in 75 cats with systemic hypertension, J Am Anim Hosp Assoc 40:359–363, 2004.
217. Brown CA, Munday JS, Mathur S, et al: Hypertensive encephalopathy in cats with reduced renal function, Vet Pathol 42:642–649, 2005.
218. Jacob F, Polzin DJ, Osborne CA, et al: Association between initial systolic blood pressure and risk of developing a uremic crisis or of dying in dogs with chronic renal failure, J Am Vet Med Assoc 222:322–329, 2003.
219. Hinchey J, Chaves C, Appignani B, et al: A reversible posterior leukoencephalopathy syndrome, N Engl J Med 334:494–500, 1996.
220 Uchino M, Haga D, Nomoto J, et al: Brainstem involvement in hypertensive encephalopathy: a report of two cases and literature review, Eur Neurol 57: 223–226, 2007.
221. Johansson BB: The blood-brain barrier and cerebral blood flow in acute hypertension, Acta Med Scand Suppl 678:107–112, 1983.
222. Bartynski WS: Posterior reversible encephalopathy syndrome, Part 1: fundamental imaging and clinical features, AJNR Am J Neuroradiol 29:1036–1042, 2008.
223. Acierno MJ, Labato MA: Hypertension in renal disease: diagnosis and treatment, Clin Tech Small Anim Pract 20:23–30, 2005.
224. O'Brien DP, Barshop BA, Faunt KK, et al: Malonic aciduria in Maltese dogs: normal methylmalonic acid concentrations and malonyl-CoA decarboxylase activity in fibroblasts, J Inherit Metab Dis 22:883–890, 1999.
225. Ruaux CG, Steiner JM, Williams DA: Metabolism of amino acids in cats with severe cobalamin deficiency, Am J Vet Res 62:1852–1858, 2001.
226. Vaden SL, Wood PA, Ledley FD, et al: Cobalamin deficiency associated with methylmalonic acidemia in a cat, J Am Vet Med Assoc 200:1101–1103, 1992.

227. Simpson KW, Fyfe J, Cornetta A, et al: Subnormal concentrations of serum cobalamin (vitamin B_{12}) in cats with gastrointestinal disease, J Vet Intern Med 15:26–32, 2001.
228. Packer RA, Cohn LA, Wohlstadter DR, et al: D-lactic acidosis secondary to exocrine pancreatic insufficiency in a cat, J Vet Intern Med 19:106–110, 2005.
229. Abramson CJ, Platt SR, Jakobs C, et al: L-2-Hydroxyglutaric aciduria in Staffordshire bull terriers, J Vet Intern Med 17:551–556, 2003.
230. Penderis J, Calvin J, Abramson C, et al: L-2-hydroxyglutaric aciduria: characterisation of the molecular defect in a spontaneous canine model, J Med Genet 44:334–340, 2007.
231. Priester WA, Glass AG, Waggoner NS: Congenital defects in domesticated animals: general considerations, Am J Vet Res 31:1871–1879, 1970.
232. McLone DG: The biological resolution of malformations of the central nervous system, Neurosurgery 43:1375–1380, 1998.
233. DeSesso JM, Scialli AR, Holson JF: Apparent lability of neural tube closure in laboratory animals and humans, Am J Med Genet 87:143–162, 1999.
234. Noden DM, deLahunta A: Central nervous system and eye. In Noden DM, deLahunta A, editors: The embryology of domestic animals: developmental mechanisms and malformations, Baltimore, 1985, Williams & Wilkins.
235. Noden DM, deLahunta A: Causes of congential malformations. In Noden DM, deLahunta A, editors: The embryology of domestic animals: developmental mechanisms and malformations, Baltimore, 1985, Williams & Wilkins.
236. Braund KG: Degenerative and developmental disorders. In Oliver JE, Hoerlein BF, Mayhew IG, editors: Veterinary neurology, Philadelphia, 1987, Saunders.
237. Wunschmann A, Oglesbee M: Periventricular changes associated with spontaneous canine hydrocephalus, Vet Pathol 38:67–73, 2001.
238. Dhein CR, Prieur DJ, Riggs MW, et al: Suspected ciliary dysfunction in Chinese Shar-Pei pups with pneumonia, Am J Vet Res 51:439–446, 1990.
239. Cox NR, Shires A, McCoy CP, et al: Obstructive hydrocephalus due to neoplasia in a Rottweiler puppy, J Am Anim Hosp Assoc 26:335–338, 1990.
240. van der Lugt JJ, Prozesky L: The pathology of blindness in new-born calves caused by hypovitaminosis A, Onderstepoort J Vet Res 56:99–109, 1989.
241. DeBowes RM, Gift L: Common malformations and congenital abnormalities of the central nervous system. In Robinson NE, editor: Current therapy in equine medicine, Philadelphia, 1992, WB Saunders.
242. Washburn KE, Streeter RN: Congenital defects of the ruminant nervous system, Vet Clin North Am Food Anim Pract 20:413–434, 2004:viii.
243. Binns W, Shupe JL, Keeler RF, et al: Chronologic evaluation of teratogenicity in sheep fed *Veratrum californicum*, J Am Vet Med Assoc 147:839–842, 1965.
244. Rousseaux CG: Congenital defects as a cause of perinatal mortality of beef calves, Vet Clin North Am Food Anim Pract 10:35–51, 1994.
245. DiBartola SP, Johnson SE, Johnson GC, et al: Hypodipsic hypernatremia in a dog with defective osmoregulation of antidiuretic hormone, J Am Vet Med Assoc 204:922–925, 1994.
246. Dow SW, Fettman MJ, LeCouteur RA, et al: Hypodipsic hypernatremia and associated myopathy in a hydrocephalic cat with transient hypopituitarism, J Am Vet Med Assoc 191:217–221, 1987.
247. Higgins RJ, Vandevelde M, Braund KB: Internal hydrocephalus and associated periventricular encephalitis in young dogs, Vet Pathol 14:236–246, 1977.
248. Selby LA, Hayes HM Jr, Becker SV: Epizootiologic features of canine hydrocephalus, Am J Vet Res 40:411–413, 1979.
249. Sahar A, Hochwald GM, Kay WJ, et al: Spontaneous canine hydrocephalus: cerebrospinal fluid dynamics, J Neurol Neurosurg Psychiatry 34:308–315, 1971.
250. Wouda W, Vandevelde M, Kihm U: Internal hydrocephalus of suspected infectious origin in young dogs, Zentralbl Veterinarmed A 28:481–493, 1981.
251. Hoerlein BF: Canine neurology: diagnosis and treatment, ed 3, Philadelphia, 1978, Saunders.
252. Simpson ST: Hydrocephalus. In Kirk RW, editor: Current veterinary therapy X, Philadelphia, 1989, WB Saunders.
253. Dodman NH, Knowles KE, Shuster L, et al: Behavioral changes associated with suspected complex partial seizures in bull terriers, J Am Vet Med Assoc 208:688–691, 1996.
254. Dewey CW: External hydrocephalus in a dog with suspected bacterial meningoencephalitis, J Am Anim Hosp Assoc 38:563–567, 2002.
255. Dewey CW, Coates JR, Ducoté JM, et al: External hydrocephalus in two cats, J Am Anim Hosp Assoc 39:567–572, 2003.
256. Hudson JA, Simpson ST, Buxton DF, et al: Ultrasonographic diagnosis of canine hydrocephalus, Vet Radiol 31:50–58, 1990.
257. Rivers WJ, Walter PA: Hydrocephalus in the dog: utility of ultrasonography as an alternate diagnostic imaging technique, J Am Anim Hosp Assoc 28:333–343, 1992.
258. Esteve-Ratsch B, Kneissl S, Gabler C: Comparative evaluation of the ventricles in the Yorkshire terrier and the German shepherd dog using low-field MRI, Vet Radiol Ultrasound 42:410–413, 2001.
259. Haan CE, Kraft SL, Gavin PR, et al: Normal variation in size of the lateral ventricles of the Labrador retriever dog as assessed by magnetic resonance imaging, Vet Radiol Ultrasound 35:83–86, 1994.
260. Kii S, Uzuka Y, Taura Y, et al: Magnetic resonance imaging of the lateral ventricles in beagle-type dogs, Vet Radiol Ultrasound 38:430–433, 1997.
261. Spaulding KA, Sharp NJH: Ultrasonographic imaging of the lateral cerebral ventricles in the dog, Vet Radiol Ultrasound 31:59–64, 1990.
262. Vite CH, Insko EK, Schotland HM, et al: Quantification of cerebral ventricular volume in English bulldogs, Vet Radiol Ultrasound 38:437–443, 1997.
263. Vullo T, Korenman E, Manzo RP, et al: Diagnosis of cerebral ventriculomegaly in normal adult beagles using quantitative MRI, Vet Radiol Ultrasound 38:277–281, 1997.
264. Jaderlund KH, Hansson K, Berg AL, et al: Cerebral ventricular size in developing normal kittens measured by ultrasonography, Vet Radiol Ultrasound 44:581–588, 2003.
265. Haskins SC, Munger RJ, Helphrey MG, et al: Effect of acetazolamide on blood acid-base and electrolyte values in dogs, J Am Vet Med Assoc 179:792–796, 1981.
266. Javaheri S, Corbett WS, Simbartl LA, et al: Different effects of omeprazole and Sch 28080 on canine cerebrospinal fluid production, Brain Res 754:321–324, 1997.
267. Browd SR, Ragel BT, Gottfried ON, et al: Failure of cerebrospinal fluid shunts: part I: obstruction and mechanical failure, Pediatr Neurol 34:83–92, 2006.

268. Filgueiras Rda R, Martins Cde S, de Almeida RM, et al: Long-term evaluation of a new ventriculoperitoneal shunt valve system in a dog, J Vet Emerg Crit Care (San Antonio) 19:623–628, 2009.
269. Summers BA, Cummings JF, DeLahunta A: Malformations of the central nervous system. Veterinary neuropathology, St Louis, 1995, Mosby.
270. Sharp NJ, Davis BJ, Guy JS, et al: Hydranencephaly and cerebellar hypoplasia in two kittens attributed to intrauterine parvovirus infection, J Comp Pathol 121:39–53, 1999.
271. Osburn BI, Johnson RT, Silverstein AM, et al: Experimental viral-induced congenital encephalopathies. II. The pathogenesis of bluetongue vaccine virus infection in fetal lambs, Lab Invest 25:206–210, 1971.
272. Osburn BI, Silverstein AM, Prendergast RA, et al: Experimental viral-induced congenital encephalopathies. I. Pathology of hydranencephaly and porencephaly caused by bluetongue vaccine virus, Lab Invest 25:197–205, 1971.
273. Trautwein G, Hewicker M, Liess B, et al: Studies on transplacental transmissibility of a bovine virus diarrhoea (BVD) vaccine virus in cattle. III. Occurrence of central nervous system malformations in calves born from vaccinated cows, Zentralbl Veterinarmed B 33:260–268, 1986.
274. Parsonson IM, Della-Porta AB, Snowdon WA, et al: Congenital abnormalities in foetal lambs after inoculation of pregnant ewes with Akabane virus, Aust Vet J 51:585–586, 1975:(letter).
275. Scott FW, deLahunta A, Schultz RD, et al: Teratogenesis in cats associated with griseofulvin therapy, Teratology 11:79–86, 1975.
276. Zook BC, Sostaric BR, Draper DJ, et al: Encephalocele and other congenital craniofacial anomalies in Burmese cats, Vet Med Small Anim Clin 78:695–701, 1983.
277. Noden DM, Evans HE: Inherited homeotic midfacial malformations in Burmese cats, J Craniofac Genet Dev Biol Suppl 2:249–266, 1986.
278. Lawler DF, Monti KL: Morbidity and mortality in neonatal kittens, Am J Vet Res 45:1455–1459, 1984.
279. Sullivan SA, Harmon BG, Purinton PT, et al: Lobar holoprosencephaly in a miniature schnauzer with hypodipsic hypernatremia, J Am Vet Med Assoc 223(1778):1783–1787, 2003.
280. Jeffery ND, Watson PJ, Abramson C, et al: Brain malformations associated with primary adipsia identified using magnetic resonance imaging, Vet Rec 152:436–438, 2003.
281. Greenfield JG, Love S, Louis DN, et al: Malformations. Greenfield's neuropathology, ed 8, London, 2008, Hodder Arnold.
282. Saito M, Sharp NJH, Kortz GD, et al: Magnetic resonance imaging features of lissencephaly in 2 Lhasa Apsos, Vet Radiol Ultrasound 43:331–337, 2002.
283. Jurney C, Haddad J, Crawford N, et al: Polymicrogyria in standard poodles, J Vet Intern Med 23:871–874, 2009.
284. Read DH: Congenital polymicrogyria in Murray Grey calves. From Proceedings, Palmerston North, New Zealand Veterinary Association, pp. 69–75, 1983.
285. Osweiler GD, Carson TL, Buck WB: Clinical and diagnostic veterinary toxicology, ed 3, Dubuque, Iowa, 1985, Kendall/Hunt.

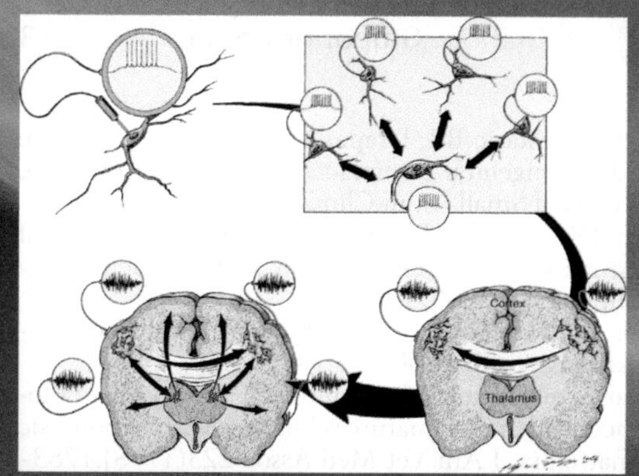

CHAPTER 13

Seizures, Narcolepsy, and Cataplexy

The term *seizure* has been broadly defined as a sudden, transient, abnormal phenomenon of a motor, sensory, autonomic, or psychic nature resulting from a transient dysfunction of part or all of the brain.[1] Additionally, a seizure can be defined as the clinical manifestation of excessive hypersynchronous neuronal activity.[2] *Epilepsy* is a disorder of the brain that is characterized by recurring, unpredictable seizures.[2] A seizure has several components. The actual seizure is called the *ictus*. The ictus usually lasts for 1 to 2 minutes, but variation is considerable. Ictus in animals involves dysfunction of one or more of the following: (1) alteration of muscle tone or involuntary movement; (2) disturbance of the autonomic nervous system (e.g., salivation, urination, defecation); (3) loss or derangement of consciousness; and (4) automatisms (repetitive movement) or paroxysms of behavior (also known as psychic disturbances). Clinically automatisms or paroxysms of behavior may be expressed clinically as repetitive, abnormal stereotypic actions or behaviors, respectively, such as aggression, restlessness or anxiety demonstrated as escaping behaviors or attention seeking, licking, chewing, and whining or shaking that demonstrate a response to anticonvulsant therapy.[3,4]

A *prodrome* (preictal) period may occur within hours preceding ictus during which the animal may display altered behavior. Animals may hide, appear nervous, or seek out their owners during this time. Also preceding ictus, an *aura*, stereotypic motor, behavioral, or autonomic changes occurring seconds to minutes before the ictus, may be observed and signifies the onset of ictus.[5] Differentiation between prodrome and aura can be difficult. After the seizure, *postictal period* the animal may return to normal in seconds to minutes or may be restless, lethargic, confused or disoriented; display hunger or thirst; urinate or defecate; or be blind for minutes to hours. The aura and the postictal phase do not have any relationship to the severity or the cause of the seizures.[5]

Most importantly seizures are defined as a "clinical manifestation" of an abnormal action or behavior. Seizures are identified and classified on observations and interpretations of behavior and activity displayed by the affected animal. Careful questioning of the owner is required to determine whether the episode described is actually a seizure. If the event is repetitive and has the same appearance each time, it is likely a seizure. Isolated motor activity such as forced turning of the head or clonic jerks of muscle groups are commonly signs of seizure activity.

Several disorders can be misinterpreted as a seizure. Owners frequently confuse syncope or acute signs of vestibular dysfunction with seizures. Syncope is a transient loss of consciousness caused by ischemia of the brain and can be difficult to differentiate from true seizures. The most common cause of syncope in animals is cardiac arrhythmia. In many cases, the history is usually indicative of syncope rather than seizures. Syncope is often precipitated by stress, excitement, pain, and exercise. In some instances, syncope may occur during urination, defecation, or coughing. Knowledge of a prior cardiac disease may raise the index of suspicion for syncope. Similarly, given the prevalence of heart disease commonly associated with syncope in certain breeds (i.e., boxer and Doberman pinscher), signalment also may help direct attention to a thorough cardiac evaluation to help exclude syncope from consideration. Auscultation of the heart combined with evaluation of an electrocardiogram, Holter monitor recordings, thoracic radiographic and echocardiographic imaging may disclose the problem. Similarly, an acute or peracute presentation of vestibular dysfunction also can be confused with seizures. Affected animals usually display persistent signs consistent with disturbances of the vestibular system (see Chapter 8).

Narcolepsy is a disorder of the brain that is marked by sudden recurring attacks of sleep. Given its abrupt onset and transient nature, confusion with a seizure is possible. Narcolepsy is discussed at the end of this chapter. Disorders of involuntary movement also need to be differentiated from a seizure, in particular, those seizures that do not alter consciousness (see Chapter 10). Likewise, certain behavioral disorders (e.g., tail chasing) are associated with stereotypic actions. If possible, having an owner record an event on video may allow for proper classification of the event. If the diagnosis of seizure cannot be made with certainty, a thorough diagnostic workup aimed at identifying an underlying etiology associated with seizures should be pursued. In cases in which diagnostic testing fails to uncover an underlying cause of seizures, a trial with an anticonvulsant drug may be warranted.

PATHOPHYSIOLOGY

Seizures are always a sign of abnormal cerebral or thalamic function. Epileptic seizures can be dichotomously divided into those that originate from discharges in a circumscribed part of the brain (a seizure focus) or those that result from discharges that appear from the very start to involve both cerebral hemispheres, bilaterally and synchronously.[6] Once initiated, focal discharges may subsequently spread to other parts of the brain resulting in a generalized cerebral disturbance. The initiation and propagation of the seizure focus is responsible for the clinical manifestation, which defines the seizure type (see Classification; Box-1). Electroencephalography (EEG) allows observation of the electrical events of the cerebral cortex occurring during a seizure or between seizures (interictal). The hallmark of a seizure focus is massive depolarization.[7] From experimental models of seizures, recordings made from microelectrodes within neurons in a seizure focus disclose activity characterized by large-amplitude, prolonged membrane depolarizations with associated high-frequency bursts of spikes, termed paroxysmal depolarization shifts.[8] Clinically, paroxysmal depolarizations may result in interictal activity, which clinically can be appreciated on the EEG.[9,10] Interictal EEG activity consists of spike discharges, spike waves, and spike-and-slow wave complexes.[11] Ictal EEG activity can take on many forms, including those observed during the interictal period or sleep, or as repetitive stereotyped waveforms such as a 3-Hz spike-and-wave pattern or paroxysms that alternate between repetitive spike discharges and spike-and-slow wave discharges.[11] In dogs with epilepsy, interictal EEG abnormalities occur in 65% to 86% of dogs, many of which display focal abnormalities.[12-14] Interpretation of EEG recordings requires considerable expertise and specialized equipment. Although not frequently performed, EEG recording may be of value in cases in which it is difficult to discern the nature of the event as a seizure or help in the assessment of anticonvulsant therapy in severely affected animals. Recent technology has improved to allow for telemetry recording so animal restraint may not be necessary.

The generation of a seizure, *epileptogenesis*, has traditionally been ascribed to a single, isolated group of neurons called a seizure focus. Epileptogenesis can also occur from hyperexcitable neurons that are a part of a group of interconnected and widely spread neurons called neural networks.[11,15] One such network, the thalamocortical network, is involved in the pathogenesis of absence seizures.[16] In cats administered large doses of penicillin intramuscularly (IM), behavioral and EEG evidence (slow wave discharges [SWDs]) of seizures develop that were thought to originate in the thalamus and subsequently spread bilaterally to the cerebral cortex in a process called the centrencephalic theory.[17] Later, this theory was challenged by studies in which identical SWDs in the thalamus could be recorded despite the induction of a seizure focus in the cerebral cortex.[18] Such experiments have led to the idea that abnormal activity of any group of neurons within a neural network may be responsible for the development and spread of a seizure (Figure 13-1). The clinical manifestation of the seizure may reflect not only the function but also the distribution of the neural network throughout the brain.

Abnormal neuronal activity causing seizures may occur secondary to a structural lesion (e.g., brain tumor) or may occur in the absence of structural lesions and simply reflect changes in neurotransmitters and their receptors.[15] Among many possible neurotransmitters, alterations in glutamate and gamma-aminobutyric acid (GABA) are fundamental to the paroxysmal depolarization shifts that initiate seizures.[19] Mechanistically, seizures may develop from an imbalance between excitatory and inhibitory mechanisms that favor the sudden onset of excitation. Glutamate and GABA are the primary excitatory and inhibitory neurotransmitters, respectively. Multiple cellular receptors exist for each agent. There are two main types of glutamate receptors, inotropic (iGluR), which function as a calcium ion channels, and metabotropic glutamate (mGluR), which work via a second messenger system that when activated increase sodium and calcium influx resulting in depolarization of neurons.[20,21] There also are two main GABA receptors, $GABA_A$ and $GABA_B$ receptors. Once activated, $GABA_A$ receptors, directly linked to an ion channel, allow the influx

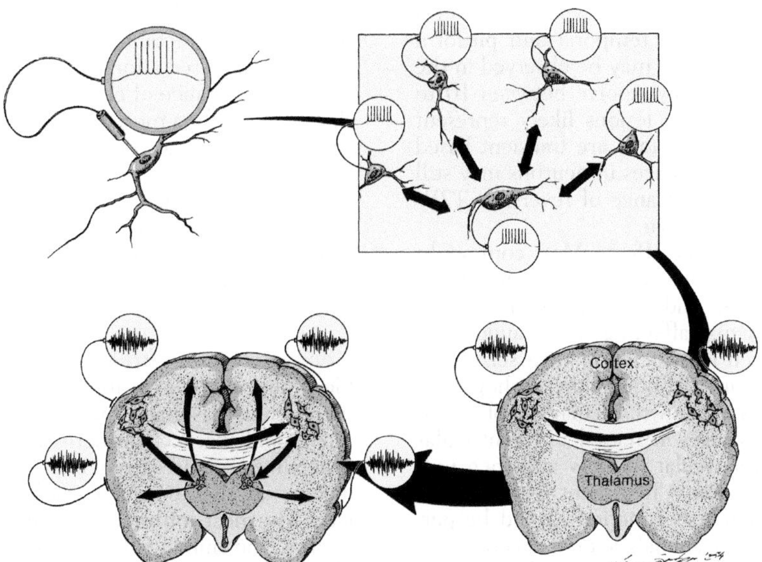

Figure 13-1 Spread of seizure activity from a focal area to the entire cerebrum. A, paroxysmal depolarization shift in a neuron. B, Spread of activity to surrounding neurons. C, propagation of seizure activity to other cortical areas by axonal conduction. D, Generalization of seizure activity through the diencephalon. (From Olive JE, Hoerlein BF, Mayhew IG, editors: Veterinary neurology, Philadelphia, 1987, WB Saunders.)

of chloride ions, which hyperpolarize neurons while $GABA_B$ receptors work via a second messenger system to increase potassium conductance and decrease calcium conductance, which also hyperpolarizes the neuron.[22,23] The end result is postsynaptic inhibition. Excessive activation of glutamate receptors or defective inhibition of $GABA_A$ and $GABA_B$ receptors plays fundamental roles in the pathogenesis of epilepsy.[24] In dogs with untreated epilepsy, cerebrospinal fluid (CSF) concentrations of GABA are reduced, whereas CSF concentrations of glutamate are increased compared with normal dogs.[25,26] Moreover, dogs with low CSF concentrations of GABA have a reduced response to anticonvulsant therapy.[27] With the advent of novel anticonvulsant drugs targeting different aspects of neurotransmission, in the future it may be possible to tailor anticonvulsant therapy based on a knowledge of seizure epileptogenesis.

Abnormalities in neurotransmitters also may cause structural pathology of the brain. Excessive amounts of glutamate are released during seizures. As a result, seizure-associated neuronal damage may occur, termed excitatory neurotoxicity, in which specific neuronal populations, such as hippocampal neurons, display a selective vulnerability.[28] Excessive glutamate causes neuronal loss by increasing intracellular calcium concentrations, which leads to apoptosis.[29] Hippocampal neuronal loss occurs even when the initiating seizure focus is located distant from the hippocampus. In the majority of humans with temporal lobe epilepsy, there is degeneration and loss of neurons in the same topography as occurs with experimentally induced glutamate excitatory neurotoxicity.[30] However, it remains unclear whether neuronal loss represents the inciting cause of temporal lobe epilepsy or a perpetuating factor once pathology is established.[31] Similar neuronal loss in the hippocampus has been observed in dogs with epilepsy.[32,33] The degree of neuronal loss in dogs with epilepsy is unknown. In one study of dogs with refractory epilepsy, neuronal loss in the hippocampus was not evident.[34] However, neuronal necrosis in the hippocampus and piriform lobe occurs in cats.[35] Abnormalities secondary to seizures may be detected clinically using magnetic resonance imaging (MRI). Seizure-related abnormalities observed on MRI consist of hyperintensities on T2-weighted images (T2W) in areas similar to those affected by excitatory neurotoxicity.[36] On MRI, the lesions have characteristics consistent with edema in a distinctive topography affecting the temporal and piriform lobes of the cerebrum.[36] Lesions also may be observed in the cingulate gyri. The changes typically resolve between 10 to 16 weeks following seizures.[36] The lesions likely represent cytotoxic edema.[37] Although the lesions are transient based on MRI, degenerative histologic changes in neurons may still be present.[38] In the end, the significance of reversible T2W hyperintensities in animals is unknown.

Seizures also may have systemic effects. Most commonly, seizures increase sympathetic tone, which leads to hypertension, tachycardia, acidosis, and hyperthermia.[39] Noncardiogenic pulmonary edema affecting the caudodorsal lung fields has been observed in association with seizures.[40] Rarely, hemoptysis may occur.[41] Although the pathogenesis of noncardiogenic edema is unknown, it may involve systemic hypertension, which causes increased left ventricular afterload, diminished left ventricular outflow and then pulmonary hypertension and edema.[40] Treatment is supportive. Frequent monitoring of respiratory function should be performed. If hypoxemic, affected animals should receive oxygen supplementation. In rare instances, mechanical ventilation may be necessary. Edema usually does not respond to diuretic therapy. In addition, myocardial infarction also has been associated with seizures in dogs; however, the clinical impact of this remains unclear.[42] Although unknown, myocardial infarction may develop as a result of increased sympathetic tone or the direct impact of excitatory neurotransmitters on the myocardium.[43]

CLASSIFICATION

The classification of seizures involves both etiology and seizure type (Box 13-1). The following discussion of classification and terminology of seizures has been adopted from those used in humans.[44,45] Some of the terminology has been modified so that terms can be more appropriately applied to animals.

Etiology-Based Classification of Seizures

Primary epilepsy is used to describe seizures that have an unknown cause. Additionally, primary epilepsy implies that there is a known or strongly suspected underlying hereditary basis predicated on a high prevalence in a specific breed.

Idiopathic epilepsy is used to describe seizures where an underlying cause cannot be identified. Idiopathic epilepsy can be used to classify seizures in a wide range of clinical scenarios. For example, idiopathic epilepsy may be used akin to primary epilepsy in some animals in which the age, neurologic examination findings are identical to those observed in primary epilepsy (see Box 13-1); however, without pedigree analysis or breeding studies, a hereditary basis cannot be established. In this case, idiopathic epilepsy implies a "disease unto itself" and not an unknown cause.[44] In other cases, an underlying disease process may be strongly suspected but is not identified through diagnostic tests. An example might be a geriatric dog in which a brain tumor may be suspected yet a lesion is not observed with cross-sectional imaging. The implication is quite different as an underlying disorder may exist and with time become evident. Consequently, depending on the signalment, history, and neurologic examination, careful monitoring may reveal changes with time that dictate further diagnostic testing.

Symptomatic epilepsy is used to describe seizures, in which an underlying pathologic or structural disease of the brain (intracranial) is identified.[44]

Reactive seizure is applied when a metabolic or toxic cause is determined and the brain itself is normal. These seizures have an extracranial cause and occur as a reaction to the insult.[46] Given that metabolic or toxic insults infrequently result in unpredictable, recurrent seizures, reactive seizures are not considered a form of epilepsy, per se.

The importance of classifying seizures based on etiology is that it allows for a more specific differential diagnosis. Specific causes of seizures are described in detailed below and in Tables 13-1 and 13-2.

In addition to an etiology-based classification, seizures can also be categorized based on the seizure type or clinical manifestation as *generalized, focal,* or *focal onset with secondary generalization.* Within each category, several clinical presentations exist (see Box 13-1).

Generalized Seizures

Generalized seizures are subdivided into tonic-clonic (formerly known as grand mal), tonic or clonic alone, myoclonic, atonic, and absence (formerly known as petit mal). Signs with generalized seizures begin bilaterally, often symmetrically, and involve an alteration in consciousness at some point during ictus. The most common generalized seizure is the tonic-clonic seizure. The animal falls and becomes unconscious.[4] The tonic phase involves rigid extension of the limbs and opisthotonos lasting a brief period of time (10 to 30 seconds) during which time respirations may stop (apnea). Following the tonic phase, the clonic phase involves uncoordinated, purposeless, jerking movements of the limbs. The clonic phase may alternate with tonic activity. Additionally, chewing movements with the lips drawn back are common. Autonomic activity may start in the tonic or clonic phase of the ictus and may include mydriasis, salivation, urination, defecation, and piloerection. Automatisms such as running or paddling movements of the limbs also may occur. During the tonic and clonic activity, most animals are unconscious. Although consciousness is difficult to determine in animals, it is frequently measured in terms of responsiveness, attentiveness, or by the presence of disorientation. The ictus usually lasts 1 to 2 minutes. The postictal phase may last a variable time period during which the animal may

BOX 13-1

Classification of Seizures Based on Clinical Signs

Etiology-Based Classification

Primary or Idiopathic Epilepsy Related to a disease process in and of itself Does not infer "cause not identified" Possibly related to imbalance of excitatory and inhibitory influences on susceptible neuronal population	*Dog:* age of onset between 1 and 5 years Normal PE and NE Normal interictal behavior No abnormalities identified on diagnostic tests Defined or suspected genetic or familial predisposition *Cats:* rare *Horses:* Arabian foals (familial juvenile onset) *Cattle:* Brown Swiss and Swedish Red cattle
Symptomatic Epilepsy (Secondary; acquired) Related to an identifiable structural or pathologic lesion	Intracranial in origin
Reactive Seizures (Extracranial; metabolic/toxic) A reaction to an extracranial cause	Extracranial in origin related to a metabolic or toxic disorder

Seizure Types—Based on Clinical Signs

Generalized:

Bilateral, symmetrical motor movements with autonomic dysfunction, and altered consciousness implicating bilateral cerebral involvement from the onset of the seizures

- *Tonic-clonic:* Most common presentation of a generalized epileptic seizure
  - Tonic phase: abrupt fall to lateral recumbency; increased extensor tone in all limbs and opisthotonos (initial phase)
  - Clonic: purposeless, jerking movements of the limbs (follows tonic phase)
  - Autonomic signs common (mydriasis, salivation, urination, defecation)
  - Altered or loss of consciousness: judged based on responsiveness and attentiveness
- *Tonic:* Uncommon; increased extensor tone and opisthotonos as the sole manifestation
- *Clonic:* Uncommon; jerking movements of the limbs as the sole manifestation
- *Atonic:* Loss of tone
- *Myoclonic:* Uncommon
  - Spontaneous or in response to stimuli (visual, light, sound); repetitive contractions of muscles
  - Most commonly affecting the head, neck, and thoracic limbs
- *Absence:* Rare
  - Altered or loss of consciousness without motor movements (need EEG recording to identify)

Focal:

Clinical manifestation limited to a focal area of the head or body implicating involvement of a focal region of the cerebral cortex

Qualified based on whether or not consciousness is altered

- *Simple*: No alterations in consciousness
- *Complex:* Altered or loss of consciousness

Characterized by one or a combination of the following:

- *Motor disturbance:* focal or isolated anatomic part or muscle group (i.e., facial muscles or single limb)
- *Autonomic disturbance:* mydriasis, vomiting, salivation, urination, defecation
- *Automatisms/paroxysms of behavior:* repetitive, stereotypic movements or behaviors
  - Licking, chewing, rubbing of the face, head turning, shaking, "fly biting"
  - Fear, anxiety, attention seeking, aimless wandering, aggression, whining

Focal seizure with secondary generalization:

Focal seizure during onset suggesting focal area of the brain involved but subsequently evolves to involve bilateral motor disturbances implicating bilateral cerebral cortical involvement

Often considered the aura; by definition, the aura is considered the onset of ictus

Most common presentation of primary epilepsy in dogs

Requires careful observations to identify partial seizure onset; often missed by owners

TABLE 13-1

*Causes of Seizures Based on Etiologic Classification**

Classification	Frequent Causes	Diagnostic Tests
Reactive seizures		The following apply to all these differentials:
	Metabolic (15)	History, PE/NE findings, potential for exposure
	Liver or renal disease	Presence of interictal abnormalities (common)
	Electrolyte (Na, Ca, Mg)	When present, neurologic deficits—*symmetric*
	Hypoglycemia	
	Endocrine	Minimum database (MDB)
	Toxic disorders (15)	CBC, chemistry profile, UA
	Heavy metals, pesticides	Based on MDB specialized testing
	rodenticides, poisonous plants, drugs, antifreeze	Blood ammonia, preprandial and postprandial bile acids
	Disinfectants, methylxanthines	Serum cholinesterase activity
	Illicit drugs, medications	Blood gas, urine, organic acids
	Animal-related poisoning (toad, spiders)	Specific testing to identify a toxin
	5-Hydroxytryptophan	Response to therapy
	Tetanus (10)	
	Nutritional (15)	
	Thiamine	
Symptomatic epilepsy		
		The following apply to all these differentials:
	Degenerative (15)	Signalment, history, PE/NE findings
	Storage diseases (A)	Presence of interictal abnormalities (common)
	Neuronal ceroid lipofucinosis	When present, neurologic deficits—*asymmetric*
	Leukodystrophies	MDB is normal
	Metachromatic leukodystrophy	Cross-sectional imaging (MRI or CT)
	Mitochondrial encephalopathy	CSF analysis
	Inborn errors of metabolism	Serology, PCR testing, microbiology—infectious
	Spongiform encephalopathy	Organic acid testing of urine—degenerative
	Multiple system neuronal degeneration	
	Developmental/anomalous (12)	
	Hydrocephalus	
	Lissencephaly	
	Porencephaly, hydranencephaly	
	Polymicrogyria	
	Agenesis of corpus callosum	
	Dandy-Walker syndrome	
	Chiari-like malformation	
	Intracranial arachnoid cyst/diverticulum	
	Inflammatory/Infectious (15)	
	Infectious	
	Bacterial: any type	
	Viral: canine distemper virus (D), FIP (C), rabies (A)	
	IBRV (B), viral encephalomyelitis (E), FIV (C)	
	Feline panleukopenia (C)	
	Protozoal: toxoplasmosis or neosporosis	
	Mycotic: cryptococcosis, coccidioidomycosis, blastomycosis, histoplasmosis	
	Rickettsial: RMSF, ehrlichiosis	
	Noninfectious (D)	
	Granulomatous meningoencephalomyelitis	
	Necrotizing encephalitides	
	Neoplastic (12)	
	Traumatic (12)	
	Vascular (12)	

TABLE 13-1

Causes of Seizures Based on Etiologic Classification*—cont'd

Classification	Frequent Causes	Diagnostic Tests
Primary or idiopathic epilepsy		Signalment, history, age of onset, familial incidence Normal PE/neurologic examination Normal interictal behavior No abnormalities identified Imaging of the brain—normal CSF analysis—normal Genetic testing or pedigree analysis

Modified from Oliver JE Jr: Seizure disorders in companion animals, Compend Contin Educ Pract Vet 2:77–86, 1980.
CBC, Complete blood cell count; *CSF*, cerebrospinal fluid; *CT*, computed tomography; *FIP*, feline infectious peritonitis; *IBRV*, infectious bovine rhinotracheitis virus; *FIV*, feline immunodeficiency virus; *MRI*, magnetic resonance imaging; *NE*, neurologic examination; *PCR*, polymerase chain reaction; *PE*, physical examination; *RMSF*, Rocky Mountain spotted fever; *UA*, urinalysis.
(A), all species; (B), bovine (C), cat; (E), equine.
*Numbers in parentheses refer to chapters in which disease classes are discussed.

TABLE 13-2

Common Causes of Seizures Based on Age of Onset

AGE†		
Younger Than 1 Year of Age	**Between 1 and 5 Years of Age**	**Older Than 5 Years of Age**
Degenerative Storage diseases (glycogen, lysosomal) Neuronal ceroid lipofuscinosis Multiple system degeneration Mitochondrial encephalopathy Inborn error of metabolism Spongiform encephalopathy Metachromic leukodystrophy Developmental/Anomalous* Hydrocephalus Lissencephaly Porencephaly, hydranencephaly Polymicrogyria Dandy-Walker syndrome Chiari-like malformation Intracranial arachnoid cyst/diverticulum Metabolic Hepatic (congenital portosystemic shunt, microvascular dysplasia) Renal (congenital disease) Hypoglycemia Neonatal asphyxia Nutritional—thiamine deficiency Infectious* Bacterial: any type Viral: canine distemper virus, FIP, rabies Protozoal, parasitic, rickettsial, fungal Toxic Trauma	Primary epilepsy* Metabolic or endocrine Electrolyte disorders Hepatic (acquired disease) Renal (acquired disease) Endocrine hypoglycemia Inflammatory/noninfectious GME, necrotizing encephalitides Infectious—any type Toxic Trauma Vascular	Neoplasia* Older age onset degenerative disorders Metabolic or endocrine Electrolyte disorders Hepatic (acquired disease) Renal (acquired disease) Endocrine—hypoglycemia Pancreatic β-islet tumor Inflammatory Toxic Trauma Vascular

Modified from Oliver JE Jr: Seizure disorders in companion animals, Compend Contin Educ Pract Vet 2:77–86, 1980.
*Denotes the most common etiologies for the age group.
†Primarily relates to dogs but can be used as a guideline for other species.

rest followed by a return to normal activity or may include confusion, disorientation, restlessness and pacing, hunger or thirst, defecation or urination, and blindness, which can persist for up to 24 hours or longer. Abnormalities that persist longer than 24 hours may reflect a structural lesion of the central nervous system (CNS).

In cats, generalized tonic-clonic seizures can be violent.[47] Cats may be propelled into the air or have such violent movements that they traumatize themselves (contusions, excoriations, avulsion of nails, and biting the tongue). Milder forms of generalized seizures in cats are characterized by mydriasis, facial twitching, and, less frequently, salivation and urination.

Tonic, atonic, or clonic seizures alone occur uncommonly.[4] Myoclonic seizures have been observed in the miniature wire haired dachshund, beagle, and basset hound dogs in association with Lafora disease.[48-53] Clinical signs involved repetitive, brief myoclonic jerking of the head, neck, and thoracic limbs and are frequently strong enough to cause the animal to fall backward into a sitting or lying position.[48,51,54] Myoclonic jerks may occur spontaneously or in response to stimuli such as visual (passing a hand in front of the face of the dog), light, or sound.[48,52] Most affected dogs are between 6 and 9 years of age at onset. Presumptive diagnosis of Lafora disease is suggested by the clinical signs; however, definitive diagnosis requires histologic identification of intracellular accumulations of polyglucosan (Lafora bodies) in muscle, liver, skin, or brain.[51] In affected miniature wire-haired dachshunds, a three copy repeat within the *Epmb2* gene resulting in a decreased expression of the laforin protein appears to underlie the disease.[55] Affected dogs respond minimally to anticonvulsant drugs. Depending on the frequency and severity, affected dogs can maintain a normal quality of life.

Absence seizures are very uncommon in animals and more likely not easily recognized. They are characterized by a brief (seconds) loss of contact with the environment and lack motor activity. Variations in humans include minor motor components such as facial twitching, loss of postural tone, and autonomic activity. As in humans, absence seizures are associated with a characteristic EEG pattern (4-Hz spike-wave complexes).[56] Unless these attacks are frequent or the owner is very observant, they go unrecognized.

Focal Seizures

A focal seizure develops in a discrete area of the brain (seizure focus) that is responsible for producing a particular clinical sign.[57] Focal seizures may or may not be associated with alterations in consciousness. *Simple* focal seizures do not affect consciousness, whereas *complex* seizures do.[58] In addition to consciousness, focal seizures are categorized based on the presence of motor, autonomic, or automatisms and paroxysms of abnormal behavior. Signs may occur alone or in various combinations. Frequently, focal seizures are recognized by motor disturbances. Movements are restricted to one part of the body, such as the face or one limb. The motor component of the seizure onset is one of the key features differentiating focal from generalized seizures. Focal motor seizures are presumed to arise from a seizure focus near a primary motor area in the frontal cortex on the contralateral side of the observed motor disturbance. Animals with focal motor seizures are more likely to have localized EEG abnormalities during interictal periods than are those with generalized seizures. Focal autonomic seizures are not commonly recognized in isolation; however, autonomic disturbance may occur in conjunction with motor movements. Autonomic disturbances may show the classical signs of mydriasis and salivation or involve visceral activity such as diarrhea, vomiting, and abdominal discomfort, which may correlate with lesions of the limbic system.[59] Rarely, hypersalivation, dysphagia, salivary gland enlargement, and esophageal spasms can occur.[60,61]

Automatisms or paroxysms of abnormal behavior are commonly observed in dogs.[3,4] When occurring minutes to seconds before ictus, these are considered an aura and by definition are part of the ictus regardless of the development of other characteristic signs of seizures.[1] However, automatisms and paroxysms of abnormal behavior can be the sole manifestation of the seizure activity without involving consciousness, motor function, or autonomic disturbances. Automatisms or paroxysms of abnormal behavior may include a wide array of repetitive activities. These include chewing, licking (into the air or directed at a specific body part), aimless wandering or restlessness, attention-seeking behavior or avoidance/escaping behavior, aggression, rage, or biting at imaging objects ("fly biting").[3,4,59,62] Animals that have repetitive episodes of fly biting may be having focal sensory seizures in the visual cortex similar to focal sensory seizures that occur in humans; however, sensory disturbances cannot be truly identified in animals. Similarly, fly biting may be considered a focal seizure involving a paroxysm of abnormal behavior.[4,63] Alternatively, fly biting may represent a form of obsessive-compulsive behavior rather than a seizure.[64]

In the bull terrier, behavioral changes such as compulsive tail chasing, rage, trances, preoccupations, fears, hyperactivity, sound sensitivities, and phobias may be seizure activity.[65] Electroencephalogram abnormalities include multiple epileptic spikes characterized by high-amplitude, low-frequency discharges. Many affected dogs have concurrent hydrocephalus demonstrated on computed tomography (CT) imaging. Clinical signs develop at 6 to 13 months of age and occasionally in older dogs. The syndrome in bull terriers may reflect an inherited form of temporal lobe epilepsy.

Focal seizures occur in cats.[47,66,67] They are characterized by lack of response to sensory stimuli and often show a trance-like state. Unilateral facial twitching, turning the head to one side, and repetitive movements of one limb can be observed. Bizarre behavior, such as inappropriate hissing, growling, running blindly into objects, and compulsive behavior, such as self-chewing, biting, and circling, have been observed in association with facial twitching and salivation.

Focal Seizures With Secondary Generalization

Focal seizures with secondary generalization is the most common presentation of seizures in dogs with primary or idiopathic epilepsy.[3-5] In several studies, focal seizures with secondary generalization were observed in 80% to 90% of primary or idiopathic epileptic dogs.[3-5,46,68-70] In most instances, the onset of ictus is marked by an aura that defines ictus as beginning with a focal seizure onset. Within seconds to minutes, the ictus evolves to include bilaterally symmetric disturbances in motor movements, autonomic dysfunction, and altered consciousness typical of generalized seizures. Most cases require close observation to recognize signs consistent with an aura, which is essential for indentifying focal seizure onset.

Status Epilepticus (SE) and Cluster Seizures

Historically, SE was defined as a condition in which a seizure persists for a sufficient length of time or is repeated frequently enough to produce a fixed and enduring epileptic condition. Current definition in veterinary medicine implies SE is a seizure that persists for more than 5 minutes or two or more sequential seizures without a full recovery to consciousness. Cluster seizure (CS) is defined as increased frequency of seizures within a day or few days. Cluster seizure also can be defined as more than two seizures in a 24-hour period. If seizures last longer than 5 minutes, emergency management to stop the seizures is needed.

DISEASES

Seizures can be caused by any process that alters normal neuronal function. The differential diagnoses are listed for each etiologic classification of seizures. The most likely diseases within each category should be considered based on signalment, physical and neurological examination findings, and results of diagnostic tests (see Tables 13-1 and 13-2).

Primary and Idiopathic Epilepsy

The gross structure of the brain in animals with primary or idiopathic epilepsy has no demonstrable pathologic lesion. The cause may be genetic (primary) or unknown (idiopathic). The incidence in dogs has been estimated at 1% to 2%.[13] Although primary and idiopathic epilepsy occurs in a number of species, the most comprehensive studies have been those of humans and dogs.[3-5,13,46,53,68-84] Most importantly, to establish a diagnosis, affected animals must have a normal neurologic examination and remain normal during the interictal period. In addition, other systemic and brain abnormalities are not detected with diagnostic tests. From a clinical perspective, idiopathic epilepsy is a diagnosis of exclusion. The breed, age, and history also provide important clues to an underlying hereditary basis especially if a familial history of seizures exists. The finding of idiopathic seizures without an underlying cause does not necessarily rule in or out a genetic cause. Only careful breeding studies or pedigree analysis can prove a pattern of inheritance.

The most common seizure type in dogs with primary and idiopathic epilepsy is a focal seizure with secondary generalization.[3-5,68,69,84] However, in some studies, generalized, tonic-clonic seizures were the most commonly observed seizure type.[14,70] An inherited basis, familial transmission, or a higher incidence has been recognized in many breeds. Domestic animals and breeds known to have a genetic basis for epilepsy are listed in Box 13-2.

In a dog with primary or idiopathic epilepsy, the first seizure usually occurs between the ages of 1 and 5 years.[4,5,14,68-70] Early onset of seizures has been described in two Labrador retriever puppies with seizures at 2 months of age born from a breeding of two Labrador retrievers with primary epilepsy.[85] Three puppies of a litter of 10 had seizures beginning at 8 to 9 weeks of age. Eventually, 5 of 8 surviving pups had seizures. In a large beagle colony, 29 dogs had their first seizure at a mean age of 30 months (range, 11 to 70 months).[72]

Based on the strict definition of primary epilepsy in which evidence of a pattern of inheritance must exist, primary epilepsy in cats is rare.[47,67] However, in 25% of cats presenting for seizures, a cause of seizures is not identified and therefore may be referred to as idiopathic epilepsy.[66]

Inherited epilepsy also has been reported in Brown Swiss and Swedish Red cattle.[86]

Primary epilepsy is uncommon in horses.[87] A juvenile onset primary epilepsy has been reported in Arabian foals.[88] The median age of onset was 2 months (range 2 days to 6 months), with affected horses spontaneously recovering between 2.5 to 9 months.[88]

BOX 13-2

Breeds With Idiopathic Epilepsy

Genetic Factor Proved or Highly Suspected

Beagle[72]
Belgian tervuren[69,71,74]
Bernese mountain dog[76]
Border collie[78]
Dachshund[13]
English springer spaniel[80]
Finnish spitz dog[83]
German shepherd dog (Alsatian)[73]
Golden retriever[82]
Irish wolfhound[77]
Keeshond[75]
Labrador retriever[70,]
Logotto Romagnolo dog[79]
Standard poodles[84]
Vizsla[81]
Arabian foal[88]
Aberdeen Angus cattle[90]
Brown Swiss cattle[86]
Swedish Red cattle[86]

High Incidence of Seizure Disorders

Boxer
Cocker spaniel
Collie
Irish setter
Miniature schnauzer
Saint Bernard
Siberian husky
Wire fox terrier

Symptomatic Epilepsy

Degenerative

Deficiency in a key enzyme can cause abnormalities in metabolic pathways with the accumulation of metabolic byproducts within the neurons. These conditions are referred to as storage diseases. Storage diseases may produce seizures as part of the clinical syndrome (see Chapters 8 and 15). Although most animals with degenerative disease have an abnormal neurologic examination or display interictal abnormalities, some affected dogs may present for seizures refractory to anticonvulsant drugs without any other abnormalities detectable on examination or routine diagnostic testing.[89]

A hereditary syndrome characterized by recurrent seizures and the gradual development of cerebellar ataxia occurs in purebred and crossbred Aberdeen Angus cattle. The seizures start in young calves but decline in frequency in those that survive to approximately 15 months of age. Most cattle are clinically normal by 2 years of age. Pathologic changes have been found in the Purkinje cells of the cerebellum.[90]

Developmental

Disorders related to neuronal migration and some forms of cranial malformations are apt to induce seizures. Brain malformations associated with seizure activity include hydrocephalus, Dandy-Walker syndrome, hydranencephaly, lissencephaly, Chiari-like malformation, intracranial intraarachnoid cyst, polymicrogyria and agenesis of the corpus callosum.[91] Disorders in this group may or may not be inherited but are distinguished from idiopathic epilepsy by the presence of demonstrable pathologic changes in the brain. Hydrocephalus is the most common developmental disorder that causes seizures (see Chapter 12; Tables 13-1 and 13-2) Lissencephaly is a developmental disorder involving a defect in neuronal migration in which there is an absence of cerebral gyri and sulci, a thickened cerebral cortex, and an absence of the corona radiata.[92,93] It has been reported in Lhasa apso dogs, wire fox terriers, and Irish setters, and in one cat.[92,93] In addition to seizures, affected animals may have behavioral abnormalities along with visual and proprioceptive deficits. MRI characteristic of the brain closely mirror gross necropsy findings.[94] Hydranencephaly/porencephaly is a malformation consisting of fluid-filled cavitations of the cerebrum that usually communicate with the lateral ventricle or the subarachnoid space. This condition is usually a consequence of viral infection in utero altering neuronal development and migration.

Inflammatory/Infectious

Any inflammatory or infectious disease has the potential to cause seizures if it affects the brain. The most prevalent diseases are listed in Tables 13-1 and 13-2. Canine distemper virus is probably the most common infectious cause of seizures in dogs. Seizures may appear without any noticeable clinical illness or may occur long after a clinical illness has been resolved.

Granulomatous meningoencephalomyelitis (GME) and the necrotizing encephalitides are a common noninfectious inflammatory cause of seizures in dogs. Pathologic features consist of a nonsuppurative, necrotizing meningoencephalitis with a predilection for the cerebrum in the pug and Maltese dogs.[95,96] Seizures also have been reported in Yorkshire terriers, but brainstem signs are more commonly manifested.[97] Young dogs are predisposed and are usually 6 months of age or older. The chronic form more often has clinical signs of generalized or focal seizures. Definitive diagnosis of the noninfectious inflammatory meningoencephalitides is based on a histopathologic diagnosis. A nonsuppurative meningoencephalomyelitis was reported as a common cause of seizures in cats from Canada.[47] The diagnosis of inflammatory or infectious CNS disease requires CSF examination, CSF serology, polymerase chain reaction (PCR) testing, and cross-sectional imaging. Inflammatory and infectious CNS diseases are discussed in Chapter 15.

Neoplastic

Intracranial neoplasia, either primary or secondary (metastatic or extension into the cranial cavity), can cause seizures. The seizure activity is caused by an abnormality in neurons adjacent to the neoplasm that are compressed or distorted or that have an insufficient blood supply. Seizures may be the first sign of brain tumor.[98] A neurologic deficit may not be apparent until weeks to months after the onset of seizures, especially if the mass is located in the rostral aspect of the cerebrum.[98,99] Neoplasia as a cause of seizures is relatively common in dogs and cats older than 5 years of age, and the incidence increases as animals age.[99-102] Older animals with a sudden onset of seizures should be considered to have a tumor until proved otherwise. MRI is the diagnostic imaging modality of choice. Neoplasia is discussed in Chapter 13.

Traumatic

Seizures may be seen immediately after acute traumatic brain injury as the result of direct neuronal injury (primary traumatic brain injury). Posttraumatic seizures may occur weeks to several years after a head injury. Posttraumatic seizures may be focal or generalized, depending on the location of the brain lesion. An epileptic focus likely develops secondary to a neuronal injury. The pathogenesis is incompletely understood but likely represents a change in neurotransmitter concentrations, modulation of neurotransmitter receptors, changes in ion channels, and the creation of aberrant neural connections at the site of the initial injury.[103] Treatment is directed at controlling the seizures.

Reactive Seizures

Metabolic

Failure of one of the major organs and a variety of endocrine disorders may produce alterations in the electrolytes or glucose or the accumulation of toxic products, which results in seizures (see Tables 13-1 and 13-2). Hypoglycemic syndromes and hepatoencephalopathy are the most common diseases in this category. The major metabolic disorders are discussed in Chapter 15.

Nutritional

Seizures may be the terminal manifestation of a number of nutritional disorders. The B complex vitamins are most frequently incriminated. Thiamine deficiency causes polioencephalomalacia in ruminants, which is discussed in Chapter 15. Thiamine deficiency in dogs and cats causes hemorrhage and necrosis of specific brainstem nuclei. Antemortem diagnosis may be established with clinicopathologic testing and MRI.[104]

Animals that are fed most commercial diets do not develop thiamine deficiencies. Dogs that are fed only cooked meat develop a variety of neurologic signs including seizures. Early treatment with thiamine reverses the clinical progression of the disease. Thiamine deficiency in cats has been attributed to fish-based cat foods that contain thiaminase or inappropriately prepared foods.[105] Supplementation with thiamine eliminates the problem. Cats typically have a syndrome that is characterized by flexion of the head and neck, ataxia, behavioral changes, mydriasis, seizures, and eventually coma. Given the absence of side effects associated with thiamine administration, supplementation should be given in suspected cases. A dose of 50 to 100 mg is given intravenously (IV) the first day; thereafter, daily intramuscular injections are given until a response is obtained or another diagnosis is established.[106]

Toxic

Many toxins affect the CNS and most can cause seizures. Toxins induce seizures through a number of different mechanisms: increased excitation, decreased inhibition, and interference with energy metabolism.[107]

The diagnosis usually depends on the history, identification of the toxic substance from analysis of body tissues, urine, or intestinal contents, and the response to treatment.

Lead toxicity is common in animals.[108] Other clinical signs may include dullness, tremor, and ataxia, which sometimes are associated with gastrointestinal signs. Seizures are often associated with behavioral signs. Peripheral blood changes may include nucleated erythrocytes (red blood cells [RBCs]) and basophilic stippling of RBCs without anemia or with mild anemia.[108] Blood lead determination is diagnostic. Calcium ethylenediamine tetraacetic acid (CaETA) may be used in treatment.[109] In some animals, CaETA can worsen neurologic signs. Succimer (meso 2,3-dimercaptosuccinic acid) has been used successfully in the treatment of lead toxicity in dogs and cats at 10 mg/kg orally every 8 hours for 10 days.[110-112]

Strychnine causes a tonic seizure that is exacerbated by stimulation. The animal remains conscious unless respiration stops. Strychnine blocks inhibitory interneurons, glycine, in the spinal cord, causing a release of motor neuron activity.

Organophosphate and chlorinated hydrocarbon insecticides are common causes of seizures.

Seizures induced by the toxin produced by the *Bufo marinus* toad have been reported.[113] Although several species of *Bufo* toads exist worldwide, most reports in the United States are from southern Florida, Colorado, Arizona, Texas, and Hawaii. The incidence was highest during warm months of the year. In addition to seizures, neurologic signs include stupor, ataxia, nystagmus, extensor rigidity, and opisthotonos. Hyperemic oral mucous membranes and ptyalism are common findings. The toxin is released from the toad's parotid glands and is readily absorbed through the oral mucosa. Intoxication may be fatal. The oral cavity should be lavaged with water. Diazepam is used to control seizures and extensor rigidity. IV fluids and diuretics are given to promote urinary excretion of the toxin. Overall mortality is low in animals treated within a few hours of intoxication.

In dogs, 5-hydroxytryptophan toxicosis has been reported as a cause of seizures.[114] It is a precursor to serotonin, a common CNS neurotransmitter. The signs in dogs are similar to the "serotonin syndrome" as described in humans. In addition to seizures, neurologic signs include depression, tremors, hyperesthesia, transient blindness, and ataxia. Gastrointestinal signs include vomiting, diarrhea, ptyalism, and abdominal pain. Hyperthermia is also a common finding. Signs develop within minutes to hours following accidental ingestion of dietary supplements containing the agent. Treatment includes decontamination (induction of emesis, gastric lavage, and oral administration of activated charcoal), IV fluid therapy, thermoregulation, and parenteral administration of anticonvulsant drugs (diazepam or phenobarbital). The serotonin antagonist cyproheptadine administered at a dose of 1.1 mg/kg administered orally or rectally every 1 to 4 hours may be useful as adjunct therapy.[114]

Disorders of toxicity are further discussed in Chapter 15.

DIAGNOSIS AND MANAGEMENT OF SEIZURES

Regardless of the underlying etiology, most affected animals have a similar history of episodic seizures. Consequently, signalment and history alone are not sufficient to identify the underlying etiology. Therefore all affected animals should undergo a similar testing protocol in an attempt to establish a definitive diagnosis that ultimately impacts on the plan for management. Ideally, diagnostics are performed in a specific order to first rule out reactive seizures (extracranial causes) followed by procedures to rule out symptomatic epilepsy (intracranial causes). Only after excluding extracranial and intracranial causes can a diagnosis of primary or idiopathic epilepsy be presumed. Ultimately, the extent to which a complete diagnostic workup is performed will depend on the desire of the animal's owner to pursue testing, financial constraints, clinicopathologic findings, and availability of diagnostic tests.

Diagnostic Evaluation

In animals with an isolated single seizure, the minimum database (MDB) should consist of a complete blood count, chemistry profile, and urinalysis to rule out extracranial causes, such as metabolic, toxic, and nutritional disorders. The diagnostic workup based on etiologic classification of seizures is presented in Box 13-3. Based on results of the MDB, specialized tests may be needed to diagnose specific metabolic conditions suggested by the MDB. For example, increased liver enzymes, hypoalbuminemia, hypoglycemia, decreased blood urea nitrogen along with microcytic, hypochromic anemia suggest hepatic dysfunction in which case measurement of serum ammonia concentration or preprandial and postprandial bile acid concentrations may be pursued. Likewise, concurrent, nonneurologic clinical signs along with a history compatible with exposure to toxins may necessitate pursuing specialized tests to identify a toxin as the underlying cause (see Chapter 15). The extent to which in-depth metabolic testing or toxin screening is pursued will vary depending on results of the MDB, clinical suspicion, and potential of exposure to toxins. Information from the MDB yields one of three findings: (1) a definitive diagnosis, (2) possible cause of the seizures that requires further tests to confirm, or (3) no suggestion of the cause.

Following exclusion of extracranial causes, diagnostics directed at identifying an intracranial cause of seizures should be pursued. Intracranial causes include degenerative diseases, anomalous or developmental disorders, encephalitis (infectious or noninfectious), neoplasia (primary or secondary brain tumors), traumatic injuries, and vascular disorders. Magnetic resonance imaging is the diagnostic imaging modality of choice for evaluation of animals with seizures. In addition to cross-sectional imaging, CSF analysis should be performed. Importantly, CSF analysis should be performed in animals with normal brain structure on imaging studies as meningoencephalitis may be present despite normal imaging. Because cats most commonly have symptomatic epilepsy, MRI and CSF analysis are important in determining the cause of seizures in this species. The most common causes of seizures in cats is structural brain disease, such as meningoencephalitis, feline ischemic encephalopathy, and neoplasia.[47,67] In large animals, diagnostic testing for intracranial disease is more limited based on availability of imaging facilities capable of performing MRI or CT; however, CSF analysis may provide insight into the seizure etiology.

Plan for Management

Seizures occur episodically. Therefore, the veterinarian frequently must evaluate an animal without ever observing the seizure. As a result, the determination of whether or not the affected animal has had a seizure is based on the veterinarian's interpretation of an owner's observations. Consequently, the history must be taken carefully and must include a thorough description of the animal's actions (movements, responsiveness, behavior, presence of autonomic signs) during the seizure and seizure frequency, duration, and severity. The first goal is to determine that the animal has had a seizure.

Animals that have had only one isolated seizure should undergo a thorough physical and neurologic examination. As detailed above, an MDB should be completed for every animal that has a seizure. However, further diagnostics beyond an MDB may not be performed based on the level of concern felt by the owner and veterinarian. For example, in dogs having had a single seizure that are between 1 and 5 years of age, with a normal physical and neurologic examination, and a normal MDB, a wait and see approach may be considered given the possibility of primary or idiopathic epilepsy. Despite the low likelihood of diagnosing a structural brain lesion, MRI should still be considered in such cases, if for no other reason than to be definitive in exclusion of an underlying brain abnormality. In dogs younger than 1 year or older than 5 years, a complete diagnostic evaluation should be performed even after a single seizure in an effort to identify a definitive etiology. All cats with seizures regardless of number, frequency, severity, or duration should undergo diagnostic testing since reactive seizures or symptomatic seizures underlie the cause of most seizures in cats.[47,67]

Recommendations for instituting administration of anticonvulsant drugs depend on factors such as the underlying etiology, seizure frequency, severity, and duration. Ultimately, the decision to initiate treatment depends on the need to control seizures to avoid detrimental secondary effects (intracranial or systemic) and improve the quality of life of the animal. This decision must be balanced to weigh in the side effects of the medications and owner's ability to comply and manage the financial constraints

In most animals with symptomatic epilepsy (intracranial disease), anticonvulsant drugs should be strongly considered.

BOX 13-3

Anamnesis and Diagnostic Testing for Animals Exhibiting Seizures

Signalment, History, Seizure Description, and Physical/Neurologic Examination

Patient profile
- Species, breed, age, sex

History
- Immunizations: type, date, by whom

Environment

Age at onset

Description of ictus
- Description of seizure: general, focal, or focal onset with secondary generalization
- Duration of ictus
- Severity

Postictal description

Other factors: time of day, association with exercise, food, sleep, or stimuli

Previous or present illness or injury

Behavioral changes

Physical examination
- Complete examination of systems, including specifically:
  - Musculoskeletal: Size, shape of skull, evidence of trauma, atrophy of any muscles
  - Cardiovascular: Color of mucous membranes, evidence of arrhythmias, murmurs
  - Funduscopic examination

Neurologic examination
- Note time of last seizure; if it was within 24-48 hr and neurologic examination is abnormal, repeat in 24 hr (may represent transient postictal disturbance)

The presence of interictal neurologic deficits excludes primary epilepsy from consideration

Symmetric deficits—more commonly associated with reactive seizures

Asymmetric deficits—more commonly associated with symptomatic seizures

Diagnostic Testing to Identify the Etiology of Reactive Seizures

Clinical pathology
- CBC
- Chemistry profile
- Urinalysis

Others as indicated (e.g., blood ammonia, preprandial and postprandial bile acid levels, endocrine testing)

Testing for specific metabolic or endocrine disorders

Testing for specific toxins

Diagnostic Testing to Identify the Etiology of Symptomatic Epilepsy

Testing is pursued *after* exclusion of reactive epilepsy

Imaging

Thoracic radiographs (in dogs and cats ≥5 years to evaluate for metastatic lesions)

Abdominal ultrasonography (based on other clinical pathologic data)

Magnetic resonance Imaging (MRI)

Computed tomography, if MRI is not available

CSF analysis: Cell count, total and differential; protein concentration

Based on suspicion, additional testing of CSF

Bacterial cultures, measurement of antibody or antigen concentrations, PCR testing

EEG (requires expertise and specialized equipment)

CBC, Complete blood cell count; *CSF,* cerebrospinal fluid.

In most cases of symptomatic epilepsy, the underlying pathology may not be reversible despite appropriate treatment. Therefore the likelihood of recurrent seizures remains high. Consequently, anticonvulsant drugs are advisable even when only a single seizure has been observed. With metabolic or toxic disorders, if the underlying condition can be eliminated, anticonvulsant therapy may not be necessary. Occasionally, short-term anticonvulsant therapy may be needed until the underlying disease is corrected. After correction of the underlying metabolic or toxic insult, anticonvulsant drugs may be slowly tapered in attempt to discontinue medication. However, when the underlying cause cannot be reversed, anticonvulsant drugs may be required long term. In the absence of a definitive diagnosis (primary or idiopathic epilepsy), anticonvulsant therapy is recommended in dogs and cats when single seizures occur more than once every 6 weeks, when cluster seizures (two seizures within 24 hours) occur, or if SE has been observed. Anticonvulsant therapy also should be initiated in animals having SE or cluster seizures even if it is represents the onset of seizures in animals without any prior history of seizures.

Reevaluation of diagnostic testing in animals undergoing appropriate therapy is warranted under several circumstances. Failure to control seizures in animals receiving adequate therapy (see Plans for Treatment section) necessitates a complete diagnostic workup to rule out an underlying etiology. This is particularly true in animals with idiopathic epilepsy in which there is a strong suspicion of an underlying pathology that was not identified with initial diagnostic testing. In these animals, reevaluations may reveal an underlying disease that originally was not evident. The development of interictal neurologic signs or any change in neurologic signs also indicates a reappraisal of the need for a complete evaluation. Similarly, animals experiencing a dramatic change in the frequency, severity, or duration of seizures that have been previously well controlled should undergo a complete diagnostic workup after determining that there have been no changes in serum concentrations of anticonvulsant drugs or drug therapy (reduction in dosing, skipped doses, or error in dose calculation). Some breeds have primary or idiopathic epilepsy that is difficult to control. The most common examples are German shepherd dogs, Saint Bernards, Labrador retrievers, and Irish setters.[115] For any animal, poor seizure control despite adequate anticonvulsant therapy suggests a guarded prognosis. The treatment can be altered by changing the amount and frequency of drug dosage or the drug type, or by combining medications.

Treatment

Successful treatment depends heavily on client education and diligence. Treatment failures are usually the result of (1) progressive disease, (2) refractory seizures, or (3) inadequate client education or poor client compliance leading to subtherapeutic drug concentrations. Clients need to understand the importance of frequent monitoring for successful seizure control.

The most important aspect of a successful outcome is the understanding by the client that successful treatment consists of (1) a reduction in the frequency of seizures, (2) a reduction in the duration of seizures, or (3) a reduction in the severity of seizures. Although complete elimination of seizures is certainly a goal, it is not a realistic expectation for most animals. This is particularly true for breeds of dogs that are commonly refractory to treatment.[115]

A realistic goal for most dogs with primary epilepsy is no more than one seizure every 6 weeks. Depending on the initial frequency of seizures, animals' tolerance to the side effects of anticonvulsant drugs, and the underlying cause, more frequent seizures may be acceptable in some animals.

The client should be given the following guidelines for treating animals with seizures regardless of cause:

1. Medication is required for life. Do not decrease dosages rapidly or too soon after seizure control is achieved. Dose adjustments should only be made in consultation with a veterinarian.
2. Do not judge the efficacy of the medication for at least 4 weeks; longer periods may be needed to assess efficacy depending on the drug half-life.
3. Do not change or discontinue the medication suddenly. SE may follow.
4. No single drug or combination of drugs works in all cases. Adjustments in the dosage, the schedule, or the combination of drugs probably will be required. Finding the right combination usually occurs by trial and error, but monitoring therapeutic serum levels helps to eliminate the guesswork.
5. Good seizure control is more difficult to achieve in some large-breed dogs.
6. The severity of seizure disorder in cats is not a good predictor of outcome.

Once the decision has been made to initiate therapy, there are several anticonvulsant drugs available for use. A protocol for the treatment of seizures is outlined in Figure 13-2. For the majority of dogs and cats with primary or idiopathic epilepsy, phenobarbital is the drug of choice based on efficacy, convenience of the dosing regimen, minimal drug side effects, and reasonable expense. Alternatively, potassium bromide may be used as an initial anticonvulsant drug in dogs. In humans, the selection of an anticonvulsant therapy is made based on seizure symptomatology, EEG, seizure mechanism, and genetic factors. Unfortunately, veterinary medicine has not achieved the same level of sophistication. While certain underlying etiologies may dictate drug choices (e.g., animals with hepatic disease should not be treated with drugs requiring hepatic metabolism), a consensus regarding treatment has not been established. Based on control of seizures, additional medications may be added. Before initiating adjunctive anticonvulsant drugs, sufficient time must be allotted to determine whether or not seizures have been controlled. Moreover, adequate serum drug concentrations should be achieved before establishing lack of efficacy and poor seizure control.

In general, anticonvulsant drugs are initiated at the low end of the dose range regardless of the medication. The need to adjust the dosage is primarily based on seizure control. Measurement of the serum drug concentration is available for some medications. For these drugs, a therapeutic serum concentration should be established. Therapeutic serum concentrations are based on studies evaluating the concentration at which the majority of affected animals experienced seizure control. As individual variation occurs, it is possible that some animals can be controlled at serum concentrations below reported therapeutic ranges while others require concentrations be maintained at the high end of the therapeutic range. Consequently, adjustments in dosage should not be made solely on serum drug concentrations. Instead, adjustments in medications should be made based on the assessment of the seizure control in addition to the serum drug concentration and drug side effects. Serum concentrations of an anticonvulsant drug only should be performed once the drug has reached steady state levels. The measurement of the serum drug concentration is important in certain circumstances. (1) Serum drug concentrations should be measured in those animals experiencing unexpected or severe side effects, particularly if the animal is receiving a low dosage. (2) Finding a high serum concentration in an animal treated with a low dosage may suggest abnormal drug metabolism. (3) Serum drug concentration also should be measured in those animals receiving high dosages yet remaining poorly controlled in which increased dosing is considered. In doing so, determining whether the serum drug concentration is in the therapeutic range is critical. In poorly controlled animals with a low serum drug concentration, the dosage should be increased to reach a therapeutic concentration. Additionally, knowing the serum drug concentrations may help predict the likelihood of developing irreversible side effects (e.g., hepatotoxicity with phenobarbital).[116]

Although anticonvulsant treatment should be considered as a lifelong therapy, discontinuation of anticonvulsant drugs may be considered in animals that are seizure free for 1 to 2 years. Gradual tapering of anticonvulsant drugs should be done over a 6-month period or longer. Owners need to be aware that as serum drug concentration declines, seizures may recur. In some instances, discontinuation of anticonvulsant drugs can be successful.

Anticonvulsant Drug Therapy

Most of the commonly used anticonvulsant drugs (phenobarbital, potassium bromide, and diazepam) increase GABA-activated chloride channels, act to modulate sodium or calcium channels, or reduce glutamate-mediated excitation.[117-120] In some instances, the exact mechanism of action remains unknown. Table 13-3 lists anticonvulsant drugs used in the treatment of seizures.

Most dogs with primary epilepsy can be controlled with a single anticonvulsant drug. Approximately 20% to 40% of dogs with primary epilepsy require a second anticonvulsant drug to control seizures.[121,122] Occasionally, severely affected dogs require a third medication. Determining an effective anticonvulsant combination is based on familiarity with the medications and their side effects combined with financial constraints of owners and the potential for synergistic adverse effects. Ultimately, no single combination of anticonvulsant drugs will provide control for every animal. In some animals, seizure control is not possible without serious adverse effects which impact health and quality of life regardless of therapy.

Phenobarbital. Phenobarbital (PB) is the initial drug of choice for treating seizures in dogs and cats.[121-124] PB is effective, inexpensive, and convenient for administration. The usual starting dosage is 2.5 mg/kg orally twice daily. The dose range is 2.2 to 4.4 mg/kg orally twice daily. The drug can be given orally or via intramuscular (IM) or IV injection. Some dogs may require 5 mg/kg orally twice a day to achieve therapeutic blood levels. Absorption and excretion differ considerably among individuals, and this is especially important in cats. A

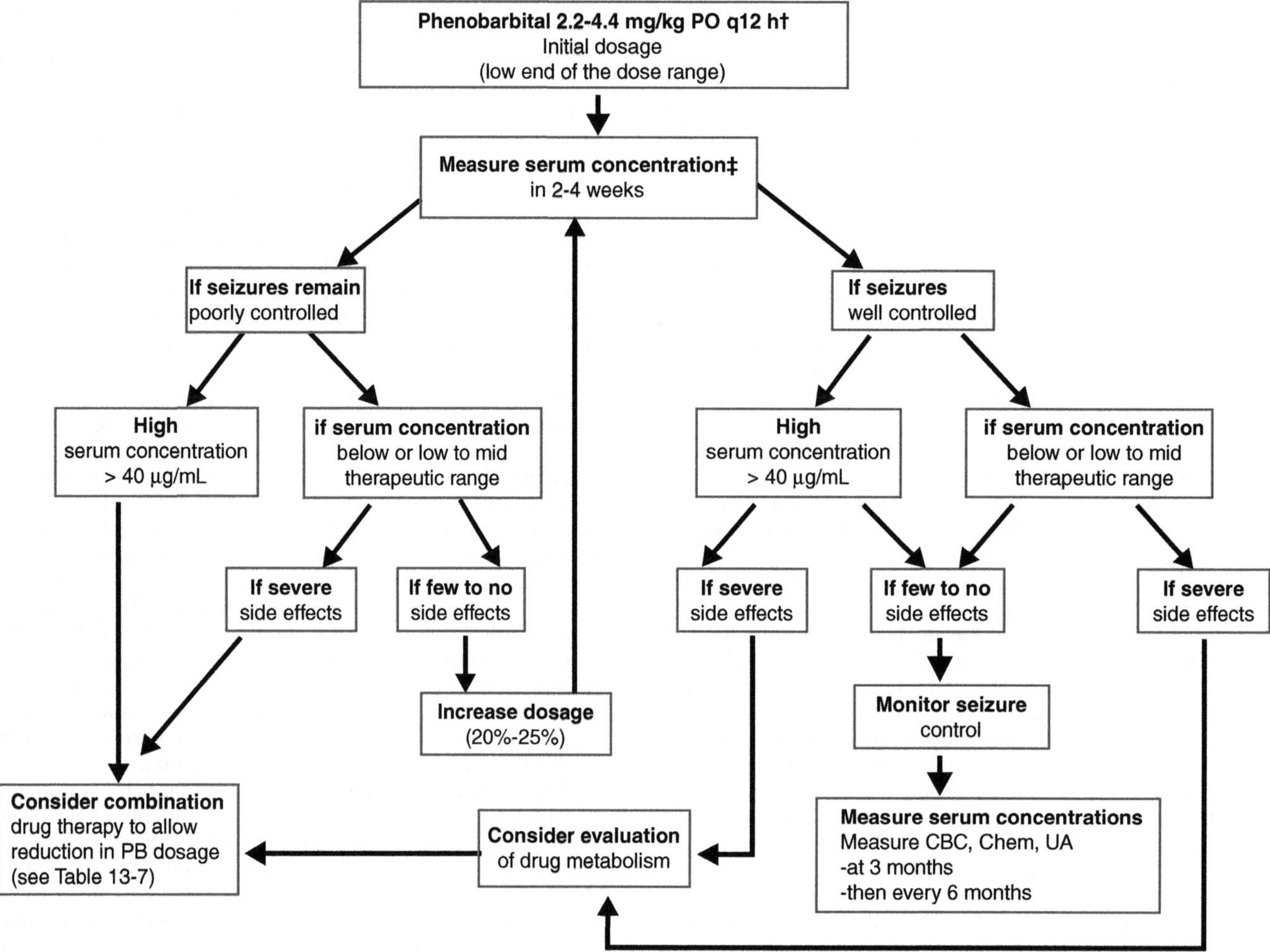

Figure 13-2 Protocol for initiating AED in dogs with suspected or confirmed primary epilepsy.
q, Every; *h*, hours; *PB*, phenobarbital; *CBC*, complete blood count.
*Similar protocol can be used in cats with suspected or confirmed idiopathic or probable symptomatic epilepsy.
†Similar protocol can be used:
If an AED other than PB is used.
If already on phenobarbital and initiating KBr therapy (see text).
If already on combination therapy and initiating third AED.
‡Timing of the measurement of serum AED concentration varies with different drugs (see Table 13-3)

lower dosage may be used if seizures are infrequent and occur as single episodes. Higher dosages are recommended if seizures are frequent or tend to occur in clusters or SE. Ultimately, the dosage is adjusted according to seizure control, side effects, and serum concentrations. After achieving seizure control on a stable dosage, PB concentrations should be monitored every 6 months to avoid toxicity.[117]

PB undergoes hepatic metabolism but approximately one third of the drug is excreted unchanged by the kidneys.[126] Peak concentration is typically reached 4 to 8 hours after oral administration.[127] Bioavailability is approximately 90%.[128] The half-life ($t_{1/2}$) of PB in dogs ranges from 32 to 89 hours.[127,129-133] Elimination $t_{1/2}$ may be more rapid in beagle dogs (32 hours).[127,134] Half-life in cats and horses is 34 to 43 hours and 14 to 25 hours, respectively.[111,135,136] As with all drugs, steady state concentration is reached after approximately 5.5 half-lives. Consequently, to ensure that the serum concentration is evaluated after achieving steady state concentrations, measurements in the dog should not be performed until approximately 3 weeks after starting the medication or after a change in dosage. Importantly, with chronic administration, a new, lower serum concentration develops over time as a result of autoinduction (more rapid metabolism due to the drug's induction of the cytochrome P450 system).[129] As a result, serum concentrations evaluated after chronic administration may be lower than those measured at the beginning of therapy. Diet may also impact PB metabolism. Dogs fed a low-protein or low-protein and low-fat diet have a more rapid elimination of PB.[132] Similarly, renal elimination of PB may be enhanced by alkalinizing the urine resulting in lower serum concentrations.[137]

In dogs and cats, the therapeutic range for PB is 15 to 45 mg/mL.[121,122,124] In most dogs, measurement of serum concentration can be performed at any point during the day. In a study of 33 dogs treated with twice daily PB, 91% of all samples taken at 0 (trough), 3, and 6 hours posttreatment were within the therapeutic range, varying less than 30% among samples.[138] Only standard blood collection tubes should be used in collection; using serum separation blood collection tubes containing a clot activator may artificially lower serum drug levels.[139] Additionally, approximately 33% of

TABLE 13-3

*Anticonvulsants Commonly Used in Domestic Animals**

Drug	Dosage (mg/kg)	Therapeutic Serum Concentration (mg/mL)	Half-Life (hr)	Time to Steady State (days)
Phenobarbital	2.2-5 q12h (D)	15-45 mg/dL (D)	32-89 h (D)	10-18 (D)
	1-2 q12h (C)	10-20 mg/dL (C)	34-43 h (C)	10-14 (C)
	5 q24h (H)		14-25 h (H)	3-6 (H)
Potassium bromide	22-40 q24h or divided	100-300 mg/dL	25 (days)	120
Levetiracetam	10-20 q8h (D,C)	5 to 45 µg/mL	2.3-4h (D,C)	1-2
Zonisamide	4-8 q12h	10 to 60 µg/mL	17 (D)	3-4
	5-10 q24h		33 (C)	7-8
Gabapentin	10 q8h	4 to16 mg/L	3-4	1
Pregabalin	4 q8h	2.8- 8.2 µg/mL	3-4	1
Felbamate	20 q8h	30-100 mg/L	4-6	1-2

q, Every; *h*, hour; D, dog, C, cat, H, horse.
*Unless specifically stated, information pertains to dogs.

dogs treated with PB alone or in conjunction with potassium bromide (KBr) develop hypertriglyceridemia, which is likely attributable to delayed clearance of chylomicron, reduced lipoprotein lipase activity, or hepatic very low density lipoprotein (VLDL) overproduction.[140] It is unclear if this is related to an overweight body condition, an idiosyncratic reaction to PB, or a multifactorial process.[140] However, caution should be exercised when interpreting PB concentrations in the presence of hypertriglyceridemia because hypertriglyceridemia may falsely elevate PB measurements.[140]

One of the main side effects is sedation. Sedation may occur within the first and second week of therapy but usually disappears in the subsequent 1 to 2 weeks of treatment. Sedation tends to be more severe in older dogs or large-breed dogs.[122] Animals with intracranial disease, particularly older dogs with brain tumors, also may experience profound sedation even with low doses. In dogs with brain tumors in which the mental state is already severely affected, initiating therapy at a lower dosage (1 mg/kg) than the normal may be advisable unless seizures are frequent. Alternatively, medications such as levetiracetam, which have minimal sedative effects, may be used instead of PB. Polyphagia, polydipsia, and polyuria are seen in most patients. Occasionally hyperactivity, restlessness, and even aggression may be noted.

Hepatotoxicity with PB can occur.[116] Whether this represents a direct dose-dependent hepatotoxicity or an idiosyncratic drug reaction is still unknown; however, dogs with serum concentrations at the high end of the therapeutic range or above (>35 µg/mL) are at greater risk. Several studies in normal dogs and dogs with epilepsy, have documented that PB induces hepatic enzyme production, primarily involving elevations in alkaline phosphatase (ALP) concentrations in the absence of liver failure.[141] When serum target levels were maintained within the range between 20 and 40 µg/mL with a dosage of 5 mg/kg every 12 hours, both ALP and alanine aminotransferase (ALT) are increased following 29 weeks of administration. These increases result in enzyme activity of ALP above the normal reference range, whereas ALT activity is at the high end of the reference range. Gamma-glutamyl transferase (GGT) may be transiently increased. Aspartate transaminase (AST), bile acids (BAs), and bilirubin are not affected. Enzyme induction does not occur in the cat. Moderate hepatomegaly may be detected on abdominal radiographs, but hepatic ultrasonography is usually normal.[142] Hepatic enzymes return to normal within 6 to 8 weeks following discontinuation of PB treatment. Hepatic enzyme induction must be taken into account when dogs are monitored for hepatotoxicity. However, presence of bilirubinuria, bilirubinemia, and hypoalbuminemia, and increased concentrations of preprandial or postprandial bile acids are the best indicators for possible hepatotoxicity. Serum ALT activity that is consistently above the normal reference range is also an indicator for possible hepatotoxicity.

Life-threatening neutropenia and thrombocytopenia have been reported in dogs receiving acute and chronic administration of PB.[143,144] Cytopenias typically resolve when the drug is discontinued. Although the exact mechanism is unknown, most likely the cytopenias reflect a toxicity of the bone marrow rather than an immune-mediated process directed at circulating cells as bone marrow necrosis and myelofibrosis also have been associated with PB administration.[145,146]

Superficial necrolytic dermatitis has been reported in association with chronic PB administration.[147] Although superficial necrolytic dermatitis is typically associated with a hepatopathy, affected dogs may not have clinicopathologic findings indicative of a hepatic disorder.[147] Although discontinuation of PB is advised, skin lesions may not resolve. Dermatologic lesions also have been reported in a cat.[148] In the cat, reported lesions resolved with discontinuation of the drug. A movement disorder has been observed in a dog receiving PB.[149] The signs consist of severe, whole body jerking movements that would cause the affected dog to fall. The affected dog displayed agitation, restlessness, and intermittent fine tremors. Resolution of signs occurred with discontinuation of the drug.

Several studies have demonstrated the effects of long-term PB treatment on the thyroid and pituitary-adrenal axis of normal and epileptic dogs.[141,150-154] Short-term use (<3 weeks) of PB is not associated with changes in total thyroxine (TT_4), free T_4 (fT_4), or thyroid-stimulating hormone (TSH) levels.[150] However, with chronic PB administration, TT_4 and fT_4 concentrations can be reduced to levels consistent with hypothyroidism, whereas TSH concentrations remain normal to slightly increased.[141,153,154] These findings support the hypothesis that PB causes increased clearance of T_4 while suppressing the secretion of TSH.[155] Complicating this is the occurrence of euthyroid sick syndrome in dogs with idiopathic epilepsy. In one study, approximately 38% of dogs with idiopathic epilepsy had thyroid testing results consistent with euthyroid sick syndrome, which was independent of the occurrence of seizure activity.[156] In another study, TT_4 concentrations were lower when measured within 24 hours of a seizure in comparison to measurements obtained at a time not associated with a seizure.[152] In summary, dogs on PB therapy may have test results consistent with hypothyroidism, despite not being hypothyroid. The effect is probably dose related because dogs with PB levels below 15 μg/mL developed few or no changes in T_4 of fT_4 concentrations. Chronic PB administration does not influence the pituitary-adrenal axis when evaluated with adenocorticotropichormone (ACTH) stimulation or low dose dexamethasone suppression testing.[154]

Animals that cannot be controlled with adequate levels of PB may require adjunctive drug therapy. In dogs, PB is commonly combined with potassium bromide. Phenobarbital is continued while other drugs are added to the regimen. Other anticonvulsant drugs can be used in combination with PB; however, their efficacy has not been thoroughly studied.

Potassium Bromide. Potassium bromide (KBr) is a safe and effective anticonvulsant in dogs. It can be used alone or in conjunction with PB.[157] In dogs with primary epilepsy refractory to phenobarbital, the addition of KBr reduces seizure frequency in approximately 50% to 70% of treated dogs with approximately 21% to 26% attaining seizure-free status.[125,158,159] Potassium bromide also can be used in dogs with unacceptable side effects or those experiencing hepatotoxicity related to PB.[157] Approximately 20% of dogs receiving KBr are able to have PB eventually discontinued while maintaining seizure control.[159] In combination with PB, 72% of dogs experience a 50% or greater reduction in PB dosage.[159] In 45% percent of these dogs, no seizures were observed with PB concentrations below 20 μg/mL thereby greatly reducing the potential for PB hepatotoxicity.[159]

The starting dose of KBr is 22 to 40 mg/kg orally per day. However, given the reversibility of side effects, the upper limit of the dosage is dictated by the animal and owner's ability to tolerate side effects.[117] In the dog, the $t_{1/2}$ of KBr is approximately 25 days (range 15 to 45 days).[117,160-162] Due to its long $t_{1/2}$ the dosage can be given once daily. Potassium bromide should be given with food to avoid nausea. If nausea occurs, the daily dosage can be divided and given twice daily. In some dogs, nausea may necessitate changing to sodium bromide, which may be less irritating to the gastric mucosa.[157] In such cases, the dosage of sodium bromide should be 15% less than potassium bromide.[157] Potassium bromide is not marketed as a drug. Instead, chemical (analytic) grade KBr can be obtained and formulated into a solution. If prepared under appropriate sterile conditions, sodium bromide can be administered intravenously. Standards for veterinarians and compounding pharmacies can be obtained from the United States Pharmacopeia at www.usp.org.

KBr is excreted unchanged in the urine predominantly by glomerular filtration. Extensive competition between bromide and chloride occurs in the renal tubules. Consequently, the rate of elimination of bromide varies directly with chloride intake. The greater the chloride intake, the greater the renal elimination rate of bromide.[161,163] As a result, diet plays an important role in maintaining appropriate serum concentrations.[161,164] Diets low in salt (NaCl) content can predispose to toxicity. Therefore, dogs should be maintained on a constant diet to prevent fluctuations in serum bromide concentrations. More importantly, KBr should be avoided in dogs with renal dysfunction to prevent toxicity related to reduced renal eliminiation.[165] If KBr therapy is necessary, dogs with renal dysfunction should be treated initially with at least half the recommended dosage with close monitoring for adverse effects along with frequent measurement of serum concentrations.[157]

As a consequence of the prolonged $t_{1/2}$, steady state concentrations may not be reached until approximately 120 days. Although measurement of serum concentration of KBr should not be performed until after reaching steady state, 75% and 95% of steady state levels are reached at 30 days and 60 days, respectively.[162] The therapeutic range for serum concentration of KBr is 100 to 300 mg/dL.[157,160,166] In one study, the mean serum concentration for dogs achieving seizure control with PB and KBr was 162 mg/dL (ranging from 50 to 288 mg/dL).[159] The mean serum concentration was higher, approximately 200 mg/dL, for those dogs in which PB could eventually be withdrawn.[159] Likewise, in dogs controlled on KBr alone, a mean serum concentration of 190 mg/dL was needed to achieve seizure control.[159] Therefore, dogs treated with KBr alone may require serum concentrations between 200 and 350 mg/dL to achieve adequate control.[157,159,162] When used in conjunction with PB, dosing at 30 to 40 mg/kg orally *once* daily should achieve a steady state concentration of 100 to 200 mg/dL; when used as a sole agent, dosing at 30 mg/kg orally *twice* daily may be needed to achieve a median concentration of 245 mg/dL.[162] As with phenobarbital, unless seizure frequency is high, initiation of therapy should begin at the low end of the dose range. Increases in dosages should be based on seizure control and serum concentrations. After achieving seizure control on a stable dosage, KBr concentrations should be monitored every 6 months to prevent toxicity.[125,167]

Similar to PB, side effects include polyphagia, polydipsia, and polyuria.[117,125,157,168] Toxicity (bromism) is associated with pelvic limb weakness.[157] Tetraparesis and paraparesis with characteristics of upper motor neuron or lower motor neuron weakness have been observed.[167] Changes in mentation ranging from sedation to stupor also can occur. In severely affected animals, mydriatic pupils with incomplete pupillary light reflexes may be observed.[167] Risk factors for developing toxicity include development of renal dysfunction, inadequate monitoring, and iatrogenic dosing errors.[167] In cases of mild signs of toxicity, the dosage of KBr should be reduced by 25% to 50%. With moderate to severe toxicity, diuresis with 0.9% NaCl is used to reduce serum concentrations; care should be exercised when reducing serum concentrations rapidly as recurrence of seizures may occur.

An association between KBr therapy and pancreatitis has been reported.[125,169-171] In one report, the prevalence of pancreatitis has been estimated to be approximately 10%.[170] It is unknown whether pancreatitis is a direct result of KBr or related to dietary indiscretion caused by polyphagia associated with anticonvulsant usage.[125] However, given the difficulty in establishing a definitive diagnosis of pancreatitis, the risk of developing pancreatitis due to KBr administration remains unknown.

Pigmentation, erythematous dermatitis, and nodular/pustular skin lesions are reported in humans.[125,157] Dermatologic toxicity is uncommonly observed in dogs. Megaesophagus also has been observed in dogs treated with KBr. In most cases, esophageal dysfunction resolves with discontinuation of KBr.

Pseudohyperchloridemia can occur depending on the analytic method used to measure serum chloride concentrations. In some methods, total halide concentration, chloride and bromide versus chloride alone, are used, which falsely elevates chloride measurements. Unfortunately, the degree of pseudohyperchloridemia cannot be used to predict bromide serum concentrations.[172]

KBr should not be used in cats. In one study, cats treated with KBr developed coughing, a bronchial pattern on thoracic radiographs, and eosinophilic inflammation alone or in combination with neutrophilic inflammation in bronchoalveolar lavage specimens.[173] Eight of 17 treated cats developed toxicity, whereas only 7 of 14 treated cats experienced seizure control.[173]

Levetiracetam (Keppra). Levetiracetam is a relatively new anticonvulsant. It has been evaluated for use in the dog and cat.[174,175] The recommended dosage for dogs and cats is 20 mg/kg orally every 8 hours. A parenteral formulation is available and safe for IV and IM injection.[176] The bioavailability of IM and oral administration is nearly 100%.[176] The maximum serum concentration following IM administration occurs in approximately 40 minutes, which combined with bioavailability and lack of tissue damage associated with IM injection suggests suitability for use in emergency situations in dogs.[176] The mechanism of action of levetiracetam is unique. It does not appear to work directly through GABAergic facilitation, inhibition of Na^+ channels, or modulation of low voltage activated Ca^{2+} currents.[177] Instead its binding site in the brain appears to be a specific synaptic vesicle protein (SVA2), which is involved in modulation of neurotransmitter release, reuptake, and recycling.[175,177] Approximately one third of the drug undergoes renal excretion related to the glomerular filtration rate. Active drug is also hydrolyzed by enzymes in a variety of tissues.[178] In the dog, the $t_{1/2}$ is short, ranging from 2.3 to 4 hours.[119,176,178,179] Half-life is similar in the cat.[174] The serum therapeutic concentration in dogs and cats is unknown; however, in humans the therapeutic concentrations are 5 to 45 μg/mL.

Few studies have been done in dogs and cats. In dogs with seizures resistant to PB and KBr therapy, approximately 9 of 15 (60%) dogs had a 50% reduction in seizure frequency at a dosage of 10 to 20 mg/kg orally three times daily.[175] Interestingly, recurrence of seizure frequency developed at 4 to 8 months in some dogs, suggesting tolerance to the drug.[175] The only reported side effect is sedation.[175,176] In a study of 10 cats, 20 mg/kg orally three times daily was associated with a 50% reduction in seizure frequency in 7 of 10 cats.[174] In those cats responding, seizure frequency decreased by 92%. Mild self-limiting anorexia and lethargy were observed in one cat.[174]

Zonisamide (Zonegran). Zonisamide is a synthetic sulfonamide-based anticonvulsant. In the dog, the recommended dosage is 10 mg/kg orally twice daily.[180] Zonisamide has several different mechanisms of action, including blockade of T-type calcium channels and voltage-gated sodium channels, enhancement of GABA function, and modulation of a number of other neurotransmitters (dopamine, serotonin, and acetylcholine).[181] Additionally, it may provide neuroprotection as a free radical scavenger.[181] The drug undergoes hepatic metabolism via microsomal enzymes with approximately 10% of the drug being excreted by the kidneys unchanged.[182] The oral bioavailability in dogs is 68%. In the dog, the $t_{1/2}$ is 17 hours with steady state concentrations reached at 7 days.[182] Once at steady state, the difference between the maximum and minimum serum concentrations is 40%.[182] Therapeutic serum concentrations range between 10 and 40 μg/mL.[180] Concurrent phenobarbital administration alters the pharmacokinetics of zonisamide, resulting in lower serum concentrations, shorter $t_{1/2}$, and less bioavailablity.[183]

In a study using zonisamide in 12 dogs treated with PB alone or in combination with KBr, 7 of 12 dogs (58%) experienced a 50% reduction in seizure frequency in which dogs responding had a median of 84% reduction in seizure frequency.[180] Two dogs became seizure free. In another study, 8 out of 10 dogs responded to zonisamide, experiencing an 82% reduction in seizure frequency.[184] Side effects were minimal. Six out of 12 dogs experienced side effects, including mild ataxia, lethargy, and keratoconjunctivitis sicca.[180] Zonisamide may also lower thyroxine levels.[182] In dogs given high dosages (75 mg/kg/day) for 1 year, side effects were limited to biochemical abnormalities such as decreased albumin and increased ALP.[184]

Gabapentin (Neurontin). Gabapentin has been used to treat seizures in dogs. The recommended dosage is 10 mg/kg orally three times daily. Although gabapentin is a structural analogue of GABA, its mechanism of action is via blockade and preventing synaptogenesis of the $\alpha_2\delta$-subunit of the voltage-gated T-type calcium channel. This thereby reduces the glutamate-mediated neurotransmission and may also increase the synthesis of GABA.[185-187] In dogs, approximately 30% to 40% of the drug is metabolized by the liver to N-methylgabapentin with the remainder being excreted unchanged by the kidneys.[188,189] The $t_{1/2}$ is about 3 to 4 hours, with a bioavailability in dogs of about 80%.[189] The serum therapeutic range is 4 to 16 mg/mL. Side effects consist of ataxia and sedation.[190]

Few studies have been done to evaluate the efficacy for gabapentin in dogs. In one study, 6 of 11 dogs experienced a 50% reduction in seizure frequency.[190] In another study, affected dogs experienced an increase in the interictal period despite no significant change in seizure frequency; 3 of 17 dogs became seizure free.[191]

Pregabalin (Lyrica). Like gabapentin, the mechanism of action of pregabalin is through blockade of $\alpha_2\delta$-subunit of voltage-gated T-type calcium channel, thereby reducing glutamate, norepinephrine, and substance P.[118] Little data are available on its use in dogs. Based on pharmacologic data, pregabalin is administered at a dosage of 4 mg/kg orally three times a day.[192] At this dosage, no side effects are observed. In a study of 11 dogs undergoing treatment with PB or KBr alone or combination, the addition of pregabalin resulted in improved seizure control with a median reduction in seizure frequency of 50%; in seven dogs with cluster seizures, all had a reduction in seizures per cluster.[193] Most dogs had serum pregabalin concentrations ranging from 2.8 to 8.2 μg/mL, which is similar to therapeutic concentrations in humans.[193] Efficacy still remains to be determined.

Felbamate. Felbamate enhances sodium channel inactivation, enhances GABA activity, and reduces glutamate-mediated excitation. Felbamate has a high bioavailability with oral administration in adult dogs, has a short $t_{1/2}$ of 4 to 6 hours, reaching steady state in 20 to 30 hours, and is excreted in urine unchanged.[194,195] In dogs, the dosage is 20 mg/kg every 8 hours. Felbamate has a wide safety margin. It has been primarily used to treat focal seizures in dogs. In a study evaluating six dogs with focal seizures, all dogs experienced improved seizure control; two dogs had complete resolution of seizures.[196] Side effects are uncommon but may include blood dyscrasias and hepatotoxicity.[196]

Benzodiazepines. Diazepam is the most commonly used drug in this class. It is used in the treatment of isolated seizures, SE, and cluster seizures. It also can be used as an add-on drug for maintenance seizure therapy. However, with better choices of anticonvulsant drugs available, benzodiazepines are not commonly used for long-term therapy. The benzodiazepines enhance the activity of GABA. Diazepam has a rapid onset of action when given parenterally to both dogs and cats. In dogs, the duration of action is very short, and tolerance can rapidly develop, making it less useful as a maintenance drug for epilepsy.[197-199] In fact, withdrawal of chronically administered benzodiazepines can precipitate seizures.[197,198,200] Diazepam has a longer half-life in cats, and tolerance is not as common in this species, making it a more effective drug for management. However, fatal idiosyncratic hepatic necrosis has been associated with oral administration of diazepam in cats.[201] Consequently, oral benzodiazepines should be carefully monitored in cats.

Clorazepate is a benzodiazepine and used as an adjunctive therapy with PB for seizure control in dogs. Clorazepate is converted to N-desmethyldiazepam in the acidic environment of the stomach.[124] Both chemicals are active components of the drug. The dosage range is 2 to 4 mg/kg orally every 12 hours. Clorazepate may increase PB concentrations in the serum, usually within 1 month after initiating therapy.[202]

Clonazepam, a longer-acting benzodiazepine, is effective for short-term control of refractory seizures. The beneficial effect seems to last for only a few months. Hepatotoxicity can be a problem in dogs receiving clonazepam for longer than a few months. The dosage is 0.5 mg/kg orally twice daily.

Vagal Nerve Stimulation. In a 13-week study evaluating 10 dogs, a 50% reduction in seizure frequency was observed in 4 of 9 dogs.[203] A reduction in frequency was only observed in the last 4 weeks of the study. Morbidity associated with surgical implantation included intraoperative bradycardia and transient Horner's syndrome postoperatively in 2 dogs.[203] The vagus nerve carries general visceral efferent and afferent axons. Afferent information projects to the solitary nucleus, which in turn diffusely projects to cerebral cortical and subcortical neurons. Experimentally, stimulation of the vagus nerve results in desynchronization of EEG patterns. It is hypothesized that stimulation of the vagus nerve may inhibit the development of hypersynchronous neuronal activity.

STATUS EPILEPTICUS AND CLUSTER SEIZURES

The most commonly accepted definition of SE is continuous seizure activity lasting 5 minutes or two or more discrete seizures where there is incomplete recovery of consciousness. In two studies, the prevalence of SE in dogs admitted to veterinary hospitals was 0.44% and 0.7%.[204,205] CS can be defined as two discrete seizures within a 24-hour period in which there is complete recovery of consciousness between seizures. SE is a serious, life-threatening emergency necessitating prompt medical attention. Likewise, CS occurring rapidly and in excessive numbers per cluster event can also have profound physiologic consequences. As a result, the approach and management of these two conditions are discussed in this section.

The basis for the development of SE involves a failure of mechanisms that normally stop a seizure.[206] This may reflect persistent and excessive excitation or a lack of recruitment of inhibition.[206] The pathologic consequences of SE can be divided into systemic and neurologic. Systemically, animals may experience hypertension (early) and hypotension (late), tachycardia, cardiac arrhythmias, hypoglycemia, acidosis, and hyperthermia.[39] Many of these abnormalities reflect increased circulating catecholamines.[39] Ultimately, these systemic disturbances can lead to disseminated intravascular coagulation (DIC) and cardiopulmonary arrest. The main neurologic consequence to SE is neuronal loss.[207] Moreover, many of the systemic abnormalities can compound neuronal damage.[206] Although there are many mechanisms by which neuronal damage occurs in SE, underlying most is excitatory neurotoxicity related to glutamate.

As with isolated seizures, the causes of SE are primary, idiopathic, and symptomatic epilepsies and reactive seizures. In addition, inadequate serum anticonvulsant concentrations also may underlie SE. In dogs with SE, primary or idiopathic epilepsy accounts for 27% to 37%, symptomatic epilepsy accounts for 32% to 39%, and reactive seizures account for 7% to 22% of cases.[204,208] In some studies, the classification of the seizure disorder was not possible in 25% to 28% of dogs.[204,205,208] Interestingly, inadequate or low anticonvulsant serum concentrations accounted for approximately 6% of cases, suggesting that SE can occur despite appropriate management.[204] In two studies, SE was the initial presentation of a seizure disorder in 42% to 44% of dogs.[204,208] In another study, the risk of developing SE was nearly three times more likely with intoxication than any other cause of epilepsy.[205] In dogs with primary or idiopathic epilepsy, the risk of developing SE was greater for dogs weighing 28.9 kg (63.6 lb) or more compared with dogs weighing 17.4 kg (28.3 lb) or less.[209] One or more episodes of SE were predictive of future episodes. The mean life-span of dogs that experienced SE was 8.3 years compared with 11.3 years in epileptic dogs with no history of SE.[209]

A protocol for the treatment of SE is presented in Figure 13-3. The same protocol can be used for treatment of cluster seizures when the seizures occur with relatively high frequency. The following proposed treatment protocol mainly pertains to animals in which the underlying etiology is known or suspected to be due to idiopathic epilepsy. A similar approach can be used in animals with other etiologies. Animals with reactive seizure treatment also should focus on correction of the underlying cause. The choice of anticonvulsant used in animals with reactive seizures is dictated based on the presence of organ dysfunction and its impact on anticonvulsant metabolism.

Concurrent with therapy directed at controlling seizures is the correction of any systemic derangements. An IV catheter is immediately placed. Following this, affected animals should have baseline physiologic parameters assessed such as heart rate, rhythm, respiratory rate and effort, temperature, blood pressure, and assessment of respiratory function (arterial blood gas or pulse oxymetry). Clinicopathologic testing should include PCV/TS, blood glucose, and electrolytes. If possible assessment of renal function and hepatic disease also should be performed. In animals in which such testing identifies or supports an underlying cause of reactive epilepsy, more specialized tests may be necessary (see previous discussion).

Benzodiazepines, propofol, and pentobarbital can be used in the treatment of SE. Diazepam is the drug of choice for initial seizure control. Diazepam can be administered at a dosage range from 0.5 to 2 mg/kg IV, per rectum (PR), or intranasally (IN).[210,211] Midazolam can also be used. The dosage of midazolam is 0.066 to 0.22 mg/kg IV or IM.[212] In animals not having received anticonvulsant drugs before SE or severe clusters, PB should be given concurrent with benzodiazepines. Initial dosage of PB is 2 to 4 mg/kg IV, which can be repeated every 30 minutes or after subsequent seizures up to a cumulative dosage of 20 mg/kg.[124] Alternatively a loading dose can be calculated using the following formula: Total mg to be given IV = Body weight (kg) × 0.9 L/kg (volume of distribution of PB) × (15 μg/mL).[117] The main drawback to bolus administration of a loading dose of phenobarbital is severe sedation. In animals already receiving phenobarbital, the amount of phenobarbital needed to reach a higher serum drug concentration can be calculated based on knowledge of the current dose and serum drug concentration. The amount of phenobarbital to be administered to reach a new higher drug concentration is based on the formula:

Desired concentration/current concentration × current total mg of PB given per day = new mg of PB needed to achieve the new higher concentration.[117]

Diazepam can also be administered as a constant rate infusion (CRI) (0.25 to 0.5 mg/kg/hr). Midazolam also can be given as a CRI. Intravenous propofol bolus also can be given to gain seizure control as an initial drug or more commonly in animals not responding to diazepam. An initial bolus of propofol at 4 to 6 mg/kg IV is administered at a rate of 25% of the dose every 30 seconds to avoid apnea.[213] In animals having recurrent seizures, a CRI of propofol at 0.1 to 0.6 mg/kg/min can be used. In general, CRI administration of diazepam or propofol should be continued for 6 to 8 hours. After a CRI is initiated and seizures are controlled, the rate can be tapered to the lowest effective rate that limits seizure. Alternatively, pentobarbital can be dosed at 3 to 15 mg/kg IV to effect.[124] However, many animals have excessive movements that mimic seizure activity while recovering from pentobarbital. Similar movements also can occur during recovery from propofol anesthesia.[214] As a result, animals recovering from

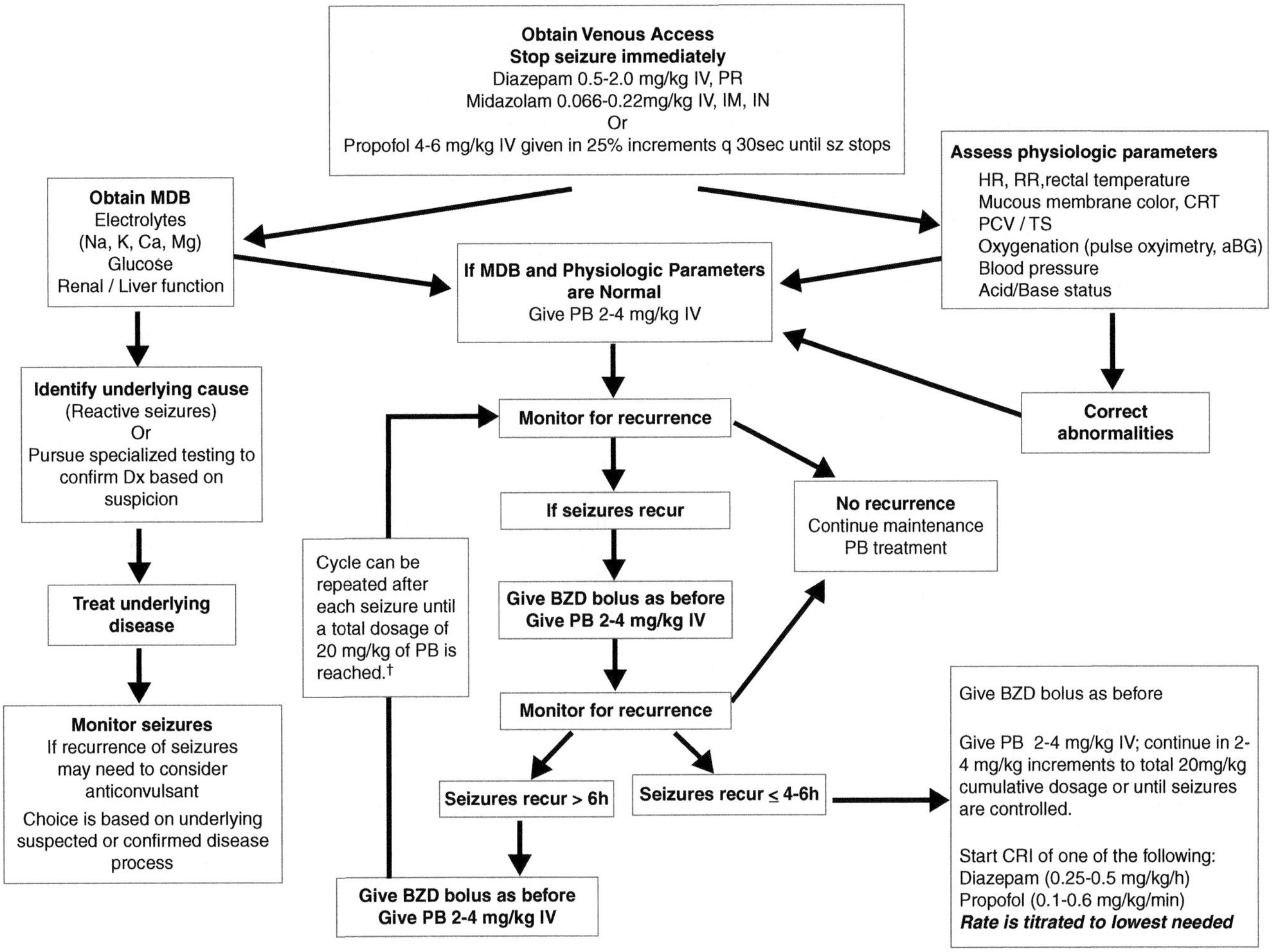

Obtain Venous Access
Stop seizure immediately
Diazepam 0.5-2.0 mg/kg IV, PR
Midazolam 0.066-0.22mg/kg IV, IM, IN
Or
Propofol 4-6 mg/kg IV given in 25% increments q 30sec until sz stops

Obtain MDB
Electrolytes
(Na, K, Ca, Mg)
Glucose
Renal / Liver function

Assess physiologic parameters
HR, RR,rectal temperature
Mucous membrane color, CRT
PCV / TS
Oxygenation (pulse oxyimetry, aBG)
Blood pressure
Acid/Base status

If MDB and Physiologic Parameters are Normal
Give PB 2-4 mg/kg IV

Correct abnormalities

Identify underlying cause
(Reactive seizures)
Or
Pursue specialized testing to confirm Dx based on suspicion

Treat underlying disease

Monitor seizures
If recurrence of seizures may need to consider anticonvulsant
Choice is based on underlying suspected or confirmed disease process

Monitor for recurrence

If seizures recur

No recurrence
Continue maintenance PB treatment

Cycle can be repeated after each seizure until a total dosage of 20 mg/kg of PB is reached.†

Give BZD bolus as before
Give PB 2-4 mg/kg IV

Monitor for recurrence

Seizures recur > 6h

Seizures recur ≤ 4-6h

Give BZD bolus as before
Give PB 2-4 mg/kg IV

Give BZD bolus as before

Give PB 2-4 mg/kg IV; continue in 2-4 mg/kg increments to total 20mg/kg cumulative dosage or until seizures are controlled.

Start CRI of one of the following:
Diazepam (0.25-0.5 mg/kg/h)
Propofol (0.1-0.6 mg/kg/min)
Rate is titrated to lowest needed

Figure 13-3 Treatment protocol for status epilepticus or an episode of frequent cluster seizures.* *IV,* Intravenously; *PR,* per rectum; *IM,* intramuscularly; *IN,* intranasally; *q,* every; *sec,* seconds; *h,* hour; *min,* minute; *sz,* seizure; *MDB,* minimum database; *Na,* sodium; *K,* potassium; *Ca,* calcium; *Mg,* magnesium; *Dx,* diagnosis; *HR,* heart rate; *RR,* respiratory rate; *CRT,* capillary refill time; *PCV,* packed cell volume; *TS,* total solids; *aBG,* arterial blood gas; *BZD,* benzodiazepine; *PB,* phenobarbital; *AED,* antiepileptic drug; *CRI,* constant rate infusion.
*Protocol is for the use in dogs not receiving AED therapy. Similar protocol could be used in dogs currently on phenobarbital. Protocol could be used in cats.
†If dog is already taking phenobarbital and serum concentration and dosage known, can calculate new higher serum concentration (see text).

pentobarbital or propofol anesthesia need to be carefully assessed to ensure that movements are related to recovery and not seizure activity. In one report, ketamine (5 mg/kg IV bolus followed by 5 mg/kg/hr CRI) was used in a dog with SE unresponsive to diazepam and propofol.[215] Ketamine caused a marked reduction in the abnormal EEG pattern suggesting efficacy. The authors postulated that the effects were due to antagonism of N-methyl-D-aspartic acid (NMDA) receptors, thereby reducing glutamate excitation.

Animals administered CRI of medications to control seizures can become excessively sedated or anesthetized. Additionally, many of these drugs often depress respiratory and cardiovascular functions. Consequently, all animals receiving CRI require intensive monitoring of the depth of sedation or anesthesia. In addition the eyes should be lubricated; manual expression, intermittent catheterization, or maintaining an indwelling urinary catheter to evacuate urine may be necessary; and padded bedding with frequent changes in recumbency is needed to prevent pressure sores. Some animals may require intubation and mechanical ventilation.

Animals undergoing treatment for SE require intensive supportive care and monitoring. Often systemic abnormalities are present and reflect the secondary effects of SE. Treatment directed at correction of derangements identified through physiologic parameters or clinicopathologic data may help protect against neuronal damage and prevent further systemic consequences. Intravenous fluid therapy should be initiated. Animals with severe obtundation, stupor, or coma, may require intubation and mechanical or hand ventilation. In animals with hypoxemia, supplemental oxygen should be provided via face mask or nasal cannula. Once the seizures are controlled and systemic abnormalities corrected, intensive supportive and nursing care is crucial for successful outcome. The median duration of hospitalization for dogs with SE is 43 hours.[204] Ultimately, in animals in which seizures are not controlled by 6 hours after admission or dogs with recurrence of seizures after 6 hours of control have a poor prognosis.[204]

Per-rectum (PR) administration of benzodiazepine drugs has been used to effectively treat cluster seizures in the hospital or home setting and to prevent the development of SE.[211]

Alternatively, midazolam can be administered IV, PR, or IN but also IM. Owners are given the injectable formulation of diazepam to give at a dose of 0.5 to 2.0 mg/kg PR or IN. Once drawn up into a syringe, the needle is removed and the drug is administered via teat cannula. Alternatively, an enteral feeding catheter can be cut short and used to administer the drug. The drug is given after an initial generalized seizure and when a second or third seizure occurs within 24 hours of the first seizure. Benzodiazepines are well absorbed from the rectum (diazepam; bioavailability of 51% to 79%) or nasal mucosa (midazolam; bioavailability of 80%) reaching peak concentration quickly (diazepam PR; approximately 15 minutes and midazolam IN; approximately 5 minutes).[210,216,217] The administration of diazepam PR at home in dogs with cluster seizures receiving adequate doses of anticonvulsant drugs reduces the total number of seizures, number of cluster seizure events, and number of seizures per cluster in affected dogs.[211]

NARCOLEPSY AND CATAPLEXY

Narcolepsy is a chronic sleep disorder characterized by excessive daytime sleepiness, sleep paralysis, hypnagogic hallucinations, and cataplexy (a sudden loss of muscle tone in response to stimulation).[218] Although hallucinations are impossible to determine in animals, excessive sleepiness and abnormal sleep patterns have been documented in dogs.[219] Despite this, most affected animals are recognized because of cataplexy (partial or complete).

The physiology of sleep has been extensively studied. The normal awake or sleep state involves interaction between the cerebrum, diencephalon, and a number of nuclei in the midbrain and pons. Sleep is characterized by two states: rapid eye movement (REM) and nonrapid eye movement (nREM) sleep.[220] Non-REM sleep is further subdivided into four categories based on EEG patterns, one of which is referred to as slow-wave sleep (SWS).[220] Normally, sleep begins with a transition from the awake state to nREM. The EEG pattern during SWS is characterized by slow, large amplitude waves. This coincides with decreased body temperature, heart rate, and respiratory rate. The EEG pattern during REM sleep is characterized by high-frequency, low-amplitude waves similar to that observed when awake. Concurrently, there is an increase in body temperature, heart rate, and respiratory rate, along with movements of the eyes. Paradoxically, there is atonia of most of the postural muscles during REM sleep.

Both adrenergic and cholinergic neurons are active during the awake state. During the transition to nREM sleep, adrenergic neurons cease activity while cholinergic neurons remain active but at a reduced activity level. With the transition to REM, adrenergic neurons remain inactive; however, cholinergic neurons increase to maximum activity level similar to that observed when awake. In addition to their diffuse projection to the thalamus and cerebrum, cholinergic neurons project to the medulla oblongata, resulting in spinal cord inhibition accounting for the atonia in REM sleep. This transition from nREM to REM occurs cyclically during periods of sleep.

Another neuronal system using a neuropeptide called hypocretin is involved in awake-sleep cycles. These neurons are located exclusively in the hypothalamus and diffusely project to the cerebrum and to the brainstem, where they have a facilitatory effect. [221] Hypocretin secretion increases during wakeful states and decreases during sleep. Thus hypocretin plays a critical role in the coordination of sleep and wakefulness.[220] In general, narcolepsy occurs as a result of either a reduced hypocretin concentration or an absence or decrease in functional receptors.[220] Without hypocretin (decreased hypocretin 1 concentrations or hypocretin receptor 1 function), narcoleptic animals are unable to stay awake and have altered responses to stimuli.[222] Hypocretin is secreted in response to emotional stimuli and feeding, which may explain the clinical presentation in affected animals.[222] In addition to the awake-sleep cycle, hypocretin modulates feeding behavior and neuroendocrine functions affecting metabolism.[220]

In the dog, both inherited and sporadic (cause unknown) cases of narcolepsy have been documented. The inherited form is the result of a mutation in the hypocretin receptor 2 gene.[223] Dogs with the inherited form have normal CSF concentrations of hypocretin 1. In sporadic cases, the clinical signs of narcolepsy are related to reduced hypocretin concentrations.[224] In the Labrador retriever and Doberman pinscher, narcolepsy is autosomal recessive with full penetrance.[225,226] A familial form also exists in the dachshund.[227] Clinical signs in dogs with the inherited form develop as early as 6 months of age. Age of onset in sporadic cases is more variable. In most sporadic cases the underlying cause is unknown. In humans, autoimmune destruction of hypocretin-secreting neurons is postulated based on the finding of low CSF hypocretin concentrations. Moreover, there is a strong association between narcolepsy and specific human leukocyte haplotypes involved in a predisposition for autoimmune disease.[228] There is no association with dog leukocyte antigen haplotypes in sporadic cases.[228] Moreover, affected dogs do not seem to respond to immunosuppression.[229] Narcolepsy/cataplexy has been reported in a young dog with distemper encephalitis.[230] Narcolepsy has been observed in a cat, a Brahman bull, horses, and ponies.[231-235]

Dogs with narcolepsy typically have episodes in which they suddenly collapse, often while excited or during emotional stimulation. Eating is the most common precipitating factor in reported cases. When the dog starts to eat, it suddenly appears weak, with the limb buckling and the head and neck drooping, which rapidly progresses to collapse and lying motionless.[236,237] Occasionally dogs may take a few steps and appear very weak and uncoordinated.[236,237] During the episodes, the animal's eye may remain open and even track objects.[236,237] Noise, shaking, or other stimuli may arouse the animal, and often it resumes eating only to fall asleep again. Continual stimulation, such as petting or shaking, may prevent the attack. The episodes often are repeated many times a day.[238,239]

A diagnosis usually is made by observation of the characteristic signs if cataplexy is a prominent part of the syndrome. In the absence of cataplexy, the disorder is difficult to recognize. EEG is the only available diagnostic test in animals not exhibiting cataplexy. A food-elicited cataplexy test can be used to identify dogs displaying mild cataplexy. The test is performed by placing 10 pieces of food in a row, 14 inches apart. Normal dogs can consume the food in less than 45 seconds; dogs with cataplexy take longer.[237] The test can also be used to monitor therapy. Additionally, pharmacologic agents can be used to elicit or inhibit attacks. A provocative test is using physostigmine (0.025 to 0.1 mg/kg IV), a cholinergic drug that crosses the blood-brain barrier. Acetylcholine concentrations increase and clinical signs are elicited.[237] Conversely, atropine (0.1 mg/kg IV) can be used to decrease the likelihood of clinical signs.[237] Similarly, yohimbine, an α_2-antagonist, suppresses cataplexy likely by increasing presynaptic adrenergic activity rather than blocking postsynaptic receptors.[240]

Treatment with tricyclic antidepressants increases adrenergic activity by inhibiting reuptake of norepinephrine. The most commonly used drugs include imipramine (0.5 to 1.0 mg/kg three times daily) or desipramine (3 mg/kg orally twice daily). In dogs demonstrating partial response, methylphenidate (Ritalin, 5 to 10 mg two or three times daily) can be used adjunctively. Although elimination of clinical signs may not always be possible, most affected dogs show improvement with therapy, enough to have a good quality of life.

CASE STUDIES

CASE 13-1 CHARLES

 veterinaryneurologycases.com

▪ Signalment
Canine, Labrador retriever, male castrated, 2 years old

▪ History
The dog has received all vaccinations on schedule and has had no major medical problems. The owner has reported that the dog had the first occurrence of a seizure approximately 2 months ago. In the past 2 weeks, the dog has had 3 more seizures. All seizures appeared similar. The last seizure was observed the night prior to examination.

The owner describes the seizures as follows: The dog seemed somewhat apprehensive and restless for approximately 30 minutes. Suddenly the dog sat down and gradually arched the head and the neck dorsally and to the right. The left thoracic and pelvic limb flexed up to the body which caused the dog to fall over. Once in lateral recumbency, all four limbs became rigid and then began making jerking movements. After about 30 seconds he started making running movements of the limbs and chewing movements of the mouth. During this time, there was excessive salivation and the dog urinated. The movements stopped after about 1 minute. In about 2-3 minutes, the dog was able to get up. He seemed a little disoriented for a few minutes, and then he gradually returned to normal.

Other than the seizures, the dog appeared healthy and normal to the owner.

▪ Physical and Neurologic Examinations
No abnormalities are found.

▪ Laboratory Examination
The complete blood cell count (CBC), chemistry profile, urinalysis (UA) was normal.

▪ Assessment
The description of the seizure is consistent a focal onset with secondary generalization. Based on the dog's signalment, normal physical and neurological examinations, normal interictal behavior, and normal MDB, idiopathic epilepsy should be considered in this dog. Primary epilepsy would necessitate demonstrating a familial history despite the documented occurrence of primary epilepsy in this breed. Moreover, consideration should be given to performing magnetic resonance imaging (MRI) of the brain to rule out symptomatic epilepsy. However, likelihood of identifying an intracranial abnormality is low.

The seizures are frequent enough necessitate therapy. The initial anticonvulsant medication of choice is phenobarbital. An initial dosage for beginning phenobarbital is 2-3 mg/kg orally twice daily. Steady state serum concentrations can be measured in 2-4 weeks after initiation of treatment. Based on steady state serum concentrations, side effects, and seizure control, the dosage of phenobarbital should be tailored to control seizures. Once control is established, routine monitoring of CBC, chemistry, urinalysis, and serum drug levels should be performed every 6 months.

CASE 13-2 BRUTUS

 veterinaryneurologycases.com

▪ Signalment
Canine, German Shepherd, male castrated, 5 years old

▪ History
The dog has a 3-year history of seizures; seizures consist of generalized and focal onset with secondary generalization seizure types. At the initial onset of the occurrence of seizures, physical and neurologic examinations were normal. An MDB was performed and was normal. The dog was initiated on phenobarbital at 3mg/kg orally twice daily. During the initial 6 months of therapy, the phenobarbital serum concentrations were monitored. Based on the serum concentration and seizure frequency, the dosage was adjusted to gain seizure control. After that time, the seizures were controlled for approximately 2 years. During those 2 years, the phenobarbital dosage was increased on two occasions. In the last 6 months, the dog has had more frequent seizures. In the last 2 months, the dog has had an average of 3-4 seizures per month. The dog's current phenobarbital dosage is 5 mg/kg orally twice daily. The dosage of phenobarbital has not changed in 6 months. The owner reports no health problems other than seizures.

▪ Physical and Neurologic Examinations
No abnormalities are found.

▪ Laboratory Examination
Chemistry profile disclosed increased alkaline phosphatase (SAP; 467 U/L; normal 12-122 IU/L) and alanine transferase (ALT; 135 IU/L; normal 8-108 IU/L).

The CBC and UA were normal.

Serum phenobarbital serum concentration was 32 mg/dL (therapeutic range 15-45 mg/dL).

▪ Assessment
At the time of onset, the dog's signalment, examination findings, and MDB results were consistent with idiopathic epilepsy. Moreover, no systemic or new neurologic abnormalities have developed which lends support to the classification of idiopathic epilepsy. Several options can be pursued in this time.

Knowledge of the phenobarbital serum concentration in this dog is extremely useful. The concentrations are within the therapeutic reference range, the dog is not exhibiting side effects (sedation, polydypsia, or polyuria, or biochemically abnormalities indicative of hepatic dysfunction); however, seizures are not controlled. Consequently, increasing the phenobarbital dosage by 20% to 25% may help regain seizure control. The main drawback is that serum concentration is approaching that which may result in hepatic injury. Alternatively, beginning adjunctive therapy with potassium bromide (KBr) may provide seizure control and ultimately allow the dosage of phenobarbital to be reduced once control is established.

Continued

CASE 13-2 BRUTUS—cont'd

Consideration should be given to performing additional diagnostic tests. The recent change in seizure frequency may herald the development of a new disease process. The changes observed on the MDB are consistent with phenobarbital-induced increased liver enzyme activity; therefore the seizures are not likely to be reactive seizures (due to an extracranial cause). To exclude the development of symptomatic epilepsy (and intracranial disorder), magnetic resonance imaging (MRI) of the brain may be pursued. As this was not a part of the initial diagnostic workup at the onset of seizures, this is not an unreasonable option. However, the owners should be made aware of the likelihood of a normal MRI study.

Treatment with KBr was initiated at 30mg/kg orally once daily. With the addition of KBr, seizure control was attained. As with phenobarbital, dose adjustments in KBr are made based on seizures control and steady state serum concentrations. Given the long half life of KBr in dogs, steady state concentrations are not reached until approximately 120 days. Despite this the drug is usually effective before reaching steady state. The owner did not choose to perform further diagnostic testing in this case. The addition of KBr helped gain control of the seizures.

CASE 13-3 MICCA

 veterinaryneurologycases.com

■ Signalment
Canine, Yorkshire Terrier, female intact, 9 months old

■ History
The owners report that in the month before presentation, the dog has had several episodes of anorexia which lasts for 1 to 1½ days each. In addition, the dog has been lethargic. Occasionally, the dog will pace aimlessly in the house or will stand and stare at the wall or out into space. During these periods, she is less responsive. Three hours before presentation, the dog ate, began pacing around the room, and had a seizure. The dog suddenly fell into lateral recumbency with its limbs paddling. The dog urinated and defecated. The seizure lasted for approximately 2 minutes. After the seizure, the dog was extremely lethargic. She bumped into objects as she walked. The dog has received all vaccinations, deworming, and heartworm prophylaxis on schedule. The dog is not allowed outside unattended.

■ Physical Examination
The dog was small in stature and had a thin body condition score.

■ Neurological Examination:
Mental Status: Dull to obtunded
Gait: Normal
Posture: Normal
Postural reactions: Normal in all four limbs
Spinal reflexes: Normal
Cranial nerves: Absence menace response OU; normal PLR and pupil size OU. Reduced response to noxious stimulation of the nasal mucosa; no other abnormalities were noted.
Sensory examination: Normal
Palpation: Normal

■ Laboratory Examination (values not listed are normal)

HCT	30%
MCV	63 fl (66-77 fl)
MCHC	30 g/dL (32-36 g/dl)

Chemistry profile

	Result	Units	Normal	Units
Urea Nitrogen	8	mg/dL	10-30	mg/dL
Creatinine	0.7	mg/dL	0.5-1.5	mg/dL
Total Protein	5.7	g/dL	5.2-7.3	g/dL
Albumin	2.2	g/dL	2.5-4.2	g/dL
Alk Phos	73	U/L	13-122	U/L
ALT	147	U/L	12-108	U/L
Glucose	68	mg/dL	77-120	mg/dL

Urinalysis
Specific gravity 1.015;
Cytological evaluation revealed ammonium biurate crystals.

■ Assessment
Lesion Location: Forebrain (based on the neurologic examination and observation of seizures)

Based on the description, the classification of the seizure type is consistent with generalized seizures. Etiologically, reactive seizures are most likely given the abnormalities identified on the laboratory examination, the abnormalities identified on neurological examination, and the presence of abnormal behavior prior to seizures. The laboratory data are highly suggestive of hepatic dysfunction. Measurement of fasting serum ammonia concentration and preprandial and postprandial bile acid levels confirmed an underlying liver disorder. Treatment for hepatic encephalopathy was initiated (see Chapter 15).

In this dog, further consideration should be given initiation of an anticonvulsant drug. Although there is no drug of choice for dogs with hepatic disease requiring anticonvulsants, phenobarbital and benzodiazepine drugs should be avoided as they undergo hepatic metabolism. Alternatively, KBr or levetiracetam can be used as these drugs do not undergo hepatic metabolism. Other drugs that undergo hepatic metabolism include zonisamide and gabapentin; therefore these drug are not recommended in dogs with hepatic disease.

In the present case, the dog was initiated on KBr along with therapy for hepatic encephalopathy. Further diagnostics disclosed a signal extrahepatic anomalous vessel arising from the portal vein. Consequently, the dog underwent surgical ligation of the portosystemic anomalous vessel. Postoperatively, the dog remained seizure-free for 6 months at which time it was gradually tapered off of KBr.

CASE 13-4 SASHA

 veterinaryneurologycases.com

■ Signalment
Canine, Mixed breed, female spayed, 4 years old

■ History
The dog has a 1 year history of generalized seizures. At the time of onset of seizures, physical and neurologic examinations and MDB were normal. Cross-sectional imaging and collection of cerebrospinal fluid (CSF) for analysis were no pursued. Initially, seizures occurred every 3-4 weeks. Based on the seizure frequency, the dog was treated with phenobarbital. In an attempt to gain control of the seizures, the dosage of phenobarbital was slowly increased to 3.2 mg/kg orally twice daily. Over the course of the last 6 months, the dog has experienced 4 episodes of cluster seizures which necessitated evaluation and hospitalization at an emergency veterinary hospital. The last cluster seizure occurred three weeks ago. At that time, phenobarbital serum concentration was 30μg/dL. There has been no change in the dosage or dosing regime of phenobarbital in the last month. No other health problems have been observed.

■ Physical and Neurologic Examinations
No abnormalities are found.

■ Laboratory Examination
With the exception of increases in SAP (351 IU/L; normal range 12-122 IU/L) no other abnormalities were identified.

■ Assessment
The likely etiologic classification for the seizures in this dog is idiopathic epilepsy. Although cross-sectional imaging and CSF analysis are necessary to rule out symptomatic epilepsy, idiopathic epilepsy remains most probable given that there has been no development of systemic or new neurologic abnormalities.

Despite what may be considered an acceptable interictal period (episodes of seizures approximately every 6 weeks) in this dog, seizure activity occurs as cluster seizures, which has required emergency evaluation and hospitalization. At the current dosage of phenobarbital, the serum concentration is within the therapeutic range. As there has not been a change in the dosage or dosing regime, this concentration represents a steady state concentration. Consequently, increasing the dosage of phenobarbital may increase the likelihood of developing toxicity without providing improved seizure control. The most probable explanation for the increase in SAP concentration is induction by phenobarbital given the lack of other findings consistent with hepatotoxicity.

There are two possible changes that can be made to improve seizure control in this dog. First, the addition of KBr therapy, may help with no only an increase in the interictal period (i.e., decrease the frequency of seizures), it may also reduce the number of seizure that occur per cluster. Therefore KBr may be initiated in this case at 30mg/kg orally per day. The dosage can be tailored based on seizure control, side effects, and serum concentrations.

Secondly, the owners can be instructed on how to administer benzodiazepines per rectum (PR) at home during a cluster seizure. The parentral formation of diazepam can be administered PR. Diazepam at a dosage of 0.5-2.0 mg/kg is drawn up and administered PR via a teat cannula or an enteral feeding catheter cut to approximately a 3-5-cm length. Alternatively midazolam can be administered at 0.2 mg/kg intranasally. Administration of a benzodiazepine is done at the time of the first seizure and can be repeated for up to 3-4 times in a 24-hour period. The use of diazepam PR in dogs is associated with a decrease in the number of cluster seizure events as well as the number of seizures that occur per cluster.

CASE 13-5 SAMMY

 veterinaryneurologycases.com

■ Signalment
Feline, DSH, female spayed, 2 years old

■ History
The cat has a 6-month history of generalized seizures. At the onset of seizures, the cat had 3 seizures in 1 week, which prompted initial evaluation. At the onset of seizures, physical and neurologic examinations, MDB, MRI of the brain, and CSF analysis were normal. Treatment with phenobarbital at 2.2 mg/kg was started. Over several months, the dosage was gradually increased based on poorly controlled seizures. The cat continues to have frequent seizures. The current seizure frequency is a single seizure every 2-3 weeks. The current dosage of phenobarbital is 4mg/kg. No changes in phenobarbital dosage or dosing regime have occurred in the last 4 weeks. The current serum phenobarbital concentration is 34 μg/dL. No other health problems have been observed. Vaccinations are current. The cat is kept strictly indoors and is the only cat in the household.

■ Physical and Neurologic Examinations
No abnormalities are found.

■ Laboratory Examination
No abnormalities are found.

■ Assessment
Symptomatic epilepsy is the most common etiologic classification for seizures in cats. Consequently, seizure activity in every cat should prompt a thorough diagnostic work up in order to rule out reactive seizures and symptomatic epilepsy. Without knowledge of a familial history or pedigree analysis, primary epilepsy is not a consideration. A specific cause of seizures was not identified in this cat, therefore the most probable etiologic classification of seizure is idiopathic epilepsy.

Treatment was started with phenobarbital, which is the initial drug of choice for most cats. Despite this, seizure control remains poor. As symptomatic epilepsy is common in cats, consideration should be given to reevaluation of diagnostic tests. However, without an acute change in seizure

Continued

CASE 13-5 SAMMY—cont'd

control or the development of systemic or neurologic deficits, repeat of previous diagnostics are likely to be normal.

To obtain seizure control, adjunctive anticonvulsant medication should be initiated. In cats, there is not routinely used adjunctive therapy. Unlike dogs in which KBr is commonly prescribed adjunctively, KBr in cats is associated with frequent adverse side effects. As a result, KBr should not be used in cats. There are limited choices of anticonvulsants to be used adjunctively with phenobarbital in cat. Choices include levetiracetam, zonisamide, gabapentin, or pregabalin. Only levetiracetam and zonisamide have been evaluated in cats. In this case, levetiracetam at 20mg/kg orally three times daily was started. The addition of levetiracetam resulted in control of seizures. The owners were advised to continue to monitor the seizure frequency, severity, and duration because in dogs the loss of seizure control has been observed 4-8 months after beginning levetiracetam suggesting tolerance to the drug. Long term control of seizures with levetiracetam has not been evaluated in cats.

CASE 13-6 TOBY

 veterinaryneurologycases.com

▪ Signalment

Canine, mixed breed, male castrated, 7 years old.

▪ History

The dog has had a recent onset of seizures. The owner describes the seizures as follows: seizure have occurred during the evenings. The dog has been at rest and without warning will extend all four limbs and develop opisthotonus that lasts for approximately 15-20 seconds. Then the dog develops violent jerking movements with its limbs. The dog typically urinates during the seizure. During the seizure, the dog is unresponsive to the owner. After the seizure the dog remains quite for 1-2 hours and then returns to normal.

The initial seizure occurred 3 months before presentation. This isolated seizure was followed 1 month later by two seizures in week. At that time an MDB was performed and was normal. The dog was initiated on phenobarbital at 2mg/kg orally twice daily. Three weeks after initiating phenobarbital, the dog experienced three seizures over 2 days.

The owner does not report any other health problems. The dog behaves normally between seizures. The dog is only allowed outside in a fenced in yard or walked on a leash. There has been no exposure to toxins.

▪ Physical and Neurologic Examinations

No abnormalities are found.

▪ Laboratory Examination

The CBC, chemistry profile, and UA were normal.

▪ Assessment

Based on the owner's description, the dog is experiencing generalized seizures. Despite the normal physical and neurologic examinations, symptomatic epilepsy should be the main consideration for this dog. The MDB and the fact that the dog appears well supervised without access to intoxicants make reactive seizures unlikely. The dog is outside of the age range that idiopathic epilepsy typically begins.

The owners should be advised that a more thorough diagnostic work-up should be pursued. Beyond the MDB, thoracic radiographs should be performed to exclude the possibility of metastatic disease. Consideration should be given evaluating the abdominal cavity (i.e., radiographs or ultrasonography). Ultimately, imaging of the brain should be performed. The gold standard imaging modality for the brain is MRI. In instances where MRI is not available, CT may be pursued.

In this dog, thoracic radiographs were normal. Abdominal imaging was not pursued. MRI of the brain disclosed an extra-axial, strongly and uniformly enhancing mass affecting the left olfactory/frontal lobes of the cerebrum. The imaging characteristics were consistent with a meningioma.

As in this dog, lesion often affects the olfactory/frontal lobes of the cerebrum with minimal impact on the dog. The most common neurologic signs related to a lesion in this area of the brain are changes in mentation and seizures. As a result, a thorough diagnostic work-up should be pursued in all dogs over the age of 5 years that develop seizures.

A transfrontal craniotomy was performed for excision of the tumor. Postoperatively, the dog underwent radiation therapy. Phenobarbital was continued throughout the dog's treatment to control seizures.

REFERENCES

1. Gastaut H: Dictionary of epilepsy, ed, Geneva, 1973, World Health Organization.
2. Fisher RS, van Emde Boas W, Blume W, et al: Epileptic seizures and epilepsy: definitions proposed by the International League Against Epilepsy (ILAE) and the International Bureau for Epilepsy (IBE), Epilepsia 46:470–472, 2005.
3. Berendt M, Gredal H, Alving J: Characteristics and phenomenology of epileptic partial seizures in dogs: similarities with human seizure semiology, Epilepsy Res 61:167–173, 2004.
4. Licht BG, Licht MH, Harper KM, et al: Clinical presentations of naturally occurring canine seizures: similarities to human seizures, Epilepsy Behav 3:460–470, 2002.
5. Berendt M, Gram L: Epilepsy and seizure classification in 63 dogs: a reappraisal of veterinary epilepsy terminology, J Vet Intern Med 13:14–20, 1999.
6. Gloor P, Fariello RG: Generalized epilepsy: some of its cellular mechanisms differ from those of focal epilepsy, Trends Neurosci 11:63–68, 1988.
7. Gorji A, Speckmann EJ: Epileptiform EEG spikes and their functional significance, Clin EEG Neurosci 40:230–233, 2009.

8. Speckmann EJ, Elger CE: Introduction to the neurophysiological basis of the EEG and DC potentials. In Niedermeyer E, Lopes da Silva FH, editors: Electroencephalography: basic principles, clinical applications, and related fields, Baltimore, 1987, Urban & Schwarzenberg.
9. Bleck TP, Klawans HL: Convulsive disorders: mechanisms of epilepsy and anticonvulsant action, Clin Neuropharmacol 13:121–128, 1990.
10. Russo ME: The pathophysiology of epilepsy, Cornell Vet 71:221–247, 1981.
11. Klass DW, Westmoreland BF: Electroencephalography: general principles and adult electroencephalograms. In Daube JR, editor: Clinical neurophysiology, Philadelphia, 1996, FA Davis.
12. Berendt M, Hogenhaven H, Flagstad A, et al: Electroencephalography in dogs with epilepsy: similarities between human and canine findings, Acta Neurol Scand 99:276–283, 1999.
13. Holliday TA, Cunningham JG, Gutnick MJ: Comparative clinical and electroencephalographic studies of canine epilepsy, Epilepsia 11:281–292, 1970.
14. Jaggy A, Bernardini M: Idiopathic epilepsy in 125 dogs: a long-term study. Clinical and electroencephalographic findings, J Small Anim Pract 39:23–29, 1998.
15. Dichter MA: Emerging concepts in the pathogenesis of epilepsy and epileptogenesis, Arch Neurol 66:443–447, 2009.
16. Blumenfeld H: The thalamus and seizures, Arch Neurol 59:135–137, 2002.
17. Futatsugi Y, Riviello JJ Jr: Mechanisms of generalized absence epilepsy, Brain Dev 20:75–79, 1998.
18. Avoli M, Gloor P: Interaction of cortex and thalamus in spike and wave discharges of feline generalized penicillin epilepsy, Exp Neurol 76:196–217, 1982.
19. Sierra-Paredes G, Sierra-Marcuno G: Extrasynaptic GABA and glutamate receptors in epilepsy, CNS Neurol Disord Drug Targets 6:288–300, 2007.
20. Bowie D: Ionotropic glutamate receptors & CNS disorders, CNS Neurol Disord Drug Targets 7:129–143, 2008.
21. Moldrich RX, Chapman AG, De Sarro G, et al: Glutamate metabotropic receptors as targets for drug therapy in epilepsy, Eur J Pharmacol 476:3–16, 2003.
22. Bormann J: The "ABC" of GABA receptors, Trends Pharmacol Sci 21:16–19, 2000.
23. Nutt D: GABAA receptors: subtypes, regional distribution, and function, J Clin Sleep Med 2:S7–S11, 2006.
24. McCormick DA, Contreras D: On the cellular and network bases of epileptic seizures, Annu Rev Physiol 63:815, 2001.
25. Ellenberger C, Mevissen M, Doherr M, et al: Inhibitory and excitatory neorotransmitters in the cerebrospinal fluid of epileptic doss, Am J Vet Res 65(8):1108–1113, 2004.
26. Loscher W, Schwartz-Porsche D: Low levels of gamma-aminobutyric acid in cerebrospinal fluid of dogs with epilepsy, J Neurochem 46:1322–1325, 1986.
27. Podell M, Hadjiconstantinou M: Low concentrations of cerebrospinal fluid GABA correlate to a reduced response to phenobarbital therapy in primary canine epilepsy, J Vet Intern Med 13:89–94, 1999.
28. Olney JW, Price MT, Samson L, et al: The role of specific ions in glutamate neurotoxicity, Neurosci Lett 65:65–71, 1986.
29. Fountain NB, Lothman EW: Pathophysiology of status epilepticus, J Clin Neurophysiol 12:326–342, 1995.
30. Sloviter RS: The functional organization of the hippocampal dentate gyrus and its relevance to the pathogenesis of temporal lobe epilepsy, Ann Neurol 35:640–654, 1994.
31. Aroniadou-Anderjaska V, Fritsch B, Qashu F, et al: Pathology and pathophysiology of the amygdala in epileptogenesis and epilepsy, Epilepsy Res 78:102–116, 2008.
32. Montgomery DL, Lee AC: Brain damage in the epileptic beagle dog, Vet Pathol 20:160–169, 1983.
33. Yamasaki H, Furuoka H, Takechi M, et al: Neuronal loss and gliosis in limbic system in an epileptic dog, Vet Pathol 28:540–542, 1991.
34. Buckmaster PS, Smith MO, Buckmaster CL, et al: Absence of temporal lobe epilepsy pathology in dogs with medically intractable epilepsy, J Vet Intern Med 16:95–99, 2002.
35. Fatzer R, Gandini G, Jaggy A, et al: Necrosis of hippocampus and piriform lobe in 38 domestic cats with seizures: a retrospective study on clinical and pathologic findings, J Vet Intern Med 14:100–104, 2000.
36. Mellema LM, Koblik PD, Kortz GD, et al: Reversible magnetic resonance imaging abnormalities in dogs following seizures, Vet Radiol Ultrasound 40:588–595, 1999.
37. Chan S, Chin SS, Kartha K, et al: Reversible signal abnormalities in the hippocampus and neocortex after prolonged seizures, AJNR Am J Neuroradiol 17:1725–1731, 1996.
38. Sloviter RS: Hippocampal epileptogenesis in animal models of mesial temporal lobe epilepsy with hippocampal sclerosis: the importance of the "latent period" and other concepts, Epilepsia 49(suppl 9):85–92, 2008.
39. Platt SR, McDonnell JJ: Status epilepticus: clinical features and pathophysiology, Compend Contin Educ Pract Vet 22:660–669, 2000.
40. Drobatz KJ, Saunders HM, Pugh CR, et al: Noncardiogenic pulmonary edema in dogs and cats: 26 cases (1987-1993), J Am Vet Med Assoc 206:1732–1736, 1995.
41. James FE, Johnson VS, Lenard ZM, et al: Severe haemoptysis associated with seizures in a dog, N Z Vet J 56:85–88, 2008.
42. King JM, Roth L, Haschek WM: Myocardial necrosis secondary to neural lesions in domestic animals, J Am Vet Med Assoc 180:144–148, 1982.
43. Kent M, Reiss C, Blas-Machado U: Elevated cardiac troponin I in a dog with an intracranial meningioma and evidence of myocardial necrosis, J Am Anim Hosp Assoc 46:48–55, 2010.
44. Engel J: A proposed diagnostic scheme for people with epileptic seizures and with epilepsy: report of the ILAE task force on classification and terminology, Epilepsia (Series 4) 42:796–803, 2001.
45. Engel J: Report of the ILAE classification core group, Epilepsia 47:1558–1568, 2006.
46. Podell M, Fenner WR, Powers JD: Seizure classification in dogs from a nonreferral-based population, J Am Vet Med Assoc 206:1721–1728, 1995.
47. Quesnel AD, Parent JM, McDonell W, et al: Diagnostic evaluation of cats with seizure disorders: 30 cases (1991-1993), J Am Vet Med Assoc 210:65–71, 1997.
48. Fitzmaurice S, Rusbridge C, Shelton GD, et al: Familial myoclonic epilepsy in the miniature wirehaired dachshund, 2001, American College of Veterinary Internal Medicine.
49. Gredal H, Berendt M, Leifsson PS: Progressive myoclonus epilepsy in a beagle, J Small Anim Pract 44:511–514, 2003.
50. Jian Z, Alley MR, Cayzer J, et al: Lafora's disease in an epileptic basset hound, N Z Vet J 38:75–79, 1990.
51. Schoeman T, Williams J, Wilpe E: Polyglucosan storage disease in a dog resembling Lafora's disease, J Vet Intern Med 16:201–207, 2002.

52. Webb AA, McMillan C, Cullen CL, et al: Lafora disease as a cause of visually exacerbated myoclonic attacks in a dog, Can Vet J 50:963–967, 2009.
53. Hegreberg GA, Padgett GA: Inherited progressive epilepsy of the dog with comparisons to Lafora's disease of man, Fed Proc 35:1202–1205, 1976.
54. Davis KE, Finnie JW, Hooper PT: Lafora's disease in a dog, Aust Vet J 67:192–193, 1990.
55. Lohi H, Young EJ, Fitzmaurice SN, et al: Expanded repeat in canine epilepsy, Science 307:81, 2005.
56. Redding RW: Electroencephalography. In Oliver JE, Hoerlein BF, Mayhew IG, editors: Veterinary neurology, Philadelphia, 1987, WB Saunders.
57. Oliver JE: Seizure disorders in companion animals, Compend Contin Educ Pract Vet 2:77–85, 1980.
58. Thomas WB: Idiopathic epilepsy in dogs, Vet Clin North Am Small Anim Pract 30:183–206, 2000:vii.
59. Breitschwerdt EB, Breazile JE, Broadhurst JJ: Clinical and electroencephalographic findings associated with ten cases of suspected limbic epilepsy in the dog, J Am Anim Hosp Assoc 15:37–50, 1979.
60. Gibbon KJ, Trepanier LA, Delaney FA: Phenobarbital-Responsive ptyalism, dysphagia, and apparent esophageal spasm in a German shepherd puppy, J Am Anim Hosp Assoc 40:230–237, 2004.
61. Stonehewer J, Mackin AJ, Tasker S, et al: Idiopathic phenobarbital-responsive hypersialosis in the dog: an unusual form of limbic epilepsy? J Small Anim Pract 41:416–421, 2000.
62. Crowell-Davis SL, Lappin M, Oliver JE: Stimulus-responsive psychomotor epilepsy in a Doberman pinscher, J Am Anim Hosp Assoc 25:57–60, 1989.
63. Cash WC, Blauch BS: Jaw snapping syndrome in eight dogs, J Am Vet Med Assoc 175:709–710, 1979.
64. Rusbridge C: Neurological diseases of the cavalier King Charles spaniel, J Small Anim Pract 46:265–272, 2005.
65. Dodman NH, Knowles KE, Shuster L, et al: Behavioral changes associated with suspected complex partial seizures in bull terriers, J Am Vet Med Assoc 208:688–691, 1996.
66. Schriefl S, Steinberg TA, Matiasek K, et al: Etiologic classification of seizures, signalment, clinical signs, and outcome in cats with seizure disorders: 91 cases (2000-2004), J Am Vet Med Assoc 233:1591–1597, 2008.
67. Barnes HL, Chrisman CL, Mariani CL, et al: Clinical signs, underlying cause, and outcome in cats with seizures: 17 cases (1997-2002), J Am Vet Med Assoc 225:1723–1726, 2004.
68. Berendt M, Gredal H, Pedersen LG, et al: A cross-sectional study of epilepsy in Danish Labrador retrievers: prevalence and selected risk factors, J Vet Intern Med 16:262–268, 2002.
69. Berendt M, Gullov CH, Christensen SL, et al: Prevalence and characteristics of epilepsy in the Belgian shepherd variants Groenendael and Tervuren born in Denmark 1995-2004, Acta Vet Scand 50:51, 2008.
70. Heynold Y, Faissler D, Steffen F, et al: Clinical, epidemiological and treatment results of idiopathic epilepsy in 54 Labrador retrievers: a long-term study, J Small Anim Pract 38:7–14, 1997.
71. Berendt M, Gullov CH, Fredholm M: Focal epilepsy in the Belgian shepherd: evidence for simple Mendelian inheritance, J Small Anim Pract 50:655–661, 2009.
72. Bielfelt SW, Redman HC, McClellan RO: Sire- and sex-related differences in rates of epileptiform seizures in a purebred beagle dog colony, Am J Vet Res 32:2039–2048, 1971.
73. Falco MJ, Barker J, Wallace ME: The genetics of epilepsy in the British Alsatian, J Small Anim Pract 15:685–692, 1974.
74. Van Der Velden NA: Fits in Tervuren shepherd dogs: a presumed hereditary trait, J Small Anim Pract 9:63–70, 1968.
75. Wallace ME: Keeshonds: a genetic study of epilepsy and EEG readings, J Small Anim Pract 16:1–10, 1975.
76. Kathmann I, Jaggy A, Busato A, et al: Clinical and genetic investigations of idiopathic epilepsy in the Bernese mountain dog, J Small Anim Pract 40:319–325, 1999.
77. Casal ML, Munuve RM, Janis MA, et al: Epilepsy in Irish wolfhounds, J Vet Intern Med 20:131–135, 2006.
78. Hülsmeyer V, Zimmermann R, Brauer C, et al: Epilepsy in border collies: clinical manifestation, outcome, and mode of inheritance, J Vet Intern Med 24:171-178, 2010.
79. Jokinen TS, Metsahonkala L, Bergamasco L, et al: Benign familial juvenile epilepsy in Lagotto Romagnolo dogs, J Vet Intern Med 21:464–471, 2007.
80. Patterson EE, Armstrong PJ, O'Brien DP, et al: Clinical description and mode of inheritance of idiopathic epilepsy in English springer spaniels, J Am Vet Med Assoc 226:54–58, 2005.
81. Patterson EE, Mickelson JR, Da Y, et al: Clinical characteristics and inheritance of idiopathic epilepsy in vizslas, J Vet Intern Med 17:319–325, 2003.
82. Srenk P, Jaggy A: Interictal electroencephalographic findings in a family of golden retrievers with idiopathic epilepsy, J Small Anim Pract 37:317–321, 1996.
83. Viitmaa R, Cizinauskas S, Bergamasco LA, et al: Magnetic resonance imaging findings in Finnish spitz dogs with focal epilepsy, J Vet Intern Med 20:305–310, 2006.
84. Licht BG, Lin S, Luo Y, et al: Clinical characteristics and mode of inheritance of familial focal seizures in standard poodles, J Am Vet Med Assoc 231:1520–1528, 2007.
85. Gerard VA, Conarck CN: Identifying the cause of an early onset of seizures in puppies with epileptic parents, Vet Med 86:1060–1061, 1991.
86. Chrisman CL: Epilepsy and seizures. In Howard JL, editor: Current veterinary therapy: food animal practice, Philadelphia, 1981, WB Saunders.
87. Mittel L: Seizures in the horse, Vet Clin North Am Equine Pract 3:323–332, 1987.
88. Aleman M, Gray LC, Williams DC, et al: Juvenile idiopathic epilepsy in Egyptian Arabian foals: 22 cases (1985-2005), J Vet Intern Med 20:1443–1449, 2006.
89. Platt S, McGrotty YL, Abramson CJ, et al: Refractory seizures associated with an organic aciduria in a dog, J Am Anim Hosp Assoc 43:163–167, 2007.
90. Barlow RM: Morphogenesis of cerebellar lesions in bovine familial convulsions and ataxia, Vet Pathol 18:151–162, 1981.
91. Coates JR, Bergman RL: Seizures in young dogs and cats: pathophysiology and diagnosis, Compend Contin Educ Pract Vet 27:447–459, 2005.
92. Greene CE, Vandevelde M, Braund K: Lissencephaly in two Lhasa Apso dogs, J Am Vet Med Assoc 169:405–410, 1976.
93. Braund K: Degenerative and developmental diseases. In Oliver JE, Hoerlein BF, Mayhew IG, editors: Veterinary neurology, Philadelphia, 1987, WB Saunders.
94. Saito M, Sharp NJH, Kortz GD, et al: Magnetic resonance imaging features of lissencephaly in 2 Lhasa Apsos, Vet Radiol Ultrasound 43:331–337, 2002.
95. Cordy DR, Holliday TA: A necrotizing meningoencephalitis of pug dogs, Vet Pathol 26:191–194, 1989.

96. Stalis IH, Chadwick B, Dayrell-Hart B, et al: Necrotizing meningoencephalitis of Maltese dogs, Vet Pathol 32:230–235, 1995.
97. Tipold A, Fatzer R, Jaggy A, et al: Necrotizing encephalitis in Yorkshire terriers, J Small Anim Pract 34:623–628, 1993.
98. Foster ES, Carrillo JM, Patnaik AK: Clinical signs of tumors affecting the rostral cerebrum in 43 dogs, J Vet Intern Med 2:71–74, 1988.
99. Bagley RS, Gavin PR, Moore MP, et al: Clinical signs associated with brain tumors in dogs: 97 cases (1992-1997), J Am Vet Med Assoc 215:818–819, 1999.
100. Snyder JM, Lipitz L, Skorupski KA, et al: Secondary intracranial neoplasia in the dog: 177 cases (1986-2003), J Vet Intern Med 22:172–177, 2008.
101. Snyder JM, Shofer FS, Van Winkle TJ, et al: Canine intracranial primary neoplasia: 173 cases (1986-2003), J Vet Intern Med 20:669–675, 2006.
102. Troxel MT, Vite CH, Van Winkle TJ, et al: Feline intracranial neoplasia: retrospective review of 160 cases (1985-2001), J Vet Intern Med 17:850–859, 2003.
103. Prince DA, Parada I, Scalise K, et al: Epilepsy following cortical injury: cellular and molecular mechanisms as targets for potential prophylaxis, Epilepsia 50(suppl 2):30–40, 2009.
104. Garosi LS, Dennis R, Platt SR, et al: Thiamine deficiency in a dog: clinical, clinicopathologic, and magnetic resonance imaging findings, J Vet Intern Med 17:719–723, 2003.
105. Singh M, Thompson M, Sullivan N, et al: Thiamine deficiency in dogs due to the feeding of sulphite preserved meat, Aust Vet J 83:412–417, 2005.
106. Oliver JE: Seizure disorders and narcolepsy. In Oliver JE, Hoerlein BF, Mayhew IG, editors: Veterinary neurology, Philadelphia, 1987, WB Saunders.
107. O'Brien D: Toxic and metabolic causes of seizures, Clin Tech Small Anim Pract 13:159–166, 1998.
108. Morgan RV, Moore FM, Pearce LK, et al: Clinical and laboratory findings in small companion animals with lead poisoning: 347 cases (1977-1986), J Am Vet Med Assoc 199:93–97, 1991.
109. Kornegay JN, Mayhew IG: Metabolic, toci, and nutritional diseases of the nervous system. In Oliver JE, Hoerlein BF, Mayhew IG, editors: Veterinary neurology, Philadelphia, 1987, Saunders.
110. Knight TE, Kent M, Junk JE: Succimer for treatment of lead toxicosis in two cats, J Am Vet Med Assoc 218(1936):1946–1948, 2001.
111. Knight TE, Kumar MS: Lead toxicosis in cats—a review, J Feline Med Surg 5:249–255, 2003.
112. Ramsey DT, Casteel SW, Faggella AM, et al: Use of orally administered succimer (meso-2,3-dimercaptosuccinic acid) for treatment of lead poisoning in dogs, J Am Vet Med Assoc 208:371–375, 1996.
113. Roberts BK, Aronsohn MG, Moses BL, et al: Bufo marinus intoxication in dogs: 94 cases (1997-1998), J Am Vet Med Assoc 216:1941–1944, 2000.
114. Gwaltney-Brant SM, Albretsen JC, Khan SA: 5-Hydroxytryptophan toxicosis in dogs: 21 cases (1989-1999), J Am Vet Med Assoc 216:1937–1940, 2000.
115. Holliday TA: Seizure disorders, Vet Clin North Am Small Anim Pract 10:3–29, 1980.
116. Dayrell-Hart B, Steinberg SA, VanWinkle TJ, et al: Hepatotoxicity of phenobarbital in dogs: 18 cases (1985-1989), J Am Vet Med Assoc 199:1060–1066, 1991.
117. Podell M: Antiepileptic drug therapy, Clin Tech Small Anim Pract 13:185–192, 1998.
118. Luszczki JJ: Third-generation antiepileptic drugs: mechanisms of action, pharmacokinetics and interactions, Pharmacol Rep 61:197–216, 2009.
119. Isoherranen N, Yagen B, Soback S, et al: Pharmacokinetics of levetiracetam and its enantiomer (R)-alpha-ethyl-2-oxo-pyrrolidine acetamide in dogs, Epilepsia 42:825–830, 2001.
120. Jensen AA, Mosbacher J, Elg S, et al: The anticonvulsant gabapentin (neurontin) does not act through gamma-aminobutyric acid-B receptors, Mol Pharmacol 61:1377–1384, 2002.
121. Farnbach GC: Serum concentrations and efficacy of phenytoin, phenobarbital, and primidone in canine epilepsy, J Am Vet Med Assoc 184:1117–1120, 1984.
122. Schwartz-Porsche D, Loscher W, Frey HH: Therapeutic efficacy of phenobarbital and primidone in canine epilepsy: a comparison, J Vet Pharmacol Ther 8:113–119, 1985.
123. Frey HH: Use of anticonvulsants in small animals, Vet Rec 118:484–486, 1986.
124. Lane SB, Bunch SE: Medical management of recurrent seizures in dogs and cats, J Vet Intern Med 4:26–39, 1990.
125. Podell M, Fenner WR: Bromide therapy in refractory canine idiopathic epilepsy, J Vet Intern Med 7:318–327, 1993.
126. Frey HH: Anticonvulsant drugs used in the treatment of epilepsy, Probl Vet Med 1:558–577, 1989.
127. Al-Tahan F, Frey HH: Absorption kinetics and bioavailability of phenobarbital after oral administration to dogs, J Vet Pharmacol Ther 8:205–207, 1985.
128. Pedersoli WM, Wike JS, Ravis WR: Pharmacokinetics of single doses of phenobarbital given intravenously and orally to dogs, Am J Vet Res 48:679–683, 1987.
129. Frey HH, Kampmann E, Nielsen CK: Study on combined treatment with phenobarbital and diphenylhydantoin, Acta Pharmacol Toxicol (Copenh) 26:284–292, 1968.
130. Frey HH, Loscher W: Pharmacokinetics of anti-epileptic drugs in the dog: a review, J Vet Pharmacol Ther 8:219–233, 1985.
131. Ravis WR, Nachreiner RF, Pedersoli WM, et al: Pharmacokinetics of phenobarbital in dogs after multiple oral administration, Am J Vet Res 45:1283–1286, 1984.
132. Maguire PJ, Fettman MJ, Smith MO, et al: Effects of diet on pharmacokinetics of phenobarbital in healthy dogs, J Am Vet Med Assoc 217:847–852, 2000.
133. Yeary RA: Serum concentrations of primidone and its metabolites, phenylethylmalonamide and phenobarbital, in the dog, Am J Vet Res 41:1643–1645, 1980.
134. Frey HH, Gobel W, Loscher W: Pharmacokinetics of primidone and its active metabolites in the dog, Arch Int Pharmacodyn Ther 242:14–30, 1979.
135. Duran SH, Ravis WR, Pedersoli WM, et al: Pharmacokinetics of phenobarbital in the horse, Am J Vet Res 48:807–810, 1987.
136. Ravis WR, Duran SH, Pedersoli WM, et al: A pharmacokinetic study of phenobarbital in mature horses after oral dosing, J Vet Pharmacol Ther 10:283–289, 1987.
137. Fukunaga K, Saito M, Muto M, et al: Effects of urine pH modification on pharmacokinetics of phenobarbital in healthy dogs, J Vet Pharmacol Ther 31:431–436, 2008.
138. Levitski RE, Trepanier LA: Effect of timing of blood collection on serum phenobarbital concentrations in dogs with epilepsy, J Am Vet Med Assoc 217:200–204, 2000.
139. Boothe DM, Simpson G, Foster T: Effects of serum separation tubes on serum benzodiazepine and phenobarbital concentrations in clinically normal and epileptic dogs, Am J Vet Res 57:1299–1303, 1996.
140. Kluger EK, Malik R, Ilkin WJ, et al: Serum triglyceride concentration in dogs with epilepsy treated with phenobarbital or with phenobarbital and bromide, J Am Vet Med Assoc 233:1270–1277, 2008.

141. Gieger TL, Hosgood G, Taboada J, et al: Thyroid function and serum hepatic enzyme activity in dogs after phenobarbital administration, J Vet Intern Med 14:277–281, 2000.
142. Muller PB, Taboada J, Hosgood G, et al: Effects of long-term phenobarbital treatment on the liver in dogs, J Vet Intern Med 14:165–171, 2000.
143. Jacobs G, Calvert C, Kaufman A: Neutropenia and thrombocytopenia in three dogs treated with anticonvulsants, J Am Vet Med Assoc 212:681–684, 1998.
144. Khoutorsky A, Bruchim Y: Transient leucopenia, thrombocytopenia and anaemia associated with severe acute phenobarbital intoxication in a dog, J Small Anim Pract 49:367–369, 2008.
145. Weiss DJ: Bone marrow necrosis in dogs: 34 cases (1996-2004), J Am Vet Med Assoc 227:263–267, 2005.
146. Weiss DJ, Smith SA: A retrospective study of 19 cases of canine myelofibrosis, J Vet Intern Med 16:174–178, 2002.
147. March PA, Hillier A, Weisbrode SE, et al: Superficial necrolytic dermatitis in 11 dogs with a history of phenobarbital administration (1995-2002), J Vet Intern Med 18:65–74, 2004.
148. Ducote JM, Coates JR, Dewey CW, et al: Suspected hypersensitivity to phenobarbital in a cat, J Feline Med Surg 1:123–126, 1999.
149. Kube SA, Vernau KM, LeCouteur RA: Dyskinesia associated with oral phenobarbital administration in a dog, J Vet Intern Med 20:1238–1240, 2006.
150. Daminet S, Paradis M, Refsal KR, et al: Short-term influence of prednisone and phenobarbital on thyroid function in euthyroid dogs, Can Vet J 40:411–415, 1999.
151. Gaskill CL, Burton SA, Gelens HC, et al: Effects of phenobarbital treatment on serum thyroxine and thyroid-stimulating hormone concentrations in epileptic dogs, J Am Vet Med Assoc 215:489–496, 1999.
152. Gaskill CL, Burton SA, Gelens HC, et al: Changes in serum thyroxine and thyroid-stimulating hormone concentrations in epileptic dogs receiving phenobarbital for one year, J Vet Pharmacol Ther 23:243–249, 2000.
153. Kantrowitz LB, Peterson ME, Trepanier LA, et al: Serum total thyroxine, total triiodothyronine, free thyroxine, and thyrotropin concentrations in epileptic dogs treated with anticonvulsants, J Am Vet Med Assoc 214:1804–1808, 1999.
154. Muller PB, Wolfsheimer KJ, Taboada J, et al: Effects of long-term phenobarbital treatment on the thyroid and adrenal axis and adrenal function tests in dogs, J Vet Intern Med 14:157–164, 2000.
155. Daminet S, Ferguson DC: Influence of drugs on thyroid function in dogs, J Vet Intern Med 17:463–472, 2003.
156. von Klopmann T, Boettcher IC, Rotermund A, et al: Euthyroid sick syndrome in dogs with idiopathic epilepsy before treatment with anticonvulsant drugs, J Vet Intern Med 20:516–522, 2006.
157. Trepanier LA: Use of bromide as an anticonvulsant for dogs with epilepsy, J Am Vet Med Assoc 207:163–166, 1995.
158. Schwartz-Porsche D, Jürgens U: Efficacy of potassium bromide against canine epilepsy unresponsive to other treatments, Tierärztl Prax 19:395–401, 1991.
159. Trepanier LA, Van Schoick A, Schwark WS, et al: Therapeutic serum drug concentrations in epileptic dogs treated with potassium bromide alone or in combination with other anticonvulsants: 122 cases (1992-1996), J Am Vet Med Assoc 213:1449–1453, 1998.
160. Ducoté JM: Potassium bromide, Compend Contin Educ Pract Vet 21:638–639, 1999.
161. Trepanier LA, Babish JG: Effect of dietary chloride content on the elimination of bromide by dogs, Res Vet Sci 58:252–255, 1995.
162. March PA, Podell M, Sams RA: Pharmacokinetics and toxicity of bromide following high-dose oral potassium bromide administration in healthy beagles, J Vet Pharmacol Ther 25:425–432, 2002.
163. Czerwinski AL: Bromide excretion as affected by chloride administration, J Am Pharm Assoc Am Pharm Assoc (Baltim) 47:467–471, 1958.
164. Shaw N, Trepanier LA, Center SA, et al: High dietary chloride content associated with loss of therapeutic serum bromide concentrations in an epileptic dog, J Am Vet Med Assoc 208:234–236, 1996.
165. Nichols ES, Trepanier LA, Linn K: Bromide toxicosis secondary to renal insufficiency in an epileptic dog, J Am Vet Med Assoc 208:231–233, 1996.
166. Boothe DM: Anticonvulsant therapy in small animals, Vet Clin North Am Small Anim Pract 28:411–448, 1998.
167. Rossmeisl JH, Inzana KD: Clinical signs, risk factors, and outcomes associated with bromide toxicosis (bromism) in dogs with idiopathic epilepsy, J Am Vet Med Assoc 234:1425–1431, 2009.
168. Podell M, Fenner WR: Use of bromide as an antiepileptic drug in dogs, Compend Contin Educ Pract Vet 16:767–774, 1994.
169. Steiner JM, Xenoulis PG, Anderson JA, et al: Serum pancreatic lipase immunoreactivity concentrations in dogs treated with potassium bromide and/or phenobarbital, Vet Ther 9:37–44, 2008.
170. Gaskill CL, Cribb AE: Pancreatitis associated with potassium bromide/phenobarbital combination therapy in epileptic dogs, Can Vet J 41:555–558, 2000.
171. Hess RS, Kass PH, Shofer FS, et al: Evaluation of risk factors for fatal acute pancreatitis in dogs, J Am Vet Med Assoc 214:46–51, 1999.
172. Rossmeisl JH Jr, Zimmerman K, Inzana KD, et al: Assessment of the use of plasma and serum chloride concentrations as indirect predictors of serum bromide concentrations in dogs with idiopathic epilepsy, Vet Clin Pathol 35:426–433, 2006.
173. Boothe DM, George KL, Couch P: Disposition and clinical use of bromide in cats, J Am Vet Med Assoc 221:1131–1135, 2002.
174. Bailey KS, Dewey CW, Boothe DM, et al: Levetiracetam as an adjunct to phenobarbital treatment in cats with suspected idiopathic epilepsy, J Am Vet Med Assoc 232:867–872, 2008.
175. Volk HA, Matiasek LA, Lujan Feliu-Pascual A, et al: The efficacy and tolerability of levetiracetam in pharmacoresistant epileptic dogs, Vet J 176:310–319, 2008.
176. Patterson EE, Goel V, Cloyd JC, et al: Intramuscular, intravenous and oral levetiracetam in dogs: safety and pharmacokinetics, J Vet Pharmacol Ther 31:253–258, 2008.
177. Lynch BA, Lambeng N, Nocka K, et al: The synaptic vesicle protein SV2A is the binding site for the antiepileptic drug levetiracetam, Proc Natl Acad Sci U S A 101:9861–9866, 2004.
178. Benedetti MS, Coupez R, Whomsley R, et al: Comparative pharmacokinetics and metabolism of levetiracetam, a new anti-epileptic agent, in mouse, rat, rabbit and dog, Xenobiotica 34:281–300, 2004.
179. Dewey CW, Bailey KS, Boothe DM, et al: Pharmacokinetics of single-dose intravenous levetiracetam administration in normal dogs, J Vet Emerg Crit Care 18:153–157, 2008.
180. Dewey CW, Guiliano R, Boothe DM, et al: Zonisamide therapy for refractory idiopathic epilepsy in dogs, J Am Anim Hosp Assoc 40:285–291, 2004.

181. Biton VMD: Clinical pharmacology and mechanism of action of zonisamide, Clin Neuropharmacol 30:230–240, 2007.
182. Boothe DM, Perkins J: Disposition and safety of zonisamide after intravenous and oral single dose and oral multiple dosing in normal hound dogs, J Vet Pharmacol Ther 31:544–553, 2008.
183. Orito K, Saito M, Fukunaga K, et al: Pharmacokinetics of zonisamide and drug interaction with phenobarbital in dogs, J Vet Pharmacol Ther 31:259–264, 2008.
184. Walker RM, DiFonzo CJ, Barsoum NJ, et al: Chronic toxicity of the anticonvulsant zonisamide in beagle dogs, Fundam Appl Toxicol 11:333–342, 1988.
185. Czapinski P, Blaszczyk B, Czuczwar S: Mechanisms of action of antiepileptic drugs, Curr Top Med Chem 5:3–14, 2005.
186. Klugbauer N, Marais E, Hofmann F: Calcium channel alpha2delta subunits: differential expression, function, and drug binding, J Bioenerg Biomembr 35:639–647, 2003.
187. Eroglu C, Allen NJ, Susman MW, et al: Gabapentin receptor alpha2delta-1 is a neuronal thrombospondin receptor responsible for excitatory CNS synaptogenesis, Cell 139:380–392, 2009.
188. Vollmer KO, von Hodenberg A, Kolle EU: Pharmacokinetics and metabolism of gabapentin in rat, dog and man, Arzneimittelforschung 36:830–839, 1986.
189. Radulovic LL, Turck D, von Hodenberg A, et al: Disposition of gabapentin (neurontin) in mice, rats, dogs, and monkeys, Drug Metab Dispos 23:441–448, 1995.
190. Platt SR, Adams V, Garosi LS, et al: Treatment with gabapentin of 11 dogs with refractory idiopathic epilepsy, Vet Rec 159:881–884, 2006.
191. Govendir M, Perkins M, Malik R: Improving seizure control in dogs with refractory epilepsy using gabapentin as an adjunctive agent, Aust Vet J 83:602–608, 2005.
192. Salazar V, Dewey CW, Schwark W, et al: Pharmacokinetics of single-dose oral pregabalin administration in normal dogs, Vet Anaesth Analg 36:574–580, 2009.
193. Dewey CW, Cerda-Gonzalez S, Levine JM, et al: Pregabalin as an adjunct to phenobarbital, potassium bromide, or a combination of phenobarbital and potassium bromide for treatment of dogs with suspected idiopathic epilepsy, J Am Vet Med Assoc 235:1442–1449, 2009.
194. Adusumalli VE, Yang JT, Wong KK, et al: Felbamate pharmacokinetics in the rat, rabbit, and dog, Drug Metab Dispos 19:1116–1125, 1991.
195. Yang JT, Adusumalli VE, Wong KK, et al: Felbamate metabolism in the rat, rabbit, and dog, Drug Metab Dispos 19:1126–1134, 1991.
196. Ruehlmann D, Podell M, March P: Treatment of partial seizures and seizure-like activity with felbamate in six dogs, J Small Anim Pract 42:403–408, 2001.
197. Frey HH, Philippin HP, Scheuler W: Development of tolerance to the anticonvulsant effect of diazepam in dogs, Eur J Pharmacol 104:27–38, 1984.
198. Scherkl R, Kurudi D, Frey HH: Clorazepate in dogs: tolerance to the anticonvulsant effect and signs of physical dependence, Epilepsy Res 3:144–150, 1989.
199. Scherkl R, Scheuler W, Frey HH: Anticonvulsant effect of clonazepam in the dog: development of tolerance and physical dependence, Arch Int Pharmacodyn Ther 278:249–260, 1985.
200. Scherkl R, Kurudi D, Frey HH: Tolerance to the anticonvulsant effect of clorazepate and clonazepam in mice, Pharmacol Toxicol 62:38–41, 1988.
201. Center SA, Elston TH, Rowland PH, et al: Fulminant hepatic failure associated with oral administration of diazepam in 11 cats, J Am Vet Med Assoc 209:618–625, 1996.
202. Dewey CW, Barone E, Smith K, et al: Alternative anticonvulsant drugs for dogs with seizure disorders, Vet Med 99:786–793, 2004.
203. Munana KR, Vitek SM, Tarver WB, et al: Use of vagal nerve stimulation as a treatment for refractory epilepsy in dogs, J Am Vet Med Assoc 221:977–983, 2002.
204. Bateman SW, Parent JM: Clinical findings, treatment, and outcome of dogs with status epilepticus or cluster seizures: 156 cases (1990-1995), J Am Vet Med Assoc 215:1463–1468, 1999.
205. Zimmermann R, Hulsmeyer VI, Sauter-Louis C, et al: Status epilepticus and epileptic seizures in dogs, J Vet Intern Med 23:970–976, 2009.
206. Lowenstein DH, Alldredge BK: Status epilepticus, N Engl J Med 338:970–976, 1998.
207. Fountain NB, Lothman EW: Pathophysiology of status epilepticus, J Clin Neurophysiol 12:326–342, 1995.
208. Platt SR, Haag M: Canine status epilepticus: a retrospective study of 50 cases, J Small Anim Pract 43:151–153, 2002.
209. Saito M, Munana KR, Sharp NJ, et al: Risk factors for development of status epilepticus in dogs with idiopathic epilepsy and effects of status epilepticus on outcome and survival time: 32 cases (1990-1996), J Am Vet Med Assoc 219:618–623, 2001.
210. Platt SR, Randell SC, Scott KC, et al: Comparison of plasma benzodiazepine concentrations following intranasal and intravenous administration of diazepam to dogs, Am J Vet Res 61:651–654, 2000.
211. Podell M: The use of diazepam per rectum at home for the acute management of cluster seizures in dogs, J Vet Intern Med 9:68–74, 1995.
212. Platt SR, McDonnell JJ: Status epilepticus: patient management and pharmacologic therapy, Compend Contin Educ Pract Vet 22:722–729, 2000.
213. Steffen F, Grasmueck S: Propofol for treatment of refractory seizures in dogs and a cat with intracranial disorders, J Small Anim Pract 41:496–499, 2000.
214. Smedile LE, Duke T, Taylor SM: Excitatory movements in a dog following propofol anesthesia, J Am Anim Hosp Assoc 32:365–368, 1996.
215. Serrano S, Hughes D, Chandler K: Use of ketamine for the management of refractory status epilepticus in a dog, J Vet Intern Med 20:194–197, 2006.
216. Mealey KL, Boothe DM: Bioavailability of benzodiazepines following rectal administration of diazepam in dogs, J Vet Pharmacol Ther 18:72–74, 1995.
217. Papich MG, Alcorn J: Absorption of diazepam after its rectal administration in dogs, Am J Vet Res 56:1629–1636, 1995.
218. Nishino S, Mignot E: Pharmacological aspects of human and canine narcolepsy, Prog Neurobiol 52:27–78, 1997.
219. Mitler MM, Dement WC: Sleep studies on canine narcolepsy: pattern and cycle comparisons between affected and normal dogs, Electroencephalogr Clin Neurophysiol 43:691–699, 1977.
220. Taheri S, Zeitzer JM, Mignot E: The role of hypocretins (orexins) in sleep regulation and narcolepsy, Annu Rev Neurosci 25:283–313, 2002.
221. Overeem S, Mignot E, van Dijk JG, et al: Narcolepsy: clinical features, new pathophysiologic insights, and future perspectives, J Clin Neurophysiol 18:78–105, 2001.
222. Nishino S: Narcolepsy: pathophysiology and pharmacology, J Clin Psychiatry 68(suppl 13)13:9–15, 2007.

223. Lin L, Faraco J, Li R, et al: The sleep disorder canine narcolepsy is caused by a mutation in the hypocretin (orexin) receptor 2 gene, Cell 98:365–376, 1999.
224. Ripley B, Fujiki N, Okura M, et al: Hypocretin levels in sporadic and familial cases of canine narcolepsy, Neurobiol Dis 8:525–534, 2001.
225. Foutz AS, Mitler MM, Cavalli-Sforza LL, et al: Genetic factors in canine narcolepsy, Sleep 1:413–421, 1979.
226. Baker TL, Foutz AS, McNerney V, et al: Canine model of narcolepsy: genetic and developmental determinants, Exp Neurol 75:729–742, 1982.
227. Hungs M, Fan J, Lin L, et al: Identification and functional analysis of mutations in the hypocretin (orexin) genes of narcoleptic canines, Genome Res 11:531–539, 2001.
228. Wagner JL, Storb R, Storer B, et al: DLA-DQB1 alleles and bone marrow transplantation experiments in narcoleptic dogs, Tissue Antigens 56:223–231, 2000.
229. Schatzberg SJ, Cutter-Schatzberg K, Nydam D, et al: The effect of hypocretin replacement therapy in a 3-year-old Weimaraner with narcolepsy, J Vet Intern Med 18: 586–588, 2004.
230. Cantile C, Baroni M, Arispici M: A case of narcolepsy-cataplexy associated with distemper encephalitis, Zentralbl Veterinarmed A 46:301–308, 1999.
231. Knecht CD, Oliver JE, Redding R, et al: Narcolepsy in a dog and a cat, J Am Vet Med Assoc 162:1052–1053, 1973.
232. Strain GM, Olcott BM, Archer RM, et al: Narcolepsy in a Brahman bull, J Am Vet Med Assoc 185:538–541, 1984.
233. Lunn DP, Cuddon PA, Shaftoe S, et al: Familial occurrence of narcolepsy in miniature horses, Equine Vet J 25:483–487, 1993.
234. Dreifuss FE, Flynn DV: Narcolepsy in a horse, J Am Vet Med Assoc 184:131–132, 1984.
235. Bathen-Nöthen A, Heider C, Fernandez AJ, et al: Hypocretin measurement in an Icelandic foal with narcolepsy, J Vet Intern Med 23:1299–1302, 2009.
236. Tonokura M, Fujita K, Nishino S: Review of pathophysiology and clinical management of narcolepsy in dogs, Vet Rec 161:375–380, 2007.
237. Coleman ES: Canine narcolepsy and the role of the nervous system, Compend Contin Educ Pract Vet 21:641–650, 1999.
238. Katherman AE: A comparative review of canine and human narcolepsy, Compend Contin Educ Pract Vet 2:818–822, 1980.
239. Mitler MM, Soave O, Dement WC: Narcolepsy in seven dogs, J Am Vet Med Assoc 168:1036–1038, 1976.
240. Nishino S, Haak L, Shepherd H, et al: Effects of central alpha-2 adrenergic compounds on canine narcolepsy, a disorder of rapid eye movement sleep, J Pharmacol Exp Ther 253:1145–1152, 1990.

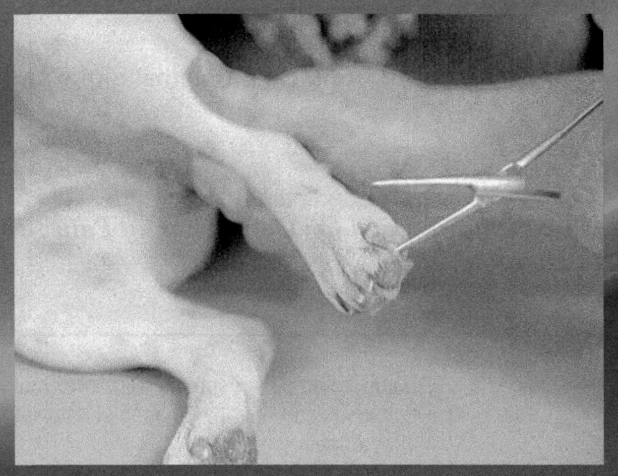

CHAPTER 14

Pain

Animals do feel pain, and yet this point has been argued for many years. For a review of the entire spectrum of animal pain, the *Colloquium on Recognition and Alleviation of Animal Pain and Distress* and the textbooks specifically addressing pain management in domestic animals are recommended.[1] This chapter reviews the pathophysiology of pain, some diseases that have pain as the primary clinical sign, and the symptomatic treatment of pain. Definitions of the terms related to the description of pain are essential to communication. Kitchell[2] has provided an excellent working definition: "Pain in animals is an aversive sensory and emotional experience (a perception), which elicits protective motor actions, results in learned avoidance, and may modify species-specific traits of behavior, including social behavior." In other words, pain is not nociception but is the conscious experience of nociception, which is only partly determined by the stimulus-induced activation of afferent neural pathways.[2,3] *Nociception* is the detection of tissue damage by specialized receptors induced by a noxious (noxious means "injurious") stimulus. It is also incorrect to refer to painful stimuli or pain receptors, pathways, or fibers. Thus we use the terms *noxious stimuli*, *nociceptors*, *nociceptive pathways*, and so on.

Formal definitions in human medicine for types of pain have been developed by the Subcommittee on Taxonomy of the International Association for the Study of Pain (Table 14-1).[4] In brief, *hyperesthesia (hyperalgesia)* denotes an increased sensitivity of nociceptive fibers to normal stimulation. It has often been used to designate an unpleasant response to a nonnoxious stimulus.[2] We use the term more generically than others because of the difficulty in truly knowing whether the animal perceives pain. Throughout this book, we use the term hyperesthesia to mean a behavioral reaction of the animal indicating that the stimulus was unpleasant despite the fact that we consider the stimulus to be nonnoxious. The most common usage is in describing an animal's response to palpation that does not evoke a reaction in a normal animal but causes an aversive reaction in an affected animal.

Hyperpathia denotes an unpleasant painful response to a noxious stimulus, especially if repeated, and is characterized by delay, overreaction, and aftersensation.[2] This term has been used frequently in veterinary medicine but is far more specific than just a "painful response." Knowing that an animal actually has the sensations associated with hyperpathia would be difficult if not impossible. *Allodynia* is pain resulting from a nonnoxious stimulus to normal skin. Because we are often assessing "painful" responses from structures other than skin, this term is not used often.

NEUROANATOMIC BASIS FOR PAIN (NOCICEPTION)

The nociceptive pathway includes peripheral nociceptors; nerve fibers; spinal cord and brain pathways; and central processing areas in the brainstem, thalamus, and cerebrum (Figure 14-1). Nociception consists of three distinct processes: (1) *transduction*, which is the translation of a noxious stimulus into electrical activity through sensory receptors; (2) *transmission*, which is the propagation of nerve impulses from the receptors into the central nervous system (CNS); (3) *modulation*, which involves facilitation or inhibition by neurons and interneurons of the spinal cord. The *perception* of a noxious stimulus is the result of integration of the projection pathways to the thalamus and cerebrum to produce the final conscious subjective and emotional experience of pain.[5] Specific pharmacologic therapies can modify the response.

There are specific types of sensory receptors: *mechanoreceptors* for touch and pressure; *nociceptors and thermoreceptors* for harmful stimuli (noxious, and heat or cold, respectively); *chemoreceptors* for detecting chemical changes (taste, smell, visceral (e.g., O_2, pH, osmolality); and *photoreceptors* (rods, cones) for light. These sensory receptors are associated with a specific sensory organ that detects the stimulus based on modality of stimulus (pressure, noxious, temperature, chemical, or light), location of the sensory unit, and the intensity and duration of the stimulus.

Impulses from mechanoreceptors for touch, vibration, and general proprioception are transmitted by large myelinated A-α and A-β fibers. These fibers ascend ipsilaterally in the dorsal columns of the spinal cord to the medulla to synapse in the gracilis and cuneate nuclei of the brainstem. The second order neurons then decussate and ascend in the medial lemniscus to end

TABLE 14-1

Nomenclature Used for Description of Pain in Humans

Term	Definition
Types of Pain	
Hyperalgesia	Exaggerated pain response from a normally noxious stimulus—increased sensitivity, lower pain threshold
Hyperpathia	Abnormally noxious and exaggerated reaction to all stimuli; related to hyperalgesia
Hyperesthesia	Exaggerated perception of touch stimulus
Allodynia*	Abnormal perception of pain from a normally nonnoxious mechanical or thermal stimulus (delay in perception)
Dysesthesia*	Any abnormal sensation described as unpleasant by patient
Paresthesia*	Spontaneous abnormal sensation that is not unpleasant
Causalgia*	Burning pain in distribution of one or more peripheral nerves
Types of Sensory Loss	
Hypoalgesia (Hypalgesia)	Decreased sensitivity and higher threshold to noxious stimuli
Anesthesia	Reduced perception of all sensation
Analgesia	Reduced perception of noxious stimulus

*Symptoms used to describe pain in humans but difficult to recognize as clinical signs in animals.

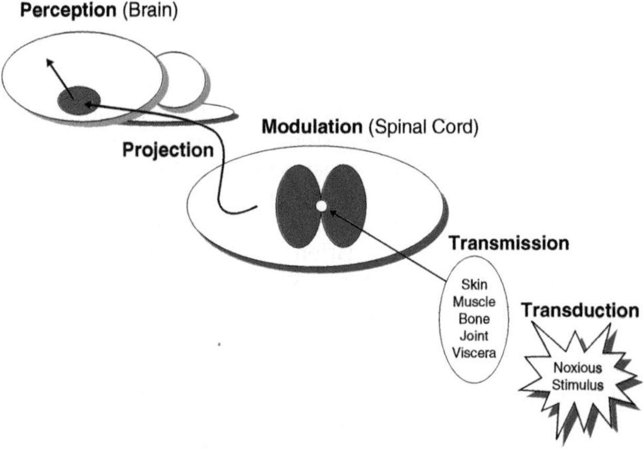

Figure 14-1 Schematic demonstrating the neural pathways for pain transduction, transmission, modulation, and perception of noxious stimuli.

in the contralateral ventral nucleus of the thalamus and from there are relayed to the somatosensory cortex at the cerebrum. Some pathways for discriminative aspects of noxious stimuli also travel in the dorsal column system. Fibers mediating touch and proprioception from the head are relayed from the main sensory and mesencephalic nuclei of the trigeminal nerve.

Nociceptive fibers are generally "free nerve endings," although the endings are never completely free of surrounding structures that terminate in the skin, subcutaneous tissue, periosteum, joints, muscles, and viscera.[3,6,7] Nociceptors and thermoreceptors may be specific to one kind of stimulus or polymodal (those responding to more than one kind of stimulus). The nociceptors of the skin have been studied in the most detail, but nociception clearly occurs from many other somatic and visceral structures. Nociceptors are usually silent unless stimulated and require more intense stimuli than do other types of receptors (e.g., those with high threshold for stimulation). Response to stimuli is proportional to the intensity of the stimulus. Impulses from nociceptors are transmitted into the CNS by A-δ fibers and C fibers. The A-δ fibers are thinly myelinated and faster conducting (12 to 30 m/sec) that transmit impulses from mechanoreceptors, nociceptors, and cold receptors that mediate the response to noxious stimuli. The A-δ fibers provide more discriminative information to the CNS. The A-δ nerve terminals can be nociceptive or nonnociceptive and are composed mainly of low-threshold mechanoreceptors. The C fibers are unmyelinated and slower conducting (0.5 to 2 m/sec) fibers that mainly transmit impulses associated with noxious stimuli and temperature. Most C fiber nociceptors are high threshold and polymodal.

Transmission of nociception also is classified as *fast* and *slow* pain.[6,7] Fast pain is associated with A-δ nociceptive fibers and slow pain is transmitted by the C nociceptive fibers. The initial noxious stimulus often causes a sharp, pricking, and localized sensation (fast pain or first pain), which is followed by a dull, intense, diffuse, burning, and unpleasant sensation (slow pain or second pain).

At the tissue level, chemical mediators act to further modulate the nociceptors. Tissue injury causes the release of bradykinin and prostaglandins that sensitize or activate nociceptors, which in turn releases substance P and calcitonin gene-related peptide. Substance P causes degranulation of mast cells and histamine release, which further activates nociceptors. Substance P and calcitonin gene-related peptide also cause extravasation of plasma and dilation of blood vessels resulting in edema.

In the CNS of domestic animals, the nociceptive pathways are multisynaptic, bilateral, and resistant to injurious processes.[3] These nociceptive fibers generally enter the spinal cord through the spinal ganglia (without synapsing) and dorsal root and synapse in the dorsal horn of the gray matter within specific laminae (Rexed laminae). This convergence of nociceptive pathways in the spinal cord may be one of the mechanisms of referred pain.[3] Importantly, the nociceptive input is "gated" by a wide variety of substances and transmitters that can increase or decrease the frequency of firing in neurons that relay the nociceptive signal. The synaptic transmitter secreted by afferent fibers of fast pain is glutamate via the N-methyl D-aspartate (NMDA) receptors and the transmitter of slow pain is substance P. The gray matter contains projection neurons, propriospinal (segmental transmission) neurons, and interneurons. Interneurons modulate and transmit information a short distance within the spinal cord. An example is interneurons for protective reflexes such as the flexor reflex in which stimulation of a single digit innervated by a few sensory fibers contained in a single spinal cord segment results in the activation of motor neurons contributing to the sciatic nerve, which are located over several spinal cord segments.

Projection neurons relay sensory information to the brain. Most axons from these neurons immediately decussate and ascend in the spinal cord, mainly in the lateral spinothalamic and spinoreticular tracts and some in the spinocervicothalamic and spinomesencephalic tracts. Some axons remain ipsilateral during their ascent. The relative significance and location of these tracts differ between species. For example, a major part of the spinothalamic tract is in the dorsal portion of the lateral funiculus in cats, compared with the ventral portion of the lateral funiculus in primates and pigs.[3] The spinoreticular and spinomesencephalic tracts probably have less discriminative capacity than the spinothalamic tracts. These spinal tracts synapse on the caudal lateral ventral nucleus of the thalamus and ultimately project to the somesthetic areas of the cerebrum. Although the majority of perceptive function for nociception lies within the cerebrum, some perception may occur within the thalamus.[8]

The majority of nociception from the head is carried in nerve branches of the trigeminal (V) nerve. The majority of these fibers synapse in the caudal aspect of the nucleus of the trigeminal nerve and then route through the trigeminal and medial lemnisci and quintothalamic tract to the ventral caudal medial nucleus of the thalamus and cerebrum.

Afferent A-δ and C fibers from visceral structures reach the CNS via the sympathetic (splanchnic) and parasympathetic nerves.[3,9] Specifically, sympathetic nerves convey visceral afferents through the thoracic and lumbar dorsal roots and parasympathetic nerves convey visceral afferents through the facial (VII), glossopharyngeal (IX), and vagus (X) nerves; the T3 to lumbar (L4-5) dorsal roots; and the sacral nerve roots. Vagal and splanchnic afferent fibers terminate in the nucleus tractus solitarius, where integration of sensory information is projected to the thalamus.

MECHANISMS OF PAIN

Stimulation of nociceptors causes two kinds of reactions. *Superficial sensation* assessed by stimulation of superficial nociceptors, such as those in the skin, is discriminative, allowing precise localization of the stimulus. Commonly referred to as *pain perception*, (deep pain perception) assessed by stimulation of nociceptors in muscle, joints, and bone is motivational, causing the animal to show a change in behavior (Figure 14-2). There are fewer A-δ fibers in the deeper structures so there is little fast or sharp pain. Superficial sensation may be difficult to assess because some animals may not respond, whereas others respond strongly. This variability is often observed in normal animals, which makes interpretation in affected animals difficult. For example, normal small and toy breed dogs such as the Chihuahua often display a vigorous response to even light touch of the skin, whereas some large breed dogs such as an older Labrador retriever or those with a docile personality such as a basset hound may not respond even to firm pinching of the skin. However, animals reliably respond to strong noxious stimulation of the periosteum such as applying pressure with a forceps across a digit.

In general, pain is clinically evaluated as acute or *physiologic* (nociceptive) pain and chronic or *pathologic*. Clinical pain also can be further classified as *inflammatory* pain or *neuropathic* pain, depending on the underlying disease and anatomic structures involved.[5] Acute pain has a sudden onset and dissipates during healing. The animal may feel a pinch, poke, or sharp pain. Acute pain is very localized and transient, and serves as a protective mechanism (e.g., perception of stimulus during the flexor withdrawal reflex). Chronic pain is described as intense and unrelenting, resulting in extended discomfort. Chronic pain is characteristic of musculoskeletal and neurologic disorders and has no beneficial role. This type of pain may persist long after recovery from the inciting injury and is often refractory to common analgesic agents (e.g., opiates, nonsteroidal antiinflammatory drugs [NSAIDs]). Neuropathic pain occurs with injury to neural tissue and represents abnormalities in transmission and somatosensory processing in the peripheral or CNS. Some disease processes encompass both nociceptive/inflammatory and neuropathic pain mechanisms. Surgical procedures and many inflammatory and ischemic disease processes create pathologic pain through one or both of these mechanisms. Neoplasms can infiltrate, and/or compress neural tissue and tissue innervated with nociceptors or cause unlocalizable pain through paraneoplastic effects.[10] Pain associated with chemotherapy and radiation may result from induced axonal injury and vascular compromise.

Inflammatory (Physiologic, Acute, or Nociceptive) Pain

Inflammatory pain is associated with tissue damage either of visceral or somatic origin.[2] Acute pain caused by tissue inflammation results in abnormal (overreactive, hyperalgesia) responses to noxious stimuli (lowered threshold to noxious stimuli). This type of pain depends on activation of high threshold receptors (nociceptors). Pain relates to ongoing

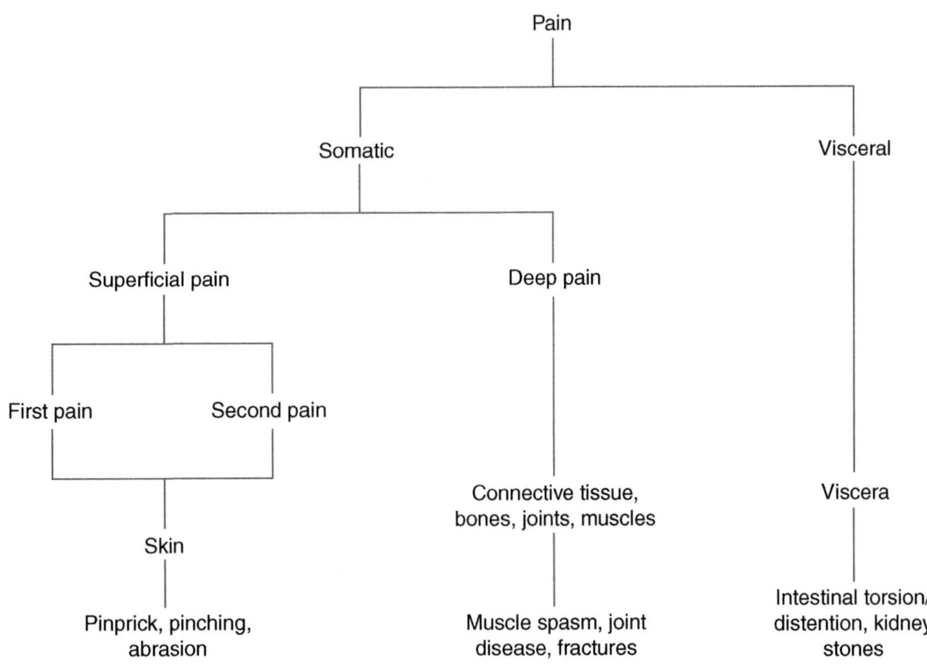

Figure 14-2 Quantities and origin of pain.

activation of primary afferents of somatic and visceral end organs. Pain arises from increased tissue swelling and tension due to fluid accumulation and presence of inflammatory mediators. Inflammation causes release of different cytokines, histamine, prostaglandins, bradykinins, nitric oxide neuropeptides, and neurotrophic factors into the inflamed area. These inflammatory mediators initiate transmission of nociception from cutaneous areas and within the dorsal horn. The vertebral column and nerve roots (radicular pain) are common sites affected by mechanical and inflammatory disorders. Nociceptors are located in the dura mater, nerve roots, outer annular fibers of the disk, periosteum and cancellous layers of bone, facet aspect of joints, joint capsule, and paraspinal ligaments, muscles, and aponeuroses. Examples of somatic pain include surgical procedures, trauma, ischemia, osteoarthritis, cancer, and abscessation. Visceral pain is associated with torsion, distention, obstruction, and ischemia of visceral structures.

Neuropathic Pain

Neuropathic pain results from disease and dysfunction of the peripheral and/or central nervous systems and represents abnormalities in transmission of nociceptive information that developed as the result of the injury.[11,12] This pathologic type of pain is described as a perception that is greater than the apparent noxious stimulus. In human medicine, notable descriptions for neuropathic pain include evidence of a sensory deficit, burning pain, pain to light stroking of the skin, and attacks of pain without provocation. Neuropathic pain occurs spontaneously and pain that is stimulus independent or stimulus-evoked.[11] In neuropathic pain, stimuli that are normally not painful are experienced as painful (allodynia) or that are normally painful but experienced as more painful than usual (hyperalgesia). Any nonnoxious sensory stimuli, enough to result in a painful response or otherwise may be perceived in a more exaggerated manner (hyperesthesia). Although unrecognized in animals, the term *causalgia* is used for severe persistent pain (burning) that results from nerve trauma. Neuropathic pain can be generated at the site of injury or referred. Common causes of neuropathic pain include nerve transection and compression of neural tissue. Nerve roots are more susceptible to compression because of lack of appreciable epineurium and perineurium, and an intact blood-nerve barrier. Nerve roots also are bathed in cerebrospinal fluid; thereby, they are exposed to inflammatory processes in the meninges.

Mechanisms of neuropathic pain evolve from a dynamic reorganization of neural circuitry following injury. Peripheral and central sensitization lower the threshold for nociception.[5] Sensitization can occur in the CNS and at peripheral sites. *Peripheral sensitization* (sensory organ) involves upregulation of sodium ion channels in primary afferents and abnormal responses to endogenous cytokines, prostaglandins, bradykinins, and neurotransmitters. This causes an overall direct excitatory effect on the nociceptive system. Inflammation or trauma may induce peripheral sensitization upon exposure of nerve terminals with reduced pain threshold to sensitizing agents.

Central sensitization occurs with increased neuronal excitation in the spinal cord arising from ongoing spontaneous activity of peripheral nociceptors and increased activity and responses in ascending nociceptive pathways. Central sensitization occurs within dorsal horn neurons secondary to several mechanisms that involve inflammatory mediators, altered gene expression, receptors, and neurotransmitters. This process, termed *wind-up*, leads to a hyperactivity in the CNS and has been proposed as an explanation of the persistent and unrelenting nature of chronic pain. The temporal and spatial summation effects of neuroexcitatory input from noxious stimuli produce a prolonged sensitization. Central sensitization enables low-intensity stimuli and low-threshold sensory fibers to thereby induce pain as a result of these changes in sensory processing within the spinal cord.[5] Central sensitization or wind-up contributes to postinjury hypersensitivity and is considered the main mechanism underlying hyperalgesia and allodynia. The perception of pain is more intense and more difficult to manage once wind-up has taken place. Moreover, a persistent nociceptive or inflammatory pain state through peripheral and central sensitization can develop into a neuropathic pain state. Since it is easier to prevent sensitization, preemptive analgesia should be used before the pain starts.

In addition, a nerve injury can contribute to acute and chronic states of neuropathic pain through disinhibition.[5] The onset of pain of nerve origin is delayed. Inhibitory interneurons within the dorsal horns modulate the transmission of nociception within the spinal cord and projection pathways to and within the brain. Gamma-aminobutyric acid (GABA) and GABA receptors modulate the inhibition. Blockage of this GABA-mediated inhibition facilitates pain transmission. In nerve injuries, opioid antagonists such as cholecystokinin are expressed that decrease the analgesic effects of endogenous and exogenous opioids.

Central Pain

Central pain is poorly understood and described as pain initiated or caused by a primary lesion or dysfunction in the CNS.[11] Central pain was originally observed with lesions of the thalamus (thalamic pain) but also can occur in lesions affecting the laminae of the dorsal horn. This phenomenon is thought to occur in animals with syringohydromyelia (see Chapter 7).[13] Humans characterize central pain as burning, aching, pricking, or radiating that is paroxysmal, varies in intensity, and is poorly localized.

Referred and Radicular Pain

Neural mechanisms underlying *referred pain* are complex. Pain can be referred from a nociceptive focus in muscle, nerve, or viscera. Radicular pain is localized to the distribution of one or more nerve roots and is often exacerbated by Valsalva maneuvers, such as coughing and sneezing, that increase intraspinal pressure or positions that stretch the affected nerve roots (see Figure 5-1). Nerve root lesions also can cause *paresthesias* and numbness localized to dermatomal distributions (see Chapter 5). Examples of paresthesias include polyradiculoneuritis and the acral mutilation seen in some sensory neuropathies (see Chapter 7). When pain is referred, it is usually to a structure that develops from the same embryonic segment or dermatome as the structure from which the pain originates. Visceral and deep somatic pain can be referred but not superficial pain. Somatic and visceral pain fibers converge on the same second-order neurons in the laminae of the dorsal horn and then project to the thalamus and cerebrum. The *convergence-projection theory* of referred pain coupled with plasticity in the CNS proposes that noxious stimuli transmitted by one group of nociceptors can increase activity in CNS neurons that receive input from another group of nociceptors, thus the brain cannot distinguish whether the origin of the stimulus came from the viscera or area of nociceptive focus.[14]

CLINICAL EXAMINATION

The methods for evaluating an animal's ability to perceive noxious stimuli are discussed in Chapter 1. Recognition of the signs of pain in animals is important for diagnosis, and for appropriate and humane care. The perception of noxious stimuli is similar in most mammalian species. However, the behavioral response to noxious stimuli depends on the species,

TABLE 14-2

Clinical Signs of Pain in Domestic Animals

Species	Clinical Signs of Pain
Canine	*Acute pain*: facial expressions (unchanged, wincing, anxious); may distance themselves; avoidance reaction or aggression; vocalization in acute pain; attempt to escape. *Chronic pain*: depression, withdrawn, reluctance to move. *Abdominal pain*: praying position, sterna recumbency, tense in abdomen, reluctance to move. *Spinal pain*: periods of recumbency, short stride, kyphosis, stiffness, reluctance to move neck or trunk. *Physiologic signs*: tachypnea, panting, tachycardia, dilated pupils, hypertension
Feline	*Acute pain*: anxious facial expression, flinching, growling, cowering, aggression, attempt to escape, hunched position. *Chronic pain*: lack of activity, inappetence, dullness, avoidance. *Abdominal pain*: sternal recumbency, hunched, tense in abdomen. *Spinal pain*: reluctance to move, stiffness, kyphosis, short stride. *Physiologic signs*: tachypnea, tachycardia, dilated pupils, hypertension
Equine	*Acute pain*: escape or attack reaction, kick or bite at source of pain, restless, distressed, agitation. *Chronic pain*: dullness, stand with head down, tucked up appearance, inappetence, avoidance behavior with other horses. *Abdominal pain*: restlessness, kicking at belly, glancing at flank, rolling, lying down and getting up. *Limb pain*: lameness, shifting of weight, lifting of leg, displacement of weight, reluctance to move. *Physiologic signs*: tachypnea, tachycardia, sweating
Bovine	*Acute*: inappetence, dullness, grunting, bellowing, teeth grinding, cessation of cudding. *Chronic*: reluctance to move, reduced grooming, separation from herd. *Abdominal pain*: flank kicking, repeat lying down and getting up
Ovine	Teeth grinding, head pressing, subtle changes in behavior
Caprine	Stop grooming, resent handling, vocalization (bleating, crying), cessation of cudding, inappetence, flank watching, kicking
Swine	Inappetence, vocalization (grunting, short high pitch), move more slowly, more tolerant to handling, shivering, piloerection

breed, age, disease, injury process, and duration.[7] Many animals give little outward indication that they are in pain, although we recognize that the physical abnormality must be painful. For example, a dog with a fractured limb often shows little outward sign of pain and suffering, but we know it must be experiencing considerable pain and suffering. Animals with severe pain show one or more of the following signs as described in Table 14-2.

When obtaining the history, the clinician should assess time of onset, temporal progression, associated behaviors and factors that relieve or provoke the pain. Determining the mode of onset for whether the pain is acute (hours to days) or chronic (weeks to months) will assist with differentials and treatment approaches. Temporally pain can be static, progressive, intermittent, and recurrent. The owners can best provide information on behavior alterations and factors that provoke pain. Loss of house training in dogs and cats may occur as pain increases.

Localization of pain is accomplished by a combination of observation, palpation, and manipulation. Localization determines whether the pain is focal, multifocal, diffuse, or referred. Diffuse or multifocal pain is usually caused by meningitis, polymyositis, polyarthritis, diffuse skeletal disease, or more rarely cancer (typically metastatic). Neurologic and orthopedic examinations of an animal with spinal or musculoskeletal hyperesthesia determine lesion localization and extent. It is important to complete the nonpainful components of these examinations before performing palpation or manipulation of an area that is painful or suspected to be painful. Both superficial sensation and pain perception (or deep pain) are used clinically to localize lesions. Testing for pain perception is the most important for assessment of prognosis in severe neural lesions.

Observation

One must recognize nonspecific behavioral indicators that are present in animals that are painful.[6,7] When possible, observation should be done from a distance. Painful animals are less likely to interact with humans and explore their environment. Some animals may become anxious, restless, and vocalize. Animals may outwardly respond with aggression or show timidness and fear. Dogs may show avoidance behavior but show aggression during attempts to handle or restrain. Cats are more likely to hide or become aggressive. Dullness or lack of interaction can be associated with acute or chronic pain in dogs and cats. In general, dogs and cats with spinal pain often show reluctance to move or change position. Reluctance to lying down is observed in dogs with acute abdominal or spinal pain. Horses often respond violently to acute pain by galloping, kicking, or biting. In cases of severe pain, the horse will be restless, tachypneic, agitated, and sweat copiously. Especially in colic, the horse will glance at the flank with frequent lying down, rolling, and getting up. With chronic and persistent pain, the horse will appear dull, stand tucked, or stand away from other horses or in the corner of a stall. In ruminants, signs of pain are often subtle. Animals may bellow or bleat, become separated from the herd, grind teeth excessively, and become dull. Ruminants with abdominal pain will have cessation of cudding, inappetence, flank watching and kicking, tachycardia, and tachypnea. Pigs in pain become more tolerant to handling. Pigs also may become inappetent, not drink, shiver, and have piloerection.

During examination the animal may manifest specific postures that may relieve pain. Posture of an animal in pain from spinal disease is typically guarded, which is reflected by muscle stiffness and spasms. Animals with thoracolumbar pain often have a kyphotic posture (see Figure 6-4). An animal with neck pain may manifest horizontal neck carriage, keep the neck in a fixed position, and show reluctance to move (see Figure 7-2). Muscle palpation can reveal increased tone and intermittent spasms/jerks. The gait of an animal in pain may be stilted or stiff and have a shortened stride length. Animals with joint, muscle, or meningeal pain often appear to be "walking on eggshells" and will shift weight to the thoracic limbs. Thoracic or pelvic limb lameness also may manifest as radicular pain (nerve root signature). Animals with low lumbar pain often have the pelvic limbs tucked under the caudal abdomen to flex the spine and lessen nerve root compression (see Figure 14-3). Other signs of myelopathy such as general proprioceptive ataxia and UMN paresis/plegia may be present concurrently with spinal hyperesthesia. Meningitis alone results in slight or no evidence of postural reaction or motor deficits. Animals with muscle and joint pain often have no neurologic deficits but physical discomfort may be associated with decreased flexor withdrawal reflexes and postural reaction deficits. In these instances, pain may be elicited with manipulation of the limbs.

Palpation

Evaluating for presence hyperesthesia is the final part of the neurologic and orthopedic examinations and useful for localization. Joint and muscle pain are assessed during palpation and evaluating range of motion. The joints of the limbs are flexed and extended to elicit a painful response. Palpation of individual muscles without pressure on bones or joints identifies muscular pain. The quadriceps, semitendinosus, semimembranosus, and gastrocnemius muscles in the pelvic limb and triceps and carpal flexor muscles in the thoracic limb are good examples of muscle groups that can be evaluated without applying pressure to the bones or joints. Palpation of the head, muscles of mastication, mandible, and opening the mouth are important in assessing cranial structures.

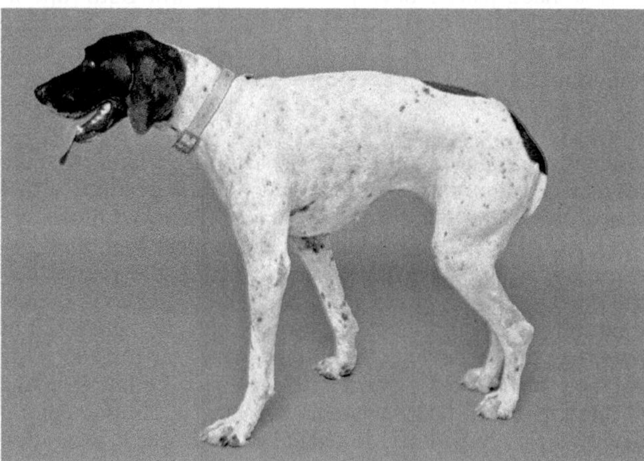

Figure 14-3 A dog with pain in the caudal lumbar vertebral column and degenerative lumbosacral stenosis. Note the slightly flexed position of the pelvis.

Paraspinal hyperesthesia is evaluated by deep palpation of the paraspinal musculature. During the palpation process, it is best for the clinician to start distally and move toward the site of the suspected lesion. Generally, spinal cord disease causes sensory deficits caudal to the lesion, hyperesthesia at the lesion site, and normal sensory function cranial to the lesion. Palpating from caudal to cranial maximizes the ability of the examiner to recognize the abnormal area. If an abnormality is identified, the palpation can be done in the reverse direction to help pinpoint the location. In large animal species, the examiner should palpate the entire dorsum, lateral neck, and trunk, starting at the head.[15,16] Due to the presence of extensive wool, palpation in sheep and camelids is challenging for detecting abnormalities. During palpation, the examiner should evaluate for symmetry, heat, swelling, atrophy, and pain. Clinical signs of hyperesthesia include flinching of the ears, twitching of the spinal musculature, and outward behavior signs of discomfort.

Palpation of the vertebral column is performed by applying pressure with one hand on the spinous processes or squeezing the articular or transverse processes, depending on the size of the animal and examiner (Figure 14-4). Placement of the other hand beneath the abdomen of small animals while palpating detects increased tension in the muscles as painful areas are approached. Placement of the hand beneath the area of the trunk being evaluated provides additional support and prevents smaller sized animals from lying down. Direct palpation of the proximal ribs may also be helpful in recognizing thoracic vertebral hyperesthesia, such as that in discospondylitis.

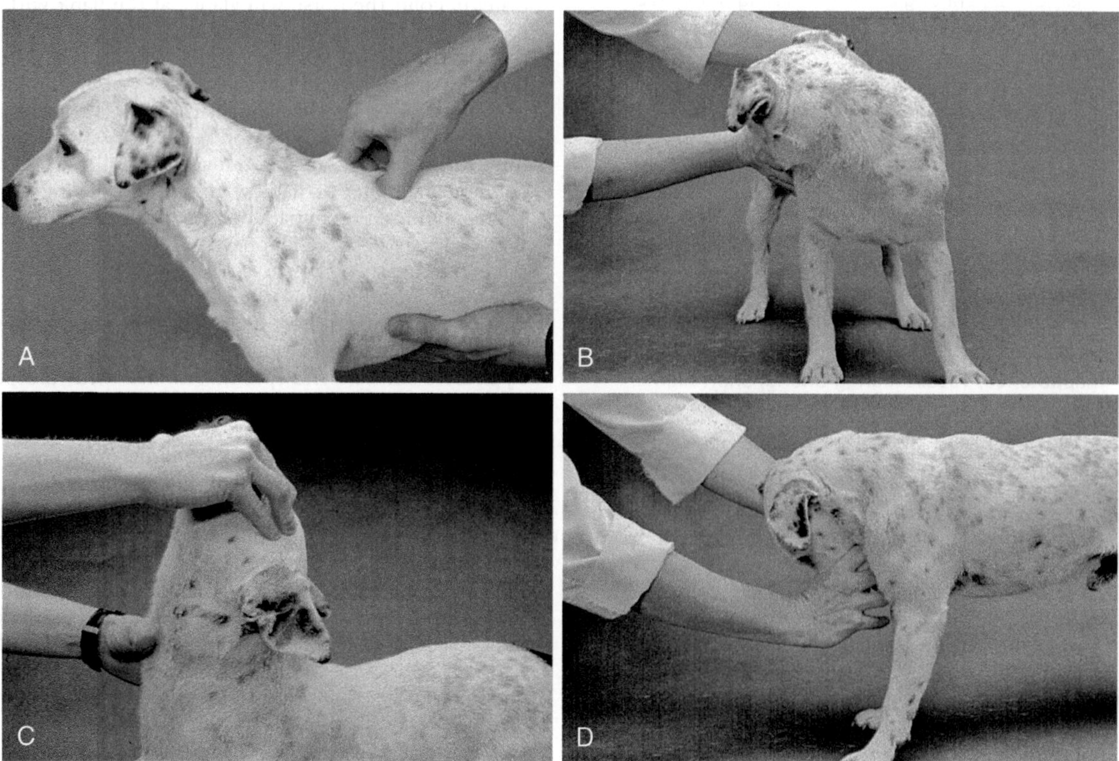

Figure 14-4 **A,** Deep palpation of the thoracic vertebral column. Manipulation of the cervical vertebral column next positioned in lateral flexion **(B)** of the neck, extended **(C)**, and flexed **(D)** positions.

The vertebral column of the cervical region is deeply located to the epaxial musculature, making it difficult to apply direction pressure to the spinous processes. When palpating the cervical vertebral column, it is best to apply pressure on the lateral aspect of the neck near the transverse processes. Diffuse paravertebral pain is a prominent finding in meningitis but may predominate in the cervical spinal region. Some animals with intracranial disease may manifest neck pain, presumably due to stretching and stimulation of nociceptors within the dura and cerebral vasculature, or to central pain mechanisms.[17]

Careful palpation can distinguish between vertebral and abdominal pain. However, some animals are so painful that localization is impossible. Sedation may allow for a more accurate examination. Visceral disorders and peritonitis cause severe abdominal pain. Vertebral or meningeal pain also causes splinting of the abdomen and a painful response when palpating the abdomen. If a painful response also occurs when palpating the vertebral column, the pain is usually not of abdominal origin.

Manipulation of the limbs and palpation of individual joints are used to identify joint pain. Careful palpation of joints that do not have superimposed muscles differentiates joint from muscle pain. The stifle, hock, elbow, and carpus are good examples.

The vertebral column can also be manipulated to elicit hyperesthesia if palpation is unsuccessful; presence of hyperesthesia may be more accurately assessed by careful flexion, extension, and lateral manipulations of the neck (see Figure 14-4). The animal may manifest a painful response and resistance to movement. Palpation of the lumbosacral joint or hyperextension of the hip accentuates canal stenosis and nerve root compression, causing a painful response. However, hip extension is not a good test for differentiating hip pain from lumbosacral pain. Extension and lateral movements of the tail also can elicit pain in an animal with disease of the caudal lumbar vertebral column. Additionally, during rectal palpation, digital presure can be applied on the ventral aspect of lumbosacral joint to elicit pain.

Assessment of the Perception of Noxious Stimuli

Superficial sensation is evaluated during cutaneous testing using a skin pinch or prick (Figure 14-5). The sensory branch of individual nerves is further assessed by mapping their dermatomal distribution (see Chapter 5). The autonomous zone is the region of skin innervated by one nerve, a specific branch of a nerve, or nerve root.[18-20] Testing of superficial sensation by stimulation of the skin of an autonomous zone helps identify dysfunction of specific nerves, nerve roots, or spinal cord segments (see Chapter 5). Superficial sensation of the limbs is perceived by the examiner as a behavioral response while performing the flexor withdrawal reflex.

If a superficial sensation is absent, and there is also an absence of voluntary motor functions, pain perception is then assessed. *Pain perception* is evaluated by placing hemostats across the digits, applying gradually increasing amounts of pressure, which stimulates nociceptors of the periosteum of the digit, and observing for a behavioral response (see Figure 14-5). Most importantly a flexor withdrawal reflex of the limbs by itself is *not* an indicator of pain perception; the animal must show a behavioral response. Stated another way, the presence or absence of pain perception is solely based on the presence or absence of a behavioral response. Loss of pain perception is considered a poor prognostic sign.

METHODS OF MEASURING PAIN

It is extremely difficult to determine the degree of pain an animal is experiencing, although it is well accepted that animals experience pain in much the same way as humans. Animal caregivers currently use scales adapted for humans. Whereas human patients have the capacity to record the intensity of their pain, in animals pain is measured by using physiologic data and subjective behavioral observation. Physiologic variables that can be studied and quantified include heart and respiratory rates; rectal temperature; packed cell volume; and serum concentrations of glucose, cortisol, norepinephrine, and epinephrine. The stress associated with pain may cause increases in heart and respiratory rates and systolic blood pressure. In cats recovering from ovariohysterectomy, increased cortisol concentrations and increased systolic blood pressure were the best indicators of postoperative pain.[21,22]

The three scales used in animals and humans are the simple descriptive scale (SDS), numeric rating scale (NRS), and visual analog scale (VAS). The SDS allows the observer to rate subjectively the degree of pain from no pain to very severe pain. The NRS is similar to the SDS, except numeric values are assigned to behavioral observations such as vocalization, movement, and agitation.[23] The NRS is commonly modified to include numeric values assigned to physiologic data. A modified NRS has been described that includes physiologic data, response to palpation, activity, mental status, posture, and vocalization.[24] The VAS is a simple scale comprising a straight line (usually 100 mm long) with the limits of the scale written at each end. The observer, or with humans, the patient, marks the line at the point that reflects the degree of pain observed or perceived. Although the VAS is subject to a great deal of variation, it is believed to be more sensitive than either the NRS or SDS in human patients. In veterinary medicine, some variations of SDS or NRS are commonly used. The accuracy of pain-rating scales is usually established by comparing scores with indicators of stress such as increased heart rate and increased concentrations of plasma cortisol.[25] Regardless of the scale used, significant variability exists among trained observers in describing the degree of pain

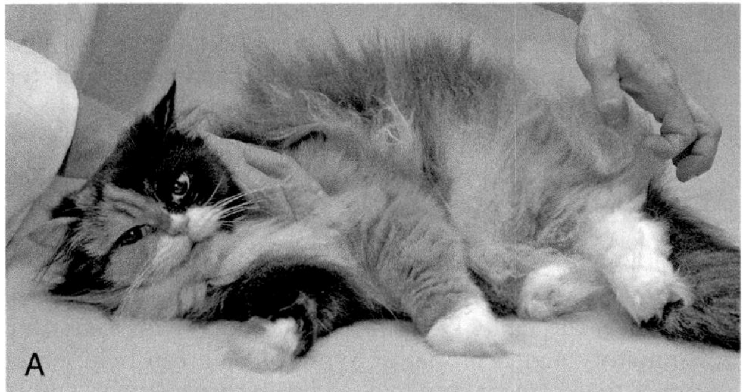

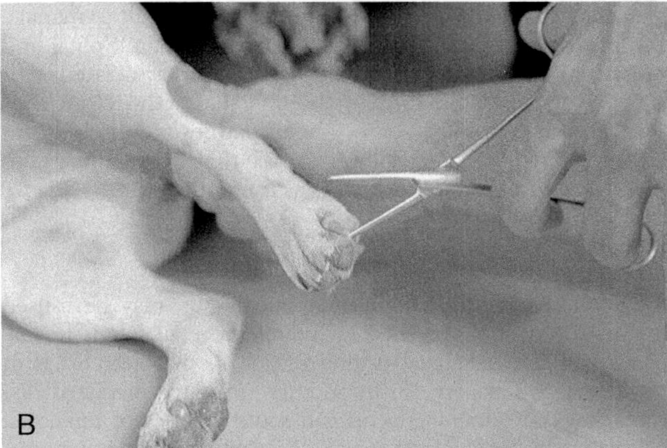

Figure 14-5 Demonstration of superficial sensation **(A)** and pain (deep) perception **(B)**.

TABLE 14-3

Differentials for Clinical Pain Associated With the Nervous and Musculoskeletal Systems in Domestic Animals

Differential Category	Nociceptive/Inflammatory Pain	Neuropathic Pain
Degenerative	Degenerative joint disease (axial and appendicular skeleton)	IVDD (Hansen type I and II), cervical spondylomyelopathy, degenerative lumbosacral stenosis, paraspinal cysts
Anomalous	Axial/appendicular skeletal malformation	Spinal malformation, caudal occipital malformation syndrome (Chiari-like malformation), syringohydromyelia, atlantoaxial instability
Metabolic	Hyperparathyroidism	Hyperparathyroidism
Neoplastic	Primary and metastatic neoplasms of bone, joint, muscle, spine, meninges	Malignant nerve sheath tumor, intracranial mass, extradural, intradural/extramedullary, intramedullary (less likely) spinal cord tumors, vertebral/cranial tumors, metastatic tumors, paraneoplastic
Nutritional	Hypervitaminosis A	
Inflammatory (Infectious/Noninfectious)	Osteoarthritis, osteomyelitis, hypertrophic osteodystrophy, infectious and noninfectious meningitis, discospondylitis, epidural empyema, myositis, polymyositis	Meningitis, epidural empyema
Immune	Osteoarthritis, myositis, systemic lupus erythema, rheumatoid disease	Chronic osteoarthritis
Idiopathic		Spinal arachnoid cyst/diverticulum Feline spinal hyperesthesia syndrome
Traumatic	Fracture, Hansen type I IVDD	Spinal fracture, Hansen type I IVD extrusion, neuroma, nerve avulsion, syrinx
Vascular	Osteonecrosis	Ischemic neuromyopathy, extradural hemorrhage

Adapted from Coates JR: Treatment of animals with spinal pain. In Bonagura JD, editor: Kirk's current veterinary therapy XIV, St Louis, 2008, Elsevier.

animals experience in the postoperative period.[26] Chronic pain such as lameness may be more accurately quantified through use of kinematic, pressure mats, and accelerometer technologies.

DISEASES

Table 14-3 lists neurologic diseases that frequently cause clinical pain. Most of these are discussed in other chapters, as indicated in the table. Determining the underlying cause for inflammatory and neuropathic types of pain can help guide appropriate treatment strategies and pain management. Disorders associated with chronic pain are often difficult to manage compared with those associated with acute pain. Spinal and musculoskeletal pain occurs in those diseases associated with compression, inflammation, or trauma that activate nociceptive receptors. Primary sensory neuropathies are discussed in Chapter 7. The only neurologic disease that frequently causes pain without other neurologic signs is meningitis.

Meningitis

Pathogenesis

Inflammation of the meninges, or meningitis, may be caused by many infectious agents, including bacterial, viral, fungal, protozoal, and rickettsial organisms.[27-30] A complete list is in the tables in Chapter 15. In addition, immune-mediated diseases can cause meningitis, as can some diseases of unknown origin, such as meningoencephalomyelitis of unknown etiology (MUE),[31,32] eosinophilic meningomyelitis characterized by an eosinophilic cerebrospinal fluid (CSF),[33,34] and a steroid-responsive meningitis-arteritis.[35-40] A vasculitis and meningitis seen in dogs, primarily beagles, has been called the canine pain syndrome.[41-43]

Regardless of the cause of meningitis, the potential for the inflammatory process to extend to the nervous tissue is always present.[27,44] Bacterial meningitis infections occur by hematogenous spread from infections in other parts of the body; by direct extension from adjacent structures including sinuses, eyes, or ears; and from direct trauma including surgery and CSF collection.[27,30] The organisms spread through the CSF to both spinal and intracranial meninges. Vasculitis is common, especially in rickettsial infections and immune-mediated disease.[31,45] The resulting encephalitis, myelitis, or encephalomyelitis causes other clinical signs such as seizures, paresis, ataxia, or altered mental status. That helps localize the disease process to a specific anatomic region of the CNS. Cranial and spinal nerves may be affected. As a consequence of inflammation, communicating hydrocephalus may develop because of reduced absorption of CSF in the subarachnoid space and through the venous sinuses.[46,47] Occlusion of the CSF flow within the ventricles may also cause obstructive hydrocephalus.

Clinical Signs

Animals with meningitis are systemically ill.[48,49] The onset is usually acute, and signs are progressive. The animals may be lethargic and reluctant to eat. Many animals, especially dogs, have rigidity with generalized pain that seems worse in the cervical spinal region. In large animals, common clinical signs include hyperesthesia, stiffness in the neck, muscle tremors, somnolence, seizures, and blindness.[16,49] Palpation of the vertebral column and head usually causes the animal to splint the muscles and appear uncomfortable, in contrast to palpation of limb musculature; however, small animals may appear to be in pain everywhere. They frequently walk as if they do not want to jar their body, as if "walking on eggshells." A fever may be present. In dogs, two thirds of the cases have focal neurologic deficits.[48]

Diagnosis

A complete blood count, biochemical profile, and urinalysis provide a minimum database. A neutrophilic leukocytosis may be evident in cases of meningitis of dogs and cats.[30,48] In large animals, neonates frequently have a neutropenia.[16] Magnetic resonance imaging of the brain can reveal meningeal enhancement and extent of meningoencephalitis.[31,50] Immunologic testing,[35,39,40,51,52] microbial culture and susceptibility testing, and polymerase chain reaction have been useful in detecting various infectious agents.[29,30,53] Please refer to Chapter 15 for further discussion of diagnostic testing results.

Treatment

Treatment of infectious diseases involves mainly antimicrobials and is discussed in Chapter 15. Treatment of noninfectious diseases requires immunosuppression and is discussed in Chapters 12 and 15.

Feline Hyperesthesia Syndrome

Pathogenesis

Feline hyperesthesia syndrome is an episodic disorder, also known as "rolling skin disease."[54,55] It is a diagnosis of exclusion and may not have a single identifying cause. Age of onset is young to middle age. Affected cats tend to be compulsive. A proposed trigger is displacement disorder, which represents an alternative to two other conflicting behaviors.[56] Environmental factors often relate to stress. Hormone alterations in compulsive disorders have been associated with increased levels of dopamine and opiates and reduced levels of serotonin.[57] Abnormal electromyography (EMG) activity and vacuolar myopathy have been associated with feline hyperesthesia syndrome.[58]

Clinical Signs

Affected cats stare at their flank and tail and then attack or excessively groom those areas. Severe alopecia and dermatitis may result. Cats may have mydriasis, hallucinate and run around the home, act irritable, and vocalize. Behavior changes include calm cats becoming aggressive and aggressive cats displaying increased affection. The episodes may be induced by stroking the cats along the trunk, which may induce seizure activity in some cats.

Diagnosis

Diagnosis is based on clinical signs and ruling out dermatologic, musculoskeletal, and other neurologic and behavioral disorders.[54] Focal seizure and underlying pain or paresthesia also need to be considered.

Treatment

Treatments are empirical. Behavior modification is focused on creating a stable and consistent home environment. Pharmacologic interventions include behavioral modifying medications such as serotonin reuptake inhibitors, tricyclic antidepressants, and benzodiazepines.[59] Anticonvulsant therapy using phenobarbital may have some effect. Gabapentin may modify neuropathic pain. Carnitine and coenzyme Q may have effects on the vacuolar myopathy. Drug trials may be necessary to determine which drug or combination has the greatest effects. Dosages should be titrated to effect to prevent side effects. Prognosis depends upon the owner's expectation and underlying cause. Successful therapy should be reduction in frequency and severity of clinical signs.

PAIN MANAGEMENT

Relief of pain in animals was often ignored in the past. Greater awareness of the signs associated with pain has resulted in more aggressive management.[1] The key component in pain management is to determine the cause of pain to the fullest extent and institute a treatment plan that has established safety and efficacy. The ultimate goals are to reduce pain and improve function and quality of life. An effective treatment plan provides acceptable analgesia with few side effects. In veterinary medicine, a treatment plan may include clinical interventions, and pharmacologic and rehabilitative approaches singly or in combination. Efficacy, tolerability, cost, and safety need consideration with any type of pharmacologic therapy. Species variability is important in selecting agents to control pain.[6,7,60,61] Routes of administration may factor into effective pain control and include oral, parenteral (intravenous, intramuscular, subcutaneous), epidural, transdermal, transmucosal, and local/regional nerve blocks.[10] Considerations should also be given for short- and long-term pain management. With lack of multicenter, randomized, controlled studies in veterinary medicine, regimens for pain management often are empirically based.

Identification of mechanisms underlying signal transduction and transmission and processing of noxious stimuli has led to the development of drugs that target chemical mediators of pain.[5] Steroidal and nonsteroidal antiinflammatory drugs (NSAIDs) are effective for inflammation; opioids, α_2-agonists modulate excitatory and inhibitory neuronal activity; and local anesthetics suppress electrical impulses. Nonopioid drugs act at the nociceptor level and alter transduction processes of pain. Opioids alter transmission and perception of pain in the CNS. Various pharmacologic regimens most often are based on complementary mechanisms of action that need to be combined in a rational fashion.[5] For chronic pain, combination therapy, or multimodality therapies may be more effective than a single agent. The NSAIDs appear to have synergistic effects with opioids and may allow for lower dosage of both.[5,62] Common analgesic agents that include glucocorticoids, NSAIDs, opioids, α_2-agonists, and other psychotropic drugs are summarized among the domestic animals in Tables 14-4 through 14-10. There are no FDA-approved analgesics for food-producing animals; all medications are extralabel use.

Corticosteroids

Inflammatory pain can be alleviated through the antiinflammatory actions of corticosteroids. These mechanisms of action suppress aspects of the inflammatory response by reduction of leukocyte numbers, phagocytosis, migration of neutrophils, and antigen presenting and processing. Effects of corticosteroids are mediated by a variety of corticosteroid receptors on target cells.[63] The main mechanism of antiinflammatory effects of corticosteroids is through inhibition of phospholipase activity, which converts membrane-released phospholipids to arachidonic acid. Prostaglandins and leukotrienes lower the nociceptive threshold, increasing sensitivity to substances that cause pain.

Specific neurologic disease processes vary widely in optimal corticosteroid usage.[63] It is important to obtain a confirmatory diagnosis before corticosteroid usage. The initial rapid improvements without a differential diagnosis can be misleading and unsupervised chronic use of corticosteroids without monitoring can lead to deleterious side effects.[64] Protocols with high-dose regimens should not be combined with other antiinflammatory regimens. For compressive spinal cord disease, dexamethasone or prednisone has been administered at antiinflammatory doses to control

TABLE 14-4

Analgesic Agents for Dogs

Drug	Trade Name	Dosage and Route	Frequency	Comments and Side Effects
Corticosteroids				
Prednisone	Generic	0.5-1.0 mg/kg PO	12-12h	PU/PD, polyphagia, weight gain, GI ulceration
Dexamethasone	Generic	0.07-0.15 mg/kg IV, SC, PO	12-24h	Same as above
NSAIDs				GI, renal, and some hepatic
Acetylsalicylic acid	Generic	10-25 mg/kg PO	12-24h	Cautiously, GI, bleeding
Acetaminophen	Generic	10-20 mg/kg PO	12h	Cautiously, GI, hepatoxicity
Deracoxib	Deramaxx	1-2 mg/kg PO	24h	GI
Etodolac	Etogesic, Lodine	10-15 mg/kg PO	24h	GI
Firocoxib	Previcox	5 mg/kg PO	24h	GI
Carprofen	Rimadyl	4 mg/kg, SC, IV once; 2-2.2 mg/kg PO	12h	GI, hepatotoxicity
Ketoprofen	Orudis KT, Ketofen	1-2 mg/kg PO, SC; IV once or q24h (max 3 days)	24h (use up to 5 days)	Extralabel use; GI, renal effects
Meloxicam	Metacam	0.1 mg/kg PO, SC; use 0.2 mg/kg IV, SC, PO for single dose loading	24h	GI
Piroxicam	Feldene	0.3 mg/kg PO	48h	GI, renal effects
Tepoxalin	Zubrin	10 mg/kg PO	24h	GI, hepatopathy, renal effects
Opioids				
Buprenorphine	Buprenex	0.005-0.02 mg/kg IV, IM, transmucosal	4-8h	Respiratory depression
Butorphanol	Torbugesic, Torbutrol, Stadol	0.2-1 mg/kg, IV, IM, SC, PO	Parenteral q2-6h; PO q4-8h	Vomiting, sedation
Codeine	Generic	0.5-1 mg/kg PO	4-6h	Sedation, dysphoria
Fentanyl citrate	Sublimaze; Duragesic; generic	10-40 µg/kg, IV, IM, SC 50 µg/10-20 kg transdermal 3-6 µg/kg/h CRI	Parenteral q2h; Transdermal q3-5 days	Respiratory depression, hypoventilation
Hydromorphone	Dilaudid; generic	0.1-0.2 mg/kg SC, IV, IM	2-6h	Vomiting
Meperidine	Demerol	3-10 mg/kg IM	PRN	Not recommended for IV use. Sedation, hypotension
Methadone	Dolophine	0.1-0.5 mg/kg IV, IM, SC	2-4h	Sedation, minimal histamine release, mild vomiting
Morphine sulfate	Generic	0.1-1.0 mg/kg IV, IM, SC	Parenteral q2-6h; PO q8h	Histamine release—hypotension, IV; respiratory and CNS depression
Nalbuphine	Nalbuphine	0.3-0.5 mg/kg IM, SC	3-4h	Sedation
Oxycodone	Percocet (with acetaminophen)	0.1-0.3 mg/kg PO	8-12h	Sedation
Oxymorphone	Numorphan	0.03-0.2 mg/kg IV, IM, SC	Repeat dosing with ½ dose q1-2h	Respiratory and CNS depression, hypotension, bradycardia, auditory sensitivity, increased intracranial pressure
Pentazocine	Talwin	1-4 mg/kg IM 2-6 mg/kg PO	2-4h	Salivation, sedation
Tramadol	Ultram	2-4 mg/kg PO	6-12h	Sedation, anorexia

TABLE 14-4

***Analgesic Agents for Dogs*—cont'd**

Drug	Trade Name	Dosage and Route	Frequency	Comments and Side Effects
α_2-Agonists				
Dexmedetomidine HCl	Dexdomitor	500 μg/m² IM; 375/m², IV	PRN	Sedation, arrhythmias, bradycardia, respiratory depression
Xylazine	Rompun; Generic	0.1-0.5 mg/kg IV, IM, SC	12h	Sedation, arrhythmias, bradycardia, respiratory depression
Local (Epidural) Anesthetics				
Bupivacaine	Marcaine	1 mL/10 cm; 1-2.5 mg/kg epidural	—	
Lidocaine	Generic, Xylocaine	3-5 mg/kg	—	
Mepivacaine	Carbocaine	3-4.5 mg/kg	q30sec until absent reflex; not to exceed 8 mg/kg	
Morphine	Generic	0.1-1 mg/kg	—	
Other Drugs				
Amitriptyline	Elavil	1-4 mg/kg PO	12-24h	Sedation, psychosis, anticholinergic, seizure
Gabapentin	Generic, Neurontin	3-10 mg/kg PO	8-24h	Sedation
Pregabalin	Lyrica	0.3-4 mg/kg PO	8h	
Ketamine (anesthetic agent)	Ketaset, Vetalar	5-7 mg/kg, IV 5 μg/kg/min, CRI	—	Usually as anesthetic agent, increased intracranial pressure, seizures

Dosages adapted from Flecknell P, Waterman-Pearson A: Pain management in animals, London, WB Saunders/Harcourt, 2000. In Gaynor JS, Muir WW: Handbook of veterinary pain management, ed 2, St Louis, Mosby/Elsevier, 2009.
PO, Per os; *SC*, subcutaneous; *IM*, intramuscular; *IV*, intravenous; *CRI*, constant rate infusion; *PRN*, as necessary.

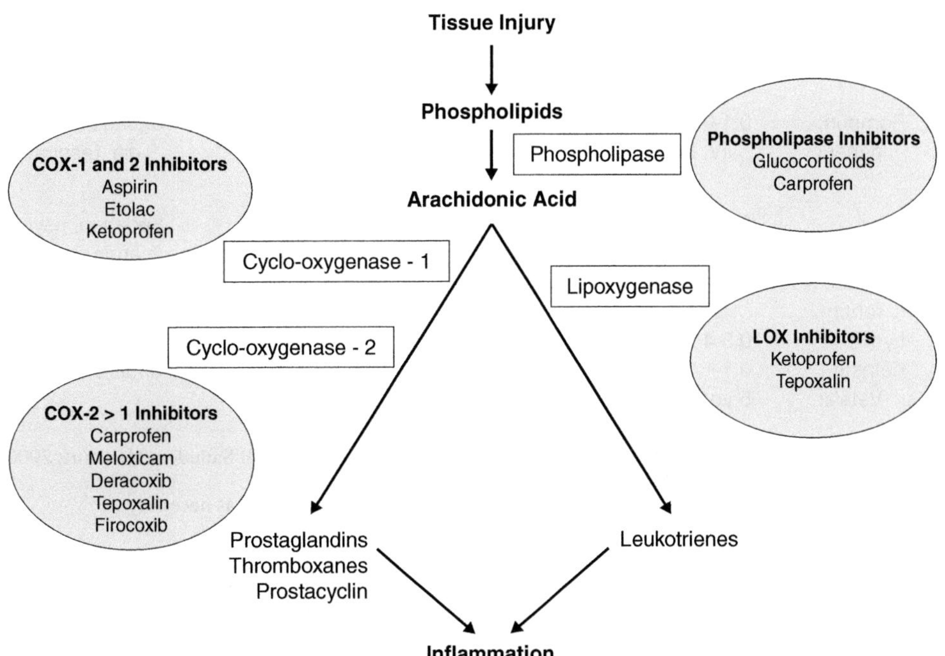

Figure 14-6 Schematic depicting pharmacologic inhibitors of arachidonic acid metabolism and the cyclo-oxygenase (COX) and lipoxygenase (LOX) pathways. (From Coates JR: Treatment of animals with spinal pain. In Bonagura JD, editor: Kirk's current veterinary therapy XIV, St Louis, 2008, Elsevier.)

TABLE 14-5

Analgesic Agents for Cats

Drug	Trade Name	Dosage and Route	Frequency	Comments and Side Effects
Corticosteroids				
Prednisolone	Generic	0.5-1.0 mg/kg PO	12-12h	Minimal, short-term
Dexamethasone	Generic	0.07-0.15 mg/kg IV, SC, PO	12-24h	Minimal, short-term
NSAIDs				GI renal, and some hepatic
Acetylsalicylic acid	Generic	40.5-81 mg/cat PO	48-72h	Anorexia, GI, bleeding
Carprofen	Rimadyl	1-4 mg/kg SC	once	Extralabel use; GI, hepatotoxicity
Ketoprofen	Orudis KT, Ketofen	1-2 mg/kg PO, SC; IV once or q24h (max 3 days)	24h (use up to 5 days)	Extralabel use; GI, renal effects
Meloxicam	Metacam	0.025 mg/kg, PO; use 0.1-0.2 mg/kg, PO, SC, IV as single dose	q24 for 1-2 days; then 0.025 mg/kg 2-3 times/ week, PO	GI, vomiting, anorexia
Opioids				Vomiting, histamine release, hypotension
Buprenorphine	Buprenex	0.005-0.02 mg/kg IV, IM, SC	4-8h	Respiratory depression
Butorphanol	Torbugesic	1.5 mg/kg IV, IM, SC, PO	Parenteral q2-4h; PO q6h	Vomiting, sedation, excitement
Fentanyl citrate	Sublimaze; Duragesic; generic	5-10 μg/kg IV, IM, SC 12.5-25 μg/cat, transdermal patch 0.3 μg/kg/min CRI	Parenteral q2h; Transdermal q3-5days	Respiratory depression and hypoventilation
Hydromorphone	Dilaudid; generic	0.1-0.2 mg/kg SC, IV, IM	2-6h	Vomiting, dysphoria, hyperthermia
Morphine	Generic	0.05-0.1 mg/kg IM, SC	Parenteral q4-6h; PO q8h	Hypotension, vomiting, CNS and respiratory depression, hyper-excitability
Oxymorphone	Numorphan	0.01-0.1 mg/kg IV, IM, SC	Repeat dosing with ½ dose q1-2h	Respiratory and CNS depression, hypotension, hyperexcitability
Tramadol	Ultram	1-4 mg/kg PO	12h	Sedation
α_2-Agonists				
Dexmedetomidine HCl	Dexdomitor	40 μg/kg IM (sedation/ analgesia) or 5-10 μg/kg IV, IM	PRN	Sedation, arrhythmias, bradycardia, respiratory depression
Xylazine	Rompun; generic	0.1-0.5 mg/kg IV, IM, SC	12h	Sedation, arrhythmias, bradycar-dia, respiratory depression
Other Drugs				
Amitriptyline	Elavil	2.5-5 mg/cat PO	24h	Sedation, psychosis, anticholin-ergic
Gabapentin	Generic, Neu-rontin	3-10 mg/kg PO	8-24h	Sedation
Pregabalin	Lyrica	0.3-4 mg/kg PO	8h	Sedation
Ketamine	Ketaset, Vetalar	0.1-1.0 mg/kg IV, IM 5 μg/min CRI	CRI for 24h	Usually as anesthetic agent

Dosages adapted from Flecknell P, Waterman-Pearson A: Pain management in animals, London, WB Saunders/Harcourt, 2000. In Gaynor JS, Muir WW: Handbook of veterinary pain management, ed 2, St Louis, 2009, Elsevier.
PO, Per os; *SC*, subcutaneous; *IM*, intramuscular; *IV*, intravenous; *CRI*, constant rate infusion; *PRN*, as necessary.

inflammatory response and pain and to reduce spinal cord edema. Concurrently, strict cage rest is important to prevent excessive activity in animals with spinal disease. Only short-term antiinflammatory regimens of prednisone are recommended. Immunosuppressive regimens are used for immune-mediated disease (e.g., polymyositis, polyarthritis, vasculitis, meningitis, encephalitis, or myelitis). The alleviation of pain is secondary to the primary goal of suppression of the immune response that underlies these diseases. Gradual taper of the drug dosage is instituted according to the patient's overall condition.

Nonsteroidal Antiinflammatory Drugs

The NSAIDs are most often used for treatment of pain associated with inflammatory conditions but may also be useful in noninflammatory conditions and chronic pain.

TABLE 14-6

Analgesic Agents for Horses

Drug	Trade Name	Dosage and Route	Frequency	Comments and Side Effects
Corticosteroids				
Dexamethasone	Generic	0.01-0.15 IV, IM	Daily	Laminitis, immunosuppression
Prednisone	Generic	0.25-1 mg/kg PO	12-24h	Laminitis, immunosuppression
NSAIDs				Minimal
Acetylsalicylic acid	Generic	25 mg/kg PO (loading); 10 mg/kg daily	12h (loading); then daily	GI ulceration, renal effects
Carprofen	Rimadyl	0.5-1.1 mg/kg PO	Daily 4-9 days	GI ulceration, renal effects
Flunixin meglumine		1.1 mg/kg PO, IV	Daily up to 5 days	GI ulceration, renal effects
Ketoprofen	Orudis KT, Ketofen	2.2 mg/kg IV, IM	Daily up to 5 days	GI ulceration, renal effects
Phenylbutazone	Butazolidin	4.4 mg/kg PO (loading); 2.2 mg/kg	After loading use q24h for 2-4 days then every other day	GI ulceration, renal effects
Opioids				
Buprenorphine	Buprenex	0.01-0.04 mg/kg IV	once	Ataxia, disorientation
Butorphanol	Torbugesic	0.02-0.1 IV; 0.04-0.2 IM	2-4h	Excitement, ataxia, disorientation
Fentanyl citrate	Sublimaze; Duragesic; Generic	0.01-0.02 mg/kg IV; 100 g/h transdermal per 450 kg	once	Excitement, increased activity
Meperidine	Demerol	0.2-1 mg/kg IM	1-2h	Anaphylaxis if given IV, excitement, increased activity
Morphine	Generic	0.03-0.1 mg/kg IV 0.1 mg/kg IM	4h	Excitement, twitching, shaking, stereotypy
Oxymorphone	Numorphan	0.001-0.002 mg/kg IV	once	Excitement, increased activity
Pentazocine	Talwin	0.5-1 mg/kg	once	Excitement, increased activity
α_2-Agonists				
Dexmedetomidine	Dexdomitor	0.005-0.01 mg/kg IV,	once	Cardiovascular depression, ataxia
Xylazine	Rompun; Generic	0.5-1.0 mg/kg IV; 1-2 mg/kg IM		Cardiovascular depression, ataxia
Local (Epidural) Anesthetics				
Lidocaine	Generic, Xylocaine	0.16-0.45 mg/kg	2-3h	Ataxia
Xylazine	Rompun	0.03-0.35	3-5h	Ataxia

Dosages adapted from Flecknell P, Waterman-Pearson A: Pain management in animals, London, WB Saunders/Harcourt, 2000. In Gaynor JS, Muir WW: Handbook of veterinary pain management, ed 2, St Louis, 2009, Elsevier.
PO, Per os; *SC*, subcutaneous; *IM*, intramuscular; *IV*, intravenous; *CRI*, constant rate infusion; *PRN*, as necessary.

The antiinflammatory properties of NSAIDs are primarily due to inhibition of cyclo-oxygenase (COX) isoenzymes 1 and 2, which synthesize prostanoids from arachidonic acid (Figure 14-6). COX-1 is constitutive, whereas COX-2 is induced by growth factors, cytokines, and tumor promoters. COX-2 is synthesized by macrophages and inflammatory cells in the presence of tissue injury and inflammation. Secondary increases in prostanoids amplify nociceptive input and transmission in the peripheral and central nervous systems. COX-2 is involved to a greater degree than COX-1 in noceceptive transmission after tissue injury.[62,65] Arachidonic acid also is metabolized by lipoxygenase to leukotrienes, which participate as inflammatory mediators.

There are now many subclasses of NSAIDs used in human and veterinary medicine. Some NSAIDs have both COX-1 and COX-2 inhibitory effects (aspirin, ketoprofen, etolac), whereas others selectively inhibit COX-2 or are COX-1 sparing (carprofen, meloxicam, deracoxib, tepoxalin, firocoxib).[65] As COX-2 appears to play a greater role in nociceptive transmission, drugs that spare COX-1 should be effective and have

TABLE 14-7

*Analgesic Agents for Cattle**

Drug	Trade Name	Dosage and Route	Frequency	Comments and Side Effects
NSAIDs				
Acetylsalicylic acid	Generic	50-100 mg PO	12h	Withdrawal: Milk—24 hr; meat—1 day
Carprofen	Rimadyl	1.4 mg/kg SC, IV	Single dose	Withdrawal: 21 days
Flunixin meglumine	Banamine	1.1-2.2 mg/kg IV	Daily for 5 days	Withdrawal: Milk—72 hr; meat—4 days
Ketoprofen	Orudis KT, Ketofen	3 mg/kg IV	Daily up to 3 days	Withdrawal: Milk—24 hr; meat—7 days
Meloxicam	Metacam	0.5 mg/kg SC, IV	Single dose	Withdrawal: milk—5 days; meat—15 days
Opioids				Bradycardia, respiratory depression; high doses cause excitement
Butorphanol	Torbugesic, Stadol	0.02-0.25 mg/kg IV, SC	4h	Withdrawal: Milk—72 hr; Meat—4 days
Morphine	Generic	0.05-0.1 mg/kg IV, SC; 0.1 mg/kg epidural q12h	4h	No withdrawal
Buprenorphine	Buprenex	0.005-0.01 mg/kg IM, SC	8-12h	
α_2-Agonists				
Xylazine	Rompun	0.1-0.2 mg/kg IM; 0.05-0.15 mg/kg IV; 0.05-0.07 mg/kg epidural	Once	Withdrawal: Milk—24 hr; meat—7 days; Brahman sensitive; FDA—not approved; analgesia short lived
Detomidine	Dormosedan	10-40 IV, IM, epidural	Once	Withdrawal: Milk—24 hr; meat—7 days
Local Anesthetics				
Lidocaine	Generic	Up to 250 mL/500 kg animal for regional blocks	Once	No withdrawal
Lidocaine	Generic	0.2 mg/kg epidural	1h	No withdrawal
Xylazine	Rompun	0.05 mg/kg	2-3h	See above

Dosages adapted from Flecknell P, Waterman-Pearson A: Pain management in animals, London, WB Saunders/Harcourt, 2000. In Gaynor JS, Muir WW: Handbook of veterinary pain management, ed 2, St Louis, 2009, Elsevier.
SC, Subcutaneous; *IM*, intramuscular; *IV*, intravenous; *FDA*, Food and drug administration.
*There are no FDA-approved pain medications for cattle, all medications are extralabel use.

fewer adverse effects. Inhibition of COX isoenzymes may cause arachidonic acid metabolites to enter the lipoxygenase (LOX) pathway and increase the inflammatory effects of leukotrienes. Some NSAIDs have been shown to inhibit both COX and LOX (ketoprofen and tepoxalin). Most NSAIDs undergo hepatic metabolism and are eliminated through the enterohepatic circulation or by renal clearance. Adverse reactions associated with NSAIDs occur in the gastrointestinal tract, liver, and kidney. Other side effects may include coagulopathy, inhibition of healing, and altered bone formation. The plethora of different NSAIDs available for use in animals, especially dogs and cats, provides the practitioner with a choice for the most appropriate NSAID that will best complement pain management while minimizing patient side effects.[65] Response to a specific NSAID may vary with each individual patient and the type of pain.[62] If one NSAID does not appear to remedy the pain, an alternative NSAID or adjunctive use of a different class of analgesic needs consideration. Concurrent use of other NSAIDs or corticosteroids provides no additional therapeutic benefit but does increase the potential for adverse reaction. A "washout" period (48 to 72 hours) should be allowed before administering a different NSAID.

Opioid Analgesics

An opioid is a natural or synthetic drug that has opiate-like activities through its interaction with opiate receptors of a target cell. Most defined opiate receptors are located in the brain and spinal cord. Various opiate receptors mediate specific opioid effects. Opioid analgesics are classified into various groups based on their pharmacologic activity, potency, and clinical use. Type and dosage of opioid selection varies upon severity of pain. Opioid analgesics modify pain perception and behavioral reactions, and relieve anxiety and distress. Pharmacologic opiates supplement the natural activity of endogenous opiates and suppress neurons in the spine and medulla that transmit pain.[61] A pure *opioid agonist* binds to one or more types of receptors to cause certain effects (e.g., analgesia, respiratory depression). A *partial agonist* binds to a receptor but gives less of an effect than a pure agonist. An *opioid agonist-antagonist* binds to more than one receptor type to cause an effect at one but no effect at another. An *opioid antagonist* binds to one or more receptor types but causes no effect or may competitively displace an agonist from the receptor. Effectiveness of pharmacologic opiates may vary with route of administration: parenteral, epidural, rectal, oral, and transdermal drug delivery (fentanyl patch). Direct delivery of opioids to

TABLE 14-8

*Analgesic Agents for Sheep and Goats**

Drug	Trade Name	Dosage and Route	Frequency	Comments and Side Effects
NSAIDs				
Acetylsalicylic acid	Generic	50-100 mg/kg PO	4-12h	Unknown for goats
Carprofen	Rimadyl	1.5-2.0 mg/kg SC, IV	24h	
Flunixin meglumine	Banamine	1-2 mg/kg SC, IV	Once or daily	
Ketoprofen	Orudis KT, Ketofen	2-3 mg/kg IV, IM	Once up to 5 days	
Opioids				Agitation, compulsive chewing at high doses
Buprenorphine	Buprenex	0.005-0.010 mg/kg IV, IM	4h—sheep; 12 hr—goat	
Butorphanol	Torbugesic, Stadol	0.5 mg/kg SC, IM	2-3h PRN	
Meperidine	Demerol	2 mg/kg IM, IV	2h	Use unknown in goats
Morphine	Generic	0.2-0.5 mg/kg IM	2h, PRN	
α_2-Agonists				
Dexmedetomidine	Dexdomitor	0.01 mg/kg IV	Once	Bradycardia, respiratory depression, reduced GI motility
Xylazine	Rompun	Sheep—0.05-0.1 mg/kg IV, 0.1-0.3 IM; Goat—0.02-0.5 IV, 0.05-0.5 IM	Once	Bradycardia, respiratory depression, reduced GI motility

Dosages adapted from Flecknell P, Waterman-Pearson A: Pain management in animals, London, WB Saunders/Harcourt, 2000. In Gaynor JS, Muir WW: Handbook of veterinary pain management, ed 2, St Louis, 2009, Elsevier.
PO, Per os; *SC,* subcutaneous; *IM,* intramuscular; *IV,* intravenous; *PRN,* as necessary.
*There are no FDA-approved pain medications for food-producing animals; all medications are extralabel use.

TABLE 14-9

Analgesic Agents for Camelids

Drug	Trade Name	Dosage and Route	Frequency	Comments and Side Effects
NSAIDs				Gastrointestinal, renal, and some hepatic
Acetylsalicylic acid	Generic	50 mg/kg, PO	12-24h	
Carprofen	Rimadyl	1-2 mg/kg, PO	24h	
Flunixin meglumine	Banamine	1-2 mg/kg, SC, IV	24h	
Ketoprofen	Orudis KT, Ketofen	2-3 mg/kg IV, IM	24h up to 3 days	
Opioids				
Morphine	Generic	0.05-0.1 mg/kg IV, IM	4h	Reduced GI motility
Butorphanol	Torbugesic	0.05-0.1 mg/kg IV, IM in alpacas; 0.02-0.05 mg/kg IV, IM in llamas	PRN	Reduced GI motility
Buprenorphine	Buprenex	0.01 mg/kg IM	PRN	Reduced GI motility
α_2-Agonists				
Dexmedetomidine	Dexdomitor	0.005-0.01 mg/kg IV	Once	Bradycardia, respiratory depression, reduced GI motility
Xylazine (standing sedation)	Rompun; generic	Llamas: 0.075-0.1 mg/kg IV; 0.15-0.2 mg/kg IM, SC. Alpacas: 0.1-0.15 mg/kg IV; 0.2-0.3 mg/kg IM, SC	Once	Bradycardia, respiratory depression, reduced GI motility

Dosages adapted from Abrahamsen EJ: Chemical restraint anesthesia, and analgesia for camelids. Vet Clin North Am Food Anim Pract 25:455–494, 2009.
PO, Per os; *SC,* subcutaneous; *IM,* intramuscular; *IV,* intravenous; *PRN,* as necessary.

TABLE 14-10

Analgesic Agents for Swine[*]

Drug	Trade Name	Dosage and Route	Frequency	Comments and Side Effects
NSAIDs				
Acetylsalicylic acid	Generic	10 mg/kg PO	4h	GI, bleeding
Carprofen	Rimadyl	2-4 mg/kg SC, IV, PO	24h	
Flunixin meglumine	Banamine	1-2 mg/kg IM, PO	24h	
Ketoprofen	Orudis KT, Ketofen	1-3 mg/kg IM	once	
Meloxicam	Metacam	0.4 mg/kg IM	Once	Withdrawal: 5 days
Opioids				Sedation
Buprenorphine	Buprenex	5-10 µg/kg IV	6-12h	—
Butorphanol	Torbugesic	0.1-0.3 mg/kg IM	4h	—
Fentanyl citrate	Sublimaze; Duragesic; generic	200 µg/kg IV	Intraoperatively	Pigs require higher doses
Morphine	Generic	0.2-1.0 mg/kg IM	4h	—
Pentazocine	Talwin	2 mg/kg IM, IV	4h	—
Meperidine	Demerol	2 mg/kg IM, IV	2-4h	—
α_2-Agonists				
Dexmedetomidine	Dexdomitor	Undetermined, epidural use in research	Once	Bradycardia, respiratory depression, reduced GI motility
Xylazine (standing sedation)	Rompun; generic	0.5-3 mg/kg IM	Once	Bradycardia, respiratory depression, reduced GI motility

Dosages adapted from Flecknell P, Waterman-Pearson A: Pain management in animals, London, WB Saunders/Harcourt, 2000. In Gaynor JS, Muir WW: Handbook of veterinary pain management, ed 2, St Louis, 2009, Elsevier.
PO, Per os; *SC*, subcutaneous; *IM*, intramuscular; *IV*, intravenous.
[*]There are no FDA-approved pain medications for pigs, all medications are extralabel use.

the spinal cord (epidural anesthesia) is used to produce effective analgesia for surgical procedures. Opioids are more effective for postsurgury or with trauma and are considered less effective for neuropathic pain.[5] Opioids that are pure agonists may provide more effective pain control than agonist-antagonist opioids. Tolerance to opiate effects may develop during repeated and chronic administration. Side effects that vary among species may include altered consciousness, including dysphoria; excitement; bradycardia; respiratory depression; autonomic signs; and panting in dogs. Some of the opioids (meperidine and morphine) can cause histamine release with IV administration. Effects of histamine release include vasodilation and hypotension. Opioids will have excitatory effects in cats and horses, and its administration should be combined with tranquilizers.

Other Analgesic Agents

α_2-Agonists

Xylazine and medetomidine are centrally acting and possess sedative, muscle relaxant, and analgesic properties. Receptors for these agents are located presynaptically and postsynaptically on the nociceptive neurons in the dorsal horn of the spinal cord. Analgesic effects are enhanced when used in combination with opioids. Cardiovascular side effects include bradycardia, hypotension, and decreased cardiac output.

Anticonvulsants

In humans, the mainstay for chronic treatment of neuropathic pain is tricyclic antidepressants and anticonvulsants.[11] Analgesic actions of antidepressant drugs are most likely related to effects on endogenous pathways that modulate nociceptive transmission.[5] The anticonvulsant, gabapentin, has been extensively investigated and proven to be effective for a variety of neuropathic pain disorders. The mechanism of action is unclear. Gabapentin and pregabalin are analogs of gamma-aminobutyric acid (GABA), the major inhibitory neurotransmitter in the CNS. Gabapentin may alter voltage-gated calcium channels. The binding action of the drug leads to a decrease in intracellular calcium ion influx, which in turn inhibits excitatory synapse formation (e.g., glutamate, substance P).[66] Unlike many analgesics, gabapentin is minimally metabolized by the liver and eliminated by renal clearance. In veterinary patients, gabapentin has been used empirically for management of refractory neuropathic pain.

Miscellaneous Agents

Muscle relaxants (e.g., diazepam, methocarbamol) can be administered for musculoskeletal pains that cause muscle spasm. Other psychotropic drugs include tranquilizers and ketamine. The tranquilizers, including phenothiazine derivatives, benzodiazepines, and butyrophenones, are primarily useful in reducing anxiety associated with pain. They may potentiate the effects of other analgesic agents but should not be given alone in the treatment of pain. Ketamine is a dissociative anesthetic and is not generally used for the management of chronic pain.

Acupuncture

Acupuncture is still controversial, although substantial evidence exists for its benefits in treating pain. If it is used for pain relief, and not as a substitute for correction of the cause of pain, it is appropriate.[67,68]

Summary

The issue of pain management is an important dimension in veterinary medicine. The willingness to provide pain intervention should be a routine practice. Considerable evidence exists that preemptive pain management can be effective in decreasing the development of chronic pain states and is beneficial to the health, recovery, and well-being of our veterinary patients.

CARE OF THE NEUROLOGIC PATIENT

Physical Rehabilitation

Physical rehabilitation in large and small animals is integral in management of medical and surgical-related neurologic diseases, enhancement of neuroregenerative processes, and providing pain relief.[69,70] Disuse and immobilization can cause loss of muscle mass and debilitating joint contracture. Physical rehabilitation during recovery from neurologic disorders is important not only for strengthening and increasing flexibility but also pain reduction and improvement in quality of life.[71] Use of physiotherapy in dogs with degenerative myelopathy suggest longer ambulatory times.[72] Rehabilitation protocols are individually tailored to meet patients' needs during the recovery process. Owners and veterinarians are encouraged to seek out facilities and certified individuals that specialize in physiotherapy and physical rehabilitation.

Passive Range of Motion

Rehabilitation in immediate postoperative and recumbent patients begins with massage and passive range of motion (ROM). Joints of limbs are extended and flexed through normal ROM 5 to 10 minutes several times a day. Active ROM includes swimming and standing exercises. The goal is to have the limbs in normal position, bearing only a portion of the body weight. Static and mechanical forms of stretching techniques are performed in conjunction with ROM exercises to prevent fibrosis and contracture of joints and muscles. This process can be initiated with carts and hydrotherapy.

Other modalities of physical therapy and supplemental therapies that complement mobility therapies include thermal, electrical stimulation, massage, ultrasonographic, acupuncture, and weight loss.[73] Superficial and deep heat therapy also can be instituted to reduce muscle spasm and improve circulation.[73] Neuromuscular stimulation is applied to selected muscle groups that undergo atrophy.[73] Neuromuscular electrical stimulation increases muscle strength, joint stability, and ROM and decreases muscle spasm and pain.

Hydrotherapy

Exercises performed in water or whirlpools are very effective for relaxing contracted muscles, maintaining joint mobility, and stimulating circulation in atrophied muscles. Hydrotherapy also will help to keep the patient clean. Water buoyancy aids in rehabilitation of weak muscles and painful joints by minimizing the amount of weight bearing on joints while generating the gait cycle. Muscles and limbs should be exercised passively. Underwater treadmills will further assist with walking motions and provide resistance to enhance muscle strengthening and proprioception.

Exercise

Exercise can be passive or active, depending on the degree of neurologic dysfunction. Gait training exercises encourages more ambulation to affected limbs. Massage and passive ROM are continued to stimulate muscle tone and delay muscle contracture. As the patient begins to ambulate without assistance, therapeutic exercises includes standing and more dynamic ambulation activities that serve to enhance ROM, muscle strength, balance, and overall daily function. Proprioceptive neuromuscular training improves the awareness and use of limbs at rest and in motion. This is facilitated using standing exercises and weight shifting using balls. Proper exercise regimen encourages dogs to walk and improves their mental status. If possible, dogs should be exercised outdoors, with a towel used as a sling. Cavaletti rails assist with limb placement and developing stride. Having the patient walk on a mattress can also improve balance and coordination. Assistive devices such as boots, dog carts, or slings may be useful for long-term rehabilitation.

Bladder Management

Many neurologic lesions disrupt voluntary micturition, resulting in urinary incontinence, retention cystitis, and bladder atony. Urinary bladders should be manually expressed or emptied by intermittent catheterization at least three times a day. Urinary tract infections should be treated with appropriate antibiotics. See Chapter 3 for details and for pharmacologic agents to assist micturition.

Supportive Care of a Recumbent Small Animal

Supportive care to involve the psychologic and physical well-being is especially important in the recumbent patient. Bedding should be supportive enough to evenly distribute the patient's weight, especially over bony prominences to prevent decubitus ulcers.[74] Absorbent materials (lamb's wool, diaper pads) need to overlie supportive materials (air, foam mattresses). The patient will need to be rotated on a frequent basis (e.g., every 4 hours). Cleanliness is critical to prevent fecal and urine scalding. Cryotherapy of the surgical incision is applied for several days until the incision is no longer warm to touch. An ice pack covered with a towel to protect the skin is applied for 10 to 20 minutes, three times daily to lessen edema and for pain management. Hydrotherapy also can play a role in increasing circulation of the limb vasculature and prevention of decubitus ulcers. Having the pet owner, veterinarian, and technicians intimately involved with the postoperative care is important in the patient's overall well-being and quality of life.

Supportive Care of a Recumbent Large Animal

Horses and cattle are especially prone to develop secondary complications caused by recumbency. Self-trauma, decubital ulceration, myopathy, neuropathy, pneumonia, malnutrition, colic, and urinary tract infections are common complications in recumbent horses. Cattle are also prone to bloat.

Horses and cattle should be protected from self-trauma. Limbs should be wrapped with thick layers of sheet cotton or quilted limb wraps. The head should be protected with a padded and properly fitted helmet. Tranquilizing agents such as chloral hydrate, detomidine, and xylazine may be required early in the course of treatment. These agents may hamper neurologic evaluation and may produce hypotension. To the greatest extent possible, large animals should be maintained in sternal recumbency because this position improves ventilation and peripheral circulation. Hay bales make good props for this purpose. Slings and overhead hoists may be helpful, but horses must be monitored continually to prevent injury and asphyxiation.

Decubital ulceration over bony prominences can be minimized by distributing pressure; applying pads over pressure points; using liberal amounts of clean, dry bedding; and turning the patient every 2 hours. Because eye injuries are common, the eyes should be examined two or three times a day. Padded helmets are useful in preventing eye injuries. Artificial tears and triple antibiotic ointment should be applied when patients cannot lubricate their corneas.

Impaction of the large or small colon and rectum is a common complication. Water should be offered frequently, and a highly digestible diet of quality hay and pelleted feeds is recommended. Pelleted feed should contain ground alfalfa, bran, and psyllium. Water should be given by nasogastric intubation if a horse has trouble drinking and swallowing. Laxative agents such as mineral oil, dioctyl sodium sulfosuccinate, and magnesium sulfate can be provided on a regular basis.

Urine retention should be evaluated by observation and rectal palpation. Urinary bladder catheterization is best accomplished using an aseptic closed system. The use of prophylactic urinary antibiotics is contraindicated. Pneumonia and pleuritis are fatal complications in recumbent horses. Frequent turning is the best way to prevent pulmonary complications.

REFERENCES

1. Colloquium on recognition and alleviation of animal pain and distress, J Am Vet Med Assoc 191:1184–1298, 1987.
2. Kitchell RL: Problems in defining pain and peripheral mechanisms of pain, J Am Vet Med Assoc 191(10):1195–1199, 1987.
3. Willis WD, Chung JM: Central mechanisms of pain, J Am Vet Med Assoc 191(10):1200–1202, 1987.
4. Mersky H, Bogduk N: Classification of chronic pain, Seattle, 1994, IASP.
5. Muir WW, Woolf CJ: Mechanisms of pain and their therapeutic implications, J Am Vet Med Assoc 219:1346–1356, 2001.
6. Flecknell P, Waterman-Pearson A: Pain management in animals, London, 2000, WB Saunders/Harcourt.
7. Gaynor JS, Muir WW: Handbook of veterinary pain management, St Louis, 2009, Mosby/Elsevier.
8. de Lahunta A, Glass E: Veterinary neuroanatomy and clinical neurology, St Louis, 2009, Saunders Elsevier.
9. Willis WD, Al-Chaer ED, Quast MJ, et al: A visceral pain pathway in the dorsal column of the spinal cord, Proc Natl Acad Sci U S A 96:7675–7679, 1999.
10. Ogilvie GK, Moore AS: Oncologic pain in dogs: prevention and treatment, Compend Contin Educ Pract Vet 28:776–785, 2006.
11. Truini A, Cruccu G: Pathophysiologic mechanisms of neuropathic pain, Neurol Sci 27:S179–S182, 2006.
12. Campbell JN, Meyer RA: Mechanisms of neuropathic pain, Neuron 52:77–92, 2006.
13. Lu D, Lamb CR, Pfeiffer NE, et al: Neurological signs and results of magnetic resonance imaging in 40 cavalier King Charles spaniels with Chiari type I-like malformations, Vet Rec 153:260–263, 2003.
14. Portenoy RK: Basic Mechanism. In Portenoy RK, Kanner RM, editors: Pain management: theory and practice (contemporary neurology series), Philadelphia, 1996, FA Davis.
15. Constable PD: Clinical examination of the ruminant nervous system, Vet Clin North Am Food Anim Pract 20:185–214, 2004.
16. Mayhew IG: Large animal neurology, ed 2, Ames, Iowa, 2009, Wiley-Blackwell.
17. Coates JR, Dewey CW: Cervical spinal hyperesthesia as a clinical sign of intracranial disease, Compend Contin Educ Pract Vet 20(9):1025–1037, 1998.
18. Kuhn RA: Organization of tactile dermatomes in cat and monkey, J Neurophysiol 16:169–182, 1953.
19. Kitchell RL, Canton DD, Johnson RD, et al: Electrophysiologic studies of cutaneous nerves of the forelimb of the cat, J Comp Neurol 210(4):400–410, 1982.
20. Bailey CS, Kitchell RL: Cutaneous sensory testing in the dog, J Vet Intern Med 1(3):128–135, 1987.
21. Smith JD, Allen SW, Quandt JE, et al: Indicators of postoperative pain in cats and correlation with clinical criteria, Am J Vet Res 57(11):1674–1678, 1996.
22. Smith JD, Allen SW, Quandt JE: Changes in cortisol concentration in response to stress and postoperative pain in client-owned cats and correlation with objective clinical variables, Am J Vet Res 60(4):432–436, 1999.
23. Conzemius MG, Hill CM: Correlation between subjective and objective measures used to determine severity of post operative pain in dogs, J Am Vet Med Assoc 210:1619–1622, 1999.
24. Firth AM, Haldane SL: Development of a scale to evaluate postoperative pain in dogs, J Am Vet Med Assoc 214(5):651–659, 1999.
25. Holton LL, Scott E, Nolan AM, et al: Relationship between physiological factors and clinical pain in dogs scored using a numerical scale, J Small Anim Pract 39:469–474, 1998.
26. Holton LL, Scott EM, Nolan AM, et al: Comparison of three methods used for assessment of pain in dogs, J Am Vet Med Assoc 212:61–66, 1998.
27. Brass DA: Pathophysiology and neuroimmunology of bacterial meningitis, Compend Contin Educ Pract Vet 16(1):45–54, 1994.
28. Meric SM: Canine meningitis. A changing emphasis, J Vet Intern Med 2(1):26–35, 1988.
29. Radaelli ST, Platt SR: Bacterial meningoencephalomyelitis in dogs: a retrospective study of 23 cases (1990-1999), J Vet Intern Med 16(2):159–163, 2002.
30. Kent M: Bacterial infections of the central nervous system. In Greene CE, editor: Infectious diseases of the dog and cat, ed 3, St Louis, 2006, Elsevier.
31. Schatzberg SJ: Idiopathic granulomatous and necrotizing inflammatory disorders of the canine central nervous system, Vet Clin North Am Small Anim Pract 40(1):101–120, 2010:(review).
32. Higginbotham MJ, Kent M, Glass EN: Noninfectious inflammatory central nervous system diseases in dogs, Comp Contin Educ Pract Vet 29(8):488–497, 2007.
33. Smith-Maxie LL, Parent JP, Rand J, et al: Cerebrospinal fluid analysis and clinical outcome of eight dogs with eosinophilic meningoencephalomyelitis, J Vet Intern Med 3(3):167–174, 1989.
34. Windsor RC, Sturges BK, Vernau KM, et al: Cerebrospinal fluid eosinophilia in dogs, J Vet Intern Med 23:275–281, 2009.
35. Bathen-Noethen A, Carlson R, Menzel D, et al: Concentrations of acute-phase proteins in dogs with steroid responsive meningitis-arteritis, J Vet Intern Med 22(5):1149–1156, 2008.
36. Schwartz M, Carlson R, Tipold A: Selective CD11a upregulation on neutrophils in the acute phase of steroid-responsive meningitis-arteritis in dogs, Vet Immunol Immunopathol 126(3/4):248–255, 2008.
37. Tipold A, Jaggy A: Steroid responsive meningitis-arteritis in dogs: long-term study of 32 cases, J Small Anim Pract 35:311–316, 1994.
38. Tipold A, Schatzberg SJ: An update on steroid responsive meningitis-arteritis, J Small Anim Pract 51(3):150–154, 2010.
39. Lowrie M, Penderis J, Eckersall PD, et al: The role of acute phase proteins in diagnosis and management of steroid-responsive meningitis arteritis in dogs, Vet J 182(1):125–130, 2009.
40. Lowrie M, Penderis J, McLaughlin M, et al: Steroid responsive meningitis-arteritis: a prospective study of potential disease markers, prednisolone treatment, and long-term outcome in 20 dogs (2006-2008), J Vet Intern Med 23(4):862–870, 2009.

41. Brooks PN: Necrotizing vasculitis in a group of beagles, Lab Anim 18:285–290, 1984.
42. Harcourt RA: Polyarteritis in a colony of beagles, Vet Rec 102(24):519–522, 1978.
43. Snyder PW, Kazacos EA, Scott-Moncrieff JC, et al: Pathologic features of naturally occurring juvenile polyarteritis in beagle dogs, Vet Pathol 32(4):337–345, 1995.
44. Webb AA, Muir GD: The blood-brain barrier and its role in inflammation, J Vet Intern Med 14(4):399–411, 2000.
45. Greene CE, Breitschwerdt EB: Rocky Mountain spotted fever, murine typhus like disease, rickettsial pox, typhus, and Q fever. In Greene CE, editor: Infectious diseases of the dog and cat, ed 3, St Louis, 2006, Elsevier.
46. Thomas WB: Hydrocephalus in dogs and cats, Vet Clin North Am Small Anim Pract 40(1):143–159, 2010.
47. Coates JR, Axlund TW, Dewey CW, et al: Hydrocephalus in dogs and cats, Compend Contin Educ Pract Vet 28(2):136–145, 2006.
48. Tipold A: Diagnosis of inflammatory and infectious diseases of the central nervous system in dogs: a retrospective study, J Vet Intern Med 9(5):304–314, 1995.
49. Fecteau G, George LW: Bacterial meningitis and encephalitis in ruminants, Vet Clin North Am Food Anim Pract 20:363–377, 2004.
50. Mellema LM, Samii VF, Vernau KM, et al: Meningeal enhancement on magnetic resonance imaging in 15 dogs and 3 cats, Vet Radiol Ultrasound 43(1):10–15, 2002.
51. Tipold A, Pfister H, Zurbriggen A, et al: Intrathecal synthesis of major immunoglobulin classes in inflammatory diseases of the canine CNS, Vet Immunol Immunopathol 42(2):149–159, 1994.
52. Tipold A, Vandevelde M, Zurbriggen A: Neuroimmunological studies in steroid-responsive meningitis-arteritis in dogs, Res Vet Sci 58(2):103–108, 1995.
53. Barber RM, Li Q, Diniz PPVP, et al: Evaluation of brain tissue or cerebrospinal fluid with broadly reactive polymerase chain reaction for *Ehrlichia*, *Anaplasma*, Spotted Fever Group *Rickettsia*, *Bartonella*, and *Borrelia* species in canine neurological diseases (109 cases), J Vet Intern Med 24(2):372–378, 2010.
54. Ciribassi J: Feline hyperesthesia syndrome, Compend Contin Educ Pract Vet (116):121, 2009.
55. Shell LG: Feline hyperesthesia syndrome, Feline Pract 22(6):10, 1994.
56. Luescher UA, McKeown DB, Halip J: Stereotypic or obsessive-compulsive disorders in dogs and cats, Vet Clin North Am Equine Pract 21(2):401–413, 1991.
57. Saxena S, Bota RG, Brody AL: Brain-behavior relationships in obsessive-compulsive disorder, Semin Clin Neuropsychiatry 6:82–101, 2001.
58. March PA, Fischer JR, Potthoff A, et al: Electromyographic and histological abnormalities in epaxial muscles of cats with feline hyperesthesia syndrome, J Vet Intern Med 13(3):238, 1999:(abstract).
59. Overall KL: Pharmacologic treatments for behavior problems, Vet Clin North Am Small Anim Pract 27(3):637–665, 1997.
60. Benson GJ, Thurmon JC: Species difference as a consideration in alleviation of animal pain and distress, J Am Vet Med Assoc 191(10):1227–1230, 1987.
61. Jenkins WL: Pharmacologic aspects of analgesic drugs in animals: an overview, J Am Vet Med Assoc 191(10):1231–1240, 1987.
62. Mathews KA: Non-steroidal anti-inflammatory analgesics: a review of current practice, J Vet Emerg Crit Care 12:89–97, 2002.
63. Platt SR, Abramson CJ, Garosi LS: Administering corticosteroids in neurologic diseases, Compend Contin Educ Pract Vet 27:210–221, 2005.
64. Behrend EN, Kemppainen RJ: Glucocorticoid therapy. Pharmacology, indications, and complications, Vet Clin North Am Small Anim Pract 27(2):187–213, 1997.
65. Curry SL, Cogar SM, Cook JL: Nonsteroidal antiinflammatory drugs: a review, J Am Anim Hosp Assoc 41:298–309, 2005.
66. Eroglu C, Allen NJ, Susman MW, et al: Gabapentin receptor alpha2 delta-1 is a neuronal thrombospondin receptor responsible for excitatory CNS synaptogenesis, Cell 139(2):380–392, 2009.
67. Janssens LAA: Acupuncture treatment for canine thoraco-lumbar disk protrusions. A review of 78 cases, Vet Med Small Anim Clin 78(10):1580–1585, 1983.
68. Martin BB Jr, Klide AM: Use of acupuncture for the treatment of chronic back pain in horses: stimulation of acupuncture points with saline solution injections, J Am Vet Med Assoc 190(9):1177–1180, 1987.
69. Olby N, Halling KB, Glick TR: Rehabilitation for the neurologic patient, Vet Clin North Am Small Anim Pract 35:1389–1409, 2005.
70. Millis DL: Physical therapy and rehabilitation of neurologic patients. In Bonagura JD, Twedt DC, editors: Kirk's current veterinary therapy XIV, St Louis, 2008, Elsevier.
71. Sherman J, Olby NJ: Nursing and rehabilitation of the neurological patient. In Platt SR, Olby NJ, editors: BSAVA manual of canine and feline neurology, ed 3, Gloucester, UK, 2004, BSAVA.
72. Kathmann I, Cizinauskas S, Doherr MG, et al: Daily controlled physiotherapy increases survival time in dogs with suspected degenerative myelopathy, J Vet Intern Med 20:927–932, 2006.
73. Steiss JE, Levine D: Physical agent modalities, Vet Clin North Am Small Anim Pract 35:1317–1333, 2005.
74. Swaim SF, Hanson RR Jr, Coates JR: Pressure wounds in animals, Compend Contin Educ Pract Vet 18(3):203–219, 1996.

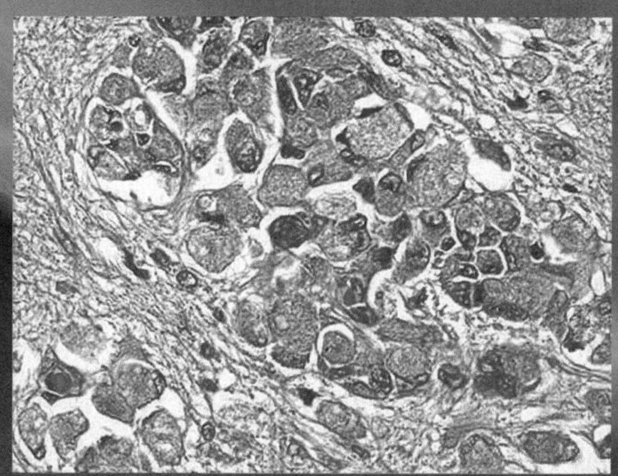

CHAPTER 15

Systemic or Multifocal Signs

There are many inflammatory, infectious, and degenerative diseases that produce multifocal central nervous system (CNS) signs and often simultaneous systemic disease. These disorders are categorized as multifocal, systemic, or diffuse diseases. Initially, some of these diseases may start with focal CNS signs, but they progress to affect other areas.

LESION LOCALIZATION

The key to recognition of these diseases is a neurologic examination that indicates the involvement of two or more parts of the nervous system that are not closely related anatomically. The most obvious example is an abnormality in both the brain and the spinal cord. All the possible combinations of signs of diffuse or multifocal diseases are too extensive to list, but Box 15-1 lists some of the more common ones.

Anytime abnormalities identified on the neurologic examination cannot be attributed to a single lesion, a multifocal neuroanatomic localization should be made. Etiologically, this group of diseases becomes more likely.

DISEASES

The major disease categories that produce systemic or multifocal signs are degenerative, metabolic, nutritional, inflammatory, toxic, and sometimes neoplastic and vascular disorders.

Diseases that are primarily skeletal in origin are mentioned but not discussed. Neoplastic and vascular disorders of the brain are further discussed in Chapter 12. Asymmetry often is associated with inflammatory, immune-mediated, neoplastic, and ischemic disorders. Diffuse and symmetric involvement is seen with degenerative, metabolic, and toxic disorders. The acute or chronic onset and the rate of progression may be of some help in establishing the diagnosis (Table 15-1).

Degenerative Diseases

Many degenerative diseases that are systemic or multifocal are either congenital and/or hereditary. However, the cause is still unknown for some of the spongiform and metabolic encephalopathies and dysautonomia. Congenital refers to a disease or malformation present at birth. It includes conditions that may be genetic or a result of exposure to toxins, malnutrition, or infection in utero. Not all congenital conditions are inherited and conversely, not all inherited conditions are congenital. The congenital malformations are discussed in Chapter 12 for the cerebrum and in Chapter 8 for the cerebellum.

Breed predilection and stereotypic clinical presentation for many of these disorders often suggest an inherited basis. Careful study of affected litters and pedigrees is required to determine the inheritance pattern. Selection processes used by breeders include inbreeding, linebreeding, and outcrossing. While selecting for a particular trait, inbreeding and linebreeding practices result in a reduction of genetic variability and an increase in homozygous and recessive traits. Simple inheritance (Mendelian) patterns have served as the basis for determining modes of inheritance of many genetic disorders. Many of these hereditary diseases have an autosomal recessive inheritance pattern. Dominant traits are more easily eliminated from the breeding pool of a breed by not breeding affected dogs. Determining inheritance pattern is more difficult for polygenetic and complex traits. Polygenetic inheritance refers to when proper development relies on sequential activation of genes or for traits of variable penetrance that result in a variety of phenotypes for a given genotype. Complex traits are determined by the interaction between environment and polygenetic predisposition. Having an understanding of the hereditary basis for these degenerative diseases is important because (1) they are genetic disorders and can be eliminated by selective breeding; (2) they may be confused with conditions of nongenetic origin, such as viral diseases; and (3) they can serve as excellent models of similar human diseases.

Differential Diagnosis

Many of these diseases have a similar clinical history and course. Clinical signs of conditions like the lysosomal storage diseases and some metabolic encephalopathies are delayed until the animal is older (usually within a few months after birth) because of the time required for build up of byproduct. Abiotrophies, disorders of premature neuronal degeneration, and other degenerative diseases affecting the axons and myelin

BOX 15-1

Examples of Systemic or Multifocal Signs

Lower motor neuron (LMN) signs (more than one location, may include cranial nerves): diffuse LMN diseases, polyneuropathy (see Chapter 7)
Brain and spinal cord signs: pelvic limb paresis and seizures
Systemic disease and CNS signs: fever, anorexia, ataxia, or seizures
Generalized pain: meningitis
Cerebral cortex and brainstem: cerebrum seizures and cranial nerve deficits, blindness, severe gait deficits, head tilt, circling
Forebrain: blindness with normal pupils (may be seen with brain swelling, hydrocephalus) (see Chapter 11)
Cerebellum and paresis: head tremor, ataxia, severe gait deficits, paresis
Ascending paralysis: pelvic limb paresis progressing to tetraparesis (focal cervical spinal cord lesion must be ruled out)

TABLE 15-1

*Etiology of Systemic Diseases**

Classification	Acute Progressive	Chronic Progressive
Degenerative	Myelinolytic disorders	Storage disease, abiotrophy
Metabolic	Hepatic encephalopathy Hypoglycemia Endocrine disease Renal disease	Hepatic encephalopathy Endocrine disease
Neoplastic	Metastatic	Primary metastatic
Nutritional	Methionine deficiency	Hypovitaminosis Hypervitaminosis
Inflammatory	Infectious and noninfectious	Infectious (usually viral) and noninfectious
Toxic	Most toxins	Heavy metals Other toxins, chrome exposure

Modified with permission from Oliver JE, Hoerlein BF, Mayhew IG: Veterinary neurology, Philadelphia, 1987, WB Saunders.

can manifest signs within a few months or late in life. These disorders are often insidious and progressive. However, some diseases such as the storage and myelin disorders can have an acute onset once the neuron or myelin reaches a critical threshold of dysfunction.

The findings on neurologic examination may indicate a predominance of signs referable to the forebrain, cerebellum, spinal cord, or neuromuscular junction. These findings, and the age and breed of the animal, should suggest a small number of possibilities. Early in the disease course, neuronal cell body diseases often can be differentiated from demyelinating diseases. Proprioceptive positioning is commonly affected in demyelinating diseases but is rarely involved in the early stages of neuronal disease. Neuronal cell body, diseases (storage disease, abiotrophy) are more likely to have forebrain or cerebellar involvement. Axonal and myelin diseases of the sensory and motor tracts of the spinal cord are more likely to have general proprioceptive (GP) ataxia and paresis of an upper motor neuron (UMN) type. If the nerve or neuronal cell body is involved, signs of LMN weakness predominate. Weakness is not a predominant feature of pure demyelinating or cerebellar disorders. However, limb and whole body tremor is a feature of myelin and cerebellar diseases.

The degenerative diseases also must be differentiated from inflammatory (infectious and noninfectious), neoplastic, and toxic disorders. Specific diagnostic tests are available for most of these conditions and are discussed later in this chapter.

This section on degenerative diseases will focus on those that are multifocal (storage disorders) or have an unknown etiology. The metabolic encephalopathies that are of primary brain origin are discussed in Chapter 12. Other degenerative disorders involving the spinal cord and brain (myeloencephalopathies), which predominate as spinal cord diseases, are discussed in Chapters 6 and 7. Those that present primarily with LMN signs that involve the axon, myelin, and the neuronal cell body (motor neuron) are discussed also in Chapter 7. Diseases that are discussed in this chapter include (1) storage disorders, (2) abiotrophies, (3) multiple system degenerations, and (4) degenerative disorders that are of unknown cause.

Storage Disorders

Storage disorders are characterized pathologically by the accumulation of metabolic products in cells (Table 15-2 and Figure 15-1).

A genetically based deficiency of a key enzyme causes accumulation of the product in neurons, glia, or other cell types. The effects of the disease may be caused by the accumulation of the product or may be a direct result of the metabolic disturbance.[1] Because the clinical signs and the progression of the disease depend on the pathologic process, many of the conditions present in a similar fashion with multifocal CNS signs and sometimes also with peripheral neuropathy. Two groups are commonly recognized: neuronal storage diseases, in which the product accumulates in neurons, and leukodystrophies.[2] In general, leukodystrophy refers to inherited conditions of younger animals in which myelin synthesis or function is defective and cannot be maintained and may include storage disease pathogenesis. Globoid cell leukodystrophy is a storage disease caused by a deficiency of galactocerebroside activity, resulting in intracellular accumulation of a metabolite toxic to myelin-forming oligodendrocytes and Schwann cells (Figure 15-2).

The storage byproducts usually can be found in the lysosomes of neurons. Lysosomal storage diseases are characterized by accumulation of sphingolipids, glycolipids, oligosaccharides, or mucopolysaccharides within lysosomes.[3] The neuronal ceroid lipofuscinoses involve the accumulation of hydrophobic proteins but the pathogenesis remains unclear (see Figure 15-1).[3]

The storage diseases are rare, but several have been reported in domestic animals.[2] Most have been recognized in specific breeds of dogs or cats.[3,4] Animals are usually normal at birth, but they fail to grow normally. Signs typically occur within the first few months of life but may be delayed until adulthood with some conditions such as some of the neuronal ceroid lipofuscinoses.[5] Many of the storage disorders affect multiple organs and regions of the nervous system. Others affect only the myelin and only neurologic signs occur. Often neurologic

TABLE 15-2

Lysosomal Storage Disorders in Domestic Animals

Disease Subgroup	Storage Disease (Human Disease)	Enzyme Deficiency	Species—Breed (age at onset)	Clinical Signs; Diagnosis	Inheritance	Reference
Glycoproteinoses						
	Fucosidosis	α-L-Fucosidase	C-*English springer spaniel* (6 mo-3 yr)	Cerebellar ataxia, behavioral change, dysphonia, dysphagia, seizures; DNA testing, enzyme assay	AR	215-219
	Mannosidosis (α-Mannosidosis)	α-D-mannosidase	F-DSH (7 mo), DLH, *Persian* (8 wk); B-Galloway, Murray gray, Aberdeen Angus (birth)	Cerebellar ataxia, tremor, corneal opacity, skeletal anomalies, neuropathy; B-cerebellar ataxia, aggressiveness; urine screening, enzyme assay, DNA testing	AR	220-226
	Mannosidosis (β-Mannosidosis)	β-D-Mannosidase	B-Salers; G-Anglo nubian (birth-1 yr)	Cerebellar ataxia, recumbency, skull and limb deformities; urine screening, enzyme assay	AR	227;228
	Lafora disease	α-Glucosidase	C-Beagle (5-9 mo), basset hound (3 yr), poodle (9-12 yr), wire-haired miniature *dachshund* (5-8 yr); F-DSH	Myoclonic seizures, dullness; muscle biopsy, DNA testing	AR	229-235
Oligosaccharidoses						
Glycogenoses						
	GSD type 1 (von Gierke disease)	Glucose-6-phosphatase	C-Silky terrier, *Maltese*, other toy breeds (weeks); F-DSH	Weakness, seizures, stupor; urine screening	AR?	236,237
	GSD type 2 (Pompe disease)	α-Glucosidase	C-Swedish Lapland dog (1.5 yr); F-DSH; B-beef shorthorn, Brahman (3-9 mo); O-Corriedale (6 mo)	Ataxia, muscle weakness, exercise intolerance, cardiac; muscle/liver biopsy, urine screening	AR	238-246
	GSD type 3 (Cori disease)	Amylo-1,6-glucosidase	C-German shepherd (2 mo), *curly-coated retriever (IIIA)* (1 yr)	Lethargy, exercise intolerance, organomegaly; muscle/liver biopsy, DNA testing	AR	247,248
	GSD type 4 (Andersen disease)	Branching enzyme	F-*Norwegian forest cat* (5 mo)	Cerebellar ataxia, muscle weakness, tremor, neuromuscular, organomegaly; muscle biopsy, enzyme assay, DNA testing	AR	249-251
	GSD type 5	Myophosphorylase	B-Charolais (weeks)	Exercise intolerance	AR	252
	GSD type7 (Tarui disease)	Phosphofructose kinase	C-*English springer spaniel* (8-12 mo)	Exercise intolerance	AR	253,254
Mucolipidosis						
	Mucolipidosis II (I-cell disease)	N-acetylglucosamine-1-phosphotransferase	F-*DSH*	Facial dysmorphism, dullness, retinal, ataxia; DNA testing	Unknown	255,256

Sphingolipidoses						
	GM1-gangliosidosis type 1 (Norman-Landing disease)	β-D-Galactosidase	C-Beagle cross (4-7 mo), Portuguese water dog (4-5 mo), English springer spaniel (4-5 mo), *Alaskan husky, Shiba dog*; F-*DSH* (2-3 mo); B-Friesian (birth); O-Coopworth Romney (1 mo), Suffolk (4 mo)	C, F-Cerebellar ataxia, corneal clouding, tremor, seizures, paralysis, skeletal, facial dysmorphism; B, O-ataxia, recumbency; enzyme assays, DNA testing	AR	257-264
	GM1-gangliosidosis type 2 (Derry disease)	β-D-Galactosidase	F-Siamese, Korat (7 mo), DSH; O-Suffolk (4-6 mo)	Same; O-rapid progression	AR	265-267
	GM2-gangliosidosis (Tay-Sachs disease) (Variant B)	β–N-acetyl hexosaminidase A (α-subunit)	C-German shorthair pointer (6-12 mo)	Cerebellar ataxia; urine screening; enzyme assay	Unknown	268,269
	GM2-gangliosidosis (Sandhoff disease) (Variant O)	β–N-acetyl hexosaminidase B (β-subunit)	C-Golden retriever; toy poodle, F-*DSH-Japan, Korat, Burmese-Europe* (2-3 mo); S-Yorkshire	Same; S-cerebellar ataxia, weakness	Unknown	270-274
	GM2AB-gangliosidosis (Bernheimer-Seitelberger disease) (Variant AB)	GM2 activator protein deficiency	C-Japanese spaniel (18 mo); F-*Korat* (18 mo)	Same	Unknown	275,276
	Galactosialidosis	Galactosialidosis with α-neuraminidase	C-Schipperke (5 yr)	Cerebellar ataxia	Unknown	278
	Glucocerebrosidosis (Gaucher disease)	β-D-Glucocerebrosidase	C-Sydney silky dog (6-8 mo); O-unknown; S-unknown	Cerebellar ataxia; enzyme assay; biopsy	AR(S)	279-281
	Globoid cell leukodystrophy (Krabbe disease)	β-D-galactosyl ceramidase (accumulation of psychosine)	C-*West Highland white terrier* (2-5 mo), *Cairn terrier* (2-5 mo), beagle (4 mo), poodle (2 yr), basset hound (1.5-2 yr), blue tick hound (4 mo), pomeranian (1.5 yr), *Irish setter* (6 mo); F-DSH, DLH (5-6 wk); O-Dorset (4-18 mo)	Cerebellar ataxia, tremor, paraparesis, neuropathy; muscle/nerve biopsy, enzyme assay; DNA testing	AR or unknown	282-292
	Metachromatic leukodystrophy	Arylsulfatase A	F-DSH (2 wk)	Progressive motor dysfunction, seizures, opisthotonus, neuropathy	Unknown	293
	Sphingomyelinosis (Niemann-Pick disease type A)	Sphingomyelinase	C-Miniature poodle (2-4 mo); F-Balinese, Siamese (2-3 mo); B-Hereford (5 mo)	Cerebellar ataxia, tremor, paraparesis, neuropathy; biopsy	Unknown, AR-Siamese	294-298

Continued

TABLE 15-2

Lysosomal Storage Disorders in Domestic Animals—cont'd

Disease Subgroup	Storage Disease (Human Disease)	Enzyme Deficiency	Species—Breed (age at onset)	Clinical Signs; Diagnosis	Inheritance	Reference
	(Niemann-Pick disease type C)	Cholesterol esterification deficiency	C-Boxer (9 mo); F-*DSH* (2-4 mo)	C-Cerebellar ataxia, hepatomegaly, neuropathy; F-cerebellar ataxia, hepatic; enzyme testing, DNA testing	Unknown	299,300
Mucopolysaccharidoses						
	MPS I (Hurler syndrome)	α-L-iduronidase	C-Plott hound (3-6 mo), *mixed-breed* (3-6 mo); F-*DSH* (10 mo)	Growth retardation, facial deformity, lameness, corneal opacity, cardiac; urine screening, enzyme testing, DNA testing	AR	301,302
	MPS II	Iduronate-2-sulfate sulfatase	C-Labrador retriever (5 yr)	Cerebellar ataxia, exercise intolerance, corneal opacity, facial dysmorphism; urine screening, enzyme assay	AR	303
	MPS III (A, B, D)	Sulfamidase A-heparin sulphamidase B-N-acetyl-alpha-D-glucosaminidase C-acetyl-CoA-alpha-glucosaminide N-acetyltransferase D-N-acetylglucosamine 6-sulphatase	C- *Huntaway dog* (IIIA) (18 mo), *Schipperke (IIIB)* (3 yr) wire-haired dachshund (IIIA) (3); B-*breed unknown-Australia (IIIB)* (2 yr); G-nubian (IIID) (birth)	Cerebellar ataxia, tremor, retinal degeneration, corneal opacity; G-weakness; urine screening, enzyme assay, DNA testing	AR	304-312
	MPS VI (Maroteaux-Lamy disease)	N-acetylgalactosamine 4-sulfase (arylsulfatase B)	C-Miniature pinscher (6 mo); F-*Siamese cat*, DSH (4-7 mo)	Growth retardation, facial deformity, corneal opacity, spinal fusion; urine screening, enzyme testing, DNA testing	AR	313-315
	MPS VII (Sly syndrome)	β–D-glucouronidase	C-Mixed breed; F-*DSH*	C-Paraparesis, cardiac; F-growth retardation, facial deformity, corneal opacity, spinal fusion, cardiac; urine screening, enzyme testing, DNA testing	AR	316,317

Proteinoses Ceroid Lipofuscinoses (Batten Disease)				All-Visual deficits, cerebellar ataxia, myoclonus, seizures of varying degree; tissue biopsy (autofluorescence)		
	CLN 1	Palmitoyl protein thioesterase I	C-Dachshund (mo)		AR(S)	Katz ML personal communication
	CLN 2	Tripeptidyl-peptidase	C-*Dachshund* (4-5 mo)		AR	318
	CLN 4 (not confirmed)	Unknown	C-*Tibetan terrier* (4-6 yr)		AR	319,320
	CLN 5	Soluble lysosomal membrane protein	C-*Border collie* (2 yr); O-*borderdale* (15 mo); B-Devon (12 mo)		AR	321-323
	CLN 6	Endoplasmic reticulum membrane protein	C-Australian shepherd (1-2 yr) O-*South Hampshire* (3 mo), *Merino* (7 mo)		Unknown or AR (O)	324-327
	CLN 8	Membrane protein of the endoplasmic reticulum	C-*English setter* (2 yr)		AR	328,329
	CSTD	Cathepsin D	C-*American bulldog* (2-4 yr); O-*White Swedish landrace*		AR	330-332
	CLN4 (Kuf's disease)	Arylsulfatase G	C-*American Staffordshire terrier* (>1 yr variable)		AR	335,334
	Unknown		C-Australian cattle dog (1-2 yr), Australian shepherd (more than one NCL), Chihuahua (2 yr), cocker spaniel (1.5-6 yr), collie, dachshund (4.5 yr), dalmatian (6 mo-1 yr), golden retriever (2 yr), Japanese retriever (3 yr), Labrador retriever, miniature schnauzer, poodle, Polish lowland sheepdog (0.5-4.5 yr), saluki (2 yr), spitz, Welsh corgi (6-8 yr); F- Siamese cat, Japanese DSH, European DSH (<1 yr); B-beefmaster (12 mo), Devon (12 mo), Holstein (adult); O-Rambouillet (4 mo); G-nubian (4 mo); E-Icelandic × Peruvian paso		Unknown	335-356

Modified from Oliver JE, Hoerlein BF, Mayhew IG: Veterinary neurology, Philadelphia, 1987, WB Saunders, Table 6-1; Mayhew IG: Large Animal Neurology, Ames, IA, 2009 Wiley-Blackwell, Table 30-2.

AR, Autosomal recessive; *AR(S)*, autosomal suspect; *CLN*, ceroid lipofuscinosis; *CTSD*, cathepsin D gene; *GSD*, glycogen storage disease; *GM*, gangliosidosis; *MPS*, mucopolysaccharidosis. Breeds in italics signify mutation discovered; C, canine; *F*, feline; *B*, bovine; O, ovine; *S*, swine; *G*, goat; *E*, equine.

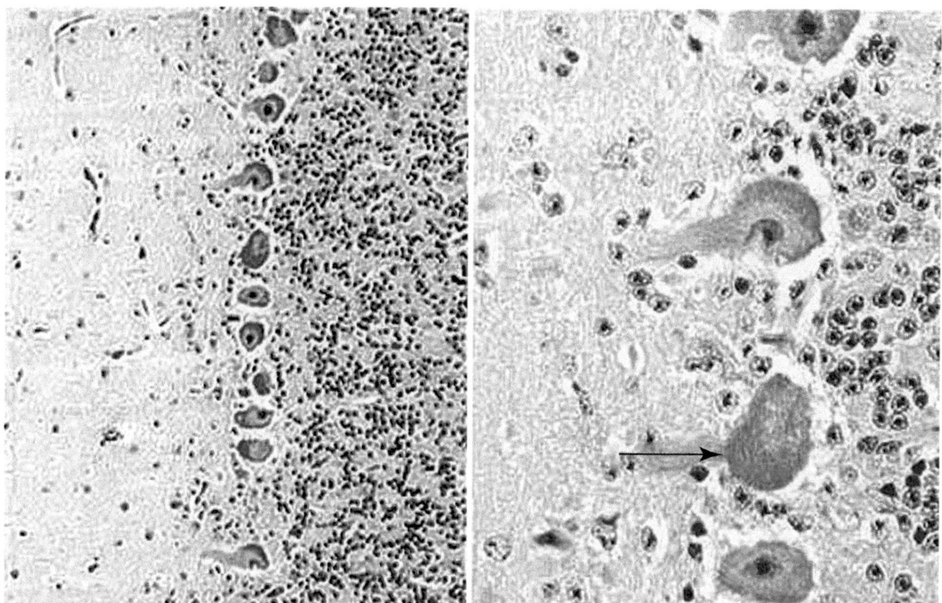

Figure 15-1 Bovine neuronal ceroid-lipofuscinosis. Luxol fast blue stain of the cerebellar cortex of a Devon cow with intense storage evident in Purkinje cells *(arrow)*. (Courtesy Cornell University College of Veterinary Medicine.)

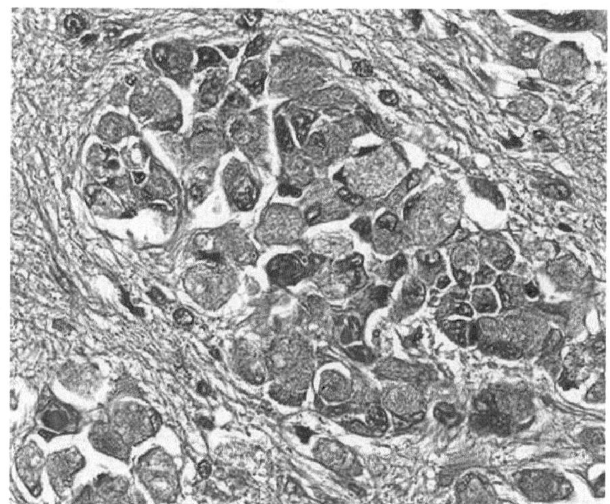

Figure 15-2 Canine globoid cell leukodystrophy. Note large globoid cells in white matter of cerebral cortex. The cells are filled with myelin breakdown products. (Courtesy Cornell University College of Veterinary Medicine.)

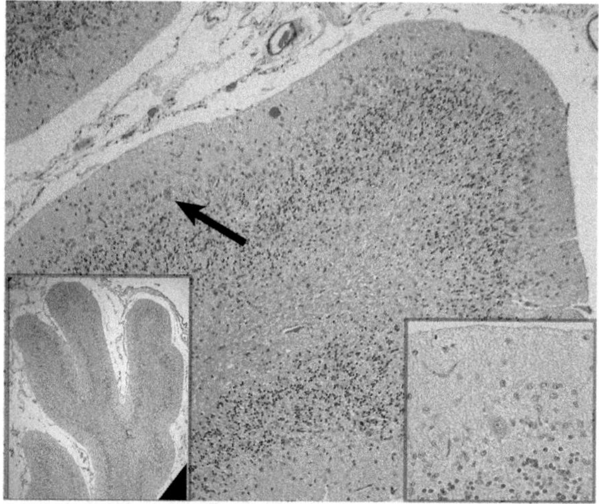

Figure 15-3 Folium from a dog with cerebellar cortical abiotrophy. The cerebellar cortex is almost devoid of Purkinje neurons. A single purkinje neuron is visible *(arrow)*. Subjectively there are few granule cell neurons than normal. Gliosis is also pressent (10× mag). *Right inset,* Higher magnification of a purkinje neuron. *Left inset,* Folia are smaller than normal.

signs include cerebellar ataxia, myelopathy, and encephalopathy. Cerebellar signs are often the first sign of storage diseases because of the complex integration of the fast conducting sensory and motor pathways (see Chapter 8).[4] The cerebellum also is particularly sensitive to disorders affecting myelin. Seizure events that occur with some storage disorders usually manifest at the end stage of the disease process. Storage disorders for which seizure activity is a predominant clinical feature include ceroid lipofuscinosis, glycoproteinoses, and leukodystrophies.[4]

Most of the diseases that have been studied have a recessive mode of inheritance, and so only a portion of the litter is affected (see Table 15-2). Lysosomal storage diseases will have signs in other organs including the retina. Skeletal and facial malformations are prominent in the mucopolysaccharidoses. In general, lysosomal storage disorders tend to be slowly progressive and lead to the animal's death.[4] Enzyme replacement, small molecule, gene, and cell-based therapies may have value in some conditions and have only been used experimentally in affected animals.[3,6] Genetic testing may be available for some of these disorders. Colonies of animals for some of these diseases have been established at research institutions.

Abiotrophies and Other Degenerative Diseases

The normal neuron is not capable of dividing and reproducing itself but has the capacity to survive for the life of the animal. Abiotrophy is a process by which cells develop normally but later degenerate due to an intrinsic cellular defect.[7] The degeneration of the neuronal cell body can primarily involve the neurons of the cerebellum, cerebrum, nerve, or multiple systems (Figure 15-3; see Chapters 7 and 8).

The multisystem disorders are further characterized as to the primary site of the degenerative process—cell body, axon, myelin, and so forth that also involve other anatomic regions of the CNS or the peripheral nervous system (PNS). Clinical signs relate to the predominant region of the nervous system affected. The motor neuron degenerations are rare and usually occur in young growing animals with an insidious and progressive clinical disease course of neuromuscular weakness and generalized LMN signs (see Chapter 7). Myelin disorders cause ataxia and tremor that progresses to paresis. Diffuse myelinopathies occur with inherited, metabolic, and toxic disorders. Primary cerebellar cortical degeneration refers to degeneration and loss of Purkinje cells and/or granule cells. Pathologic processes of cerebellar degeneration are classified microscopically as atrophy, abiotrophy, and transsynaptic neuronal degeneration. *Atrophy,* a term that lacks specificity, refers to loss of cerebellar mass often as a result of a degenerative process (Figure 15-4).[2,8]

Cerebellar degenerative disorders cause clinical signs of cerebellar ataxia and intention tremor (see Chapter 8). The progression of these abiotrophies and degenerative processes is generally slow (over months) but unrelenting. Like the storage diseases, they are rare, usually inherited, and in most instances eventually fatal. The course of disease is usually insidious but can be rapid.

Multisystem Neuronal Degenerations. These disorders often first cause cerebellar cortical degeneration and later involve other neuronal populations. A multisystem degeneration in rottweilers characterized by neuronal vacuolation has been recognized in young rottweiler dogs.[9] Affected dogs develop progressive GP ataxia, tetraparesis, cerebellar dysfunction, and laryngeal paralysis. Intracytoplasmic vacuoles are prominent in the cerebellar nuclei and other brainstem nuclei and ganglia. There is bilaterally symmetric degeneration in the spinal cord. Young Cairn terriers show a progressive GP ataxia, tetraparesis, and cerebellar signs.[10] Histopathology reveals neuron degeneration in the spinal cord, brainstem, and thalamus, and degenerative changes in the tracts of the spinal cord and brainstem. A multisystem degeneration recognized in young cocker spaniels manifests cerebellovestibular and forebrain signs.[11] Histopathology shows widespread neuronal degeneration in the cerebellum and brain with presence of swollen axons. Recently, a multisystem degeneration has been described in golden retrievers that show tremor, progressive tetraparesis, and generalized LMN signs.[12] The spinal cord had changes consistent with axonopathy; there was loss of cranial nerve motor nuclei; and nerves had evidence of Wallerian degeneration.

Multisystem degenerations also involve the basal ganglia, such as the caudate nucleus and substantia nigra, that cause movement disorders similar to Huntington and Parkinson disease in humans. These disorders have been recognized in Kerry blue terriers and Chinese crested dogs.[13,14] In these breeds, cerebellar ataxia begins between 3 and 6 months of age. As the basal nuclei degenerate, affected dogs have increasing difficulty initiating movements and maintaining balance. These disorders are autosomal recessive and have been linked to a locus on chromosome 1.[14]

Dysautonomia. In veterinary medicine, the term *dysautonomia* refers to acute or subacute idiopathic panautonomic failure involving both the parasympathetic and sympathetic systems. Dysautonomia is also described in Chapters 3, 9, and 11. It is a progressive degenerative disease of the ganglia of the autonomic nervous system. The general somatic efferent system is not affected except for involvement of the anal sphincter. Dysautonomia was first recognized in horses in Scotland (grass sickness) and then described in cats in the United Kingdom and Europe in the early 1980s.[15,16] Dysautonomia was first described in dogs from southwest Missouri and

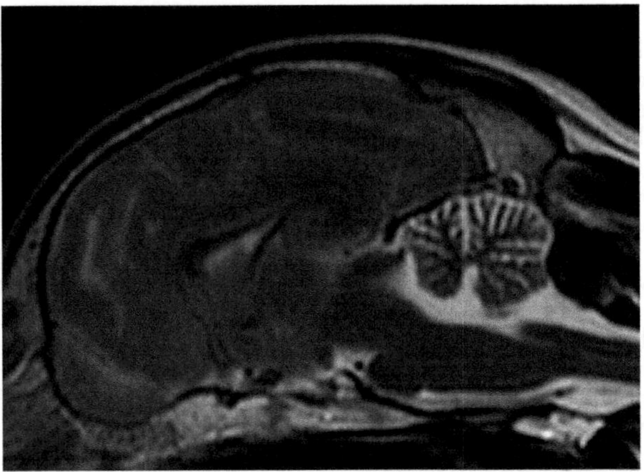

Figure 15-4 Sagittal T2W MRI from the dog in Figure 15-3. The cerebellum is small. There is atrophy of the folia as evidenced by increase amount of cerebrospinal fluid overlying the folia as well as within the fourth ventricle.

Wyoming in 1988 and continues to be reported in Missouri and surrounding states.[17-19] The etiology is still unknown but a toxico-infectious etiology resulting from *Clostridium botulinum* type CD has been proposed in horses. Acute or subacute autonomic neuropathy of people is similar to the animal forms and studies suggest an immune-mediated basis for this disease.

In dogs, dysfunction of the parasympathetic nervous system predominates, although signs related to the sympathetic nervous system may be present as well.[20] The disease is most common in young adult free-roaming dogs (median age of 18 months) and tends to affect medium- to large-breed dogs. Many affected dogs are from rural environments but the disease has been documented in dogs maintained strictly in kennel environments. The peak incidence in Missouri is from late winter to early spring. The following clinical signs develop and are progressive over 2 to 3 weeks. All signs may not be present in all dogs.

- Dysuria, distended urinary bladder: The pelvic nerve is a parasympathetic nerve that innervates the detrusor muscle. Detrusor muscle dysfunction is a common finding.
- Mydriasis and absent pupillary light reflexes: Pupillary constriction is a function of the parasympathetic fibers contained in the oculomotor nerves.
- Elevated third eyelid: This sign is present in about 50% of cases, suggesting some dysfunction of the sympathetic nervous system.
- Dry mucous membranes, decreased tear production: Dry mouth, nose, and eyes are common findings. Secretions are largely the function of the parasympathetic nervous system.
- Vomiting, regurgitation: Megaesophagus is a common finding. The vagus nerve (parasympathetic) innervates the esophagus and stomach and plays a major role in esophageal and gastric motility.
- Decreased anal (perineal) reflex: The external anal sphincter is innervated by the pudendal nerve, a general somatic efferent nerve. This is the only sign of somatic dysfunction.
- Intestinal ileus: Distention of the intestinal tract is a less common finding. Constipation and diarrhea may be seen in some dogs.
- Weight loss, muscle wasting, and decreased appetite
- Gait, postural reactions, and spinal reflexes are not affected

Dysautonomia also has been reported in cats but no clear risk factors have been identified.[21] Cats have clinical signs similar to dogs.

Dysautonomia should be suspected from the cluster of clinical signs. Although myasthenia gravis and botulism cause some of these signs, the presence of weakness in the skeletal muscles is not observed in dysautonomia. One of the best clinical procedures for confirming dysautonomia is to demonstrate denervation hypersensitivity to the pupils. Pilocarpine ophthalmic solution (1%) is diluted to a concentration of 0.05% with normal saline. One to two drops are placed in one eye and the pupils are observed every 15 minutes. Dogs with dysautonomia have rapid pupillary constriction compared with normal dogs who either do not respond at all or show delayed responses. If no response is seen in 90 minutes, the test is repeated with 1% pilocarpine. Unless parasympatholytic drugs (atropine) or toxins are present, rapid pupillary constriction should occur. Lack of innervation causes an upregulation of the postsynaptic receptors with denervation supersensitivity in neurotransmission.

Thoracic radiographs frequently show megaesophagus and abdominal radiographs reveal distention of the urinary bladder and sometimes intestinal ileus. Unless detrusor atony is present from prolonged detrusor paralysis, dogs may void urine in response to low doses of bethanechol.

No definitive treatment is available. Symptomatic therapy includes bethanechol, pilocarpine to increase tear production and to reduce photophobia from dilated pupils, metoclopramide to stimulate gastrointestinal motility, and frequent evacuation of the bladder. The mortality rate in canine dysautonomia is approximately 90%. There are isolated reports of dogs developing partial recovery.

Metabolic Disorders

Normal nervous system function depends on a closely regulated environment. Conversely, homeostasis is coordinated by the nervous system through the neuroendocrine, autonomic, and somatic systems. Systemic disorders altering homeostasis often have profound effects on the nervous system.

Hepatic Encephalopathy

Hepatic encephalopathy (HE) is a complex metabolic disorder resulting from abnormal liver function.

Pathophysiology. HE has been reported in four types of liver disease: (1) severe parenchymal liver damage, either acute or chronic (cirrhosis, neoplasia, toxicosis); (2) anomalous portal venous circulation (rare in large animals); (3) microvascular dysplasia, and (4) congenital urea-cycle enzyme deficiencies (rare).[22] Parenchymal liver diseases other than cirrhosis (fatty infiltration, chronic active hepatitis, and so forth) usually do not cause hepatic encephalopathy except in the terminal stages of the disease. Pyrrolizidine alkaloids in certain plants such as *Senecio* spp. and *Crotalaria* spp. cause parenchymal liver damage and hepatic encephalopathy in herbivores. Parenchymal disease severely reduces the capacity of the liver to perform its normal metabolic functions. Portosystemic venous shunts divert a significant portion of the portal blood past the liver into the vena cava. Potentially toxic substances that normally are absorbed from the gastrointestinal (GI) tract and detoxified in the liver enter the systemic circulation. Similar to portosystemic venous shunting, the pathophysiology in microvascular dysplasia involves shunting of portal blood into the systemic circulation but occurs within the liver vasculature on a microscopic level. Urea-cycle enzyme deficiencies prevent the metabolism of ammonia to urea.

The metabolic changes that cause the clinical syndrome of hepatic encephalopathy result from failure of the liver to (1) remove toxic products of gut metabolism and (2) synthesize factors necessary for normal brain function.[22] The exact cause of hepatic encephalopathy is unknown, but current theories of the pathogenesis include (1) ammonia as the primary putative neurotoxin, although other synergistic toxins may be involved; (2) disorders of aromatic amino acid metabolism resulting from alterations in monoamine neurotransmitters; (3) disorders of gamma-aminobutyric acid (GABA) or glutamate; and (4) increased cerebral concentrations of an endogenous benzodiazepine-like substance.[23] Ammonia is probably the most important toxic substance, although the level of ammonia in the blood does not necessarily correlate with the severity of the CNS disturbance.[24]

Clinical Signs. Most animals with liver disease severe enough to produce HE have other clinical signs indicative of hepatic failure, such as vomiting, anorexia, weight loss, retarded growth, ascites, polyuria-polydipsia, and sometimes icterus. The neurologic signs are frequently worse after feeding, especially if high-protein food is given. The release of nitrogenous materials into the portal circulation exacerbates the signs. Obtundation that may progress to stupor and coma is the most common neurologic sign. Other signs of forebrain involvement such as behavior change, continuous pacing and head pressing, blindness, and seizures also are common. Frequently, the clinical picture is that of a waxing and waning diffuse encephalopathy. The postural reactions and reflexes are only minimally involved except when the animal is nearly comatose. The cranial nerves are not markedly affected except that vision may be impaired (decreased menace response with normal pupillary light reflexes [PLRs]). Ptyalism is common, especially in cats.

A variety of factors can precipitate the neurologic signs of HE in an animal with marginal liver function (Table 15-3).

Any source of protein in the digestive tract is a common cause. Hemorrhage in the gastrointestinal (GI) tract, constipation, or increased fatty acids also may precipitate a crisis. Alterations in fluids, electrolytes, or pH may increase

TABLE 15-3

Management of Hepatic Encephalopathy (HE)

Factors That Exacerbate HE	Management of HE
Increased dietary protein and fatty acids	Low-protein, low-fat diet
Bacterial production of ammonia in large bowel	Diet, antibiotics
Constipation leading to bacterial production of ammonia in large bowel	Diet, laxatives, enemas in acute lactulose
Gastrointestinal hemorrhage	Monitoring and treatment of ulcers, bleeding disorders, hookworms, whipworms
Hypokalemia, hypovolemia, alkalosis—aggravated by diuretics	Monitoring and correction of fluid and electrolyte imbalance, use of potassium-sparing diuretics with caution or not at all
Transfusion of stored blood	Use fresh blood
Sedatives, narcotics, anesthetics	Use depressant drugs with extreme caution (in lowest possible dosages), and monitor carefully
Infections, fever	Monitoring and supportive treatment

the blood and tissue ammonia levels. Decreased renal function reduces elimination of ammonia and other metabolites. Fever and infection cause increased tissue catabolism and increased nitrogen release. Stored blood for transfusions may have an excess of ammonia. Depressant drugs directly affect the brain and frequently are metabolized in the liver. The first evidence of hepatic dysfunction often is slow recovery from anesthesia. Diuretics used to treat ascites may cause HE through their effect on potassium, renal output of ammonia, and alkalosis.

A range of clinicopathologic abnormalities may be present, depending on the cause. Microcytosis with normochromic erythrocytes, ammonium biurate crystals in the urine, and lowered cholesterol, blood glucose, and vitamin K dependent clotting factor levels may be seen with liver failure. Frequently, serum albumin and serum urea nitrogen levels are low. Parenchymal disease often causes elevations in liver enzymes, such as serum alanine aminotransferase (ALT), aspartate aminotransferase (AST), and alkaline phosphatase (ALP). These enzymes usually are not elevated significantly in portacaval shunts.[25] Hepatic dysfunction may be confirmed with tests such as the ammonia tolerance test or preprandial and postprandial serum bile acids measured after a 12-hour fast.[26,27] Hepatic ultrasonography (US) is a sensitive indicator of liver size, but the definitive diagnosis of anomalous portal vein circulation requires US, contrast-enhanced radiography or computed tomography (CT), or nuclear medicine. Depending on the experience of the operator, abdominal US has a sensitivity of about 80% and a specificity of about 65% for the detection of extrahepatic portosystemic shunts (PSS). The sensitivity for detection of intrahepatic shunts is nearly 100%.[28] Radiocolloid scintigraphy using technetium-99m sulfur colloid (TcSC) is used to evaluate liver size and shape. Transcolonic TcSC procedures have been described for the diagnosis of macrovascular shunts in dogs, cats, and potbellied pigs.[29,30] Biopsy is required for confirmation of parenchymal disease.

The successful medical management of HE depends on the cause of the liver disorder and the degree of liver malfunction. Animals with marginal liver function may be managed by reducing the sources of nitrogenous products in the GI tract (see Table 15-3). A high-carbohydrate, low-fat, low-protein diet with high biologic value is indicated. If dietary management alone is inadequate, then oral, nonabsorbable antibiotics (such as neomycin) may be given to reduce the bacterial flora that split urea. Mild laxatives or lactulose (a nonabsorbable disaccharide) may be helpful.[31,32] In addition to its laxative effects, lactulose creates an acid environment in the colon that allows NH_3 to be trapped as NH_4^+ in the gut lumen.

Acute crises of hepatic encephalopathy require more vigorous treatment. Protein sources must be removed completely. Enemas and laxatives are used to remove all nitrogenous material from the GI tract. Sedative drugs, methionine, and diuretics are discontinued. Sources of GI hemorrhage are corrected if they are present. Administration of antibiotic aimed at altering the GI bacterial flora in an attempt to reduce ammonia production should be considered. Antibiotics can be given parenterally or as a retention enema in animals unable to receive oral medications. Dehydration, hypokalemia, and alkalosis are managed with intravenous (IV) fluid therapy. Renal output must be maintained to eliminate nitrogenous products. Oxygen therapy may be necessary, especially in cases of coma. The prognosis for herbivores with hepatic encephalopathy from pyrrolizidine toxicity is poor.

Specific treatment of the cause is instituted, if possible. Unfortunately, most chronic liver diseases and the urea-cycle enzyme deficiencies cannot be treated specifically. Portosystemic shunts may be corrected surgically if portal circulation to the liver is adequate. Partial occlusion of the shunt may be effective. Seizures and neurologic complications following PSS attenuation have been well documented.[33,34] Potential risk factors for neurologic complications include older dogs and dogs with single extrahepatic and portoazygos shunts.[35] For details of the management of hepatic encephalopathy, the reader should consult the references.[23,24,32,35,36-39]

Ketonemic Syndromes

Ketosis. These diseases occur primarily in ruminants and are characterized by hypoglycemia and the accumulation of ketones in body fluids. Conditions that have been recognized include bovine ketosis (acetonemia) and pregnancy toxemia of cattle, sheep, and goats. Unlike most monogastric animals, ruminants produce most of their glucose supplies from the gluconeogenesis of volatile fatty acids (acetic, propionic, and butyric acids). Nearly 50% of the glucose in a cow is normally derived from dietary propionic acid that is converted to glucose in the gluconeogenic pathway. Reduction of propionic acid production in the rumen can result in hypoglycemia and the subsequent mobilization of free fatty acids and glycerol from fat stores. The liver has a limited ability to use these fatty acids because the levels of oxaloacetate are low. Acetyl coenzyme A therefore is not incorporated into the tricarboxylic acid cycle and is converted into the ketone bodies acetoacetate and ß-hydroxybutyrate. When the production of ketones by the liver exceeds peripheral use, pathologic ketosis results.

Both ketosis and primary hypoglycemia are involved in the development of the clinical signs. The most common signs include depression, partial to complete anorexia, weight loss, and decreased milk production. The neurologic signs present in some cows include ataxia, apparent blindness, salivation, tooth grinding, excessive licking, muscle twitching, head pressing, and hyperesthesia. Cows may charge blindly if they are disturbed.

The diagnosis of bovine ketosis is based on the presence of elevated ketone levels in blood and milk with concomitant hypoglycemia. The odor of ketones may be perceived on the breath and in the urine. The immediate therapy is an IV injection of glucose, followed by oral administration of 125 to 250 g of propylene glycol twice a day. Corticosteroids are also beneficial in cows that are not septic. Cows with severe neurologic signs can be treated with 2 to 8 g of chloral hydrate orally twice a day for 3 to 5 days.

Pregnancy/Toxemia. Pregnancy toxemia is a condition that is closely related pathophysiologically to bovine ketosis. It occurs in ewes during the last 6 weeks of pregnancy, when the demand for glucose by developing fetuses is large. Pregnancy toxemia occurs in pastured or housed beef cows during the last 2 months of pregnancy. Overweight cows or those bearing twin calves are especially susceptible. In ewes and cows, the basic cause is nutrition insufficient to maintain normal blood glucose concentrations when fetal glucose demands are high. Hypoglycemia precipitates the ketosis, as has been described earlier in this section.

In sheep, clinical signs may develop in a flock and may extend for several weeks. Ewes become depressed and develop weakness, ataxia, and loss of muscle tone. Terminally, recumbency and coma develop. Neuromuscular disturbances include fine muscle tremors of the ears and the lips. In some cases, seizures develop. "Stargazing" postures and grinding of the teeth are common. The neurologic signs in cattle include depression, excitability, and ataxia. The diagnosis of pregnancy toxemia is based on the history, clinical signs, and presence of ketosis and hypoglycemia.

In sheep, flock treatment consists of increasing the availability of glucose precursors in the diet or drenching affected ewes twice daily with 200 mL of a warm 50% glycerol solution. The anabolic steroid trenbolone acetate also is beneficial given in 30-mg doses administered intramuscularly (IM). Induction of parturition or fetal removal by cesarean section also may be needed to reduce the metabolic drain on the ewe. Cattle are treated by the method described for bovine ketosis. Pregnancy toxemia can be prevented by ensuring adequate nutrition during pregnancy.

Renal Failure

The terminal stages of renal failure may cause tetany or seizures. Chronic renal disease may be associated with vomiting, diarrhea, anorexia, muscle wasting, and weakness. Encephalopathy, polyneuropathy, and polymyopathy have been seen in humans with chronic renal disease, especially those receiving hemodialysis. Renal encephalopathy has been reported in cows and dogs.[40-42] Alterations in parathyroid hormone levels and electrolyte metabolism, especially calcium and potassium, may cause signs that are related to the nervous system (discussed later in this chapter). Parathyroid hormone can have a primary neurotoxic effect and secondarily cause hypercalcemia.

Endocrine Disorders

Endocrine disorders that affect electrolyte and glucose homeostasis may produce neurologic signs in affected animals. Hormonal excess or deficiency may affect the function of nerves or muscles directly. Pituitary lesions may cause signs of hormonal and forebrain dysfunction if the disease extends into the hypothalamus (Figure 15-5).

In this section, specific endocrine and metabolic diseases that produce prominent neurologic signs of weakness are discussed. Those that cause involuntary movements such as tetany or constant, repetitive myoclonus (tremor) are discussed in Chapter 10. Readers should seek other textbooks for in-depth descriptions of each disorder.

Many endocrine and metabolic diseases cause electrolyte disorders that result in weakness because they affect neuromuscular functions. With certain conditions, clinical signs improve with rest and are exacerbated by exercise. The term *episodic weakness* has been applied to this condition (see Chapter 7).

Hypocalcemia

Parturient Paresis. Parturient paresis, or milk fever, is a hypocalcemic metabolic disorder that occurs in mature dairy cows, sows, sheep, and, rarely, horses, usually within 48 hours of parturition. The affected cows are usually older than 5 years of age, and incidence is increased in the heavy milk producers and Jersey breed. Many dairy cows are marginally hypocalcemic at parturition, and any factor that decreases the metabolic adjustment to this hypocalcemia may cause paresis. Such factors include milk yield versus calcium mobilization from

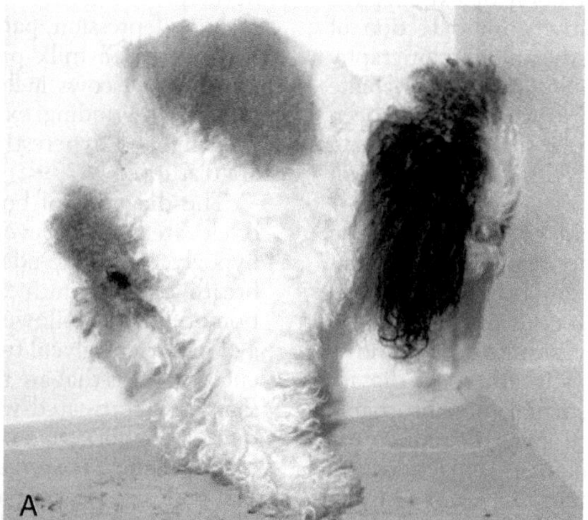

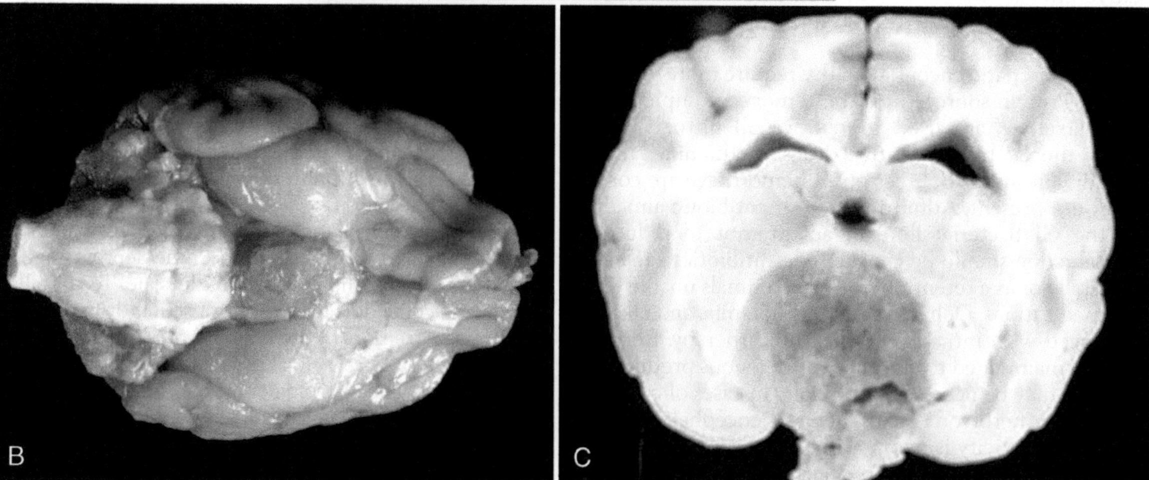

Figure 15-5 **A,** Older toy poodle showing head pressing behavior from pituitary macroadenoma. **B,** Brain from dog in **A.** Note mass at the base of the hypothalamus arising from the pituitary gland. **C,** Cross section of brain from **B.** Note the large mass invading the hypothalamus.

bone and gut, the ratios of calcium to phosphorus in the diet, anorexia and decreased intestinal motility, and dietary pH.

The onset of parturient paresis (stage 1) is often missed and is characterized by apprehension, anorexia, ataxia, and limb stiffness. Stage 2 is marked by progressive muscular weakness, recumbency, and depression. The head is usually turned to the flank, and an S-shaped curvature of the neck may be present. Other signs include dilated pupils, decreased pupillary light reflexes, reduced anal reflex, decreased defecation and urination, no ruminal motility, protrusion of the tongue, and frequent straining.

Stage 3 occurs in about 20% of cases and is characterized by lateral recumbency; severe depression or coma; subnormal temperature; a weak, irregular heart rate; and slow, irregular, shallow respirations. The pupils are dilated and unresponsive to light. Bloating may occur. Changes in serum ions include hypocalcemia, hypophosphatemia, and hypomagnesemia. With prolonged anorexia, serum sodium and potassium levels may decrease.

Intravenous calcium salts (Ca, 1 g per 45 kg of body weight) are usually effective. Calcium borogluconate is commonly used; a 25% solution contains 10.4 g of calcium per 500 mL. Milk fever can be prevented in susceptible cows or herds by the administration of vitamin D or its analogs or by the manipulation of the prepartum dietary calcium and phosphorus levels.

Dogs and Cats. Hypocalcemic syndromes are well documented in dogs and cats (also see Chapter 10).[43] In both species, primary hypoparathyroidism is a documented cause of chronic hypocalcemia. In cats, hypoparathyroidism is sometimes caused by inadvertent surgical resection of the parathyroid glands during thyroidectomy for the treatment of hyperthyroidism. Hypocalcemia may be associated with chronic renal disease in dogs and cats. It is the major biochemical abnormality in dogs with eclampsia and may be observed in animals receiving blood transfusions containing calcium-chelating anticoagulants. Enema solutions that contain phosphate may cause hypocalcemia in cats. Ionized hypocalcemia occurs in critically ill dogs; especially dogs with sepsis.[44]

When the total serum calcium concentration falls below 6 to 7 mg/dL (ionized <0.6 to 0.7 mmol/L), the clinical signs of hypocalcemia are likely to occur.[45] Hypocalcemia increases membrane hyperexcitability by decreasing the membrane threshold to more easily elicit an action potential. Tetanic muscle contractions are the most common clinical signs, but some dogs develop muscle weakness early in the disease. Hypocalcemia should be investigated when the total serum calcium concentration is less than 7.0 mg/dL and the serum albumin concentration is normal. Serum ionized calcium concentrations help to confirm the diagnosis. Once the diagnosis of hypocalcemia is confirmed, the underlying cause should be identified. The diagnosis of both eclampsia and iatrogenic hypoparathyroidism is usually obvious from the history and physical findings. Primary hypoparathyroidism may be confirmed through parathormone (PTH) assays conducted at specialized laboratories.

Animals experiencing seizures should be given 10% calcium gluconate solution IV at a dose of 0.5 to 1.5 mL/kg. The dosage should be slowly infused over a 10- to 20-minute period, and the heart rate and Q–T interval should be closely monitored with an electrocardiogram (ECG) recording. The calcium dose can be repeated every 6 to 8 hours as a bolus injection.

Oral maintenance therapy is instituted when the total serum calcium concentration is consistently less than 7.0 mg/dL. Calcium gluconate or calcium lactate is administered orally in doses of 1 to 4 g for dogs and 0.5 to 1.0 g for cats. In parathyroid deficiency, vitamin D therapy is required. Dihydrotachysterol (DHT) is a synthetic vitamin D that is active in the absence of PTH. The loading dose is 0.03 mg/kg daily administered orally for 3 to 4 days.[46] The maintenance dose is 0.01 to 0.02 mg/kg per day. Calcitriol is a vitamin D analog that is used to treat subacute and chronic hypocalcemia in dogs. The initial dose is 10 to 15 ng/kg twice a day for 3 to 4 days. Then the dose is reduced to 2.5 to 7.5 ng/mg twice a day. Animals should be closely monitored because hypercalcemia may be a complication of vitamin D therapy, especially when supplemental calcium salts are administered.[46]

Diabetes Mellitus

Diabetes mellitus may result in a variety of neurologic signs. Insulin deficiency results in failure of glucose transport into muscle and adipose tissue. An early sign of diabetes mellitus may be exercise intolerance and weakness. As insulin deficiency progresses, ketonemia develops from a marked increase in lipolysis and serum fatty acids. The ensuing metabolic acidosis results in depressed cerebral function that culminates in coma and death. In the untreated ketoacidotic dog or cat, hyperkalemia can cause flaccid muscles by depressing neuromuscular and cardiovascular functions. With therapy and correction of the acidosis, potassium ions reenter cells, and hypokalemia may be a complication that fosters muscle weakness and depression. In some animals, the hyperglycemia may be severe, even though acidosis is absent. This syndrome is called hyperosmolar nonketotic coma. Clinical signs result from the hyperosmolar effects of glucose on the cerebral cortex. Diabetic animals, especially cats, may also develop neuropathy with associated LMN signs (see Chapter 7).

The comatose diabetic animal is a difficult therapeutic challenge. The clinician must exercise great care in performing insulin, acid-base, electrolyte, and fluid therapy. Interested readers should consult other texts for an in-depth discussion of the diagnosis and management of the diabetic patient.

Hypothyroidism

Deficiencies of thyroxine result in a marked decrease in forebrain function and basal metabolic rate. Severely hypothyroid dogs may become obtunded or may appear dull and unresponsive. Coma also known as myxedema coma may occur in severe cases.[47-49] A very low voltage electroencephalogram (EEG) usually is seen. The forebrain signs improve dramatically after replacement thyroid medication. Polyneuropathy and myopathy have been recognized in dogs without the usual signs of hypothyroidism.[50,51] Clinical signs of polyneuropathy include laryngeal paralysis, vestibular dysfunction, and paresis involving various peripheral and cranial nerves (Figure 15-6).[50,52] Hypothyroidism may cause hyperlipidemia and atherosclerosis, conditions that are risk factors for CNS infarction.[50]

The fact that the animal has a polyneuropathy rather than a single problem may be defined by electromyography (EMG) or other electrodiagnostic tests. Measurement of free thyroxine and thyroid-stimulating hormone (TSH) concentrations or TSH response testing are necessary to confirm a diagnosis.[53,54] Many of these animals respond well to thyroid hormone supplementation, but weeks to months may be required for nerve function to recover.[55]

Hyperadrenocorticism

Hyperadrenocorticism (Cushing disease/syndrome) occurs in dogs, horses, and cats. In dogs and horses, pituitary adenomas that hypersecrete adrenocorticotropic hormone (ACTH) are the most common cause, but functional cortisol-secreting adrenal tumors also produce this syndrome in dogs and

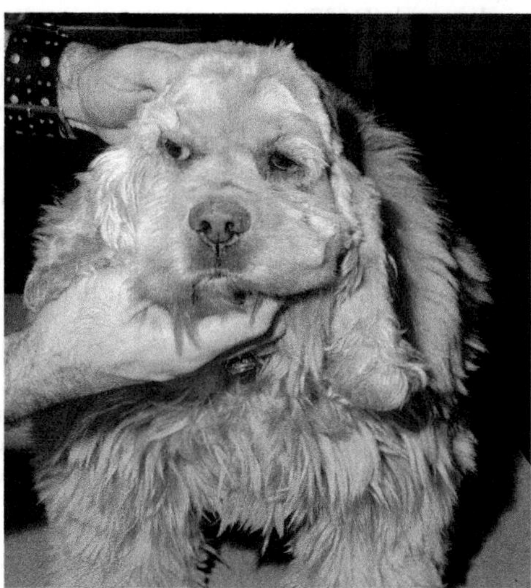

Figure 15-6 Older cocker spaniel dog with myxedematous hypothyroidism and facial nerve paralysis.

cats. The clinical signs are caused by the metabolic effects of hypercortisolemia. Generalized muscle weakness resulting from the catabolic effects of glucocorticoids is a common finding. Some dogs develop muscle degeneration, known as steroid-induced myopathy (see Chapters 7 and 10). This condition produces spontaneous muscle contractions (pseudomyotonia) and a stiff gait.

Pituitary adenomas (macroadenomas) may create neurologic signs by growth and expansion into the hypothalamus (see Figure 15-5, *A* through *C*).[56] Signs of pituitary macroadenomas are usually vague and include depression, confusion, circling, ataxia, and seizures.[57] Macroadenomas are more common in older, large-breed dogs. Pituitary tumors causing hyperadrenocorticisms may be present without causing neurologic signs.[57]

In dogs and cats, hyperadrenocorticism is confirmed with screening tests such as the low-dose dexamethasone suppression test, the ACTH stimulation test, or the urine cortisol:creatinine ratio. Pituitary-dependent hyperadrenocorticism is differentiated from functional adrenocortical tumors with the high-dose dexamethasone suppression test or ACTH assay or both. Similar tests and measurement of increased plasma ACTH concentrations are useful in the diagnosis of equine Cushing disease.[58] Abdominal US may also be helpful in the diagnosis of adrenal gland disease. Macroadenomas can be accurately diagnosed with MRI or CT.[59] In dogs, pituitary-dependent hyperadrenocorticism is usually treated medically with mitotane or trilostane.[60] Mitotane causes necrosis of the adrenal cortex, primarily the zona fasciculata and reticularis, and results in markedly decreased cortisol production. If the dosage is carefully monitored, aldosterone secretion is much less affected. Side effects include vomiting, diarrhea, anorexia, weight loss, and depression. Trilostane reduces synthesis of cortisol, aldosterone, and adrenal androgens. It also can be used in dogs, cats, and horses for pituitary and adrenal-dependent hyperadrenocorticism. It is well tolerated and has fewer side effects than mitotane. However, it may not produce long-term control of clinical signs. Readers are encouraged to consult internal medicine textbooks or veterinary drug handbooks for dosages and correct regimens for each drug. In dogs and cats with pituitary macrotumors, treatment also is directed at control of the pituitary mass (see Chapter 12). Adrenalectomy is recommended for adrenocortical neoplasia.

Hypercalcemic Syndromes

An increased concentration of serum calcium may result in neuromuscular, cardiovascular, and renal dysfunction. Hypercalcemia (>14 mg/dL) increases membrane threshold (making it more difficult to depolarize the membrane) resulting in hypoexcitability of the muscle membrane. CNS reflex and response activities and muscles become sluggish and weak. Hypercalcemia decreases the Q–T interval of the ECG and decreases myocardial function. Hypercalcemia impairs renal concentrating ability. In prolonged hypercalcemia, mineralization of soft tissue may occur. The syndrome of hypercalcemic nephropathy is well documented in animals and culminates in chronic renal failure. In dogs calcium levels above 12.5 mg/dL may result in hypercalcemic signs. Ionized calcium concentrations should be measured to confirm hypercalcemia. In some cases, muscle weakness may be worse during exercise.

Several causes of hypercalcemia exist, including primary hyperparathyroidism, paraneoplastic syndromes, vitamin D rodenticide intoxication, hypoadrenocorticism, and iatrogenic calcium therapy.[61] Primary hyperparathyroidism results from autonomously functioning parathyroid adenomas. These tumors secrete PTH in the presence of increasing serum calcium concentrations. Certain nonendocrine tumors such as lymphosarcoma, anal sac adenocarcinoma, squamous cell carcinoma, and thymoma secrete substances with PTH-like activity that results in hypercalcemia.[62-64] This syndrome is called the hypercalcemia of malignancy and is the most common cause for hypercalcemia in dogs and cats.[64] Rodenticides that contain analogues of vitamin D promote increased absorption of calcium and may produce hypercalcemia.[65]

The symptomatic therapy of hypercalcemia includes IV diuresis with 0.9% saline and furosemide. Corticosteroids also are beneficial because they promote the renal excretion of calcium. Clinicopathologic data for the diagnosis of lymphoma should be obtained before administration of corticosteroids as these drugs can induce remission confounding the diagnosis of lymphosarcoma. Salmon calcitonin may also be given to decrease serum calcium concentrations.[66]

Hyperkalemia

Increased serum concentrations of potassium (>6.5 mEq/L) decrease the resting membrane potential causing an increase in membrane excitability. Eventually, the muscle is unable to repolarize and the muscle fatigues. Excessive extracellular potassium causes cardiac flaccidity and decreases the conduction of impulses through the atrioventricular (AV) node. Thus, heart rate and cardiac output may be severely depressed. Hyperkalemia therefore manifests as generalized weakness that may worsen with exercise.

Adrenal Insufficiency. Hyperkalemia may occur secondary to severe acidosis; however, the usual cause is adrenal insufficiency. Adrenal insufficiency, a chronic immune-mediated adrenalitis, may result in aldosterone deficiency secondary to atrophy of the zona glomerulosa. Hyperkalemia and hyponatremia contribute to the typical signs of depression, anorexia, vomiting, diarrhea, weakness, bradycardia, and hypotension secondary to decreased cardiac output. The disease responds well to fluid therapy and replacement adrenocortical hormone therapy.

Hyperkalemic periodic paralysis. Hyperkalemic periodic paralysis (HPP), an episodic syndrome of muscular weakness and fasciculations, occurs in young, adult quarter horses (see Chapter 7).[67] This is an autosomal dominant inherited disease caused by a genetic mutation in the α-subunit of the equine adult sodium-channel gene.[68] It is associated with marked hyperkalemia without major acid-base imbalance or high serum activity of enzymes derived from muscle. The episodes occur spontaneously or can be induced by administration of potassium chloride orally. Electromyographic changes include fibrillation potentials, positive sharp waves, and complex repetitive discharges. Histologic changes in muscle are minimal but may include vacuolation of type-2b fibers or mild degenerative changes. Hyperkalemia or normokalemia may occur during episodes. Intravenous administration of calcium, glucose, or bicarbonate results in recovery. Administration of acetazolamide, 2.2 mg/kg orally every 8 to 12 hours, prevents the episodes. Decreasing the potassium content of the feed may also be effective. This can be done by feeding oat hay, feeding grain two to three times daily, and providing free access to salt.[67]

Hypokalemia

Decreased serum concentrations of potassium decrease the activity of skeletal muscle because the membranes are hyperpolarized. In other words, decreased extracellular potassium causes a decrease in membrane sensitivity by increasing the resting membrane potential. Muscle weakness and even paralysis may occur. The primary causes of hypokalemia include diuretic therapy, vomiting, diarrhea, alkalosis, excessive mineralocorticoid therapy for adrenal insufficiency, renal failure, and diabetic ketoacidosis. Hypokalemic myopathy is well documented in cats with renal failure, in cats with chronic anorexia, and in cats receiving low-potassium diets. Most patients respond well to potassium supplementation (see Chapter 7).

Hypoglycemia

Hypoglycemia causes altered CNS function similar to that associated with hypoxia. The blood glucose concentration is of prime importance for normal neuronal metabolism because glucose oxidation is the primary energy source. No glycogen stores are present in the CNS. Glucose enters nervous tissue by noninsulin dependent transport mechanisms. Hypoglycemia at glucose concentrations less than 40 mg/dL can precipitate signs of hypoglycemia. Neurologic signs of hypoglycemia are manifested by dullness, hypothermia, weakness, seizures, and coma. Factors responsible for clinical signs include rate of decrease, level, and duration of hypoglycemia. The severity of the CNS signs may be related more to the rate of decrease than to the actual concentration of glucose. Sudden drops in glucose levels are more likely to cause seizures, whereas slowly developing hypoglycemia may cause weakness, paresis, behavioral changes, or stupor.

Neonatal Hypoglycemia. Studies in puppies have shown that during hypoglycemia, lactic acid is not only incorporated into the perinatal brain but also consumed to the extent that the metabolite can support up to 60% total cerebral energy required for metabolic processes.[69] Although the neonatal brain can readily metabolize ketone bodies, lack of body fat and prolonged time necessary to produce ketones prevent this mechanism from protecting neonates from acute hypoglycemia. Hypoglycemia in young animals may be secondary to malnutrition, parasitism, stress, or some GI abnormality. Puppies are frequently extremely depressed or comatose. Serum glucose should be determined, and IV glucose is administered immediately (2 to 4 mL of 20% glucose per kilogram of body weight). Diazepam often will have no effect on halting hypoglycemic seizures. Continued signs of stupor or coma indicate brain swelling and are treated with hypertonic solutions (see Chapter 12). Dietary regulation, including tube feeding if necessary, must be established to maintain normoglycemia.

Hypoglycemia in puppies also occurs because of immature hepatic enzyme systems, deficiency of glucagon, and deficiency of gluconeogenic substrates. Fatty liver syndrome causes hypoglycemia in toy breed puppies at 4 to 16 weeks of age.[70] Persistent and recurrent hypoglycemia, hepatomegaly, acidosis, and ketosis suggest a glycogen storage disorder.[71] Liver and muscle biopsies are required to make a definitive diagnosis. The management of these cases is frequently unsuccessful.

Insulinoma. Adult-onset hypoglycemia usually is caused by a functional tumor of the pancreatic β-islet cells commonly called insulinomas.[72-74] Excessive insulin produces an increased transfer of blood glucose into the nonneuronal cellular compartments, resulting in hypoglycemia and abnormal CNS metabolism. Although insulinomas are relatively rare, increasing awareness has resulted in more frequent diagnosis. Most insulinomas in dogs have metastasized to the local lymph node (stage II) or liver (stage III) and other sites by the time a definitive diagnosis is made. In addition to hypoglycemia, insulinomas may also induce peripheral neuropathies (see Chapter 7). Other neoplasms (e.g., leiomyosarcoma) also may induce hypoglycemia.[75]

Seizures associated with insulinomas are more frequently related to exercise, fasting (or, conversely, eating), and excitement. Other signs such as weakness, facial and muscle tremors, disorientation, and behavioral changes are also common. The signs are episodic until irreversible neuronal damage occurs. LMN paresis can be detected in dogs with peripheral neuropathies.

Blood glucose concentrations after a 12-hour fast are usually below normal (<60 mg/dL). Longer fasts (24 to 48 hours) may be necessary in some cases, but animals should be monitored closely during this time. serum insulin levels are more specific for making a diagnosis.[76] Serum insulin concentrations are near zero when serum glucose concentrations are less than or equal to 30 mg/dL. Serum insulin levels should be measured when the blood glucose concentrations are below 60 mg/dL. Normal or increased serum insulin concentrations in hypoglycemic dogs are strongly suggestive of insulinoma. An amended insulin:glucose ratio greater than 30 is supportive of an insulinoma. The glucagon tolerance test may be used as an alternative procedure, but it carries a greater risk of profound hypoglycemia during the test. Abdominal ultrasonography, CT, or MRI may detect pancreatic masses in some cases and help localize the lesion for surgical resection.

The management of patients in coma and status epilepticus is discussed in Chapters 12 and 13, respectively. Surgical removal of the tumor is indicated when the patient's condition has stabilized. The reported incidence of malignancy ranges from 56% to 82%; therefore the prognosis is poor even with successful removal of the pancreatic focus.[72,73] Animals with insulinoma should be fed several small meals each day. Diets high in simple sugars should be avoided. Symptomatic treatment with glucocorticoids such as prednisolone, given at a dosage of 0.25 to 0.50 mg/kg per day, help to normalize the blood glucose concentration because of their antiinsulin effects. Streptozotocin is effective in dogs with even metastatic disease. Concurrent saline diuresis should be given to prevent renal toxicity. Seizures may persist because of prior neuronal injury even though serum glucose levels have been normalized.[76]

Nutritional Disorders

Nervous system disorders caused by nutritional deficiencies or excesses are uncommon in companion animals, but they are more common in food animals. Severe malnutrition can cause a variety of abnormalities that are related to multiple deficiencies.

Vitamin A Deficiency

Deficiencies in vitamin A can produce night blindness. Hypovitaminosis A in young animals may cause excessive thickening of the skull and the vertebrae with secondary compression of nervous tissue (especially of the cranial nerves as they pass through the foramina). Decreased absorption of CSF may result in communicating hydrocephalus.[77] Skull malformation and cerebellar herniation have been reported in exotic cats fed a vitamin A–deficient diet.[78] Hypovitaminosis A is rare or rarely recognized in companion animals but has been reported in food animals.[77-80] Blindness in cattle with vitamin A deficiency is caused by several pathologic mechanisms.[81] Papilledema occurs in adult animals secondary to increased CSF pressure, which is secondary to decreased absorption. Photoreceptor abnormalities, especially affecting the rods, lead to night blindness. Similar changes occur in growing calves, but, in addition, the optic nerves are compressed by narrowing of the optic canals, resulting in ischemia and direct interference with the nerve.

Vitamin E Deficiency

A noninflammatory myopathy may be produced by vitamin E deficiency; however, vitamin E deficiency is rare in companion animals. Calves and sheep have a myopathy associated with a deficiency in vitamin E and selenium. Swine may die suddenly because of degeneration of cardiac muscle. Retinal degeneration may occur secondary to vitamin E deficiency (see Chapter 11). Low vitamin E blood levels have been associated with degenerative myeloencephalopathy and motor neuron disease in horses (see Chapter 7).[82,83]

Vitamin B Complex–Thiamine Deficiency (Polioencephalomalacia)

Deficiencies in B vitamins can cause pathologic changes in both the CNS and PNS. Thiamine deficiency has been reported in dogs, cats, and ruminants.[79,84-87] The syndrome in dogs progresses from anorexia to paraparesis, tetraparesis, seizures, and coma in approximately 1 week.[87] Malacia and hemorrhage were found in multiple sites in the brain and the spinal cord, with the most severe lesions in the brainstem. Animals treated with thiamine recovered. A peripheral neuropathy with LMN paralysis can occur.[84]

Cats with thiamine deficiency often have characteristic ventral flexion of the head and the neck, sometimes causing the mandible to touch the sternum. Vestibular ataxia and seizures may be present. The pathologic lesions are similar to those that occur in dogs.[79] The deficiency in dogs was produced by a diet consisting entirely of cooked meat or a specific thiamine-deficient diet.[87] Cat foods with fish as the primary ingredient contain thiaminase, which destroys thiamine in the diet.[79]

Treatment should be instituted immediately for any animal suspected of having thiamine deficiency. In dogs and cats, 50 to 100 mg of thiamine should be given IV and then repeated IM daily until a response is obtained or another diagnosis is established.

Polioencephalomalacia (symmetric necrosis of the cerebral cortex) is caused by thiamine deficiency in young ruminants (feedlot calves and lambs). The deficiency results from increased breakdown of thiamine in the rumen by thiaminase-secreting bacteria or from sulfur toxicity. Animals have usually been moved from a marginal pasture to a lush pasture, are in a feedlot, or have had some similar change in feeding patterns. Feedlot diets high in sulfates decrease thiamine production in the rumen and may inhibit the production of ATP. Animals younger than 2 years of age are most commonly affected.[86]

Clinical signs are primarily forebrain in origin and include depression, pacing, head pressing, blindness, ataxia, teeth grinding, opisthotonos, and seizures. Dorsomedial strabismus has been attributed to trochlear nerve (cranial nerve [CN] IV) paralysis. Increased intracranial pressure is common and may lead to transtentorial herniation. Symmetric laminar cortical necrosis is the most prominent pathologic finding (Figure 15-7).

Edema of the brain with flattening of the gyri may be present. Measurement of transketolase, the thiamine-dependent coenzyme, is helpful for making a diagnosis. Autofluorescence of the cut surface of the cerebral cortex under ultraviolet light may assist diagnosis (see Figure 15-7).

The condition should be treated with thiamine, 250 to 1000 mg administered IV or IM for 3 to 5 days. Corticosteroids should be given if CNS signs are severe. Severely affected animals may have permanent cortical damage.[88]

Niacin and riboflavin deficiencies are less common, but because animals with thiamine deficiency also may have deficiencies in these vitamins, multiple B-complex preparations are indicated. The diet should be corrected to prevent recurrences.

Vitamin A Toxicity

Increased levels of vitamin A have been reported in cats fed predominantly liver diets. Hypertrophic vertebral bone formation causes ankylosing spondylosis, usually of the cervical vertebrae but in some cases extending to the lumbar region. The clinical signs relate primarily to the rigidity of the vertebral column. A compressive neuropathy occurs in severely affected cats. Dietary correction stops the progression of the spondylosis but does not significantly reduce the existing spondylosis that is present. Antiinflammatory and analgesic drugs have been recommended but must be used with caution, especially in cats.[79]

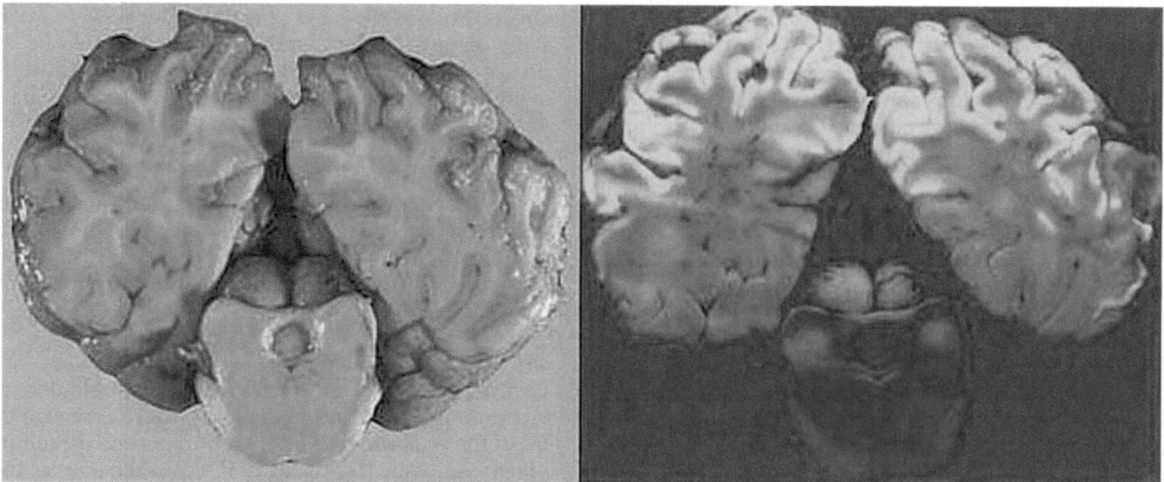

Figure 15-7 Polioencephalomalacia in a calf. There is acute cortical necrosis evidenced by locally extensive softening and discoloration *(left image)* and highlighted by fluorescence under ultraviolet light. (Courtesy Cornell University College of Veterinary Medicine.)

Toxic Disorders

Toxicities causing CNS dysfunction are common in both small and large animals. Many cause biochemical changes and are potentially reversible, whereas others produce structural damage. The more common toxicants are listed in Table 15-4.

Toxicologic disorders, including those caused by poisonous plants, are discussed in detail in several texts.[79,89,90] A helpful information resource about toxic agents and treatment protocols is the ASPCA's National Animal Poison Control Center (*http://www.napcc.aspca.org*).

Diagnosis

A history of exposure to a toxin is the most important factor in establishing the diagnosis in cases of poisoning. Neurologic signs of intoxication include (1) seizures; (2) depression or coma; (3) tremors, ataxia, and paresis; and (4) LMN signs. Animals that show any of these four signs must be considered as possible poisoning victims until proved otherwise. Metabolic and inflammatory disorders are most commonly confused with toxicosis.

Toxins can cause imbalances of neurotransmitter in the CNS to cause tremor. In particular neurotoxic agents that stimulate the CNS will manifest signs of hyperactivity, hyperesthesia, muscle tremor and fasciculation, and behavior changes. Toxicants affecting the autonomic nervous system induce clinical signs by interference with cholinergic neurotransmission. Stimulation of the cholinergic neurotransmission will result in bronchoconstriction, muscle tremors, exocrine gland stimulation, bradycardia, and other CNS effects. Toxins may exert effects at the neuromuscular junction through increased release of acetylcholine and increased receptor stimulation and subsequent muscular fatigue. Blockade of cholinergic neurotransmission depends upon the type of cholinergic receptor involved. Muscarinic receptor blockade causes CNS depression. Nicotinic receptor blockade results in skeletal muscle paralysis and often tremor. Toxins such as bromethalin and

TABLE 15-4

Common Toxicants

Use	Toxicant	Primary Effect
Pesticides	Chlorinated hydrocarbons	CNS stimulation
	Organophosphates	Binding of acetylcholinesterase
	Carbamates	Binding of acetylcholinesterase
	Pyrethrins	Blocking of nerve conduction and GABA inhibition
	Metaldehyde	CNS stimulation
	Arsenic	GI irritation
Rodenticides	Strychnine	Blocking of inhibitory interneurons (glycine)
	Thallium	GI irritation, CNS stimulation, peripheral neuropathy, skin lesions
	α-Naphthylthiourea (ANTU)	GI irritation, pulmonary edema, depression,coma
	Sodium fluoroacetate (1080)	CNS stimulation
	Warfarin	Anticoagulation
	Zinc phosphide	GI irritation, depression
	Phosphorus	GI irritation, CNS stimulation, coma
	Cholecalciferol	CNS depression, cardiac depression
	Bromethalin	Acute—CNS stimulation; chronic—CNS depression
Herbicides and fungicides	Numerous	GI irritation, CNS depression, some are stimulants
Heavy metals	Lead (see arsenic and thallium)	GI irritation, CNS stimulation or depression (see above)
Drugs	Narcotics	CNS depression
	Amphetamines	CNS stimulation
	Barbiturates	CNS depression
	Tranquilizers	CNS depression
	Aspirin	GI irritation, coma
	Marijuana	Abnormal behavior, depression
	Anthelmintics	GI irritation, CNS stimulation
	Ivermectin	Depression, tremors, ataxia, coma
Garbage	Staphylococcal toxin	GI irritation, CNS stimulation
	Botulinum toxin	LMN paralysis
Poisonous plants	Various	Various
Antifreeze	Ethylene glycol	GI irritation, CNS stimulation, renal failure
Detergents and disinfectants	Hexachlorophene	CNS stimulation or depression, tremors
	Phenols	GI irritation, CNS degeneration
Animal origin	Snake bite	Necrotizing wound, shock, CNS depression
	Toad (*Bufo* spp.)	Digitoxin-like action, CNS stimulation
	Black widow spider	Initial signs—spasms, pain tremor initally; later signs—LMN paralysis
	Lizards	GI irritation, CNS stimulation or depression
	Tick paralysis (*Dermacentor* spp. *Ixodes* in Australia)	LMN paralysis

hexachlorophene affect myelin causing intramyelinic edema and alter conduction of the action potential.

When an animal shows signs suggestive of poisoning, the owner must be questioned carefully to find a possible source. Animals in status epilepticus must be treated immediately, and the history must be obtained later (see Chapter 13). Direct questions regarding agents that are capable of producing the signs must be asked. Owners usually are aware of common agents such as insecticides and rodenticides, but they may have difficulty identifying a source of lead poisoning and may be reluctant to admit a source of illicit drug intoxication.

The clinical signs may be sufficient for the clinician to establish a presumptive diagnosis (e.g., intoxication from strychnine and organophosphates). Other agents, such as lead and drugs, may require laboratory confirmation (Tables 15-5 through 15-8) or tissue analysis.

Toxicants Causing Seizures

The most common sign of poisoning in small animals is seizures (see Table 15-5). The CNS is primarily or secondarily involved with a variety of toxic substances. Dorman reported that seizures occurred in 8.2% of all cases of suspected

TABLE 15-5

Common Toxicants Causing Seizures

Toxicants	Diagnosis	Management	Prognosis
Organochlorines	Exposure; muscle fasciculations common; laboratory confirmation difficult	Removal of toxicant—washing, gastric lavage; sedation or anesthesia with barbiturates	Poor with seizures
Organophosphates and carbamates	Exposure; salivation, diarrhea, constricted pupils, muscle weakness; blood cholinesterase level decreased; tissue analysis poor	Removal of toxicant; atropine; pralidoxime chloride (2-PAM) (not for carbamates)	Good if treated early
Pyrethrins	Exposure; tremor, salivation, ataxia, seizures; analysis of tissues	Removal of toxicant; sedation	Good if treated early
Strychnine	Exposure; tetany without loss of consciousness, increased by stimulation or noise; laboratory analysis of stomach contents, urine, tissues	Removal of toxicant—gastric lavage or emesis; sedation—barbiturates; respiratory support if needed	Good if treated early
Bromethalin	Exposure; high dose—excitement, tremor, seizures; low dose—tremor, depression, ataxia	Removal of toxicant—activated charcoal; corticosteroids, mannitol	Fair if treated vigorously for several days
Sodium fluoroacetate (1080)	Exposure; seizures are clonic and severe; laboratory confirmation difficult	Removal of toxicant; sedation—barbiturates	Poor with seizures
Thallium	Exposure; GI signs, seizures only in severe poisonings; laboratory analysis of urine and tissues	Removal of toxicant; diphenylthiocarbazone (Dithion) early, ferric ferrocyanide (Prussian blue) late late	Poor with seizures, fair with other signs, good with treatment
Lead	Exposure (may be difficult to document); chronic intoxication may cause intermittent seizures, behavioral change, tremor, GI signs; blood lead level >0.4 ppm; basophilic stippling, nucleated red blood cells (RBCs) with no anemia	Removal of toxicant; calcium ethylenediaminetetraacetic acid, 2,3-dimercaptosuccinic acid	Good with treatment
Staphylococcal toxin	Exposure to garbage; severe GI signs; isolation of toxins and testing in laboratory animals laboratory animals	Removal of toxicant; sedation	Poor with seizures; animals usually die rapidly
Toad (*Bufo* spp.—reported only in southern Florida)	Exposure; severe buccal irritation	Wash mouth; sedation—anesthesia	Fair if treated within 15-30 min, otherwise poor
Amphetamines	Exposure to prescription or "street" drugs; hyperactivity, dilated pupils; analysis of urine	Removal of toxicant; sedation or anesthesia—barbiturates	Good if treated early
Metaldehyde	Exposure to snail bait; tremor, ataxia, salivation; seizures are tonic, similar to strychnine, but not changing with stimuli; laboratory analysis of stomach contents	Removal of toxicant; sedation or anesthesia; support respiration	Fair if treated early
Caffeine and other methylxanthines	Ataxia, tachycardia, seizures, coma; laboratory analysis of stomach contents and tissues	Removal of toxicant; sedation, fluids	Fair with treatment
Zinc phosphide	Exposure to rodenticide; behavioral changes, hysteria followed by seizures; GI irritation; analysis of stomach contents and tissues	Removal of toxicant; oral and intravenous bicarbonate; sedation—barbiturates	Poor

TABLE 15-6

Common Toxicants Causing Behavioral Changes, CNS Depression, or Coma

Toxicants	Diagnosis	Management	Prognosis
Drugs—narcotics, barbiturates, tranquilizers, marijuana	Degree of depression depends on dose; source of pharmaceuticals or "street" drugs; laboratory analysis of blood or urine	Removal of toxicant, narcotic antagonists, diuresis, support respiration	Good with treatment
α-Naphthylthiourea (ANTU)	Exposure; pulmonary edema; depression and coma terminal; laboratory analysis of stomach contents and tissues	Removal of toxicant, treatment of pulmonary edema	Poor
Ethylene glycol	Exposure; GI irritation, renal failure; oxalate crystals in urine	IV ethanol (30%) with sodium bicarbonate; alternative for dogs—4-methylpyrazole	Poor with coma, fair to good if treated early
Cholecalciferol	Exposure; depression, weakness, cardiac depression, renal failure	Removal of intoxicant; IV saline diuresis, furosemide, corticosteroids	Fair with treatment
Many poisons produce coma terminally			

TABLE 15-7

Common Toxicants Causing Tremor, Ataxia, or Paresis

Toxicants	Diagnosis	Management	Prognosis
Hexachlorophene	Exposure; usually young, nursing animal; large dose causes GI irritation, severe depression; chronic exposure causes cerebellar signs and CNS edema	Removal of toxicant, supportive care; treatment for cerebral edema	Fair; may be residual effects
Lead	Chronic lead poisoning may produce cerebellar signs and dementia (see Table 15-5)	See Table 15-5	Good
Organophosphates	Chronic low doses (flea collars, dips) may produce tremor and weakness (see Table 15-5)	See Table 15-5	Good
Organochlorines	Low-dose exposure may produce weakness and muscle fasciculation (see Table 15-5)	See Table 15-5	Fair to good
Tranquilizers	Ataxia common with tranquilizers (see Table 15-5)	None needed	Good
Marijuana	Behavioral changes and ataxia common	Removal of toxicant	Good
Ergot alkaloids	Cattle and other herbivores grazing on Dallis grass or ryegrass; ataxia, uncoordinated gait	Removal from pasture	Good
Nitro-bearing plants (e.g., *Astragalus* spp., locoweed)	Cattle, sheep, horses; ataxia, weakness or hyperexcitability, death	Removal from pasture	Fair in ruminants; may be permanent CNS damage
Yellow star thistle	Horses have an acute onset of rigidity of muscles of mastication and involuntary movement of the lips; ataxia, circling, and pacing may occur; lesions are necrosis of the globus pallidus and substantia nigra	No treatment known	Poor

toxicosis.[91] Toxins induce seizures through a number of different mechanisms: increased excitation, decreased inhibition, and interference with energy metabolism.[92] The animal may show (status epilepticus) or cluster seizures (e.g., from organophosphates, strychnine) or may have a history of intermittent seizures (e.g., from lead). Animals in status epilepticus must be treated immediately (see Chapter 13).

Tetany. The tetany produced by strychnine is differentiated from the seizures produced by other agents in this group. Tetany is a period of sustained muscular contraction with intermittent periods of relaxation. Despite the severe muscle contractions, the animal is conscious. Tetany caused by strychnine may be confused with hypocalcemic tetany seen in lactating animals of all species or in tetanus. Intravenous calcium provides immediate relief in cases of hypocalcemia. The term *tetanus* is associated with the toxic effects of *Clostridium tetani*. Tetanus is much slower in onset than is strychnine poisoning and generally causes more continuous contraction of the muscles. Seizures from other agents produce clonus (alternating flexion and extension).

Insecticides. Organophosphates may be distinguished from organochlorines by their profound effect on the autonomic nervous system, producing profuse salivation, constricted pupils, and diarrhea. Organochlorines frequently

TABLE 15-8

Common Toxicants Causing LMN Signs

Toxicants	Diagnosis	Management	Prognosis
Botulinum toxin	Exposure to contaminated food, carrion, and so forth; ascending LMN paralysis (see Chapter 7)	See Chapter 7	Good
Tick paralysis (*Dermacentor* spp., *Ixodes* species in Australia)	Presence of ticks; ascending LMN paralysis (see Chapter 7)	Removal of ticks (see Chapter 7)	Good in the United States of America; poor in Australia
Drug reaction (nitrofurantoins, doxorubicin, vincristine)	Exposure; rare in animals	Removal of source	Fair
Cyanide (from *Sorghum* spp. grass)	Cauda equina syndrome with dysuria, flaccid anus and tail, prolapsed penis; may progress to paraplegia; usually occurs in horses	Removal from pasture; no treatment available	May improve after removal from source; residual deficits common
Organophosphates	Chronic exposure may cause LMN signs; axonopathy affecting pelvic limbs first	Removal of source; atropine and pralidoxime if acute signs present; no treatment for peripheral neuropathy	Fair to poor
Heavy metals (lead, arsenic, mercury, thallium)	Chronic exposure, rare in animals (see Table 15-5)	See Table 15-5	See Table 15-5
Industrial chemicals (acrylamide, carbon disulfide, polychlorinated biphenyls)	Not reported in animals; presumably could cause distal axonopathy	Removal from source	Unknown

produce fine-muscle fasciculations, even between seizures. Pyrethrins and pyrethroid insecticides alter both sodium and chloride conductance causing tremor and seizures. The seizure may be preceded by tremors, ataxia, salivation, and other signs. Class I and II pyrethrins and pyrethroid compounds act on voltage-gated sodium channels in nerve and muscle, causing persistent depolarization and failure of membrane repolarization. Class II pyrethroids also inhibit binding of GABA to the $GABA_A$ receptor, which prevents influx of chloride.

Miscellaneous Stimulants. Ingestion of products containing caffeine and other methylxanthines, including chocolate, may also cause seizures. Metaldehyde, a common snail bait, can cause continuous seizures.[91] Both bromethalin and hexachlorophene are toxins that result in intramyelinic edema and demyelination. Bromethalin is a rodenticide that uncouples oxidative phosphorylation depleting cellular ATP.[93,94] Clinical signs include ataxia; conscious proprioceptive deficits; paresis/paralysis; depression, which can progress to stupor; focal or generalized seizures; decerebrate posture; and vocalization.

Metronidazole. Central nervous system signs of lead intoxication are seen most often in cases of chronic exposure.[95-99] The seizures are intermittent. The differential diagnosis of seizure disorders is discussed in Chapter 13. Laboratory analysis of the blood for evidence of lead is diagnostic. If the blood lead values are in the high normal range and lead poisoning is suspected, treatment followed by measurement of urine lead levels is diagnostic. Other toxicants causing seizures are seen infrequently.

Metronidazole is an antimicrobial, antiprotozoal agent that is lipophilic readily penetrating the blood-brain barrier and causes neurotoxicity in dogs and cats.[100-102] The drug is also used in the chronic treatment of inflammatory bowel disease. Neurologic signs include seizures, tremors, ataxia, blindness, hyperactivity, and vestibular dysfunction. Doses of metronidazole reported to be toxic in cats ranged from 111 mg/kg of body weight per day for 9 weeks to 58 mg/kg of body weight per day for 6 months.[101] The neurologic signs resolved within days of drug withdrawal and supportive treatment. In dogs, doses as low as 67.3 mg/kg of body weight per day for 3 to 14 days caused neurotoxicity.[100] In a report of five dogs, two were euthanized because of severe CNS disease, and three recovered after several months.[100] Most dogs recover within 7 to 14 days. Diazepam may be effective in treatment of the neurologic signs because it facilitates the effects of GABA, a potent inhibitory neurotransmitter.[102] Diazepam, 0.43 mg/kg PO every 8 hours for 3 days, decreased response time from 4.25 days for untreated dogs to 13.4 hours for treated dogs. In addition, the time to recovery was reduced from 11 days to 38.8 hours.[102]

Ivermectin. Ivermectin is widely used as an antiparasitic agent and heartworm preventative. It is also used in higher doses for the treatment of sarcoptic and demodectic mange in dogs. In most breeds of dogs, ivermectin has a wide margin of safety. Collies, Australian shepherds, Shetland sheepdogs, and Old English sheepdogs have an increased sensitivity to ivermectin and related compounds. These breeds have a genetic mutation that results in a nonfunctional P-glycoprotein.[103,104] P-glycoprotein plays an important neuroprotective role in the blood-brain barrier in that it enhances the transport of drugs from the CSF back into circulation. Ivermectin is a GABA agonist that inhibits activity at presynaptic and postsynaptic neurons in the CNS. Clinical signs of ivermectin neurotoxicity include depression, disorientation, tremors, ataxia, blindness, mydriasis, retinopathy, seizures, and coma.[104-107] Clinical signs are dose dependent in that susceptible breeds rarely develop clinical signs at 6 μg/kg once a month, which is the standard dose for heartworm prevention. Doses exceeding 200 μg/kg may cause clinical signs in susceptible breeds and doses above 400 μg/kg may cause death.[105] The recovery period may take more than 3 weeks. There is no specific anecdote for ivermectin toxicity. Three adult horses developed neurologic signs 18 hours after oral administration of ivermectin paste.[108] Signs included depression, ataxia, drooping of the lips, mydriasis, decreased pupillary light reflexes, absent menace responses and muscle fasciculations. Two horses recovered following symptomatic therapy.

Toxicants Causing Behavioral Change, Stupor, or Coma

Stupor or coma may be seen with almost any poison in the terminal stages. Drugs such as narcotics, barbiturates, and tranquilizers most frequently cause stupor or coma and also may cause behavioral changes in smaller doses (see Table 15-6). Some other agents such as chlorpyrifos and lead also can produce behavioral changes with chronic intoxication.[99,109] The diagnosis may be obvious if the source is known (e.g., with accidental overdosing with an antiepileptic drugs or ingestion by an animal of its owner's tranquilizers). Reports of animals that have ingested illicit drugs are not uncommon, and the owner is usually reluctant to admit the source of the intoxication in these cases. Laboratory analysis of blood or urine may be necessary to confirm the diagnosis.

Leukoencephalomalacia (Moldy Corn Toxicity). Leukoencephalomalacia is caused by the mycotoxin fumonisin B1 found in contaminated corn. The toxin creates a severe liquefactive necrosis and degeneration of the cerebrum, brainstem, and spinal cord. The disease has a worldwide distribution and typically occurs in the late fall through early spring. Neurologic (most common) and hepatoxic syndromes are recognized. Clinical signs develop 3 to 4 weeks after daily ingestion of contaminated corn. The onset of clinical signs is rapid with death occurring in 2 to 3 days. The CNS signs are similar to other equine encephalopathies. The hepatotoxic syndrome is associated with swelling of the lips and nose, somnolence, severe icterus, petechia of mucous membranes, abnormal breathing, and cyanosis. Diagnosis is based on histopathology. Analysis for the toxin in feed is recommended. There is no treatment and mortality is high.

Toxicants Causing Tremors, Ataxia, and Paresis

Chronic organophosphate poisoning from flea collars and topical or systemic insecticides frequently causes signs that are suggestive of cerebellar disease or muscle weakness (see Table 15-8). The finding of weakness is not consistent with pure cerebellar disease, so when both are present, poisoning must be considered.[110] Organophosphates bind acetylcholinesterase to cause muscle weakness through effects on the neuromuscular junction (see Chapter 7) and have direct CNS effects causing seizure. Tremor and fasciculation associated with muscle weakness occur as a depolarizing neuromuscular junction blockade effect take place. Atropine is used to counteract the muscarinic effects of the organophosphate. Pralidoxime chloride (2-PAM) is a drug that acts specifically on the organophosphate-enzyme complex and freeing the enzyme. Hexachlorophene toxicity has been seen in puppies with signs of tremor and ataxia.[111-113] Severe depression may follow. The usual source has been repeated washing of the bitch's mammary glands with a soap containing hexachlorophene. Bathing young dogs or cats of any age in hexachlorophene soap also has produced the syndrome. Hexachlorophene is rarely available now.

Metaldehyde poisoning, which produces tremor and ataxia progressing to depression and coma, is seen frequently in areas where the substance is used for snail bait. Chronic lead poisoning (see Chapter 10) and numerous plant toxicities cause tremor and ataxia (Table 15-7). Mycotoxins also can cause severe tremors and seizures in dogs (see Chapter 10).

Toxicants Causing LMN Signs

Botulism and tick paralysis cause generalized LMN paralysis by blockade of the neuromuscular junction (see Table 15-8). These conditions are discussed in Chapter 7. Some drugs (e.g., nitrofurans and chemotherapeutic drugs and some chronic toxicities (such as lead, organophosphate, and arsenic poisoning) can produce peripheral neuropathies. Other signs usually predominate, however.

Toxic Plants

Toxic plants causing neurologic syndromes of herbivores are summarized in Table 15-9.

Treatment

Removal of the toxic substance is the most important part of the treatment for many toxicities. Agents that have entered the animal through the skin, such as insecticides, should be removed by thorough washing and rinsing. Ingested agents may be removed by inducing emesis, performing gastric lavage, or administering laxatives or enemas. Diuresis may promote excretion when absorption has occurred. Activated charcoal is an effective adsorbing agent.[114] Electrolyte imbalances and other secondary metabolic disorders are treated symptomatically and by managing the underlying disease process. Status epilepticus is a life-threatening emergency and must be treated accordingly (see Chapter 13).

Specific treatments for the various toxicities are outlined in Tables 15-5 through 15-9. The reader should consult the references for details.[79,89,90,115] Toxins causing spasticity can be counterbalanced with use of muscle relaxants. Diazepam (0.25 to 1.0 mg/kg IV or per rectum) is a centrally acting muscle relaxant and can relieve acute-onset tremor disorders. However, diazepam should be avoided in cats with organophosphate toxicity as it may potentiate muscle tremor, and other muscarinic signs. Methocarbamol also a centrally acting muscle relaxant can be administered. Often a dark, quiet room is necessary to remove external stimuli associated with CNS stimulants (strychnine, bromethalin, etc.). Frequent patient monitoring and other measures of supportive care are important. Fluid therapy maintains electrolyte concentration and normovolemia. Oxygenation, blood pressure, electrolytes, and glucose should be monitored. In severe cases of respiratory muscle weakness, assisted ventilation may be necessary.

Inflammatory Diseases

The inflammatory diseases of the nervous system are caused by infectious and parasitic organisms or are immune mediated. Canine distemper, feline infectious peritonitis, equine protozoal myeloencephalitis, West Nile encephalomyelitis, alphaviral encephalomyelitis, and bacterial infections, including thromboembolic meningoencephalitis and listeriosis, are common infectious causes of CNS inflammatory disease. Some fungal diseases are common in endemic areas. Most of the other diseases are relatively uncommon. Infectious diseases are discussed in many textbooks.[116-121] Granulomatous meningoencephalomyelitis, steroid-responsive meningoencephalitis, and other breed-specific meningoencephalitides are common noninfectious or immune causes of CNS inflammatory disease. The differential diagnosis is discussed in the next section. The more common inflammatory diseases are outlined in Tables 15-10 to 15-17.

Principles of Diagnosis

Most of the inflammatory diseases are characterized by an acute onset. All are progressive, and some are chronic-progressive. Diffuse or multifocal involvement is characteristic of most of the diseases in this group, but localized signs also occur. The minimum database (see Chapters 1 and 4) may provide evidence of systemic infection (e.g., alterations in white blood cell [WBC] count), although many primary CNS inflammatory diseases do not produce a systemic response.

Text continued on p. 462.

TABLE 15-9

Examples of Several Plant (and Fungal) Toxicoses of Domestic Herbivores That Can Result in Syndromes Characterized by Neurologic Signs

Plant	Species Affected	Neurologic Signs	Pathophysiology	Neural Legions	Treatment	Prognosis
Ryegrass	Sheep, cattle, horses	Ataxia, tremor, tetany	Penitrem and fumi tremorgenic mycotoxins from *Penicillium* spp.	Secondary Purkinje cell degeneration	Diazepam	Good
Phalaris spp.	Sheep, cattle	Ataxia, tremor, weakness, seizures	Dimethyltryptamine alkaloids act as monoamine oxidase inhibitors	Neuronal pigmentation (indole melanins)	?Diazepam	Poor
Paspalum, Dallis grass	Cattle, sheep	Ataxia, tremor	*Claviceps paspali* ergot alkaloids probably neurotoxic	None	—	Good
Swainsona spp. and locoweeds	Sheep, cattle, horses	Weight loss, ataxia, aggressiveness	Indolizidine alkaloid (swainsonine) induces α-mannosidosis	Neuroaxonal dystrophy, neurovisceral storage products	Reserpine (locoweed)	Fair to very good
Sorghum spp.	Horses, cattle, sheep	Ataxia, bladder paralysis	Possibly HCN or lathyrogenic toxins	Spinal cord degeneration	—	Poor to fair
Solanum esuriale	Sheep	Exercise intolerance, weakness, arched back (humpyback)	Unknown (suspected toxin in *S. esuriale*)	Spinal cord fiber degeneration; myopathy	—	Poor
Solanum fastigiatum, S. dimidiatum, S. kwebense	Cattle	Cerebellar ataxia, "cerebellar seizures"	Suspected induction of gangliosidosis	Purkinje cell vacuolation and degeneration	—	Poor
Cycad palms	Cattle, goats, horses	Ataxia, recumbency	Possibly toxic glycosides, cycasin and macrozamin	Spinal cord degeneration	—	Poor
Melochia pyramidata	Cattle	Ataxia, recumbency	Unknown	Spinal cord and nerve degeneration	—	Poor
Tribulus terrestris	Sheep	Asymmetric pelvic limb weakness	Possibly neuromuscular process	None	—	Poor
Karwinskia humboldtiana	Goats	Hypermetria, weakness	Unknown	Peripheral neuropathy, central neuroaxonal dystrophy, myopathy	—	Poor

Nardoo fern, *Marsilea drummondii*	Sheep	Depression, blindness, convulsions	Probably a thiaminase	Polioencephalomalacia	Thiamine	Good if early
Birdsville indigo, *Indigofera linnaei*	Horses	Weight loss, ataxia, weakness	Arginine antagonist alkaloids; indospicine, canavine	None	Arginine-rich feeds (gelatin, Lucerne)	Good
Mexican fireweed, *Kochia scoparia*	Cattle	Blindness (nephrosis, hepatitis)	Saponins, alkaloids, oxalates; possibly thiaminase	Polioencephalomalacia	—	Poor
Buckeye, *Aesculus* spp.	Cattle	Staggering, convulsions	Glycosides and alkaloids described	Unknown	—	Fair
Helichrysum argyrosphaerum	Sheep, cattle	Peripheral blindness, nystagmus, weakness	Unknown	Patchy status spongiosus, white matter	—	Fair for life, poor for vision
Yellow star thistle, Centaurea solstitialis	Horses	Depression, pacing, dystonia of muscles of prehension, mastication, and deglutition	Uknown	Nigropallidal encephalomalacia	Tube feed	Poor, starve

Modified from Kornegay JN, Mayhew IG: Metabolic, toxic, and nutritional diseases of the nervous system. In Oliver JE, Hoerlein BF, Mayhew IG, editors: Veterinary neurology, Philadelphia, 1987, WB Saunders.

TABLE 15-10

Bacterial Diseases of the Nervous System

Disease	Cause	Incidence	Clinical Signs and Pathology	Course and Prognosis	Diagnostic Tests	Treatment
Meningitis	*Staphylococcus, Pasteurella,* others	Variable, but generally uncommon	Generalized or localized (especially cervical) hyperesthesia; degree of illness variable; temperature and white blood cell (WBC) count may be normal count may be normal	Usually acute onset, but may be chronic; prognosis good with early treatment	CSF (protein often >200 mg/dL, increased cells, primarily neutrophils), culture and sensitivity testing	Antibiotics according to sensitivity: ampicillin, trimethoprim, chloramphenicol
Meningoencephalomyelitis	As in meningitis	Uncommon	As in meningitis, plus signs of brain or spinal cord disease; often includes blindness, seizures, ataxia, cranial nerve deficits	Usually acute: prognosis good with early treatment, but neurologic deficits are common	Same as meningitis; EEG may indicate encephalitis; cross-sectional imaging	Same as for meningitis; seizures—diazepam, phenobarbital; acute cerebral edema—mannitol, hypertonic saline
Abscess	As in meningitis	Rare	May have focal signs or focal signs plus signs of meningitis or meningoencephalitis	May be chronic; progression may be rapid once signs are obvious	Same as in meningoencephalitis	Same as for meningoencephalitis
Vertebral osteomyelitis, discospondylitis (see Chapter 6)	*Staphylococcus, Brucella canis,* others	Moderately frequent in dogs	Pain, usually focal; may have spinal cord compression; usually clinically ill, often over weeks to months	Chronic, may become acute when spinal cord is compressed	Radiography, cross-sectional imaging, *Brucella* serology; blood and urine culture and sensitivity	Antibiotics, preferably bactericidal; curettage, decompression if spinal cord is compressed
Tetanus	*Clostridium tetani*	Rare except in horses	Extensor rigidity of all limbs, often with opisthotonos; contraction of facial muscles, prolapsed nictitating membrane; usually infected wound; toxin blocks glycine release	Acute onset, often lasts 1-2 wk, animals may die; prognosis fair if treated	Signs, history, isolation of organism from wound	Penicillin, metronidazole, tetanus antitoxin, tranquilizers or muscle relaxants; quiet environment; treat wound, nursing
Botulism	*Clostridium botulinum*	Sporadic	LMN-type paralysis. often beginning with pelvic limbs, progressing to tetra- paresis in less than 24 hr; caused by toxin blocking neuromuscular transmission	Acute onset, lasts about 2 wk; good prognosis unless respiratory paralysis is present early	Serum, fecal analysis, history, EMG, and nerve conduction velocity	Enemas and laxatives early, supportive care, antitoxin usually not effective
Thromboembolic meningoencephalitis	*Histophilus somni*	Cattle, primarily young in feedlot	Fever, depression, blindness, lack of coordination, cranial nerve signs, seizures	Acute progressive; fair prognosis with early treatment	History, CSF (increased protein, increased neutrophils), culture	Antibiotics, vaccine available
Listeriosis	*Listeria monocytogenes*	Sporadic in ruminants	Depression, asymmetric ataxia and paresis, cranial nerve signs, central vestibular signs	Acute progressive in sheep and goats, more chronic in cattle; poor prognosis if CNS signs are present	History, signs, CSF (increased protein, increased mononuclear cells), histopathology, fluorescent antibody, isolation of organism	Antibiotics (penicillin, sulfonamides, tetracyclines) for 2-4 wk

TABLE 15-11

Mycotic and Actinomycetes Infections of the Nervous System

Disease	Cause	Incidence	Clinical Signs and Pathology	Course and Prognosis	Diagnostic Tests	Treatment
Cryptococcosis	*Cryptococcus neoformans*	Low; primarily in eastern and midwestern United States but not reported throughout United States	Nose and sinuses usually are infected, with extension to brain; ocular lesions and blindness common; CNS involvement common	Chronic; guarded prognosis	Cytology and culture of exudates, serology, antigen test, CSF (increased protein, increased cells, neutrophils and mononuclear cells, possibly organisms)	Itraconazole, fluconazole*
Blastomycosis	*Blastomyces dermatitidis*	Low; primarily in eastern and midwestern United States	Rarely involves CNS; pyogranulomatous encephalitis or single or multifocal granulomas; frequently involves lungs, skin, and eyes	Chronic; poor prognosis	PCR, serology, cytology	Amphotericin B,* 5-fluorocytosine, ketoconazole, itraconazole, fluconazole
Histoplasmosis	*Histoplasma capsulatum*	Low, primarily in central United States	CNS involvement uncommon; involves reticuloendothelial cells of most viscera	Chronic; guarded prognosis	PCR, serology, cytology	Amphotericin B,* 5-fluorocytosine, ketoconazole, itraconazole, fluconazole
Coccidioidomycosis	*Coccidioides immitis*	Can be relatively common in endemic areas of southwestern United States	CNS involvement uncommon; pulmonary infection common	Chronic; poor prognosis	PCR, serology, cytology	Amphotericin B,* 5-fluorocytosine, ketoconazole, itraconazole, fluconazole
Nocardiosis	*Nocardia* sp.	Low throughout United States	Systemic disease, signs similar to canine distemper, respiratory or cutaneous forms; CNS abscesses and vertebral osteomyelitis reported	Chronic; poor prognosis	Smears, cultures, CSF (increased protein, increased cells, neutrophils)	Penicillin, sulfonamides, trimethoprim
Actinomycosis	*Actinomyces* sp.	Low throughout United States	Similar to nocardiosis	Chronic; poor prognosis	Similar to nocardiosis	Penicillin, clindamycin, erythromycin, lincomycin
Paecilomycosis	*Paecilomyces* sp.	Rare	Disseminated form of discospondylitis	Chronic; poor prognosis	Culture, biopsy	None
Aspergillosis	*Aspergillus* sp.	Primarily in large animals	Encephalitis can develop after immunosuppression or guttural pouch infection	Chronic; poor prognosis	Culture, CSF, cytology	Amphotericin B,* 5-fluorocytosine, ketoconazole, itraconazole, fluconazole
Phaeohyphomycosis	*Cladosporium* sp.	Rare	Encephalitis with granulomas has been reported in dogs and cats	Chronic; poor prognosis	Culture, biopsy	Amphotericin B,* 5-fluorocytosine, ketoconazole, itraconazole, fluconazole

*Itraconazole and fluconazole have been used effectively in some cats with cryptococcal encephalitis and are the preferred treatment. Data for other fungal CNS infections are largely lacking.

TABLE 15-12

Protozoal Diseases of the CNS

Disease	Cause	Incidence	Clinical Signs and Pathology	Course and Prognosis	Diagnostic Tests	Treatment
Toxoplasmosis	*Toxoplasma gondii*	Common infection but infrequent clinical problem	Clinical manifestations usually associated with another disease or immunosuppression; CNS, eyes, lungs, gastrointestinal tract and skeletal muscles often affected	Chronic; fair to poor prognosis	Serology, oocysts in stool (cats), biopsy, CSF (increased protein, mononuclear cells and neutrophils)	Sulfonamides, pyrimethamine, clindamycin
Neosporosis	*Neospora caninum*	Uknown frequency, cases of toxoplasmosis reported in past were sometimes *Neospora;* reported in dogs and rarely in cats, cattle, and horses	Similar to toxoplasmosis; ascending paralysis of limbs with extension of the pelvic limbs is frequent in young pups	Chronic progressive; fair to poor prognosis	CSF, biopsy, isolation of organism, serology	Sulfonamides, pyrimethamine, clindamycin are probably effective if given early
Babesiosis	*Babesia* spp.	Rare in United States	Parasite of red blood cells; rarely causes CNS disease, hemorrhage; more severe with other infections, such as *Ehrlichia*	Acute to chronic; poor prognosis	Peripheral blood smears, serology	Diminazene, phenamidine, or imidocarb
Encephalitozoonosis	*Encephalitozoon cuniculi*	Rare; primarily affects dogs <2 mo old	Acute encephalitis, ataxia, tremors, behavioral changes	Acute; poor prognosis	Serology, culture, histopathology	None
Trypanosomiasis	*Trypanosoma cruzi*	Rare in United States	Parasite of red blood cells; rarely causes CNS disease	Chronic, fair prognosis with treatment	Peripheral blood smears	Nifurtimox
Equine protozoal myeloencephalitis	*Sarcocystis neurona (Sarcocystis falcatula)*	Fairly common in horses	Systemic, multifocal, involving almost any part of the nervous system: commonly spinal cord, cauda equina, and cranial nerve signs	Chronic, progressive; guarded prognosis; treatment may be effective	CSF: Western blot, ELISA, IFA, and PCR	Pyrimethamine, trimethoprim-sulfonamide, diclazuril, ponazuril, nitazoxanide
Coccidiosis	Several species	Common enteric, rare CNS, several species of animals affected	Enteric coccidiosis is reported to cause CNS signs in some cases; *Sarcocystis* spp. may cause myopathy	Variable	Fecal identification, organism in muscle biopsy or necropsy	Sulfonamides, amprolium
Hepatozoonosis	*Hepatozoon canis*	Rare; dogs	Muscle pain and gait abnormalities may be seen	Chronic; guarded prognosis	Biopsy, PCR	Possibly sulfonamides, pyrimethamine (efficacy not known)

TABLE 15-13
Viral Diseases of the CNS

Disease	Cause	Incidence	Clinical Signs and Pathology	Course and Prognosis	Diagnostic Tests	Treatment	Prevention
Multiple Species							
Rabies	Rhabdovirus	Variable; all mammals Rare; more common in cats	Initially behavioral changes; rapid progression to either furious or dumb form; atypical variants are common in large animals (colic in horses and tenesmus in cattle) *Furious:* restlessness, wandering, biting, aggression, seizures *Dumb:* severe depression, pharyngeal and hypoglossal paralysis, progressive paralysis *Paralytic:* Ascending paralysis; progresses to include other brain signs	Acute, progresses to death in 3-10 days from onset	Necropsy: FA of brain	None	Vaccine
			Postvaccinal: Inadequate attenuated virus; rare; progressive ascending paralysis to diffuse CNS signs	Acute, progressive, poor prognosis	Necropsy: FA	None	Use proper vaccine
Pseudorabies	Herpesvirus	Rare; eradicated in domestic swine in United States	Swine: subclinical in adults; neonates: seizures, tremors, ataxia, death Other animals: excitement, intense pruritus and self-mutilation at site of viral entry; rapid progression to coma and death; contact with swine	Acute; progression to death in 1-2 days	Necropsy: FA on brain and spinal cord	None	Avoid contact with infected swine
Dogs							
Canine distemper	Morbillivirus	Common; dogs. Also large cats, raccoons, ferrets, marine mammals	*Acute:* young dogs; systemic illness; respiratory and gastrointestinal signs; CNS: acute seizures *Chronic:* Young or mature dogs. Demyelination of cerebellum, cerebral peduncles, optic nerves and tracts, and spinal cord. May begin with focal signs and progress to multifocal lesions. CNS signs occur weeks to months after systemic illness or without systemic signs. *Old dog encephalitis:* Mature or older dogs. Necrosis of cerebral gray matter. Forebrain signs predominate.	Acute to chronic; poor prognosis	CSF, FA on CSF, serology. Histopathology	Supportive; anticonvulsants	Vaccine
			Postvaccinal: see chronic distemper	1-2 wk postvaccination; acute and progressive	See distemper		None

Continued

TABLE 15-13

Viral Diseases of the CNS—cont'd

Prevention	Cause	Incidence	Clinical Signs and Pathology	Course and Prognosis	Diagnostic Tests	Treatment	Prevention
Infectious canine hepatitis	Canine adenovirus type I	Rare	Affects vascular endothelium, which may cause CNS signs; primarily affects liver, kidney, and lung. Can cause hepatoencephalopathy	Acute to chronic	Clinical pathology profile (liver)	Supportive	Vaccine
Canine herpesvirus	Canine herpesvirus	Sporadic; neonates and young puppies	In utero or early postwhelping exposure; polysystemic signs: depression, diarrhea, rhinitis, coma, opisthotonus, seizures	Acute progressive to death	Virus isolation; histopathology	Supportive	Colostrum; hyperimmune serum
Cats							
Feline infectious peritonitis	Coronavirus	Relatively common in cats	*Effusive form (wet):* diffuse, fibrinous peritonitis *Noneffusive (dry) form:* disseminated pyogranulomatous lesions in viscera, CNS, and eye. CNS signs can be focal or disseminated. Meningeal involvement and secondary hydrocephalus are common.	Slowly progressive; eventually fatal	Neutrophilic leukocytosis; increased serum globulins; CSF; mixed pleocytosis and increased protein	Supportive	Vaccine; marginally effective. Isolate infected cats
Feline panleukopenia	Parvovirus	Sporadic; neonatal cats	In utero or early postnatal CNS infection causing cerebellar hypoplasia (see Chapter 8)	Present at birth; nonprogressive	Necropsy	None	Vaccine
Feline leukemia virus (FLV)	Retrovirus	Common; cats	Epidural lymphoma causes spinal cord signs; diffuse brain disease may be present; systemic involvement and immunosuppression are common	Chronic progressive	Imaging, CSF, ELISA, FA, PCR	Combination chemotherapy	Vaccine
Feline immunodeficiency virus (FIV)	Lentivirus	Rare for neurologic signs	Behavioral signs	Chronic	ELISA, histopathology	None	Vaccine
Feline paramyxovirus	Paramyxovirus	Rare	Similar to canine distemper; demyelination; myoclonus reported	Chronic progressive	Virus isolation	None	None
Horses							
Encephalomyelitis (Western, Eastern, Venezuelan)	Togavirus (alphaviruses)	Variable; sporadic outbreaks in United States	Depression, fever, anorexia, ataxia, pacing, and circling; cranial nerve involvement in some cases	Acute progressive; guarded prognosis	CSF; serology; virus isolation; histopathology	Supportive	Vaccine mosquito control

West Nile virus	Togavirus (flavivirus)	Variable outbreaks; horses, birds and humans; sometimes other species including dogs and cats	Fever, paresis, ataxia, and muscle fasciculations. Lesions most severe in spinal cord; usually asymmetric and multifocal. Abnormal mentation and cranial nerve abnormalities occur in 44% to 67% of affected horses.	Acute progressive; guarded prognosis	CSF; plaque reduction neutralization tests (PRNTs); IgM capture ELISA test	Supportive	Vaccine
Equine herpesvirus	Equine herpesvirus 1 (EHV 1)	Variable	Upper respiratory infection, abortion, ataxia, urinary incontinence, paresis, signs more severe in pelvic limbs, sometimes cranial nerve signs	Acute progressive; fair to good prognosis	CSF, serology	Supportive Acyclovir	Vaccine ± isolation
Equine infectious anemia (EIA)	Retrovirus	Rare CNS signs	Behavioral changes, blindness, ataxia, weakness	Chronic progressive	Coggin test	Supportive	None
Cattle							
Infectious bovine rhinotracheitis (IBR) 1 and 5	Bovine herpesvirus types 1 and 5	Rare form of IBR	Calves <6 wk of age most susceptible. Fever, depression, respiratory signs, salivation, ataxia, circling, nystagmus, blindness, coma	Acute progressive; fatal	CSF; virus isolation; FA; immunoperoxidase; histopathology	Supportive	Vaccine
Malignant catarrhal fever	Herpesvirus	Sporadic	Adult cattle: depression, blindness, pacing, seizures, death; nasal and ocular discharge	Acute progressive to death	Histopathology	Supportive	None
Swine							
Enteroviral encephalomyelitis	Enterovirus	Variable	Pelvic limb paresis and ataxia, paralysis, seizures	Acute progressive; recovery or death in 1-3 wk	Virus isolation, serology	Supportive	Vaccine
Hemagglutinating encephalomyelitis virus	Coronavirus	Sporadic	Young swine: depression, ataxia, seizures, hyperesthesia	CNS form is acute	Serology; virus isolation	None	None
Porcine paramyxovirus	Paramyxovirus	Rare	Nursing piglets: depression, ataxia, seizures, weakness, tremor, blindness, and panophthalmitis	Acute progressive; fatal	Viral isolation; histopathology	None	None

Continued

TABLE 15-13

Viral Diseases of the CNS—cont'd

Prevention	Cause	Incidence	Clinical Signs and Pathology	Course and Prognosis	Diagnostic Tests	Treatment	Prevention
Sheep and Goats							
Visna, maedi	Lentivirus	Variable; sheep >2 yr old; horizontal transmission	Visna: ataxia, pelvic limb paresis; progressive to tetraparesis; facial tremors, blindness Maedi: progressive pneumonia	Chronic progressive; fatal in 1-2 yr	CSF, virus isolation, serology, histopathology	None	Culling carriers, chronically infected sheep
Louping ill (ovine encephalomyelitis)	Togavirus	Ireland; tick vector (Ixodes). Young sheep; sometimes horses, wildlife and other ruminants	Ataxia of head, trunk, and limbs. Rabbit hopping gait, blindness, seizures	Acute progressive; 50% fatal	Serology, virus isolation, presence of ticks	Supportive	Vaccine
Caprine arthritis-encephalitis virus (CAE virus)	Retrovirus (lentivirus)	Kids 2-6 mo old (virus shed in colostrum)	Persistent asymptomatic infection in adults. Progressive ataxia and paresis worse in pelvic limbs, tremors, opisthotonus. Evidence of arthritis, pneumonia, and mastitis (hard bag) in herd.	Acute to chronic progressive; fatal in kids	Agar gel immunodiffusion (AGID) blood	None	Culling chronically infected adults; heat treat colostrum
Border disease (hairy shaker lamb)	Pestivirus (similar to BVD of cattle)	Lambs (transmission is vertical and horizontal). Can affect goats and cattle	In utero infection before 50 days of gestation. Hairy wool, tremors of head and neck, ataxia. Flock history of abortion, infertility, deformed lambs. Goats: abortion and muffied fetus. Cattle: early abortion	Chronic; persistent infections	PCR, serology	None	Remove persistently infected animals

TABLE 15-14

Rickettsial and Chlamydial Diseases of the CNS

Disease	Cause	Incidence	Clinical Signs and Pathology	Course and Prognosis	Diagnostic Tests	Treatment
Rocky Mountain spotted fever	*Rickettsia rickettsii*	Fairly common in endemic areas of United States; dogs	Meningitis, ataxia, other CNS signs, can look like canine distemper	Acute; good prognosis with treatment	History of ticks, signs; thrombocytopenia, serology	Doxycycline, chloramphenicol
Ehrlichiosis	*Ehrlichia canis*	Rarely CNS signs in dogs	Meningitis, encephalitis	Acute to chronic; good prognosis if treated early	Pancytopenia, thrombocytopenia, serology	Doxycycline, chloramphenicol
Salmon poisoning	*Neorickettsia helminthoeca*	Rare, Pacific Northwest United States	Depression and convulsions terminally; paresis of pelvic limbs less common; nonsuppurative meningoencephalitis	Acute; fair to good prognosis if treated early	History of eating salmon, fluke eggs in feces	Doxycycline, chloramphenicol
Sporadic bovine encephalomyelitis (Buss disease)	*Chlamydia psittaci*	Sporadic, young cattle	Respiratory disease, polyarthritis, diffuse cerebral signs	Acute progressive; mortality approximately 50%	History, signs, CSF (increased protein, increased mononuclear cells), serology	Tetracycline, tylosin
Neuroborreliosis (Lyme disease)	*Borrelia burgdorferi*	Rare, except in endemic areas	Depression, meningitis	Acute to chronic (poorly characterized)	Antibodies to *B. burgdorferi* (especially in CSF)	Third-generation cephalosporins, tetracyclines

TABLE 15-15

Parasitic Diseases of the CNS

Disease	Cause	Incidence	Clinical Signs and Pathology	Course and Prognosis	Diagnostic Tests	Treatment
Dirofilariasis	*Dirofilaria immitis*, microfilaria or aberrant adult	Rare, areas with heartworm disease	CNS signs rare; microfilaria or migrating adult heartworms may cause infarction; seizures and other cerebral signs	Acute onset; prognosis guarded	Blood smear or serology to confirm heartworm disease, CSF (increased eosinophils suggestive), difficult to prove antemortem	None proven
Larva migrans	*Toxocara canis* and other species	Rare	Granulomas in brain or spinal cord from migrating larvae; signs related to location of lesion	Acute or chronic; prognosis depends on severity of signs	None, necropsy	None
Cuterebrosis	*Cuterebra* spp.	Rare	CNS signs depend on location of lesion	Acute to chronic; guarded prognosis	None, necropsy	None
Coenurosis	*Coenurus* spp.	Rare; most often reported in sheep	CNS signs depend on location of lesion	Acute to chronic; poor prognosis	None, sheep have softening of skull that can be palpated or seen on radiographs	Surgical removal in sheep

TABLE 15-16

Immune-Mediated Diseases of the CNS

Disease	Cause	Incidence	Clinical Signs and Pathology	Course and Prognosis	Diagnostic Tests	Treatment
Coonhound paralysis	Probable immune reaction to transmissible agent in raccoon saliva or environment	Fairly high in some areas; dogs	Ascending LMN paralysis; may last approximately 6 wk; ventral roots and peripheral nerves have segmental demyelination and some axon loss	Acute onset, lasts approximately 6 wk; good prognosis with good nursing	History, EMG, nerve conduction studies	Supportive
Postvaccinal rabies	CNS tissues in vaccine	Rare—these vaccines are no longer used	Ascending paralysis; demyelination from immune reaction to myelin in brain-origin vaccines	Acute onset, progressive; poor prognosis	None	None

Therefore, positive findings in laboratory data are useful, but negative findings do not rule out infectious disease. Focal deficits should be investigated according to the location of the lesion (see Chapters 5 through 15).

Analysis of CSF is a useful test for establishing the diagnosis of inflammatory disease (see Chapter 4). Increases in CSF protein concentrations range from low (50 to 100 mg/dL) in chronic viral diseases to very high (>300 mg/dL) in bacterial and fungal infections. Characteristic cell changes are increased mononuclear cells in viral diseases; increased neutrophils in bacterial diseases; increased numbers of both mononuclear cells and neutrophils in mycotic and protozoal diseases and feline infectious peritonitis; and increased numbers of mononuclear cells, neutrophils, and some eosinophils in parasitic, fungal, and immune-mediated diseases. *Exceptions are common.* For example, chronic bacterial infections may cause a

TABLE 15-17

Unclassified (noninfectious) Inflammatory Diseases of the CNS in Dogs and Cats

Disease	Cause	Incidence	Clinical Signs and Pathology	Course and Prognosis	Diagnostic Tests	Treatment
Steroid-responsive Meningitis-Arteritis (SRMA)	Unknown	Uncommon. Dogs less than 2 yr of age. Large-breed dogs: boxers, Bernese mountain dogs	Severe cervical hyperesthesia from inflammation of meninges and arteries. Sometimes associated with immune-mediated polyarthritis.	Acute and progressive; fair to good prognosis	CSF: neutrophilic pleocytosis and increased protein; increase IgA in serum and CSF	Immunosuppressive doses of prednisone
Necrotizing vasculitis	Unknown	Likely a severe form of SRMA. Seen in young beagles, Bernese mountain dogs and German short-haired pointers	Severe necrotizing vasculitis of the meninges, especially in cervical region. Signs similar to SRMA but more likely to have paresis. Spinal cord infarction reported in Bernese mountain dogs	Acute progressive; guarded prognosis	CSF: see SRMA	See SRMA
Pyogranulomatosis meningoencephalomyelitis	Unknown	Rare; reported in pointers	Mixed mononuclear-neutrophil infiltration of meninges and parenchyma of brain and spinal cord. Severe cervical pain, atrophy of cervical muscles, mild ataxia	Acute progressive; guarded to poor prognosis	CSF: neutrophilic pleocytosis; histopathology	See SRMA; some dogs respond to antibiotics
Granulomatous meningoencephalomyelitis (GME)	Unknown; probably type IV hypersensitivity	Relatively common in small-breed dogs	Granulomatous infiltrates in meninges, perivascular spaces, and brain parenchyma. Lesions may be disseminated, focal, or multifocal. Signs depend on lesion distribution. Cervical pain is common.	Chronic progressive; guarded prognosis, relapses are common	CSF: presence of macrophages is useful; histopathology, MRI	Prednisone, cytosine arabinoside, cyclosporine, other immunosuppressants
Necrotizing meningoencephalitis (NME); necrotizing leukoencephalitis (NLE)	Unknown; possibly immune mediated	Rare disease reported in young pugs, Maltese, Pekingese, Chihuahua, Yorkshire terrier, shih-tzu, French bulldog; West Highland white terrier, Boston terrier, Japanese Chin, miniature pinscher	Lymphoplasmacytic perivascular infiltrates in cerebrum and meninges. Multifocal necrosis in cerebrum. Seizures and other forebrain signs. Brainstem signs occur more with NLE.	Chronic progressive; poor prognosis	CSF (lymphocytic pleocytosis, increased protein); MRI	See GME; responds poorly to immunosuppressants
Feline polioencephalomyelitis	Unknown	Rare	Pelvic limb paresis, tremors, hyperesthesia. Spinal cord neurons and white matter primarily affected; brain lesions are scattered	Chronic progressive; poor prognosis	Histopathology; some cats have leukopenia and nonregenerative anemia	None

mononuclear cell response, especially increases in macrophages, whereas some viral diseases cause increased neutrophils in the CSF. The presence of a few neutrophils in the CSF is not necessarily abnormal. The only cell whose presence in the CSF seems consistently abnormal is the macrophage. The CSF can be normal in CNS inflammation.

Clinical suspicion of an infection is an adequate indication for bacterial and fungal cultures and bacterial sensitivity tests. The presence of antibodies in the CSF to specific viruses or to other infectious agents provides evidence of infection because they are not present in normal, vaccinated animals or those with systemic infection but without CNS disease (also see Chapter 4).[92] In CSF samples contaminated by blood (hemorrhage), serum albumin and antibody concentrations should be compared with concentrations in the CSF. When the level of CSF antibodies exceeds that of serum, CNS infection is more likely. Inflammation may increase the permeability of the blood-brain barrier, allowing serum antibodies to leak into the CSF.

Principles of Medical Treatment

Medical treatment is most commonly indicated for infections involving the nervous system. Physical therapy also is necessary for rehabilitation (see Chapter 14). Seizures (see Chapter 13) and other diseases requiring specific treatment are covered in the descriptions of the diseases. The management of CNS edema resulting in increased intracranial pressure is discussed in Chapter 12 in the section on brain trauma. Management of pain is reviewed in Chapter 14.

Effective therapy for CNS infections depends on the identification of the cause and selection of the appropriate antimicrobial agent. Identification is based on CSF analysis in which the organism may be observed (albeit rarely), culture and when available, polymerase chain reaction (PCR) testing, and measurement of antibody or antigen titers. Selection of the appropriate antimicrobial agent depends on two principles: (1) the agent must be effective against the microbial target without severely injuring the patient; and (2) it must be delivered to, and must penetrate, the CNS. Unfortunately, anatomic and physiologic barriers to successful therapy for CNS infections exist, especially when certain drugs are used. The combined effects of these obstacles create a functional blood-brain barrier.

The combined functions of the CNS capillaries and the choroid plexus create a barrier to the movement of drugs from the capillary or pericapillary fluid into nervous tissue or CSF. Discrepancies between serum and CNS drug concentrations occur because of two factors: those promoting drug accumulation in the CNS (the secretory selectivity of the choroid plexus) balanced against those preventing drug accumulation (the special anatomy of CNS capillaries and drug efflux pumps such as P-glycoprotein). In capillaries outside the CNS, drugs and other agents pass from the blood through clefts between endothelial cells and through fenestrations in the capillary basement membrane. In the CNS, capillary endothelial cells are joined by tight junctions that seal the intercellular clefts. The capillary basement membrane has no fenestrations and glial cell foot processes surround the capillaries helping create a barrier to diffusion.

In the CNS, a drug must penetrate an inner bimolecular lipid membrane, the endothelial cell cytoplasm, an outer lipid membrane, and a basement membrane and then traverse the glial foot processes.[122] Penetration of a drug is largely a function of its endothelial membrane solubility. Membrane solubility is favored by (1) a low degree of ionization at physiologic pH, (2) a low degree of plasma protein binding, and (3) a high degree of lipid solubility of the unionized drug.[123,124] Certain highly lipid-soluble drugs bind strongly to tissue sites in the brain, permitting high concentrations to be achieved within nervous tissue.

Regulation of CSF solutes occurs at the choroid plexus. Plasma dialysate that filters through fenestrated capillaries is selectively secreted by choroid epithelial cells. Certain CSF constituents also are actively reabsorbed by the choroidal epithelial cell, which tends to clear these substances from the CSF and from nervous tissue. This active transport system for weak organic acids removes drugs such as penicillin and gentamicin. Inflammation may block this system, allowing drug concentrations in the nervous tissue to increase. In addition, inflammation may increase the permeability of endothelial membranes to certain antibiotics, allowing these drugs to penetrate nervous tissue in cases of disease. In the normal animal, these antibiotics penetrate poorly. As the inflammation decreases, penetration of the antibiotic also decreases.

Antimicrobial Agents in Treating Infections

Antimicrobiocidal agents are grouped by their capacity to achieve concentrations in CSF sufficient to inhibit microorganisms throughout the period of therapy.[124] Table 15-18 lists these drugs relative to achievable concentrations in CSF.

Microbicidal drugs are preferred to microbiostatic drugs whenever possible. Antibiotics such as the aminoglycosides diffuse poorly, even in the presence of inflammation. Intrathecal administration may be required for adequate CSF concentrations to be achieved, but this route is rarely used in animals because of the necessity for anesthesia with each injection. Placement of intraventricular catheters can facilitate the injection of drugs into the CSF.

Infectious Inflammatory Disease

Bacterial Infections (See Table 15-10)

Bacterial Meningoencephalomyelitis. The pathogenesis, pathophysiology, and implications of treatment of bacterial meningitis in humans and experimental animals have been reviewed.[100] Bacteria must be able to survive in the intravascular space, penetrate the blood-brain barrier, and colonize in the meninges or CSF. Breakdown of the blood-brain barrier causes exudation of albumin into the CSF and facilitates the development of brain or spinal cord edema. Experiments in rats suggest that bacteria in the CSF elicit the release of endogenous inflammatory mediators that are important in the development and progression of clinical signs.[125] Experimental studies in rabbits reveal that the inflammatory process causes brain edema, probably secondary to loss of cerebrovascular autoregulation, direct cytotoxicity, and increased CSF outflow resistance.[101]

These findings may have important therapeutic implications. Rapidly acting bactericidal therapy delivered into the CSF is mandatory because only bactericidal therapy is associated with a cure in humans and experimental animal models. Rapid destruction of bacteria could release high concentrations of inflammatory bacterial toxins (lipopolysaccharides), which might exacerbate the inflammatory process.[126-128]

These studies also suggest that adjunctive therapy with antiinflammatory agents may be beneficial in bacterial meningitis.[101] In animals with experimental *Streptococcus pneumoniae* meningitis, methylprednisolone reduced CSF outflow resistance and both methylprednisolone and dexamethasone reduced brain edema.[101] Pretreatment with dexamethasone followed in 15 to 20 minutes with third-generation cephalosporins resulted in decreased inflammatory mediator release in laboratory animals with *Haemophilus influenzae* CNS infections.[127] Several controlled studies in children with bacterial meningitis demonstrated the benefits of adjunctive corticosteroid therapy, especially when corticosteroids were administered 15 to 20 minutes before bactericidal antibiotic therapy.[128] In these studies, dexamethasone was given

TABLE 15-18

Antimicrobial Drugs: Ability to Penetrate the Blood-Brain Barrier*

	Good	Intermediate	Poor
Microbicidal	Trimethoprim	Penicillin G†	Penicillin G Benzathine
	Moxalactam	Ampicillin†	
	Cefotaxime	Methicillin†	Cephalosporins§
	Ceftazidime	Nafcillin†	Aminoglycosides
	Metronidazole	Carbenicillin†	
	Enrofloxacin	Oxacillin	
	Vancomycin		
Microbistatic	Chloramphenicol	Tetracycline	Amphotericin B
	Sulfonamides	Flucytosine	Erythromycin ‖
	Isoniazid	Clindamycin	
	Minocycline‡		
	Doxycycline‡		
	Rifampin		

*Drugs prohibited for use in all food-producing animals: Chloramphenicol, clenbuterol, diethylstibestrol (DES), dimetridazole, ipronidazole and other nitroimidazoles, furazolidone, nitrofurazone, and other nitrofuans, sulfonamide drugs in lactating dairy cattle (except approved use of sulfadimethoxine, sulfabromomethazine, sulfaethoxypyridazine), fluoroquinolones, glycopeptides (http://www.fda.gov).
†High intravenous doses are needed to achieve the maximal effect.
‡Lipid-soluble tetracyclines that achieve higher concentrations in CSF than do other tetracyclines.
§First and second generation, may be effective early in bacterial meningitis; concentrations dramatically decrease with repair of the blood-brain barrier.
‖Penetration in the face of inflammation is unpredictable.

15 to 20 minutes before cefotaxime therapy and was continued every 6 hours for 4 days.

Other antiinflammatory agents that might be useful include indomethacin, pentoxifylline, and superoxide dismutase. Specific monoclonal antibodies have shown promise in experimental models of bacterial meningitis, especially when dexamethasone is also administered.[129]

Although these studies may have therapeutic implications for bacterial meningitis in domestic animals, controlled studies regarding these species have not been published. Furthermore, these studies involve specific neurotrophic bacteria in humans that may behave differently than the agents producing meningitis in animals. Ultimately, the use of corticosteroids in animals with confirmed or suspected CNS infection should be done judiciously and with caution. Despite the obvious counterintuitive rationale for their use, corticosteroids may be beneficial to reduce edema and alleviate clinical signs. When used, the dosage of corticosteroids should be tailored to the least amount necessary to control clinical signs. When possible, rapid tapering of the dosage should be prescribed based on continued response to therapy in an effort to restrict the administration of corticosteroids to short-term usage.

Bacterial Meningoencephalomyelitis in Dogs and Cats. Bacterial meningoencephalomyelitis is not common in dogs and cats. It usually occurs in association with bacteremia secondary to endocarditis, urinary tract infections, and pulmonary infections. Critically ill patients may have added risk of CNS infection. Meningitis may also occur from extension of infection in structures adjacent to the nervous system, such as the nasal passages, sinuses, and internal ears as well as direct penetration into the CNS such as occurs with bite wounds. Aerobic bacteria associated with bacterial meningitis in dogs and cats include *Pasteurella multocida, Staphylococcus Pseudintermedius, Streptococcus* spp., *and Escherichia coli.*[124,130,131] Uncommonly, *Proteus, Pseudomonas, Salmonella,* and *Klebsiella* organisms may be the causative agents. These gram-negative organisms are more common in nosocomial infections of critically ill patients. *Bartonella* sp. may also cause CNS disease in dogs.[132] Anaerobic bacteria isolated from dogs and cats with CNS infection include *Bacteroides, Fusobacterium, Peptostreptococcus,* and *Eubacterium.*[133]

Definitive treatment of bacterial meningitis is based on isolation of the organism from the CSF and determination of its antibiotic sensitivity. Other diagnostic tests include serology and PCR testing. The identification and elimination of the source of infection are imperative to successful treatment. Blood and urine cultures may be useful to identify the causative agent. Pending the outcome of CSF cultures, the initial antibiotic therapy in small animals is based on clinical findings of concomitant infection and the most likely causative agent present. Broad-spectrum bacteriocidal antibiotics that penetrate the CSF are chosen.

Trimethoprim-sulfonamide combinations and enrofloxacin are good initial choices. Both are available to veterinarians, penetrate the CSF in good concentrations, cover a broad spectrum of bacterial agents, and are not expensive compared with third-generation cephalosporins. Enrofloxacin has greater activity against gram-negative bacteria and very little activity against anaerobes.[134] Clindamycin hydrochloride may be used concurrently to provide anaerobic and gram-positive coverage. For animals unable to receive oral medications, parenteral formulations of enrofloxacin and clindamycin hydrochloride are available. The dose for enrofloxacin in dogs is 2.5-5.0 mg/kg PO, IM, SC, IV every 12 hours. Enrofloxacin should be used with care in dogs 2 to 12 months of age to avoid cartilage damage. The dose of enrofloxacin in cats is 5 mg/kg once a day PO or 2.5 mg/kg IM every 12 hours. Rare incidence of retinal toxicity in cats have been reported at doses >15 mg.kg/day. The dose for clindamycin in dogs and cats is 3-11 mg/kg PO, IV, IM SC every 8 hours. Gastroenteritis is the most common side effect of clindamycin therapy in dogs and cats. The initial dose for trimethoprim-sulfonamides is 30 mg/kg every 12 hours for 5 to 7 days and then 15 mg/kg every 12 hours for 10 to 14 days.

Third-generation cephalosporins such as cefotaxime and ceftazidime penetrate the CSF in good concentrations and are effective against many resistant gram-negative bacteria.[135] They are usually effective against anaerobes but have reduced activity against gram-positive cocci. Ceftiofur, approved for use in animals, does not cross the blood-brain barrier unless inflammation is present, and, in this regard, is similar to the aminopenicillins. When gram-negative sepsis is suspected as the cause of the meningitis, the third-generation cephalosporins are the drugs of choice.

Meningitis caused by gram-positive bacteria may respond to high doses of aminopenicillins.[131] Many isolates of *S. Pseudintermedius* and *S. aureus* secrete beta lactamase, which inactivates most aminopenicillins. Aminopenicillins combined with clavulanic acid and lactamase-resistant penicillins such as methicillin or oxacillin are better choices for staphylococcal infections. Rifampin is bactericidal, readily penetrates the CSF, and has very good activity against staphylococci.[136] It is also effective against many gram-negative bacteria. Bacterial resistance to rifampin develops readily, especially when it is given as a single agent. For staphylococcal infections, rifampin is best combined with β-lactam antibiotics. The human dose of 10 mg/kg daily produces a concentration in canine serum four times that required in people to inhibit bacteria but also causes adverse side effects in dogs. A dose less than 10 mg/kg daily is recommended, but definitive pharmacologic studies have not been published.[136] Rifampin also may be useful in treating chronic abscesses and pyogranulomatous infections. Imipenem is a β-lactam compound that belongs to the carbapenem family of antibiotics. It has broad-spectrum activity against most gram-positive and gram-negative aerobes and anaerobes. Imipenem is useful in the treatment of nosocomial gram-negative infections that do not respond to other antibiotic regimens.[135,137] After intravenous administration, imipenem penetrates the CSF in good concentrations.

Occasionally, systemic infection with *Brucella canis* extends to the nervous system. While most animals are euthanized due to zoonotic issues, brucellosis can be treated with combination of streptomycin and minocycline. Streptomycin should be administered for 2 weeks by parenteral injection. Minocycline should be given orally for 4 weeks in combination with the 2-week course for streptomycin.[138,139] It is difficult to eradicate brucella infections in animals.

Bacterial Meningoencephalomyelitis in Horses. Bacterial meningitis occurs most commonly in septicemic foals that do not acquire passive transfer of immunity.[140-142] Common primary sites of infection include the GI tract, lung, and umbilicus. Pneumonia, peritonitis, hypopyon, septic arthritis, and omphalophlebitis are common. Extension to the brain and spinal cord frequently occurs if treatment is not aggressive.

The diagnosis of meningitis in foals is confirmed by cytologic evaluation and bacterial culture of the CSF. A neutrophilic pleocytosis is typical, and cell counts may exceed 1000 cells/uL (normal <5 cells/uL).[142,143] The total CSF protein level is usually more than 100 mg/dL. *E. coli* and *Klebsiella* spp. are the most frequently isolated organisms.[142,143]

Although definitive antibiotic therapy is based on bacterial culture and antimicrobial sensitivity testing, initial empiric therapy is based on the assumption that gram-negative enteric bacteria are the most likely cause. Third-generation cephalosporins are the antimicrobials recommended in foals. These include cefotaxime sodium (40 mg/kg IV q8h) and ceftazidime (50 mg/kg IV q12h). Ceftiofur (2 to 4 mg/kg IV q12h) is available to veterinarians but does not penetrate the CSF in normal horses. Although very expensive, these antibiotics can rapidly sterilize the CSF and may shorten the total treatment time and thus reduce overall costs of therapy.[140] Trimethoprim-sulfonamide combinations may be effective but are less so than the third-generation cephalosporins previously described.

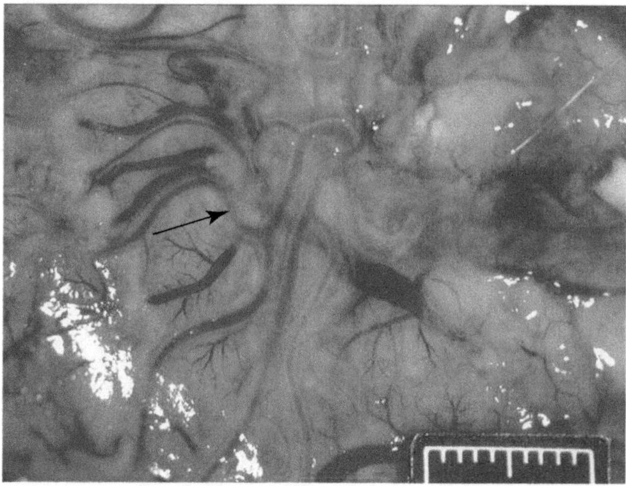

Figure 15-8 Suppurative meningitis in a calf. Note the cloudy and thickened meninges that tend to obscure engorged (inflamed) blood vessels *(arrow)*. (Courtesy Dr. Roger Panciera, Oklahoma State University College of Veterinary Medicine.)

Adjunctive antiinflammatory therapy and other supportive care are used in foals with progressive neurologic dysfunction. Corticosteroids (dexamethasone, 0.15 mg/kg q6h IV) are used with caution in septic foals because corticosteroid therapy can cause rapid bacterial dissemination.[140] Dimethyl sulfoxide (1 g/kg IV q24h) may help to reduce CNS inflammation and edema and protect against reperfusion injury when cerebral ischemia is present. Mannitol (0.25 to 1.0 g/kg IV q24h) helps reduce CNS edema. Plasma transfusions (1 to 2 L IV) and enteral hyperalimentation may be indicated. Diazepam (0.2 to 0.5 mg/kg every 15 minutes) or phenobarbital (10 to 20 mg/kg IV q8h) or both can be given to control seizures.[115]

Bacterial Meningoencephalomyelitis in Cattle. Bacterial meningitis is the most common CNS disease in neonatal calves.[119] It develops secondary to septicemia and bacteremia associated with failure of passive transfer of colostral antibodies. A presumptive diagnosis of bacterial meningitis with failure of passive transfer is based on presence of omphalophlebitis or septic arthritis, fever and signs suggestive for meningoencephalomyelitis (obtundation, tetraparesis, hyperesthesia, and multiple cranial nerve deficits) (Figure 15-8).

Neutrophilic pleocytosis and increased protein are present in the CSF of 60% to 70% of affected calves. Mononuclear pleocytosis may be present in chronic disease. The identification of bacteria in the CSF is less than 50% of cases examined. *E. coli* is the organism most frequently responsible in clinical cases.[119] Isolates may be resistant to trimethoprim-sulfonamides, and many, if not most, are now resistant to triple sulfonamide drugs. Other bacterial agents include *Salmonella* sp. and *Arcanobacterium pyogenes*. Most affected calves die or are euthanized, usually within 2 to 3 days after diagnosis and initiation of therapy.

Treatment of bacterial meningitis in calves is difficult and the mortality rate is high.[144] Selection of antimicrobial drugs is based on culture and sensitivity of bacteria from the CSF; however, their use is often empirical. The antimicrobial regimen should be broad spectrum against gram-negative and gram-positive bacteria. Although trimethoprim-sulfonamides and triple sulfonamide drugs are frequently chosen to treat bacterial meningitis in calves, studies indicate an emerging resistance of gram-negative bacteria to these drugs. Ampicillin

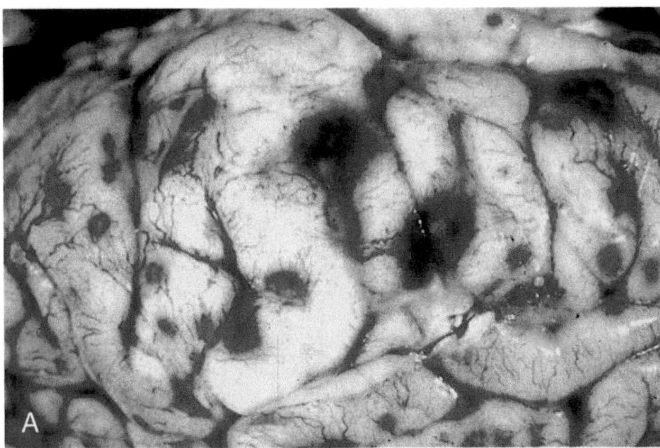

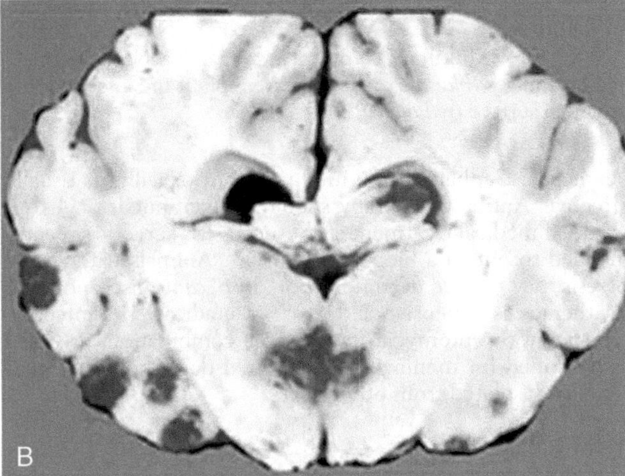

Figure 15-9 **A,** Extensive hemorrhages in the cerebral cortex are typical gross lesions of thromboembolic meningoencephalomyelitis. **B,** Note the multiple hemorrhagic lesions seen in cross section of the brain in **A.** (**A** and **B,** Courtesy Dr. Roger Panciera, Oklahoma State University College of Veterinary Medicine.)

(10 to 20 mg/kg IV q8h) has been used in combination with other antimicrobials. Although expensive, the third-generation cephalosporins (such as ceftiofur, 5 to 10 mg/kg IV or IM q12h) are rational empiric drugs for treatment. Because of their cost, the use of these drugs may not be economically feasible in many cases. Adequate amounts of colostrum and early recognition and treatment of bacterial infections is essential for prevention of bacterial meningitis in calves.

Thromboembolic Meningoencephalitis (TEME). *Histophilus somni* (formerly *Haemophilus somnus*) is the major cause of TEME in cattle.[145] Exposure to this organism is widespread, and up to 25% of cattle may harbor serum antibodies to the organism. *H. somni* persists in the urinary and reproductive tracts of cattle and is shed in urine and reproductive secretions. The disease is most common in weaned calves, and outbreaks of TEME occur 1 to 2 weeks after cattle arrive at the feedyard.[146] Bronchopneumonia is the most common form of hemophilosis, but arthritis, myelitis, retinitis, myocarditis, laryngitis, otitis media or otitis interna, and conjunctivitis also occur. TEME usually follows the occurrence of pneumonia by 1 to 2 weeks. Morbidity is low, and mortality is high. Diagnosis is based on history and physical examination. Changes in CSF reflect a bacterial infection that often is hemorrhagic. Necropsy findings provide a definitive diagnosis with presence of hemorrhagic infarcts in the brain and spinal cord. Histology reveals vasculitis, thrombosis, and neutrophilic infiltrates (Figure 15-9).

As with the neurotrophic bacteria that infect people, *H. somni* possesses several virulent factors (mucopolysaccharide capsule, outer membrane proteins, and endotoxin concentrated in the cell wall) that enhance its penetration into, and subsequent injury to, the CNS. *H. somni* colonizes the small vessels of the meninges, brain, and spinal cord. Fibrin thrombi and brain infarction cause the neurologic signs. The most effective antibiotics for TEME include the aminopenicillins, ceftiofur, oxytetracycline, and florfenicol. All are approved for use in food animals and penetrate the CSF when active inflammation is present. Parenteral oxytetracycline is used for non-CNS infections. Treatment of animals that progress to recumbency is often not effective. When a case is suspected, the other animals in contact should be closely monitored to detect and treat at the early disease stage.

Listeriosis (Circling Disease). *Listeria monocytogenes* is a resistant and ubiquitous bacterium that causes CNS disease in people and domestic animals (listeriosis, circling disease, silage disease).[147] Ruminants appear more susceptible to infection than do other domestic animals. The organism can be transmitted in silage and other feed. Food-borne infection is common in humans. Outbreaks usually occur in the winter. In cattle and sheep, the organism penetrates the oral mucosa via wounds and is transmitted to the brain in a retrograde fashion via the trigeminal nerve. Signs related to infection of the rostral medulla (trigeminal, facial, and vestibulocochlear nerve dysfunction) are common. Although meningitis and encephalitis are the classic manifestations of listeriosis in ruminants, spinal cord disease, abortion, and mastitis also occur. Clinical signs of encephalitis are often more severe in small ruminants. The most useful antemortem diagnostic test is CSF analysis. Characteristic findings include increased protein concentration and nucleated cell count with mononuclear cells predominating. Definitive diagnosis is made by histopathology. Gross necropsy findings are not very remarkable. Histopathology reveals multifocal areas of necrosis with infiltrations of macrophages and neutrophils. Diagnosis is confirmed by isolation of the organism from body fluids or tissues. Warm or cold enrichment methods are used to isolate the organism but immunohistochemistry is more successful than bacteriologic culture for detecting *L. monocytogenes* in brain tissue. Treatment is initiated early and involves long-term parenteral antibiotic therapy (penicillin, ampicillin, amoxicillin, or oxytetracycline). Prevention is aimed a limiting fecal contamination of the feed from ruminants and wildlife.

Bacterial Brain Abscess. Brain abscesses are more common in large animals than in dogs and cats. Neurologic signs relate to the specific location of the abscess and compression or necrosis of surrounding neurologic structures. Large abscesses may create signs similar to any other intracranial mass. Increased intracranial pressure, cerebral edema, and brain herniation may occur (Figure 15-10).

The pituitary abscess syndrome has been described in cattle, goats, sheep, and swine (Figure 15-11).[148]

The anatomy of the rete mirabilis and its close association to the pituitary gland may explain the predilection for pituitary abscesses in cattle. The primary clinical signs include depression, ataxia, blindness, absence of the pupillary light reflex, dysphagia, dropped jaw, head pressing, bradycardia, nystagmus, and strabismus. The CSF may contain increased total protein concentrations and pleocytosis. Bacterial cultures of CSF are usually negative. *Arcanobacterium pyogenes* and *Pasteurella multocida* are most commonly isolated from abscesses at necropsy.[148] Infection at other sites with the same organisms occurs in about 50% of cases. The mortality rate is nearly 100%, and successful therapy is rare.

In horses, brain abscesses are usually caused by *Streptococcus equi*, but other streptococci are occasionally isolated.[149]

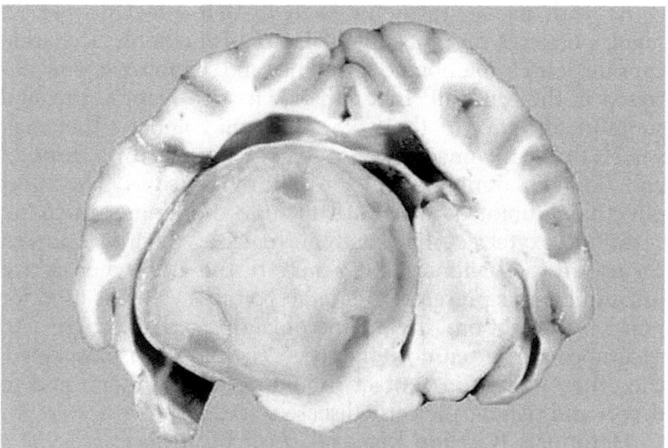

Figure 15-10 Large brain abscess in a sheep. (Courtesy Cornell University College of Veterinary Medicine.)

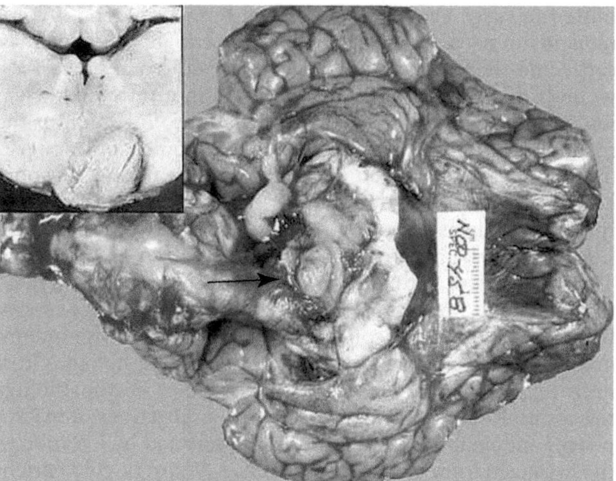

Figure 15-11 A large and destructive pituitary abscess in a cow *(black arrow)*. Inset figure shows abscess extending into the hypothalamus. (Courtesy Cornell University College of Veterinary Medicine.)

The prognosis is generally poor. If diagnosed by CT, successful surgical drainage is possible.[150] Brain abscesses are rare in dogs and cats but may result from extension of purulent otitis media/interna, rhinitis, sinusitis, open skull fractures, and foreign-body penetration of the brain. The causative agents are usually *Staphylococcus* spp., *Streptococcus* spp., and *Pasteurella* spp. Anaerobes may also be isolated in some cases. Localization of the abscess with CT or MRI may allow surgical drainage or excision. Methicillin, oxacillin, and rifampin may be useful for gram-positive infections. Clindamycin and metronidazole may be given in anaerobic infections. A guarded prognosis should be made.

Cats may have meningitis secondary to abscesses that are caused by anaerobic bacteria. Penicillin or amoxicillin is effective and reasonable in cost. Clindamycin or metronidazole is a good alternative for resistant infections.[151] If accessible, surgical drainage of intracranial infections should be considered.

Discospondylitis (also see Chapter 6)

The most common cause of bacterial discospondylitis in dogs is *Staphylococcus pseudintermedius*; occasionally *Brucella canis* organisms are the source.[152] The disease may be associated with urinary tract infection and bacteremia. In staphylococcal discospondylitis, penicillinase-resistant antibiotics should be chosen. Cephalosporin, methicillin, or oxacillin is usually effective. Antibiotic therapy should be continued for 4 to 6 weeks. If medical treatment is not successful, surgery is recommended to obtain a biopsy and culture. Animals with severe paresis may require decompression. In *B. canis* discospondylitis, therapy is expensive and may not eradicate the infection effectively. Streptomycin-minocycline combinations are used as described for meningitis.[114] Affected dogs should be neutered and isolated from other dogs.

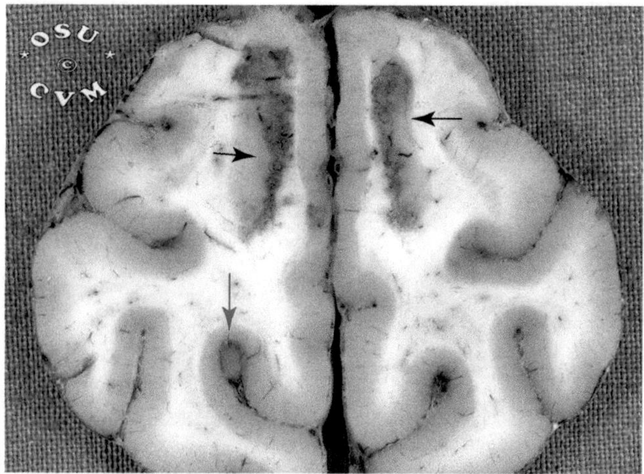

Figure 15-12 Multifocal cryptococcosis in a dog. Note the thickened meninges *(black arrows)* and extension of the infection into the brain surface *(red arrow)*.

Mycotic Infections (see Table 15-11)

The more common mycotic infections of the CNS are caused by *Cryptococcus neoformans*, *Blastomyces dermatitidis*, and *Coccidioides immitis*. They produce polysystemic disease, including granulomatous meningoencephalomyelitis or neuritis (Figure 15-12).

A definitive diagnosis is made by isolation or identification of the organism in the CSF or other body secretions. Treatment regimens are similar for the various deep mycotic agents, as discussed below.

Therapy

Cryptococcal Meningitis. For many years the mainstay of therapy for the deep mycotic pathogens has been amphotericin B. This drug is poorly absorbed from the GI tract and must be given IV for a full therapeutic effect. Amphotericin B diffuses poorly into the CSF. For this reason, although amphotericin B has value in fulminating systemic infections, agents such as itraconazole and fluconazole are preferred for cryptococcal meningitis. Several therapeutic regimens of amphotericin B have been described.

Flucytosine, when combined with amphotericin B, acts synergistically in vitro against *C. neoformans*. It achieves satisfactory concentrations in the CSF. The oral dose of flucytosine is 50 to 75 mg/kg every 8 hours.[153,154] The rate of relapse is considerably lower with the combined therapy. Side effects include leukopenia, thrombocytopenia, vomiting, and diarrhea.

Successful management of cryptococcal meningitis has been reported with the azole and triazole antifungal compounds.[130,131] At usual concentrations achieved in the plasma these compounds are considered fungistatic, but at higher concentrations they may be fungicidal.[155] The azoles and triazoles inhibit synthesis of ergosterol in the fungal cell membrane. Ketoconazole, itraconazole, and fluconazole have been studied in dogs and cats. All are well absorbed from the GI tract. Absorption of itraconazole is enhanced by food in the intestinal tract.

Ketoconazole does not penetrate the CSF in adequate concentrations to be effective, and yet reports exist of success with this agent in the treatment of cryptococcal meningitis, especially when combined with flucytosine.[157] Ketoconazole therapy is associated with hepatic dysfunction, elevated liver enzymes, and suppression of endogenous steroid synthesis. It has a slow onset of action, and in life-threatening conditions ketoconazole is often combined with amphotericin B to provide immediate fungicidal activity in all tissues except the eye and the CNS. The dose of ketoconazole for dogs and cats is 10 to 15 mg/kg daily.

Itraconazole has a broad spectrum of activity against many fungal organisms and has been effective in the treatment of cryptococcal meningitis in cats.[158] In systemic blastomycosis, itraconazole produces a cure rate equal to or greater than that of combined therapy with ketoconazole and amphotericin B. Itraconazole is less toxic than ketoconazole but is more expensive. Fluconazole is a bistriazole compound with broad-spectrum antifungal activity. It is well absorbed from the GI tract and has a bioavailability greater than 90%.[156] It penetrates into the meninges and CSF with or without inflammation. Fluconazole is the drug of choice in the treatment of cryptococcal meningitis in humans and is used in dogs and cats with mycotic infections of the CNS. Serious side effects are uncommon. The recommended dose in dogs and cats for both itraconazole and fluconazole is 10 mg/kg daily divided twice daily for 2 to 3 months beyond the resolution of all signs.[159] The successful resolution of cryptococcal meningitis and optic neuritis with fluconazole has been reported in the horse. The dose was 5 mg/kg per day and the horse was treated for 197 days.[160]

Coccidioidal Meningitis. *Coccidioides immitis* is not susceptible to the synergistic activity of combined amphotericin B and flucytosine therapy but may respond to ketoconazole administered at 10 mg/kg every 24 hours for 9 to 12 months.[136] Although in some cases treatment resolved the clinical signs, recurrences were common when treatment was discontinued. Similar results were found in a few cases treated with itraconazole and fluconazole.[161]

Other Systemic Fungal Infections. *Histoplasma capsulatum, Blastomyces dermatitidis, Aspergillus* spp., *Candida* spp., and *Sporothrix schenckii* occasionally are involved in meningitis. Treatment is the same as for cryptococcosis and coccidioidomycosis.[162-165]

Actinomycetes Infections (see Table 15-1)

Tuberculous Meningitis. Although it is nearly nonexistent in dogs and cats, tuberculous meningitis occurs occasionally in primates. Most of the antituberculous drugs readily penetrate the CNS. A combination of isoniazid and ethambutol is suggested. Other effective drugs include rifampin, ethionamide, pyrazinamide, and cycloserine.

Nocardiosis. The drugs of choice have been triple sulfonamides or trimethoprim-sulfa combinations. Their in vitro effect, however, has not been duplicated in vivo. The drugs should be given in high doses, and precautions should be taken to prevent nephrotoxicity. Alternative drugs include minocycline, amikacin, and erythromycin combined with ampicillin.[166]

Actinomycosis. The drug of choice is ampicillin given IV at 10 to 20 mg/kg every 6 hours.[166] Therapy is continued with clindamycin, chloramphenicol, or minocycline.

Protozoan Infections (see Table 15-12)

Toxoplasmosis. *Toxoplasma gondii* is an intracellular coccidian parasite that produces systemic infection in dogs and cats and occasionally in other domestic animals. Cats are the definitive host and pass oocysts in the feces. In cats infection may occur through ingestion of any of the three life stages of the organism or transplacentally.[167] The organism may infect the muscle, CNS, liver, lung, and eye. A variety of clinical signs may occur, including uveitis, retinitis, myositis, pneumonia, and encephalitis. The diagnosis of clinically active toxoplasma infection is based on suggestive clinical signs, demonstration of *T. gondii* tachyzoites or bradyzoites in tissue biopsy sections, or immune testing for antibodies or antigen in serum, ocular fluid, or CSF. Although several immunologic tests are commercially available, the *T. gondii*-specific immunoglobulin M (IgM) and IgG enzyme-linked immunosorbent assay (ELISA) are most often used in dogs and cats. IgM levels tend to increase within 2 to 4 weeks of infection but are negative by 16 weeks.[168] IgM titers more than 1:256 indicate recent or active infection. A fourfold increase in IgG titers also indicates recent or active disease. Both IgG and IgM titers can be assessed in samples of CSF and compared with serum concentrations of albumin, IgG, and IgM. When the levels in CSF exceed those in serum, active or recent CNS infection should be suspected.

Clindamycin hydrochloride is the primary antimicrobial selected to treat clinical toxoplasmosis in dogs and cats. The dose in cats is 12.5 to 25 mg/kg orally or IM every 12 hours. The dose in dogs is 10 to 20 mg/kg orally or IM every 12 hours. Although clindamycin does not adequately penetrate the CSF of humans, the drug may penetrate the CSF of cats in sufficient levels to be effective for neurologic disease.[169] Transient vomiting is a common side effect in some cats. Cats should be treated for at least 4 to 5 weeks.

Neosporosis. Neosporosis is caused by the protozoan *Neospora caninum*. Natural infections have been reported in dogs and calves. The muscles and the CNS are the most common sites of infection. Affected animals typically develop nonsuppurative encephalomyelitis, polyradiculoneuritis, and myositis. A positive diagnosis is based on demonstration of the organism in blood, CSF, or tissues. A fluorescent antibody test can detect *N. caninum*–specific antibodies. Clinical experience with treatment is limited, but treatment with clindamycin should be tried early in the course of illness. Sulfadiazine may also be effective (see also Chapter 7).[167]

Equine Protozoal Myeloencephalitis (EPM). EPM is described in Chapter 6 because clinical signs commonly manifest as spinal cord dysfunction. It is the most common neurologic disease in horses with multifocal or asymmetric neurologic deficits. Infection of the CNS may occur anywhere, but the spinal cord is most commonly affected.[170-173] EPM is most commonly caused *Sarcocystis neurona*. A small number of EPM cases have been attributed to infection by *Neospora hughesi*. The opossum is the definitive host for *S. neurona* and harbors the sexual stages of the protozoa within its gastrointestinal tract. Natural intermediate hosts for *S. neurona* that have been identified include the skunk, raccoon, cat, Pacific harbor seal, and nine-banded armadillo. The horse is an aberrant dead-end host. Horses are most likely infected by fecal-oral transmission. The diagnosis and treatment of EPM are discussed in Chapter 6.

Viral Infections

The viral diseases causing encephalomyelitis are summarized in Table 15-13. Viral infection of the CNS may fit into one of three categories: (1) viral invasions resulting in inflammation (viral meningitis, encephalitis, encephalomyelitis, or poliomyelitis); (2) postinfectious, noninflammatory encephalopathic states; and (3) postinfectious and postvaccinal inflammatory states ("old dog" encephalitis, perhaps polyradiculoneuritis, brachial plexus neuropathy).

Rabies. Rabies is caused by a rhabdovirus that results in a fatal encephalomyelitis in mammals. Common sources of infection include bites from skunks, bats, raccoons, foxes, and coyotes.

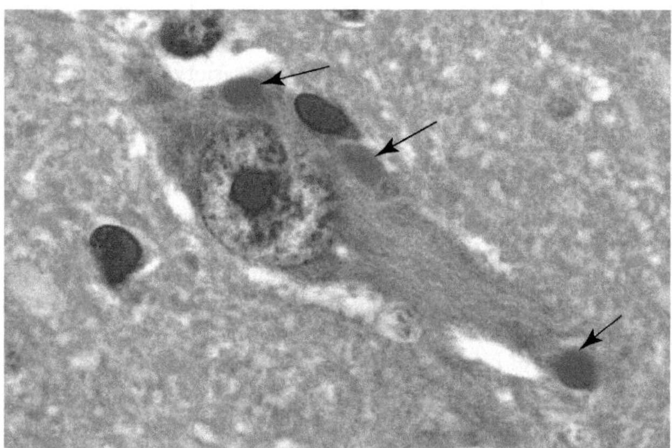

Figure 15-13 Brain from a horse with rabies. Note the prominent Negri bodies *(arrows)* in a neuron. (Courtesy Cornell University College of Veterinary Medicine.)

The virus is transmitted via infected saliva (animal bites, contamination of wounds) and is transmitted by retrograde axonal transport to the brain and spinal cord. Lesions in the nervous system are most severe in the midbrain, cervical spinal cord, and cranial nerve ganglia and include perivascular cuffs of plasma cells and lymphocytes. The Negri body, found in neurons, is the classical inclusion body of rabies virus (Figure 15-13).

Three forms of rabies have been described in domestic animals: furious, dumb, and paralytic. Initially, infected animals often develop behavioral changes with rapid progression to one of the three forms. The furious form is characterized by restlessness, wandering, aggression, and seizures. The dumb form is characterized by progressive paralysis, pharyngeal and hypoglossal paralysis, depression, and head pressing. The paralytic form occurs more commonly in large animals than in dogs and cats. It is a progressive ascending paralysis that may begin as a shifting leg lameness. In cattle, the most common clinical signs are salivation, bellowing, aggressiveness, paresis/paralysis, and straining. Colic, aggressiveness, hyperesthesia, and ataxia are common clinical signs in horses. Sheep will commonly manifest hyperesthesia, tremors, and salivation. Goats and pigs also manifest mainly aggressiveness, hyperexcitability, and squealing. It is important to keep in mind that rabies can clinically present with any neurologic sign.

Definitive diagnosis is a positive fluorescent antibody test performed on brain tissue. There is no effective treatment. Infected animals and those suspected to be infected should be euthanized and brain submitted for fluorescent antibody (FA) examination. Given the human health hazard, FA examination of the brain should be pursued in every suspected case in which there has been significant risk of exposure to humans. If uncertainty exists, a state health official should be contacted for advice. Vaccines are available and very effective in domestic animals. Despite their efficacy, rabies infection can occur in vaccinated animals.[172]

Pseudorabies. Pseudorabies (Aujeszky disease, mad itch) is caused by a neurotrophic α-herpesvirus. The virus can be latent or subclinical in adult swine and pigs are thought to be the source of infection in other animal species. After a pig bite, the virus enters the skin and travels to the brain or spinal cord by retrograde axonal transport. The incubation period is 90 to 156 days. Piglets show seizures, tremors, ataxia, and death. In other species, severe pruritus, dermal abrasions, swelling, and alopecia develop at the site of virus inoculation (Figure 15-14).

Other signs include ataxia, paresis, circling, aggression, depression, and seizures.

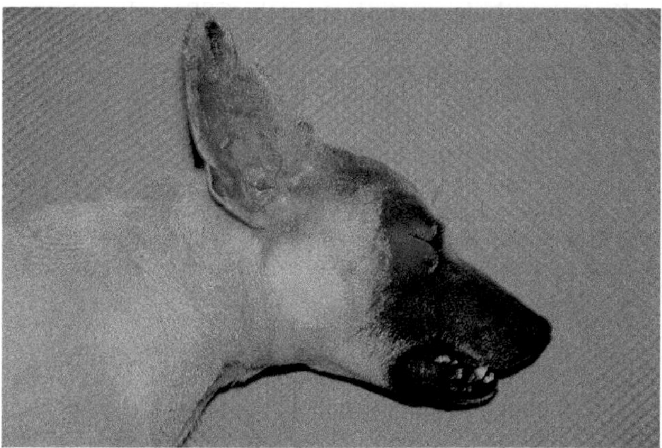

Figure 15-14 Dog with pseudorabies. Note the extensive self-mutilation of the head secondary to severe pruritus. (Courtesy Dr. Joan Coates.)

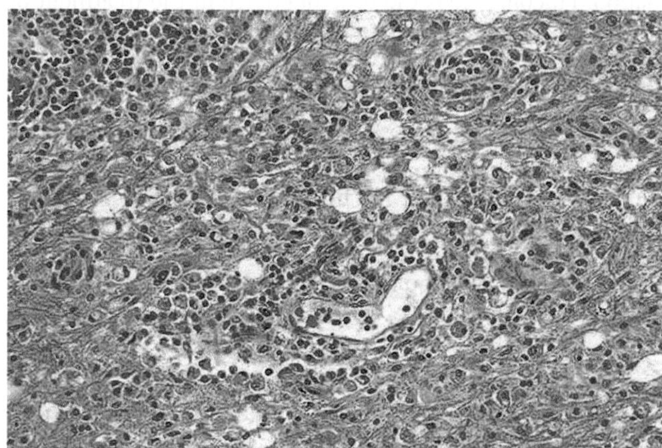

Figure 15-15 Canine distemper encephalomyelitis. Cerebellar folial white matter with perivascular lymphocytes and plasma cells, numerous macrophages and vacuolated neuroparenchyma. (Courtesy Cornell University College of Veterinary Medicine.)

Diagnosis is based on viral isolation and histopathology. There is no effective treatment. Pseudorabies has been eradicated from domestic swine in the United States.

Canine Distemper Virus. Canine distemper is a common polysystemic disease of dogs that may infect the CNS. The virus is also pathogenic in ferrets, raccoons, big cats, and other animal species. There are three neurologic syndromes. Acute distemper occurs in susceptible young dogs and respiratory and digestive signs predominate. Neurologic signs may occur later in the clinical course but many dogs die before these signs develop. Seizures are the most common neurologic manifestation. Lesions most commonly represent a polioencephalomyelitis.

Chronic distemper encephalomyelitis occurs in young dogs that survive the acute stages of the disease and in mature dogs without signs of system disease. Chronic distemper is a multifocal severe demyelinating meningoencephalomyelitis. Lesions are most common in the cerebellum, cerebellar peduncles, cervical spinal cord, optic tracts, and periventricular white matter (Figure 15-15).

Clinical signs include progressive and severe ataxia, paresis, depression, and generalized or "chewing gum" seizures (focal seizures involving biting movements of the mandible). Constant repetitive myoclonus, twitching of temporal or

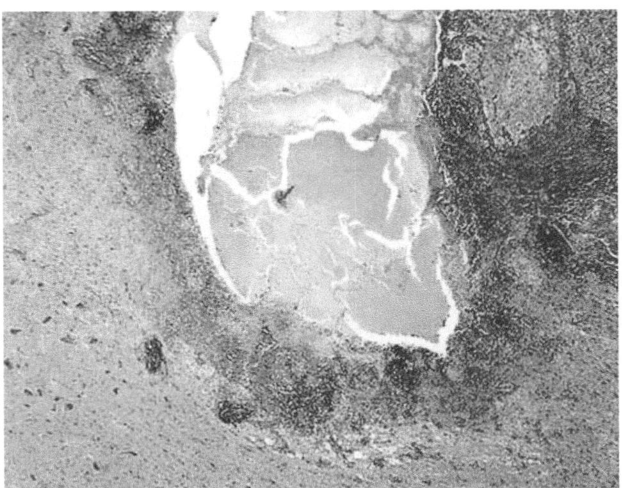

Figure 15-16 Neurologic feline infectious peritonitis with extensive periventricular inflammation and protein effusion into the ventricular lumen. (Courtesy Cornell University College of Veterinary Medicine.)

appendicular muscles, occurs in some dogs and is supportive of the diagnosis. Distemper virus may cause chorioretinitis and optic neuritis and visual deficits may develop.

Old dog encephalitis is a rare form of canine distemper that appears to be a manifestation of chronic viral infection after years of latent brain infection. The clinical signs result from necrosis of cerebral gray matter and are typical of other forebrain disorders.

The diagnosis of canine distemper is based on positive FA tests on neural tissue, cerebrospinal fluid cells (infected lymphocytes), or other lymphoid tissues. Other supporting findings include ophthalmologic evidence of chorioretinitis, increased lymphocytes and protein in CSF, and distemper myoclonus.

There is no definitive treatment. Seizures can be managed with anticonvulsants drugs such as phenobarbital but control is difficult. Vaccines are highly protective against both system and neurologic signs.

Feline Infectious Peritonitis Virus (FIP). The noneffusive (dry) form of FIP virus includes neurologic signs in some cats. The FIP virus induces a vasculitis involving the meninges, ependymal lining, and choroid plexus (Figure 15-16).

Characteristic histopathologic lesions are a pyogranulomatous meningoencephalitis and lymphoplasmacytic periventriculitis. The lesions are most severe around the third ventricle of the brain resulting in an obstructive hydrocephalus. Ataxia related to vestibular dysfunction is the most common neurologic sign. Intention tremor and fine head tremor have been associated with cerebellar and meningeal disease. Forebrain, cerebellar, and thoracolumbar spinal cord signs are also common. Signs are slowly progressive and eventually fatal. Affected cats frequently have an anterior uveitis.

Diagnosis is based on clinical signs, presence of ocular lesions, cytology of abdominal effusion if present, and CSF analysis (neutrophilic-lymphocytic pleocytosis and increased protein). There is no effective treatment.

Equine Herpesvirus-1 (EHV-1). Equine herpesvirus type 1 causes a diffuse multifocal myeloencephalopathy and is discussed in detail in Chapter 6.

West Nile Virus. West Nile virus is a flavivirus that causes acute polioencephalomyelitis in birds, horses, and humans and rarely in other animal species.[173-175] In horses the most common clinical signs are fever, paresis, ataxia, and muscle fasciculations.[173] The lesions are most severe in the spinal cord and are usually asymmetric and multifocal. Abnormal mentation and cranial nerve abnormalities occur in 44% to 67% of affected horses.[173] See Chapter 6 for discussion of diagnosis and treatment.

Western, Eastern, and Venezuelan Equine Encephalomyelitis (WEE, EEE, VEE). A group of mosquito-transmitted alphaviruses cause encephalomyelitis in horses (Eastern, Western, and Venezuelan equine encephalomyelitis). Descriptions have been mainly reported in humans, horses, and in a number of other mammalians, including dogs, cats, cattle, camelids, rodents, and pigs.[176-178] The causative agents are single-stranded enveloped RNA viruses, *Alphavirus* genus of the family Togaviridae. Birds are involved in application of the disease. Susceptible horses, usually younger, show clinical signs 2 to 3 weeks after viral infection of birds. Times for peak infection are June to August in the southern states and September in the northern states. The clinical signs include mild to severe pyrexia, anorexia, stiffness, propulsive walking, depression, hyperesthesia, aggression, and excitability.[179] Obtundation is the most common clinical sign and seizures occur in one third of the cases. Neurologic signs are variable and occur as diffuse or multifocal forebrain disease with brainstem and spinal cord involvement. The signs are peracute to acute in onset and progressive. Mortality rates are highest with EEE. Histopathology reveals gray matter predominance with multifocal to diffuse meningoencephalomyelitis. Diagnosis is made via serology (CF, HI, SN, and IgM capture ELISA). Results of CSF analysis are distinctive and reveal very high protein concentrations and severe neutrophilic pleocytosis. Treatment is mostly supportive care, which includes corticosteroids or nonsteroidal antiinflammatory agents and physical therapy. Long-term antiinflammatory therapy may be important for neurologic recovery. Efficacious vaccines are available but twice yearly vaccination is recommended. Mosquito control is important in reducing risk of infection.

Antiviral Therapy. Few reports address the use of antiviral agents in animals. Acyclovir is an antiherpes viral agent that inhibits the enzyme thymidine kinase and thus inhibits deoxyribonucleic acid (DNA) synthesis. This effect is 200 times greater for the viral enzyme than for the enzyme in mammalian cells.[180] Acyclovir can be given orally and intravenously. It penetrates into the CSF and aqueous humor at 30% to 50% of the plasma concentration. In human herpes encephalitis, the IV dose is 10 mg/kg every 8 hours. The dose should be reduced with renal failure because the drug is excreted in the urine. Encephalopathy is a rare side effect with high doses.

Foscarnet is effective against herpesvirus, cytomegalovirus, and the human immunodeficiency virus. It penetrates the CNS in good concentrations.[180]

The Transmissible Spongiform Encephalopathies (TSE)

The TSE are a group of slowly progressive, neurodegenerative diseases of the CNS. The group includes bovine spongiform encephalopathy (BSE, mad cow disease), scrapie in goats and sheep, chronic wasting disease in elk and deer, transmissible mink encephalopathy, and feline spongiform encephalopathy. The cause is a particle in which nucleic acids have not been demonstrated. These particles may represent infectious proteins derived from the normal host. Normal prion proteins (PrP) are located in nervous system membranes and are suspectable to proteases. Abnormal PrP are protease resistant (PrP-res). Protease resistant prions accumulate in the neurons and interfere with cell function and cause vacuole formation (Figure 15-17). There is a long latency period before clinical signs develop. The TSE are reportable diseases.

Bovine Spongiform Encephalopathy (BSE). BSE was first reported in dairy cattle in the United Kingdom. Infection was tied to the consumption of meat and bone meal contaminated with BSE-infected nervous tissue. BSE has been sporadically

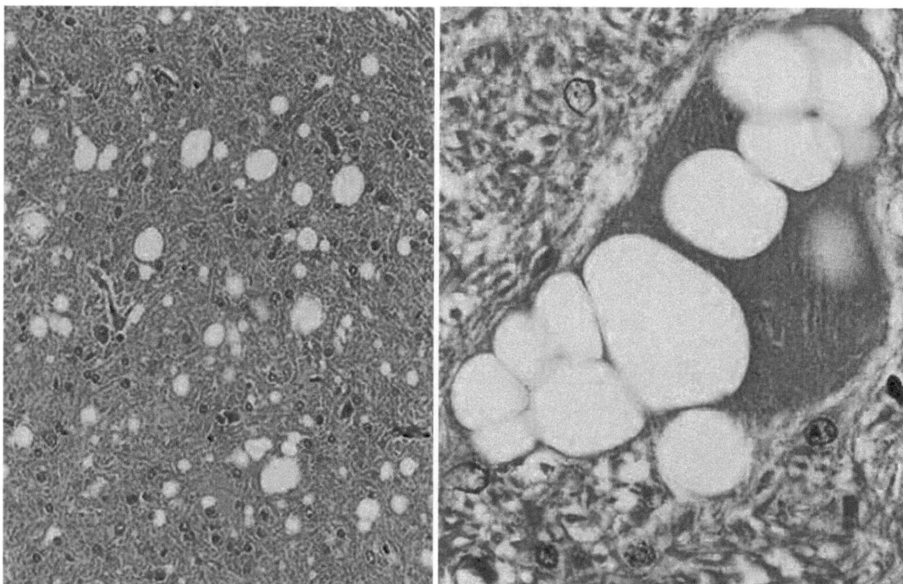

Figure 15-17 Spongiform change (vacuoles) in the caudal brainstem gray matter of a cow with bovine spongiform encephalopathy *(left image)* and large vacuoles in a large neuron (*right image*). (Courtesy Cornell University College of Veterinary Medicine.)

reported in Canada and a few cases have been reported in the United States. The incubation period can be long (2 to 8 years). The clinical signs include nervousness, aggression, frequent licking at the muzzle, muscle fasciculations, and bruxism. Cows are hypersensitive to external stimuli. Locomotor signs include ataxia, hypermetria, paresis, falling, and recumbency. There is no antemortem diagnostic test. Postmortem diagnosis includes histopathology, immunohistochemistry, and Western blot or ELISA on the brain. There is no treatment or vaccine. Human TSE, variant Creutzfeldt-Jakob disease, has been linked to consumption of brain and spinal cord tissue from BSE-infected cattle.

Scrapie. Scrapie is a TSE that affects sheep and goats. The prion is transmitted by ingestion or direct or indirect contact with infected placenta and birth fluids. The incubation is 1 to 7 years with clinical signs usually present at 2 to 5 years of age. Scrapie is most common in black-faced sheep (Suffolk, Cheviot, Hampshire). These breeds are genetically susceptible to the prion proteins. In addition to the signs described for cattle, sheep develop tremors, pruritus, wool break, and inducible nibbling reflex. When startled, sheep may tremble and fall down in a seizure. The signs progress slowly to recumbency and death (6 weeks to 1 year). The clinical signs in goats are similar. About 33% of infected goats regurgitate rumen contents.

The antemortem diagnosis of scrapie is based on clinical signs and third eyelid biopsy for immunohistochemistry of PrP-res. Postmortem diagnosis is made from histopathology of brain (vacuolation of gray matter) and immunohistochemistry of brain and/or lymphoid tissue. There is no treatment. The disease can be prevented by selecting ewes and rams that are genetically resistant to scrapie and by maintaining closed herds.

Feline Spongiform Encephalopathy. Spongiform encephalopathy has been reported to cause tremor in cats. A 7-year-old spayed female domestic shorthair cat presented for a 4-month history of progressive aggressive behavioral changes, tremor, and pelvic limb ataxia.[181] Histopathology revealed diffuse vacuolation of the neuropil and neuronal cell bodies most marked in the frontal lobe of the cerebral cortex. Due to the lack of plaques, which are associated with transmissibility, it is unclear if this is a true example of transmissible spongiform encephalopathy. Spongiform change was also reported in an 8-month-old female domestic shorthair cat that had a 2-week history of generalized ataxia and lethargy.[182] Neurologic examination also revealed head tilt, cervical spine ventroflexion, tetraparesis, tremor, and visual deficits. Histopathology revealed generalized vacuolation of the gray matter of the brain and spinal cord.

Rickettsial Infections (see Table 15-14)

The agents that cause Rocky Mountain spotted fever (RMSF) and canine ehrlichiosis may cause meningitis and encephalitis in addition to vasculitis and hematologic disorders.[183,184] Both diseases are transmitted by ticks and are limited to areas harboring the appropriate vector. Dogs with RMSF may have acute cervical pain and minimal signs related to brain or spinal cord disease. Dogs with neurologic ehrlichiosis usually have signs related to brainstem or spinal cord lesions. CSF may be normal or reveal increased protein and a mixed pleocytosis.[183] Confirmation of ehrlichiosis may be difficult in some dogs and is based on serologic tests and isolation of the organism.[185] Treatment is with tetracycline, minocycline, or doxycycline. Doxycycline is preferred because it penetrates the CSF in good concentrations. For doxycycline, a dose is 5 to 10 mg/kg every 12 hours IV or orally.

Parasitic Infections

Parasitic disease of the nervous system is uncommon. The most common parasitic diseases are summarized in Table 15-15.

Noninfectious Inflammatory Diseases

Immune Mediated Diseases

Polyradiculoneuritis (see Chapter 7) is probably an immune-mediated reaction to a transmissible agent in raccoon saliva. Postvaccinal rabies is rare (see Table 15-13). Both conditions are summarized in Table 15-16.

Meningoencephalomyelitis of Unknown Etiology (MUE) (see Table 15-17)

Several nonseptic inflammatory diseases may respond to medical therapy.[186,187,188] The causes of these diseases are

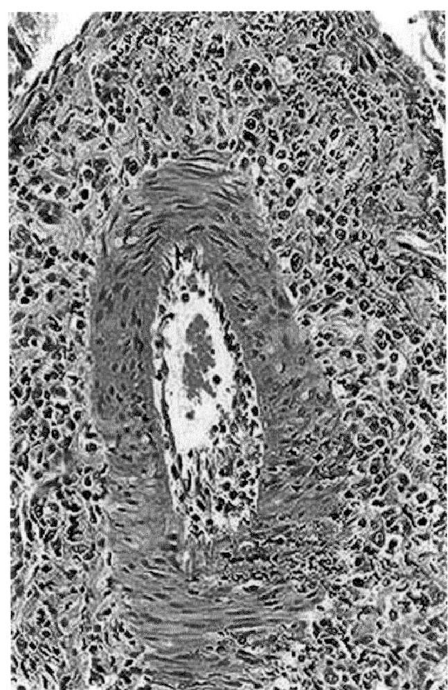

Figure 15-18 Canine juvenile polyarteritis (steroid responsive meningitis-arteritis). Note the prolific arterial inflammation with neutrophils. (Courtesy Cornell University College of Veterinary Medicine.)

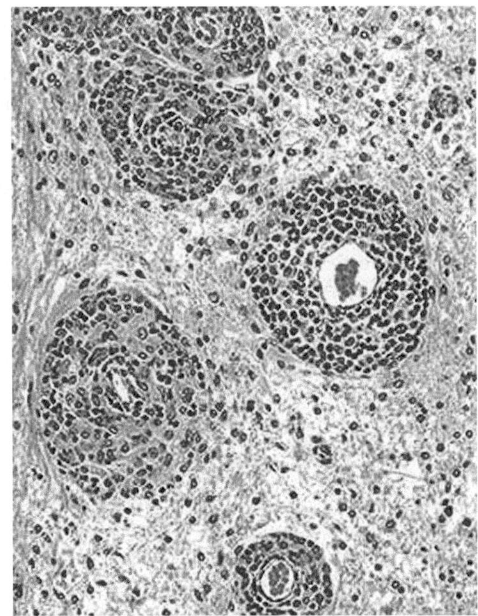

Figure 15-19 Perivascular cuffs of lymphocytes, plasma cells, and histiocytes in the cerebral white matter of a dog. These lesions are typical of granulomatous meningoencephalomyelitis. (Courtesy Cornell University College of Veterinary Medicine.)

not currently known, but immune-mediated mechanisms are suspected. Accordingly, corticosteroids and other immunosuppressive drugs may be beneficial with certain diseases. Differentiating these diseases from bacterial or viral infections is difficult because the clinical signs and CSF findings may be similar with both types of inflammation (see Chapter 4).

Steroid-Responsive Meningitis-Arteritis (SRMA)

Steroid-responsive meningitis-arteritis occurs in large-breed dogs, usually less than 2 years of age (Figure 15-18).

Cervical spinal hyperesthesia occurs in more than 90% of affected dogs. Neutrophilic leukocytosis with left shift and fever occurs in two thirds of affected dogs. Boxers, Bernese mountain dogs, beagles, weimaraners, and Nova Scotia duck tolling retriever dogs may be predisposed to this disease.[187-193] Dogs with noninfectious, nonerosive, idiopathic immune-mediated polyarthritis (IMPA) commonly have spinal pain, and about 50% of these dogs have concurrent SRMA.[188] Analysis of CSF usually reveals marked increases in protein and neutrophils. Bacterial cultures from the CSF are negative. IgA concentrations are increased in both the plasma and the CSF. Measurement of acute phase proteins in CSF may also aid in the diagnosis and management of affected dogs.[194,195] Most dogs respond dramatically to prednisone, 2 to 4 mg/kg every 24 hours.[194] In dogs not responding to prednisone alone, additional immunosuppressive therapy may be needed. Once the signs are controlled, the dose of prednisone is decreased to alternate-day therapy, and then the total dose is gradually reduced over months. Relapses are common when the corticosteroid dose is too low or is discontinued.

Necrotizing Meningeal Vasculitis

Necrotizing meningeal vasculitis is a severe form of SRMA.[186,187,194] Necrotizing vasculitis also occurs in young dogs, especially beagles, Bernese mountain dogs, and German shorthaired pointers. Although the prognosis in affected beagles is guarded, other breeds may respond well to prednisone at 2 to 4 mg/kg every 24 hours using the aforementioned reducing-dosage regimen.

Granulomatous Meningoencephalomyelitis (GME)

GME is a common nonseptic inflammatory disease that affects young to middle-aged small-breed dogs.[186,187,188,196,197] Females are more often affected.[188] The exact cause is unknown, but studies of inflammatory cells in dogs with GME suggest a T cell–mediated delayed type of hypersensitivity.[198] Neurologic signs may be acute or chronic. Clinically, GME has been characterized into three clinical presentations: focal, disseminated, or ocular.[199,200] Cervical pain is a common finding. About 50% of affected dogs have focal signs referable to the forebrain, and about 50% have forebrain and brainstem disease.[196] Central vestibular signs are common manifestations of acute disease.[197] Rarely, involvement of the peripheral nervous system may be observed.[201]

A definitive diagnosis is based on histopathologic examination of the CNS. Microscopically, the hallmark of GME is perivascular cuffs of granulomatous inflammation (Figure 15-19).[202]

Presumptive antemortem diagnosis is based on a combination of signalment, anamnesis, clinicopathologic data, and exclusion of other disease capable of producing similar clinical signs. Since the definitive diagnosis of GME necessitates histologic evaluation of CNS tissue, the term meningoencephalomyelitis of unknown etiology (MUE) has been used to describe dogs without a definitive diagnosis.

The diagnosis of MUE should be pursued in a logical manner (see Chapter 4). Briefly, minimum database (complete blood count, chemistry profile, and urinalysis) often discloses nonspecific abnormalities. Analysis of CSF is critical to establishing a presumptive antemortem diagnosis. Mononuclear pleocytosis, activated macrophages, occasionally neutrophils, and rarely mast cells with increases in protein content are common CSF abnormalities. Cross-sectional imaging also is important in the diagnostic workup. MRI of the brain is the imaging modality of choice. With MRI, multifocal hyperintensities on T2-weighted and fluid attenuated inversion recovery sequences predominantly affecting the white matter are observed. Enhancement patterns vary on T1-weighted sequences after administration of contrast media. A focal space occupying mass or abnormalities involving the optic nerves may be observed in animals with the focal or ocular forms, respectively.[203] Abnormal findings from CSF analysis and MRI of the brain can be found in other forms of MUE. Therefore, the value in pursuing these diagnostics tests is not only in documenting abnormalities but in excluding other disease processes; the greatest importance of which is eliminating infectious disease from consideration. Given the treatment of GME is centered on immunosuppression, misdiagnosis may be devastating in animals with infectious disease. Therefore, depending on the clinician's index of suspicion, further diagnostic testing aimed at the identification of an infectious etiology may be warranted. Likewise, CNS lymphoma may occur with clinical signs of multifocal signs and have MRI findings and lymphocytic pleocytosis that are difficult to differentiate from GME. PCR for the antigen receptor rearrangements may be useful in the diagnosis of CNS lymphoma.

Response to prednisone therapy is highly variable. Some dogs respond to prednisone (2 to 4 mg/kg every 24 hours, using the aforementioned reducing-dosage regimen), but relapses and progression of neurologic signs are common in many dogs. Cytosine arabinoside, given as a single agent or in combination with prednisone, is a more effective treatment.[204,205] In one study of 10 dogs treated with cytosine arabinoside and prednisone, all dogs achieved partial or complete remission and the median survival time was 531 days; five dogs were still alive at the end of the study.[206] Cytosine arabinoside is administered in cycles. Each cycle consists of administering the drug at a dose of 50 mg/m^2 given subcutaneously twice a day for 2 consecutive days. Cycles are initially repeated every 3 weeks. With time, gradual lengthening of the interval between cycles can be done. In severely affected animals, initial administration of 600 mg/m^2 given as a constant rate infusion over 2 days may be beneficial.[207] To monitor for myelosuppression, a CBC should be performed 10 to 14 days following the first course of treatment and every 2 to 3 months throughout the course of therapy. Cyclosporine may also be effective in treating GME. Two protocols have been reported.[205,208] In one, cyclosporine was administered at 10 mg/kg every 24 hours for 6 weeks. The dose was then reduced to 5 mg/kg per day. Prednisone was also administered at 2 to 4 mg/kg daily for 3 to 4 weeks. In another protocol, cyclosporine was administered at 3 to 10 mg/kg every 12 hours. Serum cyclosporine levels were followed but the drug was not detected in the CSF, even in dogs with good clinical response. In one study of 10 dogs treated with cyclosporine and prednisone, all dogs responded and the median survival time was 930 days.[208] Procarbazine has also been used as an adjunctive therapy combined with prednisone.[209] The dosage administered was 25 to 50 mg/m^2 orally once daily. The combination of procarbazine and prednisone in 21 dogs provided a median survival time of 14 months. Seven dogs experienced myelosuppression and three dogs had hemorrhagic gastroenteritis. Other immunosuppressive drugs used in the treatment of GME include mycophenolate mofetil (20 mg/kg orally twice daily) and leflunomide (1.5 to 4.0 mg/kg orally once daily).[210]

Radiation treatment is effective for dogs with focal GME.[173] The prognosis for survival is better for dogs with focal disease.[196]

Necrotizing Meningoencephalitis (NME) and Necrotizing Leukoencephalitis (NLE)

These breed-specific diseases are seen most commonly in young adult dogs. They are fatal disorders that cause a nonsuppurative inflammation and necrosis of the brain. Variants have been reported in the pug, Yorkshire terrier, Maltese, Pekingese,

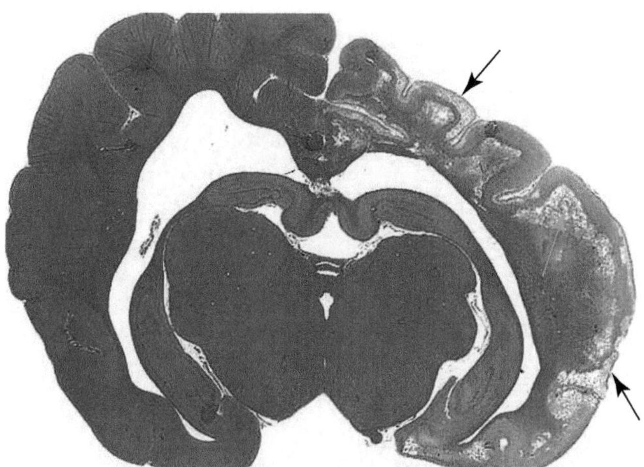

Figure 15-20 Brain from Maltese dog treated for intractable seizures. Note the laminar loss of cortical tissue *(black arrows)* and cribriform changes in the white matter *(green arrows)*. These are the lesions of necrotizing meningoencephalitis. (Courtesy Cornell University College of Veterinary Medicine via Dr. R. Higgins, University of California, Davis.)

French bulldog, Chihuahua, and shih-tzu.[211] NME is most common in the pug and Maltese and NLE is most common in Yorkshire terriers and French bulldogs. In pugs, the mean age of onset of clinical signs is 18 months (range 4 to 113 months). Females are more commonly affected than males. Most pugs with NME have a mononuclear pleocytosis.

As with GME, definitive diagnosis requires histopathologic evaluation of the brain. Gross evaluation of the brain in dogs with NME discloses abnormalities limited to the gray/white matter junction of the cerebrum (Figure 15-20).

Microscopically, the lesion affects gray and white matter, meninges, and choroid and consists of inflammatory infiltrate composed of lymphocytes, plasma cells, and macrophages. In addition, areas of liquefactive necrosis and cavitation occur. In dogs with NLE, gross lesions predominate in the deep white matter of the cerebrum and thalamus. Similar to NME, inflammation composed of lymphocytes, plasma cells, and macrophages exist along with necrosis and cavitation of the white matter. Typical white matter lesions involve the thalamus, internal capsule, centrum semiovale, and corona radiata.

Although there are gross anatomic differences in the distribution of the lesions in NME and NLE, these diseases may represent a spectrum of a single disease process rather than separate entities. In fact, although NME or NLE has been reported to affect specific breeds, occasionally NLE has been observed in a breed normally thought to be affected with NME and vice versa.[212,213]

Presumptive diagnosis can be relatively accurately established based on signalment (specifically breed), clinicopathologic data, and exclusion of other disease processes that may result in similar clinical signs. Importantly, a relatively accurate presumptive diagnosis can be made based on MRI findings. Magnetic resonance imaging characteristics and topography of the lesion mirrors the gross and histologic findings (Figure 15-21).[212,213]

Treatment is pursued using the same drug combinations as with GME. Overall, the prognosis is guarded depending on the severity of clinical signs and extent of necrosis of the brain. The mean survival time in one study was 93 days.[211]

Eosinophilic Meningoencephalomyelitis (EME)

Eosinophils are rarely found in CSF. When the percentage is less than 5%, it is a nonspecific finding and can be found in several CNS disorders. When eosinophil counts exceed 20%,

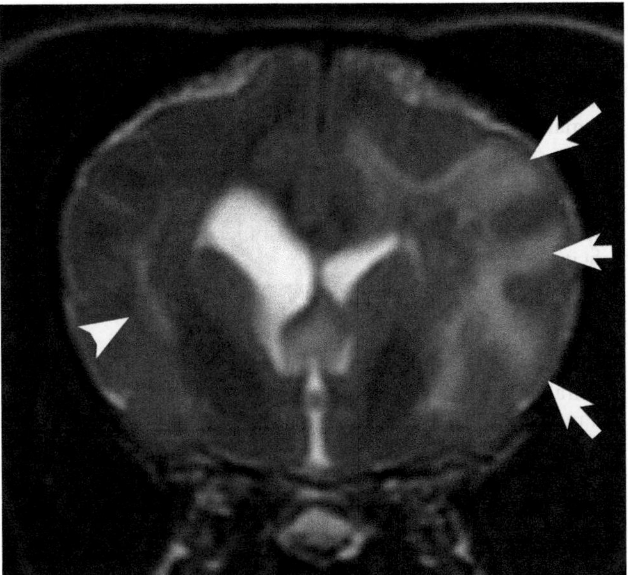

Figure 15-21 Axial T2W image of the brain of an adult Dachshund dog with meningoencephalitis of unknown origin. There is excessive hyperintensity of the white matter (internal capsule, centrum semiovale, and corona radiate) of the left cerebrum *(arrows)*. There is also edema in internal capsule of the right cerebrum *(arrowhead)*.

an eosinophilic pleocytosis exists and the most common causes are parasitic migration, cryptococcosis, neosporosis, and idiopathic EME. Idiopathic EME occurs in both large- and small-breed dogs with a median age of 3.5 years.[214] There is no gender bias and about 75% of dogs respond to prednisone therapy (0.33 to 1 1 mg/kg q12h).

CASE STUDIES

Key: *0*, Absent; *+1*, decreased; *+2*, normal; *+3*, exaggerated; *+4*, very exaggerated or clonus: *PL*, pelvic limb; *TL*, thoracic limb; *NE*, not evaluated.

CASE STUDY 15-1 *CASEY*

 veterinaryneurologycases.com

▪ Signalment
Mastiff, female spayed, 1.5 years old

▪ History
Clinical signs began several days ago. Dog has experienced vomiting, diarrhea, dry eyes and nose, urinary incontinence, and weight loss. All vaccinations are current.

▪ Physical Examination Findings
Dog is dull and dehydrated. The bladder is distended and easily expressed. Gas-filled intestinal loops can be palpated. Both eyes are very dry and the planum nasale is dry and crusted. Both pupils are widely dilated and do not respond to a strong light source. Third eyelids are prolapsed.

▪ Neurologic Examination
Mental status
Dull

Gait and posture
Normal

Postural reactions
Normal

Spinal reflexes
Normal except the perineal reflex is weak and anal tone is reduced.

Cranial nerves
Pupils are dilated and do not respond to strong light source.

Sensory evaluation
Normal

▪ Lesion Localization
Generalized disease of autonomic nervous system

▪ Differential Diagnosis
1. Dysautonomia
2. Botulism

▪ Diagnostic Plan
Dilute pilocarpine in left eye (immediate constriction); poor wheal and flare to intradermal histamine phosphate injection.

▪ Diagnosis
Dysautonomia

▪ Treatment
Dilute pilocarpine in each eye daily. Cisapride was administered twice a day to promote esophageal motility.

▪ Outcome
This case responded poorly to treatment,

CASE STUDY 15-2 MCCOY

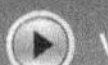 veterinaryneurologycases.com

▪ Signalment
Pus, female spayed, 3 years old

▪ History
Two months prior to presentation, the dog was brought in because of a paralyzed tail. A cauda equina syndrome was presumptively diagnosed and the dog seemed to respond to nonsteroidal antiinflammatory drugs. On this visit, the dog was seen for severe ataxia. Owner declined diagnostic testing and the dog was placed on prednisone and doxycycline. Three days later, the dog's condition had worsened and seizures developed. The dog was treated with phenobarbital and referred. All vaccinations are current.

▪ Physical Examination Findings
See neurologic examination.

▪ Neurologic Examination
Mental status
Dull and poorly responsive to auditory stimuli

Gait and posture
Unable to stand without assistance. She is very ataxic and falls both left and right. Left head tilt is present.

Postural reactions
1. Proprioceptive placing: normal in left front leg and very depressed in all other limbs
2. Hopping: +1 in thoracic limbs and 0 in pelvic limbs

Spinal reflexes
1. Patellar: +3 in both limbs
2. Withdrawal: normal

Cranial nerves
Menace response: reduced
Palpebral reflex: normal
Pupils: very dilated and no PLRs absent
Vertical nystagmus

Sensory evaluation
Normal

▪ Lesion Localization
Forebrain based on seizures
Left cranial medulla based on vestibular signs and postural deficits
Retina/optic nerves bilateral based on reduced menace responce and absent PLRO

▪ Differential Diagnosis
1. Viral encephalitis
2. Pug dog encephalitis
3. Protozoal encephalitis
4. Rickettsial encephalitis

▪ Diagnostic Plan
CSF and immunocytochemistry analysis; cross-sectional imaging and serology

▪ Results
CSF: mild increase in protein; normal cell count; CSF cells positive on immunofluorescent antibody for canine distemper; MRI and serology not performed

▪ Diagnosis
Canine distemper encephalomyelitis

▪ Treatment
Euthanasia

CASE STUDY 15-3 RASCAL

 veterinaryneurologycases.com

▪ Signalment
Abyssinian cat, male castrated, 1 year old

▪ History
The cat had severe paraparesis. Clinical signs began 3 weeks ago with lameness of the right thoracic limb that was managed with NSAIDs. Weakness and ataxia also became evident in the pelvic limbs. Muscular atrophy developed rapidly in the pelvic limbs. The cat has had two episodes of pyrexia and anorexia. Vaccinations are current.

▪ Physical Examination
The rectal temperature is normal. Cat is thin with generalized muscle atrophy. Enlarged popliteal lymph nodes are present.

▪ Neurologic Examination
Mental status
Alert and responsive

Posture
Normal

Gait
Severe paraparesis. The tail is paralyzed.

Postural reactions
Hopping and proprioceptive deficits are noted in both pelvic limbs. Hopping is decreased in the right thoracic limb.

Spinal reflexes
Spinal reflexes are increased in all limbs except the left pelvic limb where the patellar reflex is absent and hock flexion is decreased during flexion. Perineal reflex is absent.

Cranial nerves
The menace response is reduced and the pupils are widely dilated (medication to examine retinas). Pupillary light reflexes cannot be evaluated due to administration of cycloplegic drugs.

CASE STUDY 15-3 *RASCAL*—cont'd

Palpation
The urinary bladder is distended.

Sensory evaluation
Hyperesthesia is noted in the LS region. Noxious stimuli are poorly perceived from the tail.

▪ Lesion Localization
At least two and maybe three spinal cord lesions are present. In addition, disease of multiple spinal nerves (neuritis) or muscle may also be present to explain the generalized muscle atrophy.

1. T3-L3 based on paraparesis and increased spinal reflexes
2. Left L4-S2 based on absent patellar and flexor reflexes
3. Cauda equina based on sensory examination of tail and decreased perineal reflex

▪ Differential Diagnosis
There are multifocal lesions making inflammatory disease much more likely than degenerative or neoplastic processes.

1. Protozoal myelitis-neuritis (toxoplasmosis and neosporosis)
2. Mycotic myelitis-neuritis (cryptococcosis, histoplasmosis, blastomycosis, aspergillosis)
3. FIP
4. Lymphoma

▪ Diagnostic Plan
1. CBC
2. Fine-needle lymph node biopsy
3. Thoracic and LS radiographs
4. MRI
5. CSF analysis

▪ Results
Fundic examination revealed severe bilateral chorioretinitis. Lymph node aspirate isolated histoplasma organisms. Radiographs of the lumbosacral spine did not reveal any skeletal lesions. Cross-sectional imaging and CSF analysis not performed.

▪ Diagnosis
Histoplasmosis with myelitis and neuritis (likely fungal granulomas)

▪ Treatment
Itraconazole (cat greatly improved and regained ability to urinate)

CASE STUDY 15-4 *SADIE*

 veterinaryneurologycases.com

▪ Signalment
Boxer, 9-month-old female intact

▪ History
The dog has a 2-day history of anorexia, decreased activity, and stiff gait. There is no history of trauma. She lives in northeastern Kansas, is well vaccinated, and eats a premium dog food. The dog was examined in early September.

▪ Physical Examination Findings
The abnormalities include a stiff gait and rectal temperature of 104.5° F. Ticks are present on the dog.

▪ Neurologic Examination
Mental status
Responsive to her environment

Gait and posture
Discomfort evident when handled or picked up. A stiff gait and reluctance to walk are noted. There is no head tilt circling, or ataxia.

Postural reactions
Normal

Spinal reflexes
Normal

Cranial nerves
Normal

Sensory evaluation
Marked hyperesthesia is elicited upon palpation over the thoracolumbar and cervical vertebral column.

▪ Lesion Localization
There are no findings suggestive of intramedullary spinal cord disease, especially with the presence of paraspinal pain. The hyperesthesia suggests disease involving the TL and cervical vertebra or meningeal disease. Muscles and joints also have pain sensitive fibers.

▪ Differential Diagnosis
1. Steroid responsive meningitis-arteritis
2. Rickettsial (RMSF) meningitis
3. GME
4. Discospondylitis
5. Metastatic neoplasia
6. Intervertebral disk disease
7. Polymyositis
8. Polyarthritis

▪ Diagnostic Plan
1. CBC, biochemical profile, UA
2. Thoracic radiographs and abdominal ultrasound to rule-out metastatic disease; spinal radiography
3. Serology: RMSF and *Ehrlichia canis*
4. CSF analysis

CASE STUDY 15-4 *SADIE*—cont'd

▪ Results

1. The primary abnormality on the CBC was a platelet count of 90,000. The biochemical profile and UA were normal.
2. Thoracic radiographs and abdominal ultrasound within normal limits;
3. Negative serology for RMSF and *Ehrlichia canis*
4. No CSF analysis was performed

▪ Diagnosis

Given the clinical signs and the presence of ticks, RMSF meningitis was suspected.

▪ Treatment

Dog was placed on oral doxycycline. The dog dramatically responded to treatment. Convalescence RMSF titers were 1:256.

CASE STUDY 15-5 *VICTOR*

 veterinaryneurologycases.com

▪ Signalment

Miniature schnauzer, intact male, 14 months old

▪ History

The dog has been anorexic and lethargic for the past 2 days. He vomited one to two times in last 48 hours. Dog has right head tilt, circles and falls to the right, and bumps into objects on the right side. Owners report that the dog is reluctant to open his mouth and whines when his mouth is opened. Another veterinarian also found a mild fever and modest thrombocytopenia (165,000 platelets/μL).

▪ Physical Examination Findings

The liver was not palpable on abdominal palpation. Rectal temperature at admission was 103.2° F.

▪ Neurologic Examination

Mental status

Dull, confused, and disoriented

Gait and posture

Right head tilt; drifts and falls to the right, right hemiparesis, circles both directions but mostly to the right side. Visual deficits are suspected on right side.

Postural reactions

Very decreased on the right side

Spinal reflexes

All spinal reflexes are intact

Cranial nerves

Menace response: OD—absent; OS—normal
Palpebral reflex: normal
PLR: intact
Physiologic nystagmus is intact. There is no pathologic nystagmus but a ventrolateral strabismus is observed in the right eye
Facial sensation: normal
Swallowing/gag: normal
Tongue movement: normal

Sensory perception

Normal

▪ Lesion Localization

Left cerebral cortex; right brainstem (rostral medulla—central vestibular disease)

▪ Differential Diagnosis

1. Rickettsial encephalitis
2. Viral encephalitis
3. Meningoencephalomyelitis of unknown origin
4. Fungal encephalitis
5. Toxoplasmosis/neosporosis
6. Hepatoencephalopathy

▪ Diagnostic Plan

1. Fundic examination
2. CBC, biochemical profile, UA
3. Bile acids
4. Abdominal radiographs/ultrasonography
5. MRI
6. CSF analysis

▪ Results

1. CBC: platelets 162,000 (200,00 to 500,000 cells/μL); CK 501 (22 to 491); ALT 76 (3 to 69)
2. UA: normal
3. Abdominal radiographs: small liver
4. Bile acids: pre-5.3; postprandial 23.8 (5 to 23)
5. CSF: WBC—488; RBC—173; Total protein—94.39; cytology—100% lymphocytes
6. PCR and serology for *Ehrlichia*: negative
7. *Toxoplasma gondii* and *Neospora caninum*: negative titers (IFA) at 1:50
8. MRI not performed

▪ Diagnosis

Meningoencephalitis of unknown etiology; possibly GME

▪ Treatment

Initially chloramphenicol and prednisone was administered. The dog was maintained on an immunosuppressive dose of prednisone.

▪ Outcome

1. Recheck 1 month: Improved
2. Recheck 2 months: Much improved
3. Recheck 3 months: Signs in remission. The dog developed severe iatrogenic Cushing. The dose of prednisone was reduced to every other day. Other immunosuppressive agents (e.g., cytosine arabinoside) were considered.

CASE STUDY 15-6 OTTO

 veterinaryneurologycases.com

▪ Signalment

Miniature schnauzer, male, 16 weeks old

▪ History

Otto developed clinical signs at 8 weeks of age and signs have progressively worsened. There are no other clinical signs. He eats, drinks, and is growing normally. Owner describes clumsy gait and falling right and left.

▪ Physical Examination Findings

No abnormalities found except for neurologic examination findings.

▪ Neurologic Examination

Mental status

Alert and responsive

Gait and posture

There was a base wide stance. Gait showed severe cerebellal ataxia, hypermetria, and falling to right. Intention tremors were evident upon eating.

Postural reactions

+1 hopping in left thoracic and pelvic limbs.

Cranial nerves

Normal

Spinal reflexes

Patellar reflex on left side is +3. All other reflexes are normal.

Sensory evaluation

Normal

▪ Lesion Localization

The prominent clinical signs localized to the cerebellum. Dog probably has either brainstem and/or cervical spinal cord lesion to explain the postural reaction deficits.

▪ Differential Diagnosis

1. Cerebellar abiotrophy
2. Lysosomal storage disease
3. Canine distemper virus
4. Other infectious inflammatory disease

▪ Diagnostic Plan

1. CSF analysis
2. Serology for distemper, toxoplasmosis, neosporosis, and rickettsial agents.
3. MRI
4. Urine organic acid screening

▪ Results

1. CSF: Normal
2. Serology results were for negative infectious agents
3. MRI and urine screening not performed

▪ Treatment

No treatment was administered because dog most likely has a neurodegenerative disease

▪ Outcome

Dog developed rapid progression of neurologic signs and was euthanized at 6 months of age. Necropsy and histopathology confirmed cerebellar abiotrophy with degenerative lesions also in the brainstem.

REFERENCES

1. Baker HJ, et al: The gangliosidoses: comparative features and research applications, Vet Pathol 16:635–649, 1979.
2. Summers BA, Cummings JF, de Lahunta A: Degenerative diseases of the central nervous system. Veterinary neuropathology, St Louis, 1995, Mosby.
3. Jolly RD, Walkley SU: Lysosomal storage diseases of animals: an essay in comparative pathology, Vet Pathol 34:527–548, 1997.
4. Skelly BJ, Franklin RJM: Recognition and diagnosis of lysosomal storage diseases in the cat and dog, J Vet Intern Med 16:133–141, 2002.
5. Jolly RD: Comparative biology of neuronal ceroid-lipofuscinoses (NCL): an overview, Am J Med Genet 57(2):307–311, 1995.
6. Ellinwood NM, Vite CH, Haskin ME: Gene therapy for lysosomal storage diseases: the lessons and promise of animal models, J Gene Med 6:481–506, 2004.
7. de Lahunta A: Abiotrophy in domestic animals: a review, Can J Vet Res 54:65–76, 1990.
8. Kornegay JN: Ataxia of the head and limbs: cerebellar diseases in dogs and cats, Prog Vet Neurol 1:255–274, 1990.
9. Kortz GD, Meier WA, Higgins RJ, et al: Neuronal vacuolation and spinocerebellar degeneration in young Rottweiler dogs, Vet Pathol 34(4):296–302, 1997.
10. Zaal MD, van dan Ingh T, Goedegebuure SA, et al: Progressive neuronopathy in two Cairn terrier litter mates, Vet Q 19:34–36, 1997.
11. Jaggy A, Vandevelde M: Multisystem neuronal degeneration in cocker spaniels, J Vet Intern Med 2(3):117–120, 1988.
12. da Costa RC, Parent JM, Poma R, et al: Multisystem axonopathy and neuronopathy in golden retriever dogs, J Vet Intern Med 23:935–939, 2009.
13. deLahunta A, Averill DR: Hereditary cerebellar cortical and extrapyramidal nuclear abiotrophy in Kerry blue terriers, J Am Vet Med Assoc 168:1119–1124, 1976.
14. O'Brien DP, Johnson GS, Schnabel RD, et al: Genetic mapping of canine multiple system degeneration and ectodermal dysplasia loci, J Hered 96:727–734, 2005.
15. Pool WA: "Grass disease" in horses, Vet Rec 8:23–30, 1928.
16. Key TJ, Gaskell CJ: Puzzling syndrome in cats associated with pupillary dilatation, Vet Rec 110:160, 1982.
17. Wise LA, Lappin MR: A syndrome resembling feline dysautonomia (Key-Gaskell syndrome) in a dog, J Am Vet Med Assoc 198:2103–2106, 1991.
18. Berghaus RD, O'Brien DP, Thorne JG, et al: Incidence of canine dysautonomia in Missouri, USA, between January 1996 and December 2000, Prev Vet Med 54(4):291–300, 2002.

19. Harkin KR, Andrews GA, Nietfeld JC: Dysautonomia in dogs: 65 cases (1993-2000), J Am Vet Med Assoc 220(5):633–639, 2002.
20. Longshore RC, O'Brien DP, Johnson GC, et al: Dysautonomia in dogs: a retrospective study, J Vet Intern Med 10:103–109, 1996.
21. Kidder AC, Johannes C, O'Brien DP, et al: Feline dysautonomia in the Midwestern United States: a retrospective study of nine cases, J Feline Med Surg 10(2):130–136, 2008.
22. Hardy RM: Pathophysiology of hepatic encephalopathy, Semin Vet Med Surg 5:100–106, 1990.
23. Maddison JE: Hepatic encephalopathy: current concepts of the pathogenesis, J Vet Intern Med 6:341–353, 1992.
24. Bunch SE: Hepatic encephalopathy, Prog Vet Neurol 2:287–296, 1992.
25. Center SA, Magne ML: Historical, physical examination, and clinicopathologic features of portosystemic vascular anomalies in the dog and cat, Semin Vet Med Surg 5:83–93, 1990.
26. Center SA, et al: Evaluation of twelve-hour preprandial and two-hour post prandial serum bile acids concentrations for diagnosis of hepatobiliary diseases in dogs, J Am Vet Med Assoc 199:217–226, 1991.
27. Center SA, Erb HN, Joseph SA: Measurement of serum bile acids concentrations of hepatobiliary disease in cats, J Am Vet Med Assoc 207:1048–1054, 1995.
28. Holt DE, Schelling CG, Saunders HM, et al: Correlation of ultrasonographic findings with surgical, portographic, and necropsy findings in dogs and cats with portosystemic shunts: 63 cases (1987-1993), J Am Vet Med Assoc 207:1190–1193, 1995.
29. Koblik PD, et al: Use of 99m technetium-pertechnetate as a screening test for portosystemic shunts in dogs, J Am Vet Med Assoc 196:925–930, 1990.
30. Koblik PD, Hornof WJ: Transcolonic sodium pertechnetate Tc 99m scintigraphy for diagnosis of macrovascular portosystemic shunts in dogs, cats, and potbellied pigs: 176 cases (1988-1992), J Am Vet Med Assoc 207:729–733, 1995.
31. Tyler JW: Hepatoencephalopathy. Part II: pathophysiology and treatment, Compend Contin Educ Pract Vet 12:1260–1270, 1990.
32. Taboada J: Medical management of animals with portosystemic shunts, Semin Vet Med Surg 5:107–119, 1990.
33. Matushek KJ, Bjorling D, Mathews K: Generalized motor seizures after portosystemic shunt ligation in dogs: five cases (1981-1988), J Am Vet Med Assoc 196:2014–2017, 1990.
34. Hardie EM, Kornegay JN, Cullen JM: Status epilepticus after ligation of portosystemic shunts, Vet Surg 19:412–417, 1990.
35. Tisdall PL, Hunt GB, Youmans KR, et al: Neurological dysfunction indogs following attenuation of congenital extrahepatic portosystemic shunts, J Small Anim Pract 41:539–546, 2000.
36. Johnson C, Armstrong P, Hauptman J: Congenital portosystemic shunts in dogs: 46 cases (1979-1986), J Am Vet Med Assoc 191:1478–1483, 1987.
37. Matushek KJ, Bjorling D, Mathews K: Generalized motor seizures after portosystemic shunt ligation in dogs: five cases (1981-1988), J Am Vet Med Assoc 196:2014–2017, 1990.
38. Van Gundy TE, Boothe HW, Wolf A: Results of surgical management of feline portosystemic shunts, J Am Anim Hosp Assoc 25:55–62, 1990.
39. Lawrence D, Bellah JR, Diaz R: Results of surgical management of portosystemic shunts in dogs: 20 cases (1985-1990), J Am Vet Med Assoc 201:1750–1753, 1992.
40. Dunigan C, Tyler J, Valdez R, et al: Apparent renal encephalopathy in a cow, J Vet Intern Med 10:39–41, 1996.
41. Wolf AM: Canine uremic encephalopathy, J Am Anim Hosp Assoc 16:735–738, 1980.
42. Abramson CJ, et al: L-2-hydroxyglutaric aciduria in Staffordshire bull terriers, J Vet Intern Med 17:551–556, 2003.
43. Allison RW, Mienkoth JH, Rizzi TE: Abnormalities of the standard biochemical profile. In Lorenz MD, Neer TM, Demars PL, editors: Small animal medical diagnosis, ed 3, Ames, Iowa, 2009, Wiley Blackwell.
44. Holowaychuk MK, et al: Ionized calcium in critically ill dogs, J Vet Intern Med 23:509–513, 2009.
45. Kornegay JN: Hypocalcemia in dogs, Compend Contin Educ Pract Vet 4:103–110, 1982.
46. Plumb DC: Plumbs veterinary drug handbook, ed 5, Ames, Iowa, 2005, Blackwell.
47. Kelly M, Hill J: Canine myxedema stupor and coma, Compend Contin Educ Pract Vet 6:1049–1057, 1984.
48. Kelly MJ: Canine myxedema stupor and coma. In Kirk RW, editor: Current veterinary therapy X: small animal practice, Philadelphia, 1989, WB Saunders.
49. Panciera DL: Hypothyroidism in dogs: 66 cases (1987-1992), J Am Vet Med Assoc 204:761–767, 1994.
50. Vitale CL, Olby NJ: Neurologic dysfunction in hypothyroid, hyperlipidemic Labrador retrievers, J Vet Intern Med 21:1316–1322, 2007.
51. Rossmeisl JH Jr, Duncan RB, Inzana KD, et al: Longitudinal study of the effects of chronic hypothyroidism on skeletal muscle in dogs, Am J Vet Res 70(7):879–888, 2009.
52. Schwartz BC, Sallmutter T, Nell B: Keratoconjunctivitis sicca attributable to parasympathetic nerve dysfunction associated with hypothyroidism in a horse, J Am Vet Med Assoc 233:1761–1766, 2008.
53. Nelson RW, et al: Serum free thyroxine concentrations in healthy dogs, dogs with hypothyroidism, and euthyroid dogs with concurrent illness, J Am Vet Med Assoc 198:1401–1407, 1991.
54. Peterson ME, Gamble DA: Effect of nonthyroid illness on serum thyroxine concentrations in cats: 494 cases (1988), J Am Vet Med Assoc 197:1203–1208, 1990.
55. Jaggy A, et al: Neurologic manifestations of hypothyroidism: a retrospective study of 29 dogs, J Vet Intern Med 8:328–336, 1994.
56. Sarfaty DS, Carillo JM, Peterson ME: Neurologic, endocrinologic, and pathologic findings associated with large pituitary tumors in dogs: eight cases (1976-1984), J Am Vet Med Assoc 193:854–856, 1988.
57. Wood FD, et al: Diagnostic imaging findings and endocrine test results in dogs with pituitary-dependent hyperadrenocorticism that did or did not have neurologic abnormalities: 157 cases (1989-2005), J Am Vet Med Assoc 231:1081–1085, 2007.
58. Love S: Equine Cushing's disease, Br Vet J 149:139–153, 1993.
59. Duesberg CA, et al: Magnetic resonance imaging for diagnosis of pituitary macroadenomas in dogs, J Am Vet Med Assoc 206:657–662, 1995.
60. Barker EN, Campbell S, Tebb AJ, et al: A comparison of the survival times of dogs treated with mitotane or trilostane for pituitary-dependent hyperadrenocorticism, J Vet Intern Med 19(6):810–815, 2005.

61. Feldman EC, Nelson RW: Hypercalcemia and primary hyperparathyroidism. In Canine and feline endocrinology and reproduction, Philadelphia, 1996, WB Saunders.
62. Harris CL, et al: Hypercalcemia in a dog with thymoma, J Am Anim Hosp Assoc 27:281–284, 1991.
63. Klausner JS, et al: Hypercalcemia in two cats with squamous cell carcinoma, J Am Vet Med Assoc 196:103–105, 1990.
64. Messinger JS, Windham WR, Ward CR: Ionized calcium in dogs: a retrospective study of 109 cases (1998-2003), J Vet Intern Med 23:514–519, 2009.
65. Foosbee SK, Forrester SD: Hypercalcemia secondary to cholecalciferol rodenticide toxicosis in two dogs, J Am Vet Med Assoc 196:1265–1268, 1990.
66. Dougherty SA, Center SA, Dzanis DA: Salmon calcitonin as adjunct treatment for vitamin D toxicosis in a dog, J Am Vet Med Assoc 196:1269–1272, 1990.
67. Spier SJ, et al: Hyperkalemic periodic paralysis in horses, J Am Vet Med Assoc 197:1009–1017, 1990.
68. Rudolph JA, et al: Periodic paralysis in quarter horses: a sodium channel mutation disseminated by selective breeding, Nat Genet 2:144–147, 1992.
69. Atkins CE: Disorders of glucose homeostasis in neonatal and juvenile dogs:hypoglycemia (Part I), Compend Contin Educ Pract Vet 6:197–206, 1984.
70. van der Linde-Sipman JS, van den Ingh TS, van Toor AJ: Fatty liver syndrome in puppies, J Am Anim Hosp Assoc 26:9–12, 1990.
71. Atkins CE: : Disorders of glucose homeostasis in neonatal and juvenile dogs:hypoglycemia (Part II), Compend Contin Educ Pract Vet 6:353–364, 1984.
72. Elie MS, Zerbe CA: Insulinoma in dogs, cats, and ferrets, Compend Contin Educ Pract Vet 17:51–59, 1995.
73. Caywood DD, et al: Pancreatic insulin-secreting neoplasms: clinical, diagnostic, and prognostic features in 73 dogs, J Am Anim Hosp Assoc 24:577–584, 1988.
74. Hawks D, Peterson ME, Hawkins KL: Insulin-secreting pancreatic (islet cell) carcinoma in a cat, J Vet Intern Med 6:193–196, 1992.
75. Dyer DR: Hypoglycemia: a common metabolic manifestation of cancer, Vet Med 87:40–47, 1992.
76. Chrisman CL: Postoperative results and complications of insulinomas in dogs, J Am Anim Hosp Assoc 16:677–684, 1980.
77. Frier H, et al: Formation and absorption of cerebrospinal fluid in adult goats with hypo and hypervitaminosis A, Am J Vet Res 35:45–55, 1974.
78. Baker JR, Lyon DG: Skull malformation and cerebellar herniation in captive African lions, Vet Rec 19:154–156, 1977.
79. Kornegay JN, Mayhew IG: Metabolic, toxic, and nutritional diseases of the nervous system. In Oliver JE, Hoerlein BF, Mayhew IG, editors: Veterinary neurology, Philadelphia, 1987, WB Saunders.
80. van Donkersgoed J, Clark EG: Blindness caused by hypovitaminosis A in feedlot cattle, Can Vet J 29:925–927, 1988.
81. Anderson WI, et al: The ophthalmic and neuro-ophthalmic effects of a vitamin A deficiency in young steers, Vet Med 86:1143–1148, 1991.
82. Mayhew I, et al: Equine degenerative myeloencephalopathy: a vitamin E deficiency that may be familial, J Vet Intern Med 1:45–50, 1987.
83. Dill SG, et al: Serum vitamin E and blood glutathione peroxidase values of horses with degenerative myeloencephalopathy, Am J Vet Res 50:166–168, 1989.
84. Anderson WI, Morrow LA: Thiamine deficiency encephalopathy with concurrent myocardial degeneration and polyradiculoneuropathy in a cat, Cornell Vet 77:251–257, 1987.
85. Houston DM, Hulland TJ: Thiamine deficiency in a team of sled dogs, Can Vet J 29:383–385, 1988.
86. Rammell C, Hill J: A review of thiamine deficiency and its diagnosis, especially in ruminants, N Z Vet J 34:202–204, 1987.
87. Read DH, Harrington DD: Experimentally induced thiamine deficiency in beagle dogs: pathologic changes of the central nervous system, Am J Vet Res 47:2281–2289, 1986.
88. Mayhew IG: Large animal neurology, ed 2, Ames, 2009, Wiley-Blackwell.
89. Osweiler GD, Carson TL, Buck WB, et al: Clinical and diagnostic veterinary toxicology, ed 3, Dubuque, Iowa, 1985, Kendall/Hunt Publishing.
90. Grauer GF, Hjelle JJ: Toxicology. In Morgan RV, editor: Handbook of small animal practice, New York, 1988, Churchill Livingstone.
91. Dorman DC: Toxins that include seizures in small animals. In the Proceedings of the 8th ACVIM Forum, McGuirk SM ed. Washington DC, 361–364, 1990.
92. O'Brien DP: Toxic and metabolic causes of seizures, Clin Tech Small Anim Pract 13:159–166, 1998.
93. Dorman DC, Parker AJ, Buck WB: : Bromethalin toxicosis in the dog. Part I: clinical effects, J Am Anim Hosp Assoc 26:589, 1990.
94. Dorman DC, Parker AJ, Dye JA, et al: Bromethalin neurotoxicosis in the cat, Prog Vet Neurol 1:189, 1990.
95. Bratton GR, Kowalczyk DF: Lead poisoning. In Kirk RW, editor: Current veterinary therapy X: small animal practice, Philadelphia, 1989, WB Saunders.
96. Dollahite JW, et al: Chronic lead poisoning in horses, Am J Vet Res 39:961–964, 1978.
97. Zook BC, Carpenter JL, Leeds EB: Lead poisoning in dogs, J Am Vet Med Assoc 155:1329–1342, 1969.
98. Knecht CD, Crabtree J, Katherman A: Clinical, clinicopathologic, and electroencephalographic features of lead poisoning in dogs, J Am Vet Med Assoc 175:196–201, 1979.
99. Nicholls TJ, Handson PD: Behavioural change associated with chronic lead poisoning in working dogs, Vet Rec 112:607, 1983.
100. Dow SW, et al: Central nervous system toxicosis associated with metronidazole treatment of dogs: five cases (1984-1987), J Am Vet Med Assoc 195:365–368, 1989.
101. Caylor KB, Cassimatis MK: Metronidazole neurotoxicosis in two cats, J Am Anim Hosp Assoc 37:258–262, 2001.
102. Evans J, et al: Diazepam as a treatment for metronidazole toxicosis in dogs: a retrospective study of 21 cases, J Vet Intern Med 17:302–310, 2003.
103. Mealy KL: Role of P-glycoprotein in the blood-brain barrier. In the Proceedings of the 19th ACVIM Forum, Davenport D, Paradis MR, eds. Denver, 396–398, 2001
104. Nelson OL, et al: Ivermectin toxicity in an Australian shepherd dog with MDR1 mutation associated with ivermectin sensitivity in collies, J Vet Intern Med 17:354–356, 2003.
105. Hopper K, Aldrich J, Haskins SC: Ivermectin toxicity in 17 collies, J Vet Intern Med 16:89–94, 2002.
106. Kenny PJ, et al: Retinopathy associated with ivermectin toxicosis in two dogs, J Am Vet Assoc 233:279–284, 2008.

107. Merola V, Khan S, Gwaltney-Brant S: Ivermectin toxicosis in dogs: A retrospective study, J Am Anim Hosp Assoc 45:106–111, 2009.
108. Swor TM, Whittenburg JL, Chaffin MK: Ivermectin toxicosis in three adult horses, J Am Vet Med Assoc 235:558–562, 2009.
109. Jaggy A, Oliver JE: Chlorpyrifos toxicosis in two cats, J Vet Intern Med 4:135–139, 1990.
110. Farrow BRH: Tremor syndromes in dogs. In the Proceedings of the 6th ACVIM Forum, Pigeon G ed. Washington DC, 57–60, 1988.
111. Bath ML: Hexachlorophene toxicity in dogs, J Small Anim Pract 19:241–244, 1978.
112. Scott DW, Bolton GR, Lorenz MD: Hexachlorophene toxicosis in dogs, J Am Vet Med Assoc 162:947–949, 1973.
113. Thompson J, Senior D, Pinson D, et al: Neurotoxicosis associated with the use of hexachlorophene in a cat, J Am Vet Med Assoc 190:1311–1312, 1987.
114. Dorman dc: Initial management of toxicosis. In the Proceedings of the 8th ACVIM Forum, McGuirk SM ed. Washington DC, pages 419–422:1990.
115. Hamir A, Sullivan N, Handson P, et al: A comparison of calcium disodium ethylene diamine tetraacetate (Ca EDTA) by oral and subcutaneous routes as a treatment of lead poisoning in dogs, J Small Anim Pract 27:39–43, 1986.
116. Munana KR: Encephalitis and meningitis, Vet Clin North Am (Small Anim Pract) 26:857–874, 1996.
117. Kent M: Bacterial infections of the CNS. In Greene CE, editor: Infectious diseases of the dog and cat, ed 3, Philadelphia, 2006, Elsevier.
118. Tipold A, Vandevelde M: Neurologic diseases of suspected infectious origin and prion disease. In Greene CE, editor: Infectious diseases of the dog and cat, ed 3, Philadelphia, 2006, Elsevier.
119. Braund KG, Brewer BD, Mayhew IG: Inflammatory, infectious, immune, parasitic, and vascular diseases. In Oliver JE, Hoerlein BF, Mayhew IG, editors: Veterinary neurology, Philadelphia, 1987, WB Saunders.
120. Greene CE, Appel MJ: Canine distemper. In Greene CE, editor: Infectious diseases of the dog and cat, ed 3, Philadelphia, 2006, Elsevier.
121. Bagely RS: Multifocal neurological disease. In Ettinger S, Feldman E, editors: Textbook of veterinary internal medicine, ed 6, Philadelphia, 2005, Elsevier.
122. Milhorat TH: Cerebrospinal fluid and the brain edemas, New York, 1987, Neuroscience Society of New York.
123. Webb AA, Muir GD: The blood-brain barrier and its role in inflammation, J Vet Intern Med 14:399–411, 2000.
124. Fenner WR: Bacterial infections of the central nervous system. In Greene CE, editor: Infectious diseases of the dog and cat, Philadelphia, 1990, WB Saunders.
125. Quagliarello V, Scheld WM: Bacterial meningitis: pathogenesis, pathophysiology, and progress, N Engl J Med 327:864–872, 1992.
126. Scheld WM, et al: Cerebrospinal fluid outflow resistance in rabbits with experimental meningitis: alterations with penicillin and methylprednisolone, J Clin Invest 66:243–253, 1980.
127. Mustafa MM, et al: Modulation of inflammation and cachectin activity in relation to treatment of experimental Haemophilus influenzae type B meningitis, J Infect Dis 160:818–825, 1989.
128. Odio CM, et al: The beneficial effects of early dexamethasone administration in infants and children with bacterial meningitis, N Engl J Med 324:1535–1541, 1991.
129. Saez-Llorens X, Jafari HS, Severien C, et al: Enhanced attenuation of meningeal inflammation and brain edema by concomitant administration of anti-CD 18 monoclonal antibodies and dexamethasone in experimental *Haemophilus* meningitis, J Clin Invest 88:2003–2011, 1991.
130. Radaelli ST, Platt SR: Bacterial meningoencephalomyelitis in dogs: a retrospective study of 23 cases (1990-1999), J Vet Intern Med 16:159–163, 2002.
131. Kornegay JN, Lorenz MD, Zenoble RD: Bacterial meningoencephalitis in two dogs, J Am Vet Med Assoc 173:1334–1336, 1978.
132. Cross JR, et al: Bartonella-associated meningoradiculoneuritis and dermatitis or panniculitis in 3 dogs, J Vet Intern Med 22:674–678, 2008.
133. Dow SW, et al: Central nervous system infection associated with anaerobic bacteria in two dogs and two cats, J Vet Intern Med 2:171–176, 1988.
134. Bahri LE, Blouin A: Fluoroquinolones: a new family of antimicrobials, Compend Contin Educ Pract Vet 13:1429–1434, 1991.
135. Orsini JA, Perkons S: New beta-lactam antibiotics in critical care medicine, Compend Contin Educ Pract Vet 16:183–186, 1994.
136. Frank LA: Clinical pharmacology of rifampin, J Am Vet Med Assoc 197:114–117, 1990.
137. Haskins SC: Management of septic shock, J Am Vet Med Assoc 200:1915–1924, 1992.
138. Greene CE: Infectious diseases affecting the nervous system. In Kornegay JN, editor: Neurologic disorders, New York, 1986, Churchill Livingstone.
139. Carmichael LE, Greene CE: Canine brucellosis. In Greene CE, editor: Infectious diseases of the dog and cat, ed 3, Philadelphia, 2006, Elsevier.
140. Moore BR: Update on equine therapeutics: bacterial meningitis in foals, Compend Contin Educ Pract Vet 17:1417–1420, 1995.
141. Morris DD, Rutkowski J, Lloyd KC: Therapy in two cases of neonatal foal septicemia and meningitis with cefotaxim96 sodium, Equine Vet J 19:151–154, 1987.
142. Santschi EM, Foreman JH: Equine bacterial meningitis. Part I, Compend Contin Educ Pract Vet 11:479–483, 1989.
143. Foreman JH, Santschi EM: Equine bacterial meningitis, Part II, Compend Contin Educ Pract Vet 11:640–644, 1989.
144. Green SL, Smith LL: Meningitis in neonatal calves: 32 cases (1983-1990), J Am Vet Med Assoc 201:125–128, 1992.
145. Harris FW, Janzen ED: The Haemophilus somnus disease complex (Haemophilosis): a review,, Can Vet J 30:816–822, 1989.
146. Donkersgoed JV, Janzen ED, Harland RJ: Epidemiological features of calf mortality due to haemophilosis in a large feedlot, Can Vet J 31:821–825, 1990.
147. Blenden DC, Kampelmacher EH, Torres-Anjel MJ: Listeriosis (zoonosis update), J Am Vet Med Assoc 1:79–84, 1990.
148. Perdizet JA, Dinsmore P: Pituitary abscess syndrome, Compend Contin Educ Pract Vet 8:311–318, 1986.
149. Raphel CF: Brain abscess in three horses, J Am Vet Med Assoc 180:874–877, 1982.
150. Allen JR, Barbee DD, Boulton MD: Brain abscess in a horse: diagnosis by computed tomography and successful surgical treatment, Equine Vet J 19:552–555, 1987.
151. Greene CE: Abscesses and pyogranulomatous inflammation caused by bacteria. In Greene CE, editor: Infectious diseases of the dog and cat, ed 3, Philadelphia, 2006, Elsevier.

152. Kornegay JN: Diskospondylitis. In Slatter DH, editor: Textbook of small animal surgery, Philadelphia, 1993, WB Saunders.
153. Malik R, et al: Cryptococcosis. In Greene CE, editor: Infectious diseases of the dog and cat, ed 3, Philadelphia, 2006, Elsevier.
154. Cook JR, Evinger JV, Wagner LA: Successful combination chemotherapy for cryptococcal meningoencephalitis, J Am Anim Hosp Assoc 27:61–64, 1991.
155. Hill PB, Moriello KA, Shaw SE: A review of systemic antifungal agents, Vet Dermatol 6:59–66, 1995.
156. Heit MC, Riviere JE: Antifungal therapy: ketoconazole and other azole derivatives, Compend Contin Educ Pract Vet 1:21–31, 1995.
157. Mikiciuk MG, Fales WH, Schmidt DA: Successful treatment of feline cryptococcosis with ketoconazole and flucytosine, J Am Anim Hosp Assoc 26:199–201, 1990.
158. Medleau L, Jacobs GJ, Marks MA: Itraconazole for the treatment of cryptococcosis in cats, J Vet Intern Med 9:39–42, 1995.
159. Legendre A, Berthelin C: How do I treat central nervous system cryptococcosis in dogs and cats?, Prog Vet Neurol 6:32–34, 1995.
160. Hart KA, et al: Successful resolution of cryptococcal meningitis and optic neuritis in an adult horse with oral fluconazole, J Vet Intern Med 22:1436–1440, 2008.
161. Greene RT, Troy GC: Coccidioidomycosis in 48 cats: a retrospective study (1984-1993), J Vet Intern Med 2:86–91, 1995.
162. Clinkenbeard KD, Cowell RL, Tyler RD: Disseminated histoplasmosis in dogs: 12 cases (1981-1986), J Am Vet Med Assoc 193:1443–1447, 1988.
163. Sharp NJH, Sullivan M: Use of ketoconazole in the treatment of canine nasal aspergillosis, J Am Vet Med Assoc 194:782–786, 1989.
164. Miller PE, Miller LM, Schoster JV: Feline blastomycosis: a report of three cases and literature review (1961 to 1988), J Am Anim Hosp Assoc 26:417–424, 1990.
165. Hodges RD, et al: Itraconazole for the treatment of histoplasmosis in cats, J Vet Intern Med 8:409–413, 1994.
166. Edwards DF: Actinomycosis and nocardiosis. In Greene CE, editor: Infectious diseases of the dog and cat, ed 3, Philadelphia, 2006, Elsevier.
167. Dubey JP, Lappin MR: Toxoplasmosis and neosporosis. In Greene CE, editor: Infectious diseases of the dog and cat, ed 3, Philadelphia, 2006, Elsevier.
168. Lappin MR, Greene CE, Winston S, et al: Clinical feline toxoplasmosis: serologic diagnosis and therapeutic management of 15 cases, J Vet Intern Med 3:139–143, 1989.
169. Dubey JP, Lappin MR: Toxoplasmosis and neosporosis. In Greene CE, editor: Infectious diseases of the dog and cat, ed 3, Philadelphia, 2006, Elsevier.
170. Fenger CK: PCR-based detection of Sarcocystis neurona: implications for diagnosis and research. In Proceedings of the 12th American College of Veterinary Internal Medicine Forum, 550–552, 1994.
171. Fenger CK: Update on the diagnosis and treatment of equine protozoal myeloencephalitis (EPM). In the Proceedings of the 13th ACVIM Forum, DeNovo R, Hoeppner Ck eds. Lake Buena Vista, FL, 597–599, 1995.
172. Murray KO, Holmes KC, Hanlon CA: : Rabies in vaccinated dogs and cats in the United States, 1997-2001, J Am Vet Med Assoc 235:691–695, 2009.
173. Porter MB, et al: West Nile virus encephalomyelitis in horses: 46 cases (2001), J Am Vet Med Assoc 222:1241–1247, 2003.
174. Tyler JW, et al: West Nile virus encephalomyelitis in a sheep, J Vet Intern Med 17:242–244, 2003.
175. Wamsley HL, et al: Findings in cerebrospinal fluids of horses infected with West Nile virus: 30 cases (2001), J Am Vet Med Assoc 221:1303–1305, 2002.
176. Przelomski MM, O'Rourke E, Grady GF, et al: Eastern equine encephalitis in Massachusetts: a report of 16 cases, 1970-1984, Neurology 38:736–739, 1988.
177. Farrar MD, Miller DL, Baldwin CA, et al: Eastern equine encephalitis in dogs, J Vet Diagn Invest 17: 614–617, 2005.
178. Walton TE: Arboviral encephalomyelitides of livestock in the Western Hemisphere, J Am Vet Med Assoc 200:1385–1389, 2000.
179. Del Piero F, Wilkins PA, Dubovi EJ, et al: Clinical pathologic immunohistochemical, and virologic findings of eastern equine encephalomyelitis in two horses, Vet Pathol 38:451–456, 2001.
180. Gilman AG, et al: Antiviral agents. In Goodman, Gilman, editors: The pharmacological basis of therapeutics, New York, 1990, Pergamon Press.
181. Leggett MN, Dukes J, Pirie HM: A spongiform encephalopathy in a cat, Vet Rec 127:586, 1990.
182. Vidal E, Montoliu P, Anor S, et al: A novel spongiform degeneration of the grey matter in the brain of a kitten, J Comp Pathol 131:98, 2004.
183. Meinkoth JH, et al: Morphologic and molecular evidence of a dual species ehrlichial infection in a dog presenting with inflammatory central nervous system disease, J Vet Intern Med 12:389–393, 1989.
184. Maretzki CH, Fisher DJ, Greene CE: Granulocytic ehrlichiosis and meningitis in a dog, J Am Vet Med Assoc 205:1554–1556, 1994.
185. Neer TM, et al: Consensus statement on ehrlichial disease of small animals from the infectious disease study group of the ACVIM, J Vet Intern Med 16:309–315, 2002.
186. Meric SM: Canine meningitis: a changing emphasis, J Vet Intern Med 2:26–35, 1988.
187. Tipold A: Diagnosis of inflammatory and infectious diseases of the central nervous system in dogs: a retrospective study, J Vet Intern Med 9:304–314, 1995.
188. Granger N, Smith PM, Jeffery ND: Clinical findings and treatment of non-infectious meningoencephalomyelitis in dogs: a systematic review of 457 published cases from 1962-2008, Vet J , 2009.
189. Webb AA, Taylor SM, Muir GD: Steroid-responsive meningitis-arteritis in dogs with noninfectious, nonerosive, idiopathic, immune-mediated polyarthritis, J Vet Intern Med 16:269–273, 2002.
190. Tipold A, Schatzberg SJ: An update on steroid responsive meningitis-arteritis, J Small Anim Pract , 1999.
191. Behr S, Cauzinille L: Aseptic suppurative meningitis in juvenile boxer dogs: retrospective study of 12 cases, J Am Anim Hosp Assoc 42:277–282, 2006.
192. Snyder PW, Kazacos EA, Scott-Moncrieff JC, et al: Pathologic features of naturally occurring juvenile polyarteritis in beagle dogs, Vet Pathol 32:337–345, 1995.
193. Redman J: Steroid-responsive meningitis-arteritis in the Nova Scotia duck tolling retriever, Vet Rec 151:712, 2002.
194. Penderis ML, et al: Steroid responsive meningitis-arteritis: a prospective study of potential disease markers, prednisolone treatment, and long-term outcome in 20 dogs (2006-2008), J Vet Intern Med 23:862–870, 2009.
195. Bathen-Noethen A, Carlson R, Menzel D, et al: Concentrations of acute-phase proteins in dogs with steroid responsive meningitis-arteritis, J Vet Intern Med 22:1149–1156, 2008.

196. Munana K, Luttgen PJ: Prognostic factors for dogs with granulomatous meningoencephalomyelitis: 42 cases (1982-1996), J Am Vet Med Assoc 212:1902–1906, 1998.
197. Demierre S, et al: Correlation between the clinical course of granulomatous meningoencephalomyelitis in dogs and the extent of mast cell infiltration, Vet Rec 148:467–472, 2001.
198. Kipar A, Baumgartner W, Vogil C: Immunohistochemical characterization of inflammatory cells in brains of dogs with granulomatous meningoencephalitis, Vet Pathol 35:43–52, 1998.
199. Cuddon PA, Smith-Maxie L: Reticulosis of the central nervous system in the dog, Compend Contin Educ Pract Vet 6:23–29, 1984:32.
200. Smith JS, deLahunta A, Riis RC: Reticulosis of the visual system in a dog, J Small Anim Pract 18:643–652, 1977.
201. Fliegner RA, Holloway SA, Slocombe RF: Granulomatous meningoencephalomyelitis with peripheral nervous system involvement in a dog, Aust Vet J 84:358–361, 2006.
202. Braund KG, Vandevelde M, Walker TL, et al: Granulomatous meningoencephalomyelitis in six dogs, J Am Vet Med Assoc 172:1195–1200, 1978.
203. Talarico LR, Schatzberg SJ: Idiopathic granulomatous and necrotising inflammatory disorders of the canine central nervous system: a review and future perspectives, J Small Anim Pract , 2009.
204. Cuddon PA, Coates JR, Murray M: New treatments for granulomatous meningoencephalomyelitis. In the Proceedings of the 20th ACVIM Forum, Davenport D, Lester GD eds. Dallas, 319–321, 2002.
205. Smith PM, et al: Comparison of two regimens for the treatment of meningoencephalomyelitis of unknown etiology, J Vet Intern Med 23:520–526, 2009.
206. Zarfoss M, Schatzberg S, Venator K, et al: Combined cytosine arabinoside and prednisone therapy for meningoencephalitis of unknown aetiology in 10 dogs, J Small Anim Pract 47:588–595, 2006.
207. Ruslander D, Moore AS, Gliatto JM, et al: Cytosine arabinoside as a single agent for the induction of remission in canine lymphoma, J Vet Intern Med 8:299–301, 1994.
208. Adamo PF, Rylander H, Adams WM: Ciclosporin use in multi-drug therapy for meningoencephalomyelitis of unknown aetiology in dogs, J Small Anim Pract 48: 486–496, 2007.
209. Coates JR, Barone G, Dewey CW, et al: Procarbazine as adjunctive therapy for treatment of dogs with presumptive antemortem diagnosis of granulomatous meningoencephalomyelitis: 21 cases (1998-2004), J Vet Intern Med 21:100–106, 2007.
210. Schatzberg SJ: Idiopathic granulomatous and necrotizing inflammatory disorders of the canine central nervous system, Vet Clin North Am Small Anim Pract 40: 101–120, 2010.
211. Levine JM, et al: Epidemiology of necrotizing meningoencephalitis in pug dogs, J Vet Intern Med 22:961–968, 2008.
212. Higginbotham MJ, Kent M, Glass EN: Noninfectious inflammatory central nervous system diseases in dogs, Compend Contin Educ Pract Vet 29:488–497, 2007.
213. Young BD, et al: Magnetic resonance imaging characteristics of necrotizing meningoencephalitis in pug dogs, J Vet Intern Med 23:527–535, 2009.
214. Windsor RC, et al: Cerebrospinal fluid eosinophilia in dogs, J Vet Intern Med 23:274–281, 2009.
215. Herrtage ME: Canine fucosidosis, Vet Ann 28:223–227, 1988.
216. Barker CG, Herrtage ME, Shanahan F, et al: Fucosidosis in English springer spaniels: results of a trial screening programme, J Small Anim Pract 29(10):623–630, 1988.
217. Littlewood JD, Herrtage ME, Palmer AC: Neuronal storage disease in English springer spaniels, Vet Rec 112(4):86–87, 1983.
218. Skelly BJ, Sargan DR, Winchester BG, et al: Genomic screening for fucosidosis in English springer spaniels, Am J Vet Res 60(6):726–729, 1999.
219. Smith MO, Wenger DA, Hill SL, et al: Fucosidosis in a family of American-bred English springer spaniels, J Am Vet Med Assoc 209(12):2088–2090, 1996.
220. Berg T, Tollersrud OK, Walkley SU, et al: Purification of feline lysosomal α-mannosidase, determination of its cDNA sequence and identification of a mutation causing α-mannosidosis in Persian cats, Biochem J 328(3): 863–870, 1997.
221. Blakemore WF: A case of mannosidosis in the cat: clinical and histopathological findings, J Small Anim Pract 27(7):447–455, 1986.
222. Cummings JF, Wood PA, de Lahunta A, et al: The clinical and pathologic heterogeneity of feline a-mannosidosis, J Vet Intern Med 2(4):163–170, 1988.
223. Healy PJ, Harper PA, Dennis JA: Phenotypic variation in bovine a-mannosidosis, Res Vet Sci 49(1):82–84, 1990.
224. Maenhout T, Kint JA, Dacremont G, et al: Mannosidosis in a litter of Persian cats, Vet Rec 122(15):351–354, 1988.
225. Vandevelde M, Fankhauser R, Bichsel P, et al: Hereditary neurovisceral mannosidosis associated with a-mannosidase deficiency in a family of Persian cats, Acta Neuropathol 58(1):64–68, 1982.
226. Embury DH, Jerrett IV: Mannosidosis in Galloway calves, Vet Pathol 22(6):548–551, 1985.
227. Bryan L, Schmutz S, Hodges SD, et al: Bovine b-mannosidosis: pathologic and genetic findings in Salers calves, Vet Pathol 30(2):130–139, 1993.
228. Shapiro JL, Rostkowski C, Little PB, et al: Caprine b-mannosidosis in kids from an Ontario herd, Can Vet J 26(5):155–158, 1985.
229. Cusick PK, Cameron AM, Parker AJ: Canine neuronal glycoproteinosis—Lafora's disease in the dog, J Am Anim Hosp Assoc 12:518–521, 1976.
230. Gredal H, Berendt M, Leifsson PS: Progressive myoclonus epilepsy in a beagle, J Small Anim Pract 44(11): 511–514, 2003.
231. Hall DG, Steffens WL, Lassiter L: Lafora bodies associated with neurologic signs in a cat, Vet Pathol 35(3): 218–220, 1998.
232. Jian Z, Alley MR, Cayzer J, et al: Lafora's disease in an epileptic Basset hound, N Z Vet J 38(2):75–79, 1990.
233. Kaiser E, Krauser K, Schwartz-Porsche D: Lafora disease (progressive myoclonus epilepsy) in the basset hound. Early diagnosis by muscle biopsy, Tierarztl Prax 19(3):290–295, 1991.
234. Moreau PM, Vallat Jm, Hugon J, et al: Lafora's disease in basset hounds. In the Proceedings of the 8th ACVIM Forum, McGuirk SM ed. Washington DC, 1045–1049, 1990.
235. Webb AA, McMillan C, Cullen CL, et al: Lafora disease as a cause of visually exacerbated myoclonic attacks in a dog, Can Vet J 50(9):963–967, 2009.
236. Brix AE, Howerth EW, McConkie-Rosell A, et al: Glycogen storage disease type Ia in two littermate Maltese puppies, Vet Pathol 32(5):460–465, 1995.

237. Bardens JW, Bardens GW, Bardens B: Clinical observations on a Von Gierke-like syndrome in puppies, Allied Vet 32:4–7, 1961.
238. Walvoort HC, Koster JF, Reuser AJ: Heterozygote detection in a family of Lapland dogs with a recessively inherited metabolic disease: canine glycogen storage disease type II, Res Vet Sci 38(2):174–178, 1985.
239. Walvoort HC, Slee RG, Koster JF: Canine glycogen storage disease type II. A biochemical study of an acid alpha-glucosidase-deficient Lapland dog, Biochim Biophys Acta 715(1):63–69, 1982.
240. Walvoort HC: Glycogen storage disease type II in the Lapland dog, Vet Q 7(3):187–190, 1985.
241. Sandstrom B, Westman J, Ockerman PA: Glycogenosis of the central nervous system in the cat, Acta Neuropathol 14:194–200, 1969.
242. Dennis JA, Healy PJ, Reichmann KG: Genotyping Brahman cattle for generalised glycogenosis, Aust Vet J 80(5):286–291, 2002.
243. Reichmann KG, Twist JO, Thistlethwaite EJ: Clinical, diagnostic and biochemical features of generalised glycogenosis type II and Brahman cattle, Aust Vet J 70(11):405–408, 1993.
244. Dennis JA, Moran C, Healy PJ: The bovine α-glucosidase gene: coding region, genomic structure, and mutations that cause bovine generalized glycogenosis, Mammn Genome 11(3):206–212, 2000.
245. Dennis JA, Healy PJ: Genotyping shorthorn cattle for generalised glycogenosis, Aust Vet J 79(11):773–775, 2001.
246. Manktelow BW, Hartley WJ: Generalized glycogen storage disease in sheep, J Comp Pathol 85(1):139–145, 1975.
247. Gregory BL, Shelton GD, Bali DS, et al: Glycogen storage disease type IIIa in curly-coated retrievers, J Vet Intern Med 21(1):40–46, 2007.
248. Rafiquzzaman M, Svenkerud R, Strande A, et al: Glycogenosis in the dog, Acta Veterinaria Scand 17(2):196–209, 1976.
249. Coates JR, Paxton R, Cox NR, et al: A case presentation and discussion of Type IV glycogen storage disease in a Norwegian forest cat, Prog Vet Neurol 7(1):5–11, 1996.
250. Fyfe JC, Giger U, Van Winkle TJ, et al: Glycogen storage disease type IV: inherited deficiency of branching enzyme activity in cats, Pediatr Res 32(6):719–725, 1992.
251. Fyfe JC, Giger U, Van winkle TJ, et al: Familial glycogen storage disease type IV (GSD IV) in Norwegian forest cats (NWFC). In the Proceedings of the 8th ACVIM Forum, McGuirk SM ed. Washington DC, 1129, 1990.
252. Johnstone AC, McSporran KD, Kenny JE, et al: Myophosphorylase deficiency (glycogen storage disease Type V) in a herd of Charolais cattle in New Zealand: confirmation by PCR-RFLP testing. N Z Vet J 52(6):404–408, 2004.
253. Smith BF, Stedman H, Rajpurohit Y, et al: Molecular basis of canine muscle type phosphofructokinase deficiency, J Biol Chem 271(33):20070–20074, 1996.
254. Harvey JW, Calderwood MM, Gropp KE, et al: Polysaccharide storage myopathy in canine phosphofructokinase deficiency (type VII glycogen storage disease), Vet Pathol 27(1):1–8, 1990.
255. Bosshard NU, Hubler M, Arnold S, et al: Spontaneous mucolipidosis in a cat: an animal model of human I-cell disease, Vet Pathol 33(1):1–13, 1996.
256. Giger U, Tcherneva E, Caverly J, et al: A missense point mutation in N-acetylglucosamine-1-phosphotransferase causes mucolipidosis II in domestic shorthair cats, J Vet Intern Med 20:781, 2006.
257. Muller G, Alldinger S, Moritz A, et al: GM1-gangliosidosis in Alaskan huskies: clinical and pathologic findings, Vet Pathol 38(3):281–290, 2001.
258. Shell LG, Potthoff AI, Carithers R, et al: Neuronal-visceral GM_1 gangliosidosis in Portuguese water dogs, J Vet Intern Med 3(1):1–7, 1989.
259. Alroy J, Orgad U, DeGasperi R, et al: Canine G_{M1}-gangliosidosis. A clinical, morphologic, histochemical, and biochemical comparison of two different models, Am J Pathol 140(3):675–689, 1992.
260. Yamato O, Ochiai K, Masuoka Y, et al: GM1 gangliosidosis in Shiba dogs, Vet Rec 146(17):493–496, 2000.
261. Yamato O, Kobayashi A, Satoh H, et al: Comparison of polymerase chain reaction-restriction fragment length polymorphism assay and enzyme assay for diagnosis of GM1-gangliosidosis in Shiba dogs, J Vet Diagn Invest 16(4):299–304, 2004.
262. Read DH, Harrington DD, Keenan TW, et al: Neuronal-visceral GM1 gangliosidosis in a dog with beta-galactosidase deficiency, Science USA 194(4263):442–445, 1976.
263. Murnane RD, hern-Rindell AJ, Prieur DJ: Ovine GM1 gangliosidosis, Small Rumin Res 6(1-2):109–118, 1991.
264. Donnelly WJC, Sheahan BJ: Bovine, GM1 gangliosidosis: an inborn lysosomal disease, Vet Sci Commun 1(1):65–74, 1977.
265. Baker HJ Jr, Lindsey JR, McKhann GM, et al: Neuronal GM1 gangliosidosis in a Siamese cat with beta-galactosidase deficiency, Science 174(4011):838–839, 1971.
266. De Maria R, Divari S, Bo S, et al: Beta-galactosidase deficiency in a Korat cat: a new form of feline GM1-gangliosidosis, Acta Neuropathol 96(3):307–314, 1998.
267. Dial SM, Mitchell TW, LeCouteur RA, et al: GM_1-gangliosidosis (type II) in three cats, J Am Anim Hosp Assoc 30(4):355–360, 1994.
268. Singer HS, Cork LC: Canine GM2 gangliosidosis: morphological and biochemical analysis, Vet Pathol 26(2):114–120, 1989.
269. Bernheimer H, Karbe E: Morphological and neurochemical investigations of two types of amaurotic idiocy in the dog. Evidence of a GM2-gangliosidosis, Acta Neuropathol 16:243–261, 1970.
270. Neuwelt EA, Johnson WG, Blank NK, et al: Characterization of a new model of G_{M2}-gangliosidosis (Sandhoff's disease) in Korat cats, J Clin Invest 76(2):482–490, 1985.
271. Yamato O, Matsunaga S, Takata K, et al: GM2-gangliosidosis variant 0 (Sandhoff-like disease) in a family of Japanese domestic cats, Vet Rec 155(23):739–744, 2004.
272. Bradbury AM, Morrison NE, Hwang M, et al: Neurodegenerative lysosomal storage disease in European Burmese cats with hexosaminidase β-subunit deficiency, Mol Genet Metab 97(1):53–59, 2009.
273. Kosanke SD, Pierce KR, Bay WW: Clinical and biochemical abnormalities in porcine GM2-gangliosidosis, Vet Pathol 15(6):685–699, 1978.
274. Cummings JF, Wood PA, Walkley SU, et al: GM2 gangliosidosis in a Japanese spaniel, Acta Neuropathol 67(3/4):247–253, 1985.
275. Ishikawa Y, Li SC, Wood PA, et al: Biochemical basis of type AB G_{M2} gangliosidosis in a Japanese spaniel, J Neurochem 48(3):860–864, 1987.
276. Knowles K, Alroy J, Castagnaro M, et al: Adult-onset lysosomal storage disease in a Schipperke dog: clinical, morphological and biochemical studies, Acta Neuropathol 86(3):306–312, 1993.
277. Hartley WJ, Blakemore WF: Neurovisceral glucocerebroside storage (Gaucher's disease) in a dog, Vet Pathol 10(3):191–201, 1973.

278. Water NS, Jolly RD, Farrow BRH: Canine Gaucher disease: the enzymic defect, Aust J Exp Biol Med Sci 57(5):551–554, 1979.
279. Jolly RD, Walkley SU: Lysosomal storage disease of animals: an essay in comparative pathology, Vet Pathol 34(6):527–548, 1997.
280. Selcer ES, Selcer RR: Globoid cell leukodystrophy in two West Highland white terriers and one Pomeranian, Compend Contin Ed Pract Vet 6(7):621–624, 1984.
281. Victoria T, Rafi MA, Wenger DA: Cloning of the canine GALC cDNA and identification of the mutation causing globoid cell leukodystrophy in West Highland white and Cairn terriers, Genomics 33(3):457–462, 1996.
282. Wenger DA, Victoria T, Rafi MA, et al: Globoid cell leukodystrophy in Cairn and West Highland white terriers 90(1):138–142, 1999.
283. Johnson GR, Oliver JE Jr, Selcer R: Globoid cell leukodystrophy in a beagle, J Am Vet Med Assoc 167(5): 380–384, 1975.
284. Zaki FA, Kay WJ: Globoid cell leukodystrophy in a miniature poodle, J Am Vet Med Assoc 163(3):248–250, 1973.
285. Luttgen PJ, Braund KG, Storts RW: Globoid cell leukodystrophy in a basset hound, J Small Anim Pract 24: 153–160, 1983.
286. McDonnell JJ, Carmichael KP, McGraw RA, et al: Preliminary characterization of globoid cell leukodystrophy in Irish Setters, J Vet Intern Med 14(3):339, 2000.
287. McGraw RA, Carmichael KP: Molecular basis of globoid cell leukodystrophy in Irish setters, Vet J 171(2): 370–372, 2006.
288. Johnson KH: Globoid leukodystrophy in the cat, J Am Vet Med Assoc 157(12):2057–2064, 1970.
289. Pritchard DH, Naphtine DV, Sinclair AJ: Globoid cell leukodystrophy in polled Dorset sheep, Vet Pathol 17:399–405, 1980.
290. Sigurdson CJ, Basaraba RJ, Mazzaferro EM, et al: Globoid cell-like leukodystrophy in a domestic longhaired cat, Vet Pathol 39:494–496, 2002.
291. Blakemore WF: Neurolipidoses: examples of lysosomal storage diseases, Vet Clin North Am Small Anim Pract 10(1):81–90, 1980.
292. Wenger DA, Sattler M, Kudoh T, et al: Niemann-Pick disease: a genetic model in Siamese cats, Science 208:1471–1473, 1980.
293. Yamagami T, Umeda M, Kamiya S, et al: Neurovisceral sphingomyelinosis in a Siamese cat, Acta Neuropathol 79(3):330–332, 1989.
294. Baker HJ, Wood PA, Wenger DA, et al: Sphingomyelin lipidosis in a cat, Vet Pathol 24(5):386–391, 1987.
295. Somers KL, Royals MA, Carstea ED, et al: Mutation analysis of feline Niemann-Pick C1 disease, Mol Genet Metab 79(2):99–103, 2003.
296. Saunders GK, Wenger DA: Sphingomyelinase deficiency (Niemann-Pick disease) in a Hereford calf, Vet Pathol 45(2):201–202, 2008.
297. Lowenthal AC, Cummings JF, Wenger DA, et al: Feline sphingolipidosis resembling Niemann-Pick disease type C, Acta Neuropathol 81(2):189–197, 1990.
298. Kuwamura M, Awakura T, Shimada A, et al: Type C Niemann-Pick disease in a boxer dog, Acta Neuropathol 85(3):345–348, 1993.
299. Haskins ME, Aguirre GD, Jezyk PF, et al: The pathology of the feline model of mucopolysaccharidosis I, Am J Pathol 112(1):27–36, 1983.
300. Shull RM, Munger RJ, Spellacy E, et al: Canine a-L-iduronidase deficiency. A model of mucopolysaccharidosis I, Am J Pathol 109(2):244–248, 1982.
301. Wilkerson MJ, Lewis DC, Marks SL, et al: Clinical and morphologic features of mucopolysaccharidosis type II in a dog: naturally occurring model of Hunter syndrome, Vet Pathol 35(3):230–233, 1998.
302. Jolly RD, Ehrlich PC, Franklin RJM, et al: Histological diagnosis of mucopolysaccharidosis IIIA in a wire-haired dachshund, Vet Rec 148(18):564–567, 2001.
303. Jolly RD, Allan FJ, Collett MG, et al: Mucopolysaccharidosis IIIA (Sanfilippo syndrome) in a New Zealand Huntaway dog with ataxia, N Z Vet J 48(5):144–148, 2000.
304. Jolly RD, Johnstone AC, Norman EJ, et al: Pathology of mucopolysaccharidosis IIIA in Huntaway dogs, Vet Pathol 44(5):569–578, 2007.
305. Yogalingam G, Pollard T, Gliddon B, et al: Identification of a mutation causing mucopolysaccharidosis type IIIA in New Zealand Huntaway dogs, Genomics 79(2):150–153, 2002.
306. Ellinwood NM, Wang P, Skeen T, et al: A model of mucopolysaccharidosis IIIB (Sanfilippo syndrome type IIIB): N-acetyl-alpha-D-glucosaminidase deficiency in Schipperke dogs, J Inherit Metab Dis 26(5):489–504, 2003.
307. Karageorgos L, Hill B, Bawden MJ, et al: Bovine mucopolysaccharidosis type IIIB, J Inherit Metab Dis 30(3):358–364, 2007.
308. Hoard HM, Leipprandt JR, Cavanagh KT, et al: Determination of genotypic frequency of caprine mucopolysaccharidosis IIID, J Vet Diagn Invest 10(2):181–183, 1998.
309. Jones MZ, Alroy J, Boyer PJ, et al: Caprine mucopolysaccharidosis-IIID: clinical, biochemical, morphological and immunohistochemical characteristics, J Neuropathol Exp Neurol 57(2):148–157, 1998.
310. Fischer A, Carmichael KP, Munnell JF, et al: Sulfamidase deficiency in a family of dachshunds: a canine model of mucopolysaccharidosis IIIA (Sanfilippo A), Pediatr Res 44(1):74–82, 1998.
311. Neer TM, Dial SM, Pechman R, et al: Mucopolysaccharidosis VI in a miniature pinscher, J Vet Intern Med 9(6):429–433, 1995.
312. Breton L, Guérin P, Morin M: A case of mucopolysaccharidosis VI in a cat, J Am Anim Hosp Assoc 19(6): 891–896, 1983.
313. Haskins ME, Aguirre GD, Jezyk PF, et al: The pathology of the feline model of mucopolysaccharidosis VI, Am J Pathol 101(3):657–674, 1980.
314. Ray J, Haskins ME, Ray K: Molecular diagnostic tests for ascertainment of genotype at the mucopolysaccharidosis type VII locus in dogs, Am J Vet Res 59(9):1092–1095, 1998.
315. Haskins ME, Otis EJ, Hayden JE, et al: Hepatic storage of glycosaminoglycans in feline and canine models of mucopolysaccharidoses I, VI, and VII, Vet Pathol 29(2):112–119, 1992.
316. Awano T, Katz ML, O'Brien DP, et al: A frame shift mutation in canine TPP1 (the ortholog of human CLN2) in a juvenile dachshund with neuronal ceroid lipofuscinosis, Mol Genet Metab 89(3):254–260, 2006.
317. Cummings JF, de Lahunta A, Riis RC, et al: Neuropathologic changes in a young adult Tibetan terrier with subclinical neuronal ceroid-lipofuscinosis, Prog Vet Neurol 1(3):301–309, 1990.
318. Katz ML, Narfstrom K, Johnson GS, et al: Assessment of retinal function and characterization of lysosomal storage body accumulation in the retinas and brains of Tibetan terriers with ceroid-lipofuscinosis, Am J Vet Res 66:67–76, 2005.
319. Melville SA, Wilson CL, Chiang CS, et al: A mutation in canine CLN5 causes neuronal ceroid lipofuscinosis in border collie dogs, Genomics 86:287–294, 2005.

320. Taylor RM, Farrow BR: Ceroid-lipofuscinosis in border collie dogs, Acta Neuropathol 75(6):627–631, 1988.
321. Harper PA, Walker KH, Healy PJ, et al: Neurovisceral ceroid-lipofuscinosis in blind Devon cattle, Acta Neuropathol 75(6):632–636, 1988.
322. O'Brien DP, Katz ML: Neuronal ceroid lipofuscinosis in 3 Australian shepherd littermates, J Vet Intern Med 22(2):472–475, 2008.
323. Tammen I, Houweling PJ, Frugier T, et al: A missense mutation (c.184C > T) in ovine CLN6 causes neuronal ceroid lipofuscinosis in Merino sheep whereas affected South Hampshire sheep have reduced levels of CLN6 mRNA, Biochim Biophys Acta 1762(10):898–905, 2006.
324. Cook RW, Jolly RD, Palmer DN, et al: Neuronal ceroid lipofuscinosis in Merino sheep, Aust Vet J 80(5): 292–297, 2002.
325. Mayhew IG, Jolly RD, Pickett BT, et al: Ceroid-lipofuscinosis (Batten's disease): pathogenesis of blindness in the ovine model, Neuropathol Appl Neurobiol 11:273–290, 1985.
326. Katz ML, Khan S, Awano T, et al: A mutation in the CLN8 gene in English setter dogs with neuronal ceroid-lipofuscinosis, Biochem Biophys Res Commun 327: 541–547, 2005.
327. Koppang N: The English setter with ceroid-lipofuscinosis: a suitable model for the juvenile type of ceroid-lipofuscinosis, Am J Med Genet Suppl 5:117–126, 1988.
328. Awano T, Katz ML, O'Brien DP, et al: A mutation in the cathepsin D gene (CTSD) in American bulldogs with neuronal ceroid lipofuscinosis, Mol Genet Metab 87(4):341–348, 2006.
329. Evans J, Katz ML, Levesque D, et al: A variant form of neuronal ceroid lipofuscinosis in American bulldogs, J Vet Intern Med 19(1):44–51, 2005.
330. Tyynela J, Sohar I, Sleat DE, et al: A mutation in the ovine cathepsin D gene causes a congenital lysosomal storage disease with profound neurodegeneration, EMBO J 19(12):2786–2792, 2000.
331. Olby N, Blot S, Thibaud JL, et al: Cerebellar cortical degeneration in adult American Staffordshire terriers, J Vet Intern Med 18(2):201–208, 2004.
332. Abitbol M, Thibaud JL, Olby NJ, et al: A canine arylsulfatase G (ARSG) mutation leading to a sulfatase deficiency is associated with neuronal ceroid lipofuscinosis, Proceed Nat Acad Sci 107:14775–14780, 2010.
333. Jolly RD: Comparative biology of the neuronal ceroid-lipofuscinoses: an overview, Am J Med Genet 57:307–311, 1995.
334. Appleby EC, Longstaffe JA, Bell FR: Ceroid-lipofuscinosis in two Saluki dogs, J Comp Pathol 92(3):375–380, 1982.
335. Cho DY, Leipold HW, Rudolph R: Neuronal ceroidosis (ceroid-lipofuscinosis) in a blue heeler dog, Acta Neuropathol 69(1-2):161–164, 1986.
336. Cantile C, Buonaccorsi A, Pepe V, et al: Juvenile neuronal ceroid-lipofuscinosis (Batten's disease) in a poodle dog, Prog Vet Neurol 7(3):82–87, 1996.
337. Jolly RD, Sutton RH, Smith RIE, et al: Ceroid-lipofuscinosis in miniature Schnauzer dogs, Aust Vet J 75(1):67, 1997.
338. Modenato M, Marchetti V, Barsotti G, et al: Neuronal ceroid-lipofuscinosis in a Chihuahua, Annali della Facolt+á di Medicina Veterinaria di Pisa 60:215–224, 2007.
339. Sisk DB, Levesque DC, Wood PA, et al: Clinical and pathologic features of ceroid lipofuscinosis in two Australian cattle dogs, J Am Vet Med Assoc 197(3):361–364, 1990.
340. Goebel HH, Bilzer T, Dahme E, et al: Morphological studies in canine (Dalmatian) neuronal ceroid-lipofuscinosis, Am J Med Gen (Suppl 5):127–139, 1988.
341. Vandevelde M, Fatzer R: Neuronal ceroid-lipofuscinosis in older dachshunds, Vet Pathol 17(6):686–692, 1980.
342. Bildfell R, Matwichuk C, Mitchell S, et al: Neuronal ceroid-lipofuscinosis in a cat, Vet Pathol 32(5):485–488, 1995.
343. Cummings JF, de Lahunta A: An adult case of canine neuronal ceroid lipofuscinosis, Acta Neuropathol 39:43–51, 1977.
344. Kuwamura M, Nakagawa M, Nabe M, et al: Neuronal ceroid-lipofuscinosis in a Japanese domestic shorthair cat, J Vet Med Sci 71(5):665–667, 2009.
345. Green PD, Little PB: Neuronal ceroid-lipofuscin storage in Siamese cats, Can J Comp Med 38(2):207–212, 1974.
346. Harper PA, Walker KH, Healy PJ, et al: Neurovisceral ceroid-lipofuscinosisinblindDevoncattle,ActaNeuropathol 75(6):632–636, 1988.
347. Fiske RA, Storts RW: Neuronal ceroid-lipofuscinosis in Nubian goats, Vet Pathol 25(2):171–173, 1988.
348. Umemura T, Sato H, Goryo M, et al: Generalized lipofuscinosis in a dog, Jpn J Vet Sci 47(4):673–677, 1985.
349. Jolly RD, Palmer DN, Studdert VP, et al: Canine ceroid-lipofuscinoses: a review and classification, J Small Anim Pract 35:299–306, 1994.
350. Jolly RD, Walkley SU: Lysosomal storage diseases of animals; an essay in comparative pathology, Vet Pathol 34(6):527–548, 1997.
351. Pickett JP, Lindley DM, Boosinger TR, et al: Stationary night blindness in a collie, Prog Vet Comp Ophthalmol 1(4):303–308, 1991.
352. Pickett P, Dyer K, Saunders O, et al: Ocular manifestation of ceroid-lipofuscinosis in a spitz dog, Vet Pathol 29:469, 1992.
353. Edwards JF, Storts RW, Joyce JR, et al: Juvenile-onset neuronal ceroid-lipofuscinosis in Rambouillet sheep, Vet Pathol 31(1):48–54, 1994.
354. Woods PR, Storts RW, Shelton M, et al: Neuronal ceroid lipofuscinosis in Rambouillet sheep: characterization of the clinical disease, J Vet Intern Med 8(5):370–375, 1994.
355. LeGonidec G, Kuberski T, Daynes P, et al: A neurologic disease of horses in New Caledonia, Aust Vet J 57:1944–1945, 1981.
356. Url A, Bauder B, Thalhammer J, et al: Equine neuronal ceroidlipofuscinosis,ActaNeuropathol101:410–414,2001.

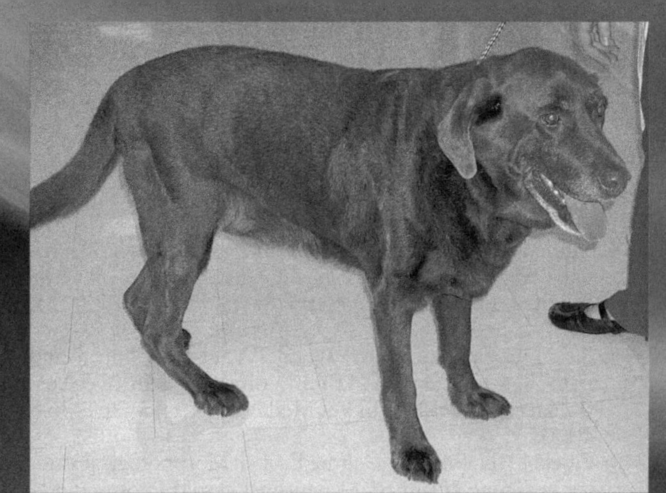

APPENDIX

Congenital, Inherited, or Breed-Associated Neurologic and Muscular Diseases in Domestic Animals

BOVINE DISEASES				
Breed	**Disease**	**Chapter**	**Inherited**	**References**
Aberdeen angus	Cerebellar degeneration/abiotrophy	8	S	1, 716
	Cerebellar hypoplasia	8	S	2, 704, 708
	Epilepsy	13	Y	3
	Mannosidosis	8, 15	Y	4-6, 787
Angus & shorthorn	Hypomyelination	10	Y	7, 8
Ayrshire	Cerebellar degeneration	8	Y	9, 10
	Cerebellar hypoplasia	8		10
	Cerebellar malformation (Dandy Walker)	8	S	701-703
Ayrshire cross	Atlanto-occipital malformation	7		11
Beefmaster	Ceroid lipofuscinosis	15		12
	Neuronal lipodystrophy	15	Y	6
Brahman	Glycogenosis (type II)	7, 15	Y	13, 803-805
	Myasthenia gravis (congenital)	7	Y	1045
	Narcolepsy/cataplexy	13		14
Brown Swiss	Cerebellar degeneration	8		15-17
	Degenerative myeloencephalopathy	7	S	15-17, 899
	Epilepsy	13	Y	18
	Spinal muscular atrophy	7	Y	934-936
Charolais	Cerebellar hypoplasia	8		19, 710, 715
	Leukodystrophy	7, 15	Y	6, 20-23
	Cerebellar degeneration and epilepsy	13		6
	Glycogenosis (type V)	7, 15	S	813, 1009
	Myelodysplasia	6	Y	24, 25
Charolais cross	Atlanto-occipital malformation	7		11
Devon	Atlanto-occipital malformation	7		26
	Ceroid lipofuscinosis	15		12, 27
Galloway	Mannosidosis	15		28
Guernsey	Narcolepsy/cataplexy	13		29
Hereford	Cerebellar degeneration	8	Y	30
	Cerebellar hypoplasia	8	Y	6, 30, 31, 705, 709
	Ceroid lipofuscinosis	15		6
	Epilepsy	13		32
	Hydrocephalus	12	Y	33-35

BOVINE DISEASES—cont'd				
Breed	**Disease**	**Chapter**	**Inherited**	**References**
	Hypomyelination	8, 10		8, 36
	Neuronal degeneration	7	Y	37, 38
	Gangliosidosis (Niemann-Pick)	8, 15	S	843
	Spinocerebellar degeneration	7		37
Holstein-Friesian	Atlanto-occipital malformation	7		39, 40
	Atlantoaxial luxation	7	S	39
	Cerebellar brainstem malformation	8		41
	Cerebellar degeneration/abiotrophy	8	Y	6, 30, 42, 712-714
	Cerebellar hypoplasia	8		43, 711
	Ceroid lipofuscinosis	8, 15	S	879
	Gangliosidosis GM_1	8, 15	Y	4, 44-47, 824
	Hypomyelination	8, 10		555
	Myopathy of diaphragmatic muscles		Y	556
	Spinal dysraphism	6		48
	Spongiform degeneration	12		49
	Vertebral malformation	6	U	647
Jersey	Cerebellar degeneration	8		6, 721, 722
	Cerebellar hypoplasia/abiotrophy	8	S	706, 707
	Hypomyelination	8, 10	Y	8, 50
Limousin	Epilepsy	13		6
Limousin cross	Neuronal degeneration	15	Y	51, 52, 717
Murray grey	Dysmyelinopathy	7, 15	Y	53, 54
	Mannosidosis	15	Y	5
Norwegian red poll	Pelvic limb paralysis	6	Y	52
Polled Hereford	Congenital myoclonus (neuraxial edema)	10, 15	Y	55-59
	Neuronal degeneration	8, 15	Y	60, 722
Polled shorthorn	Congenital myoclonus (neuraxial edema)	10, 15	Y	557
Red Danish	Congenital paralysis		Y	61
Salers	ß-Mannosidosis	15	Y	62, 63, 790
Shorthorn	Cerebellar degeneration	8, 15	Y	6
	Cerebellar hypoplasia	8	Y	6, 30, 64, 65
	Glycogenosis	7, 8, 15	Y	6, 66, 67, 806
	Hydrocephalus	12	Y	33, 34, 68
	Hypomyelination	8, 10	Y	8, 36
	Retinal dysplasia	11	Y	69
Simmental	Neuronal degeneration	15	Y	51, 52
	Spongiform myelopathy			558
Swedish red	Epilepsy	13		70
Various	Arthrogryposis	7		71
	Cerebellar brainstem malformation	8		72
	Myelodysplasia	6		73, 74
	Neurofibromatosis	15		75

Y, Yes; *S*, suspected.

CANINE DISEASES				
Breed	**Disease**	**Chapter**	**Inherited**	**References**
Afghan hound	Myelopathy	6	Y	76-79
	Retinal degeneration	11	Y	69
Airedale terrier	Cerebellar hypoplasia	8		80-82
	Cerebellar degeneration	8	Y	30, 660
	Congenital myasthenia gravis	7	Y	83
Akita	Cerebellar degeneration	8		30, 665
	Congenital vestibular disease	8	S	84
	Deafness	9	Y	730
	Glycogenosis (type III)	7, 15	S	809, 1006
	Myasthenia gravis (acquired)	7	U	1036
Alaskan husky	Encephalomyelopathy	7	Y	900
	Gangliosidosis GM_1	15	S	818
Alaskan malamute	Muscular dystrophy	7	S	985
	Peripheral neuropathy	7	Y	552, 942
	Retinal degeneration	11	Y	69
American bulldog	Ceroid lipofuscinosis	15	S	868, 869
Australian cattle dog	Ceroid lipofuscinosis	15	Y	85, 870

Continued

CANINE DISEASES—cont'd				
Breed	**Disease**	**Chapter**	**Inherited**	**References**
	Dermatomyositis	7	Y	551
	Myotonia congenita	10	Y	752
	Portosystemic shunt	13, 15		559
Australian heeler	Deafness	9	Y	86
Australian kelpie	Cerebellar degeneration	8	Y	551, 656
Australian shepherd dog	Chorioretinal dysplasia	11	Y	69
	Ceroid lipofuscinosis (CLN 6)	8, 15	S	862
	Deafness	9	Y	86, 87
Basenji	Coloboma	11	Y	69
Basset hound	Cervical malformation	7	S	88-90
	Globoid cell leukodystrophy	15	S	91
	Glycoproteinosis (LaFlora's disease)	13, 15	S	92, 795-797
Bavarian mountain dog	Cerebellar degeneration	8	S	666
Beagle	Agenesis vermis cerebellum	8	S	93, 654, 655
	Cerebellar degeneration	8	Y	30, 84, 657, 658
	Congenital vestibular disease	8		94, 95
	Deafness	9	Y	745
	Epilepsy	13	Y	81, 96-105
	Gangliosidosis GM_1	15	Y	45, 46, 106
	Globoid cell leukodystrophy	15	S	107
	Glycoproteinosis (LaFlora's disease)	13, 15	S	92, 96, 97, 108, 793
	Necrotizing vasculitis	15	Y	553
	Retinal degeneration	11	Y	69
	Retinal dysplasia	11		69
Beagle-schnauzer cross	Cerebellar degeneration	8		551
Bedlington terrier	Retinal dysplasia	11	Y	69, 81, 109
Belgian sheepdog (Groenendaeler shepherd dog)	Muscular dystrophy	7	Y	573, 984
Belgian Tervuren	Epilepsy	13	Y	81, 98, 382, 765, 767
Belgian Malinois	Lumbosacral stenosis	6	S	646
Bern running dog	Cerebellar degeneration	8	Y	30
Bernese mountain dog	Aggression			110
	Cerebellar degeneration	8	Y	84, 667, 668
	Epilepsy	13	S	768
	Hypomyelination	10		111
	Leukodystrophy	15		560
	Malignant histiocytosis	15		112
	Necrotizing vasculitis	14		561
Bichon frise	Steroid responsive tremor syndrome	10		551
Blue heeler	Ceroid lipofuscinosis	15		113, 114
Bluetick coonhound	Globoid leukodystrophy	15	Y	81, 115
Border collie	Cerebellar degeneration	8	Y	116, 669
	Ceroid lipofuscinosis	15	Y	84, 117, 118, 861
	Deafness	9		87
	Epilepsy	13	S	770
	Retinal degeneration	11	Y	69, 81, 109
	Sensory neuropathy	7, 14		119, 948
Borzoi	Cervical vertebral malformation	7		120
Boston terrier	Deafness	9	Y	86
	Gliomas	12	S	75, 121, 122
	Hemivertebrae	6	Y	81, 123, 124
	Hydrocephalus	12	P	125, 126
	Muscular dystrophy	7	S	996
	Myelodysplasia	6	Y	123
	Pituitary tumors	12, 15	S	75
	Vermian hypoplasia	8		136
Bouvier des Flandres	Laryngeal paralysis	9	Y	127, 128
	Muscular dystrophy	7	S	1001, 1002
Boxer	Axonopathy	7	Y	129, 130, 901, 902, 954
	Deafness	9	Y	86
	Degenerative myelopathy	6	S	615
	Ependymoma	12		75
	Seizures	13	H	763, 778
	Glioma	12	S	75, 121, 122
	Myositis (immune mediated)	7	U	976, 968

CANINE DISEASES—cont'd				
Breed	**Disease**	**Chapter**	**Inherited**	**References**
	Pituitary tumors	12	S	75
	Sensory neuronopathy	7	Y	551
	Sphingomyelinosis	15		562
	Spondylosis deformans	6	S	622
Briard	Retinal degeneration	11	Y	69, 109
Brittany	Cerebellar degeneration	8		131, 671, 672
	Muscular dystrophy	7		563, 995
	Motor neuropathy	7	Y	132, 133
	Retinal dysplasia	11		69
	Sensory ganglioradiculitis	14		551
Bull mastiff	Cerebellar and neuronal degeneration	8	Y	134
	Cervical vertebral malformation	7		135
	Leukodystrophy	7	U	889
Bull terrier	Cerebellar hypoplasia	8		136
	Deafness	9	Y	81, 87, 137, 138
	Hyperkinesis	10		139
	Laryngeal paralysis	9		551
Cairn terrier	Cerebellar degeneration	8		8
	Globoid cell leukodystrophy	7, 8, 15	Y	81, 140-144, 834, 835
	Hydrocephalus	12	P	126
	Neuronal degeneration (multisystem)	7, 8	S	145, 146, 692, 904, 905
Cardigan Welsh corgi	Degenerative myelopathy	7	Y	611
	Retinal degeneration	11	Y	69, 81
Catahoula	Deafness	9		551, 730
Cavalier King Charles spaniel	Caudal occipital malformation syndrome	7	Y	908-911, 913-916
	Muscular hypertonicity	7, 10	Y	147-149
	Muscular dystrophy	7	S	990
Chesapeake Bay retriever	Degenerative myelopathy	6		604, 611, 612
	Retinal degeneration	11		69
Chihuahua	Ceroid lipofuscinosis	15	Y	873
	Hydrocephalus	12	P	81, 126, 150
	Muscular dystrophy	7	S	969
	Neuroaxonal dystrophy	7		151
Chinese crested dog	Multisystem degeneration	8		691
Chondrodystrophic breeds	Intervertebral disk disease	6	S	152-158, 601
Chow chow	Cerebellar hypoplasia	8	S	30, 159
	Hypomyelination	10	Y	161-164
	Myotonia congenita	10	Y	165-171
Clumber spaniel	Cerebellar degeneration	15		30
	Mitochondrial myopathy	7		551, 1017, 1019
Cocker spaniel	Aggression			110, 172
	Cerebellar degeneration	8, 15		8
	Ceroid lipofuscinosis	15	Y	173
	Congenital vestibular disease	8	S	84, 94
	Deafness	9	S	86
	Esophageal hypomotility		Y	174, 175
	Facial paralysis	9	S	176, 177
	Hydrocephalus	12		81
	Mitochondrial myopathy	7	Y	1046
	Muscular dystrophy	7		969
	Myopathy (lipid storage)	7		1020
	Myotonia congenita	10	S	753
	Neuronal degeneration	7		178
	Phosphofructokinase deficiency myopathy	7	Y	564, 814, 815, 1010
	Portosystemic shunt	12	Y	565
	Retinal degeneration	11	Y	69, 81, 109
	Retinal dysplasia	11	Y	69, 109
	Seizures	13	H	763, 778
Collie	Cerebellar degeneration	8	Y	30, 179, 180
	Ceroid lipofuscinosis	15	S	870,
	Chorioretinal dysplasia	11	Y	69, 109
	Collie eye syndrome	11	Y	69, 109
	Deafness	9	Y	181, 729
	Dermatomyositis	7	Y	167, 182-187, 977

Continued

CANINE DISEASES—cont'd				
Breed	**Disease**	**Chapter**	**Inherited**	**References**
	Seizures	13	H	763, 778
	Myelodysplasia	6		188
	Neuroaxonal dystrophy	7	Y	180
	Neuronal degeneration	7		189
	Retinal degeneration	11	Y	109
	Sensory ganglioradiculitis	10		551
Corgi	Ceroid lipofuscinosis	15		566
Corgi, Pembroke	Degenerative myelopathy	6	S	603, 610, 611
	Dermatomyositis	7	U	978
	Muscular dystrophy	7	S	969
Coton de Tulear	Cerebellar degeneration/abiotrophy	8	S	659, 673
Corgi, Welsh	Sensory ganglioradiculitis	7		551
Curly coated retriever	Glycogenosis (type III)	7	S	808
Czech spotted dog	Epilepsy	13	Y	98, 288
Dachshund	Cerebellar hypoplasia	8		136
	Ceroid lipofuscinosis	15	Y	190
	Epilepsy	13	Y	191
	Esophageal hypomotility	13		174, 175
	Glycoproteinosis (LaFlora's disease)	15	S	798
Dachshund, dappled	Deafness	9	Y	730
Dachshund, longhaired	Ceroid lipofuscinosis	15	Y	192, 858
	Sensory neuropathy	7	Y	193, 194, 955
Dachshund, miniature	Myasthenia gravis (congenital)	7	S	1041
Dachshund, miniature, longhaired	Retinal degeneration	11	Y	69, 109
Dachshund, wire-haired	Mucopolysaccharidosis (MPS III)	8, 15	S	845, 852
Dalmatian	Ceroid lipofuscinosis	15		566, 874
	Deafness	9	Y	81, 86, 87, 137, 138, 181, 195-200, 730, 739-744, 746, 747
	Globoid cell leukodystrophy	15		81
	Hyperkinesis	10	S	201
	Hypomyelination	10	Y	202
	Leukodystrophy	7, 15	Y	203
	Myelodysplasia	6	S	204
	Polyneuropathy, laryngeal paralysis	7, 9		567
Doberman pinscher	Aggression			205
	Cervical spondylomyelopathy	7	S	88-90, 206-212, 917, 921, 922
	Congenital vestibular disease	8	S	84, 94, 95
	Deafness	9		213, 731
	Distal polyneuropathy	7		214
	Hemivertebrae	6		215
	Myositis (immune mediated)	7		971-974
	Narcolepsy/cataplexy	13	Y	216-220
	Sensory neuropathy/dancing doberman disease	7	S	221, 943
Dogo Argentino	Deafness	9	Y	727, 730
Dolichocephalic breeds	Meningioma	15		75, 222
Dutch kooiker dog	Leukoencephalomyelopathy	7	S	577, 578, 892
English bulldog	Cerebellar degeneration	8	S	674
	Deafness	9	S	86
	Hemivertebrae	6	Y	81, 123, 124
	Hydrocephalus	12	P	81, 125, 126
	Myelodysplasia	6	Y	81, 188, 223-225, 649
	Vertebral canal stenosis	6		226
English pointer	Cerebellar degeneration	8	S	675
	Hyperkinesis	10	Y	227-229
	Motor neuropathy	7	S	930
	Myopathy	7		1021
	Sensory neuropathy	7	Y	81, 194, 230-232
English setter	Ceroid lipofuscinosis	15	Y	233-236, 866, 867
	Deafness	9	Y	86, 238
English springer spaniel	Cerebellar degeneration	8		551
	Epilepsy	13	S	772
	Fucosidosis	7, 8, 15	Y	371-377, 779-783
	Gangliosidosis GM_1	15	Y	239, 820
	Myasthenia gravis (congenital)	7	S	1040

CANINE DISEASES—cont'd				
Breed	**Disease**	**Chapter**	**Inherited**	**References**
	Phosphofructokinase deficiency myopathy	7	Y	240, 241, 814, 815
	Polymyopathy, dyserythropoiesis	7		242
	Sensory neuropathy	7, 14	Y	956
Finnish harrier	Cerebellar degeneration	8	Y	30, 243
Finnish spitz	Epilepsy	13	Y	775
Foxhound	Deafness	9	Y	81, 244, 723
	Myelinopathy	6	S	609
Fox terrier	Axonopathy (central)	7	S	898
	Myasthenia gravis (congenital)	7	Y	167, 245, 246, 1044
	Deafness	9		81, 728
	Spinocerebellar degeneration	7, 8	S	81
French bulldog	Hemivertebrae	6		81, 123
French spaniel	Sensory neuropathy	7, 14	S	957
Gammel Dansk honsehund	Myasthenia gravis	7	Y	569, 1043
German shepherd dog	Aggression		S	205
	Cerebellar degeneration	8		84, 551
	Congenital vestibular disease	8	S	84, 94, 95, 247
	Degenerative myelopathy	6	S	248-257, 602-608, 611, 613, 614, 617
	Epilepsy	13	Y	81, 98, 270
	Esophageal hypomotility	9	S	174, 175, 258-260
	Giant axonal neuropathy	7	Y	261-265, 944
	Glycogenosis (type III)	7, 15	Y	551, 1006
	Lumbosacral stenosis	6	S	266-268, 624-646
	Myasthenia gravis (acquired)	7		1036
	Myelodysplasia	6		269
	Myopathy (fibrotic)	7		979
	Myopathy (mitochondrial)	7		1018
	Myositis (masticatory)	7		970
	Peripheral neuropathy	7		570
	Spondylosis deformans	6		618-624
German shorthaired pointer	Gangliosidosis GM_2	15	Y	4, 44-46, 271, 827, 828
	Hemivertebrae	6		272
	Muscular dystrophy	7		986
	Necrotizing vasculitis	14		551
	Sensory neuropathy	7, 14		959
German wire-haired pointer	Myositis (immune mediated)	7		975
Golden retriever	Ceroid lipofuscinosis	15		566, 870
	Epilepsy	13	S	774
	Gangliosidosis GM_2	15	S	828a, 828b
	Horner syndrome	11		571
	Hydrocephalus and hypertrichosis	12	S	554
	Multisystem axonopathy	7, 8		693
	Muscular dystrophy (x-linked)	7	Y	167, 273-276, 980, 981, 993, 994
	Myasthenia gravis (acquired)	7		1036
	Myotonia	10	S	166
	Peripheral hypomyelination	7		938, 939
	Retinal degeneration	11	Y	69, 81, 109
	Sensory neuropathy	7, 14		277, 960
Gordon setter	Cerebellar degeneration	8	Y	30, 278-281
	Retinal degeneration	11	Y	69, 81, 109
Great Dane	Central core myopathy	7	S	572
	Cerebellar degeneration	8		8, 652
	Cervical spondylomyelopathy	7	S	7, 88-90, 206-212, 282-284, 917, 918
	Deafness	9	Y	729
	Esophageal hypomotility	9	S	175, 258, 285, 286
	Extradural synovial cysts	7		927, 928
	Myasthenia gravis (acquired)	7		1037
	Myotonia congenita	10	S	551, 754
	Neuropathy (distal)	7		945, 946
	Retinal dysplasia	11		69, 81, 109
	Spondylosis deformans	6		618-624

Continued

CANINE DISEASES—cont'd				
Breed	**Disease**	**Chapter**	**Inherited**	**References**
Great Dane cross	Neuronal degeneration	7	Y	287
Great Pyrenees	Deafness	9	Y	726, 730
Greyhound	Exertional rhabdomyolysis	7		1027
	Esophageal hypomotility	9		260
	Retinal degeneration	11	Y	69
Griffon Bruxellois	Caudal occipital malformation syndrome	7		912, 916
Ibizan hound	Axonopathy (central and peripheral)	7	S	885
Italian greyhound	Cerebellar degeneration	8		677
Irish setter	Cerebellar degeneration	8	Y	30, 84, 661, 662
	Cerebellar hypoplasia	8	S	30
	Seizures	13	H	763, 778
	Esophageal hypomotility		S	286
	Globoid cell leukodystrophy	15	S	836, 837
	Hereditary quadriplegia and amblyopia	7	Y	30, 81, 661, 662
	Lissencephaly	13	S	30
	Retinal degeneration	11	Y	69, 81, 109
Irish terrier	Muscular dystrophy	7	Y	167, 289, 993
	Myopathy	7		982
Irish wolfound	Epilepsy	13	S	769
	Fibrocartilageous embolism	6		289a
	Portosystemic shunt	12		575
Jack Russell terrier	Cerebellar degeneration	7, 8	Y	81, 292, 676
	Deafness	9	Y	732
	Myasthenia gravis (congenital)	7	Y	167, 290, 291, 1042
	Myopathy (mitochondrial)	7		1015
	Myotonia congenita	10	S	755, 762
	Neuroaxonal dystrophy	7		576
	Sensory neuronopathy	7, 14		551, 958
	Spinocerebellar ataxia	7		292, 897
Japanese spaniel	Gangliosidosis GM_2	15		294, 833
Japanese spitz	Muscular dystrophy	7		988
Japanese retriever	Ceroid lipofuscinosis	15		293
Keeshond	Epilepsy	13	Y	81, 98, 295
Kerry blue terrier	Cerebellar degeneration	8	Y	30
	Degenerative myelopathy	6		611
	Multisystem degeneration	8		296-298
Labrador retriever	Axonopathy	7	Y	579
	Cerebellar hypoplasia	8		136
	Cerebellar degeneration	8	P	299, 678
	Centronuclear myopathy	7	Y	166, 300-306, 989, 999, 1000, 1047
	Congenital 1 tetany	10	S	309
	Epilepsy	13	S	764, 766
	Exercise intolerance-collapse syndrome	7	S	1023, 1024
	Fibrinoid encephalopathy (Alexander disease)	7, 12		551, 886
	Leukoencephalomalacia	7, 12		580
	Lumbosacral stenosis	6		631, 633-637
	Mucopolysaccharidosis (MPS II)	15	S	865
	Muscular dystrophy	7	Y	989
	Myasthenia gravis (acquired)	7		1036
	Narcolepsy/cataplexy	13	Y	216, 218-220, 307, 308
	Retinal degeneration	11	Y	69, 81, 109
	Retinal dysplasia	11	Y	69, 81, 109
	Spongiform (myelin) degeneration	12		310, 311
Lagotto Romagnolo	Cerebellar degeneration	8	S	679
	Epilepsy	13	S	771
Lapland dog	Glycogenosis (type II)	7, 15	Y	312, 313, 802
	Neuronal degeneration	7	Y	81, 314, 315
Lhaso apso	Hydrocephalus	12	P	126, 316, 317
	Lissencephaly	13	S	318, 319
Leonberger	Leukoencephalomyelopathy	6, 7		616
	Polyneuropathy	7		929, 947

CANINE DISEASES—cont'd

Breed	Disease	Chapter	Inherited	References
Lurcher	Hypomyelination	10	S	162, 164, 320
Maltese	Deafness	9	Y	726, 730
	Glycogenosis (type I)	7, 15	S	799
	Hydrocephalus	12	Y	126, 321, 322
	Portosystemic shunt	12, 15		559
	Steroid responsive tremor syndrome	10		551
Miniature pinscher	Mucopolysaccharidosis	15		551, 853
	Retinal degeneration	11	Y	69, 81, 109
Miniature schnauzer	Cerebellar degeneration	8	S	680
	Ceroid lipofuscinosis	15		566, 872
	Myotonia (congenital)	10	Y	757, 761, 762
	Seizures	13	H	763, 778
	Esophageal hypomotility	9	Y	174, 175, 323, 324
	Muscular dystrophy	7		581
Mixed-breed dogs	Cerebellar brainstem malformation	8		72, 654, 655
	Deafness	9	Y	730
	Gangliosidosis GM_2	15		325
	Mucopolysaccharidosis	15	Y	326, 856
Newfoundland	Esophageal hypomotility	9	Y	175, 327
	Myasthenia gravis (acquired)	7		1038
	Myositis (immune mediated)	7		976
New Zealand huntaway dog	Mucopolysaccharidosis (MPS III)	15	S	846-848
	Myopathy/axonopathy	7		903
Norwegian dunkerhound	Deafness	9	Y	745
Norwegian elkhound	Retinal degeneration	11	Y	69, 81, 109
Old English sheepdog	Cerebellar degeneration	8	S	681
	Deafness	9	Y	86, 328
	Myopathy (mitochondrial)	7		551, 1014
Papillon	Deafness	9	Y	730
	Neuroaxonal dystrophy	7, 8		582, 697, 698
Pekingese	Hydrocephalus	12	P	126
Plott hound	Mucopolysaccharidosis (MPS 1)	15	Y	326, 329
Pointer	Deafness	9	Y	724
	Neurogenic muscular atrophy	7	Y	330-332
	Retinal degeneration	11		69, 81, 109
Pomeranian	Globoid cell leukodystrophy	15		333
	Hydrocephalus	12	P	126
Poodle	Agenesis vermis cerebellum	8	S	334
	Cerebellar hypoplasia	8	S	334, 335
	Ceroid lipofuscinosis	15	S	871
	Degenerative myelopathy	7	S	336
	Globoid cell leukodystrophy	15	Y	81, 337
	Glycoproteinosis (Laflora's disease)	13	S	92
	Sphingomyelin lipidosis	15	Y	338
Poodle, miniature or toy	Retinal degeneration	11	Y	69, 81, 109
Poodle, miniature	Cerebellar degeneration	7		551
	Deafness	9	Y	730
	Degenerative myelopathy	6	S	611
	Fibrinoid encephalomyelopathy (Alexander disease)	15		551, 663
	Leukodystrophy	7		890
Poodle, standard	Degenerative myelopathy	6	S	611
	Epilepsy	13		776
	Neonatal encephalopathy	12, 13	Y	583b
	Polymicrogyria and hydrocephalus	12		583
Poodle, toy	Hydrocephalus	12	P	126, 322
	Sphingomyelinosis	8, 15	S	338
Portuguese Podengo	Cerebellar abiotrophy	8		684
Portuguese water dog	Gangliosidosis GM_1	15		339, 819
Pug	Degenerative myelopathy	6	S	611
	Encephalitis	15	Y	584-586
	Esophageal hypomotility			259
	Hemivertebrae	6		123
	Hydrocephalus	12	P	126, 317
Pyrenean mountain dog	Central axonopathy	7		340

Continued

CANINE DISEASES—cont'd				
Breed	**Disease**	**Chapter**	**Inherited**	**References**
	Sensory neuronopathy	7		551
Rat terrier	Muscular dystrophy	7		987
Redbone coonhound	Retinal degeneration	11	Y	69, 81, 109
Rhodesian ridgeback	Cerebellar abiotrophy	8	S	664
	Cervical spondylomyelopathy	7		917
	Deafness	9	Y	730
	Degenerative myelopathy	6	S	615a
	Myotonic myopathy	10		551
Rottweiler	Cervical spondylomyelopathy	7		917
	Deafness	9	Y	725
	Distal sensory neuropathy	7		587
	Laryngeal paralysis (polyneuropathy)	7, 9		952
	Leukoencephalomyelopathy	15	Y	341, 342, 891
	Motor neuron disease	7, 8		346-348
	Myopathy (distal)	7		1005
	Muscular dystrophy	7		551, 983
	Neuroaxonal dystrophy	7	Y	342-345, 907
	Neuronal vaculation	8	S	694
	Retinal dysplasia	11		69, 109
	Spinal dysraphism	6		349
Saint Bernard	Cerebellar hypoplasia	12	Y	653
	Seizures	13	H	763, 778
Saluki	Ceroid lipofuscinosis	15	Y	350
	Retinal degeneration	11	Y	69, 81, 109
	Spongiform degeneration	12		351
Samoyed	Cerebellar degeneration	8	Y	30, 84
	Cerebellar hypoplasia/lissencephaly	8	S	652
	Steroid responsive tremor syndrome	10		551
	Hypomyelination	10		162, 164, 352
	Muscular dystrophy	7		588
	Myasthenia gravis	7		1036
	Retinal degeneration	11	Y	69, 81, 109
	Spongiform degeneration	12	S	353
Schipperke	Galactosialidosis	15		590
	Mucopolysaccharidosis (MPS III)	15	S	849
Scottish terrier	Cerebellar degeneration	8	S	683
	Deafness	9		81, 728
	Leukodystrophy	7		354, 887
	Neuroaxonal dystrophy	7		589
	Sensory ganglioradiculitis	7		551
	Scotty cramp	10	Y	81, 355-362
Sealyham terrier	Deafness	9	Y	728
	Retinal dysplasia	11	Y	69, 81, 109
Shetland sheepdog	Dermatomyositis	7		167, 363, 977
	Leukoencephalomyelopathy	7		893, 894
	Retinal degeneration	11	Y	69, 81, 109
	Chorioretinal dysplasia	11	Y	69, 81, 109
Shiba dog	Gangliosidosis (GM_1)	15	P	821, 822
Shropshire terrier	Deafness	9		87
Siberian husky	Cerebellar hypoplasia	8		364
	Degenerative myelopathy	6		365
	Seizures	13	H	763, 778
	Laryngeal paralysis	9	Y	366
	Sensory neuropathy	7		221
Silky terrier	Agenesis vermis cerebellum	8		93
	Glucocerebrosidosis	15	Y	367, 368
	Spongiform degeneration	12	S	369
Soft-coated Wheaton terrier	Degenerative myelopathy	6	S	611
Spitz	Ceroid lipofuscinosis	15	S	880
	Steroid responsive tremor syndrome	10		551
Springer spaniel	Aggression		S	110, 205
	Congenital myasthenia gravis	7	Y	167, 370
	Fucosidosis	15	Y	371-377
	Glycogenosis	15	Y	551
	Hypomyelination	10	Y	162, 164, 378

CANINE DISEASES—cont'd				
Breed	**Disease**	**Chapter**	**Inherited**	**References**
	Retinal degeneration	11	Y	69, 81, 379
	Retinal dysplasia	11	Y	69, 109
Staffordshire terrier	Cerebellar abiotrophy	8	Y	684
	Myotonic myopathy	10		551, 756
	Deafness	9	Y	730
	Degenerative myelopathy	6	S	615a
Sussex spaniel	Myopathy (mitochondrial)	7	S	551, 1016, 1019
Swedish Lapland dog	Glycogenosis (type 2)	15	S	800-802
	Motor neuron disease	7	Y	695
Terrier cross	Ceroid lipofuscinosis	15		381, 877
Tibetan mastiff	Hypertrophic neuropathy	7	Y	383-386, 940
Tibetan spaniel	Retinal degeneration	11	Y	109
Tibetan terrier	Ceroid lipofuscinosis	15		591, 859, 860
	Retinal degeneration	11	Y	69, 109, 387
Toy breeds	Atlantoaxial luxation	7	S	81, 388-392
	Hydrocephalus	12	P	126
	Occipital dysplasia	8	S	393, 394
Various	Cartilaginous exostoses	6		395-398
Vizsla	Epilepsy	13	S	773
West Highland white terrier	Deafness	9	Y	730
	Globoid cell leukodystrophy	15	Y	81, 142-144, 333, 399, 834, 835
	Myotonic myopathy	10		551, 758
	Steroid responsive tremor syndrome	10		551
Weimaraner	Cerebellar hypoplasia	8		136
	Hypomyelination	10		162, 164, 400-402
	Spinal dysraphism	6	Y	81, 403-408, 648
Whippet	Sensory neuropathy	14		221
Wire fox terrier	Cerebellar hypoplasia	8	S	30
	Degenerative myelopathy	6	S	611
	Esophageal hypomotility		Y	174, 175, 258, 260, 286, 409
	Lissencephaly	13	S	30
	Muscular dystrophy	7		969
	Seizures	13	H	763, 778
Yorkshire terrier	Steroid responsive tremor syndrome	10		551
	Hydrocephalus	12	Y	126
	Necrotizing encephalitis	15		592
	Portosystemic shunt	12		575
	Retinal dysplasia	11		69, 81, 109
Yugoslavian sheepdog	Ceroid lipofuscinosis	15		551

Y, yes; *P*, probable; *S*, suspected, *H*, high incidence of seizures.

CAPRINE DISEASES				
Breed	**Disease**	**Chapter**	**Inherited**	**References**
Goats	Myotonia	10	Y	300, 410, 411
Nubian	Ceroid lipofuscinosis	15	Y	416, 417
	Mannosidosis	15	Y	412-414, 791
	Mucopolysaccharidosis (MPS III)	8, 15	Y	850, 851
Angora	Atlantoaxial luxation	7		415

Y, Yes.

EQUINE DISEASES				
Breed	**Disease**	**Chapter**	**Inherited**	**References**
Appaloosa	Hyperkalemic periodic paralysis	7	S	1031-1035
	Myeloencephalopathy	7, 15		418
	Night blindness	11	S	69
	Retinal degeneration, nyctalopia	11	Y	69
Arabian	Atlanto-occipital malformation	7	Y	419-421
	Cerebellar degeneration	8	Y	30, 422-424, 701
	Cerebellar dysplasia	8		422, 423
	Storage myopathy	7	S	1011, 1013

Continued

EQUINE DISEASES				
Breed	**Disease**	**Chapter**	**Inherited**	**References**
Arabian foals	Epilepsy	13	S	425, 777
Belgian	Storage myopathy	7	S	1012, 1013, 1029
Donkey	Myeloencephalopathy	7, 15		426
Gotland pony	Cerebellar degeneration	8	Y	30, 427
Horses	Atlanto-occipital malformation	7		419, 428, 429
	Cartilaginous exostoses	6		430, 431
	Cervical spondylomyelopathy	7	S	284, 419, 421, 432-436, 923-926
	Deafness	9	Y	737
	Degenerative myeloencephalopathy	7	S	418, 426, 437, 438
	Distal neuropathy	7		949-951
	Myotonia	10	S	439
Icelandic x Peruvian Paso	Ceroid lipofuscinosis	15	S	883, 884
Miniature horses	Narcolepsy	13	Y	593
Morgan	Myeloencephalopathy	7, 15		418
	Neuroaxonal dystrophy	7		440, 441
	Storage myopathy	7	S	1012, 1013, 1029
Oldberg	Cerebellar degeneration	8, 15		51
Paint	Glycogenosis (type IV)	7		1007, 1008
Paso Fino	Cerebellar hypoplasia	8		701
Percheron	Storage myopathy	7		1012, 1013
Przewalski's horse	Myeloencephalopathy	7, 15		418
Quarter horse	Glucogenosis (type IV)	7		1007, 1008
	Hyperkalemic periodic paralysis	7	S	1031-1035
	Storage myopathy	7		1011
Shetland ponies	Narcolepsy/cataplexy	13	S	421
Standardbred	Muscular dystrophy	7	Y	442
	Myeloencephalopathy	7, 15		418
Suffolk draft horses	Narcolepsy/cataplexy	13	S	421
Thoroughbred	Cerebellar dysplasia	8		443, 701
	Cervical vertebral malformation	7	S	419, 421, 435, 444-447
Tennessee walking horse	Storage myopathy	7		1012, 1013, 1027
Thoroughbred (and others)	Exertional rhabdomyolysis	7	S	1028, 1030
	Laryngeal paralysis	9	S	448-460
Various	Peripartum asphyxia syndrome	12		461
Welsh pony	Myeloencephalopathy	7, 15		462
Zebra	Cervical spondylomyelopathy	7		462
	Degenerative myeloencephalopathy	7, 15	S	418, 617

Y, Yes; *S,* suspected.

FELINE DISEASES				
Breed	**Disease**	**Chapter**	**Inherited**	**References**
Abyssinian	Glucocerebrosidosis	15	Y	463, 464
	Myasthenia gravis	7		1039
	Retinal degeneration	11	Y	109
	Retinal dysplasia	11	Y	109
Balinese	Sphingomyelin lipidosis	15		465
Birman	Distal central peripheral axonopathy	7	Y	551, 953
	Spongiform encephalopathy	12		594
Burmese	Congenital vestibular disease	8	S	84, 94, 95
	Encephalocele	12	Y	466, 467
	Gangliosidosis (GM_2)	15	S	831
Cats (white, blue eyes)	Deafness	9	Y	196, 468-475, 733-736, 738, 748-751
Devon rex	Muscular dystrophy	7	Y	574, 997
Domestic	Atlanto-occipital-axial malformation	7		476
	Cartilaginous exostoses	6		475
	Cerebellar degeneration	8		30, 84, 685-687
	Cerebellar hypoplasia	8		475, 477-479
	Ceroid lipofuscinosis	15	S	876, 878
	Degenerative myelopathy	6		480
	Gangliosidosis GM_1	15	Y	4, 44-46, 826
	Gangliosidosis GM_2	15	Y	45, 46, 481, 482, 830
	Globoid cell leukodystrophy	8, 15	Y	4, 483, 838

FELINE DISEASES				
Breed	**Disease**	**Chapter**	**Inherited**	**References**
	Glycogenosis	15	Y	4, 484
	Glycoproteinosis (LaFlora's disease)	15	S	794
	Hyperlipoproteinemia	7	S	964, 965
	Hyperoxaluria-associated polyneuropathy	7	Y	551, 967
	Hypochylomicronemia	7	S	961-963, 966
	Laryngeal paralysis	9		485-487
	Leukodystrophy	15	Y	488, 489
	Lissencephaly	13		490
	Mannosidosis	8, 15	Y	491, 492, 786
	Meningioma	15	S	75, 121, 493-495
	Motor neuron disease	7		932, 933
	Mucolipidosis	15		816, 817
	Mucopolysaccharidosis	15	Y	496, 497, 854, 855, 857
	Muscular dystrophy	7		595-597, 941, 991, 992, 998
	Myasthenia gravis	7		551, 1039
	Myotonia (congenital)	10		759, 760
	Nemaline rod myopathy	7		1003, 1004
	Neuronal ceroid lipofuscinosis	15		598
	Neuroaxonal dystrophy	7	Y	498, 699, 700
	Neuronal degeneration	7	Y	499
	Olivopontocerebellar degeneration	8		30, 696
	Retinal degeneration	11		69
	Sphingomyelin lipidosis	15	Y	500, 501, 841, 844
Egyptian Mau	Spongiform (myelin) degeneration	12	Y	502
Havana brown	Cerebellar degeneration	8	S	690
Himalayan	Esophageal hypomotility			503
	Neuropathy, hyperchylomicronemia	7	Y	962-964
Korat	Gangliosidosis GM_1	15	Y	44-46, 825, 829
	Laryngeal paralysis	9		486
Maine coon	Motor neuron disease	7	S	932
Manx	Myelodysplasia	6	Y	123, 504-507, 650, 651
Norwegian forest cat	Glycogenosis (type IV)	15	Y	508, 810-812
Persian	Cerebellar degeneration	8	S	689
	Laryngeal paralysis	9		486
	Mannosidosis	8, 15	Y	509-511, 784, 786, 788, 789
	Neuropathy, hyperlipoproteinemia	7	Y	965
Siamese	Cerebellar degeneration	8	S	688
	Ceroid lipofuscinosis	15	Y	512
	Congenital vestibular disease	8	S	84, 94, 95
	Esophageal hypomotility		S	175
	Gangliosidosis GM_1	15	Y	44-46, 77
	Hydrocephalus	12	Y	475
	Hypomyelination	10		599
	Mucopolysaccharidosis	15	Y	513-519
	Myasthenia gravis	7		551
	Myotonia congenita	10	Y	759, 760
	Muscular dystrophy	7		941, 998
	Neuroaxonal dystrophy	8		498, 700
	Neuropathy, hyperchylomicronemia	7	Y	966
	Optic pathway anomaly	11	Y	69
	Sphingomyelin lipidosis	15	Y	520, 521, 839, 840, 842, 844
	Strabismus	11		475
Somalis	Myasthenia gravis (acquired)	7		1039
Sphynx	Muscular dystrophy	7		997

Y, Yes; *S*, suspected.

OVINE DISEASES				
Breed	**Disease**	**Chapter**	**Inherited**	**References**
Border Leicester	Cerebellar degeneration	8		522
Charolais	Cerebellar degeneration	8	S	719
Coopworth	Neuroaxonal dystrophy	7	Y	523
Corriedale	Cerebellar degeneration	8	Y	30, 718
	Glycogenosis (type 1)	15	Y	524

Continued

OVINE DISEASES				
Breed	**Disease**	**Chapter**	**Inherited**	**References**
Merino	Agenesis vermis cerebellum	8		93
	Anencephaly	12		525
	Cerebellar degeneration	8		526
	Ceroid leukodystrophy (CLN 6)	15	Y	863, 864
	Muscular dystrophy	7	Y	527-529
	Neuroaxonal dystrophy	7		526
	Thalamic cerebellar neuropathy	8		600
Polled Dorset	Globoid cell leukodystrophy	15	Y	530
Rambouillet	Ceroid lipofuscinosis	15	Y	531, 881, 882
Romney lambs	Motor neuropathy	7	S	937
Sheep	Arthrogryposis	7		532, 533
	Atlantoaxial luxation	7		534
	Cerebellar hypoplasia	8		532
	Glucocerebrosidosis	15	Y	24
	Glucogenosis	15	U	807
	Hydrocephalus	12		532
	Hypomyelination	10		532
	Myelodysplasia	6		532
South Hampshire	Ceroid lipofuscinosis	15	Y	12, 865
Suffolk	Congenital myopathy	7	Y	527, 535
	Gangliosidosis GM_1, GM_2	15	Y	536, 823
	Neuroaxonal dystrophy	7	Y	523, 537
Welsh mountain	Cerebellar degeneration	8	Y	30, 703
Wiltshire	Cerebellar degeneration/abiotrophy	8	S	720
Various	Agenesis vermis cerebellum	8		532
	Cerebellar brainstem malformation	13		72, 532

Y, Yes. *S*, Suspected.

PORCINE DISEASES				
Breed	**Disease**	**Chapter**	**Inherited**	**References**
British saddleback	Hypomyelination	7, 10	Y	538
Landrace	Hypomyelination	7, 10	Y	538-540
	Malignant hyperthermia (PSS)	7	Y	541-545, 1025, 1026
Pietrain	Malignant hyperthermia (PSS)	7	Y	541, 1025, 1026
	Myopathy, hypertrophy	7	Y	546, 1022
Poland China	Malignant hyperthermia (PSS)	7	Y	541, 545, 1025, 1026
Saddleback—large white	Cerebellar degeneration	8		547
Swine	Encephalocele	12		548
	Glucocerebrosidosis	15	S	24
	Hydrocephalus	12		540
	Lissencephaly	13		548
Yorkshire	Cerebellar degeneration	8	Y	30, 701
	Gangliosidosis GM_2	8, 15	Y	44, 46, 549, 832
	Neuronal degeneration	7	S	550

Y, Yes; *S*, suspected.

REFERENCES

1. Barlow R: Morphogenesis of cerebellar lesions in bovine familial convulsions and ataxia, Vet Pathol 18:151–162, 1981.
2. Edmonds L, Crenshaw D, Selby LA: Micrognathia and cerebellar hypoplasia in an Aberdeen angus herd, J Hered 64:62–64, 1973.
3. Barlow RM, Linklater KA, Young GB: Familial convulsions and ataxia in angus calves, Vet Rec 83:60–65, 1968.
4. Jolly RD, Hartley WJ: Storage diseases of domestic animals, Aust Vet J 43:1–8, 1977.
5. Healy PJ, Cole AE: Heterozygotes for mannosidosis in angus and Murray grey cattle, Aust Vet J 52:385–386, 1976.
6. Barlow R: Genetic cerebellar disorders in cattle. In Rose FC, Behan PO, editors: Animal models of neurological disease, Kent, UK, 1980, Pitman Medical.
7. Young S: Hypomyelinogenesis congenital (cerebellar ataxia) in angus shorthorn calves, Cornell Vet 52:84–93, 1962.
8. Braund KG: Degenerative and developmental diseases. In Oliver JE, Hoerlein BF, Mayhew IG, editors: Veterinary neurology, Philadelphia, 1987, WB Saunders.
9. Jennings A, Summer G: Cortical cerebellar disease in an Ayrshire, Vet Rec 63:60, 1951.
10. Howell J, Ritchie H: Cerebellar malformations in two Ayrshire calves, Pathol Vet 3:159–168, 1966.
11. Boyd J, McNeil P: Atlanto-occipital fusion and ataxia in the calf, Vet Rec 120:34–37, 1987.

12. Mayhew I, Jolly R: Ovine ceroid lipofuscinosis. Proceedings of the Fourth ACVIM Forum, Washington, DC, 1986, American College of Veterinary Internal Medicine.
13. O'Sullivan BM, et al: Generalised glycogenosis in Brahman cattle, Aust Vet J 57:227–229, 1981.
14. Strain GM, et al: Narcolepsy in a Brahman bull, J Am Vet Med Assoc 185:538–541, 1984.
15. Aitchison S, et al: Ultrastructural alterations of motor cortex synaptic junctions in Brown Swiss cattle with weaver syndrome, Am J Vet Res 46:1733–1736, 1985.
16. Baird JD, Sarmiento UM, Basrur PK: Bovine progressive degenerative myeloencephalopathy ("weaver syndrome") in Brown Swiss cattle in Canada: a literature review and case report, Can Vet J 29:370–377, 1988.
17. Stuart LD, Leipold HW: Lesions in bovine progressive degenerative myeloencephalopathy ("weaver") of Brown Swiss cattle, Vet Pathol 22:13–23, 1985.
18. Atkeson FW, Ibsen HL, Eldridge E: Inheritance of an epileptic type character in Brown Swiss cattle, J Hered 34:45, 1944.
19. Cho DY, Leipold HW: Cerebellar cortical atrophy in a Charolais calf, Vet Pathol 15:264–266, 1978.
20. Palmer AC, et al: Progressive ataxia of Charolais cattle associated with a myelin disorder, Vet Rec 91:592–594, 1972.
21. Montgomery D, Mayer J: Progressive ataxia of Charolais cattle, Southwest Vet 37:247–250, 1986.
22. Cordy D: Progressive ataxia of Charolais cattle: an oligodendroglial dysplasia, Vet Pathol 23:78–80, 1986.
23. Zickeer SC, et al: Progressive ataxia in a Charolais bull, J Am Vet Med Assoc 192:1590–1592, 1988.
24. Done JT: Developmental disorders on the nervous system in animals, Adv Vet Sci Comp Med 21:69–114, 1977.
25. Leipold HW, et al: Spinal dysraphism, arthrogryposis and cleft palate in newborn Charolais calves, Can Vet J 10:268–273, 1969.
26. McCoy D, et al: Stabilization of atlantoaxial subluxation secondary to atlantooccipital malformation in a Devon calf, Cornell Vet 76:277–286, 1986.
27. Harper PAW, et al: Neurovisceral ceroid-lipofuscinosis in blind Devon cattle, Acta Neuropathol 75:632–636, 1988.
28. Embury DH, Jerrett IV: Mannosidosis in Galloway calves, Vet Pathol 22:548–551, 1985.
29. Palmer AC, Smith GF, Turner S: Cataplexy in a Guernsey bull, Vet Rec 106:421, 1980.
30. de Lahunta A: Comparative cerebellar disease in domestic animals, Compend Contin Educ Pract Vet 8:8–19, 1980.
31. O'Sullivan BM, McPhee CP: Cerebellar hypoplasia of genetic origin in calves, Aust Vet J 51:469–471, 1975.
32. Strain GM, Olcott BM, Turk MA: Diagnosis of primary generalized epilepsy in a cow, J Am Vet Med Assoc 191:833–836, 1987.
33. Greene HJ, Leipold HW, Hibbs CM: Bovine congenital defects: variations of internal hydrocephalus, Cornell Vet 64:596–616, 1974.
34. Leech RW, Haugse CN, Christoferson LA: Congenital hydrocephalus, Am J Pathol 92:567–570, 1978.
35. Axthelm MK, Leipold HW, Phillips RM: Congenital internal hydrocephalus in polled Hereford cattle, Vet Med Small Anim Clin 76:567–570, 1981.
36. Hulland TJ: Cerebellar ataxia in calves, Can J Comp Med 21:72–76, 1957.
37. Rousseaux CG, et al: "Shaker" calf syndrome: a newly recognized inherited neurodegenerative disorder of horned Hereford calves, Vet Pathol 22:104–111, 1985.
38. Rousseaux CG, Klavano GG, Johnson ES, et al: A newly recognized neurodegenerative disorder of horned Hereford calves, Can Vet J 24:296–297, 1983.
39. Watson AG, et al: Occipito-atlanto-axial malformation with atlanto-axial subluxation in an ataxic calf, J Am Vet Med Assoc 187:740–742, 1985.
40. Leipold HW, et al: Congenital defect of the atlanto-occipital joint in a Holstein Friesian calf, Cornell Vet 62:646–672, 1972.
41. Hiraga T, Abe M: Two calves of Arnold-Chiari malformation and their craniums, Jpn J Vet Sci 49:651–656, 1987.
42. White ME, Whitlock RH, de Lahunta A: A cerebellar abiotrophy of calves, Cornell Vet 65:476–491, 1975.
43. Umemura T, et al: Histopathology of congenital and perinatal cerebellar anomalies in twelve calves, Jpn J Vet Sci 49:95–104, 1987.
44. Baker HJ, et al: Animal models of human ganglioside storage diseases, FASEB J 35:1193–1201, 1976.
45. Baker HJ, et al: Feline gangliosidoses as models of human lysosomal storage diseases. In Desnick RJ, Patterson DF, Scarpelli DG, editors: Animal models of inherited metabolic diseases, New York, 1982, Alan R Liss.
46. Baker HJ, et al: The gangliosidoses: comparative features and research applications, Vet Pathol 16:635–649, 1979.
47. Donnelly WJC, Sheahan BJ, Rogers TA: GM_1 gangliosidosis in Friesian calves, J Pathol 111:173–179, 1973.
48. Henninger RW, Sigler RE: Spinal dysraphism in a calf, Compend Contin Educ Pract Vet 5:5488–5491, 1983.
49. Wells G, et al: A novel progressive spongiform encephalopathy in cattle, Vet Rec 121:419–420, 1987.
50. Saunders LZ, et al: Hereditary congenital ataxia in Jersey calves, Cornell Vet 42:559–591, 1952.
51. Mayhew IG: Large animal neurology: a handbook for veterinary clinicians, Philadelphia, 1989, Lea & Febiger.
52. de Lahunta A: Abiotrophy in domestic animals: a review, Can J Vet Res 54:65–76, 1990.
53. Richards R, Edwards J: A progressive spinal myelinopathy in beef cattle, Vet Pathol 23:35–41, 1986.
54. Edwards JR, Richards RB, Carrick MJ: Inherited progressive spinal myelinopathy in Murray Grey cattle, Aust Vet J 65:108–109, 1988.
55. Healy P, Harper P, Dennis J: Diagnosis of neuraxial oedema in calves, Aust Vet J 63:95–96, 1986.
56. Duffell S: Neuraxial oedema of Hereford calves with and without hypomyelinogenesis, Vet Rec 117:95–98, 1986.
57. Donaldson C, Mason R: Hereditary neuraxial oedema in a poll Hereford herd, Aust Vet J 61:188–189, 1984.
58. Healy PJ, Harper PAW, Bowler JK: Prenatal occurrence and mode of inheritance of neuraxial oedema in poll Hereford calves, Res Vet Sci 38:96–98, 1985.
59. Gundlach AL, et al: Deficit of spinal cord glycine/strychnine receptors in inherited myoclonus of poll Hereford calves, Science 241:1807–1810, 1988.
60. Harper P, et al: Maple syrup urine disease in calves: a clinical, pathological and biochemical study, Aust Vet J 66:46–49, 1989.
61. Innes JRM, Saunders LA: Comparative neuropathology, New York, 1962, Academic Press.
62. Abbitt B, et al: ß-Mannosidosis in twelve Salers calves, J Am Vet Med Assoc 198:109–113, 1991.
63. Jolly RD, et al: ß-Mannosidosis in a Salers calf: a new storage disease of cattle, N Z Vet J 38:102–105, 1990.
64. Swan R, Taylor E: Cerebellar hypoplasia in beef shorthorn calves, Aust Vet J 59:95–96, 1982.
65. O'Sullivan B, McPhee C: Cerebellar hypoplasia of genetic origin in calves, Aust Vet J 51:469–471, 1975.

66. Richards RB, et al: Bovine generalized glycogenosis, Neuropathol Appl Neurobiol 3:45–56, 1977.
67. McHowell J, et al: Infantile and late onset form of generalized glycogenosis type II in cattle, J Pathol 134:266–277, 1981.
68. Greene HJ, et al: Internal hydrocephalus and retinal dysplasia in shorthorn cattle, Ir Vet J 32:65–69, 1978.
69. Slatter D: Fundamentals of veterinary ophthalmology, Philadelphia, 1981, WB Saunders.
70. Chrisman CL: Epilepsy and seizures. In Howard JL, editor: Current veterinary therapy: food animal practice, Philadelphia, 1981, WB Saunders.
71. Russell RG, Oteruelo FT: Ultrastructural abnormalities of muscle and neuromuscular junction differentiation in a bovine congenital neuromuscular disease, Acta Neuropathol 62:112–120, 1983.
72. Van den Akker S: Arnold-Chiari malformation in animals, Acta Neuropathol (suppl 1):39–44, 1962.
73. Boyd JS: Unusual case of spina bifida in a Friesian cross calf, Vet Rec 116:203–205, 1985.
74. Wasserman C: Myelodysplasia in a calf, Mod Vet Pract 67:879–883, 1986.
75. Luginbuhl H, Fankhauser R, McGrath JT: Spontaneous neoplasms of the nervous system in animals, Prog Neurol Surg 2:85–164, 1968.
76. Averill DR, Bronson RT: Inherited necrotizing myelopathy of Afghan hounds, J Neuropathol Exp Neurol 36:734–747, 1977.
77. Baker HJ, et al: Neuronal GM1 gangliosidosis in a Siamese cat with ß-galactosidase deficiency, Science 174:838–839, 1971.
78. Cockrell BY, et al: Myelomalacia in Afghan hounds, J Am Vet Med Assoc 162:362–365, 1973.
79. Cummings JF, de Lahunta A: Hereditary myelopathy of Afghan hounds: a myelinolytic disease, Acta Neuropathol 42:173–181, 1978.
80. Cordy DR, Snelbaker HA: Cerebellar hypoplasia and degeneration in a family of Airedale dogs, J Neuropathol Exp Neurol 11:324–328, 1952.
81. Erickson F, Leipold HW, McKinley J: Congenital defects in dogs. Part 2, Canine Pract 14:51–61, 1977.
82. Dow RW: Partial agenesis of the cerebellum in dogs, J Comp Neurol 72:569–586, 1940.
83. Duncan ID, Griffiths I: Neuromuscular diseases. In Kornegay JN, editor: Neurologic disorders, New York, 1986, Churchill Livingstone.
84. de Lahunta A: Veterinary neuroanatomy and clinical neurology, ed 2, Philadelphia, 1983, WB Saunders.
85. Sisk DB, et al: Clinical and pathologic features of ceroid lipofuscinosis in two Australian cattle dogs, J Am Vet Med Assoc 197:361–364, 1990.
86. Hayes HM, et al: Canine congenital deafness: epidemiologic study of 272 cases, J Am Anim Hosp Assoc 17:473, 1981.
87. Igarashi M, et al: Inner ear anomalies in dogs, Ann Otol Rhinol Laryngol 81:249–255, 1972.
88. Shores A: Canine cervical vertebral malformation/malarticulation syndrome, Compend Contin Educ Pract Vet 6:326–333, 1984.
89. Wright F, Rest JR, Palmer AC: Ataxia of the Great Dane caused by stenosis of the cervical vertebral canal: comparison with similar conditions in the basset hound, Doberman pinscher, ridgeback and the thoroughbred horse, Vet Rec 92:1–6, 1973.
90. Denny H, Gibbs C, Gaskell C: Cervical spondylopathy in the dog: a review of thirty-five cases, J Small Anim Pract 18:117–132, 1977.
91. Luttgen PJ, Braund KG, Storts RW: Globoid cell leukodystrophy in a basset hound, J Small Anim Pract 24:153–160, 1983.
92. Cusick PK, Cameron AM, Parker AJ: Canine neuronal glycoproteinosis: Lafora's disease in the dog, J Am Anim Hosp Assoc 12:518–521, 1976.
93. Pass DA, Howell JM, Thompson RR: Cerebellar malformation in two dogs and a sheep, Vet Pathol 18:405–407, 1981.
94. Lane SB: Vestibular disease in companion animals, Pedigree Forum 6:11–16, 1987.
95. Chrisman CL: Disorders of the vestibular system, Compend Contin Educ Pract Vet 1:744–757, 1979.
96. Hegreberg GA, Padget GA: Inherited progressive epilepsy of the dog with comparisons to Lafora's disease of man, FASEB J 35:1202–1205, 1976.
97. Edmonds HL, et al: Spontaneous convulsions in beagle dogs, FASEB J 39:2424–2428, 1979.
98. Holliday TA: In Frey HH, Janz D, editors: Handbook of experimental pharmacology, Epilepsy in animals, vol. 74, Berlin, 1985, Springer-Verlag.
99. Biefelt SW, Redman HC, Broadhurst JJ: Sire and sex-related differences in rates of epileptiform seizures in a purebred beagle dog colony, Am J Vet Res 32:2039–2048, 1971.
100. Montgomery DL, Lee AC: Brain damage in the epileptic beagle dog, Vet Pathol 20:160–169, 1983.
101. Edmonds HL Jr, et al: Spontaneous convulsions in beagle dogs, FASEB J 38:2424–2428, 1979.
102. Redman HC, Wilson GL, Hogan JE: Effect of chlorpromazine combined with intermittent light stimulation on the electroencephalogram and clinical response of the beagle dog, Am J Vet Res 34:929–936, 1973.
103. Redman HC, Weir JE: Detection of naturally occurring neurologic disorders of beagle dogs by electroencephalography, Am J Vet Res 30:2075–2082, 1969.
104. Redman HC, Hogan JE, Wilson GL: Effect of intermittent light stimulation singly and combined with pentylenetetrazol on the electroencephalogram and clinical response of the beagle dog, Am J Vet Res 33:677–685, 1972.
105. Wiederholt WC: Electrophysiologic analysis of epileptic beagles, Neurology 24:149–155, 1974.
106. Read DH, et al: Neuronal-visceral GM_1 gangliosidosis in a dog with ß-galactosidase deficiency, Science 194:442–445, 1976.
107. Johnson GR, Oliver JE, Selcer R: Globoid cell leukodystrophy in a beagle, J Am Vet Med Assoc 167:380–384, 1975.
108. Tomchick T: Familial Lafora's disease in the beagle dog, FASEB J 32:8–21, 1973.
109. Barnett KC: Inherited eye disease in the dog and cat, J Small Anim Pract 29:462–475, 1988.
110. Voith VL: Diagnosis and treatment of aggressive behavior problems in dogs. In Proceedings of the 47th Annual Meeting of the American Animal Hospital Association, 1980.
111. Palmer A, et al: Recognition of "trembler," a hypomyelination condition in the Bernese mountain dog, Vet Rec 120:609–612, 1987.
112. Rosin A, Moore P, Dubielzig R: Malignant histiocytosis in Bernese mountain dogs, J Am Vet Med Assoc 188:1041–1046, 1986.
113. Cho D, Leipold H, Rudolph R: Neuronal ceroidosis (ceroid-lipofuscinosis) in a blue heeler dog, Acta Neuropathol 69:161–164, 1986.
114. Wood PA, et al: Animal model: ceroidosis (ceroid-lipofuscinosis) in Australian cattle dogs, Am J Med Genet 26:891–898, 1987.

115. Boysen BG, Tryphonas L, Harries NW: Globoid cell leukodystrophy in the bluetick hound dog. 1. Clinical manifestations, Can Vet J 15:303–308, 1974.
116. Gill JM, Hewland ML: Cerebellar degeneration in the border collie, N Z Vet J 8:170, 1980.
117. Taylor RM, Farrow BRH: Ceroid lipofuscinosis in border collie dogs, Acta Neuropathol 75:627–631, 1988.
118. Studdert VP, Mitten RW: Clinical features of ceroid lipofuscinosis in border collies, Aust Vet J 68:137–140, 1991.
119. Wheeler SJ: Sensory neuropathy in a border collie puppy, J Small Anim Pract 28:281–289, 1987.
120. Jaggy A, et al: Hereditary cervical spondylopathy (wobbler syndrome) in the borzoi dog, J Am Anim Hosp Assoc 24:453–460, 1988.
121. Hayes KC, Schiefer B: Primary tumors in the CNS of carnivores, Pathol Vet 6:94–116, 1969.
122. Hayes HM, Priester WA, Pendergrass TW: Occurrence of nervous-tissue tumors in cattle, horses, cats and dogs, Int J Cancer 15:39–47, 1975.
123. Bailey CS: An embryological approach to the clinical significance of congenital vertebral and spinal cord abnormalities, J Am Anim Hosp Assoc 11:426–434, 1975.
124. Morgan JP: Congenital anomalies of the vertebral column of the dog: a study of the incidence and significance based on a radiographic and morphometric study, J Am Vet Radiol Soc 9:21–29, 1968.
125. de Lahunta A, Cummings JF: The clinical and electroencephalographic features of hydrocephalus in three dogs, J Am Vet Med Assoc 146:954–964, 1965.
126. Selby L, Hayes H, Becker S: Epizootiologic features of canine hydrocephalus, Am J Vet Res 40:411–413, 1979.
127. Venker-van Haagen AJ, Bouw J: Hartman W: Hereditary transmission of laryngeal paralysis in young Bouviers, J Am Anim Hosp Assoc 17:75–76, 1981.
128. Venker-van Haagen AJ, Hartman W: Goedogebuure SA: Spontaneous laryngeal paralysis in young Bouviers, J Am Anim Hosp Assoc 14:714–720, 1978.
129. Griffiths I: Progressive axonopathy of boxer dogs. In Proceedings of the Fifth Annual Veterinary Medical Forum, San Diego, 1987, American College of Veterinary Internal Medicine.
130. Griffiths IR, Duncan ID, Barker J: A progressive axonopathy of boxer dogs affecting the central and peripheral nervous system, J Small Anim Pract 21:29–43, 1980.
131. LeCouteur RA, Kornegay JN, Higgins RJ: Late onset progressive cerebellar degeneration of Brittany spaniel dogs. In Proceedings of the Sixth Annual Veterinary Medical Forum, Washington, DC, 1988, American College of Veterinary Internal Medicine.
132. Cork LC, et al: Hereditary canine spinal muscular atrophy, J Neuropathol Exp Neurol 38:209–221, 1979.
133. Lorenz MD, et al: Hereditary muscular atrophy in Brittany spaniels: clinical manifestations, J Am Vet Med Assoc 175:833–839, 1979.
134. Carmichael S, Griffiths IR, Harvey MJA: Familial cerebellar ataxia with hydrocephalus in bull mastiffs, Vet Rec 112:354–358, 1983.
135. Raffe M, Knecht C: Cervical vertebral malformation in bull mastiffs, J Am Anim Hosp Assoc 14:593–594, 1978.
136. Kornegay J: Cerebellar vermian hypoplasia in dogs, Vet Pathol 23:374–379, 1986.
137. Hudson W, Ruben R: Hereditary deafness in the Dalmatian dog, Arch Otolaryngol Head Neck Surg 75:213–219, 1962.
138. Anderson H, Henricson B, Lundquist P, et al: Genetic hearing impairment in the Dalmatian dog, Acta Otolaryngol Suppl 232:1–34, 1968.
139. Brown S, et al: Naloxone-responsive compulsive tail chasing in a dog, J Am Vet Med Assoc 190:884–886, 1987.
140. Kurtz HJ, Fletcher TF: The peripheral neuropathy of canine globoid-cell leukodystrophy (Krabbe type), Acta Neuropathol 16:226–232, 1970.
141. Howell JM: Globoid cell leukodystrophy in two dogs, J Small Anim Pract 12:633–642, 1971.
142. Fletcher TF, Kurtz HJ, Low DG: Globoid cell leukodystrophy (Krabbe type) in the dog, J Am Vet Med Assoc 149:165–172, 1966.
143. McGrath JT, et al: A morphologic and biochemical study of canine globoid cell leukodystrophy, J Neuropathol Exp Neurol 28:171, 1969.
144. Suzuki Y, et al: Studies in globoid leukodystrophy: enzymatic and lipid findings in the canine form, Exp Neurol 29:65–75, 1970.
145. Palmer AC, Blakemore WF: Progressive neuronopathy in the cairn terrier, Vet Rec 123:39, 1988.
146. Cummings JF, de Lahunta A, Moore JJ: Multisystemic chromatolytic neuronal degeneration in a cairn terrier pup, Cornell Vet 78:301–314, 1988.
147. Wright J, et al: Muscle hypertonicity in the cavalier King Charles spaniel: myopathic features, Vet Rec 118:511–512, 1986.
148. Jones BR, Johnstone AC: An unusual myopathy in a dog, N Z Vet J 30:119–121, 1982.
149. Herrtage ME, Palmer AC: Episodic falling in the cavalier King Charles spaniel, Vet Rec 112:458–459, 1983.
150. Few AB: The diagnosis and surgical treatment of canine hydrocephalus, J Am Vet Med Assoc 149:286–293, 1966.
151. Blakemore W, Palmer A: Nervous disease in the Chihuahua characterised by axonal swellings, Vet Rec 117:498–499, 1985.
152. Hansen HJ: A pathologic-anatomical study on disk degeneration in the dog, Acta Orthop Scand Suppl 11, 1952.
153. Ghosh P, et al: A comparative chemical and histochemical study of the chondrodystrophoid and nonchondrodystrophoid canine intervertebral disc, Vet Pathol 13:414–427, 1976.
154. Priester W: Canine intervertebral disc disease: occurrence by age, breed, and sex among 8,117 cases, Theriogenology 6:293–303, 1976.
155. Brown N, Helphrey M, Prata R: Thoracolumbar disk disease in the dog: a retrospective analysis of 187 cases, J Am Anim Hosp Assoc 13:665–672, 1977.
156. Hoerlein B: Comparative disk disease: man and dog, J Am Anim Hosp Assoc 15:535–545, 1979.
157. Hoerlein B: Intervertebral disc protrusions in the dog. I. Incidence and pathological lesions, Am J Vet Res 51:260–283, 1953.
158. Braund KG: Intervertebral disk disease. In Kornegay JN, editor: Neurologic disorders, New York, 1986, Churchill Livingstone.
159. Knecht CD, et al: Cerebellar hypoplasia in chow chows, J Am Anim Hosp Assoc 15:51, 1979.
160. Knecht C, et al: Cerebellar hypoplasia in chow chows, J Am Anim Hosp Assoc 15:51–53, 1979.
161. Vandevelde M, et al: Dysmyelination of the central nervous system in the chow chow dog, Acta Neuropathol 42:211–215, 1978.
162. Duncan I: Congenital tremor and abnormalities of myelination. In Proceedings of the Fifth Annual Veterinary Medical Forum, San Diego, 1987, American College of Veterinary Internal Medicine.

163. Vandevelde M, et al: Dysmyelination in chow chow dogs: further studies in older dogs, Acta Neuropathol 55:81–87, 1981.
164. Duncan I: Abnormalities of myelination of the central nervous system associated with congenital tremor, J Vet Intern Med 1:10–23, 1987.
165. Shores A, et al: Myotonia congenita in a chow chow pup, J Am Vet Med Assoc 188:532–533, 1986.
166. Braund KG: Identifying degenerative and developmental myopathies, Vet Med 81:713–718, 1986.
167. Shelton G, Cardinet H: Pathophysiologic basis of canine muscle disorders, J Vet Intern Med 1:36–44, 1987.
168. Farrow BRH: Canine myotonia. In the Proceedings of the 6th ACVIM Forum. Washington, DC, 1988.
169. Nafe LA, Shires P: Myotonia in the dog. In the Proceedings of the 2nd ACVIM Forum. Washington DC, 1984.
170. Jones BR, et al: Myotonia in related chow chow dogs, N Z Vet J 25:217–220, 1977.
171. Farrow BRH, Malik R: Hereditary myotonia in the chow chow, J Small Anim Pract 22:451–465, 1981.
172. Mugford RA: Aggressive behavior in the English cocker spaniel, Vet Ann 24:310–314, 1984.
173. Nimmo Wilkie JS, Hudson EB: Neuronal and generalized ceroid-lipofuscinosis in a cocker spaniel, Vet Pathol 19:623–628, 1982.
174. Clifford DH, Malek R: Diseases of the canine esophagus due to prenatal influence, Am J Dig Dis 14:578–602, 1969.
175. Clifford DH: Esophageal achalasia, Comp Pathol Bull 10:2–3, 1978.
176. Kern TJ, Erb HN: Facial neuropathy in dogs and cats: 95 cases (1975-1985), J Am Vet Med Assoc 191:1604–1609, 1987.
177. Braund KG, et al: Idiopathic facial paralysis in the dog, Vet Rec 105:297–299, 1979.
178. Jaggy A, Vandevelde M: Multisystem neuronal degeneration in cocker spaniels, J Vet Intern Med 2:117–120, 1988.
179. Hartley WJ, et al: Inherited cerebellar degeneration in the rough coated collie, Aust Vet Pract 8:79–85, 1978.
180. Clark RG, et al: Suspected neuroaxonal dystrophy in collie sheep dogs, N Z Vet J 30:102–103, 1982.
181. Lurie M: The membranous labyrinth in the congenitally deaf collie and Dalmatian dog, Laryngoscope 58:279–287, 1948.
182. Hargis AM, Haupt KH, Hegreberg GA, et al: Familial canine dermatomyositis, Am J Pathol 116:234–244, 1984.
183. Haupt KH, et al: Familial canine dermatomyositis: clinical, electrodiagnostic, and genetic studies, Am J Vet Res 46:1861–1869, 1985.
184. Hargis A, et al: Postmortem findings in four litters of dogs with familial canine dermatomyositis, Am J Pathol 123:480–496, 1986.
185. Hargis A, et al: Prospective study of familial canine dermatomyositis, Am J Pathol 123:465–479, 1986.
186. Hargis AM, et al: Dermatomyositis: familial canine dermatomyositis, Am J Pathol 120:323–325, 1985.
187. Kunkle GA, et al: Dermatomyositis in collie dogs, Compend Contin Educ Pract Vet 7:185–192, 1985.
188. Wilson JW, et al: Spina bifida in the dog, Vet Pathol 16:165–179, 1979.
189. de Lahunta A, Shively GN: Neurofibrillary accumulation in a puppy, Cornell Vet 65:240–247, 1975.
190. Cummings JF, de Lahunta A: An adult case of canine neuronal ceroid-lipofuscinosis, Acta Neuropathol 39:43–51, 1977.
191. Holliday TA, Cunningham JG, Gutnick MJ: Comparative clinical and electroencephalographic studies of canine epilepsy, Epilepsia 11:281–292, 1971.
192. Vandevelde M, Fatzer R: Neuronal ceroid-lipofuscinosis in older dachshunds, Vet Pathol 17:686–692, 1980.
193. Duncan ID, Griffiths IR, Munz M: The pathology of a sensory neuropathy affecting long haired dachshund dogs, Acta Neruopathol 58:141–151, 1982.
194. Braund KG: Identifying degenerative peripheral neuropathies in pets, Vet Med 88:352–380, 1987.
195. Johnsson L, et al: Vascular anatomy and pathology of the cochlea in Dalmatian dogs. In Darin de Lorenzo AJ, editor: Vascular disorders and hearing defects, University Park, Md, 1973, University Park Press.
196. Suga F, Hattler K: Physiological and histopathological correlates of hereditary deafness in animals, Laryngoscope 80:80–104, 1970.
197. Marshall A: Use of brain stem auditory-evoked response to evaluate deafness in a group of Dalmatian dogs, J Am Vet Med Assoc 188:718–722, 1986.
198. Ferrara ML, Halnan CRE: Congenital brain defects in the deaf Dalmatian, Vet Rec 112:344–346, 1983.
199. Mair IWS: Hereditary deafness in the Dalmatian dog, Arch Otol 212:1–14, 1976.
200. Branis M, Burda H: Inner ear structure in the deaf and normally hearing Dalmatian dog, J Comp Pathol 95:295–299, 1985.
201. Woods CB: Hyperkinetic episodes in two Dalmatians, Am Anim Hosp Assoc 13:255–257, 1977.
202. Greene CE, Vandevelde M, Hoff EJ: Congenital cerebrospinal hypomyelinogenesis in a pup, J Am Vet Med Assoc 171:534–536, 1977.
203. Bjerkas I: Hereditary "cavitating" leukodystrophy in Dalmatian dogs, Acta Neuropathol 40:163–169, 1977.
204. Neufeld JL, Little PB: Spinal dysraphism in a Dalmatian dog, Can Vet J 15:335–336, 1974.
205. Houpt KA: Aggression in dogs, Compend Contin Educ Pract Vet 1:123–128, 1979.
206. Seim H: Ventral decompression and stabilization for the treatment of caudal cervical spondylomyelopathy in the dog. In Proceedings of the Fifth Annual Veterinary Medical Forum, San Diego, 1987, American College of Veterinary Internal Medicine.
207. Lyman R: Continuous dorsal laminectomy for treatment of Doberman pinschers with caudal cervical vertebral instability and malformation. In the Proceedings of the 5th ACVIM Forum. San Diego, 1987.
208. Seim H, Withrow S: Pathophysiology and diagnosis of caudal cervical spondylo-myelopathy with emphasis on the Doberman pinscher, J Am Anim Hosp Assoc 18:241–251, 1982.
209. Read R, Robins G, Carlisle C: Caudal cervical spondylo-myelopathy (wobbler syndrome) in the dog: a review of thirty cases, J Small Anim Pract 24:605–621, 1983.
210. Trotter E, et al: Caudal cervical vertebral malformation-malarticulation in Great Danes and Doberman pinschers, J Am Vet Med Assoc 168:917–930, 1976.
211. Mason T: Cervical vertebral instability (wobbler syndrome) in the dog, Vet Rec 104:142–145, 1979.
212. Raffe M, Knecht C: Cervical vertebral malformation: a review of 36 cases, J Am Anim Hosp Assoc 16:881–883, 1980.
213. Wilkes M, Palmer A: Congenital deafness in Dobermans, Vet Rec 118:218, 1986.
214. Chrisman CL: Distal polyneuropathy of Doberman pinschers. In the Proceedings of the 3rd ACVIM Forum. San Diego, 1985.

215. Leyland A: Ataxia in a Doberman pinscher, Vet Rec 116:414–415, 1985.
216. Baker TL, et al: Diagnosis and treatment of narcolepsy in animals. In Kirk RW, editor: Current veterinary therapy VIII: small animal practice, Philadelphia, 1983, WB Saunders.
217. Bowersox S, et al: Brain dopamine receptor levels elevated in canine narcolepsy, Brain Res 402:44–48, 1987.
218. Kaitin KI, Kilduff TS, Dement WC: Evidence for excessive sleepiness in canine narcoleptics, Electroencephalogr Clin Neurophysiol 65:447–454, 1986.
219. Foutz AS, Mitler MM, Dement WC: Narcolepsy, Vet Clin North Am 10:65–80, 1980.
220. Bakr TL, et al: Canine model of narcolepsy: genetic and developmental determinants, Exp Neurol 75:729–742, 1982.
221. Wouda W, et al: Sensory neuronopathy in dogs: a study of four cases, J Comp Pathol 93:437–450, 1983.
222. Patnaik A, Kay W, Hurvitz A: Intracranial meningioma: a comparative pathologic study of 28 dogs, Vet Pathol 23:369–373, 1986.
223. Parker AJ, et al: Spina bifida with protrusion of spinal cord tissue in a dog, J Am Vet Med Assoc 163:158–160, 1973.
224. Parker AJ, Byerly CS: Meningomyelocele in a dog, Vet Pathol 10:266–273, 1973.
225. Kornegay JN: Congenital and degenerative diseases of the central nervous system. In Kornegay JN, editor: Neurologic disorders, New York, 1986, Churchill Livingstone.
226. Knecht C, Blevins W, Raffe M: Stenosis of the thoracic spinal canal in English bulldogs, J Am Anim Hosp Assoc 15:182–183, 1979.
227. Klein E, et al: Adenosine receptor alterations in nervous pointer dogs: a preliminary report, Clin Neuropharmacol 10:462–469, 1987.
228. Murphree OD, Dykman RA: Litter patterns in the offspring of nervous and stable dogs. I. Behavioral tests, J Nerv Ment Dis 141:321–332, 1965.
229. Dykman RA, Murphree OD, Ackerman PT: Litter patterns in the offspring of nervous and stable dogs. II. Autonomic and motor conditioning, J Nerv Ment Dis 141:419–431, 1966.
230. Cummings JF, et al: Reduced substance P-like immunoreactivity in hereditary sensory neuropathy of pointer dogs, Acta Neuropathol 63:33–40, 1984.
231. Cummings JF, et al: Animal model of human disease: hereditary sensory neuropathy: nociceptive loss and acral mutilation in pointer dogs: canine hereditary sensory neuropathy, Am J Pathol 112:136–138, 1983.
232. Cummings JF, de Lahunta A, Winn SS: Acral mutilation and nociceptive loss in English pointer dogs, Acta Neuropathol 53:119–127, 1981.
233. Koppang N: Canine ceroid-lipofuscinosis in English setters, J Small Anim Pract 10:639–644, 1970.
234. Watson B, Watson G: Electroretinograms in English setters with neuronal ceroid lipofuscinosis, Invest Ophthalmol Vis Sci 19:87–90, 1980.
235. Armstrong D, Koppang N, Jolly R: Ceroid-lipofuscinosis, Comp Pathol Bull 12:2–4, 1980.
236. Armstrong D, Koppang N, Nilsson S: Canine hereditary ceroid lipofuscinosis, Eur Neurol 21:147–156, 1982.
237. Jasty V, et al: An unusual case of generalized ceroid-lipofuscinosis in a cynomolgus monkey, Vet Pathol 21:46–50, 1984.
238. Sims MH, Shull-Selcer E: Electrodiagnostic evaluation of deafness in two English setter littermates, J Am Vet Med Assoc 187:398–404, 1985.
239. Alroy J, et al: Neurovisceral and skeletal GM1 gangliosidosis in dogs with ß-galactosidase deficiency, Science 229:470–472, 1985.
240. Giger U, Argov Z: Metabolic myopathy in phosphofructokinase deficient English springer spaniels. In the Proceedings of the 5th ACVIM Forum. San Diego, 1987.
241. Giger U, Roudebush P: Inherited phosphofructokinase deficiency in English springer spaniels causes hemolytic disorder with hemolytic crises. In the Proceedings of the 5th ACVIM Forum. San Diego, 1987.
242. Holland CT, et al: Dyserythropoiesis, polymyopathy, and cardiac disease in three related English springer spaniels, J Vet Intern Med 5:151–159, 1991.
243. Tontitila P, Lindberg LA: ETT Fall av cerebellar ataxi hos finsk stovare, Svoman Elainlaakarilehti 77:135, 1971.
244. Adams EW: Hereditary deafness in a family of foxhounds, J Am Vet Med Assoc 128:302–303, 1956.
245. Jenkins WL, Van Dyk E, McDonald CB: Myasthenia gravis in a fox terrier litter, J S Afr Vet Assoc 47:59–62, 1976.
246. Miller LM, et al: Congenital myasthenia gravis in 13 smooth fox terriers, J Am Vet Med Assoc 182:694–697, 1983.
247. Lee M: Congenital vestibular disease in a German shepherd dog, Vet Rec 113:571, 1983.
248. Braund KG, Vandevelde M: German shepherd dog myelopathy: a morphologic and morphometric study, Am J Vet Res 39:1309–1315, 1978.
249. Williams DA, Sharp NJH, Batt RM: Enteropathy associated with degenerative myelopathy in German shepherd dogs. In the Proceedings of the 1st ACVIM Forum. New Orleans, 1983.
250. Waxman FJ, et al: Progressive myelopathy in older German shepherd dogs. I. Depressed response to thymus-dependent mitogens, J Immunol 124:1209–1215, 1980.
251. Waxman FJ, Clemmons RM, Hinrichs DJ: Progressive myelopathy in older German shepherd dogs. II. Presence of circulating suppressor cells, J Immunol 124:1216–1222, 1980.
252. Averill DR: Degenerative myelopathy in the aging German shepherd dog, J Am Vet Med Assoc 162:1045–1051, 1973.
253. Griffiths IR, Duncan ID: Chronic degenerative radiculomyelopathy in the dog, J Small Anim Pract 16:461–471, 1975.
254. Braund KG: Hip dysplasia and degenerative myelopathy: making the distinction in dogs, Vet Med 82:82–89, 1987.
255. Clemmons RM: Degenerative myelopathy. In Kirk RW, editor: Current veterinary therapy X: small animal practice, Philadelphia, 1989, WB Saunders.
256. Williams DA, Prymak C, Baughan J: Tocopherol (vitamin E) status in canine degenerative myelopathy. In the Proceedings of the 3rd ACVIM Forum. San Diego, 1985.
257. Amanai H: Leukomyelodegeneration in two aged German shepherd littermates: patho-morphological observations, Jpn J Vet Res 35:121, 1987.
258. Clifford DH, Pirsch JG: Myenteric ganglial cells in dogs with and without hereditary achalasia of the esophagus, Am J Vet Res 32:615–619, 1971.
259. Boudrieau RJ, Rogers WA: Megaesophagus in the dog: a review of 50 cases, J Am Anim Hosp Assoc 21:33–40, 1985.

260. Clifford DH, Gyorkey F: Myenteric ganglial cells in dogs with and without achalasia of the esophagus, J Am Vet Med Assoc 150:205–211, 1967.
261. Duncan ID, Griffiths IR: Canine giant axonal neuropathy, Vet Rec 101:438–441, 1977.
262. Duncan ID, Griffiths IR: Peripheral nervous system in a case of canine giant axonal neuropathy, Neuropathol Appl Neurobiol 5:25–39, 1979.
263. Duncan ID, Griffiths IR: Canine giant axonal neuropathy: some aspects of its clinical, pathological and comparative features, J Small Anim Pract 22:491–501, 1981.
264. Griffiths IR, et al: Further studies of the central nervous system in canine giant axonal neuropathy, Neuropathol Appl Neurobiol 6:421–432, 1980.
265. Julien JP, et al: Giant axonal neuropathy: neurofilaments isolated from diseased dogs have a normal polypeptide composition, Exp Neurol 72:619–627, 1981.
266. Jaggy A, Lang J, Schawalder P: Cauda equina syndrom beim Hund, Schweiz Arch Tierheilkd 129:171–192, 1987.
267. Oliver J, Selcer R, Simpson S: Cauda equina compression from lumbosacral malarticulation and malformation in the dog, J Am Vet Med Assoc 173:207–214, 1978.
268. Lenehan T: Canine cauda equina syndrome, Compend Contin Educ Pract Vet 5:941–951, 1983.
269. Clayton HM, Boyd JS: Spina bifida in a German shepherd puppy, Vet Rec 112:13–15, 1983.
270. Falco MJ, Barker J, Wallace ME: The genetics of epilepsy in the British Alsatian, J Small Anim Pract 15:685–692, 1974.
271. Karbe E: Animal model of human disease: GM2 gangliosidosis (amaurotic idiocies) types I, II, and III. Animal model: canine GM2 gangliosidosis, Am J Pathol 71:151–154, 1973.
272. Kramer JW, et al: Characterization of heritable thoracic hemivertebra of the German shorthaired pointer, J Am Vet Med Assoc 181:814–815, 1982.
273. Kornegay JN: Golden retriever myopathy. In the Proceedings of the 2nd ACVIM Forum. Washington, DC, 1984.
274. Kornegay JN: Golden retriever myopathy. In Kirk RW, editor: Current veterinary therapy IX: small animal practice, Philadelphia, 1986, WB Saunders.
275. Kornegay JN: Golden retriever muscular dystrophy. In the Proceedings of the 6th ACVIM Forum. Washington, DC, 1988.
276. Valentine B, et al: Progressive muscular dystrophy in a golden retriever dog: light microscope and ultrastructural features at 4 and 8 months, Acta Neuropathol 71:301–310, 1986.
277. Steiss JE, et al: Sensory neuropathy in a dog, J Am Vet Med Assoc 190:205–208, 1987.
278. Cork LC, Troncoso JC, Price DL: Canine inherited ataxia, Ann Neurol 9:492–499, 1981.
279. de Lahunta A, et al: Hereditary cerebellar cortical abiotrophy in the Gordon setter, J Am Vet Med Assoc 177:538–541, 1980.
280. Steinberg S, et al: Clinical features of inherited cerebellar degeneration in Gordon setters, J Am Vet Med Assoc 179:886–890, 1981.
281. Troncoso JC, Cork LC, Price DL: Canine inherited ataxia: ultrastructural observations, J Neuropathol Exp Neurol 44:165–175, 1985.
282. Hedhammer A, et al: Overnutrition and skeletal disease: an experimental study in growing Great Dane dogs, Cornell Vet 64(suppl 5):1–60, 1974.
283. Olsson S, Stavenhorn M, Hoppe F: Dynamic compression of the cervical spinal cord: a myelographic and pathologic investigation in Great Dane dogs, Acta Vet Scand 23:65–78, 1982.
284. Wright F, Rest J, Palmer A: Ataxia of the Great Dane caused by stenosis of the cervical vertebral canal: comparison with similar conditions in the basset hound, Doberman pinscher, ridgeback and the thoroughbred horse, Vet Rec 92:1–6, 1973.
285. Strombeck DR, Troya L: Evaluation of lower motor neuron function in two dogs with megaesophagus, J Am Vet Med Assoc 169:411–414, 1976.
286. Strombeck DR: Pathophysiology of esophageal motility disorders in the dog and cat, Vet Clin North Am 8:229–244, 1978.
287. Stockard C: An hereditary lethal factor for localized motor and preganglionic neurons, Am J Anat 59:1–53, 1936.
288. Cunningham JG, Farnbach GC: Inheritance and idiopathic canine epilepsy, J Am Anim Hosp Assoc 24:421–424, 1988.
289. Wentink GH, et al: Myopathy with a possible recessive X-linked inheritance in a litter of Irish terriers, Vet Pathol 9:328–349, 1972.
289a. Junker K, van den Ingh TSGAM, Bossard MM, et al: Fibrocartilaginous embolism of the spinal cord (FCE) in juvenile Irish Wolfhounds. Vet Q 22:154–156, 2001.
290. Palmer AC, Goodyear JV: Congenital myasthenia in the Jack Russell terrier, Vet Rec 103:433–434, 1978.
291. Wilkes MK, et al: Ultrastructure of motor endplates in canine congenital myasthenia gravis, J Comp Pathol 97:247–256, 1987.
292. Hartley WJ, Palmer AC: Ataxia in Jack Russell terriers, Acta Neuropathol 26:71–74, 1973.
293. Umemura T, et al: Generalized lipofuscinosis in a dog, Jpn J Vet Sci 47:673–677, 1985.
294. Cummings JF, et al: GM2 gangliosidosis in a Japanese spaniel, Acta Neuropathol 67:247–253, 1985.
295. Wallace ME: Keeshonds: a genetic study of epilepsy and EEG readings, J Small Anim Pract 16:1–10, 1975.
296. de Lahunta A, Averill DR: Hereditary cerebellar cortical and extrapyramidal nuclear abiotrophy in Kerry blue terriers, J Am Vet Med Assoc 168:1119–1124, 1976.
297. Montgomery D, Storts R: Hereditary striatonigral and cerebello-olivary degeneration of the Kerry blue terrier, Vet Pathol 20:143–159, 1983.
298. Montgomery D, Storts R: Hereditary striatonigral and cerebello-olivary degeneration of the Kerry blue terrier II. Ultrastructural lesions in the caudate nucleus and cerebellar cortex, J Neuropathol Exp Neurol 43:263–275, 1984.
299. Perille AL, et al: Postnatal cerebellar cortical degeneration in Labrador retriever puppies, Can Vet J 32:619–621, 1991.
300. Atkinson JB, LeQuire VS: Myotonia congenita, Comp Pathol Bull 17:3–4, 1985.
301. McKerrell RE, Braund KG: Hereditary myopathy of Labrador retrivers. In Kirk RW, editor: Current veterinary therapy X. Small animal practice. Philadelphia, 1989, WB Saunders, pp 820–822.
302. Moore M, et al: Electromyographic evaluation of adult Labrador retrievers with type II muscle fiber deficiency, Am J Vet Res 48:1332–1336, 1987.
303. Braund KG: Labrador retriever myopathy. In the Proceedings of the 6th ACVIM Forum. Washington, DC, 1988.

304. McKerrell R, Braund K: Hereditary myopathy in Labrador retrievers: clinical variations, J Small Anim Pract 28:479–489, 1987.
305. McKerrell R, Braund K: Hereditary myopathy in Labrador retrievers: a morphologic study, Vet Pathol 23:411–417, 1986.
306. Amann JF, Laughlin MH, Korthuis RJ: Muscle hemodynamics in hereditary myopathy of Labrador retrievers, Am J Vet Res 49:1127–1130, 1988.
307. Shores A, Redding R: Narcoleptic hypersomnia syndrome responsive to protriptyline in a Labrador retriever, J Am Anim Hosp Assoc 23:455–458, 1987.
308. Katherman AE: A comparative review of canine and human narcolepsy, Compend Contin Educ Pract Vet 2:818–822, 1980.
309. Fox JG, et al: Familial reflex myoclonus in Labrador retrievers, Am J Vet Res 45:2367–2370, 1984.
310. O'Brien DP, Zachary JF: Clinical features of spongy degeneration of the central nervous system in two Labrador retriever littermates, J Am Vet Med Assoc 186:1207–1210, 1985.
311. Zachary JF, O'Brien DP: Spongy degeneration of the central nervous system in two canine littermates, Vet Pathol 22:561–571, 1985.
312. Walvoort HC, et al: Canine glycogen storage disease type II: a clinical study of four affected Lapland dogs, J Am Anim Hosp Assoc 20:279–286, 1984.
313. Mostafa IE: A case of glycogenic cardiomegaly in a dog, Acta Vet Scand 11:197–208, 1970.
314. Sandefeldt E, et al: Hereditary neuronal abiotrophy in the Swedish Lapland dog, Cornell Vet 63:1–71, 1973.
315. Sandefeldt E, et al: Hereditary neuronal abiotrophy in Swedish Lapland dogs, Am J Pathol 82:649–652, 1976.
316. Schmahl W, Kaiser E: Hydrocephalus, syringomyelia, and spinal cord angiodysgenesis in a Lhasa apso dog, Vet Pathol 21:252–254, 1984.
317. Sahar A, et al: Spontaneous canine hydrocephalus: cerebrospinal fluid dynamics, J Neurol Neurosurg Psychiatry 34:308–315, 1971.
318. Greene CE, Vandevelde M, Braund K: Lissencephaly in two Lhasa apso dogs, J Am Vet Med Assoc 169:405–410, 1976.
319. Zaki FA: Lissencephaly in Lhasa apso dogs, J Am Vet Med Assoc 169:1165–1168, 1976.
320. Mayhew IG, et al: Tremor syndromes and hypomyelination in lurcher pups, J Small Anim Pract 25:551–559, 1984.
321. Simpson ST: Hydrocephalus in the Maltese dog: Electroencephalographic and C.T. correlations. In Proceedings of the 4th ACVIM Forum. Washington, DC, 1986.
322. Simpson ST, et al: Hydrocephalus. In Proceedings of the 5th ACVIM Forum. San Diego, 1987.
323. Cox VS, et al: Hereditary esophageal dysfunction in the miniature schnauzer dog, Am J Vet Res 41:326–330, 1980.
324. Clifford DH, et al: Management of esophageal achalasia in miniature schnauzers, J Am Vet Med Assoc 161:1012–1020, 1972.
325. Rotmistrovsky RA, et al: GM2 gangliosidosis in a mixed-breed dog, Prog Vet Neurol 2:203–208, 1991.
326. Shull RM, et al: Morphologic and biochemical studies of canine mucopolysaccharidosis I, Am J Pathol 114:487–495, 1984.
327. Schwartz A, et al: Congenital neuromuscular esophageal disease in a litter of Newfoundland puppies, J Am Vet Radiol Soc 17:101–105, 1976.
328. Coulter DB: A dog with a partial merle coat, white iris, and bilaterally impaired hearing, Calif Vet 12:9–11, 1982.
329. Shull RM, et al: Animal model of human disease: canine alpha-iduronidase deficiency. A model of mucopolysaccharidosis I, Am J Pathol 109:244–248, 1982.
330. Inada S, et al: Canine storage disease characterized by hereditary progressive neurogenic muscular atrophy: breeding experiments and clinical manifestation, Am J Vet Res 47:2294–2299, 1986.
331. Inada S, et al: A clinical study on hereditary progressive neurogenic muscular atrophy in pointer dogs, Jpn J Vet Sci 40:539–547, 1978.
332. Izumo S, et al: Morphological study on the hereditary neurogenic amyotrophic dogs: accumulation of lipid compound-like structures in the lower motor neuron, Acta Neuropathol 61:270–276, 1983.
333. Selcer ES, Selcer RR: Globoid cell leukodystrophy in two West Highland white terriers and one Pomeranian, Compend Contin Educ Pract Vet 6:621–624, 1984.
334. Oliver JE, Geary JC: Cerebellar anomalies: two cases, Vet Med Small Anim Clin 60:697, 1965.
335. Kay WJ, Budzilovich GN: Cerebellar hypoplasia and agenesis in the dog, J Neuropathol Exp Neurol 29:156, 1970.
336. Matthews NS, de Lahunta A: Degenerative myelopathy in an adult miniature poodle, J Am Vet Med Assoc 186:1213–1214, 1985.
337. Zaki F, Kay WJ: Globoid cell leukodystrophy in a miniature poodle, J Am Vet Med Assoc 163:248–250, 1973.
338. Bundza A, Lowden JA, Charlton KM: Niemann-Pick disease in a poodle dog, Vet Pathol 16:530–538, 1979.
339. Shell LG, et al: Neuronal visceral GM1 gangliosidosis in Portuguese water dogs. In the Proceedings of the 6th ACVIM Forum. Washington, DC, 1988.
340. Wright JA, Brownlie S: Progressive ataxia in a Pyrenean mountain dog, Vet Rec 116:410–411, 1985.
341. Gamble DA, Chrisman CL: A leukoencephalomyelopathy of Rottweiler dogs, Vet Pathol 21:274–280, 1984.
342. Chrisman C: Neuroaxonal dystrophy and leukoencephalomyelopathy of Rottweiler dogs. In Kirk RW, editor: Current veterinary therapy IX: small animal practice, Philadelphia, 1986, WB Saunders.
343. Chrisman CL, Cork LC, Gamble DA: Neuroaxonal dystrophy of Rottweiler dogs, J Am Vet Med Assoc 184:464–467, 1984.
344. Cork LC, et al: Canine neuronaxonal dystrophy, J Neuropathol Exp Neurol 42:286–296, 1983.
345. Evans MG, Mullaney TP, Lowrie CT: Neuroaxonal dystrophy in a Rottweiler pup, J Am Vet Med Assoc 192:1560–1562, 1988.
346. Shell L, Jortner B, Leib M: Familial motor neuron disease in Rottweiler dogs: neuropathologic studies, Vet Pathol 24:135–139, 1987.
347. Shell L, Jortner B, Leib M: Spinal muscular atrophy in two Rottweiler littermates, J Am Vet Med Assoc 190:878–880, 1987.
348. Shell LG: Spinal muscular atrophy in Rottweiler pups. In the Proceedings of the 6th ACVIM Forum. Washington, DC, 1988.
349. Shell LG, et al: Spinal dysraphism, hemivertebra, and stenosis of the spinal canal in a Rottweiler puppy, J Am Anim Hosp Assoc 24:341–344, 1988.
350. Appleby EC, Longstaffe JA, Bell FR: Ceroid lipofuscinosis in two Saluki dogs, J Comp Pathol 92:375–380, 1982.

351. Luttgen PJ, Storts RW: Central nervous system status spongiosus. In the Proceedings of the 5th ACVIM Forum. San Diego, 1987.
352. Cummings J, et al: Tremors in Samoyed pups with oligodendrocyte deficiencies and hypomyelination, Acta Neuropathol 71:267–277, 1986.
353. Mason RW, Hartley WJ, Randall M: Spongiform degeneration of the white matter in a Samoyed pup, Aust Vet Pract 9:11–13, 1979.
354. Sorjonen D, Cox N, Kwapien R: Myeloencephalopathy with eosinophilic refractile bodies (Rosenthal fibers) in a Scottish terrier, J Am Vet Med Assoc 190:1004–1006, 1987.
355. Meyers KM, et al: Hyperkinetic episodes in Scottish terrier dogs, J Am Vet Med Assoc 155:129–133, 1969.
356. Robert DD, Hitt ME: Methionine as a possible inducer of Scotty cramp, Canine Pract 13:29–31, 1986.
357. Meyers KM, et al: Muscular hypertonicity, Arch Neurol 25:61–67, 1971.
358. Meyers KM, Schaub RG: The relationship of serotonin to a motor disorder of Scottish terrier dogs, Life Sci 14:1895–1906, 1974.
359. Meyers KM, Padgett GA, Dickson WM: The genetic basis of a kinetic disorder of Scottish terrier dogs, J Hered 61:189–192, 1970.
360. Meyers KM, Dickson WM, Schaub RG: Serotonin involvement in a motor disorder of Scottish terrier dogs, Life Sci 13:1261–1274, 1973.
361. Andersson B, Andersson M: On the etiology of "Scotty cramp" and "splay"—two motoring disorders common in the Scottish terrier breed, Acta Vet Scand 23:550–558, 1982.
362. Clemmons RM, Peters RI, Meyers KM: Scotty cramp: a review of cause, characteristics, diagnosis and treatment, Compend Contin Educ Pract Vet 2:385–390, 1980.
363. Hargis A, et al: Post-mortem findings in a Shetland sheepdog with dermatomyositis, Vet Pathol 23:509–511, 1986.
364. Harari J, et al: Cerebellar agenesis in two canine littermates, J Am Vet Med Assoc 182:622–623, 1983.
365. Bichsel P, Vandevelde M: Degenerative myelopathy in a family of Siberian husky dogs, J Am Vet Med Assoc 183:998–1000, 1983.
366. Reinke JD, Suter PF: Laryngeal paralysis in a dog, J Am Vet Med Assoc 172:714–716, 1978.
367. Hartley WJ, Blakemore WF: Neurovisceral glucocerebroside storage (Gaucher's disease) in a dog, Vet Pathol 10:191–201, 1973.
368. Van De Water N, Jolly R, Farrow B: Canine Gaucher disease: the enzymatic defect, Aust J Exp Biol Med Sci 57:551–554, 1979.
369. Richards RB, Kakulas BA: Spongiform leukoencephalopathy associated with congenital myoclonia syndrome in the dog, J Comp Pathol 88:317–320, 1978.
370. Johnson RP, et al: Myasthenia in Springer spaniel littermates, J Small Anim Pract 16:641–647, 1975.
371. Taylor R, Farrow B, Healy P: Canine fucosidosis: clinical findings, J Small Anim Pract 28:291–300, 1987.
372. Abraham D, et al: The enzymic defect and storage products in canine fucosidosis, Biochem J 221:25–33, 1984.
373. Alroy J, Ucci AA, Warren CD: Human and canine fucosidosis: a comparative histochemistry study, Acta Neuropathol 67:265–271, 1985.
374. Hartley WJ, Canfield PJ, Donnelly TM: A suspected new canine storage disease, Acta Neuropathol 56:225–232, 1982.
375. Kelly WR, et al: Canine α-L-fucosidosis: a storage disease of Springer spaniels, Acta Neuropathol 60:9–13, 1983.
376. Littlewood JD, Herrtage ME, Palmer AC: Neuronal storage disease in English springer spaniels, Vet Rec 112:86, 1983.
377. Keller CB, Lamarre J: Inherited lysosomal storage disease in an English springer spaniel, J Am Vet Med Assoc 200:194–195, 1992.
378. Griffiths IR, et al: Shaking pups: a disorder of central myelination in the spaniel dog. Part 1. Clinical, genetic, and light microscopical observations, J Neurol Sci 50:423–433, 1981.
379. Slatter D: Fundamentals of veterinary ophthalmology, Philadelphia, 1981, WB Saunders.
380. Erickson F, Leipold HW, McKinley J: Congenital defects in dogs. Part 2, Canine Pract 14:51–61, 1977.
381. Hoover D, Little P, Cole W: Neuronal ceroid-lipofuscinosis in a mature dog, Vet Pathol 21:359–361, 1984.
382. Van der Velden A: Fits in Tervuren shepherd dogs: a presumed hereditary trait, J Small Anim Pract 9:63–70, 1968.
383. Cummings J, et al: Canine inherited hypertrophic neuropathy, Acta Neuropathol 53:137–143, 1981.
384. Cooper BJ, et al: Defective Schwann cell function in canine inherited hypertrophic neuropathy, Acta Neuropathol 63:51–56, 1984.
385. Cooper BJ, et al: Canine inherited hypertrophic neuropathy: clinical and electrodiagnostic studies, Am J Vet Res 45:1172–1177, 1984.
386. Cummings J, de Lahunta A: Hypertrophic neuropathy in a dog, Acta Neuropathol 20:325–336, 1974.
387. Millichamp NJ, Curtis R, Barnett KC: Progressive retinal atrophy in Tibetan terriers, J Am Vet Med Assoc 192:769–776, 1988.
388. Geary JC, Oliver JE, Hoerlein BF: Atlanto-axial subluxation in the canine, J Small Anim Pract 8:577–582, 1967.
389. Oliver JE, Lewis RE: Lesions of the atlas and axis in dogs, J Am Anim Hosp Assoc 9:304–313, 1973.
390. Ladds P, et al: Congenital odontoid process separation in two dogs, J Small Anim Pract 12:463–471, 1970.
391. Cook JR, Oliver JE: Atlantoaxial luxation in the dog, Compend Contin Educ Pract Vet 3:242–252, 1981.
392. Downey RS: An unusual cause of tetraplegia in a dog, Can Vet J 8:216–217, 1967.
393. Bardens JW: Congenital malformations of the foramen magnum in dogs, Southwest Vet 18:295–298, 1965.
394. Parker AJ, Park RD: Occipital dysplasia in the dog, J Am Anim Hosp Assoc 10:520–525, 1974.
395. Gee B, Doige C: Multiple cartilaginous exostoses in a litter of dogs, J Am Vet Med Assoc 156:53–59, 1970.
396. Bichsel P, et al: Solitary cartilaginous exostoses associated with spinal cord compression in three large-breed dogs, J Am Anim Hosp Assoc 21:619–622, 1985.
397. Doige C: Multiple cartilaginous exostoses in dogs, Vet Pathol 24:276–278, 1987.
398. Acton CE: Spinal cord compression in young dogs due to cartilaginous exostosis, Calif Vet 41:7–26, 1987.
399. Vicini DS, et al: Peripheral nerve biopsy for diagnosis of globoid cell leukodystrophy in a dog, J Am Vet Med Assoc 192:1087–1090, 1988.
400. Kornegay JN: Dysmyelinogenesis in dogs. In the Proceedings of the 3rd ACVIM Forum. San Diego, 1985.
401. Kornegay J: Hypomyelination in Weimaraner dogs, Acta Neuropathol 72:394–401, 1987.
402. Comont PSV, Palmer AC, Williams AE: Weakness associated with myelopathy in a Weimaraner puppy, J Small Anim Pract 29:367–372, 1988.

403. McGrath JT: Spinal dysraphism in the dog, Pathol Vet Suppl 2:1–36, 1965.
404. Gieb LW, Bistner SI: Spinal cord dysraphism in a dog, J Am Vet Med Assoc 150:618–620, 1967.
405. Engel HN, Draper DD: Comparative prenatal development of the spinal cord in normal and dysraphic dogs: embryonic stage, Am J Vet Res 43:1729–1734, 1982.
406. Engel HN, Draper DD: Comparative prenatal development of the spinal cord in normal and dysraphic dogs: fetal stage, Am J Vet Res 43:1735–1743, 1982.
407. Botelho SY, et al: Electromyography in dogs with congenital spinal cord lesions, Am J Vet Res 28:205–212, 1967.
408. Confer AW, Ward BC: Spinal dysraphism: a congenital myelodysplasia in the Weimaraner, J Am Vet Med Assoc 160:1423–1426, 1972.
409. Osborne CA, Clifford DH, Jessen C: Hereditary esophageal achalasia in dogs, J Am Vet Med Assoc 151:572–581, 1967.
410. Bryant SH: Altered membrane potentials in myotonia. In Bolis L, Hoffman JF, Leaf A, editors: Membranes and diseases, New York, 1976, Raven Press.
411. Bryant SH: Myotonia in the goat, Ann N Y Acad Sci 317:314–325, 1979.
412. Healy P, Sewell C: The use of plasma mannosidase activity for the detection of goats heterozygous for ß-mannosidosis, Aust Vet J 62:286–287, 1985.
413. Fankhauser R: Hydrocephalus Studien, Schweiz Arch Tierheilkd 101:407–416, 1959.
414. Healy PJ, et al: ß-Mannosidase deficiency in Anglo Nubian goats, Aust Vet J 57:504–507, 1981.
415. Robinson WF, et al: Atlanto-axial malarticulation in Angora goats, Aust Vet J 58:105–107, 1982.
416. Luttgen PJ, Storts RW: Ceroid lipofuscinosis in Nubian goats. In the Proceedings of the 4th ACVIM Forum, San Diego, 1987.
417. Fiske RA, Storts RW: Neuronal ceroid-lipofuscinosis in Nubian goats, Vet Pathol 25:171–173, 1988.
418. Mayhew J, Brown C, Trapp A: Equine degenerative myeloencephalopathy. In the Proceedings of the 4th ACVIM Forum, Washington, DC, 1986.
419. Mayhew IG, et al: Spinal cord disease in the horse, Cornell Vet 68(suppl 6):1–207, 1978.
420. Watson AG, Mayhew IG: Familial congenital occipitoatlantoaxial malformation (OAAM) in the Arabian horse, Spine 11:334–339, 1986.
421. Smith JM, DeBowes RM, Cox JH: Central nervous system disease in adult horses. Part II. Differential diagnosis, Compend Contin Educ Pract Vet 9:771–780, 1987.
422. Duncan I: Congenital tremor and abnormalities of myelination. In the Proceedings of the 5th ACVIM Forum, San Diego: 869–873, 1987.
423. Fraser H: Two dissimilar types of cerebellar disorder in the horse, Vet Rec 78:608–612, 1966.
424. Palmer AC, et al: Cerebellar hypoplasia and degeneration in the young Arab horse: clinical and neuropathological features, Vet Rec 93:62–66, 1973.
425. Mayhew I: Seizures disorders. In Robinson NE, editor: Current therapy in equine medicine, Philadelphia, 1983, WB Saunders.
426. Scarratt WK, et al: Degenerative myelopathy in two equids, J Equine Vet Sci 5:139–141, 1985.
427. Bjorck G, et al: Congenital cerebellar ataxia in the Gotland pony breed, Zentralbl Veterinarmed A 20(A): 341–354, 1973.
428. Mayhew IG, Watson AG, Heissan JA: Congenital occipitoatlantoaxial malformation in the horse, Equine Vet J 10:103–113, 1978.
429. Wilson WD, et al: Occipitoatlantoaxial malformation in two non-Arabian horses, J Am Vet Med Assoc 187:36–40, 1985.
430. Shupe JL, et al: Hereditary multiple exostoses, Am J Pathol 104:285–288, 1981.
431. Maciulis A, et al: High resolution chromosome banding analysis of horses with hereditary multiple exostosis, J Equine Vet Sci 5:284–286, 1985.
432. Powers B, et al: Pathology of the vertebral column of horses with cervical static stenosis, Vet Pathol 23:392–399, 1986.
433. Alitalo I, Karkkainen M: Osteochondrotic changes in the vertebrae of four ataxic horses suffering from cervical vertebral malformation, Nord Vet Med 35:468–474, 1983.
434. Wagner P, et al: Surgical stabilization of the equine cervical spine, Vet Surg 8:7–12, 1979.
435. Steel J, Whittem J, Hutchins D: Equine sensory ataxia ("wobbles"): clinical and pathological observations in Australian cases, Aust Vet J 35:442–449, 1959.
436. Wagner P, et al: Evaluation of cervical spinal fusion as a treatment in the equine "wobbler" syndrome, Vet Surg 8:84–88, 1979.
437. Mayhew I, et al: Equine degenerative myeloencephalopathy: a vitamin E deficiency that may be familial, J Vet Intern Med 1:45–50, 1987.
438. Mayhew IG, et al: Equine degenerative myeloencephalopathy, J Am Vet Med Assoc 170:195–201, 1977.
439. Steinberg S, Bothelo S: Myotonia in a horse, Science 137:979, 1962.
440. Beech J: Neuroaxonal dystrophy of the accessory cuneate nucleus in horses, Vet Pathol 21:384–393, 1984.
441. Beech J, Haskind M: Genetic studies of neuroaxonal dystrophy in the Morgan, Am J Vet Res 48:109–113, 1987.
442. Roneus B: Glutathione peroxidase and selenium in the blood of healthy horses and foals affected by muscular dystrophy, Nord Vet Med 34:350–353, 1982.
443. Poss M, Young S: Dysplastic disease of the cerebellum of an adult horse, Acta Neuropathol 75:209–211, 1987.
444. Grant B, et al: Surgical treatment of multiple level cord compression in the horse, Equine Pract 7:19–24, 1985.
445. Rooney J: Equine incoordination. I. Gross morphology, Cornell Vet 53:411–422, 1963.
446. Fraser H, Palmer A: Equine incoordination and wobbler disease of young horses, Vet Rec 80:338–355, 1967.
447. Falco M, Whitwell K, Palmer A: An investigation into the genetics of "wobbler disease" in thoroughbred horses in Britain, Equine Vet J 8:165–169, 1967.
448. Duncan I: Some aspects of the neuropathy of equine laryngeal hemiplegia. In the Proceedings of the 5th ACVIM Forum, San Diego, 1987.
449. Cole CR: Changes in the equine larynx associated with laryngeal hemiplegia, Am J Vet Res 7:69–77, 1946.
450. Duncan ID, et al: The pathology of equine laryngeal hemiplegia, Acta Neuropathol 27:337–348, 1974.
451. Hillidge C: Interpretation of laryngeal function tests in the horse, Vet Rec 118:535–536, 1986.
452. Cahill JI, Goulder B: The pathogenesis of equine laryngeal hemiplegia: a review, N Z Vet J 35:82–90, 1987.
453. Tulleners EP, Harrison IW, Raker CW: Management of arytenoid chondropathy and failed laryngoplasty in horses: 75 cases (1879-1985), J Am Vet Med Assoc 192:670–675, 1988.
454. Cahill JI, Goulden B: Equine laryngeal hemiplegia. Part II. An electron microscopic study of peripheral nerves, N Z Vet J 34:170–175, 1986.

455. Cahill JI, Goulden B: Equine laryngeal hemiplegia. Part I. A light microscopic study of peripheral nerves, N Z Vet J 34:161–169, 1986.
456. Cahill J, Goulden B: Equine laryngeal hemiplegia. Part V. Central nervous system pathology, N Z Vet J 34:191–193, 1986.
457. Cahill J, Goulden B: Equine laryngeal hemiplegia. Part IV. Muscle pathology, N Z Vet J 34:186–190, 1986.
458. Cahill J, Goulden BE: Equine laryngeal hemiplegia. Part III. A teased fibre study of peripheral nerves, N Z Vet J 34:181–185, 1986.
459. Baker GJ: Laryngeal hemiplegia in the horse, Compend Contin Educ Pract Vet 5:S61–S67, 1983.
460. Koch C: Diseases of the larynx and pharynx of the horse, Compend Contin Educ Pract Vet 2:573–580, 1980.
461. Vaala W: Diagnosis and treatment of prematurity and neonatal maladjustment syndrome in newborn foals, Compend Contin Educ Pract Vet 8:211–226, 1986.
462. Montali R, et al: Spinal ataxia in zebras: comparison with the wobbler syndrome of horses, Vet Pathol 11:68–78, 1974.
463. Van den Berg P, Baker M, Lange A: A suspected lysosomal storage disease in Abyssinian cats. Part I. Genetic, clinical and clinical pathological aspects, J S Afr Vet Assoc 48:195–199, 1977.
464. Lange AL, Brown JMM, Maree CC: Biochemical studies on a lysosomal storage disease in Abyssinian cats, Onderstepoort J Vet Res 50:149–155, 1983.
465. Baker H, et al: Sphingomyelin lipidosis in a cat, Vet Pathol 24:386–391, 1987.
466. Sponenberg DP, Graf-Webster E: Hereditary meningoencephalocele in Burmese cats, J Hered 77:60, 1986.
467. Zook B, et al: Encephalocele and other congenital craniofacial anomalies in Burmese cats, Vet Med Small Anim Clin 78:695–701, 1983.
468. Rebillard M, Rebillard G, Pujol R: Variability of the hereditary deafness in the white cat, I, Physiol Hear Res 5:179–187, 1981.
469. Rebillard M, Pujol R, Rebillard G: Variability of the hereditary deafness in the white cat, II, Histol Hear Res 5:189–200, 1981.
470. Elverland HH, Mair IWS: Hereditary deafness in the cat, Acta Otolaryngol 90:360–369, 1980.
471. Faith RE, Woodard JC: Waardenburg's syndrome, Comp Pathol Bull 5:3–4, 1973.
472. Coulter DB, Martin CL, Alvarado TP: A cat with white fur and one blue eye, Calif Vet 34:11–14, 1980.
473. Delack JB: Hereditary deafness in the white cat, Compend Contin Educ Pract Vet 6:609–616, 1984.
474. Creel D, Conlee JW, Parks TN: Auditory brainstem anomalies in albino cats. I. Evoked potential studies, Brain Res 260:1–9, 1983.
475. Saperstein G, Harris S, Leipold HW: Congenital defects in domestic cats, Feline Pract 6:18–41, 1976.
476. Watson AG, Hall MA, de Lahunta A: Congenital occipitoatlantoaxial malformation in a cat, Compend Contin Educ Pract Vet 7:245–254, 1985.
477. Carpenter M, Harter D: A study of congenital feline cerebellar malformations: an anatomic and physiologic evaluation of agenetic defects, J Comp Neurol 105:51–94, 1956.
478. Csiza C, et al: Spontaneous feline ataxia, Cornell Vet 62:300–322, 1972.
479. Herndon R, Margolis G, Kilham L: The synaptic organization of the malformed cerebellum induced by perinatal infection with the feline panleukopenia virus (PLV), J Neuropathol Exp Neurol 30:196–205, 1971.
480. Mesfin GM, Kusewitt D, Parker A: Degenerative myelopathy in a cat, J Am Vet Med Assoc 176:62–64, 1980.
481. Cork LC, Munnell JF, Lorenz MD: The pathology of feline GM2 gangliosidosis, Am J Pathol 90:723–734, 1978.
482. Cork LC, et al: GM2 ganglioside lysosomal storage disease in cats with hexosaminidase deficiency, Science 196:1014–1017, 1977.
483. Johnson KH: Globoid leukodystrophy in the cat, J Am Vet Med Assoc 157:2057–2067, 1970.
484. Sandstrom B, Westman J, Ockerman PA: Glycogenosis of the central nervous system in the cat, Acta Neuropathol 14:194–200, 1969.
485. Cribb A: Laryngeal paralysis in a mature cat, Can Vet J 27:27, 1986.
486. White R, et al: Outcome of surgery for laryngeal paralysis in four cats, Vet Rec 117:103–104, 1986.
487. Hardie EM, et al: Laryngeal paralysis in three cats, J Am Vet Med Assoc 179:879–882, 1981.
488. Fatzer R: Leukodystrophische Erschrankungen im Gehirn junger Katzen, Schweiz Arch Tierheilikd 117:641–648, 1975.
489. Hegreberg GA, Thuline HC, Francis BH: Morphologic changes in feline leukodystrophy, FASEB J 30:341, 1971.
490. Oliver JE, Hoerlein BF, Mayhew IG: Veterinary neurology, Philadelphia, 1987, WB Saunders.
491. Blakemore W: A case of mannosidosis in the cat: clinical and histopathological findings, J Small Anim Pract 27:447–455, 1986.
492. Walkley SU, Blakemore WF, Purpura DP: Alterations in neuron morphology in feline mannosidosis, Acta Neuropathol 53:75–79, 1981.
493. Braund KG, Ribas JL: Meningiomas of the central nervous system in dogs and cats. In the Proceedings of the 4th ACVIM Forum, Washington, DC, 1986.
494. Lawson DC, Burk RL, Prata RG: Cerebral meningioma in the cat: diagnosis and surgical treatment of ten cases, J Am Anim Hosp Assoc 20:333–342, 1984.
495. Braund K, Ribas J: Central nervous system meningiomas, Compend Contin Educ Pract Vet 8:241–248, 1986.
496. Haskins ME, et al: Mucopolysaccharidosis in a domestic short-haired cat: a disease distinct from that seen in the Siamese cat, J Am Vet Med Assoc 175:384–387, 1979.
497. Haskins ME, et al: The pathology of the feline model of mucopolysaccharidosis: I, Am J Pathol 112:27–36, 1983.
498. Woodard JC, Collins GH, Hessler JR: Feline hereditary neuroaxonal dystrophy, Am J Pathol 74:551–560, 1974.
499. Vandevelde M, Greene C, Hoff E: Lower motor neuron disease with accumulation of neurofilaments in a cat, Vet Pathol 13:428–435, 1976.
500. Percy DH, Jortner BS: Feline lipidosis, Arch Pathol Lab Med 92:136–143, 1971.
501. Cuddon PA, Higgins RJ, Duncan ID: Feline Niemann-Pick disease associated polyneuropathy. In the Proceedings of the 6th ACVIM Forum, Washington, DC, 1988.
502. Kelly DF, Gaskell CJ: Spongy degeneration of the central nervous system in kittens, Acta Neuropathol 35:151–158, 1976.
503. Clifford DH, et al: Congenital achalasia of the esophagus in four cats of common ancestry, J Am Vet Med Assoc 158:1554–1560, 1971.
504. Davidson AP: Congenital disorders of the Manx cat, Southwest Vet 37:115–119, 1986.

505. Kitchen H, Murray RE, Cockrell BY: Animal model for human disease, spina bifida, sacral dysgenesis and myelocele, Am J Pathol 68:203–206, 1972.
506. Hall JA, Fettman MJ, Ingram JT: Sodium chloride depletion in a cat with fistulated meningomyelocele, J Am Vet Med Assoc 192:1445–1448, 1988.
507. Leipold HW, et al: Congenital defects of the caudal vertebral column and spinal cord in Manx cats, J Am Vet Med Assoc 164:520–523, 1974.
508. Fyfe JC, et al: Familial glycogen storage disease type IV (GSD IV) in Norwegian forest cats (NWFC), J Vet Intern Med 4:127, 1990.
509. Maenhout T, et al: Mannosidosis in a litter of Persian cats, Vet Rec 122:351–354, 1988.
510. Jezyk PF, Haskins ME, Newman LR: Alpha mannosidosis in a Persian cat, J Am Vet Med Assoc 189:1483–1485, 1986.
511. Vandevelde M, et al: Hereditary neurovisceral mannosidosis with associated mannosidase deficiency in a family of Persian cats, Acta Neuropathol 58:64–68, 1982.
512. Green P, Little P: Neuronal ceroid-lipofuscin storage in Siamese cats, Can J Comp Med 38:207–212, 1974.
513. Cowell KR, et al: Mucopolysaccharidosis in a cat, J Am Vet Med Assoc 169:334–339, 1976.
514. Langweiler M, Haskins ME, Jezyk PF: Mucopolysaccharidosis in a litter of cats, J Am Anim Hosp Assoc 14:748–751, 1978.
515. Haskins ME, et al: Spinal compression and hindlimb paresis in cats with mucopolysaccharidosis: VI, J Am Vet Med Assoc 182:983–985, 1983.
516. Breton L, Guerin P, Morin M: A case of mucopolysaccharidosis VI in a cat, J Am Anim Hosp Assoc 19:891–896, 1983.
517. Jezyk P, Haskins M, Patterson DF: Mucopolysaccharidosis in a cat with arylsulfatase B deficiency: a model of Maroteaux-Lamy syndrome, Science 198:834–836, 1977.
518. Haskins ME, et al: The pathology of the feline model of mucopolysaccharidosis VI, Am J Pathol 101:657–674, 1980.
519. Haskins ME, Jezyk PF, Desnick RJ, et al: Animal model of human disease mucopolysaccharidosis VI. Maroteaux-Lamy syndrome arylsulfatase ß-deficient mucopolysaccharidosis in the Siamese cat, Am J Pathol 105:191–193, 1981.
520. Chrisp CE, et al: Lipid storage disease in a Siamese cat, J Am Vet Med Assoc 156:616–622, 1970.
521. Snyder S, Kingston R, Wenger D: Animal model of human disease: Niemann-Pick disease. sphingomyelinosis of Siamese cats, Am J Pathol 108:252–254, 1982.
522. Terlecki S, et al: A congenital disease of lambs clinically similar to "inherited cerebellar cortical atrophy" (Daft lamb disease), Br Vet J 134:299–308, 1978.
523. Nuttall WO: Ovine neuroaxonal dystrophy in New Zealand, N Z Vet J 36:5–7, 1988.
524. Manktelow CD, Hartley WJ: Generalized glycogen storage disease in sheep, J Comp Pathol 85:139–145, 1975.
525. Dennis SM, Leipold HW: Anencephaly in sheep, Cornell Vet 62:273–281, 1972.
526. Harper P, et al: Cerebellar abiotrophy and segmental axonopathy: two syndromes of progressive ataxia of merino sheep, Aust Vet J 63:18–21, 1986.
527. McGavin: Progressive ovine muscular dystrophy, Comp Pathol Bull 6:3–4, 1974.
528. Richards R, et al: Ovine congenital progressive muscular dystrophy: clinical syndrome and distribution of lesions, Aust Vet J 63:396–401, 1986.
529. Richards RB, et al: Ovine congenital progressive muscular dystrophy: mode of inheritance, Aust Vet J 65:93–94, 1988.
530. Pritchard DH, Napthine DV, Sinclair AJ: Globoid cell leukodystrophy in polled Dorset sheep, Vet Pathol 17:399–405, 1980.
531. Woods PR: Neuronal ceroid-lipofuscinosis in Rambouillet sheep. In the Proceedings of the 9th ACVIM Forum, New Orleans, 1991.
532. Saperstein G, Leipold HW, Dennis SM: Congenital defects in sheep, J Am Vet Med Assoc 167:314–322, 1974.
533. Whittington RJ, et al: Congenital hydranencephaly and arthrogryposis of Corriedale sheep, Aust Vet J 65:124–127, 1988.
534. Parish S, Gavin P, Knowles D: Quadriplegia associated with cervical deformity in a lamb, Vet Rec 114:196, 1984.
535. Nisbet DI, Renwick CC: Congenital myopathy in lambs, J Comp Pathol 71:177, 1961.
536. Prieur DJ, Ahern-Rindell AJ, Murnane RD: Animal model of human disease: ovine GM1 gangliosidosis, Am J Pathol 139:1511–1513, 1991.
537. Cordy DR, Richards WPC, Bradford GE: Systemic neuroaxonal dystrophy in Suffolk sheep, Acta Neuropathol 8:133–140, 1967.
538. Done J: The congenital tremor syndrome in pigs, Vet Ann 16:98–102, 1975.
539. Foulkes JA: Myelin and dysmyelination in domestic animals, Vet Bull 8:441–450, 1974.
540. Done JT: Congenital nervous diseases of pigs: a review, Lab Anim 2:207–217, 1968.
541. Chambers J, Hall RR: Porcine malignant hyperthermia (porcine stress syndrome), Compend Contin Educ Pract Vet 9:F317–F322, 1987.
542. Eikelenboom G, Minkema D: Prediction of pale, soft and exudative muscle with a non-lethal test for the halothane-induced porcine malignant hyperthermia syndrome, Neth J Vet Sci 99:421–426, 1974.
543. Lucke JN, Hall GM, Lister D: Malignant hyperthermia in the pig and the role of stress, Ann N Y Acad Sci 317:326–337, 1979.
544. Sybesma W, Eikelenboom G: Malignant hyperthermia in pigs, Neth J Vet Sci 2:155–160, 1969.
545. Steiss JE, Bowen JM, Williams CH: Electromyographic evaluation of malignant hyperthermia-susceptible pigs, Am J Vet Res 42:1173–1176, 1981.
546. Wells GAH, Pinsent PJN, Todd JN: A progressive, familial myopathy of the Pietrain pig: the clinical syndrome, Vet Rec 106:556–558, 1980.
547. Kidd A, et al: A new genetically-determined congenital nervous disorder in pigs, Br Vet J 142:275–285, 1986.
548. Vogt D, et al: Congenital meningocele-encephalocele in an experimental swine herd, Am J Vet Res 47:188–191, 1986.
549. Read WK, Bridges CH: Cerebrospinal lipodystrophy in swine, Pathol Vet 5:67–74, 1968.
550. Higgins RJ, et al: Spontaneous lower motor neuron disease with neurofibrillary accumulation in young pigs, Acta Neuropathol 59:288–294, 1983.
551. Coates JR, Kline KL: Congenital and inherited neurologic disorders in dogs and cats. In Kirk RW, editor: Current veterinary therapy XII: small animal practice, Philadelphia, 1995, WB Saunders.
552. Moe L: Hereditary polyneuropathy of Alaskan malamutes. In Kirk RW, editor: Current veterinary therapy XI: small animal practice, Philadelphia, 1992, WB Saunders.

553. Snyder PW, et al: Pathologic features of naturally occurring juvenile polyarteritis in beagle dogs, Vet Pathol 32:337–345, 1995.
554. Jones BR, Alley MR, Batchelor B: Hydrocephalus and hypertrichosis in golden retriever dogs, Vet J 44:38–39, 1996.
555. Bethlehem M, Gruys E, Elving L: Congenital tremor in Holstein Friesian cattle, Vet Q 14:54–56, 1992.
556. Furuoka H, et al: Hereditary myopathy of the diaphragmatic muscles in Holstein-Friesian cattle, Acta Neuropathol 90:339–346, 1995.
557. Healy PJ, et al: Maple syrup urine disease in poll shorthorn calves, Aust Vet J 69:143–144, 1992.
558. Hindmarsh M, Harper PAW: Congenital spongiform myelopathy of Simmental calves, Aust Vet J 72:193–194, 1995.
559. Tisdall PLC, et al: Congenital portosystemic shunts in Maltese and Australian cattle dogs, Aust Vet J 71:174–178, 1994.
560. Weissenbock H, Obermaier G, Dahme E: Alexander's disease in a Bernese mountain dog, Acta Neuropathol 91:200–204, 1996.
561. Meric S, Child G, Higgins R: Necrotizing vasculitis of the spinal pachyleptomeningeal arteries in three Bernese mountain dog littermates, J Am Anim Hosp Assoc 22:459–465, 1986.
562. Kuwamura M, et al: Type C Niemann-Pick disease in a boxer dog, Acta Neuropathol 85:345–348, 1993.
563. van Ham LML, Roels SMMF, Hoorens JK: Congenital dystrophy-like myopathy in a Brittany spaniel puppy, Prog Vet Neurol 6:135–138, 1995.
564. Giger U, et al: Inherited phosphofructokinase deficiency in an American cocker spaniel, J Am Vet Med Assoc 201:1569–1571, 1992.
565. Rand JS, Best SJ, Mathews KA: Portosystemic vascular shunts in a family of American cocker spaniels, J Am Anim Hosp Assoc 24:265–272, 1988.
566. Jolly RD, et al: Canine ceroid lipofuscinoses: a review and classification, J Small Anim Pract 35:299–306, 1994.
567. Braund KG, Shores A, Cochrane S, et al: Laryngeal paralysis-polyneuropathy complex in young Dalmatians, Am J Vet Res 55:534–542, 1994.
568. Holland CT, et al: Dyserythropoiesis, polymyopathy, and cardiac disease in three related English springer spaniels, J Vet Intern Med 5:151–159, 1991.
569. Flagstad A: Development of the electrophysiological pattern in congenital myasthenic syndrome, Prog Vet Neurol 4:126–134, 1993.
570. Furuoka H, et al: Peripheral neuropathy in German shepherd dogs, J Comp Pathol 107:169–177, 1992.
571. Boydell P: Idiopathic Horner's syndrome in the golden retriever, J Small Anim Pract 36:382–384, 1995.
572. Targett MP, et al: Central core myopathy in a Great Dane, J Small Anim Pract 35:100–103, 1994.
573. van Ham L, et al: A congenital myopathy resembling Duchenne muscular dystrophy in a litter of Belgian Groenedaeler shepherds. In Proceedings of the European Society of Veterinary Neurology, 6th Annual Symposium, Rome, 1992.
574. Malik R, et al: Hereditary myopathy of Devon rex cats, J Small Anim Pract 34:539–546, 1993.
575. Maddison JE: Hepatic encephalopathy, current concepts of the pathogenesis, J Vet Intern Med 6:341–353, 1992.
576. Sacre BJ, Cummings JF, de Lahunta A: Neuroaxonal dystrophy in a Jack Russell terrier pup resembling human infantile neuroaxonal dystrophy, Cornell Vet 83:133–142, 1993.
577. Mandigers PJJ, et al: Hereditary myelopathy in the Dutch Kooiker dog. In Proceedings of the European Society of Veterinary Neurology, 7th Annual Symposium, Suffolk, UK, 1993.
578. Mandigers PJJ, et al: Hereditary necrotising myelopathy in Kooiker dogs, Res Vet Sci 54:118–123, 1993.
579. de Lahunta A, et al: Labrador retriever central axonopathy, Prog Vet Neurol 5:117–122, 1994.
580. Neer TM, Kornegay JN: Leukoencephalomalacia and cerebral white matter vacuolar degeneration in two related Labrador retriever puppies, J Vet Intern Med 9:100–104, 1995.
581. Paola JP, Podell M, Shelton GD: Muscular dystrophy in miniature schnauzers, Prog Vet Neurol 4:14–18, 1993.
582. Franklin RJM, Jeffery ND, Ramsey IK: Neuroaxonal dystrophy in a litter of papillon pups, J Small Anim Pract 36:441–444, 1995.
583. van Winkle TJ, et al: Blindness due to polymicrogyria and asymmetrical dilation of the lateral ventricles in standard poodles, Prog Vet Neurol 5:66–71, 1994.
583a. Jurney C, Haddad J, Crawford N, et al: Polymicrogyria in standard poodles, J Vet Intern Med 23(4):871–874, 2009.
583b. Chen X, Johnson GS, Schnabel RD, et al: A neonatal encephalopathy with seizures in standard poodle dogs with a missense mutation in the canine ortholog of ATF2, Neurogenetics 9(1):41–49, 2008.
584. Cordy DR, Holliday TA: A necrotizing meningoencephalitis of pug dogs, Vet Pathol 26:191–194, 1989.
585. Kobayashi Y, et al: Necrotizing meningoencephalitis in pug dogs in Japan, J Comp Pathol 110:129–136, 1994.
586. Kornegay JN: Breed-associated meningitis. In the Proceedings of the 9th ACVIM Forum, New Orleans, 1991.
587. Braund KG, et al: Distal sensorimotor polyneuropathy in mature Rottweiler dogs, Vet Pathol 31:316–326, 1994.
588. Presthus J, Nordstoga K: Congenital myopathy in a litter of Samoyed dogs, Prog Vet Neurol 4:37–40, 1993.
589. van Ham L, et al: A tremor syndrome with a central axonopathy in Scottish terriers, J Vet Intern Med 8:290–292, 1994.
590. Knowles K, et al: Adult-onset lysosomal storage disease in a schipperke dog: clinical, morphological and biochemical studies, Acta Neuropathol 86:306–312, 1993.
591. Alroy J, et al: Adult onset, lysosomal storage disease in a Tibetan terrier: clinical, morphological and biochemical studies, Acta Neuropathol 84:658–663, 1992.
592. Tipold A, et al: Necrotizing encephalitis in Yorkshire terriers, J Small Anim Pract 34:623–628, 1993.
593. Lunn DP, et al: Familial occurrence of narcolepsy in miniature horses, Equine Vet J 25:483–487, 1993.
594. Jones BR, et al: An encephalomyelopathy in related Birman kittens, N Z Vet J 40:160–163, 1992.
595. Cuddon PA: Feline neuromuscular diseases. In Kirk R, Bonagura J, editors: Kirk's current veterinary therapy: small animal practice XI, Philadelphia, 1992, WB Saunders.
596. Gaschen FP, Haugh PG, Swendrowski MA: Hypertrophic feline muscular dystrophy: a unique clinical expression of dystrophin deficiency, Feline Pract 22:23–27, 1994.
597. Carpenter JL, et al: Feline muscular dystrophy with dystrophin deficiency, Am J Pathol 135:909–919, 1989.
598. Bildfell R, et al: Neuronal ceroid-lipofuscinosis in a cat, Vet Pathol 32:485–488, 1995.
599. Stoffregen DA, et al: Hypomyelination of the central nervous system of two Siamese kitten littermates, Vet Pathol 30:388–391, 1993.

600. Bourke CA, Carrigan MJ, Dent CHR: Chronic locomotor dysfunction associated with a thalamic cerebellar neuropathy in Australian Merino sheep, Aust Vet J 70:232–233, 1993.
601. Priester WA: Canine intervertebral disc disease: occurrence by age, breed, and sex among 8,117 cases, Theriogenology 6(2-3):293–303, 1976.
602. Johnston PEJ, Barrie JA, McCulloch MC, et al: Central nervous system pathology in 25 dogs with chronic degenerative radiculomyelopathy, Vet Rec 146(22):629–633, 2000.
603. March PA, Coates JR, Abyad RJ, et al: Degenerative myelopathy in 18 Pembroke Welsh corgi dogs, Vet Pathol 46:241–250, 2009.
604. Barclay KB, Haines DM: Immunohistochemical evidence for immunoglobulin and complement deposition in spinal cord lesions in degenerative myelopathy in German shepherd dogs, Can J Vet Res 58(1):20–24, 1994.
605. Williams DA, Sharp NJH, Batt RM: Enteropathy associated with degenerative myclopathy in German Shepherd dogs. In the Proceedings of the 1st ACVIM Forum, New orleans, 40, 1983.
606. Williams DA, Batt RM, Sharp NJH: Degenerative myelopathy in German shepherd dogs: an association with mucosal biochemical changes and bacterial overgrowth in the small intestine, Clin Sci 66:25, 1984:(abstract).
607. Fechner H, Johnston PE, Sharp NJH, et al: Molecular genetic and expression analysis of alpha-tocopherol transfer protein mRNA in German shepherd dogs with degenerative myelopathy, Berl Much Tierarzl Wochenschr 116:31–36, 2003.
608. Johnston PEJ, Knox K, Gettinby G, et al: Serum α-tochopherol concentrations in German shepherd dogs with chronic degenerative radiculomyelopathy, Vet Rec 148:403–407, 2001.
609. Sheahan BJ, Caffrey JF, Gunn HM, et al: Structural and biochemical changes in a spinal myelinopathy in twelve English foxhounds and two harriers, Vet Pathol 28(2):117–124, 1991.
610. Coates JR, March PA, Oglesbee M, et al: Clinical characterization of a familial degenerative myelopathy in Pembroke Welsh corgi dogs, J Vet Intern Med 21(6):1323–1331, 2007.
611. Bichsel P, Vandevelde M, Lang J, et al: Degenerative myelopathy in a family of Siberian husky dogs, J Am Vet Med Assoc 183(9):998–1000, 1983.
612. Long SN, Henthorn PS, Serpell J, et al: Degenerative myelopathy in Chesapeake Bay retrievers, J Vet Intern Med 23:401–402, 2009.
613. Clark LA, Tsai KL, Murphy KE: Alleles of DLA-DRB1 are not unique in German shepherd dogs having degenerative myelopathy, Anim Genet 39(3):332, 2008.
614. Kathmann I, Cizinauskas S, Doherr MG, et al: Daily controlled physiotherapy increases survival time in dogs with suspected degenerative myelopathy, J Vet Intern Med 20:927–932, 2006.
615. Miller AD, Barber R, Porter BF, et al: Degenerative myelopathy in two boxer dogs, Vet Pathol 46(4):684–687, 2009.
615a. Awano T, Johnson GS, WAde CM, et al: Genome-wide association analysis reveals a SOD I mutation in canine degenerative myelopathy that resembles amyotrophic lateral sclerosis. Proceedings of the National Academy of Sciences of the United States of America 106:2794–2799, 2009.
616. Oevermann A, Bley T, Konar M, et al: A novel leukoencephalomyelopathy of Leonberger dogs, J Vet Intern Med 22:467–471, 2008.
617. Toenniessen JG, Morin DE: Degenerative myelopathy: a comparative review, Compend Contin Educ Pract Vet 17(2):271–283, 1995.
618. Larsen JS, Selby LA: Spondylosis deformans in large dogs—relative risk by breed, age and sex, J Am Anim Hosp Assoc 17(4):623–625, 1981.
619. Kornegay JN: Vertebral diseases of large breed dogs. In Kornegay JN, editor: Neurologic disorders (contemporary issues in small animal practice), New York, 1986, Churchill Livingstone.
620. Romatowski J: Spondylosis deformans in the dog, Compend Contin Educ Pract Vet 8(8):531–536, 1986.
621. Morgan JP: Spondylosis deformans in the dog, Acta Orthop Scand Suppl 9:61–88, 1967.
622. Langeland M, Lingaas F: Spondylosis deformans in the boxer: estimates of heritability, J Small Anim Pract 36(4):166–169, 1995.
623. Wright JA: Spondylosis deformans of the lumbo-sacral joint in dogs, J Small Anim Pract 21(1):45–58, 1980.
624. Mattoon JS, Koblik PD: Quantitative survey radiographic evaluation of the lumbosacral spine of normal dogs and dogs with degenerative lumbosacral stenosis, Vet Radiol Ultrasound 34(3):194–206, 1993.
625. De Risio L, Thomas WB, Sharp NJH: Degenerative lumbosacral stenosis, Vet Clin North Am 30:111–132, 2000.
626. Newitt ALM, German AJ, Barr FJ: Lumbosacral transitional vertebrae in cats and their effects on morphology of adjacent joints, J Feline Med Surg 11:941–947, 2009.
627. Watt PR: Degenerative lumbosacral stenosis in 18 dogs, J Small Anim Pract 32(3):125–134, 1991.
628. Danielsson F, Sjostrom L: Surgical treatment of degenerative lumbosacral stenosis in dogs, Vet Surg 28(2):91–98, 1999.
629. Ness MG: Degenerative lumbosacral stenosis in the dog: a review of 30 cases, J Small Anim Pract 35:185–190, 1994.
630. Suwankong N, Meij BP, Voorhout G, et al: Review and retrospective analysis of degenerative lumbosacral stenosis in 156 dogs treated by dorsal laminectomy, Vet Comp Orthop Traumatol 21(3):285–293, 2008.
631. Janssens L, Beosier Y, Daems R: Lumbosacral degenerative stenosis in the dog. The results of epidural infiltration with methylprednisolone acetate: a retrospective study, Vet Comp Orthop Traumatol 22(6):486–491, 2009.
632. Chambers JN: Degenerative lumbosacral stenosis in dogs, Vet Med Rep 1(2):166–180, 1989.
633. Palmer RH, Chambers JN: Canine lumbosacral diseases. Part I. Anatomy, pathophysiology, and clinical presentation, Compend Contin Educ Pract Vet 13(1):61–69, 1991.
634. Palmer RH, Chambers JN: Canine lumbosacral diseases. Part II. Definitive diagnosis, treatment, and prognosis, Compend Contin Educ Pract Vet 13(2):213–222, 1991.
635. Chambers JN, Selcer BA, Oliver JE Jr: Results of treatment of degenerative lumbosacral stenosis in dogs by exploration and excision, Vet Comp Orthop Traumatol 3:130–133, 1988.
636. Lang J, Häni H, Schawalder P: A sacral lesion resembling osteochondrosis in the German shepherd Dog, Vet Radiol Ultrasound 33(2):69–76, 1992.

637. Morgan JP, Bailey CS: Cauda equina syndrome in the dog: radiographic evaluation, J Small Anim Pract 31:69–77, 1990.
638. Damur-Djuric N, Steffen F, Hassig M, et al: Lumbosacral transitional vertebrae in dogs: classification, prevalence, and association with the sacroiliac morphology, Vet Radiol Ultrasound 47:32–38, 2006.
639. Fluckiger MA, Damur-Djuric N, Hassig M, et al: A lumbosacral transitional vertebra in the dog predisposes to cauda equina syndrome, Vet Radiol Ultrasound 47:39–44, 2006.
640. Schmid V, Lang J: Measurements on the lumbosacral junction in normal dogs and those with cauda equina compression, J Small Anim Pract 34(9):437–442, 1993.
641. Morgan JP: Transitional lumbosacral vertebral anomaly in the dog: a radiographic study, J Small Anim Pract 40(4):167–172, 1999.
642. Morgan JP, Bahr A, Franti CE, et al: Lumbosacral transitional vertebrae as a predisposing cause of cauda equina syndrome in German shepherd dogs: 161 cases (1987-1990), J Am Vet Med Assoc 202(11):1877–1882, 1993.
643. Steffen F, Hunold K, Scharf G, et al: A follow-up study of neurologic and radiographic findings in working German shepherd dogs with and without degenerative lumbosacral stenosis, J Am Vet Med Assoc 231(10):1529–1533, 2007.
644. Godde T, Steffen F: Surgical treatment of lumbosacral foraminal stenosis, Vet Surg 36:705–713, 2007.
645. De Risio L, Sharp NJH, Olby NJ, et al: Predictors of outcome after dorsal decompressive laminectomy for degenerative lumbosacral stenosis in dogs: 69 cases (1987-1997), J Am Vet Med Assoc 219:624–628, 2001.
646. Linn LL, Bartels KE, Rochat MC, et al: Lumbosacral stenosis in 29 military working dogs: epidemiologic findings and outcome after surgical intervention, Vet Surg 2003(32):21–29, 1990-1999.
647. Agerholm JS, Bendixen C, Andersen O, et al: Complex vertebral malformation in Holstein calves, J Vet Diagn Invest 13:283–289, 2001.
648. van den Broek AHM, Else RW, Abercromby R, et al: Spinal dysraphism in the Weimaraner, J Small Anim Pract 32(5):258–260, 1991.
649. Fingeroth JM, Johnson GC, Burt JK, et al: Neuroradiographic diagnosis and surgical repair of tethered cord syndrome in an English bulldog with spina bifida and myeloschisis, J Am Vet Med Assoc 194(9):1300–1302, 1989.
650. Plummer SB, Bunch SE, Khoo LH, et al: Tethered spinal cord and an intradural lipoma associated with a meningocele in a Manx-type cat, J Am Vet Med Assoc 203(8):1159–1161, 1993.
651. Dorn AS, Joiner RW: Surgical removal of a meningocele from a Manx cat, Feline Pract 6:37–40, 1976.
652. de Lahunta A, Glass E: Veterinary neuroanatomy and clinical neurology, St Louis, 2009, Saunders Elsevier.
653. Franklin RJM, Ramsey IK, McKerrel RLE: An inherited neurological disorder of the St. Bernard dog characterised by unusual cerebellar cortical dysplasia, Vet Rec 140:656–657, 1997.
654. Dow RS: Partial agenesis of the cerebellum in dogs, J Comp Neurol 72:569–586, 1940.
655. Schmid V, Lang J, Wolf M: Dandy-Walker-like syndrome in four dogs: cisternography as a diagnostic aid, J Am Anim Hosp Assoc 28(4):355–360, 1992.
656. Thomas JB, Robertson D: Hereditary cerebellar abiotrophy in Australian kelpie dogs, Aust Vet J 66(9):301–302, 1989.
657. Kent M, Glass E, de Lahunta A: Cerebellar cortical abiotrophy in a beagle, J Small Anim Pract 41:321–323, 2000.
658. Yasuba M, Okimoto K, Iida M, et al: Cerebellar cortical degeneration in beagle dogs, Vet Pathol 25(4):315–317, 1988.
659. Coates JR, O'Brien DP, Kline KL, et al: Neonatal cerebellar ataxia in Coton de Tulear dogs, J Vet Intern Med 16:680–689, 2002.
660. Nesbit JW, Ueckermann JF: Cerebellar cortical atrophy in a puppy, J S Afr Vet Assoc 52(3):247–250, 1981.
661. Sakai T, Harashima T, Yamamura H, et al: Two cases of hereditary quadriplegia and amblyopia in a litter of Irish setters, J Small Anim Pract 35(4):221–223, 1994.
662. Palmer AC, Payne JE, Wallace ME: Hereditary quadriplegia and amblyopia in the Irish Setter, J Small Anim Pract 14(6):343–352, 1973.
663. Cummings JF, de Lahunta A: A study of cerebellar and cerebral cortical degeneration in miniature poodle pups with emphasis on the ultrastructure of Purkinje cell changes, Acta Neuropathol 75(3):261–271, 1988.
664. Chieffo C, Stalis IH, Van Winkle TJ, et al: Cerebellar Purkinje cell degeneration and coat color dilution in a family of Rhodesian ridgeback dogs, J Vet Intern Med 8(2):112–116, 1994.
665. de Lahunta A: Abiotrophy in domestic animals: a review, Can J Vet Res 54(1):65–76, 1990.
666. Flegel T, Matiasek K, Henke D, et al: Cerebellar cortical degeneration with selective granule cell loss in Bavarian mountain dogs, J Small Anim Pract 48(8):462–465, 2007.
667. Carmichael KP, Miller M, Rawlings CA, et al: Clinical, hematologic, and biochemical features of a syndrome in Bernese mountain dogs characterized by hepatocerebellar degeneration, J Am Vet Med Assoc 208(8):1277–1279, 1996.
668. Fankhauser R, Freudiger U, Vandevelde M, et al: Purkinjezellatrophie nach Masernvirus-Vakzinierung beim Hund, Schweiz Archiv Neurol Neurochir Psychiatr 112:353–363, 1973.
669. Sandy JR, Slocombe RF, Mitten RW, et al: Cerebellar abiotrophy in a family of border collie dogs, Vet Pathol 39:736–739, 2002.
670. Carmichael KP, Miller M, Rawlings CA, et al: Clinical, hematologic, and biochemical features of a syndrome in Bernese mountain dogs characterized by hepatocerebellar degeneration, J Am Vet Med Assoc 208(8):1277–1279, 1996.
671. Higgins RJ, LeCouteur RA, Kornegay JN, et al: Late-onset progressive spinocerebellar degeneration in Brittany spaniel dogs, Acta Neuropathol 96(1):97–101, 1998.
672. Tatalick LM, Marks SL, Baszler TV: Cerebellar abiotrophy characterized by granular cell loss in a Brittany, Vet Pathol 30(4):385–388, 1993.
673. Tipold A, Fatzer R, Jaggy A, et al: Presumed immune-mediated cerebellar granuloprival degeneration in the Coton de Tulear breed, J Neuroimmunol 110(1-2):130–133, 2000.
674. Gandini G, Botteron C, Brini E, et al: Cerebellar cortical degeneration in three English bulldogs: clinical and neuropathological findings, J Small Anim Pract 46(6):291–294, 2005.

675. O'Brien DP: Hereditary cerebellar ataxia. In the Proceedings of the 11th ACVIM Forum, Washington DC: 546–549, 1993.
676. Coates JR, Carmichael KP, Shelton D, et al: Preliminary characterization of a cerebellar ataxia in Jack Russell terriers, J Vet Intern Med 10(3):176, 1996.
677. Cantile C, Salvadori C, Modenato M, et al: Cerebellar granuloprival degeneration in an Italian hound, J Vet Med A Physiol Pathol Clin Med 49(10):523–525, 2002.
678. Bildfell RJ, Mitchell SK, de Lahunta AD: Cerebellar cortical degeneration in a Labrador retriever, Can Vet J 36(9):570–572, 1995.
679. Jokinen TS, Rusbridge C, Steffen F, et al: Cerebellar cortical abiotrophy in Lagotto Romagnolo dogs, J Small Anim Pract 48(8):470–473, 2007.
680. Berry ML, Blas-Machado U: Cerebellar abiotrophy in a miniature schnauzer, Can Vet J 44(8):657–659, 2003.
681. Steinberg HS, Winkle TV, Bell JS, et al: Cerebellar degeneration in Old English sheepdogs, J Am Vet Med Assoc 217(8):1162–1165, 2000.
682. van Tongeren SE, van Vonderen IK, van Nes JJ, et al: Cerebellar cortical abiotrophy in two Portuguese podengo littermates, Vet Q 22:172–174, 2001.
683. van der Merwe LL, Lane E: Diagnosis of cerebellar cortical degeneration in a Scottish terrier using magnetic resonance imaging, J Small Anim Pract 42(8):409–412, 2001.
684. Olby N, Blot S, Thibaud JL, et al: Cerebellar cortical degeneration in adult American Staffordshire terriers, J Vet Intern Med 18(2):201–208, 2004.
685. Aye MM, Izumo S, Inada S, et al: Histopathological and ultrastructural features of feline hereditary cerebellar cortical atrophy: a novel animal model of human spinocerebellar degeneration, Acta Neuropathol 96(4):379–387, 1998.
686. Inada S, Mochizuki M, Izumo S, et al: Study of hereditary cerebellar degeneration in cats, Am J Vet Res 57(3):296–301, 1996.
687. Barone G, Foureman P, de Lahunta A: Adult-onset cerebellar cortical abiotrophy and retinal degeneration in a domestic shorthair cat, J Am Anim Hosp Assoc 38:51–54, 2002.
688. Shamir M, Perl S, Sharon L: Late onset of cerebellar abiotrophy in a Siamese cat, J Small Anim Pract 40(7):343–345, 1999.
689. Negrin A, Bernardini M, Baumgärtner W, et al: Late onset cerebellar degeneration in a middle-aged cat, J Feline Med Surg 8(6):424–429, 2006.
690. Carmichael KP, Richey LJ: Cerebellar Purkinje cell degeneration and hepatic microvascular dysplasia in Havana Brown kittens, Vet Pathol 42:689, 2005:(abstract).
691. O'Brien DP, Johnson GS, Schnabel RD, et al: Genetic mapping of canine multiple system degeneration and ectodermal dysplasia loci, J Hered 96(7):727–734, 2005.
692. Cummings JF, de Lahunta A, Gasteiger EL: Multisystemic chromatolytic neuronal degeneration in cairn terriers. A case with generalized cataplectic episodes, J Vet Intern Med 5(2):91–94, 1991.
693. da Costa RC, Parent JM, Poma R, et al: Multisystem axonopathy and neuronopathy in Golden retriever dogs, J Vet Intern Med 23:935–939, 2009.
694. Kortz GD, Meier WA, Higgins RJ, et al: Neuronal vacuolation and spinocerebellar degeneration in young Rottweiler dogs, Vet Pathol 34(4):296–302, 1997.
695. Sandefeldt E, Cummings JF, de Lahunta A: Animal model of human disease. Infantile spinal muscular atrophy, Werdnig-Hoffman disease. Animal model: hereditary neuronal abiotrophy in Swedish Lapland dogs, Am J Pathol 82:649–652, 1976.
696. Resibois A, Poncelet L: Olivopontocerebellar atrophy in two adult cats, sporadic cases or new genetic entity, Vet Pathol 41(1):20–29, 2004.
697. Diaz JD, Duque C, Geisel R: Neuroaxonal dystrophy in dogs: case report in 2 litters of papillon puppies, J Vet Intern Med 21:531–534, 2007.
698. Nibe K, Kita C, Morozumi M, et al: Clinicopathological features of canine neuroaxonal dystrophy and cerebellar cortical abiotrophy in papillon and papillon-related dogs, J Vet Med Sci 69(10):1047–1052, 2007.
699. Carmichael KP, Howerth EW, Oliver JE Jr, et al: Neuroaxonal dystrophy in a group of related cats, J Vet Diagn Invest 5(4):585–590, 1993.
700. Rodriguez F, Espinosa de los Monteros A, Morales M, et al: Neuroaxonal dystrophy in two Siamese kitten littermates, Vet Res 138:548–549, 1996.
701. Mayhew IG: Large animal neurology, ed 2, Ames, Iowa, 2009, Wiley-Blackwell.
702. Jeffrey M, Preece BE, Holliman A: Dandy-Walker malformation in two calves, Vet Rec 126(20):499–501, 1990.
703. Washburn KE, Streeter RN: Congenital defects of the ruminant nervous system, Vet Clin North Am Food Anim Pract 20:413–434, 2004.
704. Wallace MA, Scarratt WK, Crisman MV, et al: Familial convulsions and ataxia in an Aberdeen angus calf, Prog Vet Neurol 7(4):145–148, 1996.
705. Innes JRM, Russel DS, Wilsdon AJ: Familial cerebellar hypoplasia and degeneration in Hereford calves, J Pathol Bacteriol 50:455–461, 1940.
706. Saunders LZ, Sweet JD, Martin SM, et al: Hereditary congenital ataxia in Jersey calves, Cornell Vet 42:559–591, 1952.
707. Allen JG: Congenital cerebellar hypoplasia in Jersey calves, Aust Vet J 53(4):173–175, 1977.
708. Edmonds L, Crenshaw D, Selby LA: Micrognathia and cerebellar hypoplasia in an Aberdeen angus herd, J Hered 64(2):62–64, 1973.
709. Innes JRM, Russell DS, Wilsdon AJ: Familial cerebellar hypoplasia and degeneration in Hereford calves, J Pathol Bacteriol 50:455–461, 1940.
710. Schild AL, Riet-Correa F, Fernandes CG, et al: Cerebellar hypoplasia and porencephaly in Charolais cattle in Southern Brazil, Ciencia Rural 31(1):149–153, 2001.
711. Finnie EP, Leaver DD: Cerebellar hypoplasia in calves, Aust Vet J 41:287–288, 1965.
712. Johnson KR, Fourt DL, Ross RH, et al: Hereditary congenital ataxia in Holstein-Friesian calves, J Dairy Sci 41:1371–1375, 1958.
713. Kemp J, McOrist S, Jeffrey M: Cerebellar abiotrophy in Holstein Friesian calves, Vet Rec 136(8):198, 1995.
714. Schild AL, Riet-Correa F, Portiansky EL, et al: Congenital cerebellar cortical degeneration in Holstein cattle in southern Brazil, Vet Res Commun 25(3):189–195, 2001.
715. Cho DY, Leipold HW: Cerebellar cortical atrophy in a Charolais calf, Vet Pathol 15(2):264–266, 1978.
716. Mitchell PJ, Reilly W, Harper PAW, et al: Cerebellar abiotrophy in angus cattle, Aust Vet J 70(2):67–68, 1993.
717. Woodman MP, Scott PR, Watt N, et al: Selective cerebellar degeneration in a Limousin cross heifer, Vet Rec 132(23):586–587, 1993.

718. Innes JRM, MacNaughton WN: Inherited cortical cerebellar atrophy in Corriedale lambs in Canada identical with daft lamb disease in Britain, Cornell Vet 40:127–135, 1950.
719. Milne EM, Schock A: Cerebellar abiotrophy in a pedigree Charolais sheep flock, Vet Rec 143:224–225, 1998.
720. Johnstone AC, Johnson CB, Malcolm KE, et al: Cerebellar cortical abiotrophy in Wiltshire sheep, N Z Vet J 53(4):242–245, 2005.
721. Gregory DW, Mead SW, Regan WM: Hereditary congenital lethal spasms in Jersey cattle, J Hered 35:195–200, 1944.
722. High JW, Kincaid CM, Smith HJ: Doddler cattle, J Hered 49:250–252, 1958.
723. Adams EW: Hereditary deafness in a family of foxhounds, J Am Vet Med Assoc 128:302–303, 1956.
724. Coppens AG, Gilbert-Gregory S, Steinberg SA, et al: Inner ear histopathology in "nervous Pointer dogs" with severe hearing loss, Hear Res 200:51–62, 2005.
725. Coppens AG, Kiss R, Heizmann CW, et al: An original inner ear neuroepithelial degeneration in a deaf Rottweiler puppy, Hear Res 161:65–71, 2001.
726. Coppens AG, Resibois A, Poncelet L: Bilateral deafness in a Maltese terrier and a great Pyrenean puppy: inner ear morphology, J Comp Pathol 122:223–228, 2000.
727. Coppens AG, Steinberg SA, Poncelet L: Inner ear morphology in a bilaterally deaf Dogo Argentino pup, J Comp Pathol 128:67–70, 2003.
728. Erickson F, Saperstein G, Leipold HW, et al: Congenital defects of dogs - Part 3, Canine Pract 4:40–53, 1977.
729. Gwin RM, Wyman M, Lim DJ, et al: Multiple ocular defects associated with partial albinism and deafness in the dog, J Am Anim Hosp Assoc 17:401–408, 1981.
730. Strain GM: Congenital deafness in dogs and cats, Compend Contin Educ Pract Vet 13:245–250, 1991:252–253.
731. Wilkes MK, Palmer AC: Congenital deafness and vestibular deficit in the Doberman, J Small Anim Pract 33:218–224, 1992.
732. Famula TR, Cargill EJ, Strain GM: Heritability and complex segregation analysis of deafness in Jack Russell terriers, BMC Vet Res 3:31, 2007.
733. Bosher SK, Hallpike CS: Observations on the histogenesis of the inner ear degeneration of the deaf white cat and its possible relationship to the aetiology of certain unexplained varieties of human congenital deafness, J Laryngol Otol 80:222–235, 1966.
734. Rebillard G, Rebillard M, Carlier E, et al: Histo-physiological relationships in the deaf white cat auditory system, Acta Otolaryngol 82:48–56, 1976.
735. Wolff D: Three generations of deaf white cats, J Hered 33:39–43, 1942.
736. Cvejic D, Steinberg TA, Kent MS, et al: Unilateral and bilateral congenital sensorineural deafness in client-owned pure-breed white cats, J Vet Intern Med 23:392–395, 2009.
737. Harland MM, Stewart AJ, Marshall AE, et al: Diagnosis of deafness in a horse by brainstem auditory evoked potential, Can Vet J 47:151–154, 2006.
738. Bosher SK, Hallpike CS: Observations on the histological features, development and pathogenesis of the inner ear degeneration of the deaf white cat, Proc R Soc Lond B Biol Sci 162:147–170, 1965.
739. Holliday TA, Nelson HJ, Williams DC, et al: Unilateral and bilateral brainstem auditory-evoked response abnormalities in 900 Dalmatian dogs, J Vet Intern Med 6:166–174, 1992.
740. Strain GM, Kearney MT, Gignac IJ, et al: Brainstem auditory-evoked potential assessment of congenital deafness in Dalmatians: associations with phenotypic markers, J Vet Intern Med 6:175–182, 1992.
741. Famula TR, Oberbauer AM, Sousa CA: A threshold model analysis of deafness in Dalmatians, Mamm Genome 7:650–653, 1996.
742. Juraschko K, Meyer-Lindenberg A, Nolte I, et al: Analysis of systematic effects on congenital sensorineural deafness in German Dalmatian dogs, Vet J 166:164–169, 2003.
743. Muhle AC, Jaggy A, Stricker C, et al: Further contributions to the genetic aspect of congenital sensorineural deafness in Dalmatians, Vet J 163:311–318, 2002.
744. Wood JLN, Lakhani KH: Prevalence and prevention of deafness in the Dalmatian: assessing the effect of parental hearing status and gender using ordinary logistic and generalized random litter effect models, Vet J 154:121–133, 1997.
745. Strain GM: Deafness prevalence and pigmentation and gender associations in dog breeds at risk, Vet J 167:23–32, 2004.
746. Famula TR, Oberbauer AM, Sousa CA: Complex segregation analysis of deafness in Dalmatians, Am J Vet Res 61:550–553, 2000.
747. Greibrokk T: Hereditary deafness in the Dalmatian: relationship to eye and coat color, J Am Anim Hosp Assoc 30:170–176, 1994.
748. Bergsma DR, Brown KS: White fur, blue eyes, and deafness in the domestic cat, J Hered 62:171–185, 1971.
749. Mair IW: Hereditary deafness in the white cat, Acta Otolaryngol Suppl 314:1–48, 1973.
750. Ryugo DK, Cahill HB, Rose LS, et al: Separate forms of pathology in the cochlea of congenitally deaf white cats, Hear Res 181:73–84, 2003.
751. Geigy CA, Heid S, Steffen F, et al: Does a pleiotropic gene explain deafness and blue irises in white cats? Vet J 173:548–553, 2007.
752. Finnigan DF, Hanna WJ, Poma R, et al: A novel mutation of the CLCN1 gene associated with myotonia hereditaria in an Australian cattle dog, J Vet Intern Med 21:458–463, 2007.
753. Hill SL, Shelton GD, Lenehan TM: Myotonia in a cocker spaniel, J Am Anim Hosp Assoc 31:506–509, 1995.
754. Honhold N, Smith DA: Myotonia in the Great Dane, Vet Rec 119:162, 1986.
755. Lobetti RG: Myotonia congenita in a Jack Russell terrier, J S Afr Vet Assoc 80:106–107, 2009.
756. Shires PK, Nafe LA, Hulse DA: Myotonia in a Staffordshire terrier, J Am Vet Med Assoc 183:229–232, 1983.
757. Vite CH, Melniczek J, Patterson D, et al: Congenital myotonic myopathy in the miniature schnauzer: an autosomal recessive trait, J Hered 90:578–580, 1999.
758. Griffiths IR, Duncan ID: Myotonia in the dog: a report of four cases, Vet Rec 93:184–188, 1973.
759. Hickford FH, Jones BR, Gething MA, et al: Congenital myotonia in related kittens, J Small Anim Pract 39:281–285, 1998.
760. Toll J, Cooper B, Altschul M: Congenital myotonia in 2 domestic cats, J Vet Intern Med 12:116–119, 1998.
761. Gracis M, Keith D, Vite CH: Dental and craniofacial findings in eight miniature schnauzer dogs affected by myotonia congenita: preliminary results, J Vet Dent 17:119–127, 2000.
762. Rhodes TH, Vite CH, Giger U, et al: A missense mutation in canine C1C-1 causes recessive myotonia congenita in the dog, FEBS Lett 456:54–58, 1999.

763. Thomas WB: Idiopathic epilepsy in dogs, Vet Clin North Am Small Anim Pract 30:183–206, 2000:vii.
764. Berendt M, Gredal H, Pedersen LG, et al: A cross-sectional study of epilepsy in Danish Labrador retrievers: prevalence and selected risk factors, J Vet Intern Med 16:262–268, 2002.
765. Berendt M, Gullov CH, Christensen SL, et al: Prevalence and characteristics of epilepsy in the Belgian shepherd variants Groenendael and Tervuren born in Denmark 1995-2004, Acta Vet Scand 50:51, 2008.
766. Heynold Y, Faissler D, Steffen F, et al: Clinical, epidemiological and treatment results of idiopathic epilepsy in 54 Labrador retrievers: a long-term study, J Small Anim Pract 38:7–14, 1997.
767. Berendt M, Gullov CH, Fredholm M: Focal epilepsy in the Belgian shepherd: evidence for simple Mendelian inheritance, J Small Anim Pract 50:655–661, 2009.
768. Kathmann I, Jaggy A, Busato A, et al: Clinical and genetic investigations of idiopathic epilepsy in the Bernese mountain dog, J Small Anim Pract 40:319–325, 1999.
769. Casal ML, Munuve RM, Janis MA, et al: Epilepsy in Irish wolfhounds, J Vet Intern Med 20:131–135, 2006.
770. Hülsmeyer V, Zimmermann R, Brauer C, et al: Epilepsy in border collies: clinical manifestation, outcome, and mode of inheritance. J Vet Intern Med 24:171-178, 2010.
771. Jokinen TS, Metsahonkala L, Bergamasco L, et al: Benign familial juvenile epilepsy in Lagotto Romagnolo dogs, J Vet Intern Med 21:464–471, 2007.
772. Patterson EE, Armstrong PJ, O'Brien DP, et al: Clinical description and mode of inheritance of idiopathic epilepsy in English springer spaniels, J Am Vet Med Assoc 226:54–58, 2005.
773. Patterson EE, Mickelson JR, Da Y, et al: Clinical characteristics and inheritance of idiopathic epilepsy in vizslas, J Vet Intern Med 17:319–325, 2003.
774. Srenk P, Jaggy A: Interictal electroencephalographic findings in a family of golden retrievers with idiopathic epilepsy, J Small Anim Pract 37:317–321, 1996.
775. Viitmaa R, Cizinauskas S, Bergamasco LA, et al: Magnetic resonance imaging findings in Finnish spitz dogs with focal epilepsy, J Vet Intern Med 20:305–310, 2006.
776. Licht BG, Lin S, Luo Y, et al: Clinical characteristics and mode of inheritance of familial focal seizures in standard poodles, J Am Vet Med Assoc 231:1520–1528, 2007.
777. Aleman M, Gray LC, Williams DC, et al: Juvenile idiopathic epilepsy in Egyptian Arabian foals: 22 cases (1985-2005), J Vet Intern Med 20:1443–1449, 2006.
778. Coates JR, Bergman RL: Seizures in young dogs and cats: pathophysiology and diagnosis, Compend Contin Educ Pract Vet 27:447–459, 2005.
779. Herrtage ME: Canine fucosidosis, Vet Ann 28:223–227, 1988.
780. Barker CG, Herrtage ME, Shanahan F, et al: Fucosidosis in English springer spaniels: results of a trial screening programme, J Small Anim Pract 29(10):623–630, 1988.
781. Littlewood JD, Herrtage ME, Palmer AC: Neuronal storage disease in English springer spaniels, Vet Rec 112(4):86–87, 1983.
782. Skelly BJ, Sargan DR, Winchester BG, et al: Genomic screening for fucosidosis in English springer spaniels, Am J Vet Res 60(6):726–729, 1999.
783. Smith MO, Wenger DA, Hill SL, et al: Fucosidosis in a family of American-bred English springer spaniels, J Am Vet Med Assoc 209(12):2088–2090, 1996.
784. Berg T, Tollersrud OK, Walkley SU, et al: Purification of feline lysosomal α-mannosidase, determination of its cDNA sequence and identification of a mutation causing α-mannosidosis in Persian cats, Biochem J 328(3):863–870, 1997.
785. Blakemore WF: A case of mannosidosis in the cat: clinical and histopathological findings, J Small Anim Pract 27(7):447–455, 1986.
786. Cummings JF, Wood PA, de Lahunta A, et al: The clinical and pathologic heterogeneity of feline a-mannosidosis, J Vet Intern Med 2(4):163–170, 1988.
787. Healy PJ, Harper PA, Dennis JA: Phenotypic variation in bovine a-mannosidosis, Res Vet Sci 49(1):82–84, 1990.
788. Maenhout T, Kint JA, Dacremont G, et al: Mannosidosis in a litter of Persian cats, Vet Rec 122(15):351–354, 1988.
789. Vandevelde M, Fankhauser R, Bichsel P, et al: Hereditary neurovisceral mannosidosis associated with α-mannosidase deficiency in a family of Persian cats, Acta Neuropathol 58(1):64–68, 1982.
790. Bryan L, Schmutz S, Hodges SD, et al: Bovine b-mannosidosis: pathologic and genetic findings in Salers calves, Vet Pathol 30(2):130–139, 1993.
791. Shapiro JL, Rostkowski C, Little PB, et al: Caprine b-mannosidosis in kids from an Ontario herd, Can Vet J 26(5):155–158, 1985.
793. Gredal H, Berendt M, Leifsson PS: Progressive myoclonus epilepsy in a beagle, J Small Anim Pract 44(11):511–514, 2003.
794. Hall DG, Steffens WL, Lassiter L: Lafora bodies associated with neurologic signs in a cat, Vet Pathol 35(3):218–220, 1998.
795. Jian Z, Alley MR, Cayzer J, et al: Lafora's disease in an epileptic basset hound, N Z Vet J 38(2):75–79, 1990.
796. Kaiser E, Krauser K, Schwartz-Porsche D: Lafora disease (progressive myoclonus epilepsy) in the basset hound. Early diagnosis by muscle biopsy, Tierarztl Prax 19(3):290–295, 1991.
797. Moreau PM, Vallat JM, Hugon J, et al: Lafora's disease in Basset hounds. In the Proceedings of 8th ACVIM Forum, Washington DC: 1045–1049, 1990.
798. Webb AA, McMillan C, Cullen CL, et al: Lafora disease as a cause of visually exacerbated myoclonic attacks in a dog, Can Vet J 50(9):963–967, 2009.
799. Brix AE, Howerth EW, McConkie-Rosell A, et al: Glycogen storage disease type Ia in two littermate Maltese puppies, Vet Pathol 32(5):460–465, 1995.
800. Walvoort HC, Koster JF, Reuser AJ: Heterozygote detection in a family of Lapland dogs with a recessively inherited metabolic disease: canine glycogen storage disease type II, Res Vet Sci 38(2):174–178, 1985.
801. Walvoort HC, Slee RG, Koster JF: Canine glycogen storage disease type II. A biochemical study of an acid alpha-glucosidase-deficient Lapland dog, Biochim Biophys Acta 715(1):63–69, 1982.
802. Walvoort HC: Glycogen storage disease type II in the Lapland dog, Vet Q 7(3):187–190, 1985.
803. Dennis JA, Healy PJ, Reichmann KG: Genotyping Brahman cattle for generalised glycogenosis, Aust Vet J 80(5):286–291, 2002.
804. Reichmann KG, Twist JO, Thistlethwaite EJ: Clinical, diagnostic and biochemical features of generalised glycogenosis type II and Brahman cattle, Aust Vet J 70(11):405–408, 1993.
805. Dennis JA, Moran C, Healy PJ: The bovine α-glucosidase gene: coding region, genomic structure, and mutations that cause bovine generalized glycogenosis, Mamm Genome 11(3):206–212, 2000.

806. Dennis JA, Healy PJ: Genotyping shorthorn cattle for generalised glycogenosis, Aust Vet J 79(11):773–775, 2001.
807. Manktelow BW, Hartley WJ: Generalized glycogen storage disease in sheep, J Comp Pathol 85(1):139–145, 1975.
808. Gregory BL, Shelton GD, Bali DS, et al: Glycogen storage disease type IIIa in curly-coated retrievers, J Vet Intern Med 21(1):40–46, 2007.
809. Rafiquzzaman M, Svenkerud R, Strande A, et al: Glycogenosis in the dog, Acta Vet Scand 17(2):196–209, 1976.
810. Coates JR, Paxton R, Cox NR, et al: A case presentation and discussion of Type IV glycogen storage disease in a Norwegian forest cat, Prog Vet Neurol 7(1):5–11, 1996.
811. Fyfe JC, Giger U, Van Winkle TJ, et al: Glycogen storage disease type IV: inherited deficiency of branching enzyme activity in cats, Pediatr Res 32(6):719–725, 1992.
812. Fyfe JC, Giger U, Van Winkle TJ, et al: Familial glycogen storage disease type IV (GSD IV) in Norwegian forest cast. In the Proceedings of the 8th ACVIM Forum, Washington DC: 1129, 1990.
813. Johnstone AC, McSporran KD, Kenny JE, et al: Myophosphorylase deficiency (glycogen storage disease Type V) in a herd of Charolais cattle in New Zealand: confirmation by PCR-RFLP testing, N Z Vet J 52(6):404–408, 2004.
814. Smith BF, Stedman H, Rajpurohit Y, et al: Molecular basis of canine muscle type phosphofructokinase deficiency, J Biol Chem 271(33):20070–20074, 1996.
815. Harvey JW, Calderwood MM, Gropp KE, et al: Polysaccharide storage myopathy in canine phosphofructokinase deficiency (type VII glycogen storage disease), Vet Pathol 27(1):1–8, 1990.
816. Bosshard NU, Hubler M, Arnold S, et al: Spontaneous mucolipidosis in a cat: an animal model of human I-cell disease, Vet Pathol 33(1):1–13, 1996.
817. Giger U, Teherneva E, Caverly J, et al: A missense point mutation in N-acetylglucosamine-1-phosphotransferase causes mucolipidosis II in domestic shorthair cats, J Vet Intern Med 20:781, 2006.
818. Muller G, Alldinger S, Moritz A, et al: GM1-gangliosidosis in Alaskan huskies: clinical and pathologic findings, Vet Pathol 38(3):281–290, 2001.
819. Shell LG, Potthoff AI, Carithers R, et al: Neuronal-visceral GM1 gangliosidosis in Portuguese water dogs, J Vet Intern Med 3(1):1–7, 1989.
820. Alroy J, Orgad U, DeGasperi R, et al: Canine GM1-gangliosidosis. A clinical, morphologic, histochemical, and biochemical comparison of two different models, Am J Pathol 140(3):675–689, 1992.
821. Yamato O, Ochiai K, Masuoka Y, et al: GM1 gangliosidosis in Shiba dogs, Vet Rec 146(17):493–496, 2000.
822. Yamato O, Kobayashi A, Satoh H, et al: Comparison of polymerase chain reaction-restriction fragment length polymorphism assay and enzyme assay for diagnosis of GM1-gangliosidosis in Shiba dogs, J Vet Diagn Invest 16(4):299–304, 2004.
823. Murnane RD, Hern-Rindell AJ, Prieur DJ: Ovine GM_1 gangliosidosis, Small Rumin Res 6(1-2):109–118, 1991.
824. Donnelly WJC, Sheahan BJ: Bovine, GM_1 gangliosidosis: an inborn lysosomal disease, Vet Sci Commun 1(1):65–74, 1977.
825. De Maria R, Divari S, Bo S, et al: Beta-galactosidase deficiency in a korat cat: a new form of feline GM_1-gangliosidosis, Acta Neuropathol 96(3):307–314, 1998.
826. Dial SM, Mitchell TW, LeCouteur RA, et al: GM_1-gangliosidosis (type II) in three cats, J Am Anim Hosp Assoc 30(4):355–360, 1994.
827. Singer HS, Cork LC: Canine GM_2 gangliosidosis: morphological and biochemical analysis, Vet Pathol 26(2):114–120, 1989.
828. Bernheimer H, Karbe E: Morphological and neurochemical investigations of two types of amaurotic idiocy in the dog. Evidence of a GM_2-gangliosidosis, Acta Neuropathol 16:243–261, 1970.
828a. Matsuki N, Yamato O, Kusuda M, et al: Magnetic resonance imaging of GM2-gangliosidosis in a golden retriever, J Vet Intern Med 46:275–278, 2005.
828b. Yamato O, Matsuki N, Satoh H, et al: Sandhoff disease in a golden retriever dog, J Inherit Metab Dis 25:319–320, 2002.
829. Neuwelt EA, Johnson WG, Blank NK, et al: Characterization of a new model of GM_2-gangliosidosis (Sandhoff's disease) in korat cats, J Clin Invest 76(2):482–490, 1985.
830. Yamato O, Matsunaga S, Takata K, et al: GM_2-gangliosidosis variant 0 (Sandhoff-like disease) in a family of Japanese domestic cats, Vet Rec 155(23):739–744, 2004.
831. Bradbury AM, Morrison NE, Hwang M, et al: Neurodegenerative lysosomal storage disease in European Burmese cats with hexosaminidase β-subunit deficiency, Mol Genet Metab 97(1):53–59, 2009.
832. Kosanke SD, Pierce KR, Bay WW: Clinical and biochemical abnormalities in porcine GM2-gangliosidosis, Vet Pathol 15(6):685–699, 1978.
833. Ishikawa Y, Li SC, Wood PA, et al: Biochemical basis of type AB GM2 gangliosidosis in a Japanese spaniel, J Neurochem 48(3):860–864, 1987.
834. Victoria T, Rafi MA, Wenger DA: Cloning of the canine GALC cDNA and identification of the mutation causing globoid cell leukodystrophy in West Highland white and cairn terriers, Genomics 33(3):457–462, 1996.
835. Wenger DA, Victoria T, Rafi MA, et al: Globoid cell leukodystrophy in Cairn and West Highland White terriers, J Hered 90(1):138–142, 1999.
836. McDonnell JJ, Carmichael KP, McGraw RA, et al: Preliminary characterization of globoid cell leukodystrophy in Irish setters, J Vet Intern Med 14(3):339, 2000.
837. McGraw RA, Carmichael KP: Molecular basis of globoid cell leukodystrophy in Irish setters, Vet J 171(2):370–372, 2006.
838. Sigurdson CJ, Basaraba RJ, Mazzaferro EM, et al: Globoid cell-like leukodystrophy in a domestic longhaired cat, Vet Pathol 39:494–496, 2002.
839. Wenger DA, Sattler M, Kudoh T, et al: Niemann-Pick disease: a genetic model in Siamese cats, Science 208:1471–1473, 1980.
840. Yamagami T, Umeda M, Kamiya S, et al: Neurovisceral sphingomyelinosis in a Siamese cat, Acta Neuropathol 79(3):330–332, 1989.
841. Baker HJ, Wood PA, Wenger DA, et al: Sphingomyelin lipidosis in a cat, Vet Pathol 24(5):386–391, 1987.
842. Somers KL, Royals MA, Carstea ED, et al: Mutation analysis of feline Niemann-Pick C1 disease, Mol Genet Metab 79(2):99–103, 2003.
843. Saunders GK, Wenger DA: Sphingomyelinase deficiency (Niemann-Pick disease) in a Hereford calf, Vet Pathol 45(2):201–202, 2008.

844. Lowenthal AC, Cummings JF, Wenger DA, et al: Feline sphingolipidosis resembling Niemann-Pick disease type C, Acta Neuropathol 81(2):189–197, 1990.
844a. Wilkerson MJ, Lewis DC, Marks SL, et al: Clinical and morphologic features of mucopolysaccharidosis type II in a dog: naturally occurring model of Hunter syndrome, Vet Pathol 35(3):230–233, 1998.
845. Jolly RD, Ehrlich PC, Franklin RJM, et al: Histological diagnosis of mucopolysaccharidosis IIIA in a wire-haired dachshund, Vet Rec 148(18):564–567, 2001.
846. Jolly RD, Allan FJ, Collett MG, et al: Mucopolysaccharidosis IIIA (Sanfilippo syndrome) in a New Zealand huntaway dog with ataxia, N Z Vet J 48(5):144–148, 2000.
847. Jolly RD, Johnstone AC, Norman EJ, et al: Pathology of mucopolysaccharidosis IIIA in huntaway dogs, Vet Pathol 44(5):569–578, 2007.
848. Yogalingam G, Pollard T, Gliddon B, et al: Identification of a mutation causing mucopolysaccharidosis type IIIA in New Zealand huntaway dogs, Genomics 79(2):150–153, 2002.
849. Ellinwood NM, Wang P, Skeen T, et al: A model of mucopolysaccharidosis IIIB (Sanfilippo syndrome type IIIB): N-acetyl-alpha-D-glucosaminidase deficiency in schipperke dogs, J Inherit Metab Dis 26(5):489–504, 2003.
850. Hoard HM, Leipprandt JR, Cavanagh KT, et al: Determination of genotypic frequency of caprine mucopolysaccharidosis IIID, J Vet Diagn Invest 10(2):181–183, 1998.
851. Jones MZ, Alroy J, Boyer PJ, et al: Caprine mucopolysaccharidosis-IIID: clinical, biochemical, morphological and immunohistochemical characteristics, J Neuropathol Exp Neurol 57(2):148–157, 1998.
852. Fischer A, Carmichael KP, Munnell JF, et al: Sulfamidase deficiency in a family of dachshunds: a canine model of mucopolysaccharidosis IIIA (Sanfilippo A), Pediatr Res 44(1):74–82, 1998.
853. Neer TM, Dial SM, Pechman R, et al: Mucopolysaccharidosis VI in a miniature pinscher, J Vet Intern Med 9(6):429–433, 1995.
854. Breton L, Guérin P, Morin M: A case of mucopolysaccharidosis VI in a cat, J Am Anim Hosp Assoc 19(6):891–896, 1983.
855. Haskins ME, Aguirre GD, Jezyk PF, et al: The pathology of the feline model of mucopolysaccharidosis VI, Am J Pathol 101(3):657–674, 1980.
856. Ray J, Haskins ME, Ray K: Molecular diagnostic tests for ascertainment of genotype at the mucopolysaccharidosis type VII locus in dogs, Am J Vet Res 59(9):1092–1095, 1998.
857. Haskins ME, Otis EJ, Hayden JE, et al: Hepatic storage of glycosaminoglycans in feline and canine models of mucopolysaccharidoses I, VI, and VII, Vet Pathol 29(2):112–119, 1992.
858. Awano T, Katz ML, O'Brien DP, et al: A frame shift mutation in canine TPP1 (the ortholog of human CLN2) in a juvenile dachshund with neuronal ceroid lipofuscinosis, Mol Genet Metab 89(3):254–260, 2006.
859. Cummings JF, de Lahunta A, Riis RC, et al: Neuropathologic changes in a young adult Tibetan terrier with subclinical neuronal ceroid-lipofuscinosis, Prog Vet Neurol 1(3):301–309, 1990.
860. Katz ML, Narfstrom K, Johnson GS, et al: Assessment of retinal function and characterization of lysosomal storage body accumulation in the retinas and brains of Tibetan terriers with ceroid-lipofuscinosis, Am J Vet Res 66:67–76, 2005.
861. Melville SA, Wilson CL, Chiang CS, et al: A mutation in canine CLN5 causes neuronal ceroid lipofuscinosis in border collie dogs, Genomics 86:287–294, 2005.
862. O'Brien DP, Katz ML: Neuronal ceroid lipofuscinosis in 3 Australian shepherd littermates, J Vet Intern Med 22(2):472–475, 2008.
863. Tammen I, Houweling PJ, Frugier T, et al: A missense mutation (c.184C > T) in ovine CLN6 causes neuronal ceroid lipofuscinosis in merino sheep whereas affected South Hampshire sheep have reduced levels of CLN6 mRNA, Biochim Biophys Acta 1762(10):898–905, 2006.
864. Cook RW, Jolly RD, Palmer DN, et al: Neuronal ceroid lipofuscinosis in merino sheep, Aust Vet J 80(5):292–297, 2002.
865. Mayhew IG, Jolly RD, Pickett BT, et al: Ceroid-lipofuscinosis (Batten's disease): pathogenesis of blindness in the ovine model, Neuropathol Appl Neurobiol 11:273–290, 1985.
866. Katz ML, Khan S, Awano T, et al: A mutation in the CLN8 gene in English setter dogs with neuronal ceroid-lipofuscinosis, Biochem Biophys Res Commun 327:541–547, 2005.
867. Koppang N: The English setter with ceroid-lipofuscinosis: a suitable model for the juvenile type of ceroid-lipofuscinosis, Am J Med Genet Suppl 5:117–126, 1988.
868. Awano T, Katz ML, O'Brien DP, et al: A mutation in the cathepsin D gene (CTSD) in American bulldogs with neuronal ceroid lipofuscinosis, Mol Genet Metab , 2006:(in press).
869. Evans J, Katz ML, Levesque D, et al: A variant form of neuronal ceroid lipofuscinosis in American bulldogs, J Vet Intern Med 19(1):44–51, 2005.
870. Jolly RD: Comparative biology of the neuronal ceroid-lipofuscinoses: an overview, Am J Med Genet 57:307–311, 1995.
871. Cantile C, Buonaccorsi A, Pepe V, et al: Juvenile neuronal ceroid-lipofuscinosis (Batten's disease) in a poodle dog, Prog Vet Neurol 7(3):82–87, 1996.
872. Jolly RD, Sutton RH, Smith RIE, et al: Ceroid-lipofuscinosis in miniature schnauzer dogs, Aust Vet J 75(1):67, 1997.
873. Modenato M, Marchetti V, Barsotti G, et al: Neuronal ceroid-lipofuscinosis in a Chihuahua, Annali della Facoltiá di Medicina Veterinaria di Pisa 60:215–224, 2007.
874. Goebel HH, Bilzer T, Dahme E, et al: Morphological studies in canine (Dalmatian) neuronal ceroid-lipofuscinosis, Am J Med Gen (suppl 5):127–139, 1988.
875. Vandevelde M, Fatzer R: Neuronal ceroid-lipofuscinosis in older dachshunds, Vet Pathol 17(6):686–692, 1980.
876. Bildfell R, Matwichuk C, Mitchell S, et al: Neuronal ceroid-lipofuscinosis in a cat, Vet Pathol 32(5):485–488, 1995.
877. Cummings JF, de Lahunta A: An adult case of canine neuronal ceroid lipofuscinosis, Acta Neuropathol 39:43–51, 1977.
878. Kuwamura M, Nakagawa M, Nabe M, et al: Neuronal ceroid-lipofuscinosis in a Japanese domestic shorthair cat, J Vet Med Sci 71(5):665–667, 2009.
879. Jolly RD, Walkley SU: Lysosomal storage diseases of animals: an essay in comparative pathology, Vet Pathol 34(6):527–548, 1997.
880. Pickett P, Dyer K, Saunders O, et al: Ocular manifestation of ceroid-lipofuscinosis in a Spitz dog, Vet Pathol 29:469, 1992.

881. Edwards JF, Storts RW, Joyce JR, et al: Juvenile-onset neuronal ceroid-lipofuscinosis in Rambouillet sheep, Vet Pathol 31(1):48–54, 1994.
882. Woods PR, Storts RW, Shelton M, et al: Neuronal ceroid lipofuscinosis in Rambouillet sheep: characterization of the clinical disease, J Vet Intern Med 8(5):370–375, 1994.
883. LeGonidec G, Kuberski T, Daynes P, et al: A neurologic disease of horses in New Caledonia, Aust Vet J 57:1944–1945, 1981.
884. Url A, Bauder B, Thalhammer J, et al: Equine neuronal ceroid lipofuscinosis, Acta Neuropathol 101:410–414, 2001.
885. Summers BA, Cummings JF, de Lahunta A: Veterinary neuropathology, St Louis, 1995, Mosby.
886. McGrath JT: In Andrews EJ, Ward BC, Altman NH, editors: Spontaneous animal models of human disease, Fibrinoid leukodystrophy (Alexander's disease), vol 2, New York, 1979, Academic Press.
887. Cox NR, Kwapien RP, Sorjonen DC, et al: Myeloencephalopathy resembling Alexander's disease in a Scottish terrier dog, Acta Neuropathol 71(1-2):163–166, 1986.
888. Sorjonen DC, Cox NR, Kwapien RP: Myeloencephalopathy with eosinophilic refractile bodies (Rosenthal fibers) in a Scottish terrier, J Am Vet Med Assoc 190(8):1004–1006, 1987.
889. Morrison JP, Schatzberg SJ, de Lahunta A, et al: Oligodendroglial dysplasia in two bull mastiff dogs, Vet Pathol 43(1):29–35, 2006.
890. Richardson JA, Tang K, Burns DK: Myeloencephalopathy with Rosenthal fiber formation in a miniature poodle, Vet Pathol 28(6):536–538, 1991.
891. Wouda W, van Nes JJ: Progressive ataxia due to central demyelination in Rottweiler dogs, Vet Q 8:89–97, 1986.
892. Mandigers PJJ, van Nes JJ, Knol BW, et al: Hereditary Kooiker dog ataxia, Res Vet Sci 54:118–123, 1993.
893. Wood SL, Patterson JS: Shetland sheepdog leukodystrophy, J Vet Intern Med 15:486–493, 2001.
894. Li FY, Cuddon PA, Song J, et al: Canine spongiform leukoencephalopathy is associated with a missense mutation in cytochrome b, Neurobiol Dis 21:35–42, 2006.
895. O'Brien DP, Zachary JF: Clinical features of spongy degeneration of the central nervous system in two Labrador retriever littermates, J Am Vet Med Assoc 186(11):1207–1210, 1985.
896. Zachary JF, O'Brien DP: Spongy degeneration of the central nervous system in two canine littermates, Vet Pathol 22:561–571, 1985.
897. Wessman A, Goedde T, Fischer A, et al: Hereditary ataxia in the Jack Russell terrier—clinical and genetic investigations, J Vet Intern Med 18:515–521, 2004.
898. Bjorck G, Mair W, Olsson SE, et al: Hereditary ataxia in fox terriers, Acta Neuropathol (suppl 1):45–48, 1962.
899. Oyster R, Leipold HW, Troyer D, et al: Clinical studies of bovine progressive degenerative myeloencephaly of Brown Swiss cattle, Prog Vet Neurol 2(3):159–164, 1991.
900. Wakshlag JJ, de Lahunta A: Hereditary encephalomyelopathy and polyneuropathy in an Alaskan husky, J Small Anim Pract 50:670–674, 2009.
901. Griffiths IR, McCulloch MC, Abrahams S: Progressive axonopathy: an inherited neuropathy of boxer dogs. 3. The peripheral axon lesion with special reference to the nerve roots, J Neurocytol 15(1):109–120, 1986.
902. Griffiths IR, McCulloch MC, Abrahams S: Progressive axonopathy: an inherited neuropathy of boxer dogs. 2. The nature and distribution of the pathological changes, Neuropathol Appl Neurobiol 11:431–446, 1985.
903. Jolly RD, Burbidge HM, Alley MR, et al: Progressive myelopathy and neuropathy in New Zealand huntaway dogs, N Z Vet J 48:188–191, 2000.
904. Palmer AC, Blakemore WF: A progressive neuronopathy in the young cairn terrier, J Small Anim Pract 30(2):101–106, 1989.
905. Zaal MD, van dan Ingh TS, Goedegebuure SA, et al: Progressive neuronopathy in two cairn terrier litter mates, Vet Q 19:34–36, 1997.
906. Cork LC, Troncoso JC, Price DL, et al: Canine neuroaxonal dystrophy, J Neuropathol Exp Neurol 42(3):286–296, 1983.
907. Chrisman CL: Neurological diseases of Rottweilers: neuroaxonal dystrophy and leukoencephalomalacia, J Small Anim Pract 33(10):500–504, 1992.
908. Bynevelt M, Rusbridge C, Britton J: Dorsal dens angulation and a Chiari type malformation in a cavalier King Charles spaniel, Vet Radiol Ultrasound 41(6):521–524, 2000.
909. Rusbridge C, MacSweeny JE, Davies JV, et al: Syringohydromyelia in cavalier King Charles spaniels, J Am Anim Hosp Assoc 36(1):34–41, 2000.
910. Rusbridge C, Knowler SP: Hereditary aspects of occipital bone hypoplasia and syringomyelia (Chiari type I malformation) in cavalier King Charles spaniels, Vet Rec 153(4):107–112, 2003.
911. Lu D, Lamb CR, Pfeiffer DU, et al: Neurological signs and results of magnetic resonance imaging in 40 cavalier King Charles spaniels with Chiari type 1-like malformations, Vet Rec 153(9):260–263, 2003.
912. Rusbridge C, Knowler SP, Pieterse L, et al: Chiari-like malformation in the Griffon Bruxellois, J Small Anim Pract 50(8):386–393, 2009.
913. Rusbridge C, Knowler SP: Hereditary aspects of occipital bone hypoplasia and syringomyelia (Chiari type I malformation) in cavalier King Charles spaniels, Vet Rec 153:107–112, 2003.
914. Couturier J, Rault D, Cauzinille L: Chiari-like malformation and syringomyelia in normal cavalier King Charles spaniels: a multiple diagnostic imaging approach, J Small Anim Pract 49(9):438–443, 2008.
915. Cerda-Gonzalez S, Olby NJ, McCullough S, et al: Morphology of the caudal fossa in cavalier King Charles spaniels, Vet Radiol Ultrasound 50(1):37–46, 2009.
916. Cerda-Gonzalez S, Dewey CW: Congenital diseases of the craniocervical junction in the dogs, Vet Clin North Am Small Anim Pract 40:121–141, 2010.
917. Lewis DG: Cervical spondylomyelopathy ("wobbler" syndrome) in the dog: a study based on 224 cases, J Small Anim Pract 30(12):657–665, 1989.
918. Olsson SE, et al: Compression of the spinal cord in Great Danes, Vet Med Small Anim Clin 77(11):1587, 1982:(abstract).
919. Baum F III, de Lahunta A, Trotter EJ: Cervical fibrotic stenosis in a young Rottweiler, J Am Vet Med Assoc 201(8):1222–1224, 1992.
920. Eagleson JS, Diaz J, Platt SR, et al: Cervical vertebral malformation-malarticulation syndrome in the Bernese mountain dog: clinical and magnetic resonance imaging features, J Small Anim Pract 50(4):186–193, 2009.
921. Costa RC, Parent JM, Holmberg DL, et al: Outcome of medical and surgical treatment in dogs with cervical spondylomyelopathy: 104 cases (1988-2004), J Am Vet Med Assoc 233(8):1284–1290, 2008.

922. Costa RC, Parent JM, Partlow G, et al: Morphologic and morphometric magnetic resonance imaging features of Doberman pinschers with and without clinical signs of cervical spondylomyelopathy, Am J Vet Res 67(9):1601–1612, 2006.
923. Moore BR, Reed SM, Biller DS, et al: Assessment of vertebral canal diameter and bony malformations of the cervical part of the spine in horses with cervical stenotic myelopathy, Am J Vet Res 55(1):5–13, 1994.
924. Hahn CN, Handel I, Green SL, et al: Assessment of the utility of using intra- and intervertebral minimum sagittal diameter ratios in the diagnosis of cervical vertebral malformation in horses, Vet Radiol Ultrasound 49(1):1–6, 2008.
925. Neuwirth L: Equine myelography, Compend Contin Educ Pract Vet 14(1):72–79, 1992.
926. Papageorges M, Gavin PR, Sande RD, et al: Radiographic and myelographic examination of the cervical vertebral column in 306 ataxic horses, Vet Radiol Ultrasound 28(2):53–59, 1987.
927. Levitski RE, Chauvet AE, Lipsitz D: Cervical myelopathy associated with extradural synovial cysts in 4 dogs, J Vet Intern Med 13(3):181–186, 1999.
928. Dickinson PJ, Sturges BK, Berry WL, et al: Extradural spinal synovial cysts in nine dogs, J Small Anim Pract 42:502–509, 2001.
929. Shelton GD, Podell M, Poncelet L, et al: Inherited polyneuropathy in Leonberger dogs: a mixed or intermediate form of Charcot-Marie-Tooth disease, Muscle Nerve 27:471–477, 2003.
930. Inada S, Sakamoto H, Haruta K, et al: A clinical study on hereditary progressive neurogenic muscular atrophy in pointer dogs, Nippon Juigaku Zasshi 40:539–547, 1978.
931. Sandefeldt E, Cummings JF, de Lahunta A: Animal model of human disease. Infantile spinal muscular atrophy, Werdnig-Hoffman diease. Animal model: hereditary neuronal abiotrophy in Swedish Lapland dogs, Am J Pathol 82:649–652, 1976.
932. He QC, Lowrie C, Shelton GD, et al: Inherited motor neuron disease in domestic cats: a model of spinal muscular atrophy, Pediatr Res 57(3):324–330, 2005.
933. Vandevelde M, Greene CE, Hoff EJ: Lower motor neuron disease with accumulation of neurofilaments in a cat, Vet Pathol 13(6):428–435, 1976.
934. Dahme E, Hafner A, Schmidt P: Spinal muscular atrophy in German Braunvieh calves - comparative neuropathological evaluation, Neuropathol Appl Neurobiol 17(6):517, 1991.
935. Nielsen JS, Andresen E, Basse A, et al: Inheritance of bovine spinal muscular atrophy, Acta Vet Scand 31(2):253–255, 1990.
936. Troyer D, Leipold HW, Cash W, et al: Upper motor neurone and descending tract pathology in bovine spinal muscular atrophy, J Comp Pathol 107(3):305–317, 1992.
937. Anderson PD, Parton KH, Collett MG, et al: A lower motor neuron disease in newborn Romney lambs, N Z Vet J 47(3):112–114, 1999.
938. Braund KG, Mehta JR, Toivio-Kinnucan M, et al: Congenital hypomyelinating polyneuropathy in two golden retriever littermates, Vet Pathol 26(3):202–208, 1989.
939. Matz ME, Shell L, Braund K: Peripheral hypomyelinization in two golden retriever littermates, J Am Vet Med Assoc 197(2):228–230, 1990.
940. Sponenberg DP, de Lahunta A: Hereditary hypertrophic neuropathy in Tibetan mastiff dogs, J Hered 72:287, 1981.
941. O'Brien DP, Johnson GC, Liu LA, et al: Laminin α2 (merosin)-deficient muscular dystrophy and demyelinating neuropathy in two cats, J Neurol Sci 189:37–43, 2001.
942. Braund KG, Shores A, Lowrie CT, et al: Idiopathic polyneuropathy in Alaskan malamutes, J Vet Intern Med 11(4):243–249, 1997.
943. Chrisman CL: Dancing Doberman disease: clinical findings and prognosis, Prog Vet Neurol 1(1):83–90, 1990.
944. Duncan ID, Griffiths IR, Carmichael S, et al: Inherited canine giant axonal neuropathy, Muscle Nerve 4(3):223–227, 1981.
945. Braund KG, Luttgen PJ, Redding RW, et al: Distal symmetrical polyneuropathy in a dog, Vet Pathol 17(4):422–435, 1980.
946. Henricks PM, Steiss J, Petterson JD: Distal peripheral polyneuropathy in a Great Dane, Can Vet J 28:165–167, 1987.
947. Shelton GD, Podell M, Sullivan S, et al: Distal, symmetrical polyneuropathy with laryngeal paralysis in young, related Leonberger dogs, J Vet Intern Med 14(3):339, 2000:(abstract).
948. Harkin KR, Cash WC, Shelton GD: Sensory and motor neuropathy in a border collie, J Am Vet Med Assoc 227(8):1263–1265, 2005.
949. Armengou L, Anor S, Climent F, et al: Antemortem diagnosis of a distal axonopathy causing severe stringhalt in a horse, J Vet Intern Med 24(1):220–223, 2010.
950. Huntington PJ, Jeffcott LB, Friend SCE, et al: Australian stringhalt—epidemiological, clinical and neurological investigations, Equine Vet J 21(4):266–273, 1989.
951. Slocombe RF, Huntington PJ, Friend SCE, et al: Pathological aspects of Australian stringhalt, Equine Vet J 24(3):174–183, 1992.
952. Mahony OM, Knowles KE, Braund KG, et al: Laryngeal paralysis-polyneuropathy complex in young Rottweilers, J Vet Intern Med 12(5):330–337, 1998.
953. Moreau PM, Vallat JM, Hugon J, et al: Peripheral and central distal axonopathy of suspected inherited origin in Birman cats, Acta Neuropathol 82(2):143–146, 1991.
954. Griffiths IR: Progressive axonopathy: an inherited neuropathy of boxer dogs. 1. Further studies of the clinical and electrophysiological features, J Small Anim Pract 26:381–392, 1985.
955. Duncan ID, Griffiths IR: A sensory neuropathy affecting long-haired dachshund dogs, J Small Anim Pract 23:381–390, 1982.
956. Mason LT: The occurrence and pedigree analysis of a hereditary sensory neuropathy in the English springer spaniel, Proc Ann Am College Vet Dermatol 15:23–24, 1999.
957. Paradis M, Jaham CD, Page N, et al: Acral mutilation and analgesia in 13 French spaniels, Vet Dermatol 16(2):87–93, 2005.
958. Franklin RJM, Olby NJ, Targett MP, et al: Sensory neuropathy in a Jack Russell terrier, J Small Anim Pract 33:402–404, 1992.
959. Sanda A, Pivnik L: Die Zehenneckrose bei kurzhaarigen Vorstehhunden, Kleintierpraxis 9:76–83, 1964.
960. Jaderlund KH, Orvind E, Johnsson E, et al: A neurologic syndrome in golden retrievers presenting as a sensory ataxic neuropathy, J Vet Intern Med 21:1307–1315, 2007.

961. Jones BR, Wallace A, Harding DRK, et al: Occurrence of idiopathic, familial hyperchylomicronaemia in a cat, Vet Rec 112(543):547, 1983.
962. Jones BR, Johnstone AC, Cahill JI, et al: Peripheral neuropathy in cats with inherited primary hyperchylomicronaemia, Vet Rec 119(11):268–272, 1986.
963. Grieshaber TL, McKeever PJ, McKeever PJ, et al: Spontaneous cutaneous (eruptive) xanthomatosis in two cats, J Am Anim Hosp Assoc 27:509–512, 1991.
964. Bauer JE, Verlander JW: Congenital lipoprotein lipase deficiency in hyperlipemic kitten siblings, Vet Clin Pathol 13:7–11, 1984.
965. Brooks KD: Idiopathic hyperlipoproteinemia in a cat, Companion Anim Pract 19:5–9, 1989.
966. Smerdon T: Hyperchylomicronaemia in a litter of Siamese kittens, Bull Feline Advisory Bureau 51–53, 1990.
967. McKerrell RE, Blakemore WF, Heath MF, et al: Primary hyperoxaluria (L-glyceric aciduria) in the cat: a newly recognised inherited disease, Vet Rec 125(2):31–34, 1989.
968. Podell M: Inflammatory myopathies, Vet Clin North Am Small Anim Pract 32:147–167, 2002.
969. Schatzberg SJ, Shelton GD: Newly identified neuromuscular disorders, Vet Clin North Am Small Anim Pract 34(6):1497–1524, 2004:(review).
970. Evans J, Levesque D, Shelton GD: Canine inflammatory myopathies: a clinicopathologic review of 200 cases, J Vet Intern Med 18(5):679–691, 2004.
971. Werner LL, Bright JM: Drug-induced immune hypersensitivity disorders in two dogs treated with trimethoprim sulfadiazine: case reports and drug challenge studies, J Am Anim Hosp Assoc 19:783–790, 1983.
972. Giger U, Werner LL, Millichamp NJ, et al: Sulfadiazine-induced allergy in six Doberman pinschers, J Am Vet Med Assoc 186(5):479–484, 1985.
973. Krum SH, Cardinet GH, Anderson BC, et al: Polymyositis and polyarthritis associated with systemic lupus erythematosus in a dog, J Am Vet Med Assoc 170(1):61–64, 1977.
974. Grindem CB, Johnson KH: Systemic lupus erythematosus: literature review and report of 42 new canine cases, J Am Anim Hosp Assoc 19(4):489–503, 1983.
975. Presthus J, Lindboe CF: Polymyositis in two German wirehaired pointer littermates, J Small Anim Pract 29(4):239–248, 1988.
976. Hankel S, Shelton GD, Engvall E: Sarcolemma-specific autoantibodies in canine inflammatory myopathy, Vet Immunol Immunopathol 113(1/2):1–10, 2006.
977. Hargis AM, Haupt KH, Prieur DJ, et al: A skin disorder in three Shetland sheepdogs: comparison with familial canine dermatomyositis in collies, Compend Contin Educ Pract Vet 7(4):306–315, 1985.
978. White SD, Shelton GD, Sisson A, et al: Dermatomyositis in an adult Pembroke Welsh corgi, J Am Anim Hosp Assoc 28(5):398–401, 1992.
979. Lewis DD, Shelton GD, Piras A, et al: Gracilis or semitendinosus myopathy in 18 dogs, J Am Anim Hosp Assoc 33(2):177–188, 1997.
980. Kornegay JN, Sharp NJH, Camp SD, et al: Early pathologic features of golden retriever muscular dystrophy: a model of Duchenne muscular dystrophy 48(3):348, 1989.
981. Kornegay JN, Tuler S, Miller D, et al: Muscular dystrophy in a litter of golden retriever dogs, Muscle Nerve 11:1056–1064, 1988.
982. Wentink GH, Meijer AEFH, Linde-Sipman JS, et al: Myopathy in an Irish terrier with a metabolic defect of the isolated mitochondria, Zentralbl Veterinarmed 21A:62–74, 1974.
983. Winand N, Pradham D, Cooper B: Molecular characterization of severe Duchenne-type muscular dystrophy in a family of Rottweiler dogs. Molecular mechanisms of neuromuscular disease, Tucson, 1994, Muscular Dystrophy Association.
984. Ham LML, Desmidt M, Tshamala M, et al: Canine X-linked muscular dystrophy in Belgian Groenendaeler shepherds, Vlaams Diergeneeskundig Tijdschrift 64(3):102–106, 1995.
985. Cardinet GH III, Holliday TA: Neuromuscular diseases of domestic animals: a summary of muscle biopsies from 159 cases, Ann N Y Acad Sci 317:290–313, 1979.
986. Schatzberg SJ, Olby NJ, Breen M, et al: Molecular analysis of a spontaneous dystrophin "knockout" dog, Neuromuscul Disord 9(5):289–295, 1999.
987. Wetterman CA, Harkin KR, Cash WC, et al: Hypertrophic muscular dystrophy in a young dog, J Am Vet Med Assoc 216(6):878–881, 2000.
988. Jones BR, Brennan S, Mooney CT, et al: Muscular dystrophy with truncated dystrophin in a family of Japanese spitz dogs, J Neurol Sci 217(2):143–149, 2004.
989. Bergman RL, Inzana KD, Monroe WE, et al: Dystrophin-deficient muscular dystrophy in a Labrador retriever, J Am Anim Hosp Assoc 38(3):255–261, 2002.
990. Piercy RJ, Walmsley G: Muscular dystrophy in cavalier King Charles spaniels, Vet Rec 165(2):62, 2009.
991. Gaschen F, Gaschen L, Burgunder JM: Clinical study of a breeding colony affected with hypertrophic feline muscular dystrophy, J Vet Intern Med 9(3):207, 1995:(abstract).
992. Vos JH, van der Linde-Sipman JS, Goedegebuure SA: Dystrophy-like myopathy in the cat, J Comp Pathol 96(3):335–341, 1986.
993. Meier H: Myopathies in the dog, Cornell Vet 48:313–330, 1958.
994. Sharp NJH, Kornegay JN, Camp SD, et al: An error in dystrophin mRNA processing in golden retriever muscular dystrophy, an animal homologue of Duchenne muscular dystrophy, Genomics 13(1):115–121, 1992.
995. Shelton GD, Ling LA, Guo LT, et al: Muscular dystrophy in female dogs, J Vet Intern Med 15:240–244, 2001.
996. Deitz K, Morrison JA, Kline K, et al: Sarcoglycan-deficient muscular dystrophy in a Boston terrier, J Vet Intern Med 22(2):476–480, 2008.
997. Martin PT, Shelton GD, Dickinson PJ, et al: Muscular dystrophy associated with alpha-dystroglycan deficiency in Sphynx and Devon rex cats, Neuromuscul Disord 18(12):942–952, 2008.
998. Poncelet L, Resibois A, Engvall E, et al: Laminin alpha2 deficiency-associated muscular dystrophy in a Maine coon cat, J Small Anim Pract 44(12):550–552, 2003:(review).
999. Kramer JW, Hegreberg GA, Hamilton MJ: Inheritance of a neuromuscular disorder of Labrador retriever dogs, J Am Vet Med Assoc 179(4):380–381, 1981.
1000. Kramer JW, Hegreberg GA, Bryan GM, et al: A muscle disorder of Labrador retrievers characterized by deficiency of type II muscle fibers, J Am Vet Med Assoc 169(8):817–820, 1976.
1001. Peeters ME, Ubbink GJ: Dysphagia-associated muscular dystrophy, Prog Vet Neurol 5(3):124, 1994:(abstract).

1002. Peeters ME, Ubbink GJ: Dysphagia-associated muscular dystrophy: a familial trait in the Bouvier des Flandres, Vet Rec 134(17):444–446, 1994.
1003. Cooper BJ, de Lahunta A, Gallagher EA: Nemaline myopathy of cats, Muscle Nerve 9:618–625, 1986.
1004. Delauche AJ, Cuddon PA, Podell M, et al: Nemaline rods in canine myopathies: 4 case reports and literature review, J Vet Intern Med 12(6):424–430, 1998.
1005. Hanson SM, Smith MO, Walker TL, et al: Juvenile-onset distal myopathy in Rottweiler dogs, J Vet Intern Med 12(2):103–108, 1998.
1006. Ceh L, Hauge JG, Svenkerud R, et al: Glycogenosis type III in the dog, Acta Vet Scand 17(2):210–222, 1976.
1007. Ward TL, Valberg SJ, Adelson DL, et al: Glycogen branching enzyme (GBE1) mutation causing equine glycogen storage disease IV, Mamm Genome 15(7):570–577, 2004.
1008. Valberg SJ, Ward TL, Rush B, et al: Glycogen branching enzyme deficiency in quarter horse foals, J Vet Intern Med 15(6):572–580, 2001.
1009. Angelos S, Valberg SJ, Smith BP, et al: Myophosphorylase deficiency associated with rhabdomyolysis and exercise intolerance in 6 related Charolais cattle, Muscle Nerve 18(7):736–740, 1995.
1010. Giger U, Argov Z, Schnall M, et al: Metabolic myopathy in canine muscle-type phosphofructokinase deficiency, Muscle Nerve 11(12):1260–1265, 1988.
1011. Valberg SJ, Cardinet GH, Carlson GP, et al: Polysaccharide storage myopathy associated with recurrent exertional rhabdomyolysis in horses, Neuromuscul Disord 2:351–359, 1992.
1012. Valentine BA, Credille KM, Lavoie JP, et al: Severe polysaccharide storage myopathy in Belgian and Percheron draught horses, Equine Vet J 29:220–225, 1997.
1013. Valentine BA, Cooper BJ: Incidence of polysaccharide storage myopathy, Vet Pathol 42:823–827, 2005.
1014. Breitschwerdt EB, Kornegay JN, Wheeler SJ, et al: Episodic weakness associated with exertional lactic acidosis and myopathy in Old English sheepdog littermates, J Am Vet Med Assoc 201(5):731–736, 1992.
1015. Olby NJ, Chan KK, Targett MP, et al: Suspected mitochondrial myopathy in a Jack Russell terrier, J Small Anim Pract 38(5):213–216, 1997.
1016. Houlton JE, Herrtage ME: Mitochondrial myopathy in the Sussex spaniel, Vet Rec 106(9):206, 1980.
1017. Herrtage ME, Houlton JEF: Collapsing clumber spaniels, Vet Rec 105(14):334, 1979.
1018. Paciello O, Maiolino P, Fatone G, et al: Mitochondrial myopathy in a German shepherd dog, Vet Pathol 40(5):507–511, 2003.
1019. Shelton GD, van Ham L, Bhatti S, et al: Pyruvate dehydrogenase deficiency in clumber and Sussex spaniels in the United States and Belgium, J Vet Intern Med 14(3):342, 2000.
1020. Platt SR, Chrisman CL, Shelton GD: Lipid storage myopathy in a cocker spaniel, J Small Anim Pract 40:31–34, 1999.
1021. Inada S, Yamauchi C, Igata A, et al: Canine storage disease characterized by hereditary progressive neurogenic muscular atrophy: breeding experiments and clinical manifestation, Am J Vet Res 47(10):2294–2299, 1986.
1022. Wells GAH, Bradley R: Pietrain creeper syndrome: a primary myopathy of the pig? Neuropathol Appl Neurobiol 4(3):237–238, 1978.
1023. Taylor SM, Shmon CL, Shelton GD, et al: Exercise-induced collapse of Labrador retrievers: survey results and preliminary investigation of heritability, J Am Anim Hosp Assoc 44(6):295–301, 2008.
1024. Taylor SM, Shmon CL, Adams VJ, et al: Evaluations of Labrador retrievers with exercise-induced collapse, including response to a standardized strenuous exercise protocol, J Am Anim Hosp Assoc 45(1):3–13, 2009.
1025. Berman MC, Harrison GG, Bull AB, et al: Changes underlying halothane induced malignant hyperpyrexia in Landrace pigs, Nature 225:653–655, 1970.
1026. Fujii J, Otsu K, Zorzato F, et al: Identification of a mutation in porcine ryanodine receptor associated with malignant hyperthermia, Science 253(5018):448–451, 1991.
1027. Gannon JR: Exertional rhabdomyolysis (myoglobinuria) in the racing greyhound. In Kirk RW, editor: Current veterinary therapy VII, ed 7, St Louis, 1980, WB Saunders.
1028. Dranchak PK, Valberg SJ, Onan GW, et al: Inheritance of recurrent exertional rhabdomyolysis in thoroughbreds, J Am Vet Med Assoc 227:762–767, 2005.
1029. Valberg SJ, MacLeay JM, Mickelson JR: Exertional rhabdomyolysis and polysaccharide storage myopathy in horses, Compend Contin Educ Pract Vet 19(9):1077–1086, 1997.
1030. MacLeay JM, Sorum SA, Valberg SJ, et al: Epidemiologic analysis of factors influencing exertional rhabdomyolysis in thoroughbreds, Am J Vet Res 60:1562–1566, 1999.
1031. Spier SJ, Carlson GP, Holliday TA, et al: Hyperkalemic periodic paralysis in horses, J Am Vet Med Assoc 197(8):1009–1017, 1990.
1032. Spier SJ, Carlson GP, Harrold D, et al: Genetic study of hyperkalemic periodic paralysis in horses, J Am Vet Med Assoc 202(6):933–937, 1993.
1033. Naylor JM, Robinson JA, Bertone J: Familial incidence of hyperkalemic periodic paralysis in quarter horses, J Am Vet Med Assoc 200(3):340–343, 1992.
1034. Rudolph JA, Spier SJ, Byrns G, et al: Periodic paralysis in quarter horses: a sodium channel mutation disseminated by selective breeding, Nat Genet 2(2):144–147, 1992.
1035. Cannon SC, Hayward LJ, Beech J, et al: Sodium channel inactivation is impaired in equine hyperkalemic periodic paralysis, J Neurophysiol 73(5):1892–1899, 1995.
1036. Shelton GD, Schule A, Kass PH: Risk factors for acquired myasthenia gravis in dogs: 1,154 cases (1991-1995), J Am Vet Med Assoc 211(11):1428–1431, 1997.
1037. Kent M, Glass EN, Acierno M, et al: Adult onset acquired myasthenia gravis in three Great Dane littermates, J Small Anim Pract 49(12):647–650, 2008.
1038. Lipsitz D, Berry JL, Shelton GD: Inherited predisposition to myasthenia gravis in Newfoundlands, J Am Vet Med Assoc 215(7):956–958, 1999.
1039. Shelton GD, Ho M, Kass PH: Risk factors for acquired myasthenia gravis in cats: 105 cases (1986-1998), J Am Vet Med Assoc 216(1):55–57, 2000.
1040. Johnson RP, Watson ADJ, Smith J, et al: Myasthenia in springer Spaniel littermates, J Small Anim Pract 16(10):641–647, 1975.
1041. Dickinson PJ, Sturges BK, Shelton GD, et al: Congenital myasthenia gravis in smooth-haired miniature dachshund dogs, J Vet Intern Med 19(6):920–923, 2005.
1042. Wallace ME, Palmer AC: Recessive mode of inheritance in myasthenia gravis in the Jack Russell terrier, Vet Rec 114(14):350, 1984.
1043. Flagstad A, Trojaborg W, Gammeltoft S: Congenital myasthenic syndrome in the dog breed Gammel Dansk Honsehund: clinical, electrophysiological, pharmacological and immunological comparison with acquired myasthenia gravis, Acta Vet Scand 30(1):89–102, 1989.

1044. Miller LM, Hegreberg GA, Prieur DJ, et al: Inheritance of congenital myasthenia gravis in smooth fox terrier dogs, J Hered 75(3):163–166, 1984.
1045. Thompson PN, Steinlein OK, Harper CK, et al: Congenital myasthenic syndrome of Brahman cattle in South Africa, Vet Rec 153(25):779–781, 2003.
1046. Cameron JM, Maj MC, Levandovskiy V, et al: Identification of a canine model of pyruvate dehydrogenase phosphatase 1 deficiency, Mol Genet Metab 90(1):15–23, 2007.
1047. Pele M, Tiret L, Kessler JL, et al: SINE exonic insertion in the PTPLA gene leads to multiple splicing defects and segregates with the autosomal recessive centronuclear myopathy in dogs, Hum Mol Genet 14(13):1905–1906, 2005.

INDEX

Page numbers followed by f indicate figures; t, tables; b, boxes.

9781437706512